John B. Davis.

A SHORT PRACTICE
OF SURGERY

By

HAMILTON BAILEY
F.R.C.S. (Eng)., F.A.C.S., F.I.C.S., F.R.S.E.

*Emeritus Surgeon, Royal Northern Hospital, London ; Senior Surgeon,
St. Vincent's Clinic and the Italian Hospital ; Formerly External Exam-
iner in Surgery, University of Bristol*

AND

R. J. McNEILL LOVE
M.S. (Lond.), F.R.C.S. (Eng.), F.A.C.S., F.I.C.S.

*Surgeon, Royal Northern, Mildmay Mission, and Metropolitan
Hospitals ; Consulting Surgeon, City of London Maternity Hospital ;
Consulting Surgeon, Potter's Bar Hospital ; Associate for General Sur-
gery, West End Hospital for Nervous Diseases ; Member of Council
and Court of Examiners, Erasmus Wilson Demonstrator, and Hunterian
Professor, Royal College of Surgeons*

With Pathological Illustrations by
L. C. D. HERMITTE
M.B., Ch.B. (Edin.)

Pathologist, Royal Infirmary, Sheffield

NINTH EDITION
(65th *thousand*)

WITH 1234 ILLUSTRATIONS
OF WHICH 272 ARE COLOURED

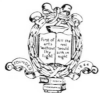

LONDON
H. K. LEWIS & Co. Ltd.
1952

First Edition	.	.	.	October 1932
Second Edition		.	.	January 1935
Reprinted	.	.	.	.	July 1935
Third Edition		.	.	.	June 1936
Reprinted	.	.	.	.	June 1937
Fourth Edition		.	.	.	August 1938
Reprinted	.	.	.	.	January 1940
Fifth Edition	.		.	.	January 1941
Reprinted	.	.	.	.	March 1942
Sixth Edition	.		.	.	March 1943
Reprinted	.	.	.	.	July 1944
Seventh Edition		.	.	.	March 1946
Reprinted	.	.	.	.	January 1948
Eighth Edition		.	.	.	1948–9
Ninth Edition		.	.	.	May 1952
Italian Edition		.	.	.	.	1952

PRINTED IN GREAT BRITAIN FOR
H. K. LEWIS AND CO. LTD. BY
HAZELL, WATSON AND VINEY LTD., AYLESBURY AND LONDON

A SHORT PRACTICE
OF SURGERY

PREFACE TO NINTH EDITION

In presenting the ninth edition of this survey of general surgery, we again wish to convey our sincere appreciation to many friends who have offered us welcome suggestions and kindly criticisms. Although only three years have elapsed since the last edition appeared, surgical practice changes so rapidly that all the chapters have been revised or rewritten.

We have endeavoured to include only such material as is completely up to date and yet generally acceptable. Following our former practice, advanced surgery and rare conditions are relegated to small type. The Chinese proverb " one picture is worth a million words " may be an exaggeration, but we feel confident of the value of illustrations to interest the reader and to shorten the text. We have therefore replaced some of the former illustrations by new ones, and have included 135 additional figures, which we believe will be appreciated by the reader. On numerous occasions we have been urged to refrain from enlarging this work, but some increase in the size of this volume was inevitable if it is to maintain its reputation as a comprehensive textbook of surgery.

Those familiar with the previous editions will observe that many new illustrations have been incorporated. For the loan of clinical photographs and illustrations, which have been acknowledged throughout the book, we here record our gratitude to Sir Reginald Watson-Jones (London), Sir John Fraser (Edinburgh), Professors W. Gemmill (Birmingham), Karl Krebs (Aarhus), Manzanilla (Mexico City), E. P. Pybus (Newcastle), A. Rendle Short (Bristol), Max Thorek (Chicago), Messrs. T. A. Bouchier-Hayes (Dublin), Alexander Law (London), W. V. Lodge (Halifax), A. A. McConnell (Dublin), G. D. F. McFadden (Belfast), E. T. C. Milligan (London), Joseph Minton (London), A. H. Southam (Manchester), Hermon Taylor (London), Mr. J. R. M. Whigham (London), and Dr. M. Kinawy (Egypt). We are also very grateful to Mr. G. C. Knight for some valuable illustrations concerning cerebral surgery from the West End Hospital for Nervous Diseases.

For constructive criticism and help in other directions we have benefited from the advice of Professor Ernest Finch (Sheffield), Mr. C. G. S. Milne (Deal), Dr. C. Allan Birch (London), Mr. Alan McLeod (London), Mr. Thomas Mackesy Prossor

(London), Dr. Dennis Dooley (London), Professor Harold Dew (Sydney), Mr. Norman C. Tanner (London), Professor Charles Wells (Liverpool), and the late Professor Grey Turner (London). The proofs have been read by Mr. A. C. King, M.B.E., Mr. Allan Clain, Mr. J. R. Elder, Mr. Leicester Atkinson, Mr. Ian Gibson, Mr. Swift Joly, and Dr. P. B. Early, and without the conscientious scrutiny of these readers, not only would our labours have been multiplied, but assuredly some errors would have escaped correction.

We tender our thanks to Mr. Le Fanu, Mr. W. J. Bishop, and Dr. W. R. Bett for their valuable assistance in verifying the historical annotations, and to Mr. J. Shields for compiling the index. We are also obliged to the Curator of the Museum of the Royal College of Surgeons, Professor Geoffrey Hadfield, for illustrations of specimens, to Mr. F. P. Fitzgerald for photographs concerning the treatment of fractures, and to Dr. S. M. Rivlin for illustrations concerning varicose veins.

This edition includes a glossary of anatomical names, which will prevent any confusion that might arise as a result of different nomenclatures.

For permission to use various blocks we are indebted also to the following publishers : Messrs. John Wright & Sons ; Cassell & Co. ; Oxford Medical Publications ; Oliver & Boyd ; J. & A. Churchill, Ltd. ; Bale, Sons & Danielsson ; University of London Press ; W. Heinemann (Medical Books) Ltd. ; D. Appleton-Century Co. ; Jackson, Wylie & Co. ; The Blakiston Co. ; W. B. Saunders Co. ; E. & S. Livingstone ; Lea & Febiger ; and also to the Editors of *The Lancet, British Medical Journal, Practitioner, British Journal of Urology, British Journal of Surgery, British Dental Journal, Journal of the American Medical Association,* and *Surgery, Gynæcology, and Obstetrics.*

Finally, we wish to express our continued indebtedness to the Publishers for their ever helpful co-operation and careful preparation of this volume for the press.

THE AUTHORS.

ROYAL NORTHERN HOSPITAL,
LONDON.
February, 1952.

CONTENTS

A SHORT PRACTICE OF SURGERY

CHAPTER I

NON-SPECIFIC INFECTIONS AND WOUNDS

The more important pyogenic organisms are :

1. **Staphylococci,** which commonly cause infection of the skin and subcutaneous tissues, such as boils, and also carbuncles. They are also responsible for some varieties of deep-seated suppuration, e.g. osteomyelitis or perinephric abscess. In these cases the organisms are usually conveyed from the skin or respiratory passages to the deeper tissues by the blood-stream.

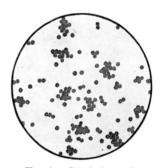

Fig. 1.—Staphylococci.

Staphylococci occur in characteristic clusters (fig. 1), are Gram-positive, and grow readily on culture media. Cultures vary in colour, and are named accordingly, e.g. albus, aureus, citreus, but the latter is non-pathogenic.

2. **Streptococci** are Gram-positive organisms, which grow in chains (fig. 11), and comprise many different strains. Also members of the same strain often develop varying degrees of virulence. Two main groups of streptococci are the hæmolytic and non-hæmolytic varieties, the former being the more virulent, and producing the spreading types of infection, such as erysipelas, cellulitis, lymphangitis, and occasionally gaining access to the blood-stream and causing ulcerative endocarditis or puerperal fever.

Non-hæmolytic streptococci are more commonly concerned with infection of the tonsils, gall bladder, etc.

3. **Pneumococci** are arranged in pairs, the individual coccus being oval in shape. These organisms are the common cause

Hans Christian Joachim Gram, 1853–1938. Professor of Medicine, Copenhagen.

of pneumonia, and are usually found either alone or in association with other organisms, e.g. in pus from empyemata. Acute arthritis, meningitis, otitis media, and peritonitis, particularly in young girls, are also sometimes caused by pneumococci.

4. **Bacilli coli** are Gram-negative, and normally inhabit the healthy intestine. They are distinguished from the typhoid group of bacilli by their action on various sugars. In intestinal obstruction and other pathological conditions of the intestine the organisms are liable to become extremely virulent. Peritonitis, cholecystitis, and urinary infections are commonly due to B. coli.

5. **Bacilli typhosi** may cause acute osteomyelitis, or acute or chronic cholecystitis, sometimes years after the original infection. Some patients after recovery continue to excrete bacilli in the urine, bile, and fæces. These " carriers " occasionally cause epidemics, as in the Aberystwyth epidemic of 1946, which was traced to an infected ice-cream vendor.

6. **Bacilli pyocyanei** occasionally infect wounds as secondary invaders, and delay healing. The pus is bluish green, with a musty odour. Applications of gauze moistened with perchloride of mercury, 1 : 8,000, usually overcome the infection. More resistant cases usually respond to a 2·2 per cent. dressing of phenoxetol (the monophenylether of ethylene glycol), applied daily.

7. **Gonococci** are Gram-negative organisms arranged in pairs. Each coccus is kidney-shaped, and the two lie with their concave sides adjacent (fig. 30). When gonococcal pus is examined, some of the polymorphonuclear cells are seen to be crowded with gonococci. The most characteristic lesion produced by gonococci is urethritis. Direct transmission is responsible for conjunctivitis (p. 45) or proctitis in the female, and organisms in the blood-stream sometimes cause arthritis, fibrositis, or endocarditis.

ACUTE ABSCESS

Organisms which cause pus formation reach the infected area by one of three routes :

(i) Direct infection from without, e.g. penetrating wounds.

(ii) Local extension from some adjacent focus of infection, such as an alveolar abscess from an infected tooth root.

(iii) Blood-stream or lymphatic vessels.

Antony van Leeuwenhoek of Delft, Holland, invented the microscope, and was the first to see bacteria in 1675. He made over 400 microscopes with his own hands.

In the case of hæmatogenous infection, some predisposing factor may operate, e.g. a torn muscle causes an extravasation of blood which forms a suitable nidus for pyogenic organisms, or debilitating disease lowers the general resistance and allows infection to arise, as occasionally occurs in the perinephric cellular tissue.

The bacteria, having gained access to the tissues, multiply and produce toxins, and so cause acute inflammation. The vitality of the tissues is lowered, and the area is surrounded by a peripheral inflammatory zone of acute inflammation, which is infiltrated with leucocytes and bacteria. The central necrotic mass undergoes liquefaction, and the tension within the cavity is raised by exudation of plasma, the resulting fluid containing leucocytes and bacteria. The abscess, if it enlarges, spreads along the paths of least resistance, usually towards the surface of the body or a hollow viscus, and eventually discharges its contents.

Occasionally the resistance of the body is sufficient to destroy the bacteria before pus finds its way to the surface, in which case the fluid is absorbed, and either fibrosis follows, or a cavity remains containing inspissated pus. In some cases, as in staphylococcal abscesses of bone (Brodie's abscess), infection remains latent, but gives rise to exacerbations of inflammation consequent on local injury or impaired general health.

Symptoms.—The patient complains of malaise, the degree depending to some extent upon the size of the abscess, the virulence of the organism, and the tension within the cavity. Throbbing pain is characteristic of suppuration, the pain becoming more acute if the affected part is dependent.

Signs.—(a) *General.*—The signs of infection are present to a varying extent. In severe cases rigors may occur.

(b) *Local.*—The signs of inflammation are present, the readiness with which they can be detected depending on the size of the abscess and its proximity to the surface. The swelling is at first brawny and œdematous ; later softening and fluctuation are manifest. In some cases increasing œdema is very characteristic of deep pus, as in acute mastitis. If untreated an abscess tends to point, the skin or membrane covering it gives way, and the contents are discharged, usually with marked amelioration of symptoms.

Sir Benjamin Brodie, 1783–1861. Surgeon, St. George's Hospital, London.

Treatment.—When an abscess threatens to form it can sometimes be aborted by rest, and elevation of the affected part will relieve pain. Kaolin poultices promote hyperæmia, and constitutional treatment, including chemotherapy and penicillin, is instituted.

If pus is suspected steps are usually taken to evacuate the abscess by incision and drainage. In regions where incisions are fraught with danger to important anatomical structures, as in the parotid gland or axilla, the method of Hilton should be used. This consists of incising the skin and fascia, and opening the abscess by thrusting a pair of sinus forceps into the cavity. By separating the blades, a sufficiently large opening can be made to insert, if necessary, a finger in order to convert loculi into a single cavity, followed by a drainage tube. Pus from an abscess should be examined bacteriologically, and, if considered advisable, its sensitivity to antibiotics is ascertained (p. 9).

If an abscess is opened incompletely, a sinus or fistula may result. A *sinus* is a narrow track lined with granulations which opens on the surface, whereas a *fistula* is an abnormal communication between two cavities, or between a cavity and the body surface. Thus, a perianal abscess may burst on the surface and lead to a sinus, erroneously termed a blind external " fistula." In other cases, the abscess opens both into the anal canal and on to the surface, resulting in a true fistula.

SINUSES and FISTULÆ often heal slowly, for the following reasons :

(i) A foreign body or necrosed tissue may be present.

(ii) The walls become lined with epithelium.

(iii) Dense fibrosis prevents contraction.

(iv) Irritating discharges, such as urine or fæces, maintain continuous inflammation.

(v) Inefficient or non-dependent drainage.

(vi) Absence of rest, such as repeated sphincteric contractions in the case of fistula-in-ano.

(vii) Type of infection, e.g. tuberculosis or actinomycosis.

Treatment consists of removal of any cause, and provision of adequate drainage, if necessary by counter-openings. Packing with gauze moistened with suitable disinfectants will encourage healing from the bottom of the cavity. Disinfectants should

John Hilton, 1805–1878. Surgeon to Guy's Hospital. One of the original 300 Fellows of the Royal College of Surgeons. Wrote a classic on " Rest and Pain."

occasionally be changed, as organisms appear to become partially immune to long-continued use of the same dressing. Rest is provided as efficiently as possible, and scraping or cautery is sometimes necessary to destroy any lining of epithelium.

AMYLOID DISEASE

This results from persistent suppuration and is becoming increasingly rare. It is most commonly seen nowadays as a result of chronic empyema, or sinuses in connection with the hip joint. The term "amyloid disease" is a misleading one, as the infiltration of tissues is not due to any starchy substance, but to chondroitin-sulphuric acid in combination with a protein. Infiltration commences in the walls of the smaller arterioles, and later spreads to larger vessels, and even to connective-tissue stroma. The substance is stained a mahogany brown by tincture of iodine, and microscopically, methyl violet stains the infiltrated tissues a rose pink, while normal structures are stained blue.

Affected organs show a regular, smooth enlargement. The first changes in the liver occur in the intermediate zone of the lobule. Polyuria is present owing to infiltration of the kidneys, which first commences in the glomeruli. Diarrhœa ensues owing to infiltration of the capillaries in the villi of the small intestine, and splenic enlargement occurs, the Malpighian bodies being chiefly affected. If the source of infection can be eradicated, early amyloid disease will resolve.

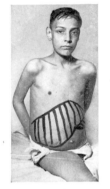

FIG. 2.—Enlargement of the liver and spleen due to amyloid disease. Amputation was performed through the left hip joint for osteomyelitis of the upper end of the femur, but sinuses persisted. He succumbed six months later.

CELLULITIS

Cellulitis is due to spreading inflammation of the subcutaneous and cellular tissue which sometimes progresses to suppuration or gangrene. In the latter case widespread sloughing of tissues occasionally results (fig. 3). The condition was formerly known as "hospital gangrene," and may progress to a fatal issue. If extension occurs in spite of treatment, the affected part should be widely excised with a diathermy knife.

The streptococcus is usually the causative organism, and often gains admission to the tissues through an accidental wound, trivial in nature, such as a graze or scratch, or possibly as the result of an operation. If the general resistance of the patient is undermined as by such conditions as diabetes, alcoholism, or renal inefficiency, cellulitis is likely to spread rapidly and extensively.

Marcello Malpighi, 1628–1694. An Italian physiologist.

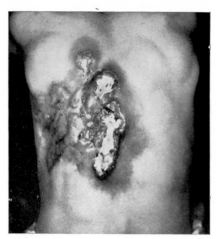

FIG. 3.—Extensive subcutaneous gangrene following operation for empyema.
(*Callam and Duff.*)

The clinical condition depends upon the virulence of the organism and the extent of infection. Redness and itching or stiffness commence at the site of inoculation, to be followed by tenderness and induration (fig. 4). The general features of infection are usually well marked, and septicaemia or pyaemia sometimes develops.

Treatment consists in attending to the general health of the patient, and a course of penicillin or other chemotherapy is prescribed. If pus is suspected, free incisions are made in the axis of the limb, down to the deep fascia. Baths of hypertonic saline (5 per cent.), to encourage lymphatic drainage, alternating with antiseptic dressings, are useful.

CELLULITIS IN SPECIAL SITUATIONS

Scalp.—This is due to infection of the sub-aponeurotic layer of the areolar tissue. Pus may extend to the attachment of the epicranial aponeurosis, so that the whole scalp is lifted off the calvarium. Necrosis of bone, or thrombosis of emissary veins spreading to intracranial sinuses, may follow. Early incisions, parallel to the arteries, are necessary when pus is suspected.

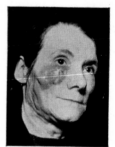

FIG. 4.—Cellulitis of the face.

Orbit.—This follows wounds or spread of infection from air sinuses in the vicinity (p. 141). Proptosis and impairment of ocular movements follow, and infection may spread to the meninges, or thrombosis extend along the ophthalmic veins to the cavernous sinus. The eyeball itself occasionally becomes infected (panophthalmitis).

Owing to risk of cellulitis, all wounds of the orbit demand

careful attention. If infection supervenes, drainage is provided by incisions in the eyelids or conjunctival fornix. Panophthalmitis is treated by evisceration of the eye ; this procedure is safer than excision, which is liable to be followed by meningitis, owing to infection extending along the open sheath of the optic nerve.

Neck.—Complicates wounds, tonsillitis, or mastoiditis. Ludwig's angina is a term applied to submaxillary cellulitis (p. 196). The two main dangers of cervical cellulitis are œdema of the glottis with possible asphyxia and mediastinitis.

Pelvis.—Not infrequently follows lacerations of the cervix uteri, or less commonly results from disease or injury to any of the pelvic organs, such as extraperitoneal rupture of the bladder. Infection frequently creeps up the side of the pelvis, in which case an indurated swelling appears above Poupart's ligament. In the first two or three weeks, on rectal or vaginal examination, a firm, tender pelvic mass can be palpated, but often by the time the swelling appears above Poupart's ligament resolution of the mass in the pelvis results in its disappearance.

In the early stages, hypogastric fomentations and vaginal douches are useful. If the swelling appears above Poupart's ligament and deep œdema or softening is detected, the abscess is incised and drained extraperitoneally. Posterior colpotomy is sometimes indicated.

WOUND INFECTION

Infection of accidental wounds is often unavoidable, although early and thorough treatment frequently prevents the development of the infection. Surgical wounds in " clean " cases may become infected owing to some flaw in technique, or faulty sterilisation of instruments or material.

LOCAL changes are those of inflammation, which, if superficial, manifests itself as a cellulitis of varying extent. If infection is deep in a wound, swelling occurs, so that the stitches appear to be under tension ; tenderness and induration follow. If suppuration occurs, the abscess is liable to burst superficially, and perhaps a knot or ligature is discharged.

GENERAL evidence of infection is due to toxæmia, septicæmia, or pyæmia, or a combination of two or all of these conditions.

TOXÆMIA is due to absorption of toxins, and a small collection

Wilhelm von Ludwig, 1790–1865. Professor of Surgery and Midwifery, Tübingen.
François Poupart, 1661–1709. French anatomist.
Lord Lister, 1827–1912, of Glasgow University, Edinburgh University, and King's College
Hospital, London, introduced antiseptic surgery in 1867.

of pus under tension, as in the mastoid antrum, often causes profound toxæmia. The general features of infection are present, although in severe cases the temperature may be subnormal, with increased pulse-rate. Headaches or even delirium, gastro-intestinal disturbances, or pulmonary symptoms are present according to the system chiefly affected.

SEPTICÆMIA and BACTERIÆMIA are due to the presence of organisms in the blood. In the former condition the organisms are not only present in the circulation, but actually proliferate therein. Streptococci are the commonest organisms to be found in the blood culture.

The condition is that of severe infection, frequently preceded by a rigor. The temperature is commonly intermittent, and rigors may continue. Icterus occasionally occurs from hæmolysis, and the degree of polymorpho-leucocytosis present is an indication of the patient's power of resistance.

Treatment consists of dealing promptly and efficiently with the causative focus of infection. Antibiotic therapy often yields striking results, especially in the case of streptococcal infections, and organisms should be isolated and tested regarding their sensitivity to penicillin. Blood transfusion is often valuable.

Sulphonamides.—Sulphatriad is commonly used, and has a wide application. It is composed of sulphathiazole, sulphadiazine and sulphamerazine. Toxic symptoms and crystalluria are uncommon with this preparation. Sulphasuxadine or sulphathalidine are usually prescribed as an intestinal disinfectant. Vomiting necessitates intravenous or intramuscular injection of a suitable preparation. If injected subcutaneously sloughing is likely to occur.

Adequate chemotherapy depends on maintaining a suitable concentration of the chemical in the blood, and the usual course of treatment lasts four or five days. During administration fluid intake must be increased, due allowance being made for loss due to increased temperature and perspiration. Potassium citrate is prescribed so as to maintain alkalinity of the urine.

Severe toxic reactions are nearly always due to an excessively long course, even though doses are small. Crystals derived from the drug may form in the renal tubules, causing renal colic, hæmaturia, and even fatal suppression. Hæmolytic anæmia and agranulocytosis are especially apt to occur during a second course of treatment. Agranulocytosis may respond to intramuscular sodium pentose nucleotide (" pentnucleotide "), 20 ml. being administered daily, and hæmatinic agents, such as liver extracts, should also be given. No course of sulpha drugs should last longer than one week, and a second course is only prescribed after a break of three days, and provided that the blood picture is satisfactory. Toxic hepatitis, skin rashes, and optic neuritis also occasionally occur.

When suppuration has occurred, care must be taken that subclinical evidence of pus does not cause deferment of a necessary operation ; this is particularly true of mastoid infection, and abscesses in any situation.

Ambulant patients are apt to suffer from lack of mental concentration, and should be warned that this may affect such intricate manœuvres as car driving.

Penicillin is a valuable antibacterial agent, which, in contradistinction to the sulphonamides, retains its activity in the presence of blood, pus, and autolysed tissues. It is particularly valuable in combating streptococcal and staphylococcal infections, and Cl. tetani and the organisms responsible for gas gangrene are sensitive to its action. Cases of gonococcal infection which are resistant to sulphonamides respond to penicillin (p. 44), which is also valuable in the treatment of syphilis. If circumstances permit, the organism is tested for sensitivity to penicillin. If the organism is sensitive, no growth occurs on a suitable medium in the vicinity of the penicillin fungus (fig. 5).

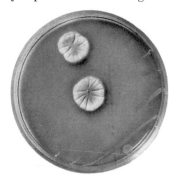

Penicillin is usually administered by intramuscular or intravenous injection and adequate blood concentration is necessary, as it is rapidly excreted by the kidneys; or it can be applied locally provided that the whole of the infected area is accessible. Oral administration is precluded, as penicillin is destroyed by acid, although some absorption occurs if large amounts are taken on a fasting stomach. The early administration of penicillin is a valuable prophylactic measure against infection of contaminated wounds, e.g. industrial injuries and road accidents.

Fig. 5.—Penicillin-sensitive staphylococci—growth is inhibited in the vicinity of the fungus.
(Glaxo Laboratories.)

Streptomycin is produced from a mould culture—Streptomyces griseus. It possesses a bacteriostatic effect on some Gram-negative organisms which are penicillin resistant. The method of administration is similar to that of penicillin, but dosage and cost of treatment are greater. As organisms tend to become resistant a short and intensive course is advisable. Streptomycin is valuable in meningeal and urinary infections due to Gram-negative bacilli, but is of little use in intestinal infections caused by typhoid or salmonella organisms. Pulmonary tuberculosis is inhibited as long as administration is continued, and some cases of tuberculous meningitis have been cured, but toxic effects occasionally follow prolonged treatment.

Aureomycin is obtained from a mould, Streptomyces aureofaciens. It is potent against a wide range of Gram-negative and Gram-positive organisms. At present its use is restricted to combat organisms which are resistant to other antibiotics. It is comparatively non-toxic, and organisms do not become resistant to it. It can be administered in the form of oral capsules.

Chloromycetin can be administered orally, and is specially useful in urinary infections, and in bowel conditions such as typhoid fever and bacillary dysentery.

PYÆMIA is due to the circulation in the blood-stream of infective emboli composed of masses of organisms, vegetations, or infected clot. Common causes of pyæmia include acute infective osteomyelitis, infection of an intracranial sinus, infective phlebitis, and ulcerative endocarditis.

When the infected embolus is arrested in a vessel, thrombosis occurs round it, and infection spreads into the adjacent tissues. If the embolus arises in connection with the systemic circulation, it is likely to be arrested in the lung, so that a wedge-shaped hæmorrhagic infarct results, which may later form an abscess. From these abscesses fresh emboli may arise and reach the left side of the heart, and thus be widely disseminated. If the focus of infection is in the portal area, the emboli are carried to the liver, giving rise to pylephlebitis (*syn.* portal pyæmia).

Clinically, in addition to the features of infection, pyæmia is characterised by rigors, an intermittent temperature, and the formation of abscesses. Abscesses occur in any part of the body, and are commonly painless ; thus an abscess in the back may be accidentally discovered as a swelling by a nurse while washing the patient. Joints are occasionally affected, and sometimes become quietly disorganised. Death usually follows abscess formation in vital structures, such as heart or brain.

The treatment of pyæmia consists in endeavouring to prevent further emboli from reaching the blood-stream. Thus, in the case of pyæmia due to suppurative arthritis of the knee joint, amputation is indicated, or if the condition is caused by thrombosis of the lateral sinus, then ligation and division of the internal jugular vein may be successful in interrupting the stream of emboli. In portal pyæmia successful cases have been reported following ligation of the superior mesenteric vein, combined with penicillin. Otherwise, abscesses are dealt with as they occur, and general treatment is instituted as for septicæmia.

WOUNDS

The treatment of an extensive wound is primarily concerned with prevention of infection. A secondary consideration is the repair of damaged structures, which are considered in their appropriate chapters. In the case of recent wounds, e.g. due to accidents, an emergency operation is performed in order to cleanse the wound as completely as possible, and every hour adds to the risk of the infection becoming established. An anæsthetic is usually necessary, and the surrounding skin is purified. The edges of the wound are excised, and damaged tissue and foreign bodies removed. Sulphonamide and penicillin

powder (5–15 gm., according to the size of the wound) is insufflated into every recess, and suitable doses are administered
orally. If a large nerve is exposed, light dusting is harmless, but
any excess is liable to result in toxic neuritis. Unless loss of skin
is excessive, closure can usually be obtained with the help of a
relaxation incision (fig. 6). Hæmorrhage from small vessels is
controlled by torsion, ligation with catgut being reserved for
larger vessels. Catgut is dead protein, and as such encourages

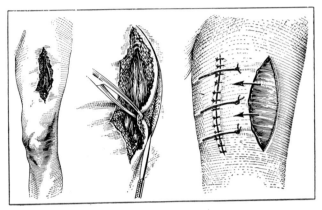

Fig. 6.—Excision of an extensive wound. Closure is facilitated
with the help of tension sutures and a relaxation incision.

infection. A plaster cast is applied, which in the case of the leg
must extend to the toes, otherwise œdema of the foot will tend to
cause ulceration where the edge of the plaster presses on the
swollen tissues. The plaster provides adequate rest to the
damaged structures ; it is removed in about three weeks, and is
reapplied if necessary. Prophylactic penicillin may be advisable
(p. 9). In some cases secondary suture is required at a later date.
In the case of a dangerous punctured wound, such as might occur
during a post-mortem or operation, acriflavine (1 ml. of 1 : 500)
should be injected immediately with a hypodermic needle
around the track of the wound.

The following points should be borne in mind concerning other antiseptics which are commonly used in the treatment of wounds. Those
which depend on oxygen or chlorine as active principles are inactivated by
blood or serum, and chlorine is driven off if the solution is heated. Iodine
also is inactivated by blood. Such substances as lysol, cyllin, and carbolic
acid devitalise tissues if used in sufficient strength to act as efficient
antiseptics. Mercury compounds are rendered inert by combination with
proteins in the serum, and are incompatible with iodine.

In all cases in which tetanus *might* develop, a prophylactic dose of A.T.S. *must* be given (p. 27). If tissues are lacerated, especially deep structures such as muscles, anti-gas-gangrene serum is also administered (p. 74). Single vials combining a suitable dose of both A.T.S. and A.G.G.S. are obtainable.

SERUM REACTIONS

Patients who have had previous serum injections, and especially those who are subject to asthma or allergic diseases, are prone to local or general reaction. To test for sensitivity a small amount of normal horse serum, or the serum to be used, should be diluted with ten times the amount of saline, and 0·1 ml. is injected intradermally. In sensitised patients a local reaction occurs within fifteen minutes, in which case the serum must be administered in fractional doses, e.g. 0·5 ml. is injected subcutaneously and the dose doubled at half-hourly intervals, until the full dose is given. After this desensitisation, further doses can be given safely.

Acute anaphylaxis may develop in sensitised patients if the above precautions are not observed. The symptoms, notably respiratory distress, usually appear in a few minutes. A tourniquet should be applied immediately, and adrenalin hydrochloride 1 ml. (1 : 1,000) injected subcutaneously at hourly intervals.

Local anaphylaxis is occasionally seen if reinjections are given at the same site after the interval of a week. An acute inflammatory reaction occurs, which in rare cases progresses to sloughing of tissues.

Serum sickness is the commonest manifestation, and may occur in any patient. Urticaria, œdema, pains or effusion in joints, and elevated temperature are usual features, which frequently occur seven to ten days after the injection. Anti-histamine compounds, e.g. Benadryl, should be administered. Otherwise cold applications applied locally, and injection of adrenalin, minimise the discomfort.

BITES

Insect bites in this country are usually inflicted by wasps or bees, although anthrax has followed the bite of a horsefly. Anaphylaxis can follow a bee or wasp sting in sensitised people. Vasomotor collapse, coma, and death have followed within twenty minutes. If anaphylactic symptoms arise, a subcutaneous injection of adrenalin (1 ml. of 1 : 1,000) is urgently required. Bees and wasps (including hornets) are easily distinguished if seen, otherwise most bees, as distinct from wasps, suffer avulsion of their sting, which is left protruding from the wound. Bee venom is acid, and should be neutralised by the application of ammonia, soda, or methylene-blue. On the contrary, the venom of the wasp is alkaline, and requires an acid, such as vinegar or lemon juice, for its neutralisation. Anti-histamine drugs given orally or applied locally are of value in allaying local irritation.

Bites of animals such as the horse, cat, and dog require the usual treatment of wounds. When there is the slightest suspicion that the animal is suffering from rabies, the bite should be freely excised or cauterised with carbolic acid, solid silver nitrate, or the cautery. If possible the responsible animal should be kept under observation, or if it has been killed Negri bodies should be sought for in the brain. Prophylactic treatment can be obtained only at a special institute.

Snake bites should be treated by the immediate application of a tourniquet, and, if the patient is co-operative, two incisions are made through the puncture wounds at right angles to a line connecting them (fig. 7). A snake's fang is curved, so poison may be deposited on either side of the puncture wounds according to the position of the reptile on biting. If available, permanganate of potassium is then applied. If incision is impracticable the patient, or a friend, sucks the wound ; any poison which may be swallowed is harmless. Stimulants are given generously, and antivenom neutralises the poison of some varieties. If possible the reptile should be killed or captured for identification purposes. In England the only poisonous reptile is the adder, or viper, but a fatal result is unlikely unless the victim is very young or debilitated. During the decade 1938–47 only two fatal cases occurred in England and Wales.

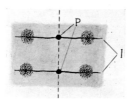

FIG. 7.—P = punctures, I = incisions. The shaded areas indicate possible deposits of venom.

Human bites should be cauterised with fuming nitric acid, and subsequently dressed with a chlorine-containing solution.

FOREIGN BODIES IN THE TISSUES

In every case of suspected foreign body which is opaque to X-rays, a radiograph must be taken in at least two planes. Other aids at X-ray localisation are the insertion of straight needles or Kirschner wires aimed at the foreign body, or Michel's clips applied to the skin over the presumed site. We have found that, in the case of comparatively superficial foreign bodies, personal observation and palpation in the X-ray room is of great assistance. When removal is attempted, a good light, ample time, and exsanguination of the limb are all highly desirable. Exsanguination assists by rendering the field bloodless, and in recent cases a reddish or brown track, due to extravasated blood, indicates the path of the foreign body.

Hypodermic needles not infrequently break at the neck, where corrosion easily occurs. Stainless needles are advisable, and should be tested frequently. The most difficult needle to recover

Adelchi Negri, 1876–1912. Professor of Bacteriology, Pavia, Italy.
Martin Kirschner, Contemporary. Professor of Surgery, University of Heidelberg.
Gaston Michel, 1874–1937. Professor of Clinical Surgery, Nancy.

is one situated in the internal pterygoid muscle, which has broken when a dental surgeon has attempted a mandibular block. The glistening tendinous intersections in the muscle continually raise the surgeon's hopes, and he is fortunate if the needle is recovered within an hour, but a good anæsthetic, adequate light, and patience bring their due reward.

Domestic needles commonly become impacted between the small bones of the hand or foot. The patient may be entirely unaware of their entry. Unless a small fragment is lodged deeply, removal is advisable, as infection may otherwise develop, and startling cases are on record in which a needle has entered the venous circulation and become embedded in the heart muscle, or travelled to some distant part of the body.

Sewing-machine needles occasionally transfix the terminal phalanx and nail, and then break. After injecting a local anæsthetic the finger should be forcibly pressed on to a hard surface, so that the fragment retraces its path. The end then projects through the nail and is removed with forceps.

Indelible-pencil fragments occasionally become lodged in the subcutaneous tissue of the hand, particularly in children. The treatment is immediate excision of the fragment and adjacent tissue. If allowed to remain, a pigmented discharge will persist for months, and exuberant granulations require constant attention.

Fish hooks, and similar articles which possess barbs, are removed by pushing the hook in such a direction that it emerges through the skin at the nearest point. The barb is then nipped off, and the hook withdrawn along the path of entry. Local anæsthesia is desirable.

Gravel is not uncommonly driven into the subcutaneous tissues of the face, hands, or knees. Ugly scars are the penalty of incomplete removal—a particularly distressing sequel if occurring on the face—"tattoo marks." In all but minor cases an anæsthetic and patient extraction are indicated. Brisk rubbing with a nail brush is sometimes helpful. Any small remaining fragments are encouraged to extrude themselves by the application of hot compresses of hypertonic saline, or 10 per cent. sodium sulphate.

Glass splinters as a rule contain sufficient lead to render them opaque to X-rays. Every lacerated or punctured wound caused by glass must be examined radiographically, as it is surprising how often fragments of glass are otherwise missed (fig. 8). In the majority of cases removal is indicated.

Punctured wounds, see p. 11.

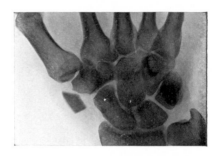

FIG. 8.—A piece of glass at the outer side of the wrist joint. Its presence was unsuspected for three weeks.

TRAUMATIC SHOCK

Shock has been defined as " a state of collapse of the circulation." It is either primary or secondary and is associated with :

(i) Diminished force of the heart beat, which is governed chiefly by the venous inflow. Death usually follows if the systolic pressure falls to 60 mm. Hg., unless speedy measures are taken to counteract the condition.

(ii) Increased permeability of the capillaries, which allows the exudation of plasma into the tissues.

(iii) Diminished blood volume, which is encouraged by hæmorrhage, vomiting, sweating, diarrhœa, and exudation of plasma into the tissues (especially in the case of burns).

(iv) Increased viscosity of the blood, owing to loss of fluid from the circulation. Hæmoconcentration follows, and is particularly liable to occur in the case of burns, owing to excessive loss of plasma (p. 79). If hæmoconcentration rises to over 150 per cent. of hæmoglobin, recovery is unlikely.

Primary shock occurs immediately as a result of over-stimulation of the medullary centres by either psychogenic or neurogenic impulses, or a combination of both.

Psychogenic shock is due to apprehension, fear, or terror. Nervous patients are much more prone to post-operative shock than those of a philosophical temperament. Thus patients who suffer an injury while their minds are engrossed, such as soldiers in the heat of battle, are sometimes entirely un-affected, even though their wounds are serious. One of the authors has seen a soldier, who was shot through the chest, entirely oblivious of the wound until a comrade enquired why his shirt was bloody. Conversely, nervous people are apt to suffer from severe primary shock from the most trivial injury. The expression " I nearly died of fright " is not necessarily hyperbolical.

Neurogenic shock follows over-stimulation of the medullary centres as a result of excessive somatic or autonomic impulses ; thus a blow on the testicle or over the solar plexus may be immediately fatal. Neurogenic shock is often associated with severe burns or multiple injuries, and may complicate abdominal operations, especially if viscera do not receive gentle treatment.

Secondary shock develops within two to a few hours after injury. It is predisposed to by exposure, pain, starvation, loss of fluid, especially blood, absorption of products from damaged tissue, and toxæmia. The psychogenic factor also plays a part, but to a lesser extent than in the case of primary shock.

The obvious clinical features of secondary shock are pallor, sweating or clamminess, an anxious expression, and often vomiting. The patient complains of thirst, but becomes increasingly apathetic if the condition progresses. Respirations are shallow, and the pulse-rate increases, while the blood-pressure diminishes. Repeated blood-pressure recordings are some indication of the progress of the case, bearing in mind that individual blood-pressures vary within wide limits. A more important guide is variations in the degree of hæmoconcentration, which should be checked at intervals.

Treatment.—*First-aid.* " What first-aid treatment is administered by the ear ? " was a question in an oral examination. The answer required was " Words of comfort ! " Cheerful confidence on the part of first-aid personnel, by counteracting the natural fear of an injured person, is not only humane but also a valuable therapeutic measure. Hæmorrhage is controlled, fractures are immobilised if necessary, a hot drink is given if available, and the patient is transported to hospital, bearing in mind that he must be protected from cold and the head kept low.

Resuscitation.—A *resuscitation room* should be available at every hospital which caters for the treatment of seriously injured patients. The room should be warm, a radiant-heat cage available, scissors, etc., at hand to remove dirty clothes, and infusion and transfusion apparatus ready for immediate use. An anæsthetic trolley, drugs, syringes, etc., are also available. After cleansing and resuscitation the patient can be transported to the operating theatre if his injuries require any major surgical procedure.

Warmth.—Overheating is harmful, more so than over-cooling, and care must be exercised in the use of such appliances as electric blankets or cradles. The patient's temperature should be raised to normal, and unless special heat-providing appliances are thermostatically controlled, it is better to resort to the old-fashioned method of blankets and covered hot-water bottles.

Morphia.—This drug has no specific anti-shock value and may indeed be harmful in increasing respiratory depression, as in the case of head injuries. Therefore, if the patient is comfortable in body and tranquil in mind, it should be withheld until some definite indication arises which requires its administration. If relief of pain is urgent, an intravenous injection of $\frac{1}{6}$ to $\frac{1}{4}$ gr. in 1 ml. of sterile water is advisable. In the case of patients with low blood-pressures, a subcutaneous or intramuscular injection is tardily absorbed, and if repeated doses are injudiciously administered, an excessive amount is liable to be absorbed when the condition of the patient improves.

Maintenance of Body Fluid.—If the patient is conscious and can retain fluid by the mouth, thirst is relieved and the fluid balance more or less restored by the administration of fluid by the mouth. Warm sweet tea is excellent for this purpose. In more severe cases infusion or transfusion is urgently required. In the shock-hæmorrhage syndrome blood transfusion is necessary, but if shock is unassociated with hæmorrhage, plasma is administered either intravenously or into the marrow of a suitable bone.

In severe cases frequent hæmoglobin readings are taken, so that dangerous hæmoconcentration can be counteracted by increased infusions.

Posture.—Raising the foot of the bed helps to maintain adequate cerebral circulation, especially in cases of primary shock. Firm bandages applied to the limbs are useful in suitable cases. Rocking a patient has been found to be a valuable resuscitative measure, which depends on the " pull and push " exerted on the diaphragm by the abdominal viscera. The patient is tied to a stretcher, face downwards in the case of drowning, and the stretcher is then rocked through about 50 degrees from ten to fifteen times a minute. Special rocking stretchers, fitted with a timing device, are now available.

Oxygen Therapy.—Routine administration of oxygen is not indicated in cases of uncomplicated shock, but oxygen therapy is useful in patients who are heavily morphinised, suffer from pulmonary complications, or who have been exposed to coal gas.

Toxæmia.—Severe injury to tissues results in the production of some toxic substance which encourages the production of shock. Whether histamine is the causative agent is doubtful, but that some toxic body is produced is beyond doubt, as the removal of a tourniquet from a crushed limb may be immediately succeeded by an exacerbation of shock. Therefore, in the case of a severe injury some surgeons amputate above the tourniquet, and include it in the part removed. Should it be decided that removal of the tourniquet is advisable, the appliance should be loosened gradually.

Pressor Substances.—Deoxycortone (D.O.C.A.) may be useful in encouraging peripheral vasoconstriction. It is also alleged to diminish the permeability of the capillaries, but further evidence is necessary before its value can be established.

OXYGEN THERAPY

The administration of oxygen is of value in many conditions, e.g. some cases of shock, pulmonary complications after operations, injuries to the chest, following operations on the thyroid gland, or in cases of fat embolism. The simplest, but very inefficient, method is to attach a funnel to the rubber tube which is fixed to the oxygen cylinder, and place the funnel in such a position that the patient inhales the gas. The pressure of gas can be estimated roughly by pinching the rubber tube and listening to the " pop " which occurs when the obstruction is released. An elaboration of this method is to bubble the oxygen through brandy (diluted if need be!). Some of the brandy volatilises and is inhaled by the patient, but, what is more important, the bubbling can be regulated to the needs of the patient, and when bubbles cease it is obvious that the cylinder is empty !

Oxygen spectacles are an improvement on the funnel, in that the oxygen passes directly into the nose, and if the patient moves the flow of gas is uninterrupted. The apparatus is comfortable and easily adjusted (fig. 9). The gas can be passed through a Woulfe's bottle, which acts as a flowmeter.

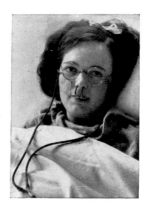

FIG. 9.—Oxygen " spectacles."

The *injector mask* (fig. 10) is a modification of the Boothby mask with an expiratory valve placed in the nose-piece. This relieves the patient from being forced to breathe against pressure of high rates of oxygen flow, and the mouth can be kept partially closed in comfort. Also the flowmeter is incorporated in the oxygen cylinder head. (A similar mask is used by airmen, when high-altitude flying necessitates an additional supply of oxygen.)

Oxygen tents are valuable, and the oxygen content is easily estimated by chemical means. Children should be reassured, as they are likely to be frightened by confinement in an enclosed space, and, if possible, nervous patients should be accustomed to a tent before its necessity arises. Nurses are warned against the risk of explosion, and naked lights are forbidden in the proximity of the tent.

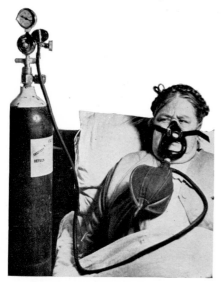

FIG. 10.—The injector mask.

CRUSH SYNDROME

This syndrome, which was commonly associated with air-raids, sometimes occurs in connection with mining or industrial accidents. As a result of massive crushing of muscles some substance gains access to the circulation which exerts a depressive effect on the renal tubules. The degree of shock associated with the injury has no relation to the development of the crush syndrome. The patient usually appears

Peter Woulfe, 1727–1803, English Chemist.
Walter Meredith Boothby, Contemporary. Director, Section on Metabolism, Mayo Clinic.
The Boothby mask is sometimes referred to as the B.L.B. mask (Boothby, Lovelace, and Bulbulian).

to be comparatively well for two or three days following the accident, although his excretion of urine is scanty. Apathy, restlessness, and possibly mild delirium indicate deficient renal function, and uræmia supervenes. First-aid treatment may necessitate the application of a tourniquet to the affected limb. The tourniquet is gradually released so that deleterious substances are admitted to the circulation in small quantities. If oliguria develops, the fluid intake must be maintained, if necessary intravenously or intramuscularly, but the risk of pulmonary œdema must be borne in mind. The urine should be rendered alkaline by the administration of sodium citrate and sodium bicarbonate. In severe cases intravenous isotonic sodium sulphate (4·285 per cent.) is urgently required.

Recent researches show that there is an alternative circulation in the kidney. The blood, instead of flowing through the vasa afferentia to the glomeruli in the cortex, may be shunted via the vasa recti to the medulla, and hence little or no urine is secreted. This medullary circulation opens up in such cases as incompatible blood transfusion, crush syndrome, and blackwater fever, and protects the cortex from damage by noxious elements. In established cases sympathetic block abolishes the reflex which initiates this secondary renal circulation.

CHAPTER II

SPECIFIC INFECTIOUS DISEASES

ERYSIPELAS

ERYSIPELAS is a spreading inflammation of the skin and subcutaneous tissues, due to infection by one of the hæmolytic streptococcus group (fig. 11). The organisms frequently gain entry to the tissues through a small or neglected wound, but in some cases no breach in the skin is discoverable. The general health of the patient is usually below par, and debilitating diseases, the extremes of life, and poor hygiene are predisposing conditions.

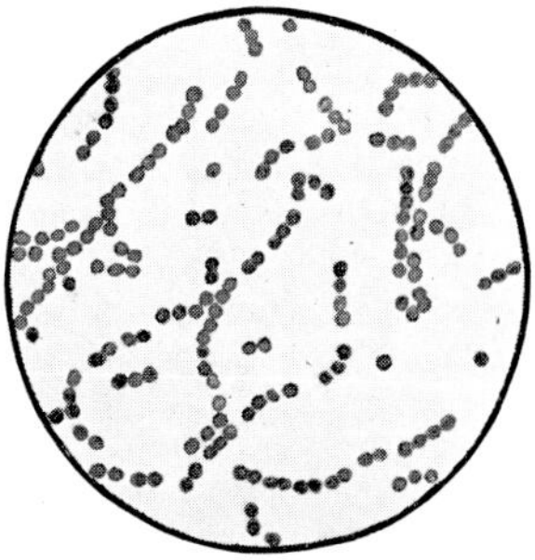

Symptoms.—The patient notices that the skin in the vicinity of a scratch or abrasion has become irritable and feels stiff. After a few hours symptoms of toxæmia supervene, which usually increase in severity until the patient is obviously ill, or even delirious.

FIG. 11.—Streptococci.

Signs.—If the infection commences in a wound, this will exhibit an inflamed or sloughing appearance, and from the margins a rose-pink rash extends over the adjacent skin (fig. 12). The edge of the rash is raised, a feature which is often more easily appreciated with the finger than the eye. The colour of the rash and its obvious edge are important points in distinguishing a true erysipelas from cellulitis. As the rash extends, vesicles appear, which burst and discharge serum. Considerable swelling occurs when

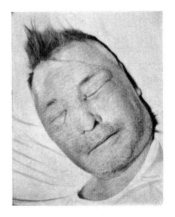

FIG. 12.—Extensive erysipelas of the face.

lax tissues are involved, particularly the orbit and the scrotum, owing to extensive œdema of the subcutaneous layers. The scrotum is liable to become as large as a melon, and is often of a peculiar waxy colour. The rash gradually fades, and for some weeks a brown discoloration of the skin remains, due to pigment set free as a result of destruction of red corpuscles. Inflammation of regional lymph nodes invariably accompanies the infection, but suppuration is unusual.

In some cases the infection wanders about the body, perhaps for months (*erysipelas migrans*).

An uncommon, but very troublesome, form of the disease is the *recurrent type*, which usually affects the face and head. Periodically, for no apparent reason, the patient suffers from an outbreak of the disease, in spite of every prophylactic measure. Lymphatic obstruction is likely to follow

COMPLICATIONS

Severe Toxæmia.—Is liable to be fatal in debilitated subjects.

Gangrene.—Sloughing of skin and subcutaneous tissues occasionally occurs, particularly of lax tissues in patients of poor resistance. Septicæmia or pyæmia may follow.

Lymphatic Obstruction.—A severe attack of erysipelas is sometimes followed by fibrosis of the lymphatic vessels and nodes, so that lymphatic drainage is impaired. The eyelids are not uncommonly affected, greatly to the detriment of the patient's appearance and comfort (fig. 13).

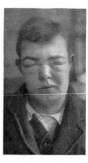

Intercurrent Disease.—It is not uncommon, particularly in the elderly, for some fatal complication to develop during an attack of erysipelas, especially pulmonary or renal complications.

Treatment.—Erysipelas is a contagious disease, and therefore the patient should be isolated or, at least, removed from a surgical ward. Care must be taken during dressings to prevent contamination, and those who dress the wound must use gloves for their own, as well as others', safety. Surgeons and accoucheurs must be particularly careful, as organisms are apt to be conveyed to other patients.

Fig. 13.—Lymphatic œdema of face and eyelids, following erysipelas. The patient was unable to open his eyes.

General treatment is directed towards improving the health of the patient in every possible way. A suitable diet, mild aperients, adequate ventilation, sulphonamide, penicillin, and stimulants all receive due consideration. Anti-streptococcal serum, prepared against the specific streptococcus of erysipelas, is now obsolescent, as penicillin usually gives speedy relief. Collosol manganese injections are useful in recurrent or long-standing cases.

Local treatment appears to exert little effect upon the spread of the disease, but ichthyol ointment is useful for relieving pain and stiffness. We have found gauze soaked in a saturated aqueous solution of magnesium sulphate to be a very satisfactory dressing. Ultra-violet irradiation is useful in arresting the spread of inflammation.

Incisions for the relief of tension are occasionally necessary, especially in lax tissues, and may obviate the onset of gangrene.

ERYSIPELOID

Erysipeloid[1] is caused by the Gram-positive bacillus Erysipelothrix rhusiopathiæ (the organism of swine fever) which is introduced into the tissues by a punctured wound, usually as a result of a prick or scratch by a fish bone or scale, or, less commonly, a splintered meat bone. Thus the disease is occupational, and it is also seasonal, being most common in late summer and early autumn. The incubation period is from two to seven days, following which a purplish induration appears, usually on a finger. Induration and dusky discoloration gradually extend to the palm and adjacent fingers (fig. 14). Discomfort and stiffness may be sufficiently severe to disable the patient, but general symptoms of infection are slight, and regional lymph nodes are not affected. Temporary improvement is commonly followed by relapses, but after a period of from three to six weeks the condition gradually subsides.

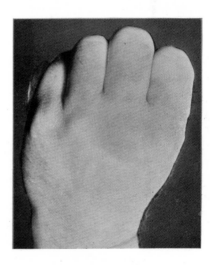

FIG. 14.—Erysipeloid.

Sulphonamides are useless. Treatment consists in keeping

[1] Described by Morrant Baker, of St. Bartholomew's Hospital, in 1873 as Erythema serpens, and now commonly known as fish-handler's disease.

the affected hand at rest, and intramuscular penicillin.   Under this régime the condition subsides in a few days.   The disease is more common than is generally recognised.

ANTHRAX

B. anthracis are large, rectangular organisms which tend to arrange themselves in chains (fig. 15).   They are Gram-positive,

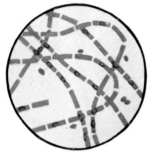

facultative anaerobes, and form spores which are very resistant to antiseptics. The disease causes epidemics in cattle, and is likely to occur in men who handle cattle, carcases, wool, hides, and hair.   A few years ago many cases were traced to contaminated Japanese shaving brushes.

Fig. 15.—B. anthracis, large rectangular bacilli in chains, with central spores.

TYPES

Cutaneous.—This is the commonest human variety ; the incubation period is from three to four days.   The lesion usually commences on an exposed portion of the body, such as the hands, forearms, or face (p. 143). An itching papule occurs, around which a patch of induration soon becomes evident.   The papule suppurates and is replaced by a black slough, and a ring of vesicles appears on the surrounding indurated area.   This stage comprises the typical " malignant pustule " (fig. 16).   The induration extends subcutaneously, so that a brawny, congested patch develops around the site of infection.   The regional lymph nodes are invariably involved.   Toxæmia is always in evidence, and an elevated temperature and raised pulse-rate are important evidences in the diagnosis of an early case of anthrax.   The diagnosis is confirmed by examining a smear of the fluid from a vesicle, as the organisms are easy to stain and recognise.

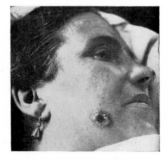

Fig. 16.—Anthrax pustule.

(*A. E Hodgson.*)

In a few cases œdema develops without any obvious primary focus. The œdema rapidly spreads, and somewhat resembles erysipelas, but

Dr. Guillotin, 1738–1814, who advocated the use of the guillotine so that executions should be speedy and painless, died from an anthrax pustule.

toxæmia is more profound. This feature, in conjunction with the patient's occupation, should arouse suspicion, which can be confirmed by the examination of fluid from a vesicle.

Treatment.—Official regulations have done much to reduce the incidence of the disease, and prophylactic measures should be followed rigidly.

Excision was formerly a favourite method of local treatment, but is no guarantee against the onset of septicæmia. A protective barrier of serum injected subcutaneously around the pustule is a safer and more rational procedure. Ipecacuanha paste appears to be of decided benefit, but otherwise antiseptic compresses, such as 1 : 1,000 oxycyanide of mercury, should be used.

Neo-salvarsan can be regarded as a specific for anthrax, and has practically replaced serum therapy. It should be given intravenously in doses of 0·6 gm. daily, or on alternate days, according to the severity of the infection. Neo-salvarsan is used extensively in South Africa, where anthrax is comparatively common, and we have used this preparation with excellent results. Successful results have also followed the administration of streptomycin.

Pulmonary (*syn.* Woolsorter's disease).—Caused by the inhalation of spores, and characterised by a virulent bronchitis and broncho-pneumonia, with toxæmia, dyspnœa, and blood-stained sputum. The organisms are found in the sputum. Immediate and intensive antibiotic therapy may save the patient.

Alimentary.—Follows the ingestion of spores, provided they escape destruction by the acid in the stomach. Severe enteritis follows, which resembles cholera. The patient collapses and suffers from severe abdominal pain and blood-stained diarrhœa.

TETANUS

This disease can be associated with any type of wound, but particularly those contaminated with cultivated soil, or of a punctured and infected nature. The popular impression that tetanus is especially liable to follow a wound between the thumb and index finger is due to the fact that those who dig much, such as gardeners and gravediggers, are likely to excoriate the skin in that area and contaminate it with soil.

The Cl. tetani is Gram-positive, and occurs as straight rods which develop a terminal spore, so that the name " drumstick "

The Clostridium tetani was first cultivated by Kitasato in Berlin in 1889.

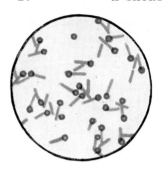

FIG. 17.—Cl. tetani (Ziehl-Neilson's stain).

spore has been aptly applied (fig. 17). The clostridium is anaerobic, hence its partiality to deep or punctured wounds, or if pyogenic organisms are also present. In some cases the wound through which the organisms gained admittance has healed before symptoms are evident. The reopening of an old wound, even years after infliction, occasionally stimulates dormant organisms into activity.

Other occasional causes are penetration of the sole by a nail in the shoe, wounds caused by wads of toy pistols, felt applied to a pressure sore, and infected catgut.

CLINICAL TYPES

Acute Tetanus.—Occurs within fifteen days of inoculation, and the shorter the incubation period the higher the mortality. The first symptoms are psychical. The patient becomes restless and uneasy, he is unable to concentrate or even keep still, and he experiences a dread of some impending evil. The temperature and pulse-rate are above normal. Within twenty-four hours muscular spasm supervenes, usually first affecting the muscles at the back of the neck, and then the jaw muscles. Risus sardonicus appears later, due to contraction of the facial muscles (fig. 18). Spasms follow, which extend to all the skeletal muscles, and during severe exacerbations the patient rests on his head and heels (opisthotonus). The psoas or rectus abdominis muscles are sometimes ruptured (fig. 19). The spasms are tonic as well as clonic, so relaxation is incomplete during the intervals. This feature distinguishes tetanus from strychnine poisoning; also in the latter case spasms commence in the extremities. Death occurs from cardiac failure following exhaustion, pulmonary œdema, or occasionally from asphyxia during a vice-like spasm of the respiratory muscles. A post-mortem rise of temperature follows.

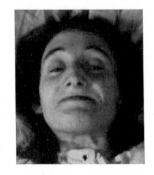

FIG. 18.—Risus sardonicus.
(*Photo by Dr. R. Blunden.*)

Chronic Tetanus.—The incubation period is over fifteen days, and may be as long as six weeks. The symptoms are similar to those of acute tetanus, but much less severe. The prognosis is favourable.

Delayed Tetanus.—Organisms are capable of remaining latent in a wound for years, and causing tetanus when the wound is reopened. A prophylactic dose of serum must always be given if a potentially infected wound requires reopening.

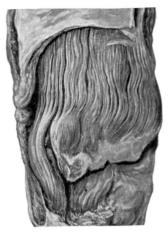

Fig. 19.—A torn rectus abdominis muscle from a case of tetanus, which followed a small wound of a toe.

Local Tetanus occurs in the muscles around the initial wound. It is usually seen when the prophylactic dose of serum has counteracted general infection, but was insufficient to prevent local nerve involvement.

Head tetanus follows a wound in the distribution of the facial nerve. This is a rare type, not many more than one hundred cases have been reported. The toxin reaches the central nervous system via the lymphatics in the sheath of a nerve, and so swelling of the nerve results. In the case of the facial nerve, which is enclosed in the rigid stylo-mastoid foramen, swelling compresses the nerve and causes paresis of the muscles of expression instead of risus sardonicus.

Bulbar tetanus is a rare and fatal form, which follows visceral infection. Involvement of the muscles of deglutition and respiration results in dysphagia and fatal dyspnœa. This type may be confused with hydrophobia.

Tetanus Neonatorum is due to infection of the newborn child via the wound left after separation of the umbilical cord. This type is fatal.

TREATMENT

Prophylactic.—Immunity conferred by injections of toxoid is of extreme importance, particularly with regard to the fighting forces. It seems that permanent immunity is obtained if 1 ml. of toxoid is administered, and repeated at intervals of eight weeks and nine months, and followed up with a " recall " dose every four years.

Unless active immunity has been obtained, it is of the utmost importance that every patient with a potentially infected wound should receive an intramuscular injection of 3,000 International units of anti-tetanic serum. Surgical treatment of the wound should be postponed until at least one hour after the injection. A smaller dose of serum may be repeated, with advantage, at weekly intervals for a month. Also, should old wounds require reopening, as for the removal of a foreign body, serum is given prior to the operation.

Symptomatic.—The patient is isolated in quiet surroundings. Anæsthetics are required to permit of nasal feeding, catheterisation, and the injection of antitoxin, and during the first anæsthetic it is advisable to pass a Ryle's stomach tube intranasally. Chloretone, chloral, and bromides are given by the mouth or rectally, and avertin or paraldehyde by the latter route is strongly recommended. Muscular spasms not only exhaust the patient, but possibly increase the amount of toxin entering the spinal cord by compressing the motor nerves, and also, under avertin anæsthesia, the patient is spared the terror which otherwise heralds the onset of a spasm. Myanesin (which has a less depressing effect on respiration than curare) is valuable in controlling spasms, and can be given in doses of 1 gr. (0·065 gm.) at intervals of two to four hours.

Sweating results in chloride depletion, so normal saline should be given through the nasal tube as necessary. Tetanus is an exhausting disease, and careful consideration must be given to ensure an adequate intake of food and fluid. Oxygen is administered through a Boothby's mask to counteract cyanosis or respiratory failure.

Therapeutic.—200,000 I.U. should be given intravenously as soon as possible, and one hour later the wound is dealt with surgically, if such treatment is required. It is shown that ample antitoxins are still in the circulation seven days later, and one massive dose obviates further disturbance of the patient which would be caused by repeated injections. Penicillin is used in conjunction with serum, and should be administered in a slow-release medium in order to minimise the number of injections required. If the condition of the patient is unsatisfactory seven days after the initial injection, a further 50,000 units of antitoxins should be administered intravenously. Intrathecal injections through a lumbar puncture have now been abandoned. This route offers no advantage over intravenous injection, and the serous meningitis which follows merely causes further irritation of the spinal nerves and cord.

Prognosis depends on the following factors :

(i) *Period of Incubation.*—If less than seven days elapses between the infliction of the wound and the first symptom, a fatal termination is to be expected. Prognosis improves with the length of the incubation period.

John Ryle (1889–1950). Nuffield Professor of Social Medicine, Oxford.
The American unit of antitoxin (A.U.) is double the potency of the International unit (I.U.).

(ii) *Period of Onset.*—This is the time which elapses between the first evidence of rigidity and the onset of reflex spasms. If this period is less than forty-eight hours death is likely, but if four days or more elapse recovery will probably ensue if adequate treatment is available.

ACTINOMYCOSIS

This disease is alleged to affect those whose work brings them into contact with corn and grain, but accumulating statistics seem to indicate that the disease affects all members of the community equally, whatever their occupation may be. Probably the actinomyces are present normally in the mouth, tonsils, and alimentary canal, and become pathogenic when some local injury abrades or reduces the vitality of the mucous membrane. The oral manifestations of the disease are certainly commoner in patients who neglect dental hygiene.

Small granules, which are sometimes sulphur-coloured, are found in the pus, which results from secondary infection. The granules are colonies of the streptothrix, and microscopically are seen to consist of masses of Gram-positive filaments, or mycelia. These

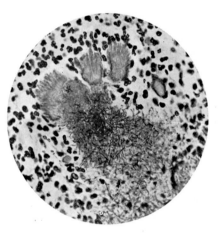

Fig. 20.—Ray fungus × 500 microphotograph. From material excised from the neck of a girl of eighteen.

filaments radiate from the central part of the granule, this arrangement accounting for the term " ray fungus." These mycelial threads are sometimes seen to have an expanded end, or " club " (fig. 20). The clubs are Gram-negative, and are only found in the body, and not in cultures. The commonest type of streptothrix is anaerobic, but an aerobic form occasionally occurs.

Actinomycotic lesions are characterised by the formation of a firm, indurated mass, the edges of which are indefinite, and infection spreads by direct invasion of adjacent tissues. Lymph nodes are not affected, but if a vein is invaded, pyæmic infection is likely to follow.

The following are the usual sites of infection :

(i) *Facio-cervical.*—The lower jaw is more frequently affected,

Otto von Bollinger, 1843–1909. Professor of Pathology at the Veterinary School, Munich, first recognised the ray fungus.

often adjacent to a carious tooth. The gum becomes so indurated that it simulates a bony swelling. As extension occurs, nodules appear, which soften and burst. The overlying skin of the face and neck is indurated and bluish in colour, softening occurs in patches, and eventually abscesses burst through the skin (see fig. 219). The characteristic features of the condition are chronicity, dense induration, and sinuses surrounded by bluish skin (see p. 201).

(ii) *Thorax.*—The lungs and pleura are infected either by aspiration of the fungus, or, occasionally, by direct spread downwards from the pharynx or neck, or upwards through the diaphragm.

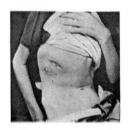

Fig. 21.—Actinomycosis of the lung involving the chest wall.

The disease extends through the lungs to the pleura and chest wall, which, in the late stages, is riddled with sinuses (fig. 21). An empyema is not uncommon, and the infection sometimes spreads through the diaphragm to the liver or subphrenic spaces. Clinically, the condition resembles tuberculosis, and in the early stages is only distinguished by the discovery of mycelial threads in the sputum.

(iii) *Abdomen.*—The ileo-cæcal region is most commonly affected, owing to the considerable stasis which occurs in this part of the bowel. Possibly for the same reason, the sigmoid colon is occasionally involved.

Ileo-cæcal actinomycosis usually occurs in one of two forms. Either an indurated mass forms in the iliac fossa, or the disease resembles appendicitis. In the latter case the true nature of the infection is usually unsuspected until the wound breaks down a few weeks or months later. In many cases the appendix shows no naked-eye evidence of inflammation.

The liver is not infrequently affected. The disease may be primary, but nearly always it arises as a pyæmic infection from the ileo-cæcal angle. The liver becomes adherent to adjacent structures, and on section the abscesses present a " honeycomb " appearance due to interlacing strands of fibrous tissue. Occasionally, infection spreads through the diaphragm from the pleura.

Treatment.—Extirpation of the infected tissues should be attempted whenever possible, as in the case of early infection of the ileo-cæcal angle. Owing to the difficulty of excision, cervical infection is usually treated conservatively. Should sinuses occur, they are scraped and packed with gauze smeared with zinc peroxide paste.

Conservative measures include the administration of massive doses of potassium iodide, up to ʒii thrice a day. Iodised milk is often beneficial, and is administered as described on p. 202. Some cases have been reported in which sulphonamide therapy has caused remarkable improvement, when iodine has had but little effect. An intensive course of penicillin is advisable, although results are variable. Streptomycin is sometimes more effective than penicillin. Deep X-ray therapy is worthy of trial in obstinate cases.

LEPROSY

This disease was formerly world wide in its distribution. Nowadays, owing to the ease and rapidity of modern travel, cases are apt to present themselves when least expected.

Prodromal features include irregular temperature, loss of eyelashes and eyebrows, skin eruptions, pruritus, and sweating. The disease then develops into one of two forms, although some features are often common to both.

Nerve Leprosy.—Nerves become thickened, and those near the surface are easily palpable or even visible. Early sensory changes include pain, formication, and later anæsthesia, and subsequently atrophy occurs of the corresponding soft tissues and bones, so that toes and fingers are destroyed. Perforating ulcers of the feet, and stenosis of the larynx (leper's cough), are later manifestations. Death commonly results from some intercurrent infection.

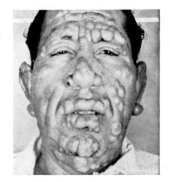

Fig. 22.—Nodular leprosy.

Nodular Leprosy.—Infiltration of the skin occurs, which begins as small nodules and eventually extends until large plaques are evident. These often coalesce so that on the face natural folds are obliterated, and the appearance becomes leonine (fig. 22). The nasal septum and the conjunctivæ are affected in the later stages. Some of the nodules gradually absorb and leave an anæsthetic area, others ulcerate and become secondarily infected.

Treatment.—Lepers should be segregated in organised colonies. When the disease is recognised, chaulmoogra oil or one of its preparations is administered. Sulphetrone has recently been used with encouraging results. Co-existing syphilis is not uncommon and demands recognition. Burdensome and useless limbs should be amputated, and a tracheotomy is sometimes required for stenosis of the larynx.

SYPHILIS

A detailed description of syphilis and gonorrhœa is outside the scope
of this work, and those requiring such should refer to one of the many
textbooks on venereal diseases. We include here a general summary of
these diseases, and affections of the various individual organs and structures
are considered in their appropriate chapters.

The usual incubation period of acquired syphilis is from
fifteen to twenty-one days, although variations of from seven to
seventy days have been noted. Diagnosis was revolutionised
by the discovery in 1905, by Schaudinn, of the causative
organism, the Treponema pallidum (*syn.* spirochæta pallida).
The treponema can be discovered in serum or scrapings from
most surface lesions. If enlarged lymph nodes are present,
lymph can be aspirated with a fine
needle, and examination will often
reveal spirochætes.

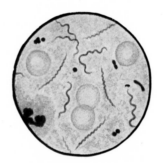

By means of dark-ground illumination an organism is seen as a
spiral organism resembling a corkscrew in appearance. On the average eight spirals are present, and the
organism is about 8 microns in
length (fig. 23).

Fig. 23.—Treponema pallidum
(corkscrew) and Spirochæta re-
fringens (spiral). Smear preparation from hard chancre.

The complement-fixation test, or
Wassermann reaction, is usually
positive in untreated cases, about
two weeks after the appearance
of the primary sore. Treatment should not be delayed
until the test is positive, but commenced immediately the
treponema is demonstrated. Treatment instituted while the
serum is negative yields excellent prospects of permanent
cure. In untreated late primary and secondary syphilis the
W.R. is almost always positive. In the tertiary stage a positive result is obtained in about 80 per cent. of cases. If the
central nervous system is affected, the cerebrospinal fluid may
give a positive reaction, although the blood serum is negative.
In some cases a doubtful reaction is rendered positive by
a small " provocative " dose of arsenic. In addition to its
diagnostic value, the W.R. is also a valuable control regarding
the efficacy and result of treatment.

*Syphilis derives its name from a poem by a physician, Girolamo Fracastor, published in
    Venice in 1530. The poem tells of the shepherd Syphilus, who was struck down by the
    disease as a punishment for neglecting the worship of Apollo.*
Fritz Schaudinn, 1871–1906. A Prussian zoologist.
*August von Wassermann, 1866–1925. Director of the Institute for Experimental Therapy
    Berlin.*

Other conditions which render the serum positive to the W.R. are yaws, glandular fever, and leprosy. Weak reactions are sometimes obtained in miliary tuberculosis, malaria, typhus, vaccinia, relapsing fever, and advanced malignant disease.

Precipitation tests are useful when elaborate technique is impossible, or curtailment of time is necessary. These tests depend upon the development of a flocculent precipitate when antigen and syphilitic serum are mixed and incubated. Although probably not quite as accurate as the W.R., these tests are of great practical value as a rapid confirmation before commencing treatment.

Clinical Features.—Acquired syphilitic manifestations are roughly divisible into three stages.

Primary Stage.—In 96 per cent. of cases the primary sore or chancre is situated on the genital organs.

In the male the chancre is usually obvious, but in the female a primary sore on the inner aspect of the vulva or on the cervix is often unnoticed by the patient, and the infection is likely to progress well into the second stage before its real nature is recognised. Extragenital chancres occur on the lips, usually the upper (fig. 104), the tongue (fig. 24), the tonsil, the anal margin, the nipple, the fingers, and rarely in other situations.

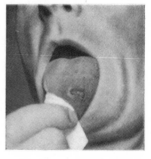

FIG. 24.—Primary chancre of the tongue. On palpation its edges felt hard. The submaxillary lymphatic nodes are enlarged. A scraping revealed treponema pallidum

Primary sores on the lips usually result from kissing, and one case is recorded in which a gentleman with secondary ulceration of the mouth infected five young ladies at a dance, each of whom developed a chancre on the lip. Dental surgeons and accoucheurs are particularly prone to inoculation on the fingers, but "syphilitic onychiæ" are less common than formerly owing to the routine use of rubber gloves and more rigorous surgical cleanliness.

A primary sore is due to inoculation of an abrasion, and is first noticed as an indurated papule, which is somewhat irritable. Secondary infection causes ulceration, and a typical Hunterian chancre develops (fig. 25). The ulcer presents a definite margin, and fibrosis of the base leads to characteristic induration. In the case of vascular structures, such as the lip, considerable œdema of the underlying tissues is present. In about 20 per

John Hunter, 1728–1793. Surgeon to St. George's Hospital. To further his knowledge of venereal disease he inoculated himself with syphilis in 1767.

cent. of cases chancres are multiple, either as a result of infection of two or more abrasions, or owing to auto-inoculation of an apposing surface by the primary sore. The regional lymph nodes become enlarged and firm, and are aptly described as " shotty." In the case of a penile chancre, the dorsal lymphatics can often be felt to be " wiry " when the subcutaneous tissue is rolled between the finger and thumb.

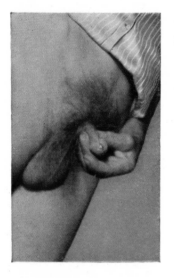

Fig. 25.—A typical hard chancre.

In some cases the initial papule disappears without ulceration, and the patient is genuinely totally unaware of its presence. On the other hand, virulent secondary infection sometimes supervenes and the ulcer becomes acutely inflamed, with secondary acute lymphangitis and enlarged and tender lymph nodes. Phagedena may supervene if phimosis is present.

A primary chancre must be distinguished from a traumatic ulcer (which follows irritation of an abrasion), a soft sore (p. 45), an early epithelioma, and herpes, which is painful and commences as a crop of vesicles on an inflamed base.

Secondary Stage.—This commences when infection is disseminated by the blood-stream, and lasts for an arbitrary period of about six months. When blood infection occurs, any organ or tissue in the body is liable to be affected.

The general manifestations of the secondary stage include malaise, anæmia, a varying degree of pyrexia, and generalised enlargement of the lymph nodes. The epitrochlear, sub-occipital, and posterior cervical nodes are especially liable to be affected. Alopecia is not uncommon (the " rat-bitten " type).

Cutaneous eruptions, although varying widely in their natures, are usually characteristic. A syphilitic rash appears, as a rule, about eight weeks after infection, and is commonly widely distributed in a symmetrical manner. The earliest manifestation is a roseolar rash due to hyperæmia of the cutaneous capillaries. Cellular infiltration and fibrosis may follow, with the formation of papules. If the infection is virulent or the patient debilitated, pustules and ulceration are likely to develop. In some cases the rash exhibits a scaly appearance, somewhat resembling psoriasis, but differing from that condition in that the flexor surfaces are chiefly, if not entirely, affected.

The main characteristics of a syphilitic eruption are the dull red or coppery colour, the absence of irritation, the symmetrical distribution, and the polymorphic nature, i.e. two or three types of rash are often present simultaneously.

Muco-cutaneous junctions and mucous membranes are commonly affected during the secondary stage. Papules appear at such muco-cutaneous junctions as the anal margin, vulva, or angle of the mouth, or where cutaneous surfaces are constantly in apposition. As a result of their situation these papules become sodden, and frequently form large, foul, greyish masses, which are termed condylomata. Condylomata are intensely infectious, but disappear rapidly with general treatment and local cleanliness.

Moist papules or mucous patches occasionally occur in the mouth as circular raised areas, greyish in colour, and surrounded by hyperæmic mucosa. Ulceration occasionally occurs. Mucous patches are sometimes so large that they resemble condylomata, and those on the dorsum of the tongue were formerly described as " Hutchinson's warts."

" Snail-track " ulcers particularly affect the mucosa covering the soft palate and tonsils. These characteristic ulcers are shallow, greyish in colour, and exhibit well-defined edges. The mucous membrane of the nose is occasionally affected in a similar manner.

Warning.—The saliva in these cases is teeming with spirochætes. Gloves should always be worn, and tongue depressors either burnt or rigorously sterilised.

At a later period of the secondary stage, fleeting bone pains or periosteal nodes are often in evidence. Transitory and usually symmetrical effusions may occur in the larger joints. Epididymitis occasionally develops and is sometimes associated with nephritis and albuminuria. Iritis sometimes occurs, and gives rise to pain, lachrymation, circumcorneal congestion, and a sluggish and irregular pupil. The colour of the iris may alter owing to œdema. At a later date such conditions as choroido-

Sir Jonathan Hutchinson, 1828–1913. Surgeon to the London Hospital.

retinitis may develop.   Perivascular infiltration and mesarteritis are likely to manifest themselves, especially in connection with the brain or cord, and neurological phenomena may result.

Rupia occasionally occurs as a late secondary manifestation, particularly in virulent or neglected cases.   The discharge from cutaneous ulcers dries in successive layers, so that an excrescence of dried pus and débris gradually accumulates, and somewhat resembles a limpet.

Tertiary Stage.—This arbitrarily commences from six months to three years after infection, and may last throughout the patient's lifetime.   The characteristic pathological changes are either diffuse gummatous infiltration, or local gumma formation, and almost any structure in the body is liable to be affected. In some organs both changes occur ; thus a gummatous orchitis is sometimes associated with a local gumma, and a cirrhotic liver may harbour gummata.

A gumma is a mass of necrotic tissue, which is surrounded by a zone of cellular infiltration.   Plasma cells, endothelial cells, giant cells, and fibroblasts are usually recognisable.   Necrosis

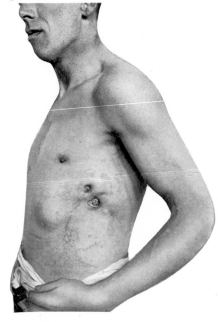

of tissue is partly due to toxins, and also to deficient blood-supply resulting from endarteritis and surrounding fibrosis.   If untreated, a gumma tends to enlarge and soften as the necrosis extends. If near the skin, hyperæmia and induration are evident. The centre of the indurated area then softens and eventually breaks down. The gumma discharges, and typically a wash-leather slough is seen at the bottom of the cavity, or on the floor of the ulcer, which is painless. The edges are characteristically sharply cut and circular in outline (fig. 26).

FIG. 26.—Gummata of the thoracic wall.

Under appropriate treatment a gumma usually absorbs with surprising rapidity, but occasionally it becomes walled-off by fibrous tissue, and eventually calcification may occur. In certain situations, notably the testes and bones, long-standing gummata are resistant to medical treatment owing to the density of the surrounding fibrosis or sclerosis, which prevents remedial agents in the blood from reaching the diseased tissues. In these circumstances, orchidectomy is advisable in the case of the testes, while guttering or trephining of bone is necessary for the relief of pain caused by an endosteal gumma (see fig. 27).

Gummatous ulcers, following subcutaneous gummata, are especially common in the upper portion of the leg, the backs of the thighs and forearms, and the face. A healed gumma leaves a " tissue-paper " scar, which is typically silvery, supple, and serpiginous, and often surrounded by a pigmented area.

A gummatous ulcer of the leg has sometimes been mistaken for a varicose ulcer (see fig. 84). The following are the main points of distinction.

Varicose Ulcer	*Gummatous Ulcer*
Usually lower third of leg.	Upper part of leg.
Irregular shape, rounded edges, and granular base.	Circular or serpiginous in shape, sharply cut edge, and sloughing base.
Single and painful.	Often multiple and painless.
History of years.	History of weeks or months.
Varicose veins present.	Other signs of syphilis.

The surgical manifestations of parasyphilis are considered in their appropriate chapters.

Treatment.—Public Health Regulations of recent years have greatly reduced the incidence of syphilis. Clinics are available in all large towns for treatment and tracing contacts, and notices to this effect are posted in suitable public places. Also laboratory facilities and remedies are at the disposal of medical practitioners, free of charge. In addition, lectures, diminished inebriety, propaganda work, and increased self-respect which is engendered by better education, all encourage sufferers to seek treatment.

The TREATMENT of syphilis falls into three groups—general, local, and specific.

(i) *General.*—As with any infection, the general resistance of the

s.p.—2

patient is an important consideration. Hygienic surroundings, adequate food, and suitable tonics are necessary ; iron is useful in order to combat anæmia during the secondary stage. Alcohol interferes with specific treatment and must be avoided. Tobacco is allowed in moderation provided mercury or bismuth has not caused stomatitis or gingivitis.

(ii) *Local.*—No antiseptic of any description should be applied to a suspected chancre until the serum has been examined bacteriologically. Pending the examination a saline compress is applied. After the diagnosis is made, the chancre is bathed twice daily with a weak antiseptic, and calomel ointment, 15–30 per cent., is applied.

Condylomata are treated by ordinary cleanliness and suitable dusting powders, such as one containing calomel, starch, and boracic acid. Gummatous ulcers and sores are kept surgically clean and dressed with mercurial lotion.

(iii) *Specific.*—In 1909, Ehrlich, at his 606th attempt, produced an arsenical preparation—*salvarsan*—suitable for intravenous injection. Subsequently, neo-salvarsan (N.A.B. or " 914 ") appeared and is more convenient than " 606," as it can be given in a more concentrated solution. Additional preparations are now available which are more stable to exposure and less painful when injected.

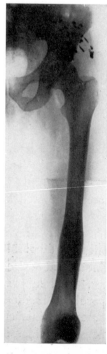

The patient should be carefully examined before embarking on a course of arsenical medication. Cardiovascular lesions in particular are excluded, and the urine is examined for bile and albumin. Intramuscular injections are conveniently given into the upper and outer portion of the buttock, and must be injected sufficiently deep to reach the muscle, as arsenic causes necrosis of the subcutaneous fat, with subsequent likelihood of an abscess. Owing to the risk of toxic effects, especially on the liver, arsenical preparations have been abandoned in many clinics in favour of penicillin and bismuth.

Penicillin is now used as a routine in addition to other measures. The usual course is 600,000 units of procaine penicillin daily until 6 mega units have been administered.

Bismuth preparations are used in conjunction with or following a course of penicillin, 0·2 gm. being injected intramuscularly weekly for ten weeks. As a matter of interest, bismuth remains locally in the tissues for years, and unless this point is remembered, confusion may result in the interpretation of radiographs (fig. 27). Dental hygiene is important before a course of bismuth is commenced, and the gums should be inspected at intervals. Blue lines occasionally occur on the gum margins following absorption of bismuth.

Mercury preparations, formerly the recognised treatment, have been largely supplanted by bismuth medication.

FIG. 27.—Bismuth injections in the gluteal muscles, in a patient with an endosteal gumma of the femoral shaft.

Dover's powder (pulv. ipec. co.) is prescribed if diarrhœa results.

Potassium iodide is indicated in the late secondary and tertiary stages. Its action is to stimulate the absorption of fibrous tissue, and thus expose infected areas to the influence of remedies previously

Paul Ehrlich, 1854–1915. Director of Experimental Therapy, Frankfurt-on-Main (" 606 " indicated the number of attempts to produce a suitable substance).
Thomas Dover, 1660–1742. Physician and buccaneer. Rescued Alexander Selkirk (Robinson Crusoe) from Juan Fernandez in 1709, and practised medicine in Bristol.

mentioned. Potassium iodide (gr. x–gr. xx) should be combined with an alkali, such as bicarbonate of soda, in order to obviate gastric disturbance. Aromatic spirit of ammonia combats depression, and liquor arsenicalis is included if the patient evinces a tendency to iodide eruptions. The mixture should be well diluted, and taken after meals, in order to promote absorption.

Various " courses " of treatment are advocated, but no hard-and-fast rules are permissible—each patient should be treated individually, as degrees of tolerance vary widely. For details regarding courses, textbooks dealing with this speciality should be consulted.

CONGENITAL (*Syn.* INHERITED) SYPHILIS

This disease is arbitrarily divided into four grades of severity :

(i) Miscarriage during the early months.

(ii) Birth of a stillborn and often macerated fœtus.

(iii) The infant presents obvious syphilitic features, such as wasting, snuffles, skin eruptions.

(iv) The child is apparently healthy, but subsequently develops syphilitic stigmata.

The following are the more important lesions in connection with inherited syphilis :

Mucous Membranes.—Inflammation of the muco-periosteum of the nose causes a purulent discharge—known as " snuffles." Mucous patches, gummatous ulceration of mucous membranes and adjacent skin, and condylomata occur. Radiating scars or rhagades are sometimes left at the angles of the mouth.

Skin.—A roseolar rash is not uncommon in the early months, especially on the buttocks. Papular or pustular eruptions, usually arranged in circles or crescents, appear on the flexor surfaces. Nodular infiltration of the skin, especially that of the face, sometimes occurs in older children, and resembles lupus vulgaris, but extends with greater rapidity and is much more destructive.

Teeth.—The milk teeth erupt late and are ill-formed. The permanent incisors are peg-shaped, so that the base is wider than the edge, and present a well-marked notch—Hutchinson's teeth. The central part of the crown of the first permanent molar is maldeveloped, a feature more

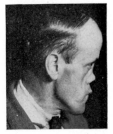

FIG. 28.—Frontal bosses and depressed nose of congenital syphilis.

obvious in the lower jaw, and known as "Moon's turreted molar."

Eye.—Iritis, sometimes accompanied by cyclitis, occurs in young children. The most characteristic lesion is interstitial keratitis, which usually appears between the ages of eight and sixteen years. The first indication is a "ground-glass" appearance of the cornea, associated with photophobia and lachrymation. "Salmon patches" occur later, due to leashes of newly formed vessels. One eye only is affected at first, but the second eye is subsequently involved. Prognosis should be guarded, as although most cases gradually subside, opacities may remain in the cornea, or deeper-seated mischief, which owing to corneal opacity cannot be seen with the ophthalmoscope, may have occurred.

Ear.—Acute otitis media may result from nasal infection. Nerve deafness sometimes develops about puberty, and is often associated with interstitial keratitis.

Bones.—Osteochondritis occasionally appears about the sixth month and gives rise to pain and swelling of the large epiphysis, the "pseudo-paralysis" of infants. The epiphysis is broad and irregular, yellow in colour, and the adjacent periosteum is thickened. Separation of the epiphysis sometimes occurs.

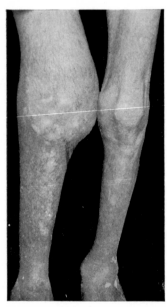

FIG. 29.—Clutton's knee (boy aged fourteen years).

From the sixth year onwards periostitis and sclerosis occur. The tibia is characteristically affected. Hyperæmia causes overgrowth of the bone, and, as the anterior aspect is mainly involved, a "sabre-shaped" tibia results.

Parrot's nodes, caused by localised areas of pericranitis, sometimes appear on the skull, especially in the frontal region.

Breaking-down gummata lead to necrosis of the palate and nasal septum. In the latter case the typical depression of the bridge results (fig. 28).

Joints.—The characteristic affec-

Henry Moon, 1845–1892. Dental Surgeon to Guy's Hospital.
Jules Marie Parrot, 1829–1883. Professor of Diseases of Children, Paris.
Henry Clutton, 1850–1909. Surgeon, St. Thomas's Hospital.

tion is Clutton's joint, which typically presents itself as a painless effusion into a large joint, most commonly the knee (fig. 29). It is frequently bilateral, although involvement of one joint may precede the other.

Central Nervous System.—Some degree of mental deficiency is common. At puberty juvenile tabes, or more rarely general paralysis, occasionally develops.

Other Organs.—A diffuse interstitial fibrosis occasionally involves the lungs. Syphilitic cirrhosis of the liver and splenic enlargement are not uncommon. Orchitis may be bilateral, and if occurring before puberty results in impotence.

Four typical lesions which shortly precede or occur at puberty are Clutton's joints, interstitial keratitis, otitis interna, and orchitis. Sufferers from these conditions were epitomised by Jonathan Hutchinson as " the halt, the blind, the deaf, and the impotent."

Treatment.—Prophylactic treatment is essential, and as a rule the mother is very tolerant to treatment during pregnancy. A healthy child is usually the reward of efficient ante-natal treatment. Treatment of an infected child should be instituted immediately after birth. A prolonged course of penicillin is prescribed in conjunction with or followed by bismuth therapy. The child should be kept under observation until growth ceases.

GONORRHŒA

In 1879 Neisser discovered the specific kidney-shaped coccus which occurs in pairs, and which is Gram-negative. On examination of suspected pus only a few polymorphonuclear cells are found to be affected (fig. 30). The probable explanation of this characteristic feature is that the cell has been killed by toxins and so the organisms have multiplied without hindrance. As a rule organisms are readily identified by the usual methods of staining, but in doubtful cases culture is necessary. The complement-fixation test may be the only means of confirming the diagnosis in chronic and systemic infections, e.g. arthritis.

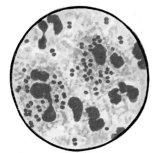

Fig. 30.—Gonococci (Gram's stain).

Albert Neisser, 1855–1916, of Breslau, recognised the gonococcus in 1879.

Acute Stage.—The incubation period is from two to ten days. The early symptoms are itching and redness of the meatus, the lips of which are sticky. A viscid discharge appears, which soon becomes thick and yellowish. Anterior urethritis develops within a day or two, with the characteristic symptoms of scalding pain on micturition, a narrowed stream, or even acute retention. Malaise and slight elevation of temperature are present during the acute stage, and the inguinal lymph nodes are sometimes tender. After ten to fourteen days acute symptoms abate, but the discharge persists.

Posterior urethritis is liable to occur at any time, either from extension of the infection or ill-advised treatment, such as inefficient irrigation or the passage of instruments.

Posterior urethritis is recognised by the frequency or urgency of micturition, with slight hæmaturia at the end of the act, aching in the perineum, painful erections, and turbidity of a second specimen of urine after the first flow has washed out the anterior urethra. When the posterior urethra is first infected, symptoms of toxæmia are usually pronounced.

LOCAL COMPLICATIONS.— *Anterior Urethritis.*—Folliculitis following infection of glands of Littré is a common complication. Balanitis is sometimes troublesome, and chordee may result from œdema of the corpus spongiosum or corpora cavernosa. Cowperitis occasionally occurs on one or both sides. Œdema of the skin is liable to cause paraphimosis, and in some cases lymphatic œdema persists.

Posterior Urethritis.—Acute prostatitis causes rectal and perineal pain which is worse on defæcation. Retention of urine is likely to occur if suppuration ensues. The inflamed prostate is easily palpable per rectum. Acute vesiculitis causes frequent and painful emissions of purulent or blood-stained semen. Epididymitis usually occurs from the third to the fifth week, and is preceded by pain in the groin due to inflammation of the spermatic cord (funiculitis). Basal cystitis is common and causes frequency and pain at the end of micturition.

Chronic or Latent Stage.—The discharge is often very inconsistent and may only occur after such events as undue exercise or alcoholic excess. Typically, a " morning dewdrop " appears, which is thick and whitish in colour. Massage of the

Alexis Littré, 1658–1725.   A teacher of anatomy in Paris.
William Cowper, 1666–1709.   London surgeon.

prostate and vesicles and examination of any expressed fluid will probably reveal latent infection. Partial emptying of the bladder followed by prostatic massage and completion of the act is a valuable test for posterior urethritis and prostatitis. Any threads which appear should be examined bacteriologically.

Urethroscopic examination requires considerable experience, but readily exposes folliculitis, erosions, abscesses, and other abnormalities, and also allows the application of local treatment.

LOCAL COMPLICATIONS.—Chronic prostatitis, with which is associated chronic vesiculitis, is a common cause of persistence of infection. Inflammation of the glands of Littré or lacunæ is also a frequent cause of relapse. Epididymitis is encouraged by the passage of bougies and rectal examinations before the disappearance of symptoms of acute urethritis. Strictures, formerly common, are becoming increasingly rare. They are due to such conditions as local infiltration of the wall of the urethra, or chronic folliculitis, and are encouraged by undue zeal in treatment, such as irrigation with excessively strong antiseptics. Gonorrhœal warts occasionally occur on the glans or prepuce.

Metastatic Complications.—Infection of joints and fibrositis are common. Endocarditis occurs as a rare complication, and is associated with pyæmic abscesses. Iridocyclitis sometimes occurs, especially in chronic cases, and necessitates repeated instillation of atropine.

IN THE FEMALE

The early symptoms are much less acute than in the male, and the incubation period is shorter, being only two to four days. Infection usually commences in the urethra or cervix, and Bartholin's glands are infected in 2 per cent. of cases. A vaginal speculum should not be passed in the acute stage, otherwise an uninfected cervix is liable to be contaminated.

The symptoms of acute infection include a sensation of heat and discomfort of the vulva, and pain on micturition. Should the cervix be infected, a blood-stained discharge is noticed and backache follows.

Complications.—Vaginitis is common in children who are accidentally infected, but adults usually escape. Cervicitis sometimes occurs spontaneously, or is encouraged by unwise instrumentation. Salpingitis, which is sometimes accompanied by oöphoritis or peritonitis, is a dreaded complication which is apt to cause sterility. Proctitis occasionally occurs, and is commoner than in males owing to the greater ease of infection.

Chronic or Latent Stage.—Chronic gonorrhœa is due to urethritis, cervicitis, or infection of Bartholin's glands, and any discharge from these organs must be meticulously examined in suspected cases. The symptoms accruing from chronic infection are very slight and the patient may merely notice an occasional yellowish discharge.

Local Complications.—Chronic endometritis occasionally occurs, and results in menorrhagia, metrorrhagia, and mild dysmenorrhœa, associated with backache. Salpingitis is often quiescent, but exacerbations are liable to follow sexual excess, debility, or labour. Warts are not uncommon and are sometimes large and numerous.

Treatment.—Prophylactic treatment largely depends on better education and preventive measures. Inunction with 30 per cent. calomel ointment before exposure to infection, and subsequent washing with 1 : 2,000 potassium permanganate solution, is almost certainly efficient. Prophylactic outfits, with directions for use, are readily obtainable. For the female, antiseptic tablets or jellies are available and should be supplemented by a vaginal douche of permanganate after exposure.

Acute gonorrhœa and its complications usually respond very satisfactorily to adequate doses of sulphonamide. It is necessary to maintain a high blood concentration for five days. About 6 per cent. of cases are resistant to sulphonamides, but most of these readily react to penicillin. As a rule procaine penicillin is used immediately the diagnosis is assured, and 300,000 units is usually curative. The patient is warned of the risks of conjunctivitis and transmission of infection, and he is kept under observation for three months, the blood being tested monthly for syphilis, as penicillin may mask a syphilitic infection or prolong the incubation period.

Chronic gonorrhœa (*syn.* gleet) often improves following a course of sulphonamide, but relapses are apt to occur, in which case penicillin should be administered. Persistent posterior urethritis can sometimes be combated by weekly instillations of silver nitrate (2 per cent.) into the prostatic urethra. Periodic dilatation by metal sounds, once or twice weekly, squeezes out infected material from the glands and crypts. With the assist-

Thomas Bartholin, 1616–1680. A Danish anatomist.

ance of an operating urethroscope such local conditions as follicular abscesses and ulcers receive appropriate treatment. Rectal diathermy of the prostate is useful in skilled hands, but is rarely necessary.

OPHTHALMIA NEONATORUM

Infection at birth is a common cause of blindness. The incubation period is twenty-four to forty-eight hours, and is followed by chemosis, lachrymation, and purulent discharge. Corneal ulceration and sloughing are liable to follow in neglected cases. Prophylactic measures include a vaginal douche at the onset of labour, and instillation into the infant's eyes of some organic preparation of silver, such as two or three drops of 20 per cent. argyrol.

Should infection occur, the eye must be irrigated with penicillin (2,500 units in 1 ml.) at frequent intervals, and sulphamezathine or penicillin is prescribed. In unilateral cases the child lies on the affected side, the sound eye being protected by a Buller's shield.

SOFT CHANCRE (*Syn.* SOFT SORE, CHANCROID)

This type of venereal disease is caused by the specific bacillus of Ducrey (page 588). The incubation period is short, and in two or three days a vesicle appears, which becomes infected and breaks down to form an ulcer about a week after infection. The sores are commonly multiple and painful, and are associated with enlargement of the inguinal lymph nodes. Suppuration usually follows (bubo), and if the nodes are infected with Ducrey's bacillus, considerable periadenitis results, and months may elapse before the wounds heal. Venereal sores are sometimes due to both Ducrey's bacillus and spirochætes, so in all cases a search must be made for the latter organisms.

An uncomplicated soft sore persists and enlarges unless adequate treatment is prescribed. As the organism is penicillin resistant, a course of sulphonamide is prescribed, and a five-days' course usually suffices. Mild antiseptics are applied locally, and balanitis receives appropriate treatment. If the diagnosis is doubtful an intradermic test is useful. Enough emulsion of the bacilli (Dmelcos is a useful preparation) is injected to raise a wheal, and in two days' time a papule with surrounding erythema indicates a positive reaction. Dmelcos curative vaccine is also useful in protracted cases.

Frank Buller, 1844–1905. Canadian ophthalmic surgeon.
Augusto Ducrey, 1860–1931. Professor of Dermatology, Pisa, isolated the bacillus in 1889.

CHAPTER III
TUMOURS

A TUMOUR is a new formation of cells of independent growth which fulfils no useful function. The term "tumour" should be reserved for new-growths, and its loose application to inflammatory swellings, such as Pott's puffy "tumour," or enlargement of an organ due to hypertrophy, is to be condemned.

CAUSATION

Over 300 years ago it was stated that "any kind of external irritation, whether from motion, heat, or acrimony, may cause cancer," and in spite of an enormous amount of research work and expenditure of money we have added little to our knowledge. Many years ago it was observed that the natives of Kashmir were prone to develop carcinoma of the skin on the inner sides of the thighs and lower abdomen (fig. 31). This is due to their habit of endeavouring to keep warm by squatting and hugging earthenware pots which contain glowing charcoal (the pot being termed a kangri), with the result that the adjacent skin is irritated by heat and fumes. It is also common knowledge that women can swallow in comfort fluids at a considerably higher temperature than men can tolerate, which fact may explain the greater incidence of post-cricoid carcinoma in females.

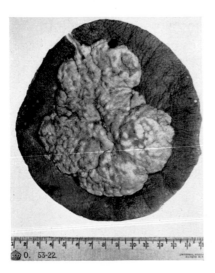

Fig. 31.—Kangri carcinoma of the abdominal wall.
(*R.C.S. Museum.*)

"Chimney-sweeps'" cancer of the scrotum was due to the chronic irritation produced by soot, which collected in the rugæ of the scrotum. Owing to the growing custom of taking regular baths, this variety of cancer is nearly obsolete, but chronic irritation from chemicals, tar, etc., occasionally produces squamous-celled carcinoma of the exposed skin in those who work among these irritants. Again, carcinoma of the lower lip was prevalent when clay pipes were popular, and carcinoma is occasionally seen at the site where tobacco smoke continually impinges on the tongue.

Regeneration of tissue appears to encourage malignant changes in the newly formed cells, which are presumably in a state of instability. Primary carcinoma of the liver is sometimes seen in cases of cirrhosis, and apparently arises from the liver cells which are endeavouring to regenerate. Similarly, squamous-celled carcinoma occasionally occurs in a chronic ulcer (fig. 32) and a fibro-sarcoma arising in a scar is not uncommon. In some situations the site of fusion of embryonic elements constitutes a favourite position for the development of carcinoma. On the tongue, for example, carcinoma is prone to occur at the junction of the anterior two-thirds and the posterior third, also carcinoma is not uncommon at the junction of the anal canal and the rectum.

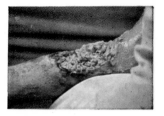

FIG. 32. — Squamous-celled carcinoma which has developed in a varicose ulcer.

Is carcinoma hereditary ? In many cases it is difficult to exclude coincidence, but in our experience the disease appears to " run in families."

Tumours reproduce cells which are similar to those from which they arise, although if the tumour grows rapidly the resemblance becomes less obvious (anaplasia). It sometimes happens that the epithelium from which the tumour grows has already changed its characteristics. The gall-bladder is normally lined by columnar epithelium, but the advent of cholecystitis eventually results in the epithelium undergoing cuboidal or even squamous-celled metaplasia.

CLASSIFICATION

The classification of tumours is fraught with difficulty owing to their varied and sometimes atypical appearances. Following the suggestion of Adami, tumours can be subdivided into two groups, teratomata and blastomata.

Teratomata are composed of cells of one individual within the tissues of a second individual (fig. 33). These tumours may arise from " totipotent " cells, or contain representative cells from all three embryonic layers ; for example, a dermoid sometimes contains hair, teeth, muscle, gland tissue, etc. Included in this group is the chorion-epithelioma, which, very occasionally, occurs in the testicle.

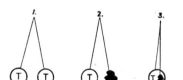

FIG. 33.—Twins and teratoma.

1. Normal twins. 2. One normal twin, the other an acardiac, anencephalic monster. 3. A teratoma — the twin brother's remnants are included in his normal brother.

Teratoid tumours are a subdivision of teratomata. They are composed of cells of the same individual, and these apparently become displaced during development (Cohnheim's theory). Until recently, the mixed parotid tumour was considered to be a teratoid tumour, but apparently it should be regarded as a new-growth of

John George Adami, 1861–1926. Professor of Pathology, McGill University.
Julius Cohnheim, 1839–1884. Professor of Pathology, Leipzig.

a parotid duct and therefore epithelial in origin. Refinements of staining indicate that the substance formerly considered to be cartilage is in reality altered mucin secreted by the gland. Sequestration dermoids are a variety of teratoid tumour.

Blastomata are produced by abnormal growth of component cells of the individual, and they may arise from any of the three embryonic layers.

From the clinical standpoint tumours thus formed are either innocent or malignant.

An *innocent* or *benign* tumour is usually encapsulated, and does not disseminate. Symptoms are due to its size and position. Frequently they are multiple.

Malignant tumours are usually single, and are liable to infiltrate surrounding tissue. They nearly always continue to grow, and prove fatal in the absence of adequate treatment. The tumour is supposed to have disappeared in patients who succumb to malignant lymph nodes of the neck, when no primary growth is discovered at necropsy. Possibly a very small growth in some obscure position, such as the naso-pharynx, had been overlooked. Very malignant tumours, such as secondary deposits of chorion-epithelioma, are apt to destroy adjacent blood-vessels with such avidity that they become surrounded by clot. They are thus isolated from their source of nutriment, and consequently perish.

The commonest forms of malignant tumours are carcinoma, sarcoma, and melanoma malignum.

METHODS OF SPREAD OF MALIGNANT TUMOURS

(i) *Local Extension.*—Carcinomata and sarcomata both infiltrate adjacent tissues and spread by direct invasion. This feature is the most reliable evidence of malignancy when the tumour is examined microscopically. Tissues are not always invaded in a uniform manner. Invasion takes place most readily along connective-tissue planes, whereas fascia or aponeurosis forms a temporary barrier. An avascular structure, such as articular cartilage, resists invasion to a remarkable extent. Other factors influence local extension ; thus it is alleged that the spread of a rodent ulcer is checked when the growing edge reaches an area of skin supplied by a different sensory nerve. Also a carcinoma of the pyloric end of the stomach rarely extends into the duodenum.

(ii) *Blood-stream.*—This is the most common method of dissemination of a sarcoma, as the venous clefts, so typical of a sarcoma, readily permit malignant cells to enter the blood-stream. These malignant emboli are liable to be arrested in

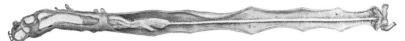

FIG. 34.—Intravenous spread of sarcoma. (*British Journal of Surgery.*)

the lungs, where they form secondary deposits, sometimes accompanied by a blood-stained pleural effusion. It is probable that in some cases malignant cells grow along the pulmonary capillaries into the veins, and so reach the systemic circulation.

Large veins are sometimes extensively invaded by sarcoma (fig. 34).

Dissemination by the blood-stream is usually a late feature of carcinoma. However, for example, a carcinoma of the kidney not infrequently invades the renal vein, with the result that secondary deposits are found in the lungs.

(iii) *Lymphatics.*—The spread of carcinoma along lymphatics occurs both by permeation and by embolism. In the former case the malignant cells grow along the lymphatic vessels from the primary growth, sometimes in a retrograde direction. The presence of the cells in the lymphatics stimulates a perilymphatic fibrosis, which compresses and destroys the malignant cells, but this destruction does not keep pace with the rate of malignant cell growth. A few cells are always ahead of the fibrosis, and so reach the shelter of a lymph node, where they multiply in safety. Other structures, such as bones, are sometimes affected by lymphatic permeation.

In some instances, notably melanoma malignum, occasional groups of cells over-

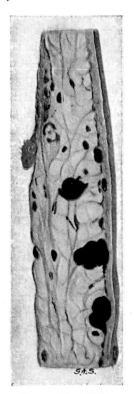

FIG. 35. — Melanomatous deposits in subcutaneous lymphatics of the abdominal wall.

come the surrounding fibrosis, and give rise to intermediate deposits between the primary growth and the lymph nodes (fig. 35).

In the case of embolism, cancer cells invade a lymphatic vessel and are carried by the lymph circulation to the regional node, so that nodes comparatively distant from the tumour are liable to be involved in the early stages.

(iv) *Inoculation.*—Inoculation of carcinoma has been observed in situations where skin or mucous membrane is closely in contact with a primary growth. Examples of this " kiss cancer " are carcinoma of the lower lip affecting the upper, and carcinoma of the labium major, giving rise to a similar growth on the opposite side of the vulva.

Recurrence after operation is, in some cases, due to implantation in the wound of malignant cells. Examples of this mischance are the appearance of a papilloma in the bladder scar after suprapubic removal of a primary growth, and nodules of carcinoma in the scar of the incision after radical mastectomy.

(v) *Gravity.*—Cells from a carcinoma in the upper abdomen sometimes become detached and gravitate to the pelvis or ovaries. This transcœlomic method of spread occasionally gives rise to malignant ovarian tumours (Krukenberg's tumour), which may mask the presence of the primary growth.

(vi) *Physiological Propulsion.*—A papilloma of the kidney pelvis is commonly associated with similar tumours in the ureter or bladder. Also it is alleged that carcinoma cells from the colon can pass along the alimentary canal and give rise to a further growth at a lower level.

BENIGN TUMOURS

PAPILLOMA

A papilloma consists of a central axis of connective tissue, blood-vessels, and lymphatics ; the surface is covered by epithelium, either squamous, transitional, cuboidal, or columnar.

The surface of a papilloma may be merely roughened, or composed of innumerable delicate villous processes, as in the case of the kidney, bladder, and rectum. In these situations papillomata resemble malignant tumours, in that they tend to recur after apparently complete removal, and secondary growths arise by implantation.

Also, as in the case of a papilloma in a duct of the breast, or

---

Friedrich Krukenberg, Contemporary. Ophthalmologist of Halle. Wrote a classical thesis in 1895 (at the age of twenty-four) on malignant ovarian tumours.

a papilloma of the bladder or rectum, obvious malignant changes are likely to supervene.

Other common sites for papillomata are the skin, the colon, the tongue and cheek, the vocal cords, and the walls of cysts, particularly those in connection with the breast and ovary. Papillomata affecting the vocal cords often disappear spontaneously.

Papillomata are sometimes due to infection, as in the case of venereal " warts," which affect the skin or mucosa of the genital organs. Papillomata in special situations are dealt with in the appropriate chapters.

FIBROMA

Fibromata occur in connection with fascia, aponeurosis, muscle and nerve sheaths, or connective tissue of organs. They are therefore widely distributed throughout the body.

In some situations, notably the breast, glandular tissue is incorporated amongst the fibrous stroma, so that the tumour is in reality a fibro-adenoma.

Fibromata are occasionally multiple, as in the case of von Recklinghausen's disease (vide p. 56).

The following types of fibromata are described :

Hard.—These tumours grow slowly, and do not attain a large size. All grades of hardness exist, according to the relative proportion of fibrous and cellular tissue. They not infrequently occur on nerve sheaths.

Soft.—These may be so cellular that a section closely resembles a sarcoma, and as they occasionally become sarcomatous, the innocent tumour imperceptibly undergoes malignant changes. Soft fibromata are common in the subcutaneous tissue of the face, and appear as soft brownish swellings. Oliver Cromwell was disfigured by one of these tumours, which he referred to as a " wart."

Recurrent.—Examples of this type are the fibroma of muscle sheaths (fig. 36) (described by Paget as a " recurrent fibroid "), the fibrous

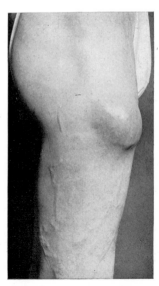

Fig. 36. — Fibro-sarcoma growing from the sheath of the tensor fasciæ femoris muscle.

Friedrich von Recklinghausen, 1833–1910. Professor of Pathology, Strasburg.
Sir James Paget, 1814–1899. Surgeon, St. Bartholomew's Hospital, London.

polyp of the nose, and the fibrous epulis (p. 154). The tumours either commence as true fibromata, and gradually become sarcomatous, or are actually of low-grade malignancy from the beginning. In any case malignant changes are hastened by incomplete efforts at removal. The moral is that wide excision should be practised in all cases, so that the tumour will not be "recurrent."

Desmoid.—This is an unusual type of fibroma occurring in the abdominal wall of middle-aged females, particularly in those who have borne children. The tumour is a typical fibroma, with the exception that it has no capsule and invades the abdominal muscles, so much so that islands of muscular tissue become incorporated in the tumour. X-rays usually cause regression of the desmoid, but if this is ineffectual, and if disability ensues, excision may be considered.

Keloid.—These tumours occur in scars, particularly those following burns. The tendency to develop a keloid is inherited, and is particularly in evidence in tuberculous and negroid families. In appearance a keloid is smooth, sometimes lobulated or even claw-like, and many invade the subcutaneous or subfascial tissues. Microscopically, the structure is similar to that of a soft fibroma. A keloid never becomes malignant, and though it may persist for years, the ultimate tendency is to disappear gradually.

Mere excision of a keloid should never be performed, as recurrence is the rule. Good results have followed excision and exposure to deep X-ray therapy before suture of the wound. If unsightly, the application of radium or low-voltage X-ray therapy causes retrogression.

LIPOMA

Diffuse lipoma occasionally occurs in the subcutaneous tissue of the neck, from which it spreads on to the preauricular region of the face (fig. 37). It is associated with excessive beer drinking, and therefore is less common than formerly, owing to the rise in price and inferior quality of this commodity. The tumour is not obviously encapsulated, and gives rise to no trouble beyond being unsightly. The tumour should be excised if the patient wishes to improve his appearance (fig. 38).

Multiple lipomata are not uncommon. The tumours remain small or moderate in size, and are sometimes painful, in which case the condition is probably one of *neuro-lipomatosis*. Dercum's disease is an associated condition.

Circumscribed lipomata are among the commonest of tumours. The characteristic features are painlessness, the presence of a definite edge, and lobulation. If the proportion of fibrous

Francis X. Dercum, 1856–1931. Neurologist, Jefferson Medical College, Philadelphia.

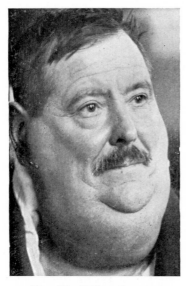

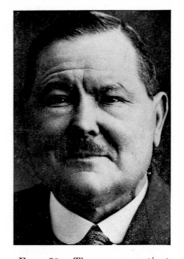

FIG. 38.—The same patient after excision of the tumour in stages. He then married, and the above photo was taken on the wedding day.

FIG. 37.—Diffuse lipoma of neck.

tissue is not excessive, a sense of fluctuation may be obtained. These tumours have a widespread distribution, as they can occur in any part of the body where fat is found. As would be expected, a lipoma deeply situated is liable to be mistaken for other swellings, as difficulty arises in recognising the typical signs.

Should the lipoma contain an excessive amount of fibrous tissue it is termed a *fibro-lipoma*. In other cases considerable vascularity is present, often with telangiectasis of the overlying skin, in which case the tumour is a *nævo-lipoma*. Myxomatous degeneration and calcification (fig. 39) sometimes occur in lipomata of long duration.

A retroperitoneal lipoma occasionally undergoes sarcomatous changes.

Clinically, circumscribed lipomata are conveniently classified according to their situation :

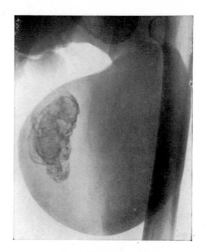

FIG. 39.—Calcification in a large pedunculated lipoma of the thigh which had been present for over twenty years.

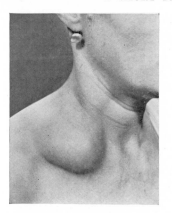

FIG. 40.—A lobulated, sub-cutaneous lipoma.

(i) *Subcutaneous* are most commonly found in the shoulders or back (fig. 40), although no part of the body is immune. Usually the characteristic features are readily ascertained. It must be remembered that a lipoma is occasionally present over the site of a spina bifida. A careful examination should distinguish such conditions as a tuberculous abscess or a sebaceous cyst, which may superficially resemble a lipoma. Subcutaneous lipomata occasionally become pedunculated, or the influence of gravity may cause the tumour gradually to change its position.

(ii) *Subfascial.*—Lipomata occurring under the palmar or plantar fascia are liable to be mistaken for tuberculous tenosynovitis, as the dense, overlying fascia masks the definite edge and lobulation of the tumour. However, the swelling is circumscribed, and wasting of muscles is negligible. Difficulty is encountered in complete removal as pressure encourages the tumour to ramify. Subfascial lipomata also occur in the areolar layer under the epicranial aponeurosis, and if of long duration they erode the underlying bone, so that a depression is palpable on pushing the tumour to one side (fig. 41).

(iii) *Subsynovial* arise from the fatty padding around joints, especially the knee. They are apt to be mistaken for Baker's cysts, but are easily distinguished as, in distinction to a cyst or bursa, their consistency is constant whether the joint is in extension or flexion.

(iv) *Intra-articular.*—The term "lipoma arborescens" is somewhat misleading, as the condition is, strictly speaking, not neoplastic, but rather a fatty and fibrous infiltration of synovial tags.

FIG. 41.—Erosion of the skull due to a subaponeurotic lipoma.

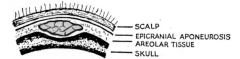

SCALP
EPICRANIAL APONEUROSIS
AREOLAR TISSUE
SKULL

(v) *Intermuscular.*—These occur particularly in the thigh or around the shoulder. Owing to transmitted pressure the tumour becomes firmer when the adjacent muscles are contracted. Weakness or aching results, owing to mechanical interference with muscular action. The condition is often difficult to distinguish from a fibro-sarcoma, and exploration is usually necessary in order to determine the actual nature of the swelling.

(vi) *Parosteal* occasionally occur under the periosteum of a bone, and are difficult to diagnose with confidence if deeply situated.

(vii) *Subserous* are not common, but are sometimes found beneath the pleura, where they constitute one variety of innocent thoracic tumour. A retroperitoneal lipoma may grow to enormous dimensions, and simulate a hydronephrosis or pancreatic cyst. A lipomatous mass is frequently found at the fundus of the sac of a femoral hernia, but this is a condensation of retroperitoneal fat rather than a neoplasm.

(viii) *Submucous* occur under the mucous membrane of the respiratory or alimentary tracts. Very rarely a submucous lipoma in the larynx causes respiratory obstruction. A submucous lipoma occasionally occurs

William Morant Baker, 1839–1896. Surgeon, St. Bartholomew's Hospital, London.

in the tongue. One situated in the intestine is likely to cause an intussusception, which is the first indication of its presence (fig. 42).

(ix) *Extradural.*—A lipoma is a rare variety of spinal tumour. Owing to the absence of fat within the skull intracranial lipomata do not occur.

(x) *Intraglandular.*—Lipomata occasionally arise from the fat within the lobules of the breast, and they have been described as occurring in the pancreas, under the renal capsule, and in connection with other organs.

Treatment.—If a lipoma is causing trouble on account of its site, size, or position, removal is indicated. Owing to its definite capsule and comparative avascularity, excision is usually easy.

ADENOMA

Adenomata arise in connection with secretory glands, and resemble to a greater or lesser extent the structure from which they arise. They are encapsulated tumours, and sometimes profoundly influence the metabolism, as in the case of the thyroid, parathyroid, and pancreas. Occasionally an adenoma contains a

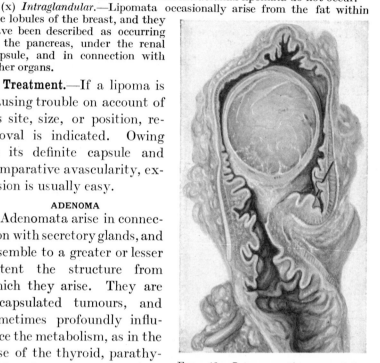

Fig. 42.—Intussusception caused by a submucous lipoma of the cæcum.

large proportion of fibrous tissue, e.g. the hard fibro-adenoma in the breast, while in other situations, notably the pancreas and thyroid gland, cystic degeneration is common. Adenomata arising from secretory glands of mucous membrane are liable to pedunculation, as in the case of a rectal " polyp." Simple enlargement of the prostate is due to a diffuse hyperplasia of glandular tissue, usually associated with multiple adenomata. Adenomata in certain situations tend to undergo malignant changes, e.g. those occurring in the prostate and thyroid gland.

NEUROMA

True neuromata are rare tumours, and occur in connection with the sympathetic system. They comprise the following types :

(*a*) *Ganglioneuroma*, which consists of ganglion cells and nerve fibres. It arises in connection with the sympathetic cord, and therefore is found in the retroperitoneal tissue, or in the neck or thorax. It usually occurs after the first decade, and is entirely innocent, causing symptoms merely by its size and position.

(b) *Neuroblastoma*, which is less differentiated than the ganglioneuroma, the cells being of an embryonic type. The tumour somewhat resembles a round-celled sarcoma, and disseminates by the blood-stream. It occurs in infants and young children.

(c) *Myelinic neuroma*, composed only of nerve fibres, ganglion cells being absent. The very few tumours which have been reported have arisen in connection with the spinal cord or pia mater.

False neuromata arise from the connective tissue of the nerve sheath. The following varieties are described :

LOCAL.—A single neuroma is usually found in the sub-cutaneous tissue, although occasionally a " trunk neuroma " grows from a large cranial or peripheral nerve, the acoustic tumour being an example. The "painful subcutaneous nodule" forms a smooth firm swelling, which may be moved in a lateral direction, but is otherwise fixed by the nerve from which it arises. Paræsthesia or pain is likely to occur from pressure of the tumour on the nerve fibres which are spread over its surface. Cystic degeneration or sarcomatous changes occasionally occur.

The tumour should be removed with the minimum of damage to the nerve. If it is necessary to resect a portion of an important nerve, the cut ends are sutured.

DIFFUSE neuromata occur in the following varieties :

Molluscum Fibrosum.—This condition consists of numerous soft fibromata, which grow from the terminal twigs of cutaneous nerves (fig. 43). They are usually distributed freely over the body, with the exception of the palms and soles. The tumours vary in size from a pin's head to a hen's egg. Pigmentation of the skin is sometimes present, and tumours are occasionally present on deeper nerves. Sarcoma may develop, and should be suspected if one of the tumours enlarges rapidly and exhibits signs of increased vascularity.

This condition is distinguished from molluscum contagiosum, in that the swellings are not confined to exposed surfaces, umbilication is absent, and the tumours of neurofibromatosis become pedunculated.

Generalised Neurofibromatosis (*syn.* von Recklinghausen's Disease of Nerves).—Cranial, spinal, and peripheral nerves may all be diffusely or nodularly thickened (fig. 44). The overgrowth occurs in connection with the endoneurium. As in the case of molluscum fibrosum, associated pigmentation of the skin is common, and sarcomatous changes occasionally occur.

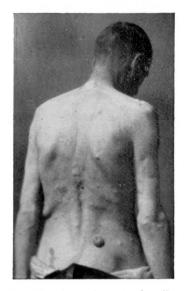

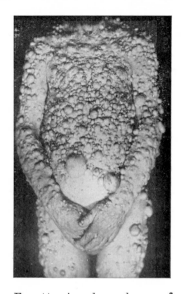

Fig. 43.—An early case of molluscum fibrosum.

Fig. 44.—An advanced case of
generalised neurofibromatosis.

Plexiform Neurofibromatosis.—This rare condition usually occurs in connection with branches of the fifth cranial nerve (fig. 45), although examples have been met with in the extremities. The affected nerves become enormously thickened as a result of myxo-fibromatous degeneration of the endoneurium. If occurring in the scalp, the underlying skull may be eroded, and in other situations the involved skin sometimes hangs down in pendulous folds. Plexiform neurofibromatosis is sometimes associated with the generalised type of neurofibromatosis. Sarcoma rarely develops.

Elephantiasis Neuromatosa.—This rare condition is congenital in origin, and usually affects one leg. The skin and subcutaneous tissues become greatly thickened, so that the patient finds walking increasingly difficult. The skin is coarse, dry, and thickened, resembling an elephant's hide. Other types of neurofibromatosis are sometimes associated. Amputation is usually necessary.

Amputation "Neuromata."—Fusi-form swellings occur at the ends of divided nerves after amputation of a limb. These swellings consist of fibrous tissue and coiled nerve fibres, and are a physiological rather than a pathological phenomenon.

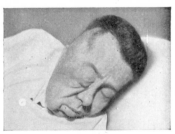

Fig. 45.—Plexiform neurofibromatosis affecting the second division
of the trigeminal nerve on the right
side. The subcutaneous tissues are
thickened, and the patient was unable to open the eye.

(*J. R. M. Whigham.*)

GLOMANGIOMA (*Syn.* GLOMUS TUMOUR)

These tumours arise from a cutaneous glomus. The glomera are composed of a tortuous arteriole which communicates directly with a venule, the vessels being surrounded with a network of small nerves. These specialised organs regulate the temperature of the skin, and are found in the limbs, especially the nail-beds. The tumour resembles a nævus, and is compressible. The associated pain is out of all proportion to the size of the tumour, which may be only a few millimetres in diameter. The pain is burning in nature, and radiates peripherally, and is often more noticeable when the limb is exposed to sudden changes of temperature.

On section the tumour consists of a mixture of blood spaces, nerve tissue and muscle fibres derived from the wall of the arteriole (angioneuroma). Large cuboidal cells are frequently seen (glomal cells). Glomal tumours grow very slowly, and do not undergo malignant changes. They should be destroyed with an electric cautery, or excised.

MALIGNANT TUMOURS

CARCINOMA

Carcinoma, which arises from tissues of ectodermal and endodermal origin, is the commonest form of malignant new-growth, and is alleged to be increasing in frequency. This increase is probably apparent rather than real, and is explained by more accurate methods of diagnosis and the greater number of people who now survive to riper years. In some situations, such as the alimentary canal and bronchi, an actual increase has occurred during recent years. Greater petrol consumption, with consequent contamination of air by irritating fumes, and increased cigarette smoking are alleged explanations of the frequency of bronchial carcinoma, which has increased tenfold in the past twenty years. Fortunately, owing to increasing avoidance of predisposing causes, other types of carcinoma are less frequent than formerly, notably that of the skin, lip, and tongue.

Carcinomata are conveniently classified according to the type of cell from which they arise, as, for example, glandular, squamous, or basal-celled.

(i) GLANDULAR is widely distributed, and commonly occurs in the alimentary tract, breast, and uterus, and less frequently in the kidney, prostate, gall-bladder, thyroid, and other organs.

Glandular carcinomata not only arise from secreting columnar epithelium, but also from ducts when the cells are cubical. The three pathological types of glandular carcinoma are as follows :

Carcinoma simplex, in which the cells are arranged in circumscribed groups or alveoli, no glandular structure being recognisable. This type commonly occurs in the breast, and the majority of cells are spheroidal in shape.

Adeno-carcinoma, so called from the tendency of the cells to form acini, which resemble those of the gland from which they are derived. The alveoli are ductless, and the walls are composed of layers of cells which invade the surrounding tissues. This type is common in the stomach and colon. The cells of the primary growth, and even of the metastases, sometimes retain secretory powers.

Colloid, which develops in tumours arising from cells which secrete mucin, and is a degenerative process. The mucin permeates the stroma of the growth, which appears as a gelatinous or semi-translucent mass. This type is typically seen in growths of the colon and stomach.

Glandular carcinoma is also subdivided into various types, e.g. encephaloid, scirrhus, and atrophic scirrhus. These distinctions depend clinically on their rate of growth, and pathologically on the relative proportions of fibrous tissue and gland elements. Examples occur in connection with the breast, and are described in Chapter xxxvii.

(ii) SQUAMOUS—which arise either from surfaces covered by squamous epithelium, or as a result of metaplasia. Thus, prolonged irritation of the gall-bladder by stones causes the normal columnar epithelium to revert to a less differentiated type, so that cuboidal or even squamous-celled carcinoma develops.

Squamous-celled carcinoma is particularly liable to occur as a result of chronic irritation (p. 46). The regional lymph nodes are likely to be invaded, but blood-borne metastases are rare. The lymph nodes occasionally undergo mucoid degeneration, to which secondary infection from the primary growth may be superadded, so that, if the skin gives way over the softened node, a glairy, semi-purulent fluid is discharged.

Macroscopically, squamous-celled carcinomata are either papilliferous or ulcerative. On section solid masses of polyhedral cells are seen, which invade the deeper structures.

" Cell-nests " are usually apparent in slowly growing cases, and are due to deeper cells becoming flattened and undergoing keratinisation.   " Prickle " cells are characteristic, and resemble the prickle cells present in the epidermis.

Squamous-celled carcinomata of different tissues are discussed in their appropriate chapters.

(iii) BASAL-CELLED (*syn.* Rodent Ulcer, p. 821).

SARCOMA

Sarcomata occur in connection with structures of mesoblastic origin.   Many tumours formerly labelled " sarcoma " are now very properly excluded from this group.   Thus a " myeloid sarcoma " is more accurately described as a " giant-celled " tumour of bone, and the " melanotic sarcoma " is now referred to as a malignant melanoma.

Sarcomata differ from carcinomata, not only in their derivation, but also in their age incidence, as sarcomata are most common during the first and second decades.   Moreover, sarcomata often grow with greater rapidity, and dissemination occurs mainly by the blood-stream.   Microscopically, the cells of a carcinoma are arranged in masses or columns, whereas sarcoma cells are always separated from each other.   In some cases a sarcoma develops in pre-existing benign tumours, such as a fibroma, or a uterine fibroid, and in bones which are affected by osteitis deformans.   A few instances are on record in which a sarcoma, usually of bone, apparently resulted from an injury. If the tumour grows slowly the sarcomatous cells reproduce tissue from which the tumour originated, e.g. osteo-sarcoma or chondro-sarcoma.

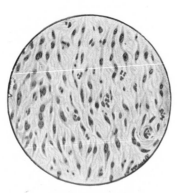

FIG. 46.—Spindle-celled sarcoma, arising from a muscle sheath (Paget's " recurrent fibroid ").

Fibro-sarcomata are composed of spindle cells of varying lengths (fig. 46).   In many cases it is difficult to distinguish with certainty, even microscopically, between a simple fibroma and a fibro-sarcoma of low-grade malignancy.   It is probable that some fibromata imperceptibly become sarcomatous, particularly after incomplete attempts at removal, e.g. Paget's recurrent fibroid (p. 51). A fibrous epulis and a fibrous polyp of the nose are further examples of fibro-sarcomata of low malignancy, but the degree of malignancy increases with each ineffectual attempt at excision.

Fibro-sarcomata not uncommonly arise in scar tissue, sometimes many years after the scar developed. Owing to the relative avascularity of scar tissue, an associated sarcoma grows slowly, but eventually causes extensive destruction of adjacent structures.

If untreated, or if local excision is unsuccessful, a fibro-sarcoma eventually fungates through the skin (fig. 47). Metastases are widely scattered, and, unfortunately, radiotherapy has no permanent effect on either the primary growth or on the secondary deposits.

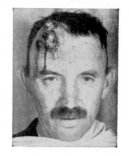

FIG. 47.—Fungating fibro-sarcoma of the scalp.
(*T. A. Bouchier-Hayes.*)

Reticulo-sarcoma (syn. lympho-sarcoma) arises in lymph nodes, tonsils, Peyer's patches, or lymph nodules in the intestines. Lymph nodes of the neck or mediastinum are most commonly affected. This variety of sarcoma grows rapidly, and gives rise to metastases in adjacent lymphoid tissue, and later in distant organs via the blood-stream. The tumour is composed of small round cells which stain deeply, and which are highly radio-sensitive, but owing to early dissemination the chance of cure is negligible.

The terms round-celled, spindle-celled, etc., are applied to tumours which contain no differentiated cells.

The macroscopic appearance of a sarcoma varies considerably. As the word implies, most tumours appear as a fleshy mass, but their consistency depends on the relative proportion of fibrous and vascular tissue. An avascular fibro-sarcoma appears as a hard, almost white tumour, whereas a sarcoma of the breast is frequently soft, hæmorrhagic, and often cystic, owing to mucoid degeneration. Hæmorrhage commonly occurs in a sarcoma, owing to the very thin walls of the veins, which in some places are represented merely by venous spaces. The absorption of fibrin ferment from extravasated blood accounts for the irregularities of temperature which are so characteristic of a rapidly growing sarcoma.

Johann Peyer, 1653–1712. Anatomist of Shauffhausen, Switzerland.

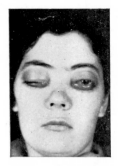

FIG. 48.—Chloroma.
(*A. A. M'Connell.*)

Sarcomata of separate organs are considered in their appropriate chapters.

Chloroma (*syn.* myeloblastic reticulosarcoma) is a rare condition in which the bones of the face, and especially those of the orbits, are involved by a growth resembling sarcoma (fig. 48). It is a leukæmic condition, and at post-mortem the tumours present a bright green colour. Blood examination shows a lymphocytosis, and no treatment is of avail.

MELANOMA

Melanotic tumours usually arise in the skin or pigmented layers of the eye.

Benign melanomata occur as congenital pigmented nævi or moles, or as pigmented warts. These tumours usually remain unaltered, but occasionally malignant changes supervene.

A *melanoma malignum* most commonly is secondary to a benign pigmented tumour. To answer the question " When is a mole not a mole ? " is often difficult, but ulceration, a tendency to bleed, or induration should give rise to the gravest suspicions. In case of any doubt the mole must be excised and scrutinised by a pathologist. The primary growth may remain quite small, and yet give rise to large secondary deposits. Occasionally a melanoma malignum arises spontaneously in the nail-bed, in the uveal tract (fig. 49), or, especially in negroes, on the sole of the foot (fig. 50).

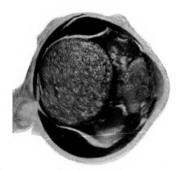

FIG. 49.—Advanced melanoma arising in the choroid.

Unless radically treated in the manner suggested by Hogarth Pringle (vide infra), a melanoma malignum is virtually a death-warrant, as these growths give rise to early and widespread dissemination. Tumours arising in the skin permeate lymphatics, and intermediate deposits commonly occur between the primary growth and regional nodes (fig. 35). At a later stage bones and viscera are likely to be involved. Melanomata occurring in the uveal tract frequently give rise to visceral deposits, which may be enormous in size, particularly in the liver (see

J. *Hogarth Pringle, 1863–1941. Surgeon, Glasgow Royal Infirmary.*

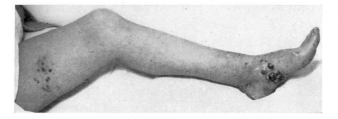

Fig. 50.—Melanoma malignum of the foot, with secondary deposits in the lymphatics of the thigh.

fig. 126). After removal of an eye on account of a melanoma a latent period of many years may elapse, but secondary deposits almost inevitably appear.

Histologically, melanomata arising in the skin usually show an alveolar arrangement. The pigment granules vary in colour from black to yellow, and are situated both in the cells and in the stroma. Secondary deposits are typically black (fig. 93, Chapter vi), but sometimes contain very little pigment or even none at all. In advanced cases melanuria occurs. It is now generally agreed that melanomata should be regarded as carcinomata—an epithelial melanocarcinoma of the skin, or a neuroectodermal carcinoma in the case of the eye.

The *treatment* of a melanoma malignum, if the site permits, consists in wide local excision, followed by an incision over the course of the lymphatic drainage. Skin flaps are turned back and a wide strip of deep fascia, containing the lymphatics, is excised until the regional lymph nodes are reached, when they are also removed. If possible the tumour, fascia, and nodes are removed in one continuous strip (Pringle). Radiotherapy is disappointing.

An unusual variety of *melanosis* is occasionally seen, in which the pigment from a congenital mole slowly spreads in the surrounding skin, with no immediate evidence of malignancy. After a period of months or even years malignant changes supervene, therefore the pigmented patch should be excised freely.

ENDOTHELIOMA

The endothelial linings of blood-vessels, lymphatic spaces, and serous membranes occasionally give rise to neoplasms. Endotheliomata, therefore, enjoy a wide range of distribution. Although the original cells are flattened, they become spheroidal or cuboidal when neoplastic changes occur. Endotheliomata are not usually highly malignant and dissemination occurs in a minority of tumours.

Endotheliomata occasionally arise from the pleura and rarely from the pericardium or peritoneum. The "endothelioma" (meningioma) of the dura mater is thought by some to arise from the arachnoid membrane, which is not an endothelial structure. Calcification occasionally occurs in these tumours, in which case it is termed a "psammoma."

Peritheliomata are tumours arising in connection with the endothelial lining of small blood-vessels or lymphatics. Carotid body tumours are probably of this nature (p. 205).

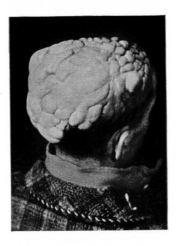

Fig. 51.—A typical "turban" tumour.

Cylindroma (*syn.* " Turban " tumour) is so called from the arrangement of the stroma in peculiar transparent cylinders. It is considered by some to be a basal-celled carcinoma, although other authorities classify the tumour as an endothelioma. The tumour gradually forms an extensive turban-like swelling extending over the scalp (fig. 51). Ulceration is uncommon, and the tumour is relatively benign.

Tumours arising in connection with special structures or organs are considered in their appropriate chapters.

BENIGN —→ MALIGNANT

Certain innocent neoplasms are prone to undergo malignant changes, and it is important, both for treatment and prognosis, to realise when the malignant characters supervene. Some or all of the following changes may be recognised :

(i) *Increase in size*—comparatively rapid enlargement is always suspicious, as in the case of a soft fibro-adenoma of the breast which is becoming sarcomatous.

(ii) *Increased vascularity*—as evinced by dilated cutaneous veins, or palpable pulsation in the tumour.

(iii) *Fixity*—due to invasion of surrounding structures, e.g. carcinomatous changes in a prostatic adenoma may cause " tethering " of the rectal mucosa.

(iv) *Involvement of adjacent structures*—carcinomatous changes in an adenoma of the thyroid should be suspected if the recurrent laryngeal nerve is implicated, and facial palsy associated with a parotid tumour suggests malignancy.

(v) *Dissemination*—discovery of secondary deposits is occasionally the clue which exposes malignancy. Thus the true nature of a doubtful lump in the breast is rendered evident if involvement of lymph nodes or osseous metastases are detected, or the discovery of a secondary deposit in a bone may lead to recognition of a hypernephroma.

RADIOTHERAPY

Very briefly, some of the principles of the therapeutic uses of radium and deep X-rays are as follows:

Radium.—

APPLICATION

(i) On the surface, as for rodent ulcers.

(ii) In cavities, e.g. the maxillary antrum.

(iii) Interstitial by means of needles, as for some cases of carcinoma of the tongue.

(iv) Teleradium or radium bomb, e.g. for malignant cervical lymph nodes.

(v) Radon seeds, which remain permanently in the tissues, e.g. cerebral tumours.

Deep X-rays.—

(i) Low voltage which act superficially.

(ii) High voltage for deeply seated structures, e.g. mediastinal tumours

PRINCIPLES OF TREATMENT

Neoplasms vary in their sensitivity to irradiation. Some tumours, such as lympho-sarcoma, are highly radio-sensitive, others, including carcinoma of the skin, are moderately sensitive. Melanomata belong to the group of radio-resistant tumours.

Indications.—

(i) Accessible tumours which are radio-sensitive, e.g. rodent ulcer.

(ii) As a preoperative measure to facilitate a surgical operation, e.g. advanced carcinoma of the breast.

(iii) Post-operatively as a precautionary measure, as after a radical mastectomy.

(iv) Inoperable cases as a palliative, or possibly curative, measure, e.g. fixed cervical lymph nodes secondary to carcinoma of the tongue.

(v) If operation is refused, or is contraindicated owing to the extent or site of the tumour, or the general health of the patient.

DANGERS

Immediate burn due to overdosage.

Necrosis of tissue or bone due to overdose or inadequate screening.

Hæmorrhage due to erosion of a vessel by the action of the radium, or secondary hæmorrhage following sloughing of necrosed tissue.

Injury by needles, e.g. puncture of the pleura or pericardium.

Loss of a needle, usually due to the thread breaking when withdrawal of the needle is attempted. The needle must be sought and removed without undue delay, otherwise prolonged action of radium will cause necrosis of adjacent tissue.

Fibrosis of adjacent structures, e.g. the rectum following radium treatment for carcinoma of the cervix.

CHAPTER IV

ULCERATION AND GANGRENE

ULCERATION

AN ULCER is caused by progressive destruction of surface tissue, i.e. cell by cell, as distinct from death of macroscopic portions.

Ulcers are classified as non-specific, specific, and malignant : the two latter groups are discussed in appropriate chapters.

Non-specific ulcers are due to infection of wounds caused by injury or physical irritants. Local irritation, as in the case of a dental ulcer, or interference with the circulation, e.g. varicose veins, are predisposing causes. Trophic ulcers are associated with derangement of vaso-motor control, and any debilitating condition predisposes to and hinders the healing of an ulcer.

The life-history of an ulcer consists of three phases; these are extension, transition, and repair. During the stage of extension the floor is covered with exudate and sloughs, while the base is indurated. The edge is sharply defined, and discharge is then purulent, and perhaps sanious. The transition stage is occupied in preparation for healing. The floor becomes cleaner and sloughs separate. Induration of the base diminishes, and the discharge becomes more serous. Small reddish areas of granulation tissue appear on the floor, and these link up until the whole surface is covered. The stage of healing consists in

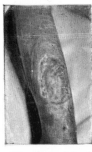

FIG. 52.—A healing varicose ulcer involving the lower third of the leg.

the transformation of granulation to fibrous tissue, which gradually contracts to form a scar (fig. 52). The edge of the ulcer becomes more shelving, and epithelium gradually extends from it to cover the floor. This healing edge consists of three zones—the outer of epithelium, which appears white, the middle one bluish in colour, where granulation tissue is covered by a few layers of epithelium, and the inner reddish zone of granulation tissue covered by a single layer of epithelial cells. Excessive granulations, commonly known as " proud flesh," need to be discouraged by scraping, or by the application of a caustic, such as silver nitrate.

CLINICAL EXAMINATION OF AN ULCER

This should be conducted in a systematic manner. The following are, with brief examples, the points which should be noted :

Site, e.g. 95 per cent. of rodent ulcers occur on the upper part of the face. Carcinoma typically affects the lower lip, while a primary chancre is usually on the upper.

Size, particularly in relation to the length of history, e.g. a carcinoma extends more rapidly than a rodent ulcer, but more slowly than an inflammatory ulcer.

Shape, e.g. a rodent ulcer remains circular until of a larger size than a carcinoma. It is stated that a rodent ulcer only becomes irregular when it encroaches on an area of skin possessing a different sensory nerve supply, when temporary arrest is said to occur. A gummatous ulcer is typically circular, or serpiginous, due to the fusion of multiple circles.

A square or angular ulcer is the result of " dermatitis artefacta." This condition is due to self-mutilation, e.g. by the application of irritants, such as corrosives. The patient has a neurotic or neuropathic temperament. The ulcer readily heals if protected by a dressing which cannot be disturbed by the patient.

Edge, a rodent ulcer is rolled or rampart, an epithelioma everted, while a tuberculous ulcer has an undermined edge (fig. 53).

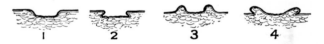

Fig. 53.—1. Healing ulcer, edges shelving. 2. Tuberculous ulcer. 3. Rodent ulcer. 4. Epithelioma.

Floor, a " wash-leather " slough may cover the floor of a gummatous ulcer, while a tuberculous ulcer often exhibits watery or greyish granulations.

Base, whether indurated, e.g. infiltration of carcinoma, or attached to deep structures, e.g. a varicose ulcer to the tibia.

Lymph nodes, not enlarged in the case of a rodent ulcer, unless due to secondary infection. May be enlarged and hard in the case of carcinoma, or shotty if their enlargement is due to a primary chancre.

Discharge, whether purulent, watery, or sanious. Organisms may be detected, e.g. spirochætes, tubercle bacilli, actinomyces.

Section, e.g. may confirm suspicions of carcinoma.

SKIN GRAFTING

This procedure is useful in hastening the healing of an extensive ulcer, and provides a more or less supple scar. The method recommended by Thiersch is most commonly used. The operation consists of scraping away the granulations on the floor of the ulcer, and securing hæmostasis by pressure with hot saline pads. Areas of cuticle are removed from healthy skin, usually from the thigh, with a non-bevelled razor, or, if available, a Padgett's dermatome. The line of section just reaches the papillæ, which appear as tiny oozing spots on removal of the graft. The grafts are transferred by a spatula to the prepared ulcer, so that they overlap each other, and a protective dressing is all that is necessary. Tulle gras is excellent for this purpose, and is composed of sterilised mesh gauze saturated with soft paraffin and impregnated with balsam of Peru.

Reverdin's method is simple, but less reliable than that of Thiersch. The skin is elevated by means of a needle or mosquito forceps, and a tiny area is snipped off and transferred to the raw area. This procedure is repeated as often as necessary.

Wolfe's method of using whole skin is useful when normal suppleness is desired, as in the palm. Tessellated grafts are a refinement of this method. The skin to be used is denuded of fat, cut into small squares, and arranged as desired.

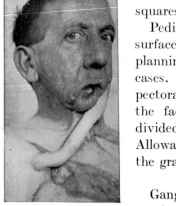

FIG. 54.—A pedicle graft.
(*Sir Archibald McIndoe.*)

Pedicle grafts are used to cover large raw surfaces, and scope for ingenuity exists in planning the precise method for individual cases. Thus a flap may be raised from the pectoral region and turned upwards on to the face, the base of the pedicle being divided when the graft has taken (fig. 54). Allowance must be made for shrinkage of the graft.

GANGRENE

Gangrene implies death of macroscopic portions of tissue combined with putrefaction.

Karl Thiersch, 1822–1895. *Professor of Surgery, Leipzig.*
Earl Calvin Padgett, Contemporary. *Associate Professor of Clinical Surgery, Kansas University, U.S.A.*

The features of gangrene are as follows :

(i) Cessation of circulation, i.e. loss of pulsation, and pressure on the skin causes no alteration of colour, indicating absence of capillary circulation.

(ii) Loss of heat.

(iii) Loss of sensation in the affected part.

(iv) Loss of function.

(v) Change of colour, depending on the type of gangrene.

Gangrene manifests itself clinically in one of two types :

Dry gangrene occurs when the tissues are desiccated by gradual slowing of the blood-stream, and typically occurs as a result of arterial degeneration, e.g. senile gangrene, or Möncke-berg's mesial degeneration in diabetes. The affected part becomes dry and wrinkled, discoloured from disintegration of hæmoglobin, and greasy to the touch.

Moist gangrene occurs when venous as well as arterial obstruction occurs, or when the artery is suddenly occluded, as by a ligature or embolus. Infection and putrefaction usually follow, and the affected part becomes swollen, discoloured, and the epidermis may be raised in blebs. Crepitus can sometimes be detected on palpation, due to infection by saprophytic gas-forming organisms.

When gangrene occurs, the local changes depend on the size of the affected tissue and the degree of infection present. Small amounts of gangrenous tissue are absorbed ; larger amounts, if aseptic, are cast off as a slough. This separation of the slough is accomplished by a layer of granulation tissue which forms between the dead and living tissue. These granulations extend into the dead tissue, until those which have penetrated farthest are unable to derive adequate nourishment owing to fibrosis occurring behind them. This defective nutrition results in ulceration, and thus a " line of demarcation " forms which separates the gangrenous mass from healthy tissue.

If the gangrenous tissue is infected, separation occurs as a result of inflammatory changes in the adjacent healthy structures. In addition to the toxins produced by infection, irritating chemical substances are formed by disintegration of the dead tissue, and the consequent inflammatory reaction in neighbouring living tissue results in suppuration. A layer of granulation tissue then forms on the surface of the healthy tissue, forming a

Johann Georg Mönckeberg (1878–1925). Professor of Pathology and Morbid Anatomy, Bonn.

line of separation. Infection may extend beyond the line of separation along lymphatic vessels or cellular tissue into healthy parts, and extensive inflammation then results.

The general treatment of gangrene consists of dealing with any predisposing causes, e.g. diabetes, and in relieving pain, ordering nutritious diet and stimulants if necessary. Locally, when gangrene threatens, the part should be kept dry, dusted with sulphanilamide powder and wrapped in cottonwool. In the case of a limb, elevation will encourage venous return. Treatment of different varieties is discussed later.

VARIETIES OF GANGRENE

The varieties of gangrene may be classified as follows :

i. *Symptomatic :*

(*a*) Raynaud's disease.

(*b*) Ergot.

(*c*) Senile.

(*d*) Thrombosis and thrombo-angiitis obliterans.

(*e*) Embolism.

(*f*) Diabetes.

ii. *Infective :*

(*a*) Gas gangrene.

(*b*) Phagedena, and cancrum oris *et* noma.

(*c*) Carbuncles and boils.

iii. *Traumatic :*

(*a*) Direct, which includes crushes, pressure sores, and the constriction groove of strangulated bowel.

(*b*) Indirect, due to injury of vessels at some distance from the site of gangrene, e.g. pressure on the popliteal artery by the lower end of a fractured femur, or the gangrenous contents of a hernial sac.

iv. *Physical*, e.g. burns, scalds, frost-bite, trench feet, chemicals, radium, X-rays, and electricity (fig. 55).

SYMPTOMATIC GANGRENE

Raynaud's disease is discussed in Chapter xxxvi.

Ergot is a common cause of gangrene among

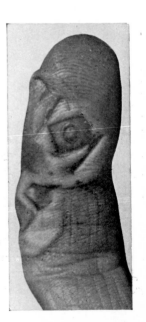

FIG. 55.—A post-mortem photograph of an electric burn, second degree. The victim touched a live terminal.

Maurice Raynaud, 1834–1881. Physician, Hôpital Laribosière, Paris.

dwellers on the shores of the Mediterranean Sea and in the Russian steppes who eat rye bread infected with Claviceps purpurea. The extremities, and sometimes the nose and ears, are affected (fig. 56).

Senile gangrene is predisposed to by arterial degeneration, the vessels becoming calcified and narrowed. Myocardial weakness causes slowing of the circulation, and slight injury causing local thrombosis may determine the onset of gangrene. Constitutional

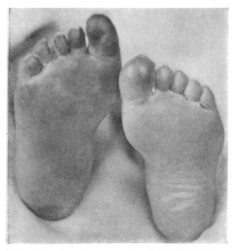

Fig. 56.—Ergot poisoning following treatment for post-partum hæmorrhage. (*R. Kennon.*)

conditions, such as nephritis or diabetes, lower the vitality of the tissues, and encourage the development of gangrene.

Treatment first consists in the prevention of minor injuries in patients who suffer from painful cramps and tingling in the legs, or other evidence of impaired circulation. Warm clothing, careful chiropody, and attention to the general health receive due consideration. If gangrene threatens, lumbar ganglionectomy is considered, but is unlikely to improve many cases, as actual degeneration rather than spasm of the arteries is the causative factor. If gangrene develops (fig. 57), amputation is usually necessary, and should be performed at a level where the blood-supply is adequate. If there is no pulsation in the tibial arteries, it is often necessary to amputate through the lower third of the thigh. An arteriogram is sometimes of value in assessing the level at which amputation may be performed in safety. Owing to the calcareous state of the vessels, hæmorrhage is controlled by digital pressure rather than by a tourniquet, and surprisingly little bleeding occurs. Flaps should be planned so as to be no longer than necessary and equal in length, as

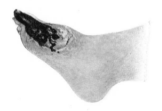

Fig. 57.—Senile gangrene.
(*British Journal of Surgery.*)

sloughing is otherwise encouraged. If calcification renders ligation of a large artery difficult on account of brittleness, some of the adjacent muscle is included in the ligature.

Thrombosis is an uncommon cause of gangrene, but occasionally occurs as a complication of specific fevers, notably enteric, or following thrombosis of deep veins, e.g. as a result of injection of varicose veins. Thrombo-angiitis obliterans is a common cause of gangrene of the leg.

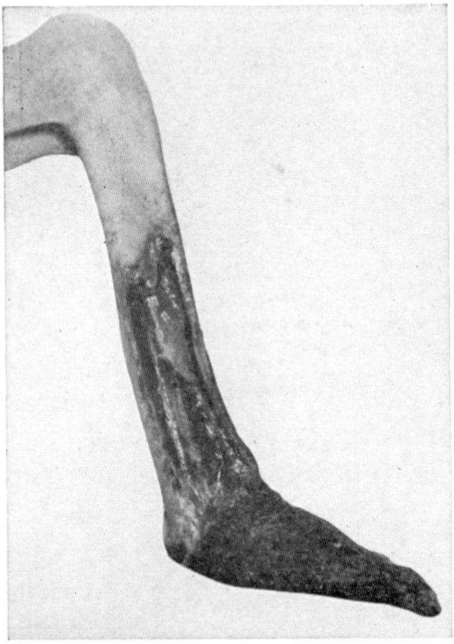

FIG. 58.—Moist gangrene due to an embolus at the bifurcation of the popliteal artery.

Embolic gangrene either arises in connection with cardiac lesions, e.g. endocarditis or mitral stenosis, or follows separation of an atheromatous plaque. Emboli are arrested at the site of bifurcation of an artery (fig. 58), or where sudden narrowing occurs owing to a large branch leaving the parent vessel. Sudden, severe pain is experienced, both at the site of impaction and along the distal course of the vessel. Circulatory changes speedily follow, pulsation is lost, and the limb becomes painful and pallid. Gangrene commences peripherally, and extends upwards until it reaches a level of adequate circulation, which usually coincides with a joint.

Treatment is discussed on p. 103.

Diabetic gangrene is due to three factors. These are : mesial calcification of the arteries, trophic changes resulting from peripheral neuritis, and the presence of sugar in the tissues, which lowers their power of resistance to infection. As in the senile type, gangrene is usually preceded by some slight trauma, and is either of the moist or dry variety.

Treatment consists in combating the diabetes by means of insulin and diet, and as the blood-supply is probably not so seriously curtailed as in senile gangrene, less extensive surgical measures are often successful. Expectant treatment is adopted, and if the spread of gangrene is arrested, removal of dead tissues may be sufficient. If amputation is imperative, it often can be carried out at a lower level than in the case of senile gangrene, e.g. at the site of election below the knee rather than through the lower third of the thigh.

INFECTIVE GANGRENE

Gas gangrene, although uncommon, is a regular contributory cause of death in the case of accidents. It is now considered that the anaerobes are introduced into the wound from infected clothing rather than carried in with soil, hence wounds of the thighs and buttocks are especially liable to infection. Excessive hæmorrhage and the use of a tourniquet are predisposing causes, and, as in all cases of gangrene, the leg is more prone to be affected than the arm. The causative organisms fall into two groups— those which break down starch, and those which break down protein. Cl. welchii (aerogenes capsulatus or perfringens) is the most important member of the saccharolytic group ; it is a Gram-positive anaerobe with a definite capsule. The proteolytic group include Cl. sporogenes, which splits protein into ammonia and sulphuretted hydrogen.

The diagnosis of true gas gangrene or clostridial myositis, i.e. gas in the tissues combined with gangrene, is essentially clinical. Gas-forming organisms are often cultivated from wounds in which they produce little or no evil results, and energetic surgical intervention is not indicated in these cases. Clostridial myositis is associated with pain, swelling, œdema, and toxæmia, which usually develop within forty-eight hours. The patient is often mentally alert and apprehensive, and complains of severe pain in the region of the wound. Later signs include rapid increase in the pulse-rate, a slight rise, or, in severe cases, a fall of temperature, and vomiting. It has been suggested that the toxins produced by the infection exert a selective and depressing action on the suprarenals, causing marked lowering of the blood-pressure and hence vomiting. The mental condition usually remains clear, and death occurs suddenly. We have seen a patient die while engaged in completing a football forecast. On examination of the wound, stitches are seen to be under tension, and, through the pouting edges, thin brownish fluid exudes, which possesses a mouldy or " mousy " odour. The limb is tense and swollen, and palpation

William Henry Welch, 1850–1934. Professor of Pathology at the Johns Hopkins University, Baltimore.

often reveals crepitus. A radiograph will demonstrate the presence of gas in intermuscular planes, and is very useful in the diagnosis of early cases.

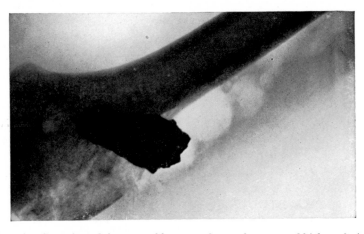

Fig. 59.—Comminuted fracture of humerus due to fragment of high-explosive. Bubbles of gas are present under the triceps muscle.

Ampoules are obtainable which contain 22,500 I.U. of poly-valent antitoxin (9,000 units Cl. welchii, 9,000 units Cl. œdema-tiens, 4,500 units Cl. septicum). One such dose should be given intravenously, or into healthy muscle, in all cases where the onset of gas infection is likely. Prophylactic penicillin should also be administered.

The next essential prophylactic measure is adequate surgical intervention. Meticulous excision of dead and dying tissue within six hours, and encasing the limb in plaster of Paris, prac-tically abolishes gas-gangrene infections. Partial suturing is sufficient, and secondary suture can be undertaken at a later date. If infection is already established, free incisions, local excision of a muscle, groups of muscles, or amputation may be necessary, according to the extent and virulence of infection. Gas and foul fluid are found in the cellular spaces ; contractility of the muscle is soon lost, and its colour changes successively from the dull red of boiled ham to green and then black. For therapeutic measures three ampoules (see above) of polyvalent serum should be given without delay, and repeated at six-hourly intervals as necessary (or combined in an intravenous drip). Neutralisation of toxin is a quantitative reaction, and early

delay cannot be compensated for by the subsequent administration of an excess of serum. Sulphonamide and penicillin should be administered at the earliest opportunity. If septicæmia occurs, gas is produced in many organs, notably the liver, which, at necropsy, drips with frothy blood, and is well named a "foaming liver."

Less severe forms of gas infection occasionally occur :

(i) *Local type*, invasion is sometimes limited to a single muscle, which becomes necrotic while adjacent muscles escape.

(ii) A *gas abscess* frequently occurs if a contaminated foreign body is present in a wound, and infection subsides when the wound is opened and the foreign body removed.

(iii) *Subcutaneous infection* is sometimes seen spreading for a considerable distance around a wound. Crepitus is easily palpable, and the skin becomes khaki-coloured as a result of hæmolysis. *Unless this condition is recognised, a needless amputation may be performed.* The only surgical treatment required is excision of the wound, combined with multiple incisions into the affected subcutaneous tissues, down to, but not including, the deep fascia, otherwise infection may be carried into the underlying fascial planes or muscles.

Cancrum oris et noma is a virulent type of infective gangrene which sometimes occurs in children who are debilitated and possibly recovering from some infectious disease (p. 157).

Carbuncles and boils are considered in connection with diseases of the skin.

TRAUMATIC GANGRENE

This variety of gangrene follows either local injury or occlusion of blood-vessels, and thus is either direct or indirect.

(i) **Direct traumatic gangrene** is due to local injury of the affected tissue, and may arise as a result of crushes, or pressure as in the case of splints, plasters, or bedsores.

Gangrene following a direct and severe injury, e.g. a street accident in which a heavy vehicle passes over a limb, is of the moist variety, and if the affected part is devitalised, removal without delay is indicated. As the tissues are presumably healthy, amputation is performed as close to the affected part as will leave the most useful limb.

BEDSORES (*syn.* decubitus ulcers) are either acute or chronic. The acute or *trophic* variety is associated with disease or injury of the spinal cord, and often progresses with alarming rapidity in spite of every care and attention.

The chronic or *postural bedsore* is predisposed to by four factors—pressure, injury, malnutrition, and moisture (fig. 60). Prophylactic treatment is of the utmost importance. Thus pressure over bony prominences is counteracted by change of posture and protection by cottonwool " nests " or sorbo-rubber rings. A water-bed is sometimes desirable. Injury due to wrinkled drawsheets, biscuit crumbs, or grit in the dusting

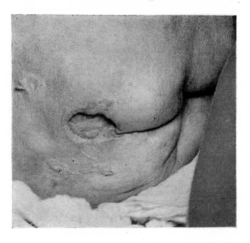

Fig. 60.—Postural bedsores over the sacrum.

powder is obviated by careful nursing. The nutrition of the skin is maintained by the application of astringent and stimulating preparations, such as eau-de-Cologne or surgical spirit. Maceration of the skin by sweat, urine, or pus is combated by skilled nursing.

A bedsore is to be expected if erythema appears which is unaffected by pressure. The application of tannic acid, or protection by strips of elastoplast, will reduce ulceration to a minimum. Actual bedsores during the stage of extension are best treated by the application of gauze moistened with anti-septics, such as dettol or flavine. When healing has commenced, 10 per cent. ichthyol in glycerine usually gives good results, and further stimulation is obtained by the use of red lotion. If the patient is young and otherwise healthy, free excision and sliding skin grafts are often successful.

(ii) **Indirect traumatic gangrene** is due to interference with blood-vessels, and some of the more important causes of this condition are as follows :

(*a*) Obstruction to artery and vein, as occurs in the loop of bowel contained in a strangulated hernia, or following pressure by a fractured bone on the main vessels of a limb.

(*b*) Thrombosis of a large artery, following injury or embolus.

(*c*) Ligation of the main artery of a limb, as after division by injury. The likelihood of gangrene then depends upon the efficiency of the collateral circulation, the elasticity of the arteries, and whether the arm or leg is affected. It is now generally agreed that in the case of a limb the accompanying vein should also be ligated, as thereby the risk of gangrene is diminished, although this procedure applied to the lower limb is likely to be followed by prolonged œdema.

Treatment is first directed to the cause, thus embolectomy, or closed or open reduction of a fracture, will sometimes prevent the onset of gangrene. A divided artery may be sutured, possibly with the aid of a vein graft, or united temporarily by a vitallium tube so that collateral circulation is allowed a few days in which to develop, and heparin is administered. In other cases, where gangrene is slow in its development, delay is sometimes advantageous in that a line of demarcation will indicate the level of vitality, but if moist gangrene rapidly spreads then amputation must be performed in order to safeguard healthy tissue. In cases of threatened gangrene the limb must be kept cool, so as to reduce metabolism to the minimum.

PHYSICAL AND CHEMICAL CAUSES

Frostbite is due to exposure to cold (fig. 61), especially if exposure is associated with wind or high altitudes (e.g. explorers and airmen). Oxygen deficiency results in tachycardia and weak cardiac contraction, also the low oxygen content of the blood diminishes the vitality of the tissues. The sufferer notices severe burning pain in the affected part, after which it assumes a waxy appearance and is pain less. Pathologically, the condition is due to damage to the vessel walls, which is followed by transudation and œdema, hence the waxy appearance of the frostbitten part. In severe cases, or if unwise treatment is adopted, vessels rupture and extravasation of blood-stained serum follows.

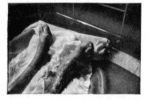

FIG. 61.—Frostbite. The patient was a farm-labourer, and sustained this condition in southern England.

Treatment demands adequate clothing, and oxygen for altitudes. Frostbitten parts must be warmed *very gradually*. The circulation is temporarily in abeyance, and it is therefore obvious that any temperature higher than that of the body will be detrimental, as the affected part will merely rise in temperature equal to that of its surroundings. Many frostbitten limbs have been either stewed or roasted in ignorance, and gangrene thereby rendered inevitable. The affected part should be wrapped in cottonwool and kept at rest. Friction, e.g. rubbing with snow, is contraindicated, as it damages the already devitalised tissues. Warm drinks and clothing are provided, and powerful analgesics are required to relieve the pain which heralds the return of circulation. Alcohol, although comforting, is contraindicated, as it causes peripheral dilatation and thus embarrasses the slowly returning circulation. If gangrene develops, the deeper structures are affected to a less extent than the skin, which naturally bears the brunt of the exposure.

Trench foot is due to cold, damp, and muscular inactivity, and is predisposed to by unsuitable clothing, such as garters, puttees, or ill-fitting boots. Other factors which encourage the condition are exhaustion, inadequate food, and cardiac or vascular disease. Prophylaxis is therefore of paramount importance. Numbness is followed by pain, which is often excruciating when boots are removed. The skin is mottled like marble, and in severe cases blisters containing blood-stained serum develop, and moist gangrene follows. The pathology is similar to that of frostbite, and treatment is the same.

BURNS AND SCALDS

Burns are due to dry heat and scalds to moist heat.

Dupuytren described six degrees of burns. The first consists of superficial congestion, whereas in the second degree the epidermis is raised by a blister. The third degree is the most painful, as the epidermis is destroyed, and the sensitive nerve terminals are exposed. In the fourth degree the whole skin is destroyed, the fifth degree includes muscles, and in the sixth degree the whole limb is charred.

General Treatment.—Severe burns are best treated in special wards or cubicles, which are now available in many of the larger hospitals. On admission, the burnt area is covered with a sterile towel or dressing, and a plasma drip is set up as soon as possible. Intravenous morphia is given in full doses. Hæmatocrit readings are taken three-hourly until hæmo-concentration is controlled (see below).

Those responsible for treatment should take precautions against infecting the burn, and they should wear a mask when the area is exposed. Increased katabolism of protein is reflected in excessive amounts of nitrogen excreted in the urine. In addition, outpouring of exudate results in further loss of protein, therefore a high protein intake is necessary, and an adequate supply of vitamins is essential. During convalescence attention must be paid to rehabilitation, and associated anæmia will require treatment.

FATAL RESULTS are due to one of three causes :

1. *Primary shock* (p. 15), which occurs simultaneously with the injury. Reassurance, warmth, and morphia nearly always tide the patient over the condition.

2. *Secondary shock* (p. 16) is responsible for 80 per cent. of

Baron Guillaume Dupuytren, 1777–1835. Surgeon, Hôtel Dieu, Paris.

deaths from burns; children are particularly susceptible, especially if the face or abdomen is involved. Plasma is lost from the circulation, some of which escapes on to the burnt surface, but probably a large amount exudes from the capillaries into surrounding tissues.

It is possible that this exudation is encouraged by toxins derived from injured tissue, which damage the endothelium of the capillaries and so render them more permeable.

Therefore, in the case of a severe burn the essential treatment is to compensate for deficiency of plasma protein by an intravenous infusion of plasma. Several pints may be necessary before hæmoconcentration approaches to normal. Blood transfusion is contraindicated, since capillaries become blocked by excess of corpuscles, while intravenous saline merely increases the œdema. Plasma loss is greatest in third-degree burns, and amounts to nearly three-quarters of the total blood volume when one-sixth of the surface of the body has been burnt.

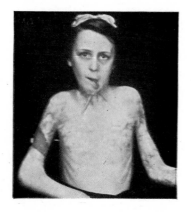

Fig. 62.—Scarring of neck and left elbow following severe burns.

3. *Toxæmia* occurs after forty-eight hours, and is augmented if secondary infection occurs. Severe cases are only likely to occur if prompt and efficient treatment of the burn is neglected, or if circumstances rendered such treatment impossible.

The infected area is treated by the application of suitable antiseptics, and as a rule a course of chemotherapy and penicillin is prescribed. Ichthyol (10 per cent.) in glycerine is a very useful preparation for eradicating prolonged infection of an extensive surface. When the condition of the wound permits, skin grafting will prevent scarring and subsequent contracture (fig. 62).

Toxins are alleged to be excreted by the bile, with consequent irritation of the second part of the duodenum and possible ulceration (Curling's ulcer). We have witnessed only one doubtful case of this nature.

Local Treatment.—*Minor Burns.*—These are commonly treated by the application of antiseptic ointments or picric acid. Tannafax, which is a non-greasy, water-soluble jelly, is a useful

Thomas Curling, 1811–1888. Surgeon to the London Hospital.

first-aid dressing. A satisfactory method is to clean the area with Cetavlon (1 per cent.), and to apply penicillin cream. The dressing of gauze and wool is retained in place with a firm crêpe bandage. In more serious cases a generous dose of morphia, suitable to the age and sex of the patient, should be administered. Intravenous injection of half the normal dose is valuable if rapid response is desirable.

Extensive Burns.—Although formerly popular, it is now agreed that the application of tannic acid to large denuded areas is dangerous. Absorption of tannic acid is apt to cause degeneration of the liver, and even necrosis. It also delays healing by coagulating healthy cells in addition to damaged tissues. As a result of these observations it is now realised that while tannic acid is suitable for minor burns, it is dangerous in the more severe cases. Extensive burns occur, more or less, in one of three distributions : localised on the neck or trunk, on one or more limbs, or widespread and perhaps multiple. Suitable methods of treatment according to the distribution, and which may be modified or combined, are as follows : pressure dressings for the neck or trunk, Bunyan's bag for the limbs, and saline baths for widespread areas.

Pressure Dressings.—Under anæsthesia the burnt area is carefully cleansed with swabs soaked in saline, and dead and severely damaged tissue is removed with scalpel or scissors. The wound is dusted with sulphonamide and penicillin powder and covered with petroleum jelly gauze. Further layers of dry gauze are applied, followed by a copious layer of cottonwool. The dressing is secured in position by an adhesive bandage firmly applied, so as to exert even pressure over the wound, as a result of which capillary exudation is diminished. The dressing is untouched for some days, and on removal burns of the third degree are found to be granulating. Deeper burns are likely to be covered with a slough, which is either excised or allowed to separate. The use of medicated preparations, such as boric acid or tulle gras, instead of petroleum jelly, does not appear to hasten healing. When the wound is clean and granulating (usually about the third week), skin grafts are applied (p. 68).

Bunyan Bag.—After cleansing, the limb is encased in a special watertight envelope, which is transparent (fig. 63). The envelope is filled with electrolytic sodium hypochlorite

John Bunyan, Contemporary. Surgeon Lieut.-Commander (D), R.N.V.R.

solution (Milton 5 per cent.), so that the limb is bathed in the fluid, which is changed twice a day. An entry and an exit are provided for this

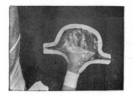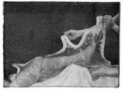

FIG. 63.—Bunyan bag applied to the hand and leg.

purpose. The burn heals rapidly with a minimum of scarring, and contractures are prevented by active movement of the parts affected. This method is especially useful for extensive burns of the hand and fingers.

Saline Baths.—In cases in which the burn is very extensive, and possibly the clothes are charred and adherent to the tissues, the patient may, with advantage, be put in a saline bath at a temperature of 98° to 100° F. This combats the shock, and allows the clothes to be soaked off. If facilities exist, baths repeated twice daily yield excellent results. After the bath the patient is placed on a sterile sheet, the affected surface is dried under a lamp, and insufflated with sulphonamide and penicillin powder. The burnt area is then covered with vaselined gauze and a saline dressing, which is remoistened two-hourly. These dressings are removed by soaking in the next bath.

Plaster of Paris applied as a splint is useful in maintaining the optimum position for burns of digits or limbs. A plaster cast should be applied if the burn is associated with a fracture, or if prolonged transport is necessary. After cleansing, the affected area is covered with tulle gras and a thick layer of cottonwool, so that swelling can occur without risk to the circulation. Unless circulatory changes occur the plaster is undisturbed for two weeks, and is then reapplied as necessary.

Burns of the face and external genitalia are conveniently treated by the application of gauze impregnated with a sulphonamide ointment.

Amputation is necessary if a limb is charred.

Chemicals sometimes cause gangrene, the most dangerous being carbolic acid, as anæsthesia occurs before gangrene supervenes. *Carbolic compresses should never be used,* and fingers have been lost by the application of compresses even as dilute as 1 : 80. Gangrene is due to local arterial spasm.

The accidental injection of pentothal into a branch of the

brachial artery may cause gangrene of the fingers. Scalding pain accompanies the injection, and should act as a warning, but the anæsthetist should have observed that the blood in the syringe was bright red in colour. The needle should be left *in situ* and procaine injected into the artery in order to relieve spasm.

Phosphorus burns require special treatment. Particles continue to burn until neutralised, the best preparation for this purpose being 2 per cent. aqueous solution of copper sulphate. Oil dissolves phosphorus and extends the scope of the burn. After the phosphorus has been rendered inert and any macroscopic particles removed, triple dye should be applied.

Electrical burns are usually deep and localised, and are best treated by early excision.

CHAPTER V
BLOOD AND BLOOD-VESSELS
BLOOD TRANSFUSION

THE indications are briefly as follows :

(1) Hæmorrhage, either acute or chronic. Transfusion is imperative if the hæmoglobin falls below 40 per cent. (Haldane), or the systolic pressure below 90 mm. Hg.

(2) Shock, in order to increase the blood volume, which is diminished by the transudation of serum through the capillaries into the surrounding tissues. In most cases plasma is preferable to whole blood, as unwanted corpuscles increase the hæmo-concentration, and impose a strain on an embarrassed heart.

(3) To increase coagulability, especially in such conditions as hæmophilia, purpuric diseases, as a pre-operative measure in obstructive jaundice, and after excessive administration of heparin.

(4) To obtain temporary improvement in certain blood diseases, such as aplastic anæmia, leukæmia, and occasionally in Hodgkin's disease.

(5) Severe infections, especially if the hæmoglobin falls below 60 per cent. Transfusion raises the patient's resistance, and anæmia is improved. Immuno-transfusion is now superseded by chemotherapy.

(6) Carbon monoxide poisoning. Venesection removes the inert carboxyhæmoglobin, and transfusion provides a fresh supply of oxyhæmoglobin.

(7) Certain cases of erythroblastosis (Rh. factor, p. 85).

Human blood falls into one of four main groups, described by the International Classification as AB, A, B, and O, although sub-groups exist. Incompatibility gives rise to the following phenomena :

(I) The red cells of the donor are agglutinated by the recipient's plasma.

(II) This agglutination is followed by hæmolysis. Hæmolysis is always preceded by agglutination, and advantage is taken of this fact in testing for compatibility.

Members of Group AB are universal recipients, and those of Group O are universal donors, but can only receive blood from their own group.

Non-paternity.—This test assists only a limited number (about 25 per cent.) of men falsely accused, i.e. it is of positive value only. If the test is negative it is of no assistance, as other men of the same group are not excluded. The Court has no power to compel the test to be made. Probably in the future use will be made of sub-groups (Roche Lynch).

Technique of Grouping.—Stock sera from Group A and Group B are placed side by side on a slide. A drop of blood obtained by a prick with a sterile cutting needle is added to each, and after five minutes is exam-

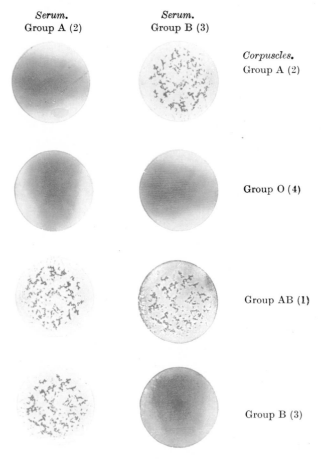

Fig. 64.—Blood grouping.

ined microscopically. If clumping of corpuscles is seen in the serum of Group A, then the corpuscles are those of an individual of Group B. If clumping occurs only in the serum of Group B, then the corpuscles are from Group A. If clumping is present in both, then the corpuscles are from Group AB, and if in neither, they belong to Group O (fig. 64).

Cross-matching.—In all cases a cross-matching test is advisable, as members of the same group sometimes show varying degrees of incompatibility. A few drops of the recipient's serum is tested with the donor's corpuscles, in the same manner as for grouping, and the donor's cells are

G. Roche Lynch, Contemporary. Senior Official Analyst, Home Office, London.

tested against the recipient's serum. Even after the extra precaution of cross-matching some degree of reaction occasionally occurs, and is sometimes due to lack of care in cleansing the equipment.

THE RH FACTOR

In 1940 the discovery of a blood agglutinogen explained some hitherto mysterious diseases which affected mothers and their offspring. The agglutinogen was termed Rh because it forms in the blood of some mammals, e.g. the rabbit, into which blood of the rhesus monkey is injected. The physiological complexities of the factor are somewhat involved, but for practical purposes the following points must be borne in mind :

Mother.—Unless facilities exist for Rh examinations a pregnant woman, (or any female under 45) should only be transfused with Rh-negative blood (of the compatible ABO group). If no Rh-negative blood of the appropriate group is available, plasma or serum should be used for transfusion.

Child.—The diseases which arise from the Rh-antigen-agglutinin reactions are :

    (i) Macerated fœtus.
    (ii) Hydrops fœtalis.
    (iii) Icterus gravis neonatorum.
    (iv) Congenital hæmolytic anæmia.

These diseases are included in the general term erythroblastosis fœtalis, and the treatment, in suitable cases, consists in blood transfusion with Group O blood of the same Rh sub-group, or the mother's washed red cells can be used. Desensitisation of the mother is not possible. If the infant at birth shows evidence of erythroblastosis, withdrawal and replacement of suitable blood via the umbilical vein should be considered.

METHODS OF TRANSFUSION

(1) *Direct Transfusion.*—A special syringe fitted with two nozzles is necessary, and each of which is connected by rubber tubing to a needle in the donor's and recipient's veins respectively. This method is obsolescent.

(2) *Drip transfusion* is utilised as a means of combating loss of blood or shock, as after a severe accident or during a formidable operation. The use of anticoagulants has greatly simplified transfusion, and sodium citrate is efficacious in preventing clotting, and innocuous to the patient. A solution of sodium citrate of 3·8 per cent. prevents clotting of six times the volume of blood, so that 80 to 100 ml. are necessary for the transfusion of one pint of blood. The donor lies on a table, and a rubber tube is tied round the arm above the elbow, or a sphygmomanometer is

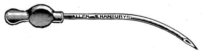

FIG. 65.—Lockhart-Mummery's needle.

applied, the pressure being raised to 70 to 80 mm. Hg. A small-bore needle (fig. 65), carrying about 10 inches (25 cm.) of rubber tubing, is inserted into a suitable vein, and the desired quantity of blood is allowed to flow into a 1,000-ml. flask, which contains the necessary amount of citrate solution. The flask is partially immersed in water at a temperature of 105° F., and an assistant agitates it in order to encourage thorough mixing. Screw-cap bottles, fitted with rubber corks, are provided by the Blood Transfusion Service for the collection of blood (fig. 66). Two glass tubes pass through the cork, one to act as an air vent and the other to admit the tube which withdraws blood from the donor. The risk of contamination is thus minimised, and the blood can be stored in the bottle pending usage.

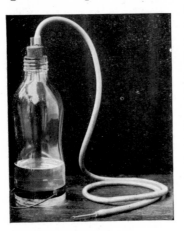

When prolonged transfusion is required, some apparatus which includes an interceptor is necessary, so that the flow of blood can be regulated. By means of two flasks blood and saline can be administered simultaneously in such proportions as are most expedient, and empty flasks can be replaced without interruption of flow (fig. 70).

Fig. 66.—Blood Transfusion Service bottle for collecting blood.

The two tubes from the containers, fitted with interceptors, are connected by a Y-shaped junction, and a single exit below leads to the patient's vein. The desired flow of blood or saline can thus be regulated.

In traumatic cases the amount of blood which should be given varies with the amount lost and the reaction of the patient. As a general rule, enough blood or fluid should be transfused to raise the systolic pressure to 100 mm. A shocked patient can safely be given two pints in a quarter of an hour, followed, if necessary, by further amounts at a slower rate, but hæmoglobinometer readings are necessary to regulate dosage.

(3) *Marrow Infusion.*—This method is valuable in patients whose veins are collapsed as a result of severe shock, or in small children whose veins are too small to admit an adequate cannula. The sternum or the tibia are the bones of choice, as they are subcutaneous, and the latter is readily immobilised. Under local anæsthesia the compact bone is pierced with a special trocar and cannula directed towards the patient's head ; sudden lack of

Richard Lewisohn, Contemporary. Surgeon at Mount Sinai Hospital, New York. Devised the citrate method in 1915.

resistance indicates that the
marrow cavity is reached.
The cannula is connected to
the transfusion apparatus, and
blood, plasma, or other fluid
is rapidly absorbed (fig. 67).

Accidents.—(1) *Due to wrong
group :*
(*a*) Immediate Reaction.—Before 100 ml. of blood have been
given the patient complains of
severe backache, constriction of
the chest, and throbbing in the
head. Cyanosis, collapse, tachycardia, and unconsciousness follow,
and death may occur immediately
or in a few hours, owing to circulatory failure. Possibly, as a result
of hæmolysis, the foreign protein
acts as an acute capillary poison.

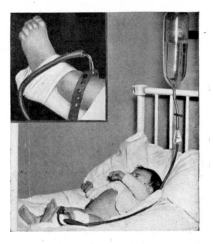

Fig. 67.—Marrow infusion into the tibia of an infant.

In milder cases recovery is preceded by jaundice and hæmoglobinuria.
(*b*) Renal Reaction.—Due to hæmolysis of the donor's cells. Collapse
occurs during transfusion, and jaundice and uræmia follow. Alkalis should
be administered, but in severe cases death from uræmia occurs in six to
ten days (fig. 68). Treatment is conducted on similar lines as for the
crush syndrome (p. 19).
(2) *After apparent accurate cross-matching :*

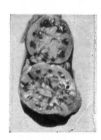

Fig. 68.—Bisected
kidney—the tub-
ules are choked
with disintegrating
red cells. Incom-
patible blood caused
fatal anuria.

(*a*) Myocardial Failure.—Elderly people and those
with myocardial degeneration may be endangered
by the reaction which is apt to follow any transfusion.
Symptoms of myocardial failure appear one or two
hours after transfusion. As a precaution, patients
with long-standing anæmia, or those over the age of
sixty, should not be given more than 300 ml. If
anæmia is severe, packed cells should be used, i.e. the
concentrated blood which remains after supernatent
plasma is removed (the plasma is stored for use in
other patients).
(*b*) Anaphylaxis, especially if the same donor is used
a second time, as sensitisation is liable to develop.
Cross-matching must therefore be performed to ensure
that the donor's blood has not become incompatible.
Also frequent transfusions render a patient increasingly liable to reactions.
(*c*) Rh factor (p. 85).

Untoward after-effects, e.g. rigors, fever, etc., are
due to particles of débris or dead bacteria; therefore all solutions must
be triply distilled before sterilisation, and the apparatus and rubber tubing
must be thoroughly washed with distilled water.

BLOOD-BANKS

The increased demand for blood has led to the establishment in suitable
centres of blood-banks. The first change which occurs in stored blood is

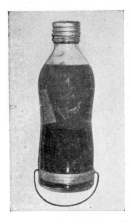

FIG. 69.—Bottle of preserved blood showing separation into corpuscular and plasma layers.

destruction of the granular cells, probably owing to proteolytic ferments which they contain, and after a week nearly all granulocytes are replaced by amorphous masses. After about a week leakage of hæmoglobin occurs from the erythrocytes, but although the red cells shrink they are not destroyed, and the vital property of ability to combine with oxygen is not seriously impaired (fig. 69). Stored blood can be transfused with safety within a month of storage, and transfusions within two months have not been followed by serious reactions.

INTRAVENOUS SALINE INFUSION

The safest and most generally useful solution for continuous intravenous infusion is one containing 0·18 per cent. sodium chloride and 4·3 per cent. dextrose.[1] The prolonged use of normal saline (0·85 per cent.) has a deleterious effect on the kidneys, and should only be used when serious chloride depletion exists.

Temporary infusion, either subcutaneous or intravenous, of saline is occasionally indicated in circumstances of urgency. If the infusion is subcutaneous the rapidity with which saline is absorbed into the tissues depends upon the adequacy of the circulation, which is a variable factor. Unless special facilities are at hand, intravenous infusion of saline has a limited application. A rapid flooding of the circulation with an excessive amount of fluid is apt to cause œdema of the lungs.

Hypertonic intravenous solutions are occasionally indicated in such conditions as excessive vomiting, when hypertonic saline replenishes the extreme deficiency of sodium chloride, and as a palliative measure in some cases of cerebral tumour.

Continuous infusion of saline and dextrose is a very valuable and sometimes life-saving method of combating dehydration, as the precise amount of fluid which actually enters the circulation can be measured with accuracy. By means of continuous infusion the solution can be administered for days, and other substances can be added, such as glucose, sera, soluble sulphonamide or sodium sulphate (4·285 per cent.) for uræmia.

The apparatus necessary for continuous infusion comprises a reservoir and tube, which is interrupted by an interceptor,

[1] In pyrogen-free water.

and a gold-plated cannula to avoid corrosion. The inter-ceptor indicates the rate at which the fluid is flowing into the vein, which can be ad-justed by screw pressure. Forty drops a minute ap-proximates to a pint in four hours. The neck of the cannula can be bent to any angle so as to adapt itself to varying thicknesses of sub-cutaneous fat, and the collar facilitates fixation in the vein by a ligature. The cannula

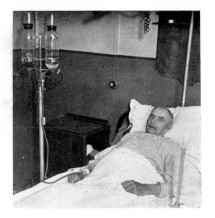

Fig. 70.—Intravenous infusion into the radial vein.

should be immersed in citrate solution before being introduced and tied into the vein.

For continuous infusion it is usually preferable to use the internal saphenous vein rather than one in the arm, as prolonged fixation of the upper limb is irksome to the patient, and move-ments are liable to dislodge the cannula. If the patient is restless, it is advisable to fix the leg in a splint. However, in aged or bed-ridden patients phlebitis and extending thrombosis are liable to follow infusion in the leg, and the arm should then be used (fig. 70). If a hot-water bottle is in contact with the proximal part of the tube, an adequate temperature of the fluid is assured. The nurse must keep the flask at least half-full, so as to avoid the risk of bubbles of air being carried along the tube into the patient's vein.

Contraindications to intravenous infusion :

(1) Myocardial weakness, as a relatively sudden increase in the circulating fluid, is apt to impose excessive strain.

(2) Renal incompetence, owing to excretory difficulty.

(3) Hypertension, as the cardio-vascular system is already embarrassed.

(4) Pulmonary congestion, as œdema of the lungs is liable to be increased.

If intravenous infusion is to be used for more than twenty-four hours, the fluid intake and output should be checked by a balance sheet.

In order to maintain chloride balance the proportion of dextrose to chloride should be varied according to the amount of urinary chlorides.

RECTAL SALINE INFUSION

Intermittent rectal saline infusion has the advantage of simplicity ; it requires neither special apparatus nor asepsis. The disadvantages are that it is somewhat slow, and fluid may be retained in the bowels. A drachm of salt to a pint of water, at a temperature of 115° F. (47°C.) is allowed to gravitate into the rectum through a funnel and tube connected to a catheter. The patient's hips are elevated, and the funnel is held at a height of not more than 2 feet (60 cm.). The usual rate of infusion is half a pint every four hours.

Murphy introduced *continuous* rectal saline infusion (proctoclysis), which was a distinct advance, especially in cases of peritonitis. Slow, continuous delivery of the saline aided its absorption and caused less disturbance to the patient (fig. 71).

In cases of mere dehydration, without chloride depletion, plain tap-water is absorbed more rapidly than saline, and is a more speedy method of relieving thirst.

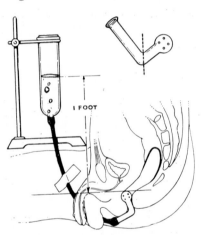

Fig. 71.—The principles of proctoclysis. Inset : Murphy's glass cannula (a rectal tube is an efficient substitute). The part to the right of the dotted line lies within the rectum.

I FOOT

BLOOD

A brief summary of the *normal constituents* is included here. Examination of marrow obtained by sternal puncture has added much to our knowledge of pathological conditions. For further details the reader should refer to a work on hæmatology.

Red Corpuscles.—The number varies between 5 and 6 million per c.mm. In conjunction with the number of red corpuscles present the proportion of hæmoglobin is usually estimated. The " Colour Index " is then obtained by dividing the percentage of hæmoglobin by the number of corpuscles expressed as a percentage of the normal, and should therefore be approximately 1.

Within a few hours of a severe hæmorrhage, the volume of the blood is restored by absorption of fluid from the tissues. The red cells are replaced

John Benjamin Murphy, 1857–1916. Professor of Surgery, North-Western University, Chicago.

more rapidly than the hæmoglobin, consequently the " Colour Index " is below 1. Hæmoglobin is replaced at an average rate of 1 per cent. each day.

Leucocytes.—Normally, 7,000 to 10,000 leucocytes are present per c.mm., and they comprise five different types :

(*a*) The Polymorphonuclear Leucocyte (63 to 72 per cent.), containing a lobed nucleus. It is formed in bone marrow, and is larger than a red corpuscle.

(*b*) The Lymphocyte (20 to 25 per cent.), with a single deeply staining nucleus smaller than a red corpuscle, and derived from lymphoid tissue.

(*c*) The large Mononuclear cell (2 per cent.), probably endothelial in origin.

(*d*) The Eosinophile Leucocyte (1 to 3 per cent.), derived from bone marrow, and has a bilobed nucleus and coarse granules.

(*e*) The Basophile, or mast cell ($\frac{1}{2}$ per cent.), constant in number and produces heparin.

Blood Platelets.—These minute bodies are formed in the bone marrow, and their normal minimum content is 230,000 per c.mm. If diminished in number, clotting is defective.

Chemical Constituents.—Calcium, phosphorus, sugar, cholesterol, and urea are all present in definite quantities.

INVESTIGATIONS OF SURGICAL IMPORTANCE

(1) **Cytological.**—(*a*) *Red Cells.*—The number of cells is increased in polycythæmia and diminished in many conditions, e.g. hæmorrhage or infection. The envelope of the cell normally withstands dilution to 0·47 per cent. saline. Excessive fragility is associated with acholuric jaundice.

(*b*) *White Cells.*—Increase of polymorphonuclear cells to an extent of 15,000 per c.mm. or more is strongly indicative of suppuration, and may be of diagnostic value. Leucopœnia may be associated with typhoid fever and tuberculosis.

A relative lymphocytosis occurs in uncomplicated tuberculosis, and an absolute and sometimes enormous increase occurs in lymphatic leukæmia.

A relative eosinophilia may occur in parasitic infections, such as trichiniasis, hydatid disease, certain skin lesions, and also in anaphylactic conditions.

(*c*) *Blood platelets* (250,000 to 300,000 per c.mm.) are diminished in thrombocytopænic purpura. In other varieties of purpura, the number may be increased, in which case the risk of thrombosis is present.

(2) **Colour Index.**—This is important in testing types of anæmia, e.g. it is increased in anæmia of the pernicious type and diminished in secondary anæmia.

(3) **Serological.**—This includes Widal's test, the W.R., and

Fernand Widal, 1862–1929. A native of Algiers, and Professor of Medicine in Paris.

other complement fixation tests, and blood grouping in connection with blood transfusion.

(4) **Bacteriological.**—In septicæmic conditions the organism may be isolated from the blood by culture. In connection with the examination of films, the diagnosis of malaria and filariasis may be made.

(5) **Chemical.**—The percentage of urea is an indication of the renal efficiency, and the blood-sugar curve distinguishes the true diabetic from renal glycosuria. Estimations of calcium, phosphorus, and phosphatase are of importance in the diagnosis and treatment of certain bone diseases. Hypocalcæmia occurs in acute pancreatitis.

(6) **Coagulation Time** (*syn.* Clotting Time).—This is prolonged in hæmophilia, and may be an important preliminary consideration when an operation is contemplated in the presence of jaundice. The normal coagulation time (Wright's method) is ten to fifteen minutes at room temperature. Clotting time is controlled mainly by the concentration of thromboplastin. It is an essential examination to control the dosage of heparin.

(7) **Blood Sedimentation Rate.**—Many pathological conditions cause an increase in the sedimentation rate, as normal cells, when damaged, act as foreign proteins. The main surgical value is that the S.R. is increased in inflammatory conditions, e.g. it may assist in distinguishing abdominal colic from acute appendicitis. It is also useful as an indication of the progress of chronic infections, such as tuberculosis. The test is unreliable during infancy, pregnancy, menstruation, and if the patient is undergoing treatment by vaccines or colloidal metals. The normal sedimentation rate is 3 to 7 mm. after one hour (Westergren method).

(8) **Prothrombin.**—Daily estimations of the prothrombin time (normally 18 seconds) of the blood are essential if tromexan is administered.

ANTI-COAGULANT THERAPY

Clotting of the blood necessitates, firstly, the formation of thrombin, and, secondly, the conversion of fibrinogen into fibrin by the preformed thrombin. The various steps concerned with the formation of blood-clot can be simplified as follows :

(1) Thromboplastinogen in presence of platelet enzyme → thromboplastin.

Helen Payling Wright, Contemporary. Department of Pathology, Guy's Hospital Medical School.
Alf W. A. Westergren, born 1891. Lecturer in Medicine, Medico-kirurgiska Instituet, Stockholm.

(2) Prothrombin complex + thromboplastin = thrombin.

(3) Fibrinogen in presence of thrombin → fibrin.

The first and third reactions are enzymatic. The second is stoichiometric, i.e. the components react in fixed proportions as in any ordinary chemical reaction (E. J. Wayne).

At the present time the two anti-coagulants of clinical importance are heparin and tromexan. Both have their disadvantages, and doubtless within a short time our colleagues, the biochemists, will produce substances which are superior to either of these preparations.

Anti-coagulants are contraindicated in pregnancy, hepatic or renal deficiency, or when there is risk of hæmorrhage, e.g. within six hours of an operation, or in cases of peptic ulceration.

Heparin.—This substance is present in body tissues, especially the liver and lung. It is produced by the mast-cells and prolongs the clotting time of blood. Heparin can be administered intravenously (50 mg. which equals 5,000 units) either at four-hourly intervals (as it is rapidly excreted) or by continuous infusion. In the former case polythene tubing is inserted into an arm vein, and the tube is strapped to the arm. A needle with a rubber diaphragm is attached to the free end of the tube, through which the heparin is injected every four hours. Preparations of " retard heparin " which can be given intramuscularly are under trial. Clotting time must be estimated twice daily. If this is unduly prolonged, a small blood transfusion should be given, or intravenous protamine sulphate, 5 ml. of a 1 per cent. solution will neutralise 50 mg. of heparin. Owing to the rapid excretion of heparin, antidotes are seldom required. Heparin is an expensive drug which requires parenteral therapy.

Tromexan is a safer preparation than dicoumarol, as on withdrawal the prothrombin time returns to normal within twenty-four hours. It acts by retarding the production of prothrombin in the liver, but as there is a physiological reserve its action is delayed for some twenty-four hours. On the first day of treatment four 300 mg. tablets are administered. Efficient laboratory control is all-important, and the dose is varied so as to maintain the prothrombin time at a little over double the normal, i.e. about 40 seconds. Should ecchymoses or hæmaturia occur

E. J. Wayne, Contemporary. *Physician, Royal Infirmary, Sheffield.*

fresh blood is immediately transfused, reinforced, if necessary, with vitamin K intravenously.

HÆMORRHAGE

Hæmorrhage is arterial, venous, or capillary ; the first variety is either primary, reactionary, or secondary in nature. If hæmorrhage is severe, the blood-pressure falls, although it is partially maintained by absorption of body fluids, and vaso-motor constriction of the arterioles. A further result is loss of the oxygen-carrying hæmoglobin, so that tissues are deprived of oxygen. In severe cases the patient complains of thirst and impending suffocation (air hunger), and later of tinnitus (buzzing in the ears), and blindness. The pulse is rapid and easily com-pressible, and increasingly dicrotic as the arteries empty. The patient is restless, clammy, and pallid.

Natural arrest of hæmorrhage is encouraged by increased coagulability of the blood, diminution in the force of the heart's action, and changes in the divided vessel. Thus, in the case of a completely divided artery, the elastic coat retracts within the sheath, and partially blocks the lumen, and clotting occurs as far as the distal branch, but if an artery is incompletely divided this retraction cannot occur and bleeding is encouraged. Per-manent occlusion follows organisation of this intravascular clot.

ARTERIAL HÆMORRHAGE

Primary.—In cases of emergency, the external hæmorrhage can be arrested temporarily by direct digital pressure, and if from a limb, a tourniquet can then be applied. This should not be allowed to remain in position for an interval of more than thirty minutes without being loosened, and it is then tightened again if necessary. If hæmorrhage occurs from a limb, eleva-tion discourages the loss of blood. Arrangements are then made for transport to a hospital, where the wound is explored, and every effort made to ligate both ends of the divided artery.

Two exceptions to this procedure are :

(1) Punctured wounds of the hands and feet. If the bleeding artery cannot be found, or if the wound is so contaminated that extensive exploration would spread infection, then the brachial or superficial femoral artery should be ligated.

(2) Bleeding from deep branches of the external carotid artery, e.g. a penetrating wound of the spheno-maxillary fossa. Exposure is impracticable, and the external carotid artery is ligated between its superior thyroid and lingual branches.

Reactionary hæmorrhage occurs within twenty-four hours, and is due to " slipping " of a ligature, or dislodgment of a clot which occludes a divided vessel, owing to rising blood-pressure concomitant upon recovery from shock. It is more likely to arise from small vessels (as bleeding from large vessels has probably been adequately arrested). If persistent, the vessel must be sought and ligated, or controlled by a stitch, otherwise the wound is cauterised, packed, or resutured. Reactionary venous hæmorrhage is apt to occur within a few hours of operations on the thyroid gland, as coughing or vomiting causes acute engorgement of the deep veins of the neck.

Secondary hæmorrhage is due to infection and sloughing of part of the wall of an artery. It is predisposed to by pressure of a drainage tube or fragment of bone, or excessive separation of the sheath of an artery during ligation. Internal secondary hæmorrhage occurs in connection with a chronic peptic or typhoid ulcer, and phthisis.

In an infected wound or amputation stump, " warning " hæmorrhages usually occur in the form of bright red stains on the dressing about the tenth day. Repeated losses, or a sudden severe hæmorrhage, may prove fatal.

When a definite warning hæmorrhage occurs, the wound should be freely opened, sloughs removed, and an attempt made to recognise and ligate the bleeding vessel. Failing this, the wound is packed with oxycel or other absorbable gauze, or with gauze moistened with turpentine. Should hæmorrhage recur, then the main vessel of the limb is ligated (ligation in continuity), or amputation performed.

This " warning " hæmorrhage often occurs in the case of peptic ulcers, and is a danger signal which it is imprudent to ignore.

Venous bleeding is troublesome in certain situations, e.g. during dissection of nodes of the neck, as the welling blood obscures the precise source of hæmorrhage. It is important to divide no tissue under traction, as veins are thereby emptied and rendered unrecognisable. If large veins are injured, a lateral ligature can sometimes be applied without occluding the

Ambroise Paré, 1509–1590. French surgeon; first to ligate severed arteries. Stated, " I dressed his wounds, but God healed them."

whole lumen. The entrance of air into veins is a rare event, but can occur in connection with large veins in which the pressure is below that of the atmosphere, e.g. the axillary vein, or if veins are attached to deep fascia and consequently cannot collapse when divided, notably the external jugular. The aspiration of air may be audible, and is followed by collapse of the patient, as the air is churned up with blood in the right side of the heart and impedes the circulation. Treatment consists in the immediate arrest of further entry by digital pressure, or flooding the wound with saline, and combating the collapse by posture and anti-shock measures.

ARTERIES

Injury.—An artery is sometimes ruptured subcutaneously, e.g. the popliteal in the case of a dislocated knee, or divided in a penetrating or incised wound.

In the former case a rapidly increasing swelling occurs, which may pulsate. The distal signs depend upon the degree of circulatory disturbance, and pressure on nerves may cause paræsthesia or pain. Distal pulsation is commonly absent.

If swelling increases, local infection or distal gangrene is liable to supervene. If coagulation occludes the rent, and collateral circulation is efficient, the extravasated blood may organise, and the limb retain its vitality.

In the case of injury to a large artery, operation should be performed, and the vessel exposed. A temporary tape ligature, or preferably a Crile's clamp (fig. 77), controls the circulation, and if possible the rent is sutured with fine vaselined silk. The judicious administration of heparin discourages intravascular clotting. End-to-end suture or grafting (p. 98) have been successfully accomplished, relaxation being obtained by posture. If the laceration is extensive, a Tuffier's tube can be introduced into the two ends as a temporary measure, in order to allow collateral circulation to become established. If these measures are impracticable, the vessel is completely divided if it is not already severed, and the ends are ligated.

ANEURISM

An aneurism is a sac filled with blood in direct communication with the interior of an artery. A *true* aneurism is due to dilatation of an artery, whereas a *false* aneurism is a sac lined by condensed cellular tissue which communicates with the artery through an aperture in its wall.

1. **True aneurisms** are fusiform, saccular, or dissecting.

A *fusiform* aneurism is one in which the lumen is more or less equally expanded, and is usually due to syphilitic mesarteritis.

George W. Crile, born 1864. Professor of Clinical Surgery at the Western Reserve Hospital, Cleveland, Ohio.
T. Tuffier, 1857–1929. Surgeon, Pitié Hospital, Paris.

A *saccular* aneurism is due to stretching of part of the arterial wall, and more commonly follows injury.

Dissecting aneurisms occur in the abdominal aorta, and are due to separation of an atheromatous plaque, which allows blood to insinuate itself between the inner and outer parts of the muscular coat. It is usually a post-mortem finding, unless leakage causes symptoms suggestive of an abdominal catastrophe, when laparotomy discloses an extensive retroperitoneal hæmorrhagic effusion.

Clinical Features.—(*a*) *Intrinsic.*—A swelling exhibiting expansile pulsation is present in the course of an artery (fig. 72). The pulsation diminishes if proximal pressure can be applied, and the sac itself is compressible, filling again in two or three beats if proximal pressure is released. A thrill may be palpable, and auscultation sometimes reveals a bruit.

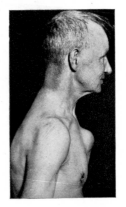

FIG. 72. — Aortic aneurism which has eroded the sternum.

(*b*) *Extrinsic.*—Neighbouring or distal structures are affected. Thus pressure on veins or nerves causes distal œdema or altered sensation, and the pulse is delayed or smaller in volume. Bones, joints, or tubes, such as the trachea or œsophagus, are sometimes affected, but structures which are resilient, such as the intervertebral discs, often withstand prolonged pressure.

Differential Diagnosis.—(i) *Swelling Under an Artery.*—An artery may be pushed forwards, e.g. the subclavian, by a cervical rib, and thus rendered prominent. Careful palpation distinguishes this condition.

(ii) *Swelling Over an Artery.*—In this case transmitted pulsation is liable to be mistaken for that caused by expansion. However, proximal pressure does not reduce the size of the tumour, and posture may diminish pulsation; thus a pancreatic cyst examined in the genupectoral position falls away from the aorta, and consequently pulsation is less definite.

(iii) *Pulsating tumours*, such as secondary carcinoma of bone, or an osteo-clastoma.—The swelling is irregular in consistency, and indefinite in outline.

(iv) *Other Causes of Deep-seated Pain.*—Cases of alleged intractable neuralgia, sciatica, etc., are occasionally due to aneurism.

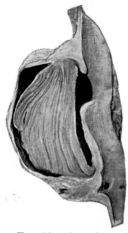

FIG. 73.—Aneurism of the aorta. Extensive clotting in the sac has almost resulted in spontaneous healing.

Natural Terminations.—1. *Spontaneous Cure.*—This sometimes occurs in cases of saccular aneurism, due to gradual clotting in the sac (fig. **73**).

2. *Infection.*—Occasionally follows operation, or arises from organisms in the blood-stream. Signs of inflammation supervene, and if untreated, suppuration and rupture follow.

3. *Rupture.*—This occurs either slowly as a leakage, or suddenly, in which case death follows in a few moments if a large vessel is involved.

Treatment.—*General.*—The patient's habits must be regulated, so as to avoid all physical and mental strain. A limited nitrogenous diet and minimum of fluid is allowed. Potassium iodide is given, as many aneurisms are associated with syphilis, and the drug frequently relieves pain associated with an aneurism.

Local.—

(*a*) Matas's operation. In selected cases of saccular aneurism, reconstruction has been attempted. The sac is opened, and the margins of the aperture approximated by stitches. Obliteration of the artery usually follows, but if the vessel remains patent, there is a risk that the weak fibrous suture line will subsequently yield, leading to recurrence.

In cases of fusiform aneurism the sac is sometimes obliterated by opening the sac, ligating the main vessel above and below from within, and inserting purse-string sutures to approximate the walls.

(*b*) Excision and grafting. Cases have been reported in which it has been possible to excise the affected arterial segment, and restore continuity by means of a venous graft, e.g. a portion of the external jugular vein. Heparin is injected proximally into the artery at the time of operation, and is subsequently administered intravenously for some days.

(*c*) Excision of the sac. This is usually satisfactory when access can be obtained. The artery is ligated above and below, and the intervening sac removed by dissection. If adhesions cause difficulty, the sac should be opened in order to define its limits more clearly. Even if part of the accompanying vein is removed, gangrene is unlikely, as both venous as well as arterial collateral circulations are probably efficiently established.

(*d*) Encouragement of clotting. Deposition of fibrin within

Rudolph Matas, born 1860, of New Orleans, introduced aneurismorrhaphy in 1902.

the sac and subsequent organisation will result in cure of the aneurism. Intermittent proximal pressure was formerly much used, either digital or by a bag of shot, but this method is very uncertain.

If practicable, proximal ligation is the common method now pursued if excision is impracticable. Anel's operation (fig. 74) consists in tying the artery immediately on the cardiac side of the aneurism, whereas Hunter placed his ligature so that one branch intervened between it and the aneurism ; e.g. if the femoral artery is tied in Hunter's canal, the anastomotica magna artery intervenes between the ligature and a popliteal aneurism. Hunter's operation necessitates the development of two systems of collateral vessels, i.e. one system to circumvent the ligature and a second to carry blood past the aneurism. This method therefore imposes a greater strain on the nutrition of the limb, and should not be used if gangrene threatens, or if marked arterial degeneration is present. On the other hand, the flow of blood through the aneurism is slowed more gradually than by Anel's method, and therefore the resultant clot will be firmer.

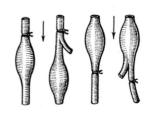

Fig. 74.—Operations on aneurisms. 1. Anel. 2. Hunter. 3. Brasdor. 4. Wardrop.

Distal ligation is practised for aneurisms anatomically situated so that proximal ligation is impossible, e.g. the vessels at the root of the neck. Brasdor ligated the artery close to the sac. In Wardrop's operation the ligature is placed so that one or more branches remain between the aneurism and the ligature (fig. 74).

After ligation the pulsation of the aneurism usually disappears. Temporary return in two or three days indicates establishment of collateral circulation. If the pulsation persists or appears at a later date, further operative interference will probably be necessary.

(e) When the above methods are impracticable, the introduction of foreign bodies into the sac should be considered. For example, cœliac aneurisms have been cured by the introduction of wire through a special cannula.

Dominique Anel, 1679–1730. Surgeon, Toulouse, France.
John Hunter, 1728–1793. Surgeon, St. George's Hospital, London. Founder of the Hunterian Museum.
Pierre Brasdor, 1721–1797. Professor of Surgery and Anatomy, Paris.
James Wardrop, 1782–1869. An Edinburgh graduate who settled in London.

(*f*) Amputation is required if infection or hæmorrhage occurs, or if gangrene supervenes. This procedure is also advisable if the function of the limb is seriously impaired by erosion of bones or joints, and amputation through the shoulder has been undertaken in the hope of curing a subclavian aneurism, a procedure akin to Brasdor's operation.

2. False Aneurisms

These are traumatic in origin, and the extravasated blood is enclosed in a false sac of condensed cellular tissue. In the case of large vessels, unless infection threatens, or the aneurism rapidly increases in size, palliative measures should be adopted temporarily, so that collateral circulation can develop. Subsequently, the sac is opened and emptied, and the injured artery tied above and below the site of trauma.

Arterio-venous Aneurism.—This condition is usually due to a penetrating wound injuring an artery and vein lying in close contact, e.g. the common carotid artery and internal jugular vein. A communication between the internal carotid artery and the cavernous sinus sometimes follows a fractured base of the skull. Two conditions may result :

(*a*) *Aneurismal Varix.*—This consists of a communication between an artery and vein, the latter becoming dilated and varicose as a result of the abnormal intravenous pressure. On palpation a thrill is usually detected, and auscultation reveals a buzzing bruit. This condition often remains stationary.

(*b*) *Varicose aneurism,* which differs from the above in that

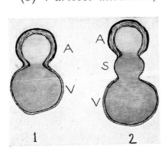

a sac exists between the two vessels (fig. 75). This sac is merely composed of condensed cellular tissue and organised clot, so that it tends to enlarge and become diffuse. The physical signs resemble those of an aneurismal varix, with the addition that the intervening sac may be palpable. In both conditions some degree of tachycardia is usually present, owing to the mixing of venous with arterial blood.

Fig. 75.—1. Aneurismal varix. 2. Varicose aneurism. A = artery, V = vein, S = sac.

As this condition is progressive, surgical treatment is indicated. The vessels are separated, and, if possible, repaired by suturing, the intervening sac being excised. More frequently quadruple ligation is necessary.

In the case of arterio-venous aneurism of the internal carotid artery and cavernous sinus, ligation and division of the common carotid artery may diminish the pulsating exophthalmos and relieve the continuous buzzing, provided that these features are improved by compression of the common carotid artery against Chassaignac's tubercle, which is situated on the transverse process of the sixth cervical vertebra.

Ligation and division of the common carotid artery is a much safer procedure than the formerly recommended operation of ligation of the internal carotid, which procedure is likely to be followed by cerebral embolism. Lambert Rogers collected a series of thirty cases in which the common carotid was ligated, with no mortality. Severance of the artery after double ligation diminishes the risk of thrombosis and embolism and also of spasm of the distal part of the artery.

EMBOLISM

An embolus is a foreign body which circulates in the blood-stream, becoming finally lodged in a vessel and so causing obstruction. Their effects vary according to their size, type, efficiency of the collateral circulation, and the nature of the organ in which they are arrested, highly specialised structures, such as the brain or retina, being readily affected by circulatory changes. Emboli are simple, infective, malignant, or parasitic.

Simple emboli are due to blood-clot, vegetations from cardiac valves, an atheromatous plaque, air bubbles (p. 108), or globules of fat. Clots of blood originate in thrombosed veins or the auricular appendage. In the latter site, mitral stenosis or auricular fibrillation predisposes to their formation, which is also encouraged if fibrillation is treated with quinidine.

FAT EMBOLISM occasionally follows severe injury to bone marrow or adipose tissue. It is especially liable to occur after fracture of atrophic bones, as these bones contain more than the normal amount of fat. Cases have been recorded following convulsive therapy. Symptoms supervene three or four days after injury, and two more or less distinct types, cerebral and pulmonary, are recognised. In the cerebral type the patient becomes drowsy, restless, and disorientated (delirium tremens may be suspected). Subsequently he is comatose, the pupils become small and pyrexia ensues. The pulmonary type is ushered in with cyanosis, which increases in intensity, and signs of right heart failure.

In suspected cases the sputum should be examined for fat droplets, and later fat may be excreted in the urine. Petechial hæmorrhages sometimes occur. Oxygen therapy is valuable, and intravenous sodium desoxycholate (10 ml. of 20 per cent. solution), in a drip infusion every two hours, is worthy of trial. This increases the emulsifying power of the blood, and reduces the size of fat globules. Larger doses cause hæmolysis.

Marie Chassaignac, 1805–1879. Professor of Surgery and Anatomy, Paris.
Lambert Rogers, Contemporary. Professor of Surgery, University of Wales.

Infective emboli consist of masses of bacteria, or infected clot, and may cause pyæmia or infected infarcts.

Malignant emboli are more commonly sarcomatous than carcinomatous, and give rise to secondary deposits, unless sufficient blood is extravasated to isolate the malignant cells from normal tissue, a phenomenon which sometimes occurs in connection with chorion-epithelioma.

Parasitic emboli are due to the ova of Tænia echinococcus and Filaria sanguinis hominis.

In some situations the results of embolism are characteristic, e.g. :

BRAIN.—The middle cerebral artery is most commonly affected, resulting in hemiplegia, temporary or permanent.

RETINA.—Occlusion of the central artery causes a momentary flash of light, followed by total and permanent blindness.

SPLEEN.—This organ is commonly affected, in which case local pain and enlargement follow.

KIDNEYS.—Resulting in pain in the loin and hæmaturia.

MESENTERIC VESSELS.—Causing engorgement and gangrene of the corresponding loop of intestine.

ABDOMINAL AORTA.—Resulting in loss of power and anæsthesia in the legs.

LUNG.—Pulmonary embolism (p. 989) is a catastrophe which may fatally interrupt convalescence after operation. Fortunately the incidence is diminished by anti-coagulation therapy.

LIMBS.—An embolus is arrested at the bifurcation of a main vessel (fig. 76), causing pain, pallor, paralysis, and loss of pulsation, followed in most cases by transient congestion and, commonly, moist gangrene ; very occasionally spontaneous

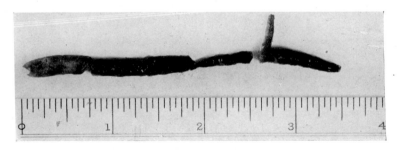

FIG. 76.—Embolus removed successfully at the bifurcation of the popliteal artery. (*A. H. Southam, Manchester.*)

recovery ensues. More than half the cases involve the femoral artery, after which, in probable order, the common iliac, brachial, popliteal, and aorta are affected. Heparin (100 mg.) should be given intravenously as a first-aid measure, and if there is no improvement after two hours embolectomy must be performed.

Embolectomy.—Local or spinal anæsthesia is to be preferred because of the condition of the patient's cardio-vascular system. The artery is exposed and occluded above the site of the embolus either by a Crile's clamp (fig. 77), or by a tape saturated in 3 per cent. sodium citrate. A half twist of the tape occludes the flow of blood, and traction on the tape steadies the vessel. The adventitia is carefully removed, otherwise strands are apt to be drawn into the lumen during suture, and so encourage thrombosis. A longitudinal incision is made just above the obstruction, care being taken not to injure the intima on the opposite wall. The embolus is removed by "milking" the artery upwards, and the incision is closed with fine needles threaded with waxed Chinese silk (size 0), the stitches passing through all coats of the vessel. During the operation the surgeon's hands and instruments are frequently rinsed in citrate solution, and afterwards the limb is kept warm and at rest for a week. Operations in the first four hours result in 62 per cent. of cures, the second four hours 50 per cent., but the third four hours only 24 per cent. Embolectomy gives better results in the arm than in the leg. Intravenous injection of heparin (50 mg. four-hourly for three doses) helps to obviate post-operative thrombosis.

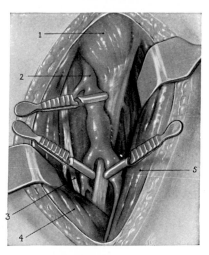

FIG. 77.—Embolectomy of the brachial artery. Crile's clamps have been applied to the brachial, radial, and ulnar arteries. 1. Biceps muscle. 2. Brachial artery. 3. Median nerve. 4. Pronator radii teres. 5. Supinator longus.

AIR EMBOLISM

Venous.—Air is occasionally sucked into an open vein or accidentally injected into the venous circulation. Thus venous air embolism occasionally complicates operations on the neck or axilla if a large vein is inadvertently opened, and it may be an accessory cause of death following a cut throat. The risks associated with intravenous infusion are so well known that this cause is uncommon, especially if a drip chamber is used containing a conical glass float which plugs the exit when fluid falls to a dangerous level.

If sufficient air enters the systemic circulation, the right side of the heart becomes filled with air so that entry of blood from the systemic veins is impeded, and the patient dies of acute right-sided heart failure.

Arterial.—During artificial pneumothorax air may be injected into a pulmonary vein, and so gain entrance to the left side of the heart, and this complication occasionally follows operation on the lungs. Paradoxical embolism is due to a patent foramen ovale, as no appreciable amount of air from the right side of the heart can pass through the capillaries of the lungs. Air which enters the systemic circulation is liable to cause coronary or cerebral symptoms.

Clinical Features.—Acute heart failure from obstruction of the pulmonary artery has already been referred to. Air in the left heart may gain entry to the coronary arteries and cause acute myocardial failure. Cerebral embolism results in dizziness, visual disturbances, and unconsciousness. Mottling of the skin of the head and shoulders is often noticed in cases of arterial air embolism.

Treatment.—The foot of the bed is raised in order to hinder bubbles of air from reaching the cerebral vessels, and the patient is turned on to his left side, because, in the case of left-sided air embolus, owing to the site of origin of the coronary arteries, air is less likely to enter these vessels if the patient is reclining on the left side. Again, in cases of right-sided air embolism this position encourages an air bubble to float into the apex of the right ventricle and cease to obstruct the flow of blood along the pulmonary artery. Attempts have been made to aspirate air from the ventricles, and this is worth attempting in desperate cases.

Inhalation of pure oxygen should be administered in order to counteract anoxæmia and assist in the excretion of nitrogen.

VEINS

Thrombosis of veins is predisposed to by :

(1) Change in the vessel wall, causing desquamation of endothelium, e.g. injury[1] or inflammation.

(2) Diminished rate of blood flow, as in debilitating conditions, such as typhoid fever.

(3) Increased coagulability of the blood, such as occurs in infective conditions, or after hæmorrhage. This blood change

---

[1] "Effort" thrombosis occasionally occurs in the axillary vein after unaccustomed use of the arm.

is the probable explanation of Trousseau's sign—thrombosis of superficial veins in association with visceral carcinoma.

The *results* of thrombosis are as follows :

(1) *Locally.*—The clot may organise into fibrous tissue, which possibly later becomes canalised. Suppuration sometimes occurs, forming a localised abscess, or giving rise to pyæmia. Calcification occasionally follows, resulting in the formation of a phlebolith, so commonly seen in pelvic veins.

(2) *Distally.*—Œdema may occur, the degree depending on the size of the vessel affected. The collateral circulation is soon established, as evinced by widespread varicosity of the superficial veins.

(3) *Proximally.*—Thrombosis may extend upwards to larger veins, and portions of clot are liable to become detached, particularly if infected. The resultant emboli may cause pulmonary infarcts, or, if the portal area is affected, multiple foci of infection will riddle the liver.

Thrombosis of deep veins is a troublesome post-operative complication which is sometimes the forerunner of pulmonary embolism (p. 989). In suspected or established cases anti-coagulants should be employed (p. 92).

Thrombophlebitis migrans, as the name implies, is a condition in which successive thrombosis occurs in veins in many parts of the body. Pulmonary veins may be involved, and local congestion of the lung results in pleurisy and possibly an effusion. Symptoms sometimes suggest that a coronary vein is implicated. As in the case of thrombosis of deep veins, some elevation of temperature is to be expected. In one case under our observation the disease lasted for over a year before subsiding. As already mentioned, multiple thromboses are sometimes associated with visceral carcinoma.

VARICOSE VEINS

A vein is stated to be varicose when it is dilated, lengthened, and tortuous. The condition commonly occurs in connection with the veins of the leg, also the spermatic, œsophageal, and hæmorrhoidal veins are frequently affected. The three latter conditions are dealt with elsewhere.

Ætiology.—Varicose veins are part of the penalty we pay for the adoption of the erect posture. Animals do not suffer from this condition. The precipitating cause is a failure of one of the valves guarding the many communications between the superficial and deep venous systems of the leg, most commonly the sapheno-femoral valve lying at the junction of the internal saphenous and common femoral veins, one inch distal to the mid-inguinal point. Next in order of frequency comes the

Armand Trousseau, 1801–1867. Physician, Hôpital St. Antoine, Paris. Noted this sign as his own death warrant, as it confirmed his suspicion of gastric carcinoma.

sapheno-popliteal valve, leading to dilatation of the external saphenous system. It must be emphasised that varices may commence at the site of any incompetent communicating vein, either alone, or in conjunction with one of the above (fig. 78).

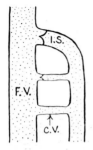

FIG. 78. — A valveless communicating vein (C.V.).

Varicose veins of the leg are sometimes associated with a congenital deficiency of the valves, or muscular coat, the condition occurring early in life and involving the same group of veins in members of the same family. Varicosity is predisposed to by any obstruction which hampers venous return, e.g. tumours and pregnancy. The condition may be widespread in both legs, or a single ampulla is sometimes present. If this is situated close to the saphenous opening, it is readily distinguished from a femoral hernia on account of the characteristic thrill when the patient coughs.

Symptoms.—The word " saphenous " is of Arabic derivation, and means " easily seen." Thus a number of patients present themselves for treatment for cosmetic reasons alone, and examination reveals a centripetal venous flow with no incompetent superficial-deep valves. These cases, in general, are better left untreated, but if considered desirable, injection is the method of choice.

Symptoms only occur in connection with varicose veins when there is a retrograde flow, and they depend on the extent of the back pressure. They may consist of a tired and aching sensation, felt in the whole of the lower leg, and especially in the calf, towards the end of the day. Sharp pains, when present, are localised to the site of the varices, and are especially noticeable in grossly dilated thigh veins. The ankle may swell towards evening, or the skin of the leg may itch. Some patients suffer from cramp in the calf shortly after retiring to bed ; this is due to a sudden change in the calibre of the communicating veins which stimulates the muscles between which they pass.

Examination.—The examination of the varices is most important, for upon it depends the success, or failure, of treatment. The aim is to locate the site of the incompetent superficial-deep valves, remembering that with an incompetent valve present the venous flow is retrograde, so that veins, when emptied, fill from above, whereas normally they fill from below. The examination is based upon the principles enunciated by Trendelenburg in 1890, and involves what has aptly been described as "the intelligent use of the tourniquet."

Briefly, the patient lies upon his back and raises his leg to empty the veins (fig. 79A). A venous tourniquet is applied just below the saphenous opening (fig. 79B), and he stands up (79C). The constriction is then released (79D). If the sapheno-femoral valve is incompetent, the veins fill immediately from above ; if not, the veins fill slowly from below. The veins may fill rapidly from above, even though the tourniquet has not been

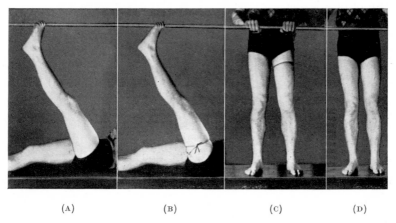

(A)   (B)   (C)   (D)

Fig. 79.—Trendelenburg's test (see text). (*S. M. Rivlin.*)

released ; this means that the varices are commencing, totally or in part, from an incompetent communicating valve, or the sapheno-popliteal valve, lower down. In this case, the tourniquet test must be repeated, with application at successively lower sites on the thigh and leg, until the point of origin is shown by prevention of the abnormal direction of flow.

Treatment.—(i) *Palliative* treatment consists of removing any possible cause. The veins are supported by crêpe or elastic bandages, or elastic stockings ; rubber bandages interfere with the evaporation of perspiration and predispose to eczema, so they should be worn only for limited periods of physical stress, e.g. an important golf match.

(ii) *Injection.*—At one time the injection method was widely practised as the primary treatment for all types of varicose veins, but experience showed that in the presence of an incompetent sapheno-femoral and/or communicating valve, the recurrence rate was of the order of 80 per cent. This does not

Friedrich Trendelenburg, 1844–1924. Professor of Surgery, Leipzig.

apply to external saphenous veins, for which, except in advanced cases, injection is still the method of choice.

Injection (or sclerosant) treatment is therefore limited to the following :

(*a*) Following ligation at the site of the incompetent valve(s), in order to thrombose the remaining varices.

(*b*) For external saphenous varices.

(*c*) Possibly for cosmetic reasons, as described above.

Sclerosants act by damaging the intima of the vein, so that a firm thrombosis, and later sclerosis, develops. Intimal damage will only take place whilst the sclerosant is able to act in suffi- cient concentration ; as soon as it is diluted by the blood in the deep veins the effect is lost, and it passes into the blood-stream to be excreted as an inert substance. If, however, a large quantity of the sclerosant is injected at one site, it may reach the deep veins in sufficient concentration to initiate a thrombosis at that point before it becomes sufficiently diluted to render it harmless. *The minimum fully effective dose* for a sclerosant should always be known, and should not be exceeded by injection at any one point. The artificial thrombus formed is remarkable for its tenacity, so that the possibility of fragments becoming detached to form emboli is extremely remote.

General Technique of Injection.—The patient stands as in fig. 79D. The site is cleaned with spirit and the injection made with a 5-ml. all-glass Luer-mount syringe using a ½-inch (1·25 c.m.) 27 needle. The needle is with- drawn from the vein and firm digital pressure applied with a sterile swab for two minutes. If the " empty vein " technique is used, the patient sits down after the introduction of the needle, and the leg is carefully elevated. The injection is then made and smaller quantities of sclerosants are adequate, with less risk of a " spill-over " into a deep vein. An adhesive dressing is applied and the patient instructed to continue his normal work. Further injections are given at weekly intervals.

Sclerosant Solutions.—

(*a*) Sodium salicylate.	⎧ These solutions were very popular during the heyday of injection treatment. Their main disadvantage lies in their liability to produce an injection ulcer, should some of the injection leak from the vein. Sodium morrhuate can produce dangerous anaphy- lactic effects, and should be abandoned.
(*b*) Quinine and urethane.	
(*c*) Sodium morrhuate.	

(*d*) Monoethylolamine oleate (5 per cent.) with benzyl alcohol (2 per cent.) (Ethamolin, Glaxo), is the most satisfactory sclerosant for out- patient use. Injection ulcers are extremely rare. Allergy can occur, but only after a prolonged course which, with modern treatment, should not be necessary ; nevertheless, a solution of 1 : 1,000 adrenalin should always be to hand in case of emergency. The maximum dose at any one point is

2 ml., and no more than 6 ml. should be given at a sitting. It is usual to commence treatment with a test dose of ½ ml. so that the extent of the local reaction may be gauged, and the dose modified as necessary.

(*e*) Phenol (2 per cent.), glucose (30 per cent.), glycerin (2 per cent.), known as " P2G," is a relatively new sclerosant. It is not as suitable as ethamolin for outpatient use, owing to the larger volume required and the poorer local thrombosis. It is, however, the solution of choice for retrograde injection at operation, where a relatively large volume (10 ml.) is needed. Its use is pain free, which is important when the operation is performed under local anæsthesia.

(iii) *Operative.*—This consists essentially of ligation and division of the internal saphenous vein at the site of the incompetent

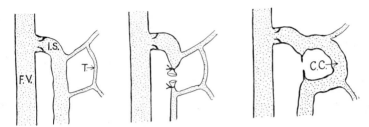

Fig. 80.—Tributaries (T.) must be ligated as well as the internal saphenous vein (I.S.), otherwise a collateral circulation (C.C.) subsequently develops.

sapheno-femoral and/or communicating valve, as previously determined by examination (fig. 79). Most cases will be found to require sapheno-femoral ligation, the operation being termed " Juxa-femoral Ligation." This implies that the internal saphenous vein should be ligated and divided at its junction with the femoral vein, and all the tributaries are ligated (fig. 80). Although there are only three named tributaries in this region, the anatomy is inconstant, and commonly five or six may be encountered. The operation may be performed under local anæsthesia. Some surgeons practise retrograde injection of the vein at the time of operation, as it greatly reduces the number of post-operative injections

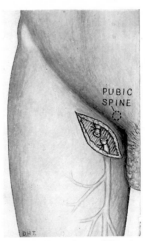

Fig. 81.—Juxtafemoral ligation of internal saphenous vein.

required. Additional ligations in the region of the knee are sometimes desirable.

Technique.—An oblique incision is made just below the groin, commencing over the pulsation of the femoral artery and extending $2\frac{1}{2}$ to 3 inches (6 to 7 cm.) medially (fig. 81). The vein is exposed by gauze dissection, and divided between forceps. If retrograde injection is to be carried out, the distal segment is opened, under traction, and either 12 inches (30 cm.) of a ureteric catheter or a 12-inch cannulated needle with a smooth olivary

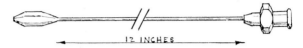

12 INCHES

Fig. 82.—Cannulated smooth olivary-tipped needle for retrograde injection.

head (fig. 82) made specially for the purpose, is introduced, and 10 ml. of P2G is injected whilst the needle is slowly withdrawn. The vein is then ligated below the opening. The proximal portion of the vein is traced to the femoral junction, which may lie $\frac{1}{2}$ inch (1·25 cm.) deep to the fossa ovalis, dividing and ligating all tributaries encountered on the way. It is then tied flush with the femoral vein. It is wise to place a second ligature on the distal side of the first in order to obviate the risk of a slipped ligature, as the proximal end of the vein is in direct communication with the right auricle.

Before commencing ligation of a communicating vein, its site is carefully determined and marked upon the skin. Under local anæsthesia, the vein is exposed at that point and the communicating vein will be seen passing through the deep fascia. It should be divided and ligated. The superficial vein should be ligated and divided too, and, if required, retrograde injection may be carried out through its distal end.

Contraindications to Injection and Operative Treatment

(*a*) *Acute Infective Thrombophlebitis.*—At least three months should be allowed to pass, after this has completely subsided, before injecting.

(*b*) *Deep Thrombosis.*—Due to any cause and revealed by a history of prolonged confinement to bed with a painful swollen leg. Perthes' test is informative if doubt exists regarding the patency of the femoral vein. The saphenous vein is occluded by a tourniquet applied immediately below the saphenous opening, and the patient walks 15 to 20 yards. Normally, the veins below the constriction become less obvious, but if the communicating veins or the femoral vein is obliterated, these subcutaneous veins become engorged.

COMPLICATIONS OF VARICOSE VEINS

Thrombophlebitis of superficial veins reveals itself as a reddened, tender cord in the subcutaneous tissues. Ambulatory treatment is easy, safe, and convenient. Strips of sorbo-rubber or dunlopillo, the edges of which are bevelled, are laid over the inflamed vein, and an inch above it a double thickness is placed transversely. The pressure so obtained obviates the risk of embolism. The leg is then bandaged with flexible adhesive plaster from above downwards (fig. 83). The strapping is removed after a fortnight. This procedure gives immediate relief, and it need only be renewed if tenderness persists.

Georg Perthes, 1869–1927. Professor of Surgery, Tübingen, Germany.

Eczema, or, more correctly, chronic infective dermatitis, is usually due to minor trauma or to the patient scratching his

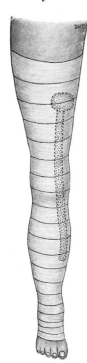

itching skin, but may be an allergic manifestation resulting from ointment or strapping applied for treatment. The condition should be treated *before* dealing with the varices, and this is easily accomplished by the application, twice daily, of an ointment consisting of Lassar's Paste with crude coal tar. As soon as the skin is healthy, the varices should be treated, otherwise a recurrence of the itching predisposes to a further exacerbation of the eczematous condition.

Ulceration.—It must be remembered that ulceration of the leg (fig. 84) may be due to other factors than varicose veins, and that an ulcer occurring on the lower half of the leg should not automatically be termed "varicose." The next most common cause of leg ulcers, after varices, is a previous thrombosis of deep

FIG. 83.—Ambulatory treatment of thrombophlebitis.

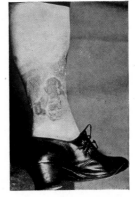

FIG. 84.—Varicose ulcers, with pigmentation of skin.

veins, e.g. "white leg" following parturition, and an ulcer arising as a result of this may take some years to develop. Venous stasis is the fundamental cause of both types, and consequently they may be grouped together under the term "Gravitational Ulcers." It is important to differentiate between these two main types, for, whereas a varicose ulcer responds promptly and satisfactorily to ambulatory treatment by compression with adhesive elastic plaster, post-thrombotic ulcers are refractory to treatment and require bed rest with possibly excision and skin grafting. Syphilitic ulcers of the leg, which are serpiginous and sometimes multiple, are far less common. Factitious or artificial ulcers commonly exhibit straight edges. Carcinomatous changes may occur in a chronic ulcer (fig. 47).

O. Lassar, 1849–1907. Dermatologist, Berlin.

Treatment of Varicose Ulcer.—The treatment of this distressing condition, usually occurring in the lower third of the leg, is the application of elastoplast or similar bandages. The method of application of these bandages is most important, as a badly applied bandage is very uncomfortable.

The response of the long-standing ulcer to this treatment often appears miraculous to the patient, but in the early stages they often look askance at the application of an adhesive bandage to the ulcer without any underlying dressing.

Technique of Application.—One or two vertical strips are laid upon the leg from the level of the tibial tubercle to the foot, so as to cover the surface of the ulcer (fig. 85 (*a*)). This is to prevent the spiral turns of bandage, to be applied later,

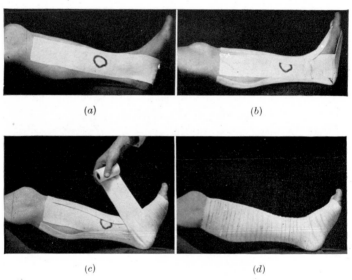

(*a*)   (*b*)

(*c*)   (*d*)

Fig. 85.—The application of elastoplast bandage for a varicose ulcer.
(*S. M. Rivlin.*)

from cutting into the healing ulcer. It is unnecessary either to clean the ulcer or to apply any dressing over it.

Two more vertical strips are now applied (fig. 85 (*b*)). The first stretches from the tibial tubercle to the base of the toes along the anterior surface of the leg. The second, along the posterior surface from behind the knee, over the calf and behind the heel to the base of the toes on the sole. These, too, are to prevent cutting in of the bandage when walking. Both these strips should be nicked transversely at various points so that the plaster lies snugly in apposition with the skin.

The main portion of the bandage is now applied as a series of continuous circular turns, from the base of the toes to the tibial tubercle and enclosing the heel (fig. 85 (c)). Each turn should overlap the one preceding by two-thirds of its width. The whole bandage should be applied tightly (fig. 85 (d)). It is essential that there should be no ruckling of the bandage on application, as each imperfection is faithfully reproduced upon the underlying skin, and may give rise to discomfort. Upon removal of a well-applied bandage, no marks or lines are visible upon the skin.

The patient is instructed to continue his usual work, and to wash off any discharge which may percolate through the bandage.

The first application is removed after one week, and thereafter the bandage is renewed at fortnightly intervals until the ulcer is healed. The area of the ulcer should be measured at each visit, so that the decrease in size may be noted. Even a large ulcer is usually healed in three months.

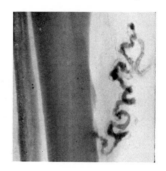

FIG. 86.—Calcified varicose veins, with periostitis of the tibia.

As soon as the ulcer is healed, the associated veins are treated by the methods outlined in the previous section.

Hæmorrhage follows rupture, usually of a thin-walled ampulla. Bleeding occurs from both ends of the vein, and is usually profuse. Fatalities have occurred when the patient was asleep or drunk. Elevation of the leg and the application of a firm pad and bandage easily control the bleeding.

Calcification occasionally occurs in veins which have been tolerated for many years (fig. 86).

Periostitis occurs in long-standing cases if the ulcer is situated over the tibia. Osteitis of the bone, and ossification of the interosseous membrane are liable to follow.

Talipes equinus may result from a long-standing ulcer. The patient finds that walking on the toes relieves the pain, and after some years the tendo achilles becomes contracted

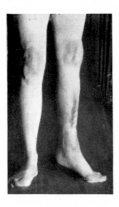

FIG. 86A.—Talipes equinus following prolonged ulceration.

(fig. 86A). Treatment should be prophylactic, and consists of remedial exercises in the early stages.

HÆMANGIOMA

Hæmangiomata are tumours composed of blood-vessels, and are congenital in origin. They sometimes remain insignificant for a prolonged period, but are apt to enlarge in size at any time.

Capillary nævi are composed of dilated capillaries, and are most common on the face and scalp. Occasionally they are submucous, in which case bleeding often occurs. The term " spider " nævus is applied when portions of the tumour radiate into surrounding tissues. Applications of carbonic-acid snow are efficacious in destroying small capillary nævi, but larger ones sometimes require radium or excision.

Cavernous angiomata consist of masses of dilated veins into which arteries open more or less directly. They occasionally occur in viscera, but are more commonly submucous or subcutaneous. Frequently capillary nævi are found in the overlying skin. Submucous nævi are prone to hæmorrhage, which is sometimes alarming (fig. 164). A characteristic feature of a cavernous angioma is its compressibility. If possible the tumour should be excised by means of an electric cautery. Otherwise diathermy, or injections of boiling water, causes thrombosis of vessels and consequent shrinkage.

Plexiform angiomata consist mainly of arteries, and consequently pulsate. The usual form is a cirsoid aneurism (p. 829). Very rarely similar tumours are found in bones, in which case a pulsating tumour appears when the compact bone is eroded

CHAPTER VI
LYMPHATICS AND LYMPHATIC NODES

Acute lymphangitis is due to infection of lymphatics from a wound in the area drained by the involved vessels. The infection is usually limited to the nodes immediately proximal to the site of infection ; these nodes become inflamed, but occasionally infection " jumps " a group of lymphatic nodes and affects those at a higher level. Thus, as a result of an infected wound of the leg, the external iliac nodes occasionally become inflamed, and form a mass in the corresponding iliac fossa. Errors in diagnosis are likely to arise, especially as the wound is sometimes healed and forgotten by the time the mass appears.

Acute lymphangitis is characterised by the appearance of subcutaneous red streaks, which correspond to the inflamed lymphatics (fig. 87). If large trunks are affected they are

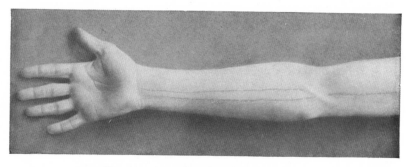

Fig. 87.—Acute lymphangitis of the arm.

sometimes palpable as tender cords. Toxæmia is often severe, and depends upon the virulence of the causative organism and the resistance of the patient. As a rule chemotherapy or antibiotic therapy speedily checks infection. Local suppuration may occur in the course of the inflamed lymphatics. Permanent occlusion sometimes follows acute lymphangitis, leading to persistent lymphatic œdema (fig. 13).

Treatment consists of dealing with the wound, unless, as is frequently the case, it is insignificant or already healed. If a limb is affected, it must be kept at rest, slightly elevated, and fomented or immersed in a hot saline or antiseptic bath for a few minutes three or four times a day. Excessive moisture causes the skin to become sodden, and this encourages infection. General measures are taken to combat infection.

Chronic lymphangitis may follow acute lymphangitis, or is, more commonly, due to repeated subacute attacks of infection. The " wiry " lymphatics passing along the dorsal aspect of the penis are characteristic of a primary chancre, and may be associated with œdema of the prepuce. Tuberculous lymphangitis occasionally occurs, notably in the periureteric lymphatics ; the resulting fibrosis and contraction leads to the ureter pursuing a straighter course than normal, and to the characteristic " golf-hole " ureteric orifice.

LYMPHATIC OBSTRUCTION

1. **Congenital,** giving rise to lymphangiectasis (p. 118).

2. **Trauma** as a result of excision of lymph nodes, e.g. lymphatic œdema of the arm, which occurs shortly after removal of the axillary nodes. It is sometimes due to division of lymphatics, as by an incision along the lower and outer margin of the orbit, which divides lymphatics passing to the preauricular nodes, and leads to œdema of the lower eyelid (fig. 13).

3. **Inflammation,** due to fibrosis of lymphatics, which may follow an acute lymphangitis, such as erysipelas (fig. 13), or result from persistent chronic infection, e.g. tropical ulcer.

4. **Neoplasm,** as typified by the " peau d'orange," due to permeation of lymphatics by carcinoma, and resultant obstruction. The " brawny arm " which develops some months or years after a radical removal of the breast for carcinoma is due to lymphatic permeation by malignant cells.

5. **Parasites.**—The Filaria sanguinis hominis is transmitted by a mosquito (Culex fatigans). Water containing ova is imbibed, and the ova pass through the gastric mucosa to enter the lymphatics. The female worm enters and obstructs the inguinal lymph vessels. The legs and scrotum are chiefly affected and enormous thickening of the subcutaneous tissue may result. Chemotherapy has a beneficial effect on the associated cellulitis and lymphadenitis.

In addition to these recognised causes, elephantiasis of the lower limbs occasionally occurs for no apparent reason (fig. 88).

Sir Patrick Manson, 1844–1922, discovered the filaria in China in 1877.

As a result of lymphatic obstruction, a solid œdema occurs, the subcutaneous tissue becomes brawny and shows little pitting on pressure. At a later stage the skin becomes coarse and rough, and the limb is often enormously swollen, a condition referred to as elephantiasis. Lymphatic vesicles sometimes appear and tend to rupture, thus leading to ulceration and recurrent infection.

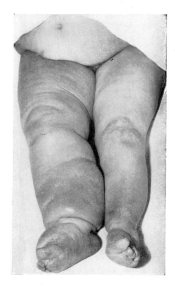

FIG. 88.—Solid œdema of the right leg, due to lymphatic obstruction of unknown origin.

Treatment.—Lymphatic obstruction is usually an unsatisfactory condition as regards surgical treatment. Elevation and elastic pressure often relieve early cases. The introduction into the subcutaneous tissues of sterilised silk (lymphangioplasty) sometimes gives temporary relief in the arm, but is useless in the leg on account of gravity. Excision of long strips of deep fascia (Kondoléon's operation) is occasionally followed by some improvement, but more often results are disappointing. The object of this operation is to remove the fascial barrier between superficial and deep lymphatics, so that lymph is returned by the latter channel. Amputation is occasionally necessary if the patient is anchored to the bed by weight of the limb, or if ulceration and infection supervene. Filariasis has been benefited by removal of the parent filariæ when their situation has been recognised. Usually the condition progresses, and removal of the scrotum or affected limb is eventually necessary.

Idiopathic Œdema.—An intractable, idiopathic œdema occasionally occurs in the legs and feet, especially in young women. Possibly this is due to abnormal permeability of lymphatic vessels and capillaries. Elastic pressure and elevation yield little relief, but improvement usually follows increased alkalisation of the blood by large doses of potassium citrate and carbonate.

DILATATION OF LYMPHATIC VESSELS

Congenital types include the following varieties :

(*a*) *Capillary Lymphangioma.*—When this condition occurs in the skin, it is known as lymphatic nævus, and consists of

Emmerich Kondoléon 1879-1943. Professor of Surgery, Athens.

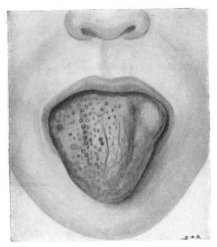

FIG. 89.—Cavernous lymphangioma of the tongue, the surface of which is covered with lymphatic nævi.

brownish papules or wart-like excrescences. On examination with a lens small vesicles can be seen.

(*b*) *Cavernous lymphangioma* is often associated with the preceding variety (fig. 89), and consists of masses of lymphatic cysts, particularly in the neck or axilla, the condition being termed a cystic hygroma (p. 187). An ill-defined spongy mass results, the skin over which may be semi-translucent, a condition which was formerly described as " hydrocele of the breast " when occurring in that organ.

(*c*) *Lymphangiectasis* usually occurs as a congenital condition, and gives rise to enlargement of different parts, e.g. tongue (macroglossia) or lip (macrocheilia). The condition occasionally affects the subcutaneous lymphatics of a limb (Milroy's disease), and amputation may then be required.

Acquired lymphatic dilatation is due to obstruction of main lymphatics. Thus, pressure on the thoracic duct may cause engorgement of the alimentary lymphatics and chylous ascites, also cases of chylous hydrocele have been described, due to obstruction of lymph drainage.

LYMPH NODES

Acute inflammation follows infection of the appropriate lymphatics, although, as already mentioned, a group of lymph nodes may escape obvious infection, whereas a more proximal group may evince a marked reaction. The affected nodes become enlarged, firm, and tender. Resolution, fibrosis, or suppuration follows.

Treatment consists of dealing with any cause, the application of warmth locally, and chemotherapy. If suppuration occurs, pus is evacuated.

William F. Milroy, 1855–1942. Emeritus Professor of Clinical Medicine, University of Nebraska, described the condition in 1892.

Chronic inflammation is either simple or specific :

1. *Simple,* or non-specific adenitis, is due to intermittent or prolonged infection of low virulence, e.g. infected tonsils or pediculi capitis, or sometimes follows incomplete resolution of acute adenitis. The nodes become enlarged, firm, and slightly tender, and occasionally quietly suppurate. This condition probably predisposes to tuberculous adenitis, the simple infection preparing the soil for the seed.

Treatment consists of removal of any local focus of infection and attention to the general health.

2. *Specific adenitis*

(*a*) Tuberculous infection of nodes is common in children and adolescents, particularly among those who live in unhygienic surroundings, or who inherit a predisposition to tuberculosis. Some chronic or intermittent focus of infection is commonly present, e.g. tonsils, teeth, or scalp, and chronic simple inflammation is converted into tuberculous by the deposition of tubercle bacilli. The cervical nodes are the commonest to be affected, at least as far as clinical evidence is concerned, although the bronchial or mesenteric nodes are commonly invaded, and calcification is frequently noted in an X-ray. The axillary or inguinal nodes sometimes suffer, particularly if there is some tuberculous focus in the area of lymphatic drainage, such as lupus verrucosa.

Tubercle bacilli most commonly reach the node by lymphatics, tubercles first forming in the cortex, but blood-borne infection sometimes occurs, in which case the medulla of the node is the first part to be affected. Microscopically, endothelial cells are in evidence, and giant cells are commonly seen with many nuclei arranged around the periphery (fig. 90).

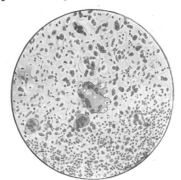

FIG. 90.—A tuberculous node, showing typical giant cells.

Clinically, the affected nodes enlarge, and become characteristically matted together owing to periadenitis. Caseation may follow, to be succeeded by suppuration. Pus is no respecter of fascia, and often burrows through the deep fascia, so that the pus is superficial and the causative node deep to this structure, forming a " collar-stud " abscess (fig. 207). If the condition progresses, the skin becomes blue and thin, eventually giving way, a tuberculous sinus resulting. Occasionally under appropriate treatment, caseous material is absorbed

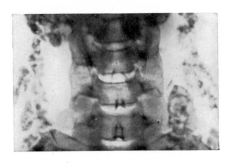

and replaced by fibrous tissue or calcification (fig. 91), in which case the nodes are stony hard on palpation.

Treatment consists of dealing with any possible source of infection, combined with care of the general health. If improvement does not occur within one month, then accessible nodes should be

FIG. 91.—Extensive calcification of cervical lymphatic nodes.

removed, otherwise suppuration is likely to supervene. Thus, in the case of cervical nodes, collar incisions are made, and infected nodes, often surprisingly large, are removed. This is a tedious operation, needing patience and a good light. Normal anatomy is distorted, and no tissue should be divided under traction, as veins are thus rendered unrecognisable and liable to injury. The welling blood obscures the actual site of hæmorrhage, and groping with artery forceps is likely to damage important structures. The hypoglossal and spinal accessory nerves are commonly embedded in a mass of nodes, and are therefore particularly prone to injury.

If abscesses are present they are aspirated, and possibly iodoform emulsion is injected. If suppuration persists, then operation should be undertaken, as otherwise the skin will give way, and sinuses and secondary infection follow. On opening the superficial abscess pus is evacuated, and granulation tissue gently curetted ; the track through the deep fascia is then enlarged so that the deeper nodes can be exposed and removed. The operation field is smeared with iodoform paste, and a glove drain inserted for twelve to twenty-four hours on account of the oozing.

If sinuses are present, excision should be performed, and the extensive wounds heal in a remarkable manner. Any small sinuses are packed with malachite green and corrosive sublimate, 1 per cent. of each, in surgical spirit, an application which gives particularly gratifying results with tuberculous sinuses in any situation.

The ideal treatment, which in our opinion should be followed more frequently, is to remove tuberculous nodes if a short course of general treatment results in no improvement. Early removal diminishes the risk of sinuses and resulting scars, of prolonged convalescence, and of dissemination elsewhere from the active focus.

(b) Syphilitic adenitis can occur in any stage of the acquired infection. " Shotty " nodes associated with a genital chancre are characteristic. During the secondary stage a generalised enlargement of nodes occurs, especially those above the internal epicondyles and along the posterior border of the sterno-mastoid (nodulæ concatenatæ). In the tertiary stage a gumma may occur in a lymph node, but is rare. More commonly the nodes enlarge as a result of secondary infection from a broken-down gumma.

CHRONIC ENLARGEMENT OF LYMPH NODES

Chronic enlargement is due to the following causes :
Inflammation (p. 119).
Reticulosis.
New-growth.

THE RETICULOSES

Various diseases which were formerly considered to be separate clinical entities are now known to arise as a result of proliferative conditions of the lymphoid or lympho-reticular tissue, with subsequent differentiation. Proliferation may begin in the follicles, medulla, or sinuses, and in most cases, as would be expected, the lymph nodes are first affected. Sooner or later other lymphoid tissue is involved, such as the spleen, liver, Peyer's patches, and the bone marrow. Histological examination is usually required in order to establish the diagnosis, and most of the conditions are radio-sensitive.

The reticuloses comprise a very complex group of conditions, but the more important ones of surgical interest can be classified as follows :
Hæmic.—The leukæmias.
Metabolic.—Gaucher's disease (p. 317).
　　　　　　Schuller-Christian's disease (p. 1103).

Neoplastic.—Benign—Boeck's sarcoid (p. 183).

Malignant—Lymphadenoma.

Lymphosarcoma (p. 123).

Reticulosarcoma.

Multiple myeloma (p. 1110).

Ewing's tumour (p. 1115).

Lymphatic leukæmia is of little surgical interest except from the point of view of differential diagnosis. Cytological examination is diagnostic— the leucocytes are enormously increased, and may number 150,000 per c.mm., of which 90 to 99 per cent. are lymphocytes. Splenic enlargement is more characteristic of chronic lymphatic leukæmia than of Hodgkin's disease.

LYMPHADENOMA (*Syn.* HODGKIN'S DISEASE)

Histologically, the picture varies with the stage of the disease. At first there is a proliferation of leucocytes, which is followed by the appearance of pale round endothelial cells. Characteristic giant cells are often in

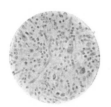

evidence (fig. 92); these contain two or more pale nuclei which overlap each other. Plasma and eosinophil cells, the latter often in large numbers, are usually to be seen. In the later stages fibroblasts and fibrous tissue are the predominant features.

Gordon's Test.—Occasionally the histological appearances are inconclusive. In such instances Gordon's test is helpful. A suspension of an affected lymph node produces encephalitis when injected into the cerebrum of a rabbit.

FIG. 92.—Section of an enlarged lymph node removed from the neck for purposes of diagnosis. Dorothy Reed giant cells are a characteristic feature of Hodgkin's disease.

Clinical Features.—It is commoner in males, and usually affects young adults, but cases vary widely as regards age incidence and virulence. Occasionally, and especially in children, the course of the disease is merely a matter of weeks, the associated irregular and often high temperature leading to errors of diagnosis. More commonly the patient first notices a painless swelling in the supraclavicular region, associated with malaise and an irregular temperature. Pressure effects, due to deep nodes, especially mediastinal, may follow, or occasionally cause the first symptoms. On examination the nodes are discrete, painless, and rubbery in consistency. The spleen is enlarged, but rarely enough to be palpable. The enlargement may be diffuse, or whitish nodules may project from the surface, the organ then bearing some resemblance to toffee studded with almonds, known as "hard-bake." In the late stages most organs in the body become affected, and periodic bouts of

Thomas Hodgkin, 1798–1866. Sometime Curator to the Museum, he failed in the election for the office of Physician at Guy's Hospital, London.

Mervin H. Gordon, Contemporary. Consulting Bacteriologist, St. Bartholomew's Hospital, London. Described his test in 1932.

Dorothy Reed (Mrs. Mendenhall), Contemporary. Formerly Fellow in Pathology, Johns Hopkins Hospital, Baltimore, U.S.A.

temperature occur at intervals of two or three weeks (Pel-Ebstein). Osseous involvement is not uncommon, and an X-ray reveals "punched-out" areas in the affected bone which resemble multiple myelomata.

Blood examination reveals a secondary anæmia, with occasionally slight eosinophilia, and serves to distinguish other conditions, e.g. lymphatic leukæmia. Excision of an appropriate node clinches the diagnosis.

Treatment consists of the administration of arsenic to combat anæmia, and intravenous injections have a more potent effect than oral administration. Nitrogen mustard is sometimes beneficial. X-rays cause a temporary reduction in the size of the nodes. Excision may be considered if a localised group of nodes only are affected, or when pressure symptoms are caused by nodes which have become tolerant to X-rays. The disease is characterised by remissions and exacerbations, but inevitably runs a fatal course.

Lymphadenoma and Leukæmia.—There seems to be some relationship between these two diseases, as some cases of Hodgkin's disease develop leukæmia. Also cases have been reported in which patients have suffered from both diseases at the same time. Irradiation of Hodgkin's nodes does not appear to encourage leukæmic changes.

NEW-GROWTH

(a) *Primary lymphosarcoma* can commence in any adenoid tissue, e.g. nodes, tonsils, or Peyer's patches. When affecting the nodes, those most commonly involved are the cervical group. Rapid, steadily progressive enlargement occurs, and later the growth erodes the capsule of the node and infiltrates surrounding structures. Dissemination occurs to other lymphoid tissue in the neighbourhood.

Excision is sometimes practicable in early cases. Radium or X-ray therapy causes retrogression, but unfortunately dissemination is only too likely to have occurred already.

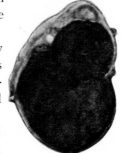

FIG. 93.—Melanomatous deposits in a lymphatic node.

(b) *Secondary Growths.*—Carcinoma and melanoma typically disseminate to lymph nodes (fig. 93). Lymphosarcoma, e.g. from lymphatic nodes or the tonsil, is likely

Pieter K. Pel, 1852–1916. Professor of Medicine, Amsterdam.
Wilhelm Ebstein, 1836–1912. Professor of Medicine, Göttingen, Germany.
Johann Peyer, 1653–1712. Anatomist of Schaffhausen, Switzerland.

to spread along regional lymphatics to adjacent nodes. Sarcomata of the testis and thyroid are alleged to disseminate by lymphatic vessels ; probably earlier observers confused these varieties of testicular neoplasms which were probably undifferentiated seminomata, while sarcoma of the thyroid gland must be regarded as a curiosity.

CHAPTER VII

FACE AND JAWS, INCLUDING THE PALATE

EMBRYOLOGY OF THE FACE

ABOUT the sixth week of fœtal life a depression appears in front of the head. Around this depression, called the stomatodœum or primitive mouth, five processes appear: a single one at the cephalic end, the fronto-nasal process, and on each side a maxillary and a mandibular process (fig. 94). Soon the frontonasal process becomes subdivided, by the appearance of the olfactory pits, into a solitary median nasal process and two lateral nasal processes. The median nasal process becomes bluntly bifurcated, and the excrescence so formed is known as the processus globularis. Thus it comes about that finally there are seven processes. These coalesce to form the face. The process of budding and cohesion is a rapid one, for it is commenced and completed in the brief space of three weeks. Thus every congenital deformity of the face has existed from the ninth week of fœtal life.

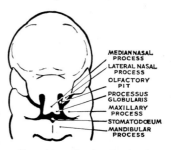

FIG. 94.—The head of an embryo. (*After His.*)

Failure of union of the median nasal process with the maxillary process and/or the maxillary process with its fellow accounts for most of the congenital facial abnormalities, which are:

1. Hare-lip.
2. Cleft-palate.
3. Facial cleft.
4. Macrostoma.

Too much union results in microstoma. Facial cleft, micro- and macrostoma are so rare that they need no further consideration in this work. The pinna is developed from six tubercles situated around the posterior end of the first branchial cleft.

PREAURICULAR SINUS

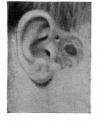

FIG. 95.—Pre-auricular sinus with ulcer. Note the sinus in the root of the helix.

Imperfect fusion of the tubercles which form the pinna results in a preauricular sinus, the opening of which is usually found at the root of the helix or on the tragus. The tract runs downwards and slightly forwards, and ends blindly. A preauricular sinus gives rise to no symptoms unless the tiny opening becomes occluded, when a cyst is prone to develop. If the cyst becomes infected, and it bursts or is opened, a cutaneous preauric-ular ulcer is liable to follow. This ulcer (fig. 95) refuses to heal, for infection is maintained from the sinus (Stammers).

The condition is often misdiagnosed. Treatment is excision of the sinus.

Francis A. R. Stammers, Contemporary. Professor of Surgery, University of Birmingham

HARE-LIP AND CLEFT-PALATE

Hare-lip and cleft-palate are but variations of one and the same congenital defect. Failure of normal union of the developing processes (see fig. 94) results in either (a) a cleft of the lip alone, (b) a cleft of the lip and alveolus, or (c) a cleft of the lip, alveolus, and palate.

These abnormalities are more common in males (3 : 2). An infant with a large opening between the mouth and the nose, as occurs with a cleft-palate (fig. 96), is unable to suck properly, for

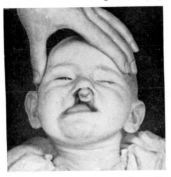

Fig. 96.—Bilateral hare-lip associated with a premaxilla and cleft-palate. (*T. A. Bouchier-Hayes.*)

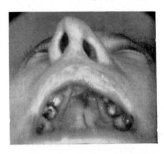

Fig. 97.—Twenty-five years after operation for bilateral hare-lip and complete cleft-palate. Operation by the late Sir James Berry.

sufficient negative pressure cannot be established. If, as is often the case, there is a hare-lip in addition, sucking is impossible. At first sight this would seem a serious matter, but it is overcome by a simple expedient. If the puncture in the rubber teat of a feeding-bottle is enlarged, or an ether dropper is substituted, milk can be made to drip evenly into the babe's open mouth, and in a few days he learns to receive his nourishment at regular intervals in this way. Alternatively, spoon-feeding can be employed.

CLEFT-PALATE

There are three degrees of cleft-palate—the tripartite, the bipartite, and the intermaxillary cleft (fig. 98, A, B, C).

In the tripartite, and to a lesser extent the bipartite, varieties of cleft-palate (fig. 98), the premaxilla, which is derived from the processi globulares, and which is, morphologically, the prognathos or snout of lower animals, juts out, causing a hideous deformity.

Treatment.—Successful operative treatment was by no means unknown before the Listerian era. For details of operative technique the reader is referred to works on operative surgery ; general principles only are

Sir James Berry, 1860–1946. Surgeon, Royal Free Hospital, London.
Sir William Fergusson, 1808–1877. Surgeon, Royal Infirmary, Edinburgh, later Professor of Surgery, King's College Hospital, London. Performed 134 cleft-palate operations with only five failures.
Lord Lister, 1827–1912. Professor of Surgery at Glasgow, Edinburgh, and London.

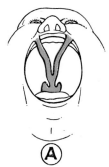
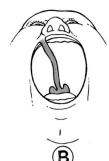
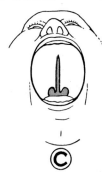

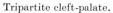

(A) Tripartite cleft-palate.   (B) Bipartite cleft-palate.   (C) Intermaxillary cleft.

Fig. 98.

considered here. The majority of surgeons prefer to operate when the child is about a year old, that is, just before it begins to speak; others advocate operation when the child has reached 10 lb. (4·5 Kgm.) in weight. When the operation is undertaken after speech is established, it is not always satisfactory from a phonetic point of view, although considerable improvement often accrues from speech training.

Pre-operative Treatment.—It is a great advantage for the child to get accustomed to its nurse, who teaches it to be spoon-fed before the operation. As the most usual cause of failure is sepsis, infected teeth and tonsils must be eradicated. Another excellent precaution is to get the child accustomed to mouth-spraying before the operation.

Operation.—Endotracheal anæsthesia is employed, and the head is well extended.

Denis Browne conducts the operation in two stages. At the first the tonsils are dissected out and the posterior palatine artery is divided between ligatures. At the second operation long lateral incisions are made from the anterior pillars of the fauces to the incisor teeth. The hamular processes are broken to relax the tensores palati. The muco-periosteum is separated from the hard palate and the attachment of the soft palate to the posterior margin of the hard palate is divided. The edges of the cleft are freshened and united by two layers of sutures. The first layer unites the nasal mucosa. The second layer unites the palatal periosteum and its attached buccal mucous membrane (fig. 99).

In every operation for cleft-palate an ideal to be aimed at is that eventually the patient will be able to speak clearly. To accomplish this, it is necessary to provide a soft palate capable of occluding the naso-pharynx.

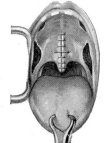

Fig. 99.—Operation for cleft-palate completed.

Browne achieves this objective by splinting the pharyngeal musculature in a position of rest while the sutured palate is healing. This he accomplishes by passing a thick catgut suture around the back of the pharynx and through the soft palate and tying it at the appropriate tension.

Denis Browne, Contemporary. Surgeon, Hospital for Sick Children, London.

Wardill reaches the same goal in another way. He commences by performing preliminary pharyngoplasty, a transverse incision being made across the posterior pharyngeal wall through the superior constrictor muscle. This incision is sewn up longitudinally. Only after this step has been completed does he commence to fashion flaps from the palate, and close the cleft.

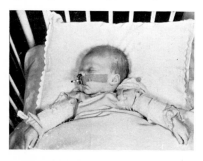

FIG. 100.—The arms are kept extended with cardboard splints. Note Logan's bow in position. (*W. E. M. Wardill.*)

POST-OPERATIVE TREATMENT

In order to prevent excessive crying, constant petting and attention are necessary. Cardboard splinting of the arms is advisable (fig. 100). Spoon-feeds of sterilised foods are given. Irrigation and spraying of the mouth with mild antiseptics are carried out every four hours or more often. Ten to twelve days after the operation the stitches are removed under an anæsthetic. When the suture line has healed sufficiently the palate is massaged. Post-operative speech training is necessary if the operation is performed after the child has commenced to talk.

HARE-LIP

Lateral hare-lip (fig. 101) is the most frequent congenital facial deformity ; it occurs once in 2,500 births. In about 15 per cent. hare-lip exists on both sides. Cases of true median hare-lip (fig. 102) are exceedingly rare, and are due to absence of the fronto-nasal process (see fig. 94).

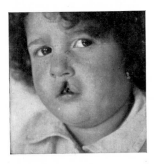

FIG. 101.—Lateral hare-lip.

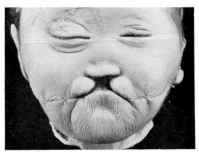

FIG. 102.—Median hare-lip in a still-born Mongol infant.

Treatment.—Repair is usually undertaken early ; about the second week of life is the popular time.

In all cases of complete hare-lip it is important to observe the nostrils. If, as is commonly the case, the naris of the affected

William E. M. Wardill, Contemporary. Surgeon, Royal Victoria Infirmary, Newcastle upon Tyne.

side is flattened, this should be corrected by a plastic procedure to the naris at the same time as the repair of the lip is undertaken.

The two main operative procedures for the repair of a hare-lip are as follows :

Rose's operation consists in freshening and uniting the edges of the cleft.

Owen's operation.—One side of the cleft is used to make a vermilion border for the newly constructed lip.

The essential objective in any operation for hare-lip is to restore the continuity of the orbicularis oris by approximating the edges of its defect with sutures.

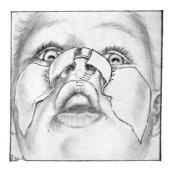

FIG. 103.—Logan's tension bow.

After the operation, the application of Logan's bow (fig. 103) is an extremely useful adjunct.

A well-performed hare-lip operation should render the patient's lips in after-life indistinguishable from normal, even on close inspection.

Double Hare-lip associated with a Premaxilla.—The premaxilla (see figs. 96 and 98A) must not on any account be removed, for the subsequent deformity is hideous. When the premaxilla juts out considerably, a V-shaped piece can be removed from the front of the nasal septum, to which the premaxilla is attached. This allows the protuberant process to be pressed back sufficiently for the lip to be reconstructed.

CONGENITAL FISTULÆ OF THE LOWER LIP

Congenital fistulæ of the lower lip is a condition unexplained by embryology. It occurs in certain families. There are two blind pits, one on either side of the middle line of the lower lip.

MACROCHEILIA

Chronic enlargement of the lip, usually the lower, may arise from inflammatory causes, but true macrocheilia is due to a lymphangioma, akin to lymphangiomatous macroglossia (p. 167). Its treatment is similar to that condition.

CRACKED LIPS

Chapping of the lips is very common, and a definite crack in the middle of the lower lip is a frequent complaint in cold weather. The crack is deep and bleeds readily. It is liable to be associated with an infection which produces a degree of swelling of the lip.

Treatment consists in the local application of aqueous silver nitrate (one per cent.), and, if necessary, strapping together the two halves of the lip for several weeks. In obstinate cases excision of the crack followed by suture should be considered.

CRACKS AT THE CORNERS OF THE MOUTH (*Syn.* RHAGADES)

Cracks at the *corners* of the mouth are a recognised manifestation of congenital or tertiary syphilis. Radiating scars in this situation should

William Rose, Jnr., 1847–1910. Surgeon, King's College Hospital, London.
Edmund Owen, 1847–1915. Surgeon, St. Mary's Hospital and the Hospital for Sick Children, London.
William Hoffman Gardiner Logan, Contemporary. Professor of Oral Surgery, Loyola University, Chicago.

arouse at once a suspicion of previous syphilitic ulceration.   On the other hand, cracks at the corners of the mouth may be due to simple infection, or to riboflavine deficiency, in which case the cracks are small and transient. Many examples of the last variety were observed in those subjected to the privations of war, and the lesions quickly responded to appropriate treatment, including the ingestion of marmite and eggs.

CHANCRE OF THE LIP

A Hunterian chancre may appear on the lip (fig. 104).   Unlike a similar lesion on the genitals, the neighbouring lymphatic nodes become *greatly* enlarged.

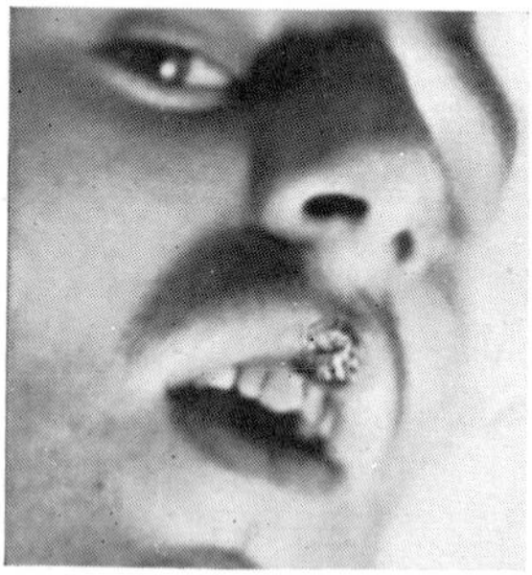

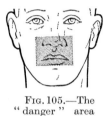

CARBUNCLE OF THE LIP

Carbuncle of the face has a sinister reputation, and the upper

FIG. 104.—Chancre of the lip.
(*A. E. W. McLachlan.*)

FIG. 105.—The " danger " area of the face.

lip is the most frequent site of this dreaded lesion (fig. 105). The public should be warned not to prick, squeeze, or otherwise tamper with a pimple in this area, for such a practice favours

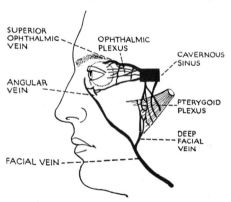

FIG. 106.—The cavernous sinus and its connections.

this dangerous condition.   It is particularly dangerous, because infection can spread along the angular vein to the ophthalmic plexus, and thence to the cavernous sinus (fig. 106).   Formerly

John Hunter, 1728–1793. Surgeon, St. George's Hospital, London.

thrombophlebitis of the cavernous sinus was regarded as inevitably fatal, but penicillin therapy, combined with treatment by heparin or dicoumarol, has reduced the number of fatalities from this cause.   A carbuncle of the lip should never be incised. A good method of local treatment is hot applications of gauze soaked in a saturated solution of magnesium sulphate until the slough separates.   At the earliest possible moment the patient is placed on penicillin therapy, which has revolutionised the outlook in cases of carbuncle of the lip.

NEOPLASMS OF THE LIP

The existence of lymphangioma in this situation has been referred to under " Macrocheilia."   Cavernous hæmangioma is another rare, innocent neoplasm in this region.

Carcinoma of the lip is usually seen in men between sixty and seventy years of age who have followed an outdoor occupation. This carcinoma, nearly always of the squamous-celled variety, usually takes the form of a shallow ulcer with the typical everted edge.   Any ulcer of the lip which refuses to heal should always be viewed with suspicion. The lower lip is affected in 93 per cent., the upper lip in 5 per cent., and 2 per cent. occur at one of the angles of the mouth. Rutherford Morison was the first to point out that a carcinoma occurring at the angle of the mouth and involving *both* lips, however slightly, is far more malignant than the more usual varieties.   In its typical form (fig. 107) carcinoma of the lip is a compara-

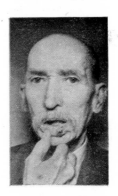

FIG. 107.—Carcinoma of the lower lip.

tively slow-growing neoplasm and a particularly favourable lesion to treat.

Treatment.—(*a*) *Excision.*—For early growths, V-shaped excision with a margin of ½ inch (1·25 cm.) of healthy tissue, gives good results.   The operation can be conducted under infiltration anæsthesia.   For larger neoplasms a quadrilateral resection of the lip is to be preferred.   In neglected cases, resection of the whole of the lip with plastic reconstruction is sometimes necessary.

(*b*) *Radium* also gives excellent results.   The needles are placed above, below, and through the lesion parallel to each

Rutherford Morison, 1853–1939. Professor of Surgery, University of Durham.

other and in two blocks. They are left in position for six to seven days, the aim being to deliver a dose of approximately 7,000 r.[1] to the growth.

(c) In some clinics X-ray treatment is preferred, and excellent cosmetic results, combined with long-term cures, are reported.

Except in elderly patients with comparatively early lesions, it is advisable to perform a suprahyoid block dissection of the neck (see p. 203) some weeks after the treatment of the primary lesion has been completed.

THE JAWS

OSTEOMYELITIS OF THE JAWS

Acute osteomyelitis of the jaw is not common.

In the upper jaw. The patient is usually an infant. The first sign is a puffiness of the face under the eyes due to suppuration involving the maxillary antra. Fortunately, sinuses opening into the mouth usually develop spontaneously, but abscesses may require opening. As a rule these patients recover with surprisingly little deformity.

In the lower jaw acute osteomyelitis is not so rare, and it is usually seen in children between the ages of five and ten years of age. While it may complicate any alveolar abscess, it is particularly liable to do so when an offending tooth is extracted during the acute stage of inflammation.

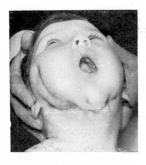

Fig. 108.—Osteomyelitis of the lower jaw shortly after a very large sequestrum had been removed.

Treatment.—In suspected cases penicillin should be commenced forthwith, and necrosis of the jaw with consequent sequestration may be avoided thereby. The necessary incision should be made, if possible, within the mouth, and carious teeth in the inflamed area are extracted only after the acute stage of the infection has abated. Suitable mouth washes are ordered until the sequestrum separates. These sequestra are often comparatively large (fig. 108). Involucrum formation in the jaws is decidedly poor, but it does occur when the patient is young. After middle life there is practically no regeneration.

[1] The letter "r." is the symbol used to denote the roentgen, which is the unit employed for measuring X-ray or gamma-ray dosage for medical purposes.

Chronic osteomyelitis (*syn.* necrosis of the jaw) is seen particularly in the lower jaw, and it occurs in a number of ways :

1. *Following a fracture,* for fractures of the jaw are so commonly compound into the mouth.

2. *As a sequel to extension of an alveolar abscess.*

3. *Tuberculous, syphilitic, and actinomycotic necrosis* of the jaws can
occur.   The well-known clinical entity of a hole in the hard palate following
a gumma is an example of syphilitic necrosis.

4. *Chemical necrosis* is now very rare.   In days gone by " phossy jaw "
was common in match-workers when yellow phosphorus was used.   A
more recent industrial cause has been disclosed in luminous paint, such as
that applied to watch dials.   Mercurial necrosis occurred when massive
doses of mercury were administered in the treatment of syphilis, and is
sometimes seen in those who work with this metal.   Occasionally chemical
necrosis is seen after arsenic has been used injudiciously in dental practice
to kill the nerves of teeth.   Radium necrosis was encountered fairly often
in the earlier days of the radium treatment of carcinoma of the floor
of the mouth.   It is occasionally met with in industrial practice where
workers with radium salts moisten their brushes with saliva.

Necrosis of the mandible is often a very chronic condition.
Radiography is helpful, particularly in indicating the presence
of sequestra.

Treatment.—Comparatively early dependent drainage gives
the best results.   A suitable incision is made beneath the
mandible, and a trough is chiselled in the bone, any sequestrum
present being removed.   The wound is left open and packed
with vaseline gauze.   Penicillin therapy is instituted.

Syphilis of the hard palate (see Chapter lxi).

MEDIAN MENTAL SINUS

Median mental sinus (fig. 109) is a clinical entity which is often diagnosed
and treated incorrectly.   It is produced by a periodontal abscess when pus
has tracked between the two halves of the lower
jaw to the point of the chin.   The patient has a
discharging sinus on, or less frequently, just
below, the chin, but always in the middle line.
He usually states that it has been scraped and
packed many times.   A radiograph of the bone
in the immediate neighbourhood reveals nothing,
but a radiograph of the lower incisor teeth,
which on clinical examination often appear to be
sound, shows areas of rarefaction around the
roots.   After extraction of the affected teeth the
sinus heals within a fortnight.

NEOPLASMS OF THE UPPER JAW

Benign.—Tumours of the alveolus are
considered on page 153.   While benign

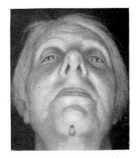

Fig.   109. — Median
mental sinus.   A drop
of pus can be seen.

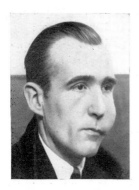

FIG. 110.—Ivory osteoma of the left maxilla. The tumour has been growing slowly for eight years.

giant-celled tumours may arise in the upper jaw proper, they nearly always commence in the alveolus. With this exception an ivory osteoma (fig. 110) is the only tumour falling into this category.

MALIGNANT DISEASE OF THE UPPER JAW

The clinical diagnosis of " malignant upper jaw " embraces a number of pathological conditions :

1. *Sarcoma.*

2. *Squamous-celled carcinoma*—derived from a tooth socket or from the gum.

3. *Columnar-celled carcinoma*—arising from the maxillary antrum or nasal cavities.

4. *Malignant odontome*—according to Eve, not a few cases of malignant upper jaw belong to this group.

5. *Invasion of the upper jaw* by a sarcoma of the ethmoid or a naso-pharyngeal tumour.

SARCOMA OF THE UPPER JAW

While neither sex nor any age is exempt, curiously, this disease has a distinct predilection for women (fig. 111) about the age of forty-five. When of the periosteal variety—and this is the more usual—it is the *anterior* aspect of the jaw which is maximally affected, but the condition soon shows itself on the inferior or palatal wall. Until perhaps the terminal stages of the disease, there is no nasal obstruction and no epiphora (blockage of the tear-duct). Pain is a late symptom. Unlike many forms of bone sarcomata, metastasis is delayed for many months.

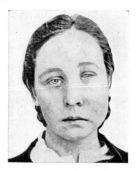

FIG. 111.—Sarcoma of the upper jaw. (*Macewen.*)

GROWTHS ARISING FROM WITHIN THE ANTRUM OR ITS WALLS

Growths arising from within the antrum or its walls (fig. 112) include both cases of carcinoma and osteogenic sarcoma, and are, in contradistinction to the above, characterised by early unilateral nasal obstruction. Sometimes osteogenic sarcoma is accompanied by foul or blood-stained discharge

Sir Frederick Eve, 1853–1916, Surgeon, London Hospital.

from one nostril. Epiphora is common, and trigeminal neuralgia may be a symptom.

DIFFERENTIAL DIAGNOSIS OF MALIGNANT UPPER JAW

Cysts, especially large follicular odontomata, present difficulty. The possibility of the swelling in question being due to an osteoclastoma must receive consideration. A closed empyema antri with polypi must also be excluded. In all these conditions much help can be derived

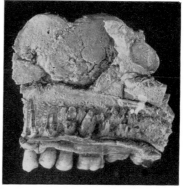

Fig. 112.—Malignant growth of upper jaw invading antrum.

from an X-ray examination. The bilateral character of leontiasis ossea (see Chapter xli) makes the segregation of this rare condition tolerably simple.

TREATMENT OF MALIGNANT UPPER JAW

Excision.—Even in pre-anæsthetic days complete excision of the upper jaw (fig. 113) was practised. It was for this purpose

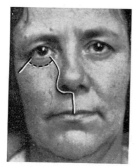

Fig. 113.—Trotter's incision for removal of the upper jaw. Ugly œdema of the lower eyelid is avoided by carrying the incision through the eyelid just outside the punctum lacrymale, along the orbital margin inside the lid, and thence as shown in the figure, avoiding the outer canthus.

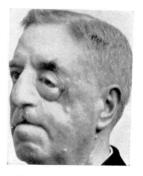

Fig. 114.—Patient two years after excision of the upper jaw and the eyeball for a carcinoma springing from the antrum and invading the orbit.

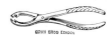

Fig. 115—Fergusson's lion forceps.

that Fergusson invented lion forceps (fig. 115). Since the introduction of intratracheal anæsthesia the operative mortality

Joseph Gensoul, 1797–1858, of Lyons. Performed the first successful resection of the upper jaw for malignant disease in 1827.
Wilfred Trotter, 1872–1939. Surgeon, University College Hospital, London.

is low. There is surprisingly little deformity after this formidable operation, especially if a prosthesis is constructed by a dental expert as soon as the wound has granulated. Such treatment offers hope of a cure (fig. 114).

Somervell (1944), after a vast experience of malignant disease of the jaws in Southern India, considers surgical removal superior to radiotherapy for this condition.

Radiotherapy.—*Combined diathermy excision and radiotherapy* is favoured by many. In this connection, carcinoma or sarcoma of the antrum must be distinguished from carcinoma of the upper alveolar margin or the hard palate spreading into the maxilla.

Carcinoma of the upper alveolar margin or hard palate.—In early cases diathermy excision is performed, combined with removing the necessary amount of bone with a chisel. Within a few days a dental plate is made of acrilic resin, in which are placed radium needles in such a way that the walls of the cavity receive a uniform dose of irradiation. In addition, external irradiation by teleradium or X-rays can be employed. In inoperable cases external irradiation by teleradium, or with high-voltage X-rays through multiple ports, gives palliative results.

Carcinoma of the antrum.—Pre-operative irradiation with high-voltage X-rays or teleradium in doses up to 4,000 r. is given anteriorly and laterally. This usually results in a temporary shrinkage of the tumour. The appropriate alveolar margin is cut away with the diathermy knife, and the floor of the antrum removed with a chisel. The growth is then removed with the diathermy loop, the ethmoidal cells being excised if they are found to be involved. The whole cavity is packed with gauze into which are inserted radium needles, and up to 40 mgm. may be required. These are removed in approximately two to three days, depending upon the amount of radium used. Two weeks later the cavity is irradiated by means of an acrilic resin obturator in which radium needles are incorporated in a manner similar to that described above.

Sarcoma.—Irradiation with high-voltage X-rays, or gamma-rays from a teleradium unit, cause temporary regression of the growth, but recurrences and metastases to the lungs are usual.

NASO-PHARYNGEAL TUMOUR

Naso-pharyngeal tumour is peculiar to patients in their teens. It is a fibro-sarcoma arising from the mucoperiosteum of the under-surface of the

Theodore Howard Somervell, Contemporary. Surgeon, Travancore, Southern India.

body of the sphenoid. It grows into, and plugs, one or both nasal fossæ, and is liable to produce epistaxis. The three leading symptoms are deafness (usually unilateral and due to obstruction of the Eustachian tube), neuralgia from pressure on the second division of the fifth cranial nerve, and displacement downwards of the soft palate. Although the tumour neither metastasises nor infiltrates in the manner of a sarcoma, its spread is destructive by reason of pressure necrosis. Microscopically it is made up principally of connective tissue.

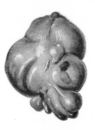

Treatment.—In the past, for the above reasons and because these tumours are essentially pedunculated, they proved both removable and curable by a bold surgical operation (fig. 116), comprising temporary resection of the upper jaw (which is swung outwards) and erasure of the pedicle from the under-surface of the body of the sphenoid. After the tumour had been removed the maxilla was replaced and the skin sutured. The operation was accompanied by torrential hæmorrhage. Preliminary irradiation, which reduces the extreme vascularity of the tumour, and the employment of surgical diathermy have robbed the extirpation of these tumours of much of their terror (Friedberg).

FIG. 116.—Nasopharyngeal tumour removed by operation. One - third scale. (*Dighton.*) (*British Journal of Surgery.*)

SARCOMA OF THE ETHMOID

Sarcoma of the ethmoid is rare. As it expands it greatly widens the space between the orbits and flattens out the nasal bones, producing that well-known clinical entity, the " frog-faced man " (fig. 117). Still later the superior maxillæ are invaded.

Treatment.—When the air sinus is infected, drainage is essential before irradiation is commenced. High-voltage X-rays or gamma-rays from a teleradium unit are employed. When the tumour does not disappear entirely as a result of irradiation, the remains should be destroyed by diathermy coagulation and removed piecemeal with a diathermy loop.

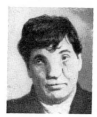

FIG. 117.—Frog-faced man. (*Musgrave Woodman.*) (*British Journal of Surgery.*)

CYSTS ABOUT THE ORBIT

From the point of view of clinical surgery it is convenient to group together certain conditions which have but one point in common —they form cystic swellings in the neighbourhood of the orbital margin. Passing latero-medially (figs. 118, 119, 120, and 121) we may recognise :

1. External Angular Dermoid.

—This is perhaps the commonest situation for a dermoid cyst (fig. 118), and its position is so constant that it allows the diagnosis to be made with irrefutable accuracy. The treatment is excision.

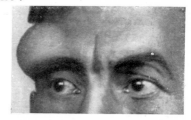

FIG. 118.—External angular dermoid.

Bartolommeo Eustacchio, 1524–1574. Professor of Anatomy, Rome.
Stanton Abeles Friedberg, Contemporary. Assistant in Otolaryngology, Presbyterian Hospital, Chicago.

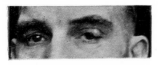

Fig. 119.—A Meibomian cyst.

2. **Meibomian cyst** usually occurs in the upper eyelid (fig. 119). It is due to a staphylococcal infection of a Meibomian gland, the swelling being, for the most part, retained Meibomian secretion. It must be distinguished from a hordeolum (stye) (fig. 120), which is due to an infection of an eyelash follicle.

Treatment of a Meibomian cyst consists in making an incision into the cyst from its conjunctival aspect, at right angles to the margin of the

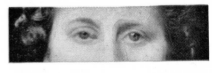

Fig. 120.—Hordeolum (stye).

lid, and scraping out the sac wall with a small spoon.

3. **Mucocele of the lachrymal sac** (fig. 121) is the result of lachrymal obstruction with distension of the sac and secondary infection of its walls (dacryocystitis).

Treatment consists in washing out the sac by means of a lachrymal syringe and removing the cause of the obstruction.

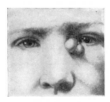

Fig. 121.—A muco-
cele of the lachrymal
sac. (*Mayou.*)

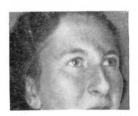

Fig. 122.—Dermoid
cyst at the root of the
nose.

4. **Cyst over the Root of the Nose.**—If the swelling is beneath the skin and does not empty with pressure, it is almost certainly a dermoid cyst. If it can be made to empty, a meningocele is probable, but a sinus pericranii, connected with one of the intracranial venous sinuses, must receive due diagnostic consideration. Especially when the swelling is not strictly median, the possibility of a mucocele of the frontal sinus or ethmoidal cells should be borne in mind.

TUMOURS OF THE ORBIT

Clinical Features.—Proptosis is the cardinal symptom. The eye is seldom pushed directly forward except when the tumour

Heinrich Meibom, 1638–1700. Professor of Medicine, Helmstädt. Resigned the Chair for that of History and Poetic Art.

is growing from the optic nerve or its sheath. Visual disturbances are complained of, and the lids are prone to become œdematous. In advanced cases the cornea becomes inflamed (keratitis) or ulcerated because it is exposed unduly.

CLASSIFICATION.—Tumours of the orbit are primary or secondary. The principal primary tumours are :

1. **Osteoma.**—It will be recalled that ivory osteomata grow from membrane bones, particularly the lachrymal bone.

2. **Carcinoma** from the lachrymal gland.

3. **Glioma** from the optic chiasma or the optic nerve (very rare).

4. **Retino-blastoma** of the optic nerve.

5. **Melanoma** of the uveal tract (p. 62).

6. **Sarcoma** (fig. 123).

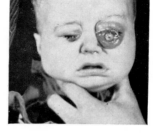

FIG. 123.—Sarcoma of the orbit. (*A. A. McConnell.*)

While it is undesirable here to enter into the particular features of each of these tumours, in a general way they may be divided into two important clinical groups :

(*a*) Those occurring in children ;

(*b*) Those occurring in adults.

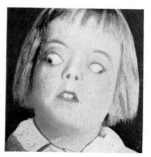

FIG. 124.—Child suffering from retrobulbar tumour. (*J. Minton.*)

In the child retino-blastoma of the optic nerve is the commonest (fig. 124). It is frequently bilateral, and occurs before the age of four years. Proptosis is considerable, and early blindness the rule. This tumour is highly malignant, and it soon breaks down and bleeds. The prognosis is hopeless.

In the adult melanoma is the principal primary tumour. It is derived from the neuro-ectodermal nerve endings. A melanoma commences in the posterior part of the choroid, and it is always unilateral. It generally occurs in individuals between forty and sixty years of age. An orbital melanoma shows little tendency to spread into the cranium, but metastases are carried to the liver

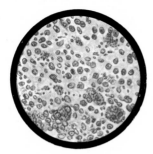

Fig. 125.—Section of liver showing secondary melanoma.

(fig. 125) and bones by the blood-stream, and to lymph nodes via the lymphatic vessels. If the globe is removed early in the course of the disease, this dissemination may be limited, but rarely is the expectation of life more than three years. Sometimes, after early diagnosis and excision of the globe, the dissemination of metastases is delayed for many years, and then arises a classical pitfall for the unwary diagnostician. Wherefore it has been remarked, with much wisdom, that the clinician should " beware the patient with a large liver and a glass eye " (fig. 126).

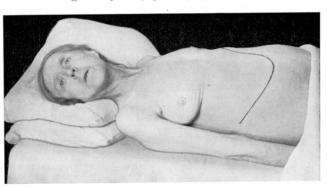

Fig. 126.—Patient with a greatly enlarged liver, who for many years had worn a glass eye.

Secondary tumours of the orbit are uncommon. A well-known example is the metastasis of neurocytoma of the adrenal gland (Hutchison's tumour) (see p. 232), but the orbit is frequently invaded by a primary carcinoma of the antrum and a very advanced rodent ulcer.

PULSATING EXOPHTHALMOS

Unilateral pulsating exophthalmos is a rare condition which always excites clinical interest. The principal causes are as follows :

1. An arterio-venous aneurism between the internal carotid artery and the cavernous sinus (fig. 127) ; invariably traumatic in origin.

2. An aneurism of the ophthalmic artery.

3. A cirsoid aneurism involving the orbit.

4. Thrombosis of the cavernous sinus. However, pulsation is not a usual feature of this condition.

5. A rapidly growing vascular intraorbital neoplasm.

Sir Robert Hutchison, Contemporary. Consulting Physician, London Hospital.

Subjective Symptoms.—In the first three conditions the patient notices a buzzing noise in the head and failing of vision.

Treatment.—The first variety, which is the commonest, is the most amenable to treatment. Ligation of the orbital veins is often successful. Adson recommends two small incisions, one over the inner canthus (angular vein) and one under the inner end of the eyebrow (superior ophthalmic vein). Loops of the veins are freed and resected. When this fails, ligation of the common carotid artery is resorted to. This combined operation cures a reasonable percentage of the patients belonging to the first three groups. Should this fail, the advisability of ligation of the internal carotid artery must receive full consideration. Liga-

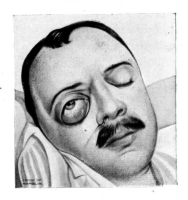

FIG. 127.—Pulsating exophthalmos due to an intracranial arteriovenous aneurism. (*British Journal of Surgery.*)

tion and division of the common carotid artery, although a hazardous undertaking (see p. 101), is considerably safer than ligation of the internal carotid artery (Lambert Rogers). For the other varieties of aneurism the reader is referred to p. 96.

ORBITAL CELLULITIS

Cellulitis of the orbit (fig. 128) gives rise to proptosis, œdema of the eyelids, and œdema of the conjunctiva (chemosis). The

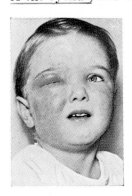

FIG. 128.—Orbital cellulitis.

most frequent cause of the condition is a spread of infection from one of the paranasal sinuses. The constitutional symptoms are often severe. There are two outstanding dangers of infection of this space. Firstly, thrombophlebitis of the cavernous sinus may follow via the ophthalmic plexus of veins, and, secondly, the globe of the eye may become infected.

Treatment.—In early cases, penicillin therapy, which should be instituted at once, sometimes results in resolution of the infection. Unless full response to chemotherapy is undoubted, an incision following the orbital margin should not be delayed; this will relieve tension in the orbit and provide drainage.

INJURIES OF THE EYE

Injuries of the eye belong properly to the domain of Ophthalmology. It is necessary here to call attention to a peculiar

A. W. Adson, *Contemporary. Professor of Neuro-Surgery, Mayo Clinic, Rochester, U.S.A.* Lambert Charles Rogers, *Contemporary. Professor of Surgery, University of Wales.*

danger of perforating wounds of the globe.   After a penetrating wound of the eye, particularly when a portion of the uveal tract prolapses, there is always a danger of sympathetic ophthalmitis occurring in the sound eye.   When this occurs, the sight of both eyes may be lost.   The only certain way of avoiding sympathetic ophthalmia is to remove the injured eye promptly.

EXCISION OF AN EYEBALL

Indications
- Trauma.
- Foreign bodies.
- Iridocyclitis.
- Phthisis bulbi.
- Neoplasms.
- Anterior staphyloma.
- Irremediable Glaucoma.

The Operation.—The speculum is introduced between the lids, and opened.   The conjunctiva is picked up with toothed forceps and divided completely all round as near as possible to the cornea.   Tenon's capsule is entered, and each of the rectus tendons is hooked up on a strabismus hook and divided close to the sclerotic (fig. 129).   The speculum is now pressed backwards and the eyeball starts forwards. Blunt scissors, curved on the flat, are insinuated on the inner side of the globe, and these are used to sever the optic nerve. The eyeball can now be drawn forward with the fingers, and the oblique muscles, together with any other strands of tissue which are still attaching the globe to the orbit, are divided.   A swab moistened with a little adrenalin and pressed into the orbit will control the hæmorrhage.

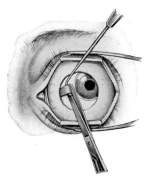

FIG. 129.—Excision of an eyeball.   Medial rectus tendon being divided, aided by a strabismus hook.

EVISCERATION OF THE EYEBALL

Owing to the danger of opening up lymphatic spaces at the back of the globe and thus favouring meningitis and sympathetic ophthalmitis, evisceration is much to be preferred to excision in panophthalmitis. The sclera is transfixed with a pointed knife a little behind the corneo-sclerotic junction, and the cornea is removed entirely by completing the encircling incision in the sclera.   The contents of the globe are then scraped out by means of a spoon, care being exercised to remove all the uveal tract.   At the end of the operation the interior must appear perfectly white.

THE FACE

WOUNDS

Thanks to its abundant blood-supply, wounds of the face heal readily.   Very accurate approximation of the skin edges is desirable to prevent an unsightly scar.

Jacques R. Tenon, 1724–1816.   Surgeon, Hôpital Saltpetrière, Paris.

Extensive Wounds with Loss of Substance.—The primary treatment is to suture skin to mucous membrane, in order to prepare for plastic procedures later.

ACUTE INFECTIONS OF THE FACE

Boils are more dangerous in this area than similar lesions elsewhere. A furuncle or carbuncle of the lip or nose is particularly dangerous, and the former has been referred to in some detail on p. 130.

Anthrax.—While cutaneous anthrax can occur in any part of the body exposed to infection, the face is the commonest site for the so-called " malignant pustule," prompt recognition of which is so important. A differential diagnosis must be made between anthrax and two conditions easily mistaken for it. The first is a virulent furuncle, and the second accidental vaccinia. The contagion in accidental vaccinia often takes place in the following way. The recently vaccinated child with the cutaneous lesion on its arm in full activity, while being carried by its mother or nurse, places the vaccinated area against her cheek (fig. 130). Final and absolute diagnosis of anthrax rests in demonstrating the anthrax bacillus (see p. 24).

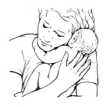

Fig. 130.—The commonest cause of accidental vaccinia.

Chronic Infections.—See Lupus, Chapter xxxii.

NEOPLASMS

Simple nævi (cutaneous hæmangiomata) are often found on the face. Small tumours can be satisfactorily removed by an application of carbon-dioxide snow. Larger ones may yield to treatment by radium, but the very extensive variety calls for the highest efforts of plastic surgery.

Pigmented and Hairy Moles.—The face is a common situation for pigmented or hairy moles, a condition for which the patient seeks relief on account of disfigurement. Their removal is also to be urged on account of the danger of a melanoma developing in the pigmented area. Hairy moles are treated successfully by excision followed by skin grafting.

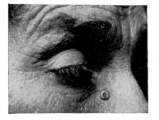

Fig. 131.—An early rodent ulcer. (*Sir Charles Paul.*)

Rodent Ulcer (Basal-celled carcinoma).—Rodent ulcers are almost confined to that portion of the face situated above a line joining the tip of the lobule of the ear with the angle of the mouth, the site of election being near the inner canthus (fig. 131).

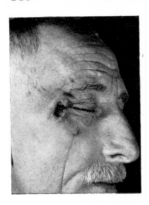

FIG. 132.—Rodent ulcer.
(*T. A. Bouchier-Hayes.*)

Ætiology.—Exposure to bright sunlight appears to be a causative factor. In parts of Australia where sunlight is powerful, the condition is very common, especially in the fair-skinned (as opposed to the darker Italian) members of the labouring population (Boyd).

The ulcer (fig. 132) appears as an irregular sclerotic scar surrounded by an area of small grey elevations, traversed here and there by a fine capillary vessel. Rodent ulcer is essentially very chronic, but usually steadily progressive. In process of time it does, as its name implies, eat into muscle, cartilage, and bone, producing ghastly disfigurement, the interior of the orbit, nose, and even the brain being exposed by the ulcer. Death releases the victim by erosion of a large artery, or by inhalation broncho-pneumonia. Even in advanced cases metastases never occur unless, as rarely happens, the rodent ulcer takes on a squamous-cell carcinomatous change.

Treatment in the early stages by X-ray is, on the whole, satisfactory, but recurrences are rather frequent.

Small early superficial lesions can be treated with beta-radiation by means of a plaque containing 6 to 10 mgm. of radium ; this is placed over the lesion for one hour on alternate days for four days. Such lesions are also treated with X-ray therapy by low-voltage (60 kV.) machines. The dose given is approximately 5,000 r. to 6,000 r., delivered in a period of a week or ten days, i.e. 500 r. a day. Inadequate treatment by X-rays may induce carcinomatous changes.

In advanced cases where the underlying bone is involved, diathermy excision is probably the most effective method of attempting to arrest the progress of the disease.

Squamous-celled Carcinoma (*syn*. epithelioma).—As opposed to rodent ulcer, squamous-celled carcinoma rather commonly attacks the pinna (fig. 133). If diagnosed and treated early, favourable results accrue from excision of the pinna. Although the lesion is obvious, for some obscure reason the condition is often comparatively far advanced before the patient seeks relief.

William Boyd, Contemporary. Professor of Pathology and Bacteriology, University of Toronto.

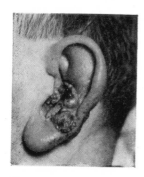

FIG. 133.—Carcinoma of
the pinna.

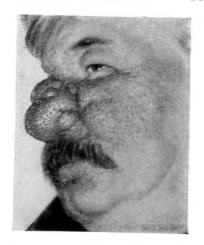

FIG. 134.—Rhinophyma.
(*Dr. E. B. Ash.*)

RHINOPHYMA (*Syn.* POTATO NOSE)

The skin of the nose, particularly the distal part, becomes surmounted with irregular bosses (fig. 134), on which the openings
of the sebaceous follicles are easily discerned. The capillaries
become dilated and the nose assumes a bluish-red colour.
Histologically, the condition appears to be due to sebaceous
adenomata.

Treatment.—Paring away the protruding masses with a
scalpel until the nose is of normal dimensions gives pleasing
results. Care must be taken not to encroach upon the cartilages
or the nostrils. The brisk hæmorrhage is controlled by hot
applications, after which a dressing of tulle gras is all that is
necessary. Skin grafting is not required.

CHAPTER VIII

THE TEETH AND GUMS

THE occurrence of supernumerary teeth is fairly common ; occasionally clusters of them are present. Teeth commonly congenitally absent are the third molars and upper second incisors.

IMPACTION OF A TOOTH

A tooth is prevented from normal eruption by the presence of other fully erupted teeth (fig. 135). Much the commonest

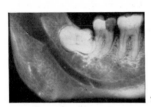

FIG. 135. — Radiograph showing impacted third molar. (*S. Blackman.*)

tooth to be affected in this way is the third lower molar. If a partially erupted tooth is in communication with the mouth, there will be a pocket in the gum in which food debris collects, resulting in infection, which tends to spread to the cheek and the neck. In such cases trismus is often present.

Treatment.—In the acute stage reliance should be placed on penicillin therapy and suitable mouth-washes. When the acute symptoms have subsided, the impacted tooth should be removed.

In order to accomplish extraction it may be necessary to sacrifice one of the teeth immediately adjacent. In cases of extreme difficulty the bony alveolus must be chiselled away before the impacted tooth can be removed.

DENTAL CARIES[1]

Necrosis of a tooth begins, as a rule, in the enamel, and extends through the dentine to the pulp. As it reaches the nerve endings within the pulp the familiar pain of toothache is produced.

Untreated, infection is liable to pass through the apical canal into the peridental tissues and the adjacent bone, when an acute or chronic abscess results.

ALVEOLAR ABSCESS

Alveolar abscess is rather more common in the lower jaw, and is usually the result of an infection carried to the tooth

[1] Evidence of dental caries was found in an herbivorous dinosaur of the estimated antiquity of 100,000 years.

socket by the process described above.   Throbbing pain, swelling of the cheek (fig. 136), redness and œdema of the gum in the
neighbourhood of the tooth which is the seat of the trouble, are
the leading symptoms.   The general reaction to the infective
process may be considerable, and a tender enlargement of the
regional lymph nodes is usual.   The pus may break through
the periodontal membrane or burrow beneath the periosteum,
causing a swelling on the labial or on the lingual aspect of the
alveolus, the former being more common.   Occasionally, in

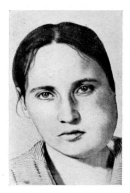

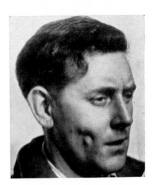

Fig. 136. — Extensive
alveolar abscess.

Fig. 137.—Sinus following
bursting of an alveolar abscess externally.

relevant cases, the abscess bursts into the maxillary antrum.
In either jaw, if the abscess is not drained promptly and effec-
tively, some degree of necrosis of the alveolus is to be expected.
Osteomyelitis of the jaw sometimes results (see p. 132).

Perforation of the alveolus of the lower jaw on the inner
side can give rise to a very acute variety of Ludwig's angina
(see p. 196).

Treatment.—Hot fomentations and poultices of all kinds should
be avoided, for they tend to promote the pointing of an alveolar
abscess externally (fig. 137), which, for cosmetic reasons, is the
very thing to be prevented, if possible.   It is dangerous to extract the offending tooth during the acute attack of inflammation, for this favours spreading osteomyelitis of the jaw and
its attendant evils.   Antiseptic mouth-washes are ordered, and
chemotherapy, together with suitable drugs to relieve pain and
induce sleep, are prescribed.   As soon as some softening of the
brawny mucoperiosteum can be palpated (usually after forty-eight

*Wilhelm von Ludwig, 1790–1865. Professor of Surgery and Midwifery, University of
    Tübingen.*

hours), the abscess is opened into the mouth.   Local anæsthetic
should never be injected into inflamed tissues for fear of disseminating the infection.

In ultra-acute and neglected cases, especially when a large
abscess has invaded the submaxillary region, a dependent external incision is indicated.   As soon as the acute symptoms have
abated, the tooth responsible for the abscess is extracted.

ROOT ABSCESSES

While alveolar abscesses are usually acute, root abscesses are
nearly always chronic.   They arise by extension of infection

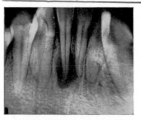

from the pulp through the apical canal.
Only too often there are no external
signs of a root abscess, which is only
revealed by a dental radiograph (fig.
138).   The causative bacteria are for
the most part non-hæmolytic streptococci, and the absorption of their toxic
products is often the cause of ill health.
Remarkable cures of some forms of
arthritis, fibrositis, and neuritis by ex-

Fig. 138.—Dental radio-
graph showing root abscesses
of the lower incisor teeth.
(S. Blackman.)

traction of infected teeth have been fully established.

ALVEOLAR CYSTS

It is necessary, first, to define two confusing terms—dentigerous and dental cysts.

Dentigerous cyst (*syn.* follicular odontome) arises in connection with a non-erupted permanent tooth.   The
swelling consists of a tooth, most commonly a canine
or the lower third molar, ———————————— . ——→
often well developed except for a truncated root,
lying obliquely in a cavity filled with viscid fluid.
In the case of a dentigerous cyst connected with a canine
tooth, the patient complains of the swelling during
adolescence or early adult life, while in the molar region
the symptoms are frequently more delayed.

Dental (root) cyst occurs in connection with the root
of a normally erupted, but chronically infected, usually
pulpless, tooth ——————————————————→
Epithelial cells, believed to be connected with the
enamel-organ, proliferate and break down, forming a

cyst. The cyst enlarges, causing expansion of the alveolus (fig. 139), and eventually most of the epithelial lining disappears. These cysts, which can appear at any age, are more frequent in

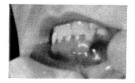

FIG. 139.—Dental (root) cyst expanding the alveolus.

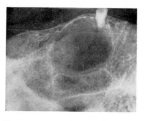

FIG. 140.—Dental (root) cyst.

the upper jaw, and when they attain a large size they encroach upon the antra or the nasal fossæ, but rarely open into these cavities. The fluid in the cyst (fig. 139) is usually clear, and it often contains cholesterol crystals. This fluid is usually sterile, but secondary infection can occur. When not infected the condition is painless.

Naso-palatine Cyst.—Cysts simulating dental root cysts, but unconnected with the teeth and seldom containing cholesterol, occur in the premaxillary region (fig. 141). They arise in connection with the naso-palatine canal. The importance of segregating this class of cyst is that as it is not connected with the incisor teeth, the latter need not necessarily be sacrificed (Roper-Hall).

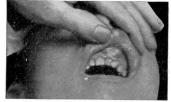

FIG. 141.—Naso-palatine cyst.

Adamantinoma (*syn.* multilocular cystic disease of the jaw) is a rare epithelial tumour of the jaw, probably arising either from enameloblasts or the gum epithelium. An adamantinoma is a slowly growing neoplasm, remaining locally malignant for years. Only occasionally does the tumour metastasise to other bones. The condition occurs more frequently in the mandible than in the maxilla, and it usually commences in the region of the second or third molar tooth. While it is found at any age, it is most common between thirty and fifty. As the condition progresses it expands the jaw, and in advanced cases eggshell crackling can be elicited. In the absence of secondary infection it is quite painless.

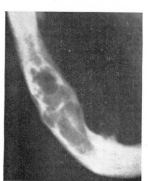

FIG. 142.—Radiograph showing an adamantinoma.

Pathology.—Within a firm, fibrous capsule are a number of cystic and solid areas, varying greatly in size and separated by fibrous septa (fig. 142). The solid areas consist of fibrous tissue, stroma, and epithelial cells.

H. T. Roper-Hall, Contemporary. Dental Surgeon, Birmingham and Midland Eye Hospital.

The cysts are filled with viscid brownish fluid, and lined by epithelial cells. In the larger cysts the epithelial wall frequently becomes obliterated.

The Treatment of Alveolar Cysts.—As a preliminary measure the teeth not in the immediate vicinity of the swelling are scaled, and should any be carious they receive suitable attention. About a week later the lesion itself is dealt with.   Both dental and dentigerous cysts are approached by turning back a flap of the mucoperiosteum overlying the external wall of the expanded alveolus.   Having evacuated the mucoid contents, every particle of the cyst lining is excised and the tooth or teeth implicated in the cyst are extracted.   After the requisite amount of the expanded alveolus has been removed with nibbling forceps, the flap of mucoperiosteum can be stitched back into position. This form of treatment is only practicable in the upper jaw, where, provided the hygiene of the mouth is attended to carefully, the wound usually heals by first intention.   In the lower jaw, and in cases which are infected, after the lining membrane has been removed (vide supra), the bone, if greatly expanded, is crushed so as to reduce the size of the cavity, which is then packed.   When packing has to be resorted to, healing is comparatively slow.

In non-infected cysts of the lower jaw, we have made a suitable external incision.   After removing the lining membrane of the cyst without entering the mouth, the cavity in the mandible has been packed with absorbable gauze, and the incision closed without drainage.   Thus the patient is spared weeks of intrabuccal packing and repacking.

The position regarding the treatment of adamantinoma is entirely different.   Evacuation and curettage of the cysts in a manner similar to that described above is invariably followed by recurrence.   X-ray or radium therapy is without value.   Therefore resection of that portion of the jaw bearing the tumour, together with a margin of healthy bone, is essential.   So long as the tumour is not encroached upon, adequate partial excision of the jaw is followed by a lasting cure.   The defect in the mandible is remedied later by bone grafting, or by an epithelial inlay followed by a suitable dental prosthesis.

ODONTOMES

An odontome is a tumour composed of the constituents of dental tissue in varying proportions and different degrees of development, arising from teeth germs or from teeth still in the

process of growth.   An easily remembered classification which
embraces all the types is as follows :

1. *Follicular odontome* is another name for dentigerous cyst (p. 148) ; the swelling contains a
tooth,................................ viz. :—→ — Fluid.

2. *Fibrous odontome* is identical with the above,
except that the unerupted tooth is surrounded by
fibrous tissue instead of fluid,..............viz. :—→ Fibrous tissue.

3. *Cementome* occurs usually in horses, and only
rarely in man.   Around the unerupted tooth there is
cement, ... viz. :—→ Cement.

4. *Compound follicular odontome.*—The capsule
surrounding the tooth ossifies sporadically, and contains cement, dentine, and enamel in varying proportions.   Sometimes these dental elements are so well
formed and arranged as to be dignified by the name
of denticules, or tiny teeth, ... viz. :—→ Denti-cules.

5. *Composite odontome.*—The three dental elements
—dentine, enamel, and cement—are mixed in a con-
glomerate fashion within the capsule, which contains
no recognisable tooth, ... viz. :— → Conglo-merate mass.

6. *Radicular odontome* occurs in connection with
the root of an *erupted* tooth, and causes difficulty in
extraction, ... viz. :—→

It follows that in all types of odontomata, except the radicular,
which is very rare, the accompanying expansion of the alveolus is
associated with a missing tooth not accounted for by extraction.

It is probable that certain odontomata can become malignant, and they are referred to in connection with malignant
upper jaw (see p. 134).

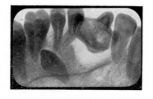

FIG. 143.—Dental radio-
graph showing both a com-
posite odontome and an
unerupted tooth.

Treatment.—Excision of the cyst as
opposed to excision of a portion of
the jaw is indicated.   It is advisable
to display the radiograph (fig. 143)
during the operation.   In the follicular
variety it is usually sufficient to remove
one bony wall and to scrape out the
contents (see treatment of alveolar
cysts, p. 150).

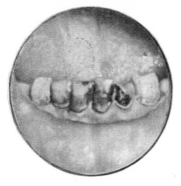

Fig. 144.—The lead line. The patient was a painter, and he was sent to the out-patient department complaining of attacks of colicky abdominal pain.

THE GUMS

GINGIVITIS

Inflammation of the gums is usually associated with generalised stomatitis (p. 156). The gums are swollen, spongy, and bleed readily. Fœtor oris is often extreme. The teeth become loose and sometimes fall out. These symptoms are in evidence in scurvy and in chronic mercurial poisoning. In chronic lead, and also bismuth, poisoning there is a characteristic narrow line of blue-black dots on the gums near the dental margin (fig. 144).

Treatment consists in removing the cause, and in dental hygiene. The administration of vitamin C is specific in the case of scurvy and sub-scurvy states.

Vincent's gingivitis (see also p. 157).—Modern investigation tends to show that a streptococcus plays the prior rôle, while the Vincent's organisms are secondary invaders. Prodromal symptoms of the acute cases are general malaise, pyrexia, and increased salivation. Constant signs are fœtor oris and hæmorrhage from the gingival margin. After swabbing the inflamed bleeding gums, small ulcers will be seen on the interdental papillæ.

Treatment.—*Acute Stage.* (1) Penicillin therapy. (2) Bland mouth-washes. (3) Local application of diluted hydrogen peroxide.

Subacute Stage. (1) Irrigation by a dental hygienator. (2) Dental scaling. (3) Local applications to the gingival margin by means of small pellets of cottonwool held in dressing forceps.

The gums in the neighbourhood of the ulcers are cleansed, particular attention being paid to the removal of the peculiarly sticky saliva that is a feature of this condition. A topical application (pure carbolic acid, trichloracetic acid, or penicillin solution 1,000 units per ml., are the most popular) is then applied to the ulcers. The mouth having been rinsed with diluted hot hydrogen peroxide, the interdental spaces are packed with a thick paste of zinc oxide, oil of cloves, and cotton fibres. This prevents débris collecting in the gum pockets. Although the treatment is painful,

Jean Hyacinthe Vincent, 1862–1950, Professor of Medicine, Val-de-Grâce (Military) Hospital, France.

once the pack is in place the patient is comfortable. The packing is renewed in about forty-eight hours. Alternatively, a pack of dental wool mixed with fresh penicillin cream can be used.

When signs of ulceration have disappeared, usually in about five days, necessary extractions are undertaken and odontal pockets are eradicated with the diathermy, or by gingivectomy. Penicillin therapy has not proved specific, but it is very useful. The administration of large doses will allow extractions to be undertaken in the presence of acute or subacute Vincent's infection, whereas, in the past, this was contraindicated. Penicillin lozenges are usually beneficial in the treatment of this disease. A lozenge is given every two hours while the patient is awake. It should dissolve slowly in the mouth. Occasionally B. coli stomatitis supervenes, and is apparently encouraged by the use of the lozenges.

PYORRHŒA ALVEOLARIS (Syn. RIGGS' DISEASE)

Pyorrhœa alveolaris is a very chronic form of gingivitis. The fundamental predisposing cause of the condition is an excessive deposit of tartar. Unless this is removed regularly, it tends to push the gum away from the teeth. Consequently, the gum recedes more and more, until the periodontal membrane is broken through. Once this has occurred, particles of food can accumulate between the gum and the tooth, and suppuration ensues. The gums bleed when touched, and in advanced cases beads of pus can be expressed by pressure. In comparatively early cases regular attendance for the removal of tartar and other conservative measures, together with gingivectomy, may be effective. Once the condition is fully established, treatment is difficult, if not impossible, without removing the teeth. In dirty mouths clearing the jaws of teeth is not to be undertaken lightly, for myriads of virulent bacteria are released both into the mouth and possibly into the circulation ; in addition, broncho-pneumonia is liable to follow. Prophylactic penicillin therapy considerably minimises these untoward possibilities. As a rule the teeth should be removed a few at a time, and if a major surgical operation—for instance, laparotomy for peptic ulcer—is contemplated, the operation, when possible, should be postponed until the gums have healed.

TUMOURS OF THE ALVEOLUS

It is customary to aggregate these under the general heading of " Epulis," an ancient term which has no pathological

John M. Riggs, 1811–1885. Lecturer in Dental Surgery, Harvard University, U.S.A.

significance, merely signifying that such swellings are "situated on the gum." There are four varieties of epulides :

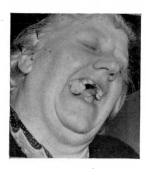

Fig. 145.—Fibro-sarcomatous epulis.

1. *Granulomatous Epulis.*—A mass of granulomatous tissue forms around a carious tooth.

Treatment consists in extraction of the tooth and scraping away the granulations.

2. *Fibro-sarcomatous Epulis* (fig. 145).—The majority of epulides belong to this group. They vary greatly in malignancy. At one end of the scale the fibromatous element predominates, and the tumour is practically benign. At the other end the tumour is almost a pure sarcoma. The more sarcomatous element there is present, the softer does the tumour feel and the more readily does it bleed.

Treatment.—After removal of the tooth or teeth in the immediate neighbourhood, a wedge of bone, including the portion of the gum containing the growth, is excised.

3. *Myelomatous Epulis.*—Benign giant-celled growths occur in the alveolar margin, particularly in the upper jaw.

Treatment.—Local excision, swabbing out the cavity with antiseptics, followed by packing, is usually satisfactory. This should be followed by deep X-ray therapy.

4. *Carcinomatous epulis* is a particularly undesirable term, as it is but another way of saying that the carcinoma begins on the gum. The treatment of a carcinomatous epulis follows that described for carcinoma of the tongue and the floor of the mouth. (See p. 170.)

HYPERTROPHY OF THE GUMS

General hypertrophy of the gums (fig. 146) is occasionally met with in children and young adults. The patients are usually, but not necessarily, mentally defective. The gum almost buries the teeth, and large polypoid masses form.

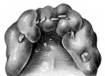

Fig. 146.—General hypertrophy of the gums.

Treatment consists in gingivectomy or, if a radiograph shows the bone to be hyper-trophoid, alveolectomy.

Local hypertrophy is more common, and is due to pressure from an ill-fitting prosthesis. When well established, the condition is indistinguishable from a fibro-sarcomatous epulis.

When removal of the cause does not remedy matters in a fortnight, the hypertrophied area should be treated as a fibro-sarcomatous epulis, and examined histologically.

The administration of soluble phenytoin (e.g. epanutin (Parke Davis)) leads to hypertrophy of the gums in some individuals who are susceptible to the toxic influence of the substance—which is used in the treatment of epilepsy. The hypertrophy is most pronounced between the front teeth and usually more in the upper jaw than the lower.

GINGIVECTOMY

Indications.—Hypertrophy of the gums and irregularities thereof, the underlying bone being normal.

Operation.—The operation can be carried out under local anæsthesia. The excess of gum is removed with a sharp scalpel and the raw surface is covered for three or four days with a sedative paste of zinc oxide and eugenol. Granulation soon occurs and epithelialisation follows.

ALVEOLECTOMY

Indications.—In addition to hypertrophy of the gums associated with hypertrophy of the underlying bone, alveolectomy is advisable before fitting a denture in certain cases of prominent gums. Alveolectomy is also necessary when the alveolus has been mutilated by dental extractions and gross irregularities of the bony contour exist. Occasionally, the operation is advisable in cases of extensive epulis.

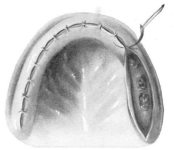

Fig. 147.—Alveolectomy.

Operation.—With a stout scalpel an incision is made right down to the bone a few millimetres from the teeth. A flap is raised with a periosteal elevator. Any teeth which require removal are extracted. Similarly, a flap is raised on the palatal aspect.

The bone is removed with a hammer and chisel. Any excess of mucosa is trimmed with scissors before suturing the cut edges over the now attenuated alveolus (fig. 147).

CHAPTER IX

THE MOUTH IN GENERAL. THE TONGUE, THE FLOOR OF THE MOUTH, AND THE CHEEK

INFECTIONS

STOMATITIS is a general term which embraces all infections of the mouth. A few of these can be distinguished as specific disorders.

Acute Catarrhal Stomatitis.—The mucous membrane is swollen and of a dusky red colour. There is an increased secretion of mucus. Eating is painful, and small superficial ulcers frequently occur. Acute stomatitis may be associated with the cutting of teeth in infancy, with carious teeth in later life, with the abuse of spirits or tobacco, with poisoning by iodides, lead, mercury, or bismuth, or in general toxæmia.

Treatment consists in removal of the cause and the use of a simple alkaline mouth-wash.

Aphthous stomatitis (*syn.* Thrush) occurs in infants and debilitated persons. It is due to the oïdium albicans, which is a saprophyte found in sour milk. The disease appears as spots on the buccal mucous membrane, varying in size from a pin's head to a pea. They are at first red, and later become covered with a yellow exudate. Pain and salivation are constant accompaniments. The condition gradually subsides without treatment, but the mouth should be kept clean with boroglycerol, and precautions taken to see that the milk is fresh and the utensils in which it is served scrupulously clean.

Ulcero-membranous stomatitis (*syn.* Vincent's [1] Stomatitis) is, at any rate in part, due to infection by Vincent's spirillum. Of 90 cases investigated bacteriologically by Henry, Vincent's spirillum was found in 87. Essentially a disease of early adult life, it is exceptional to find it after the age of thirty-five. The mouth, tonsils, and gums become inflamed, and covered with grey patches surrounded by a red zone. Ulcero-membranous stomatitis is often resistant to treatment, but the eventual

---

[1] Sometimes (incorrectly) called Vincent's *Angina*. Angina means choking.

Jean Hyacinthe Vincent, 1862–1950. Professor of Medicine, Val-de-Grâce (Military) Hospital, France.
Thomas Cradock Henry, Contemporary. Dental Surgeon, Hospital for Sick Children, Great Ormond Street, London.

prognosis is good. Vitamin C in large doses (50 mg. t.d.s.) should be prescribed. Penicillin therapy has proved helpful. The local treatment is similar to that recommended for Vincent's gingivitis (see p. 152), which is often the principal lesion.

Cancrum Oris.—This very fatal condition is now seldom seen except as a complication of kala-azar. It was perhaps related to the now extinct " hospital gangrene," and attacked children debilitated by acute infectious fevers. Various bacteria have been isolated, but there is no conclusive proof that cancrum oris is due to any one organism. The lesion first appears as an indurated area on the under-surface of a lip. This soon becomes an ulcer, and is followed by a gangrenous process destroying the lips, cheeks, and gums (fig. 148). In a few days the whole face sometimes becomes a black, putrefying mass. The treatment recommended in the past was to excise the area in the early stages with a cautery. Sulphonamides or penicillin have proved of value.

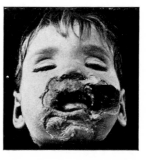

Fig. 148.—Cancrum oris.

Foot and Mouth Disease.—This well-known disease of cattle is occasionally transmitted to man by direct contact or through infected milk. A virus present in the fluid of the vesicles transmits the disease. The incubation period is from two to five days. In man the constitutional symptoms are usually of moderate severity. The buccal mucosa becomes congested and swollen, and two or three days later vesicles appear on the lips, tongue, cheek, and pharyngeal wall. Later the vesicles rupture, leaving tender, reddish, shallow ulcers, which soon heal. Similar lesions on the hands and feet, particularly round the nails, are usual. The attack confers no lasting immunity, and the same patient may have several visitations of the condition.

Treatment consists in potassium permanganate mouth-washes.

CYSTS

Retention cyst of the buccal mucous glands occurs from time to time in any part of the mucous surface of the mouth. It forms a translucent globular swelling which should be dissected out under local anæsthesia.

RANULA

A ranula[1] implies a *transparent* cystic swelling in the floor of the mouth, mainly, if not entirely, unilateral.

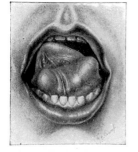

Fig. 149.—A large ranula.

Simple Ranula.—The patient may state that the swelling has come up before and burst, perhaps several times. If the swelling (fig. 149) is observed closely, tortuous veins are seen coursing over it, and at

---

[1] So named by Hippocrates, who likened this swelling to the belly of a little frog.

one point towards the apex the buccal mucosa seems deficient, as though the cyst was bursting through its covering. An opaque strand can often be made out traversing the anterior wall of the cyst ; this is Wharton's duct, which, although displaced by the cyst, takes no active part in the pathological process. Before concluding the examination the possibility of a deep prolongation of the cyst must be excluded by palpating beneath the jaw. The diagnosis of simple ranula is, as Butlin remarked, " plainly written on the face of the tumour."

Pathologically, a simple ranula is to be regarded as a myxomatous degeneration of a mucous gland. The gland at fault may be the sublingual, the gland of Blandin and Nuhn, or one of the solitary glands studded over the buccal mucous membrane. The gland of Blandin and Nuhn is a variable structure, which is situated in the inferior surface of the tongue (fig. 150).

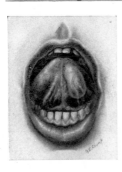

Fig. 150. — Myxomatous degeneration of the gland of Blandin and Nuhn.

Treatment.—*Complete Excision.*—A difficulty hindering ideal treatment is that the cyst bursts before dissection can be completed. If some of the fluid within the cyst can be aspirated before commencing enucleation, complete dissection is usually possible. Often, however, the contents are of the consistency of jelly, and will not flow through a hollow needle.

Partial Excision with Marsupialisation.—A considerable portion of the cyst wall, together with its superimposed mucous membrane, is removed. The cut edge of the cyst wall is then united by sutures to the cut edge of the mucous membrane; thus the cavity becomes part of the floor of the mouth.

Whichever method is practised, it is necessary to preserve the integrity of Wharton's duct.

DEEP OR PLUNGING RANULA

There still remains a group of cases which, from the mouth, appear to be typical ranulæ, but when the neck is examined a cervical prolongation is found continuous with the intrabuccal one. Possibly these cysts are derived from the cervical sinus—an embryological structure. At any rate, this hypothesis furnishes a logical basis for adequate surgery ; this type of ranula must be approached through the neck. Sometimes by this route complete extirpation is possible but, occasionally, the ramifications of the cyst render its complete removal impossible.

SUBLINGUAL DERMOID

Although congenital, sublingual dermoids are seldom noticed under the age of ten. The patient usually seeks advice between the ages of thirteen and twenty-five. These swellings are

Thomas Wharton, 1614–1673. Physician, St. Thomas's Hospital, London.
Phillipe Blandin, 1798–1849. Surgeon, Hôtel Dieu Hospital, Paris.
Anton Nuhn, 1814–1884. Professor of Anatomy, Heidelberg.

divided into two varieties, median and lateral. Each is again subdivided into those situated above and those situated below the diaphragm of the mouth (the mylo-hyoid muscles).

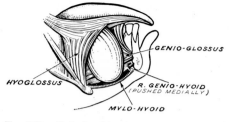

GENIO-GLOSSUS

HYOGLOSSUS

R. GENIO-HYOID (PUSHED MEDIALLY)

MYLO-HYOID

FIG. 151.—Relationships of a lateral sublingual dermoid situated above the mylo-hyoid.

Lateral variety.—*When situated above the mylo-hyoid* (fig. 151) there is an opaque, as opposed to a transparent, swelling (ranula) in the floor of the mouth to one side of the middle line.

When situated below the mylo-hyoid, a cystic swelling in the region of the submaxillary salivary gland is present.

Median variety.—*When situated above the mylo-hyoid*, the cyst often attains considerable dimensions (fig. 152) with, apparently, but little inconvenience.

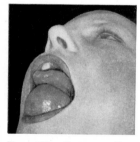

FIG. 152.—Large median sublingual dermoid.

When situated below the mylo-hyoid, the patient, if a female, often seeks advice because of a double chin. In this situation considerable care must be exercised in making a differential diagnosis, for it is not possible to rule out with certainty a supra-hyoid thyroglossal cyst. An ectopic thyroid must also be taken into consideration.

Lateral sublingual dermoids are probably derived from the second branchial cleft. The median variety, most probably, are derived from the mesobranchial field of His.

In all cases the swelling is a thin-walled cyst filled with sebaceous material, and, unlike other dermoid cysts, never contains hair.

Treatment of all varieties is removal by dissection through an external incision beneath the mandible.

TUMOURS

Hæmangioma sometimes occurs under the mucous membrane of the cheek and the floor of the mouth (see p. 114).

Wilhelm His, 1831–1904. Professor of Anatomy, Leipzig.

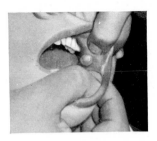

FIG. 153. — Papilloma of the mucous membrane of the cheek.

Papilloma is not uncommon, particularly on the mucous lining of the cheek (fig. 153).

Carcinoma may arise in any part of the mucous lining of the mouth. It is often the aftermath of some form of chronic irritation. Thus, in those Eastern races who indulge in chewing the betel-nut and store the quid thereof in their cheek, carcinoma of the mucous aspect of the cheek is a common occurrence. In Western races carcinoma of the mouth usually attacks the tongue and the floor of the mouth, and it will be considered fully in that section (see p. 167).

Mixed Tumour of a Molar Gland.—The molar glands are four or five in number. They lie on the outer side of the buccinator, their ducts piercing that muscle to open into the vestibule of the mouth. Cysts and mixed tumours, morphologically akin to the well-known mixed parotid tumour, occasionally occur in these glands. This is a convenient point to discuss briefly the differential diagnosis of other localised swellings of the cheek not arising in the integument or the mucous membrane.

A Lipoma developing in the Sucking Pad of the Infant.—The sucking pad is a ball of fat situated between the masseter and the buccinator. Well developed in infancy (fig. 154), it atrophies during childhood. On occasions a lipoma arises in the vestige which remains.

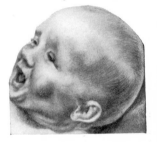

FIG. 154.—Well-developed sucking pad.

Adenitis of the Facial Lymph Node.—Few individuals possess a facial lymph node ; consequently infection coursing along the lymphatics of the cheek usually passes direct to the submaxillary nodes. When a facial lymph node is present its enlargement will perplex the diagnostician unaware of its existence.

THE TONGUE

TONGUE-TIE

Tongue-tie is really very rare, though nearly every mother fears that her firstborn is tongue-tied. A former generation of surgeons must have agreed

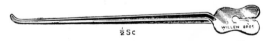

FIG. 155.—Director with guard and frænum slit.

with the mothers ; for witness, the grooved director (fig. 155) is even to-day fitted with a guard for use when dividing the frænum linguæ. This shield is held against the uplifted tongue and the frænum snipped near the floor of the mouth, the better to avoid the frænal artery. The operation must be done with prudence, for if the frænum is divided too deeply, the over-mobile tongue may be " swallowed " and asphyxia result.

MUSCULAR MACROGLOSSIA

This condition is practically confined to idiots and cretins (see p. 221). The large tongue protrudes from the mouth, and is liable to become dry and cracked. It is constantly being bitten, and there is no doubt that if the patient has attained the age of three the protruding portion should be excised.

Macroglossia may also be due to acute inflammation, syphilis, lymph-angioma, and chronic mercurial poisoning. The first three of these will receive consideration in their appropriate sections.

CONGENITAL FISSURED TONGUE (Syn. CONGENITAL FURROWING)

When a patient presents a fissured tongue, too often it is assumed that he or she is suffering from hereditary or acquired syphilis. Fissures, even deep fissures, are often due to congenital furrowing. John Thomson, after a study of a large number of cases, showed that the furrowing of the tongue was not present at birth, but was acquired in early childhood, and in his opinion it was due to tongue sucking. What is very important is that in congenital fissured tongue the fissures are *always transverse* (fig. 156), whereas in syphilitic fissured tongue they are inclined to be longitudinal.

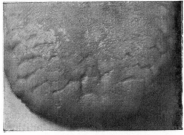

Fig. 156.—Congenital fissured tongue. Note the transverse direction of the fissures.

INJURIES

Anæsthetists are familiar with the possibility of the unconscious patient biting his tongue, and so commonly does this accident occur in epileptics that attendants are provided with rubber gags to put between the patient's teeth when a seizure is imminent. The most common deep wound of the tongue follows a blow or a fall while the patient is smoking a pipe, which breaks and is driven into the musculature of the tongue.

As a means of checking severe hæmorrhage from the posterior part of the tongue, Heath recommended passing the finger as far back as possible and hooking the tongue forward on to the jaw, and so applying pressure on the lingual artery.

Sutured wounds of the tongue heal readily with simple mouth-washes, and an almost completely divided segment, if sutured into position, will often remain viable and unite.

ACUTE SUPERFICIAL GLOSSITIS

This condition may follow scalds or other injuries. Under this heading may be included herpes of the tongue. Healing

John Thomson, 1856–1926. Physician, Hospital for Sick Children, Edinburgh.
Christopher Heath, 1835–1905. Surgeon, University College Hospital, London.

occurs readily under treatment by weak antiseptic alkaline mouth-washes. Acute superficial glossitis may also be due to an

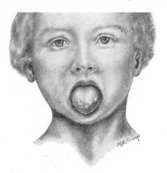

FIG. 157.—Acute glossitis. Vincent's spirillum was isolated from a specimen of serum removed from one of the vesicles.

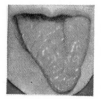

FIG. 158.— "Smooth sore tongue" due to vitamin B (riboflavin) deficiency.

infection by Vincent's spirillum (fig. 157) and to riboflavin deficiency (fig. 158).

ACUTE PARENCHYMATOUS GLOSSITIS

In well-marked cases the tongue swells enormously, protrudes from the mouth, and threatens life by asphyxiation. The patient often becomes extremely toxic. The condition, which is rare, arises in a number of different ways :

1. Classically, a wasp inserts its sting into the tongue of a holiday-maker who is quaffing ginger-beer from a bottle which has been left open.

2. From pyogenic infection of a deep lingual wound.

3. As a part of Ludwig's angina (see p. 196).

In severe cases it is necessary to be prepared for tracheotomy, which, however, is seldom actually required if the patient is treated as follows. Ice is applied to the tongue, oxygen inhaled as required, and the patient is reassured. In ultra-acute cases the œdematous tongue must be incised.

CHRONIC SUPERFICIAL GLOSSITIS (Syn. LEUKOPLAKIA GLOSSITIS)

Ætiology.—90 per cent. of patients with well-marked leukoplakia glossitis have a positive Wassermann reaction. Syphilis, in addition to some local irritation, is a frequent predisposing cause. The ætiological factors can be well summarised as *S*moking, *S*yphilis, *S*harp tooth, *S*epsis, *S*pirits, and *S*pices.

Clinical Features.—Chronic superficial glossitis passes through five stages :

Stage 1.—Enlargement of the papillæ is noticeable.

Stage 2.—There is an overgrowth of epithelium, which becomes sodden. It is during the second stage that the classical picture develops. The tongue is " as though covered with

Wilhelm von Ludwig, 1790–1865. *Professor of Surgery and Midwifery, University of Tübingen.*
August von Wassermann, 1866–1925. *Director, Institute for Experimental Therapy, Berlin.*

white paint which has hardened, dried, and cracked " (Butlin)
(fig. 159). The condition is painless.

Stage 3.—The epithelium is shed, sometimes over a considerable area. The " red glazed tongue " becomes an easily

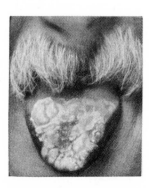

FIG. 159. — Leukoplakia,
second stage of glossitis.

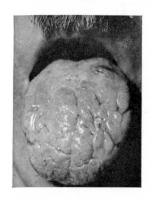

FIG. 160.—Chronic super-
ficial glossitis, fourth stage.
(*Dr. Crawford.*)

recognised clinical entity. Nerve terminals are exposed and
the tongue is painful.

Stage 4.—Submucous fibrosis occurs, causing cracks and
fissures (fig. 160).

Stage 5.—Chronic superficial glossitis is an established pre-
cancerous condition, and by the time the fifth stage has appeared
the development of a carcinoma in one of the warty projections,
ulcers, or fissures is not far distant, if it has not occurred already.

Treatment.—Remove the cause. Institute thorough anti-
syphilitic and dental treatment in necessary cases. Stop pipe
smoking altogether. Spirit drinking must be given up. A mild
antiseptic alkaline mouth-wash is prescribed, and the patient
is advised to smear some white vaseline over his tongue before
he retires. " Touching up " the patches with caustics of any
kind should be eschewed rigorously, as the development of
carcinoma is thereby encouraged. It is essential for the patient
to report once a fortnight, when the clinician reviews the
case, watching for the possible development of malignancy.
If, after a reasonable time, the condition is not improving, or
if it is getting worse, the affected portion of mucous membrane,
together with a thin slice of the underlying muscle, is removed.

Sir Henry Butlin, 1845–1912.   Surgeon, St. Bartholomew's Hospital, London.

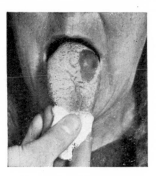

FIG. 161.—" Dyspeptic " tongue.

GEOGRAPHICAL TONGUE OF CHILDREN

Red rings with a yellow border are characteristic. The distribution is, as the name implies, irregular, and the disease runs a very chronic course. Itching and salivation are the leading symptoms. The treatment follows general lines.

RAW TONGUE (*Syn.* DYSPEPTIC TONGUE)

On some part of the dorsum there is a sore red surface deprived of its filiform papillæ (fig. 161). The area is not ulcerated ; it is partially denuded of epithelium. Raw tongue must be distinguished from a scald ; the history of a burn or scald is too well engraved on the patient's memory to make the differential diagnosis obscure. Again, the red tongue of pernicious anæmia is easily differentiated, as in the latter the redness is not localised to one area.

Treatment.—The soreness is lessened by painting with 2 per cent. chromic acid. With simple mouth-washes and attention to dental hygiene gradual improvement can be expected, but the condition is apt to recur.

BLACK OR "HAIRY" TONGUE

is an interesting, but rare, condition. Usually the " hair " is mainly confined to the centre of the tongue in front of the lingual V (sulcus terminalis) (fig. 162). The cause of the elongation and blackening of the filiform papillæ (hair) is unknown. Some consider the condition is due to bacteria, others to a fungus, the Aspergillus niger, spores of which are black.

Treatment by painting, mouth-washes, and so on has proved to be unsatisfactory. We have removed the affected area by electro-coagulation in two cases with satisfactory results.

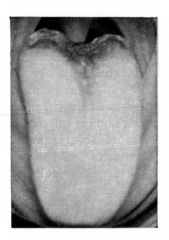

FIG. 162. — Black or hairy tongue.

GLOSSITIS RHOMBICA MEDIANA

There is a rhomboid mass situated in the middle line of the dorsum of the tongue, just anterior to the foramen cæcum. The condition may be due to a persistence of the tuberculum impar, but is more likely to be an inflammatory mass. The Wassermann reaction is negative, and those unfamiliar with the condition usually mistake it for a carcinoma. Biopsy shows epithelial thickening and sub-epithelial lymphocytic infiltration. When there is doubt as to the nature of the disease or cancerphobia exists, the lesion should be excised.

LINGUAL TUBERCULOSIS

The only tuberculous lesion of the tongue which is at all common is **tuberculous ulceration.** These shallow ulcers, often multiple and situated on the edges of the tongue near the tip, are extremely painful. In the majority of cases the patient has advanced phthisis, and the infection is carried to the tongue by the sputum. The main object of treatment is to relieve the intense pain. A decicain tablet quickly renders the area insensitive for about an hour. Painting the ulcers with a 50 per cent. solution of lactic acid sometimes improves matters, but as long as infected sputum is coughed up, the condition is liable to recur.

Very rarely, tuberculous nodes are present on the dorsum. Another exceptional tuberculous manifestation is an ulcer of considerable dimensions, which, without histological aid, is unlikely to be diagnosed correctly.

ACTINOMYCOSIS OF THE TONGUE

is rarely encountered. It gives rise to an indurated intralingual lesion, which later may go on to abscess formation. The condition has been compared with the " wooden tongue " of cattle, but, as Zachary Cope has pointed out, such a simile is erroneous, for " wooden tongue " of cattle is due to an infection with a bacillus and not to the ray fungus.

SYPHILIS OF THE TONGUE

Primary Syphilis.—An extra-genital chancre can occur on the tongue (see fig. 24). The submaxillary and submental lymph nodes become greatly enlarged, as in the case of a similar lesion on the lip.

Secondary Syphilis :

1. *Multiple shallow* (" *snail track* ") *ulcers* may be present on the sides and under-surface, and they have to be distinguished from tuberculous ulcers (vide supra).

2. *Mucous patches* occur on the tongue as well as on the fauces.

3. *Hutchinson's wart*, really a condyloma, is a strictly median " wart," and has to be distinguished from an ordinary simple papilloma which happens to occupy the middle line.

Tertiary Syphilis :

1. *Gumma of the tongue* nearly always occupies the middle line (fig. 163). It possesses the characteristics of gummata elsewhere and does not tether the tongue.

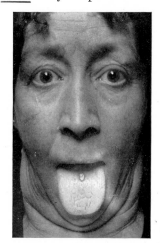

FIG. 163.—Gumma of the tongue.

*V. Zachary Cope, Contemporary. Consulting Surgeon, St. Mary's Hospital, London.
Sir Jonathan Hutchinson, 1828–1913. Surgeon, London Hospital.*

2. *Parenchymatous Gummatous Infiltration.*—The whole tongue is enlarged—indeed, it may be called syphilitic macroglossia. The tongue eventually becomes fibrotic.

3. The frequency of chronic superficial glossitis in syphilitic patients has been noted already.

ULCERS OF THE TONGUE

It is advisable at this stage to review briefly the more common types of ulcers of the tongue, as their differential diagnosis is so important in the practical application of clinical surgery.

Non-specific.—**Dyspeptic ulcer** is a small rounded painful erosion with a white centre. It often occurs near the tip of the tongue, and is more common, not in the " chronic dyspeptic individual," but during adolescent life.

Dental ulcer occurs always at the side of the tongue. It is inclined to be rather elongated, after the nature of a scratch or crack. It is usually painful, but not necessarily so. A decayed or broken tooth, or the clasp of a denture, will be found to be the causative agent.

Post-pertussis ulcer is seen at the frænum linguæ. Of necessity, this occurs only in children with whooping-cough.

Specific.—**Tuberculous ulcers** are usually multiple, and situated at the edges and the tip of the tongue. The leading characteristic is that they are agonisingly painful.

Syphilitic Ulcer.—The most typical is the gumma situated in the middle line of the dorsum rather nearer the base than the tip of the tongue.

Malignant.—**Carcinomatous ulcer** has typically the clinical features of a squamous-celled carcinoma—viz. an everted edge and an indurated base.

If doubt exists as to the nature of an ulcer—and it is sometimes difficult to be certain when dealing with cases of early carcinoma—a fragment should be removed under local anæsthesia and submitted to histological examination. In this instance a Wassermann reaction is not of much value in establishing a confident diagnosis, for so commonly a patient with carcinoma of the tongue has a positive reaction.

NEOPLASMS OF THE TONGUE

Benign neoplasms are comparatively rare. They are completely overshadowed by the appalling frequency of carcinoma of this organ. Lipomata, fibromata, plexiform neuromata, and even osteomata occur from time to time.

Papilloma is the commonest benign tumour of the tongue. It may be sessile or pedunculated. To ensure non-recurrence, it should be excised, preferably with a diathermy knife, together with a small wedge of normal tissue about its base.

Lymphangioma.—When noticed soon after birth there is usually only a small circumscribed patch of dilated lymph-vessels. This may remain stationary in size for long periods, but more often increases rapidly. Attacks of inflammation occur at irregular intervals. At last the swollen tongue permanently protrudes from the mouth—lymphangiomatous macroglossia. Treatment by radium has given encouraging results. When this fails, partial glossectomy must be performed.

Angioma in this situation is usually venous (fig. 164). The veins which form the tumour are liable to become wounded and bleed. Such hæmorrhage may be so persistent as to render the patient severely anæmic, as we have witnessed. The treatment is excision of the tumour : a diathermy knife is particularly useful in this instance.

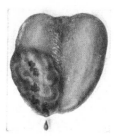

Fig. 164.—Venous hæmangioma of the tongue in a woman of twenty-three.

Lingual thyroid (see p. 207).

MALIGNANT TUMOURS

Carcinoma of the Tongue is less frequent than it was a generation or two ago. More thorough treatment of syphilis, the passing of the clay pipe and the price of tobacco, the welcome activity of our dental colleagues, and possibly the decrease in the consumption of spirituous liquors, are the chief reasons for this decline. Notwithstanding, the disease is still common.

Site.—" The whole tongue is not affected with cancer to the same degree ; the root and back part is seldom attacked, the tip itself is also very free ; next comes the under-surface of the tongue, while the dorsum is peculiarly liable to the disease, especially at the borders " (Fitzwilliams).

Clinical Features.—The patient is nearly always a middle-aged or elderly man ; the condition is rarely encountered in women. If he is observant, the patient seeks advice because of the actual lesion on his tongue. The carcinoma, which is squamous-celled, may take the form of—

1. An ulcer (fig. 165).
2. A warty outgrowth.
3. A fissure.

Duncan C. L. Fitzwilliams, Contemporary. Consulting Surgeon, St. Mary's Hospital, London.

4. An indurated mass. This variety is exceptional.

It is a sad fact that a large number of patients fail to notice or else disregard the lesion in its early stages, and report because of one or more of the later symptoms, which are :

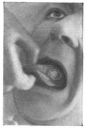

FIG. 165.—Carcinomatous ulcer of the tongue.

1. *Pain.*—This may be in the tongue or referred to the ear. The latter is not unusual, and many a patient with carcinoma of the tongue comes with a wad of cottonwool in his ear, complaining solely of earache. The explanation of this phenomenon is that the lingual nerve is irritated, and the pain is referred to another branch of the third division of the fifth cranial nerve, to wit, the auriculotemporal.

2. *Salivation.*—Profuse salivary secretion is common in lingual carcinoma. It is well known that if an elderly man, sitting in the surgical out-patient department, is seen to be constantly spitting into his handkerchief, it is highly probable that his case is one of carcinoma of the tongue. In late stages the saliva is blood-stained.

3. *Ankyloglossia.*—The tongue cannot protrude fully and deviates to the affected side. This bespeaks extensive carcinomatous infiltration of the lingual musculature or the floor of the mouth.

4. *Dysphagia.*—The patient experiences difficulty in swallowing. This symptom is more pronounced when the growth is in the posterior third of the tongue.

5. *Inability to Articulate Clearly.*—Factors 2, 3, and 4 may all play a part (fig. 166).

6. *Fœtor.*—The patient becomes offensive to his associates because of the secondary bacterial stomatitis.

7. *A lump in the neck,* due to secondary deposits in the cervical lymphatic nodes.

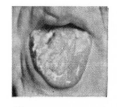

FIG. 166. — The patient sought advice because of difficulty in speaking and swallowing. Referred from a radiotherapist as growth unsuitable for radiotherapy. (See fig. 168, p. 171.)

A growth situated right at the back of the tongue may not unreasonably escape the notice of an intelligent patient and even of his careful medical adviser. *Early alteration of the voice* is often a feature of these cases. Palpation of the posterior part of the tongue and laryngoscopic examination are cardinal methods in arriving at the diagnosis.

Before leaving the subject of clinical features of carcinoma of the tongue, the reader's attention is drawn to the importance of precarcinomatous conditions, particularly chronic superficial glossitis (p. 162), chronic dental ulcer (p. 166), papilloma (p. 167), and occasionally (in women) the Plummer-Vinson syndrome (see p. 259). The thorough treatment of these conditions would doubtless prevent many cases of lingual carcinoma.

Spread of the Disease.—Carcinoma of the *anterior two-thirds of the tongue* tends to invade the floor of the mouth but seldom spreads across the middle line. The regional lymph nodes soon become invaded (fig. 167). There is often microscopical evidence of carcinomatous infiltration in the upper jugular chain of lymph nodes. In a case of some standing the stony-hard enlargement of this group is found only too often. Carcinoma of the *posterior third of the tongue* tends to spread to the soft palate and the pharynx. Metastatic involvement of the lymphatic nodes of the jugular chain of each side occurs early.

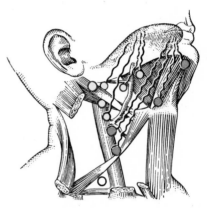

FIG. 167.—The primary lymph nodes of the tongue. Green—drain the tip and anterior third. Yellow—drain the dorsum and posterior two-thirds.

(After Taylor and Nathanson.)

Carcinoma of the tongue is a disease which is essentially confined to the mouth and neck. Untreated, it runs a variable, but inevitably fatal, course. Death occurs usually in one of the following ways :

1. *Inhalation broncho-pneumonia,* from the superadded oral sepsis.

2. *Combined cancerous cachexia and starvation.*

3. *Hæmorrhage,* from the primary growth, or secondary lymph nodes, eroding an artery.

4. *Asphyxia,* which is due either to secondary carcinomatous cervical lymph nodes pressing upon the air passages or to œdema

Henry S. Plummer, 1874–1936. Physician, Mayo Clinic, Rochester, U.S.A.
Porter P. Vinson, Contemporary. Physician, Mayo Clinic, Rochester, U.S.A.

of the glottis. The latter is rare, and occurs as an extension of lymphatic œdema around a growth at the back of the tongue.

Treatment.—There is no doubt that a primary growth situated in the anterior two-thirds of the tongue should be treated by interstitial irradiation with radium needles implanted into the tongue, unless :

(*a*) The growth is no longer confined to the tongue, but involves the mandible.

(*b*) The growth is of the scirrhous, infiltrating type with œdema and sepsis.

(*c*) The surface area occupied by the growth is very extensive.

(*d*) Irradiation has failed. (Sir Stanford Cade.)

Interstitial Irradiation.—Most patients should be rendered edentulous, certainly all carious teeth should be removed. Radiation can be started within a few days, the necessary dental extractions having been undertaken. Radium needles containing from 0·6 mg. to 2 mg. of radium, screened by 0·5 mm. of platinum, are inserted into and around the growth, parallel to each other and 1 cm. apart. The eye ends of the needles should be just below the mucous membrane.

For a lesion the diameter of 2·5 cm. and 1·5 cm. depth, 6 needles containing 1·3 mg. each and 2 needles containing 2 mg. each would be used, containing in all 11·8 mg. A dose of between 6,000 r. and 9,000 r. is thus delivered in seven days.

In cases of Carcinoma of the posterior third of the Tongue and of the Vallecula it is difficult to place needles in position accurately ; the treatment of choice is external irradiation with large masses of radium, i.e. teleradium or X-rays, or a combination of both these methods of radiation.

Several ports of entry are used in order to bring the tumour dose to 6,000 r.–7,000 r., which is the dose required to destroy the growth, and at the same time cause as little damage as possible to the skin.

Partial Glossectomy.—The growth is excised with a diathermy knife. When possible the incision should include three-quarters of an inch (2 cm.) of healthy tissue upon all sides of the neoplasm. Preliminary ligation of the external carotid artery is usually advisable. It is convenient to dissect the lymph nodes of the neck and at the same time tie this artery before removing the primary growth.

Sir Stanford Cade, Contemporary. Surgeon, Westminster Hospital, London.

Total glossectomy, in cases where radium is unsuitable or is not available, sometimes gives surprisingly good results (fig. 168). After splitting the lower lip in the mid-line, the incision is carried down to the level of the hyoid bone. The mandible is bisected, and the whole tongue removed.

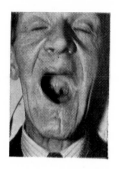

FIG. 168.—Total glossectomy. The patient, who had lived in France, can converse freely in French as well as English.

THE CERVICAL LYMPHATIC NODES IN RELATION TO TREATMENT OF CARCINOMA OF THE TONGUE

In about 50 per cent. of cases of carcinoma of the tongue, there is no palpable involvement of the cervical lymph nodes when the patient comes under observation for the first time. As a complete block dissection of the neck (see p. 203) is a very severe undertaking, it should only be employed when absolutely necessary. A practical method is to examine the patient at monthly intervals after the primary lesion has been treated. If, after the second month, enlarged lymphatic nodes are palpable, it must be presumed that they are not inflammatory, and a block dissection on the side of the original lesion is undertaken. The patient is then once more examined at monthly intervals, and should palpable lymph nodes appear on the contralateral side, a block dissection must be advised as soon as the patient is in a fit condition to withstand it. With slight modifications to suit individual cases, this plan has been found to be in the best interests of these patients, who are usually elderly.

In debilitated and old patients a block dissection of the neck is out of the question, and reliance must be placed on deep X-ray therapy.

SARCOMA OF THE TONGUE

Sarcoma of the tongue is very rare, and almost invariably fatal. An example came under our observation. The patient was a man of twenty-eight, who complained of a lump in the left side of the tongue. Deep X-ray therapy caused the lump to disappear, and the nodes of the left side of the neck were removed. Two months later enlarged lymph nodes appeared in the right side and a block dissection was carried out. A few months later the sarcoma became widely disseminated, and death resulted.

CHAPTER X

THE SALIVARY GLANDS

THE PAROTID GLAND

Acute Parotitis.—Acute inflammation of the parotid gland is now comparatively rare.

In the early days of abdominal surgery the importance of oral hygiene (i.e. cleansing the mouth and swabbing the buccal mucous membrane with boroglycerol by the nurse at regular intervals) was not appreciated ; furthermore, after laparotomy the patient was forbidden to drink for several days. These circumstances favoured an ascending infection from the parched infected mouth along Stensen's duct to the parotid gland, and *acute post-operative parotitis* was a frequent and dreaded complication of abdominal operations.

Acute parotitis is sometimes a complication of intercurrent debilitating disease, e.g. typhoid, but many cases occur spontaneously. In contradistinction to epidemic parotitis (mumps), usually one parotid gland alone is affected.

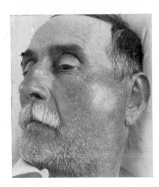

FIG. 169.—Acute parotitis.

As a rule bacteria reach the gland by retrograde infection from the mouth. In fulminating cases the causative organism is nearly always the staphylococcus aureus. In some of the less severe examples the pneumococcus is responsible.

Clinical Features.—There is a brawny swelling of the side of the face, as is well shown in fig. 169. General signs of toxæmia are variable. When they are in evidence, early decompression of the gland is called for urgently. Examination of the orifice of Stensen's duct may reveal pus or purulent saliva being discharged.

Treatment.—If acute parotitis threatens, no effort should be spared to cleanse the mouth. Boroglycerol is a useful adjunct in this respect. A sialogogue, in the form of chewing-gum or penicillin lozenges, is also valuable.

Early unilateral cases may respond to penicillin therapy.

Niels Stensen, 1638–1686. Copenhagen anatomist, physiologist, and a bishop.

Deep X-ray therapy has also been found effective when resorted to early. Exposures to the affected gland are given daily for five or six days.

Fulminating Cases.—When the response to the above measures is not obvious within forty-eight hours, and particularly in bilateral cases, early decompression of the gland or glands is strongly recommended. It should be noted that penicillin may mask the general symptoms, but the glandular swelling will still be in evidence.

Decompression of the Parotid Salivary Gland.—Local anæsthesia is entirely satisfactory. Blair's method should be employed. A vertical incision is made down to the capsule of the gland. With suitable undercutting of the skin nearly the whole of the parotid gland can be exposed (fig. 170). In order to spare the branches of the facial nerve, the capsule is incised transversely, if necessary in several places. The skin is closed with a few interrupted sutures and drainage is provided at the lower end of the wound. Thirteen consecutive patients treated by us in this way recovered. In the fourteenth case, which was bilateral, too much confidence was placed in penicillin therapy, and decompression of the glands was undertaken too late.

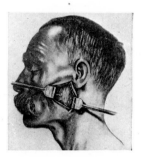

Fig. 170.—Blair's incision for exposing the parotid gland.

If decompression is not performed, provided the patient is not overwhelmed by toxæmia, suppurative parotitis goes on to abscess formation. The abscess may burst externally, usually between the bony and cartilaginous parts of the external auditory meatus.

Recurrent sub-acute and chronic parotitis are rather more common conditions. In more severe forms the pneumococcus is often responsible (Payne). The streptococcus viridans is commonly found in chronic cases. Children and young women (fig. 171) are the usual sufferers. Inspection of the orifice of Stensen's duct while gentle pressure is exerted over the gland often reveals a gush of purulent saliva in process of ejection (fig. 172), and the diagnosis, which up to that time is often in doubt, becomes indisputable. Parotid calculus (p. 175) must be elimin-

Vilray P. Blair, Contemporary. Professor of Oral Surgery, University of Washington.
Reginald T. Payne, Contemporary. Attached to British Post-graduate Hospital, London.

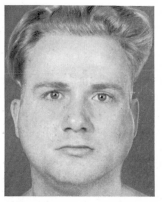

FIG. 171.—Bilateral chronic bacterial parotitis. Present for nine months. Slight variations in the size of the swellings noticed.

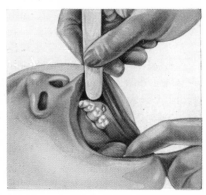

FIG. 172.—Purulent saliva being ejected from Stensen's duct.

ated. Ill-fitting dentures, by pressing on the orifices of Stensen's ducts, can cause symptoms similar to those of chronic parotitis ; indeed, by obstructing salivary secretion they predispose to actual infection.

Sialography is an important method of investigation in chronic cases. A watery (not thick and oily) solution of lipiodol, such as Neo-Hydriol (May & Baker), is injected into Stensen's duct and an enlightening radiograph of the parotid tree is often

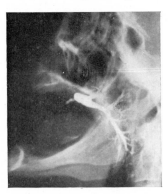

obtained. By this means obstruction by a parotid calculus is eliminated. In chronic parotitis the ducts and acini are dilated (fig. 173).

Treatment.—Oral hygiene and chemotherapy can be tried, but are usually disappointing. In our experience, patients with chronic parotitis are benefited, often dramatically, by catheterising Stensen's duct with a fine ureteric catheter and injecting a bland antiseptic fluid, such as 1 per cent. mercurochrome.

FIG. 173.—Sialograph in a case of chronic parotitis.

CONGENITAL PAROTID SIALECTASIS

Sialectasis means literally a state of dilatation of the ductules and alveoli of any salivary gland, but it is the parotid that is always affected. The condition is usually unilateral, and the symptoms commence in infancy or in very early life, but are seldom diagnosed correctly until the patient has at least reached puberty. Attacks of painful swelling of the gland, often accompanied by considerable pyrexia, are usually diagnosed as anomalous mumps until their repetition makes such a diagnosis absurd. Sialography reveals no obstruction to Stensen's duct or the main

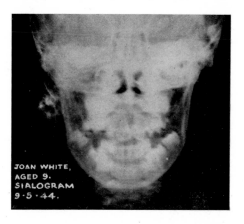

JOAN WHITE,
AGED 9.
SIALOGRAM
9·5·44.

Fig. 174.—Sialogram displaying sialectasis.

branches of the parotid tree, but the ductules and alveoli are grossly dilated (fig. 174).

Five cases failing to respond to any form of conservative measures have been treated by one of us by complete parotidectomy, with satisfactory results.

PAROTID CALCULUS

Compared with submaxillary, parotid calculi occur infrequently. The symptoms are those one would expect—a painful swelling of the gland, especially at meal-times. To suspect a parotid calculus is easier than to establish the diagnosis conclusively, for a small calculus is often difficult to visualise by radiography. It is in this condition that sialography is particularly valuable.

Fig. 175.—Stones in the parotid gland.

If the stone can be palpated from within the mouth it can be removed by slitting up Stensen's duct, but we are seldom so favoured. More often it is deeply placed within the parotid tree. In our experience the best method of treatment is to expose the gland by Blair's incision (see fig. 170) and remove the calculus through a transverse incision in the gland substance. This method has proved eminently satisfactory, and in no case has a parotid fistula developed. Many of the scars are difficult to discern after a year.

SALIVARY FISTULA

A salivary fistula may be <u>internal or external</u>. As an internal fistula does not give rise to symptoms, and as an external fistula of the sub-maxillary gland is both rare and cured readily by removal of that gland, the subject resolves itself into a consideration of the troublesome condition *external fistula of the parotid.*

Parotid Fistula.—Every time the patient has a meal, smells food, or even thinks of it, there is an outpouring of parotid secretion on to the cheek. Apart from the annoyance of such a phenomenon, the skin in the neighbourhood tends to become excoriated. These fistulæ usually follow a badly placed incision for the opening of a parotid abscess, but may be an aftermath of a penetrating wound. A salivary fistula which has persisted for several months seldom closes spontaneously.

Sialography is invaluable in these cases. It will indicate whether a main duct has been severed or if it is a ductule which is communicating with the surface. From the information gained by sialography the proper course to adopt for the cure of the fistula can be formulated.

Treatment.—In those cases in which the fistula is proved by sialography to be connected with a minor branch of the parotid tree, X-ray treatment is valuable. In other circumstances operative measures must be invoked. Of many plans suggested, Newman and Seabrook's is the most satisfactory.

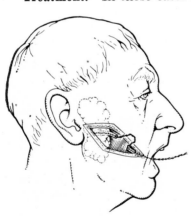

FIG. 176.—Newman and Seabrook's operation for parotid fistula.

<u>Prophylactic general penicillin therapy is administered twenty-four hours before the operation.</u> One <u>probe</u> is introduced through the orifice of Stensen's duct and another through <u>the external fistula.</u> With the probes in position, a suitable incision is made in the cheek, so as to display Stensen's duct and the area of gland containing the probes. After a tedious dissection to free the severed conducting mechanism of the gland, No. 10 <u>tantalum wire</u>, which is twisted on itself, <u>is passed as shown in fig. 176.</u> Any portion of the twisted wire that lies exposed is buried with fine catgut sutures, and the skin is closed. The distal end of the wire is suitably bent around the corner of the mouth, and anchored there by adhesive plaster.

Saul Charles Newman, Contemporary. Assistant in Otolaryngology, New York Post-Graduate Hospital.
Dean Baynard Seabrook, Contemporary. Assistant Clinical Professor of Surgery, Oregon University, U.S.A.

Post-operative Treatment.—Penicillin therapy is continued for several days.   Oral hygiene is most important, and each day the wire splint is moved very gently ; it should remain in place for three and a half weeks.

Division of the auriculo-temporal nerve has been recommended for the cure of parotid fistula, but we know of no first-hand case where this measure has been followed by a successful result.

AURICULO-TEMPORAL SYNDROME (FREY'S SYNDROME)

Most examples of this condition have followed damage of the auriculo-temporal nerve as a result of suppurative parotitis.   When the patient eats, the cheek becomes red, hot, and painful, and beads of perspiration appear upon it.   There is also hyperæsthesia of the face, especially during shaving.   The only effective treatment in severe cases is avulsion of the nerve.

NEOPLASMS

" **Mixed parotid tumour** " is a well-known clinical entity.   A hard, somewhat rounded, slowly growing neoplasm, nearly always commencing in that part of the parotid gland overlying the angle of the jaw (fig. 178), renders the diagnosis tolerably simple.   Usually benign for a varying period from several months up to ten or twenty years (fig. 177), it sooner or later breaks its confines, and exhibits characteristics of malignancy.   It now

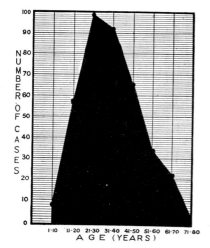

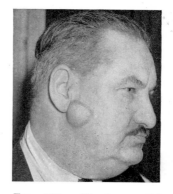

Fig. 177.—Ages at which mixed tumours of the parotid gland first appeared.

Fig. 178. — Mixed parotid tumour, typical location.

tends to invade the pterygoid fossa and the upper part of the neck, and sometimes causes facial paralysis from involvement of the seventh nerve.   When first seen in a comparatively advanced state it is difficult to diagnose from other malignant tumours of the region.

Lucie Frey, Contemporary.   Polish physician.

Pathology.—These tumours show varying histological characters (fig. 179), and from time to time have been found to contain fibrous, myxomatous, epithelial, and pseudo-cartilaginous tissue. Willis classifies them as follows :

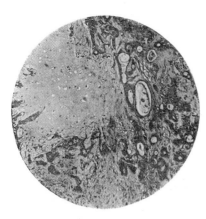

1. Pleomorphic adenoma = a localised mixed parotid tumour.

2. Pleomorphic adeno-carcinoma = a mixed parotid tumour with malignant change.

3. Anaplastic carcinoma = a highly malignant neoplasm from the commencement.

Fig. 179.—Microphotograph of a typical section of a mixed parotid tumour.

Adenolymphoma (*syn.* papillary cystadenoma lymphomatosum ; Warthin's tumour) is a well-encapsulated neoplasm filled with semisolid material. Histologically it consists of columnar epithelial cells with an underlying lymphoid stroma. This tumour feels less hard than most mixed parotid tumours, but it cannot be diagnosed clinically with any degree of certainty unless the tumour is bilateral. Elderly males are most often affected.

Treatment of Tumours of the Parotid Gland.

—While it is true that all tumours of the parotid gland tend to remain benign for long periods, a number become malignant in a comparatively short time. Unless *extracapsular excision* is carried out, recurrence usually takes place within two years. It is of paramount importance to realise that most of these tumours are radio-resistant. Consequently, if the tumour does not respond rapidly to deep X-ray therapy, the patient should be urged to have the tumour extirpated. The aim must be to excise the tumour, together with its capsule, without opening the latter.

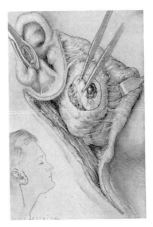

Fig. 180. — Extracapsular excision of a moderate-sized parotid tumour. The tumour must be removed with a layer of healthy parotid tissue without encroaching upon the capsule. Inset shows the skin incision.

R. A. Willis, Contemporary. *Professor of Pathology, Leeds.*
Aldred Scott Warthin, 1866–1931. *Professor of Pathology, University of Michigan.*

In order to accomplish this, good exposure (fig. 180) is essential. To enucleate the tumour and leave the capsule invites early recurrence and extension of the neoplasm, because tumour cells are spilled during the operation and many are left attached to the walls of the capsule which remains.

Parotidectomy is indicated (1) where the tumour has broken its confines and has commenced to enlarge comparatively rapidly, and (2) when the tumour has recurred after local excision.

Surgical Anatomy.—In many cases the branches of the seventh nerve do not traverse the substance of the parotid gland, but rather the parotid gland may be looked upon as having a large superficial and a smaller deep lobe, connected by an isthmus. The main trunks of the facial nerve, viz. the temporo-facial and cervico-facial divisions, embrace the isthmus (fig. 181) lying between the deep and superficial lobes. The outlying subdivisions of the nerve rest between the superficial lobe and the masseter muscle.

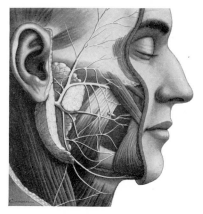

The possibility of excising the whole, or the greater part, of the parotid gland, which offers an excellent prospect of a lasting cure in an otherwise progressive condition, is too often dismissed in favour of palliative measures. The principal deterrent is the fear of facial palsy.

FIG. 181.—Showing the disposition of the seventh nerve in a case when the greater part of the superficial lobe has been removed.

It is difficult to understand why the possibility of facial palsy has deterred surgical enterprise, for the seventh nerve is so often implicated if the tumour is allowed to grow. As will be shown, facial paralysis is not an inevitable sequel to the operation, and even if it occurs, its baneful results, which are immeasurably less than those produced by a hideous tumour, can, in part, be mitigated.

While the patient must be warned that it may be impossible to preserve the facial nerve, provided the dissection is conducted with due regard to the disposition of the seventh nerve, it is often possible to resect a large portion or all of the parotid gland without permanent facial palsy ensuing (fig. 182). When the tumour belongs to type three, or is recurrent, it is often impossible,

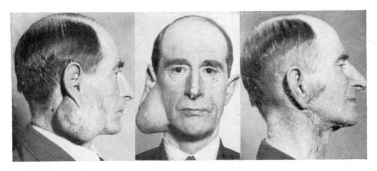

Fig. 182.—Mixed parotid tumour of over twenty years' duration, latterly increasing rapidly in size. Complete parotidectomy under local anæsthesia with preliminary ligation of the external carotid artery. The facial nerve was preserved, as can be seen from the photograph taken three weeks after the operation. The patient was free from recurrence four years later.

and indeed inadvisable, to spare the seventh nerve at the expense of complete extirpation of the growth.

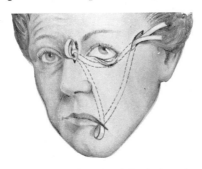

Fig. 183.—A strip of fascia lata inserted subcutaneously as shown helps to overcome the deformity of facial palsy.

(*After Lodge.*)

If, during parotidectomy, it is found impracticable to preserve the seventh cranial nerve, the resulting deformity can be mitigated later, to a large extent, by a plastic procedure such as that illustrated in fig. 183, or by substituting tantalum wire for the fascia.

THE SUBMAXILLARY SALIVARY GLAND

Calculus.—The submaxillary salivary gland and Wharton's duct are the most common sites for a salivary calculus. Indeed, they are more than fifty times more frequent here than in the parotid gland and its duct. These stones vary in size (fig. 184). One no larger than a millet seed may give rise to troublesome symptoms. At the other end of the scale relatively enormous specimens ($1\frac{1}{2} \times 1$ inch ($3 \cdot 75 \times 2 \cdot 5$ cm.)) have been recorded.

Composition.—By chemical analysis it has been demonstrated that salivary calculi and the " tartar " which collects upon teeth are almost identical. Berzelius gave the composition as follows :

Phosphates of lime and magnesia	.	.	79·0
Salivary mucus	.	.	.	.	12·5
Ptyalin .	.	.	.	.	1·0
Animal matter soluble in HCl	.	.	7·5

William O. Lodge, Contemporary. Ophthalmic Surgeon, Royal Halifax Infirmary.
Thomas Wharton, 1614–1673. Physician, St. Thomas's Hospital, London.
Jön Jakob Berzelius, 1779–1848. Professor of Chemistry, Berlin.

Swelling of the gland before or during meals is pathognomonic of the condition. Enlargement of the submaxillary
gland (fig. 185) can often be seen in these cases when the patient

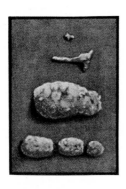

FIG. 184. — Various
types of submaxillary
salivary calculi (actual
size).

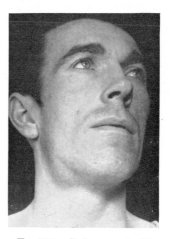

FIG. 185.—Enlargement of the
submaxillary salivary gland due
to a calculus in Wharton's duct.

is given something sour to taste. The orifice of Wharton's duct
should be examined in a strong light, comparing the two sides.
If the stone is in Wharton's duct, it can be detected by direct
palpation.

Salivary colic sometimes occurs, typically at the commencement of a
meal. The pain is described by the patient as like toothache ; on this
account he is liable to be referred to the dentist. The pain is also sometimes referred to the tongue ; this is due to irritation of the lingual nerve as
it hooks around Wharton's duct.

Radiology.—Submaxillary calculi, being rich in mineral salts,
usually cast a good X-ray shadow (fig. 186), but their density
varies. Stones, particularly in the
gland itself, are sometimes difficult or
impossible to demonstrate by X-rays.

Treatment.—A stone in Wharton's
duct can be removed under local
anæsthesia by fixing the stone and then
making an incision on to it in the long
axis of the duct. Alternatively, the
duct can be split up. There is no need
to suture the incision.

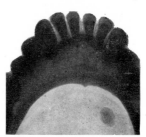

FIG. 186.—Radiograph of
stone in Wharton's duct.

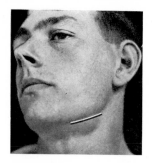

Fig. 187. — Incision for excising the submaxillary salivary gland.

For cases of calculi within the gland, extirpation of the submaxillary gland through an incision beneath the mandible is to be advised, and it will be found best to undertake the latter measure in all cases of recurrent submaxillary stones. The patient is in no way affected by the loss of one submaxillary salivary gland. The skin incision should be made in the position indicated in fig. 187. The lower edge of the incision is dissected from the mylohyoid muscle, which is incised at a lower level and retracted upwards. In this way the mandibular branch of the seventh nerve is protected from injury.

Neoplasms.—Mixed tumours of the submaxillary salivary gland (fig. 188) are not excessively rare. If diagnosed reasonably early, the treatment is eminently satisfactory, for the submaxillary salivary gland can be readily excised *in toto*. In this

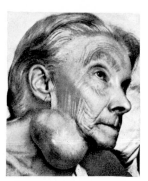

Fig. 188.—Mixed tumour of the submaxillary salivary gland. Duration forty years.

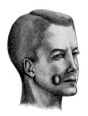

Fig. 189.—Characteristic swelling of a mixed tumour of a molar gland. It lies superficial to the buccinator muscle.
(*After Fifield.*)

connection it should be noted that from time to time mixed tumours occur in a buccal (*syn.* molar) (fig. 189) or a palatal gland. This is not extraordinary, for are not these glands which are scattered throughout the buccal mucous lining of the mouth tiny accessory salivary glands ?

Carcinoma of the submaxillary salivary gland also occurs, and in our experience it is not so rare as is generally supposed.

MIKULICZ'S DISEASE

All the salivary glands become enlarged and the lachrymal glands participate also (fig. 190). Mikulicz's disease is a rare condition, the cause of which is still obscure. There is no pain, and the condition does not endanger life. X-ray treatment is sometimes beneficial. To minimise the deformity, the affected glands can be removed, but the lachrymals are usually better left alone.

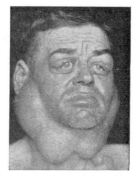

FIG. 190.—Mikulicz's disease. (*Fisher.*)

UVEO-PAROTID MANIFESTATION OF BOECK'S DISEASE (*Syn.* SARCOID)

Boeck's disease can attack any tissue. It is usually, but not necessarily, associated with skin lesions. Sarcoid of the skin resembles lupus pernio, so-called because of its likeness to a chilblain. More deeply placed lesions take the form of tumours. When both parotid glands are attacked, Boeck's disease simulates in several respects Mikulicz's disease. If one parotid is alone involved, the swelling is usually diagnosed as a mixed parotid tumour. Sarcoid of the parotid, which is perhaps the most characteristic manifestation of Boeck's disease, is frequently associated with inflammation of the uveal tract (iridocyclitis) ; the iridocyclitis may precede the parotid swelling, or vice versa.

Johannes von Mikulicz-Radecki, 1850–1905. Professor of Surgery, Breslau.
Carl William Boeck, 1808–1875. Professor of Surgery and Dermatology, Christiania (Oslo),
*   Norway.*

CHAPTER XI
THE NECK

ANOMALIES OF THE BRANCHIAL APPARATUS

In a fœtus approximately thirty-five days old, four grooves can be seen in the side of the neck. These are the branchial clefts, and the intervening bars are the branchial arches. The clefts in human embryos are, more correctly speaking, grooves—grooves on the outside (fig. 191) and on the inside (pharynx). The first cleft persists as the external auditory meatus, the second, third, and fourth clefts normally disappear. The whole, or a portion of one of these vestigial structures, may persist and give rise to one of the following anomalies :

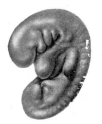

Fig. 191.—
Fœtus, showing branchial grooves and arches.

BRANCHIAL CYST

This is the most common and the most important of these vestigial anomalies. The cyst usually makes its first appearance between the twentieth and twenty-fifth years, but may be postponed until the patient is over fifty. Its position is very constant, viz. in the upper part of the neck beneath the upper third of the sternomastoid, protruding beneath its anterior border (fig. 192). Nearly always lined by squamous epithelium, its

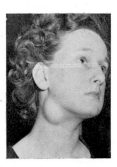

Fig. 192.—Typical branchial cyst.

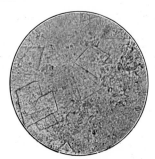

Fig. 193.—Branchial fluid. Note the abundance of cholesterol crystals.

contents bear a striking resemblance to tuberculous pus. If, however, a few drops of branchial fluid are examined in a fresh state under the microscope with a one-sixth power lens, an abundance of cholesterol crystals (fig. 193) can usually be seen. In this

way a branchial cyst can be differentiated
from a tuberculous collar-stud abscess (see
p. 198), a condition which it simulates very
closely.

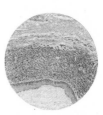

There is a rare variety of branchial cyst which is
found lying closely related to the pharynx. It is
lined by columnar epithelium, and filled with mucus.
Small cysts of this type are sometimes found at
necropsy, having given rise to no symptoms during life.

Fig. 194.—Section
of a branchial fistula
showing the lining
of the wall.

Treatment.—Excision of a branchial cyst through
an incision following one of the creases of the neck
gives uniformly satisfactory results. After the anterior
wall of the cyst has been exposed, the contents are
partially aspirated. This procedure aids in the dissection of the deeper
portions of the cyst, which may extend as far as the pharyngeal wall.

Branchiogenic carcinoma undoubtedly occurs, but such a diagnosis
is unjustifiable until every possible source of a primary growth in the
mouth, pharynx, and external auditory meatus has been scrutinised with a
negative result (p. 203).

BRANCHIAL FISTULA

Branchial fistulæ may be unilateral or bilateral. The orifice
of the fistula is nearly always to be found in the lower third of
the neck near the anterior border of the sternomastoid (fig. 195).

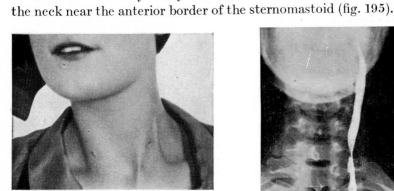

Fig. 195.—Bilateral branchial fistulæ ; left
side inflamed.

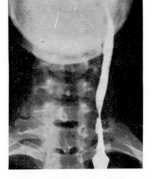

Fig. 196.—Complete
branchial fistula. External
opening in the lower third of
the neck ; internal opening
in the fossa of Rosenmüller.
Injected with uropac. A
portion of the syringe is seen
outlined in the radiograph.

Branchial fistulæ are lined by columnar
ciliated epithelium (fig. 194), discharge
mucus, and are often the seat of recurrent attacks of inflammation. When
complete, the internal orifice of the
fistula often opens into the pharyngeal recess (fossa of Rosenmüller) (fig. 196). Almost always the track is incomplete and
ends blindly in the region of the lateral pharyngeal wall. A
branchial fistula is frequently a congenital condition, but it

Johann Rosenmüller, 1771–1820. Professor of Anatomy and Surgery, Leipzig.

can be acquired. If a branchial cyst in an inflamed state is incised, the resulting sinus continues to discharge sometimes continuously and sometimes intermittently. The extent of the fistula can be determined by radiography following the injection of a radio-opaque medium.

Treatment.—When causing troublesome symptoms, branchial fistulæ should be removed completely by dissection. In fistulæ without an internal opening, dissection is facilitated by inserting a subcutaneous ligature around the external orifice a few days prior to the lipiodol injection. X-ray examination determines the extent of the fistula, the pent-up secretion serves to distend the tract, which is thus more easily followed in the depths of the wound. The operation should be conducted through a transverse incision, and the dissection of the fistula proceeds in an upward direction as far as the limits of the wound permit. A second transverse incision is then made at a higher level, and the mobilised portion of the fistula is brought out of it. The dissection of the fistula is then recommenced. The fistula is followed to its termination ; it usually passes through the fork of the common carotid artery and extends to the lateral pharyngeal wall.

BRANCHIAL CARTILAGE

A small, elongated piece of cartilage connected to the deep surface of a cutaneous dimple in the position of an external orifice of a branchial fistula is occasionally met with. The patient usually finds it accidentally, and often thinks that it is a foreign body.

CERVICAL AURICLE

So named because of its morphological significance, this cutaneous projection is almost invariably found in the position of the external orifice of a fistula (fig. 197). Cervical auricles were recognised in the days of the Romans, and are represented in some of the statuary of that period.

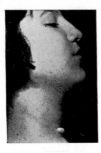

FIG. 197.—Cervical auricle.

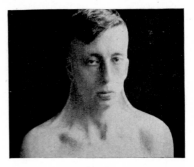

FIG. 198.—Webbing of the neck.
(*Flavell.*) (*British Journal of Surgery.*)

WEBBING OF THE NECK

This rare condition is usually associated with Turner's syndrome, which comprises webbing of the neck (fig. 198), an increased carrying angle of the elbow joints, and sexual infantilism. No satisfactory embryological explanation of the abnormality has been put forward. It may well be it is an example of atavism, for it occurs naturally in the chimpanzee.

CYSTIC HYGROMA (*Syn.* HYDROCELE OF THE NECK)

Ætiology.—About the sixth week of embryonic life the primitive lymph sacs develop in mesoblast, the principal pair being situated in the neck between the jugular and subclavian veins ; these correspond to the lymphatic hearts of amphibians. Failure of an important tributary of the primitive lymphatic system to link up with other lymphatic vessels or with the venous system would account for the appearance of these swellings.

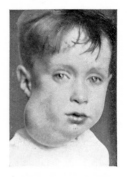

Fig. 199.—Cystic hygroma. The swelling is brilliantly translucent. (*Sir John Fraser.*)

Cystic hygromata usually appear during early infancy. Occasionally they are present at birth, and have been known to be so large as to obstruct labour. Typically, the swelling occupies the lower third of the neck, and as it enlarges it passes upwards towards the ear (fig. 199). It often extends downwards behind the clavicle to lie upon the dome of the pleura. The axilla is another, though less frequent, site for a cystic hygroma.

On pathological examination the swelling is found to consist of an aggregation of cysts like a mass of soap bubbles ; the larger cysts are near the surface, while the smaller ones lie deeply (fig. 200) and tend to infiltrate muscle planes. Each cyst is lined by a single layer of endothelium having the appearance of mosaic and is filled with clear lymph.

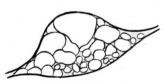

Fig. 200.—A cystic hygroma consists of an aggregation of cysts filled with lymph. The larger cysts are nearer the surface. The spaces are lined by a single layer of endothelial cells.

Clinical Course.—The behaviour of cystic hygromata is uncertain, so much so that it is impossible to prognosticate as to what will happen in a given case. Sometimes growth is rapid, after which the cyst may burst subcutaneously and disappear within forty-eight hours. At other times these cysts become the seat of recurrent inflammation, which often resolves without special treatment. In many cases the cyst continues to enlarge slowly for some months, and then appears to remain stationary in size.

Henry Hubert Turner, Contemporary. Associate Professor of Medicine, Oklahoma University, U.S.A.

Treatment.—During very early life inactivity is the best course. When the mass increases rapidly in size, spontaneous rupture can be awaited with some confidence. When the condition seems to be at a standstill, X-ray therapy is worthy

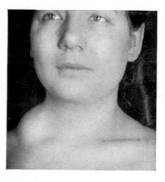

of trial, and in some cases this treatment is followed by retrogression of the swelling. If this fails, the injection of sclerosing solutions may be tried, but owing to the multilocular nature of the swelling, this form of therapy is unlikely to do more than produce some diminution in the size of the swelling. When the swelling persists in spite of these measures, and the child has reached the age of two years, provided it is strong and healthy, complete dissection of the whole mass should be attempted.

FIG. 201.—Solitary lymph cyst of the neck.

Solitary lymph cyst is a condition akin to the foregoing, but differs in that it is nearly always first seen in adult life. As its name implies, it is a single cyst filled with lymph, and it is usually found in the supraclavicular triangle (fig. 201).

Treatment by excision is eminently satisfactory.

Deep Cavernous Hæmangioma of the Neck.—Like lymphatic cysts, hæmangiomata can be emptied by pressure, but of course they are non-translucent.

Excision may be a difficult and dangerous undertaking. Porter's treatment (injecting boiling water into the veins) is not very satisfactory. X-ray treatment and the injection of sclerosing agents have also been tried.

PHARYNGEAL POUCH

When large, a pharyngeal pouch causes a swelling in the lower part of the neck, usually on the left side. Pharyngeal pouch is discussed in the chapter on the pharynx, p. 239.

STERNOMASTOID " TUMOUR "

Formerly this swelling was incorrectly considered to be a hæmatoma, due to an injury during difficult labour. It is seldom that the lump is noticed before the third week of life (fig. 202).

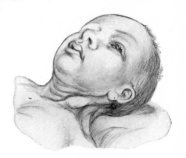

FIG. 202.—Sternomastoid "tumour."

F. Miles Porter, 1856–1933.   Professor of Surgery, Indiana University, U.S.A.

Most authorities assert that the lump is not present at birth. Twistington Higgins, from his experience, says that this is not true; in fact, these "tumours" are sometimes to be seen in babies delivered by Cæsarean section.

Histologically the mass in the sternomastoid muscle is composed of white fibrous tissue (fig. 203), and Middleton showed that it arises from thrombosis of some of the veins draining the sternomastoid.

Treatment.—There is no immediate treatment; the lump gradually disappears, but the clinician has an important duty, and that is to warn the parents that the child will probably need an operation for the correction of torticollis at the age of four. Although manipulation can be tried in order to avoid the necessity for this operation, sternomastoid "tumour" is often a precursor of torticollis. If steps are taken in time, the handicapping deformity and facial asymmetry which follows neglected torticollis can be prevented.

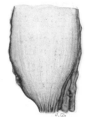

Fig. 203.— A sternomastoid "tumour" excised from an infant aged six weeks, showing replacement of the muscle by fibrous tissue. (*Middleton.*) (*British Journal o Surgery.*)

THE SCALENE SYNDROME

To understand the scalene syndrome, it must be realised that at their exit from the neck the brachial plexus and the subclavian artery pass through a narrow triangle (fig. 204). In this triangle the first dorsal nerve, together with the main aggregation of sympathetic fibres supplying the arteries of the upper limb, are in a vulnerable position; they may be looked upon as in a vice, the ventral jaw of which is the scalenus anticus, while the particular structure forming the dorsal jaw varies (fig. 205).

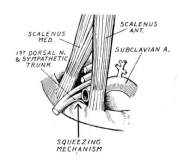

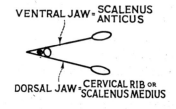

SCALENUS MED.

SCALENUS ANT.

1ST DORSAL N. & SYMPATHETIC TRUNK

SUBCLAVIAN A.

SQUEEZING MECHANISM

VENTRAL JAW = SCALENUS ANTICUS

DORSAL JAW = CERVICAL RIB OR SCALENUS MEDIUS

Fig. 204.—Explaining the scalene syndrome.

Fig. 205.—The constitution of jaws of the metaphorical vice.

Thomas Twistington Higgins, Contemporary. Surgeon, Hospital for Sick Children, Great Ormond Street, London.
Brigadier Donald Stewart Middleton, 1899–1942. Assistant Surgeon, Royal Infirmary, Edinburgh. (Died on Active Service.)

Pre-eminent among structures that constitute the dorsal jaw is a cervical rib.

It is paradoxical that frequently symptoms of the scalene syndrome are present when a cervical rib cannot be demonstrated, and an obviously fully ossified cervical rib or ribs is often unaccompanied by nerve-pressure symptoms.

Extra ribs usually spring from the seventh cervical vertebra. They are more common in women, and are bilateral more often than unilateral. When unilateral, a cervical rib occurs more frequently on the left side, but symptoms are four times more common on the right side owing to greater use of the right arm.

Five main varieties of cervical rib exist :—

(*a*) A complete rib often containing a false joint in its length, articulates anteriorly with the manubrium or the first rib. ⟶

(*b*) The free end of rib expands into a large bony mass. ⟶

(*c*) A rib ending in a tapering point, which is connected by a fibrous band to the scalene tubercle of the first rib. ⟶

(*d*) A fibrous band which develops in, or is part of, the scalenus medius alone is present. This variety, of course, cannot be demonstrated by X-rays. ⟶

(*e*) When there is "postfixation" of the brachial plexus (by which is meant that the brachial plexus receives a contribution from the second thoracic nerve), by causing pressure on the lower trunk of the brachial plexus, a normal first rib can act in a similar manner to a cervical rib.

Clinical Features.—In this condition patients usually present themselves in middle life, although it is sometimes seen at puberty and after any debilitating illness. The symptoms are no doubt due to sagging of the musculature of the shoulder girdle. Some temporary relief is effected by bracing the shoulders.

The symptoms may be divided into two categories. Usually one only is in evidence :

1. Nerve-pressure symptoms, due to squeezing of the first dorsal nerve. They are subdivided into sensory and motor.

Sensory.—There is tingling, numbness, and later pain over the ulnar border of the forearm. These symptoms are relieved temporarily by elevation of the arm.

Motor.—The muscles of the thenar eminence are first affected, and wasting is often limited to the abductor and opponens pollicis, a distribution which is in contrast to progressive muscular atrophy. In long-standing cases a claw hand can result.

Differential Diagnosis.—In the motor variety of nerve pressure symptoms, a differential diagnosis must be made from progressive muscular atrophy, syringomyelia, peripheral nerve injury, and brachial neuritis in all its various forms. Brachial neuritis due to a herniated intervertebral disc, usually between C5 and C6, is a clinical entity which must be taken into consideration. A clear lateral radiograph will help to establish or eliminate this possibility.

2. Vaso-motor symptoms are less frequent. Again, they are due to squeezing, this time of the aggregation of sympathetic fibres which lies beneath the first dorsal nerve. They are divided into vascular symptoms and hyperhidrosis of the hand.

Vascular symptoms are those of increasing circulatory impairment in the affected limb, and eventually this may go on to gangrene. The pulse is diminished, but its volume increases on raising the arm. When gangrene develops, the index finger is affected maximally (fig. 206). Formerly these vascular symptoms were attributed to kinking and compression of the subclavian artery. Telford has shown that such a view is absurd, for even in the elderly, ligation of the subclavian artery is not

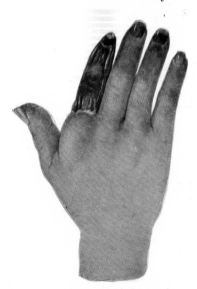

FIG. 206.—Cervical rib with vaso-motor symptoms, culminating in gangrene of the index finger. (*Telford and Stopford.*) (*British Journal of Surgery.*)

Evelyn Davison Telford, Contemporary. Emeritus Professor of Surgery, University of Manchester.

followed by gangrene. The vascular symptoms are due to pressure irritation of sympathetic nerve fibres passing to supply the brachial artery and the arteries of the forearm. These sympathetic nerve fibres form an isolated bundle beneath the first dorsal nerve.

Differential Diagnosis.—In the vascular variety a differential diagnosis must be made from Raynaud's disease, chilblains, and subclavian aneurism.

Hyperhidrosis (excessive sweating) of the hand is occasionally the main complaint.

Treatment.—In mild cases the use of a sling and exercises aimed at strengthening the muscles of the shoulder girdle may alleviate the symptoms, at least temporarily. Even in cases where a cervical rib can be demonstrated, Adson has shown that in a large percentage of cases it is unnecessary to excise the rib ; the symptoms are often relieved by dividing the scalenus anticus muscle (fig. 207), indeed this operation cures about 75 per cent. of patients with the scalene syndrome. Because in all probability the first dorsal nerve is angulated over a cervical rib, a band, or the scalenus medius, the remainder require further operative

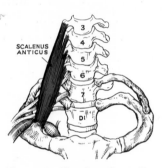

Fig. 207.—Showing the rationale of scalenotomy.

treatment. The second operation is therefore directed to removing the *dorsal* jaw of the vice (see fig. 205).

Unfortunately there remain 3 to 5 per cent. of patients who are still unrelieved, or are incompletely relieved, by the second operation. Possibly a few of these have a prolapsed cervical intervertebral disc that has been missed ; more often they belong to the category of what is known as the costo-clavicular syndrome.

THE COSTO-CLAVICULAR SYNDROME

The modes by which the lowest cord of the brachial plexus and the subclavian artery become compressed between the clavicle and the first rib (fig. 208) are various. According to Weddell, congenital narrowing of the interval between the clavicle and the first rib is the principal factor in the production of the symptoms. His explanation

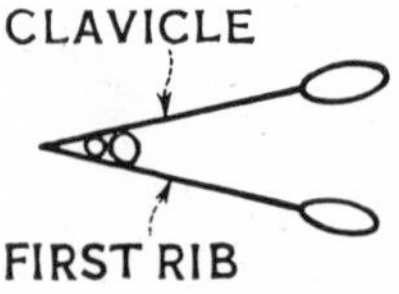

CLAVICLE

FIRST RIB

Fig. 208.—The costoclavicular vice.

Maurice Raynaud, 1834–1881. Physician, Hôpital Lariboisière, Paris.
Alfred Washington Adson, Contemporary. Neuro-Surgeon, Mayo Clinic, Rochester, U.S.A.
Alexander Graham McDonnell Weddell, Contemporary. Anatomist, Oxford.

also accounts for aneurysmal dilatation of the subclavian artery, which occasionally occurs distal to the first rib, and which hitherto has not been explained satisfactorily.

Walshe brings evidence to show that the subclavian artery is itself sometimes compressed in the costo-clavicular vice, and the symptoms are not due to compression of the sympathetic fibres in the scalene vice. Alderson finds that stress fractures of the first rib, although rare, nearly always occur in the subclavian groove, and such fractures might easily account for compression of structures in relation to the first rib.

Even two vices are insufficient to account for the symptoms in every case. Telford appears to have proved conclusively that the axillary artery can be squeezed between the two heads of the median nerve.

Treatment.—In most instances excision of the major portion of the first rib will relieve the symptoms.

CUT THROAT

In more than half the cases of cut throat which reach surgical aid the wound does not involve any vital structure—only the skin, platysma, and perhaps the sternomastoid or other muscles are severed. Even the external jugular vein does not often come under the category of a vital structure in this respect. The treatment of these superficial injuries follows elementary surgical principles.

Serious Cases.—Self-inflicted wounds of the neck are usually perpetrated with the head extended, the wound being more or less transverse. In this extended position the great vessels of the neck are protected by the sternomastoids and the larynx. So it comes about that the great vessels of the neck are comparatively rarely injured, while the air passages bear the brunt.

Treatment.—Attention is directed, firstly, to arresting hæmorrhage ; secondly, to dealing with the wounded air passage ; and, thirdly, to the repair of other structures.

Various moderate-sized arteries and veins will require ligation. Hæmorrhage from an inaccessible branch of the external carotid is best dealt with by ligating that trunk near its origin. It has been stated already that injury to the main vessels is comparatively rare, and when it occurs death usually supervenes before surgical aid is forthcoming.

The principal sites of wounds of the air passages are indicated in fig. 209.

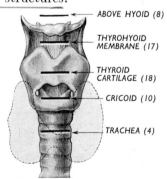

ABOVE HYOID (8)

THYROHYOID MEMBRANE (17)

THYROID CARTILAGE (18)

CRICOID (10)

TRACHEA (4)

FIG. 209.—Position of the wound into the air passages of 57 cases of suicidal cut throat with a deep wound.

Francis Martin Rouse Walshe, Contemporary. Physician, National Hospital for Nervous Diseases, Queen Square, London.
Basil Roxby Alderson, Contemporary. Surgeon-Lieutenant Commander, Royal Navy.

Wounds above the Hyoid Bone.—After cleansing the area the wound is explored with a finger. Quite often it will be found that the cavity of the mouth has been entered. The epiglottis is often partially divided near its base. This should be repaired with catgut sutures. The mucosa of the pharynx is trimmed and united. The wound is dusted with sulphanilamide powder, and loosely packed with vaseline gauze.

Wounds of the Thyrohyoid Membrane.—Again the epiglottis is often damaged. The severed thyrohyoid membrane can usually be sutured. If there is respiratory distress, it is advisable to perform tracheotomy.

Division of the Thyroid Cartilage.—The thyroid cartilage can be repaired with sutures, provided these are not tied tightly, for a stitch through cartilage tends to cut out. Laryngotomy or tracheotomy is usually indicated.

Wounds about the Cricoid Cartilage.—After the wound has been trimmed, a laryngotomy tube can be inserted via the artificial opening in the windpipe, and the tissues approximated around it.

Division of the Trachea.—Wounds of the trachea are comparatively rare. In order to obtain adequate exposure it is usually necessary to divide the thyroid isthmus between hæmostats. In most instances it is advisable to perform tracheotomy below the wound, and then to proceed to repair the latter with sutures.

Injury to Nerves.—It is remarkable how rarely important nerves are injured in self-inflicted wounds. In stab wounds any nerve may be involved. In one of our patients, a sailor, the most inaccessible nerve in the neck, the cervical sympathetic, was divided in this way, the assailant's weapon being a small penknife.

COMPLICATIONS OF CUT THROAT

1. **Loss of Blood.**—If the hæmorrhage has been severe, blood or plasma transfusion is indicated.

2. **Infection of the Wound.**—This is not very frequent, but these wounds should always be drained, as they have been inflicted with a potentially infected instrument. Cellulitis sometimes supervenes, and this may spread to the mediastinum.

3. **Pneumonia.**—Pneumonia is a frequent and lethal complication, especially in those cases where the air passages have been opened.

4. **Stenosis of the Larynx or Trachea.**—Due to cicatrisation : it may necessitate permanent tracheotomy.

5. **Œsophageal Fistula.**—Œsophageal or pharyngeal fistula is a very rare occurrence, and it tends to heal spontaneously.

6. **Surgical emphysema** is another rare complication, and it usually occurs when a laryngotomy or tracheotomy tube has been omitted in the treatment of the case.

7. **Aerial Fistula.**—A persistent communication between the air passages and the exterior is likely to occur when there has been actual loss of substance of the larynx or trachea. In certain cases a plastic operation may be undertaken.

8. **Aphonia or dysphonia** may follow injury to the vocal cords, or division of a recurrent laryngeal nerve.

9. **Air embolus** may ensue if the internal jugular vein has been incised.

WOUNDS OF THE CERVICAL PORTION OF THE THORACIC DUCT

Wounds of the thoracic duct are rare, and usually occur during dissection of lymph nodes in the left supraclavicular fossa. When the accident is not recognised at the time, chyle pours from the wound—as much as two or three pints in twenty-four hours—and, as a result, the patient wastes rapidly.

Treatment.—Should the accident be recognised during an operation, it may be possible to repair the duct. Failing this, its proximal end has been implanted successfully into the cut end of a suitable adjacent vein. Ligation of the duct is not harmful, for there are a number of anastomotic channels between the lymphatic and the venous systems in the neighbourhood. Usually the first intimation of a severed thoracic duct is a copious serous discharge from the wound on the day following the operation. Firm pressure by a pad and bandage should be applied, but this simple expedient is seldom successful. More often the wound must be re-opened. If the patient is given cream to drink an hour before the operation, there is seldom any difficulty in locating a cut thoracic duct, which is about the size of a straw and an immediate external relation of the last $1\frac{1}{2}$ inches (3·75 cm.) of the left internal jugular vein (fig. 210). If the duct is found, it should be ligated, but in any case the wound should be firmly packed and allowed to heal by granulation. Thanks to subsidiary anastomotic channels, these measures are regularly satisfactory.

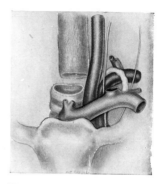

FIG. 210.—The termination of the thoracic duct.

CELLULITIS OF THE NECK

Acute cellulitis may be superficial or deep to the deep cervical fascia. The former is common, and methods of treatment follow that of cellulitis elsewhere. The latter is rare, but is especially dangerous, because not only is the infection liable to spread beneath the dense cervical fascia to the mediastinum, but sudden asphyxia from œdema of the glottis is an ever-present possibility. Therefore sterilised tracheotomy instruments should be by the bedside, and if the response to penicillin therapy is not rapid and undoubted, the deep cervical fascia must be incised in one or more places.

The question of anæsthesia is highly important in these cases. An inhalation anæsthetic is contraindicated. Intravenous anæsthesia is not without danger, for should spasm of the glottis occur, it is difficult or impossible to clear the airway. A cervical block with local anæsthetic, after suitable preliminary medication, is usually the best. It should be noted that this infiltration does not implicate the infected tissues. Alternatively an endotracheal anæsthetic can be employed.

Chronic cellulitis (*syn.* woody phlegmon of Réclus) is uncommon. One side of the neck becomes swollen and extremely indurated ; the supple integument of the neck becomes like a hide. There may be pitting on pressure, and some erythematous blush in the overlying skin. Woody

Paul Réclus, 1847–1914. Surgeon to the hospitals of Paris.

phlegmon, which is probably due to an infection by an attenuated staphylo-coccus, runs a chronic course, is almost painless, and produces few or no constitutional symptoms. The condition has to be distinguished from actinomycosis and advanced malignant disease.

Treatment.—Penicillin therapy should effect a cure ; if it fails to do so, fomentations followed by suitable incisions are indicated. Once a flow of pus has been established, the neck regains its suppleness, and the condition clears up.

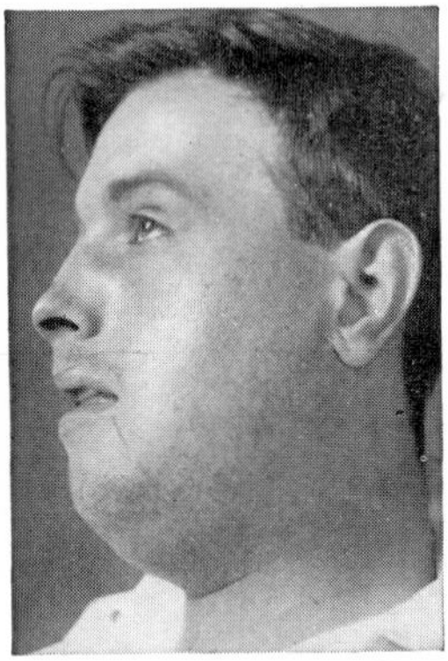

LUDWIG'S ANGINA

Ludwig described a clinical entity characterised by a brawny swelling of the submaxillary region combined with in-flammatory œdema of the mouth. It is the *combined* cervical and intrabuccal signs which constitute the characteristic feature of the lesion (fig. 211). The cause of the condition is a virulent (usually streptococcal) infection of the cellular tissues about the submaxillary salivary gland.

FIG. 211. — Ludwig's angina. The brawny swelling beneath the jaw and the œdema of the floor of the mouth are charac-teristic features of the condition.

Clinical Course.—Unless the infection is controlled, certain cases rapidly assume a grave aspect. The swollen tongue is pushed towards the palate and forwards through the open mouth, while the cellulitis extends down the neck in that most dangerous plane—deep to the deep fascia.

Ludwig's angina is an infection of a closed fascial space, and untreated the inflammatory exudate often passes via the tunnel occupied by the stylohyoid to the submucosa of the glottis, when the patient is in imminent danger of death from œdema of the glottis.

Treatment.—As in the case of cellulitis beneath the deep cervical fascia, trach-eotomy instruments should always be at hand. When the condition is diag-nosed early, the results of penicillin therapy are often dramatic. In cases where the swelling, both cervical and intrabuccal, does not subside rapidly with penicillin, a curved incision beneath the jaw, as is shown in fig. 212, is made. The incision is deepened, and after dis-

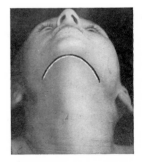

FIG. 212.—Incision for decompressing thoroughly the space beneath the mylohyoid muscle.

Wilhelm von Ludwig, 1790–1865. Professor of Surgery and Midwifery, Tübingen ; also Court Physician.

placing the superficial lobes of the submaxillary salivary gland, the mylohyoid muscles are divided. This decompresses the closed fascial space referred to. The wound is left open. The same precautions regarding the anæsthetic as detailed in the section dealing with acute cellulitis deep to the cervical fascia appertain for Ludwig's angina. After the operation penicillin therapy is continued.

CERVICAL LYMPHADENITIS

There are approximately 800 lymph nodes in the body ; no less than 300 of them lie in the neck. Inflammation of the lymph nodes of the neck is exceedingly common. Infection occurs from the oral and nasal cavities, the ear, the scalp, and face. The source of infection must be sought for systematically.

Acute Lymphadenitis.—The affected nodes are enlarged and tender, and there is a varying degree of pyrexia. The treatment, in the first instance, is directed to the general condition and to the focus of infection, the neck itself being simply protected by a bandage over wool. If, in spite of chemotherapy, pain continues or certain nodes appear to be getting larger, fomentations are applied locally. Abscess formation calls for adequate drainage.

Chronic Lymphadenitis.—In the early stages it is extremely difficult to distinguish chronic tuberculous adenitis from chronic non-tuberculous adenitis, but clinical experience shows that chronically inflamed nodes which do not resolve in the space of a few weeks are nearly always tuberculous. Tuberculin skin tests (see p. 821) are helpful in confirming a diagnosis.

Tuberculous Cervical Adenitis.—Tuberculous cervical adenitis is very common in the British Isles. The majority of patients affected are children or young adults, but the condition can occur for the first time at any age. Usually one group of cervical nodes is at first infected. Thus the patient seeks advice because of a swelling in the upper jugular chain (fig. 213), the submaxillary region, the supraclavicular or posterior triangles of the neck, the first and second situations being exceedingly common. More rarely there is widespread cervical lymphadenitis, and it is in these cases particularly that periadenitis or matting of the lymph nodes is in evidence.

Source of Infection.—In the majority of instances tubercle bacilli gain entrance through the tonsil of the corresponding side.

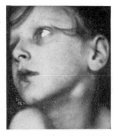

Fig. 213.—Tuberculous cervical adenitis. Tonsillar lymph node chiefly involved.

Sometimes tubercle bacilli can be demonstrated in carious teeth, and here is a possible portal which should be suspected when the submaxillary or submental groups of lymph nodes are principally affected. Contrary to what is generally believed, it is the human, and not the bovine, bacillus which is responsible for tuberculous cervical adenitis in about 70 per cent. of cases. In fully 80 per cent. of cases the tuberculous process is virtually limited to the clinically affected group of nodes, but especially in widespread adenitis, and that occurring in the base of the neck, a primary focus in the lungs must be excluded.

In the event of the patient developing a natural resistance to the infection or (more often) as a result of appropriate general

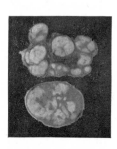

Fig. 214.—Caseating tuberculous lymph nodes.

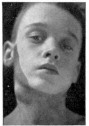

Fig. 215.—Tuberculous collar-stud abscess. (Iodine has been applied to the skin prior to the operation.)

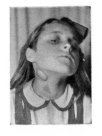

Fig. 216. — If a collar-stud abscess is neglected, the skin becomes involved and finally a discharging sinus results, sometimes, as in this case, at a distance from the original lesion.

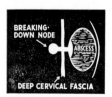

Fig. 217.—Blackboard sketch of a collar-stud abscess.

treatment, resolution or calcification may occur. In other circumstances the caseating material (fig. 214) liquefies, breaks through the capsules of the nodes, and a " cold abscess " forms. The pus is at first confined by the deep cervical fascia. This soon becomes eroded at one point, and the pus flows through the small opening into that more commodious space beneath the superficial fascia. This is the stage of collar-stud abscess (figs. 215 and 217). Unless skilful treatment is adopted, the skin will soon become reddened over the centre of the fluctuating swelling (fig. 216), and before long a discharging sinus, with its attendant evils, is at hand.

DIFFERENTIAL DIAGNOSIS

When the swelling is solid, from
1. Chronic non-tuberculous lymphadenitis which fails to resolve.
2. Hodgkin's disease.
3. Reticulo-sarcoma.
4. Secondary malignant disease

When the swelling is cystic, from
1. Branchial cyst.
2. Extension of an abscess connected with a tuberculous cervical vertebra.

When a sinus or sinuses have formed, from
1. Actinomycosis.
2. An acquired branchial fistula.

Gummata of lymphatic nodes should also be included, but it is so rare that it is almost a pathological curiosity. Absolute symmetry is a feature of the condition, and in such cases other clinical evidence is sought, and a Wassermann reaction is performed if necessary.

TREATMENT OF TUBERCULOUS LYMPHADENITIS

General Treatment.—All agree that the patient should be placed under the best dietetic and hygienic conditions possible, the most important being open air, together with natural or artificial sunlight. No matter what line of treatment is adopted, infected tonsils and carious teeth must receive appropriate attention.

Contraindications to Operative Treatment.—When there is active tuberculosis of another system, e.g. pulmonary tuberculosis, removal of the tuberculous lymph nodes in the neck is obviously contraindicated. In cases where the infected nodes are not confined to one region of the neck, when there is much periadenitis or a number of discharging sinuses, and particularly when the patient is debilitated, operative treatment is best avoided, at any rate for several months, during which time heliotherapy, if possible in a sanatorium, is undertaken. Repeated aspiration of a collar-stud abscess cannot be recommended, because so frequently aspiration leads to sinus formation and secondary infection. It is better to incise the abscess with a tenotomy knife, evacuate the pus, and suture the wound. To prevent or treat the secondary infection, chemotherapy is employed. In addition to these measures, administration of tuberculin, calciferol or, possibly, streptomycin may prove

August von Wassermann, 1866–1925. Director Institute for Experimental Therapy, Berlin.

helpful. When the massive adenitis fails to resolve, or multiple sinuses continue to discharge, deep X-ray therapy sometimes helps to cure the condition.

Operative treatment.—In the majority of cases, the tuberculous process is limited to one group of lymph nodes. For this type extirpation of the affected nodes through an oblique incision, following a crease of the neck, gives rapid and eminently satisfactory results.

Even the presence of a collar-stud abscess does not jeopardise healing by first intention if the underlying diseased lymph nodes are dissected completely, provided the overlying skin is healthy and hæmatoma formation is guarded against by careful hæmostasis and a pressure dressing.

When the overlying skin is involved, or there are several sinuses, after a course of chemotherapy designed to eradicate the secondary infection, the unhealthy area of skin may be excised completely, and the diseased nodes dissected. If it is found impracticable to bring the skin together without undue tension, after sprinkling the interior of the wound freely with sulphanilamide powder, it is packed with vaseline gauze. A viscopaste bandage is then applied. Repacking is undertaken in the operating theatre at weekly intervals, until the wound granulates. A linear scar often results (fig. 218A and B).

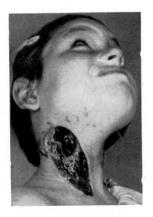 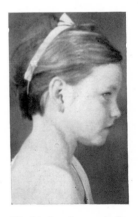

Fig. 218A and B.—Large collar-stud abscess with skin involvement. Involved skin excised, sternomastoid divided. Mass of nodes excised. Portion of internal jugular vein resected. Wound packed with vaseline gauze. (a) Photograph taken one week after operation. (b) Unretouched photograph taken four and a half months later.

During the dissection of cervical lymphatic nodes no effort should be spared to preserve :

The spinal accessory nerve ;
The mandibular branch of the facial nerve ;
The hypoglossal nerve ;

which are the nerves most likely to be injured.

To minimise unnecessary injury to large veins, no tissue should be divided when stretched taut. Should the internal jugular vein prove to be involved in the pathological process to such an extent that freeing it is difficult or impossible, this great vessel can be ligated, or a portion of it can be resected, without any untoward effect at any age (cf. ligation of the common carotid artery, p. 101).

ACTINOMYCOSIS OF THE NECK

Two-thirds of all human cases of actinomycosis occur in the neck and face. There is increasing evidence that the ray fungus gains entrance through a wound of the buccal mucosa, particularly after tooth extraction. A sinus or sinuses about the upper part of the neck, particularly indurated sinuses, should arouse suspicion immediately. The skin about the sinus may appear somewhat blue and mottled. On palpation each burrow feels hard, like a strand of whipcord. Lymph nodes are not enlarged except as the result of secondary infection. There is no pain unless the disease is advanced and nerves have become implicated in fibrous tissue. As the disease progresses the patient becomes increasingly anæmic. The discharge is thin and watery. Finding the characteristic " sulphur granules " in this discharge is the key to the diagnosis.

Modes of Spread.—The disease spreads by burrowing in the connective tissues, upwards towards the scalp and downwards into the supraclavicular region, from thence the mediastinum and pleural cavities become involved. Spread by the lymphatic stream is practically unknown, and it is truly remarkable that this favourite channel for the dissemination of all other infective processes should enjoy such a degree of immunity in the case of the ray fungus. The usual explanation of this is that the streptothrix actinomyces is too large to pass along a lymphatic vessel. Late in the course of the disease blood-borne metastases are not very rare, the liver and the brain being the two regions most commonly invaded in this way. Untreated, the disease runs a rather chronic but surely fatal course.

Treatment.—The dental surgeon attends to carious teeth, erring on the side of extraction rather than repair. In cases where the infection is limited to a circumscribed area in the neck,

James Israel, 1848–1926. First found " sulphur granules " in pus from a discharging sinus of the neck in man. He afterwards became a famous Berlin urologist.

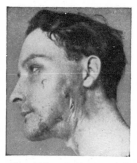

FIG. 219.—Actinomycosis. Indurated sinuses extend from the neck to the orbit.

excision of all the infected tissues and packing of the resulting cavity, combined with general treatment, gives good results. When, as is often the case, the condition is widespread, such as that shown in fig. 219, excision is impracticable, and recourse must be made to laying open and packing the sinuses. Penicillin therapy, which clears up the secondary infection inseparable from this condition, is seldom curative, but it should be given in conjunction with intensive iodine therapy, which is best administered as follows :

Thrice daily the patient drinks iodised milk prepared in the following way : 5 minims (0·3 ml.) of fresh 2 per cent. tincture of iodine are stirred into a cupful of milk. As shown by Chitty, the iodine forms a colourless organic compound with the cream. The dose is gradually increased until 10 minims (0·6 ml.) are taken t.d.s. If the sinuses fail to heal after two months of such treatment, deep X-ray therapy sometimes proves effective, provided the condition is still confined to the facio-cervical region. In rebellious cases streptomycin has proved effective.

MALIGNANT LYMPH NODES OF THE NECK

Carcinomatous infiltration of the cervical lymphatic nodes is only too common. When a patient presents himself with enlargement of the cervical lymph nodes which are suspiciously indurated, the search for a primary growth should commence. Often the primary growth lies within the buccal cavity ; when this is not the case, the search must continue. Among the sites which are prone to be overlooked are the hypo-pharynx, the external auditory meatus, the middle ear, the œsophagus, the stomach, and the testes.

Sometimes the primary growth lies hidden in the depths of the naso-pharynx. Carcinoma of the ethmoid is a case in point. Usually by the time the lymph nodes of the neck are involved, the neoplasm has grown into the sphenoidal fissure and implicated the third, fourth, ophthalmic division of the fifth, and the sixth nerves which pass through that fissure.

When the lump in question is undoubtedly malignant, but, in spite of a thorough search, no primary growth can be discovered, the possibility

Hubert Chitty, Contemporary. Surgeon, Royal Infirmary, Bristol.

of *branchiogenic carcinoma* (p. 185) can be entertained. In early cases the neoplasm is encapsulated and can be removed by dissection.

Treatment.—In order to eradicate the malignant process, most thorough excision of the lymphatic nodes and the associated fascial planes is indicated. Operation is usually undertaken a few weeks after treatment of the primary growth by radium.

" Block " dissections of the neck are of two varieties :

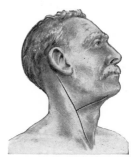

FIG. 220.—An incision for block dissection of the neck.

1. *Crile's block dissection* is conducted through the wide display afforded by skin incisions, such as are shown in fig. 220.

The skin flaps having been dissected up, the sternomastoid is divided about 1 inch above the clavicle. The muscle is freed and retracted upwards. Next, the internal jugular vein is divided between ligatures low down in the neck. The dissection proceeds upwards methodically and the muscle, fascia, fat, lymphatic nodes, the internal jugular vein, together with the submaxillary salivary gland, are dissected and removed *en bloc*. Attention must be directed to clearing the space between the parotid and the great vessels, and also the submental triangle between the geniohyoglossi, for it is in these areas that a lymphatic node can be easily overlooked. Bleeding vessels are ligated as they occur. When completed, the carotid artery is laid bare, and lying with it is the vagus nerve which has been preserved carefully. The operation aims at removing the whole of the lymphatic-bearing tissues on the affected side of the neck. The skin flaps are approximated and the wound drained. Surprisingly little deformity follows this extensive dissection, but the neck is stiff, and there is drooping of the corner of the mouth.

In necessary cases the operation must be bilateral, but it is usual to operate upon one side at a time, with an interval of several weeks.

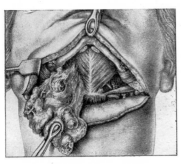

FIG. 221.—Suprahyoid block dissection of the neck.

2. *Suprahyoid block dissection of the neck* is indicated in cases of carcinoma of the lower lip, early cases of carcinoma of the tip of the tongue, and carcinoma of the floor of the mouth. Its advantage is that both sides of the neck can be attended to at one operation (fig. 221).

HODGKIN'S DISEASE (Syn. LYMPHADENOMA)

Clinical Features.—In an overwhelming proportion of cases the cervical lymph nodes are the first to be attacked. Never-

George W. Crile, 1864–1943. *Professor of Clinical Surgery, Western Reserve University, Cleveland, U.S.A.*
Thomas Hodgkin, 1798–1866. *Some time Curator to the Museum, he failed in the election or the office of Physician at Guy's Hospital, London.*

theless, the lymphatic nodes of the axilla and groin (fig. 222) must be examined in all cases. A clinical diagnosis of lymphadenoma is suggested by elastic, discrete enlargement of the

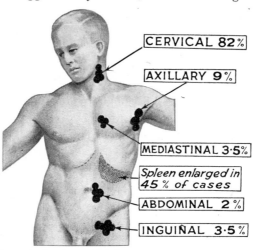

CERVICAL 82%

AXILLARY 9%

MEDIASTINAL 3·5%

Spleen enlarged in 45% of cases

ABDOMINAL 2%

INGUINAL 3·5%

Fig. 222.—Hodgkin's disease usually, but not necessarily, commences in the cervical nodes. Showing the position of the lesion when the patient was seen first. In 14 per cent. of cases more than one region was involved.
(*Baker and Mann's statistics.*)

involved nodes (fig. 223), but the clinical fallacies are so great that it should be an unwavering rule to excise a single node under

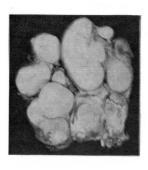

Fig. 223.—Mass of lymph nodes removed from the neck. Hodgkin's disease,

local anæsthesia and submit it to microscopical scrutiny before pronouncing the diagnosis. Later the spleen is involved (hard-bake spleen). The enlargements are progressive, though temporary remissions occur. The disease is much more common in males, the incidence being at least 3 : 1. While no age is exempt, more than half the cases occur during the second and third decades of life (Baker and Mann). Secondary anæmia is a regular accompaniment of Hodgkin's disease. Fever is a comparatively rare and late symptom, and it occurs only when the deep, i.e. abdominal or mediastinal, lymph nodes are involved. A Pel-Ebstein temperature (see p. 123) is observed in a large proportion of the febrile cases.

Charles Baker, Contemporary. Physician, Selly Oak Hospital, Birmingham, England.
William Neville Mann, Contemporary. Assistant Physician, Guy's Hospital, London.
Pieter K. Pel, 1852–1916. Professor of Medicine, Amsterdam.
Wilhelm Ebstein, 1836–1912. Professor of Medicine, Göttingen, Germany.

Treatment.—When the disease is still confined to one group of lymph nodes, eradication by excision is more than justified, because very occasionally a cure has resulted. Deep X-ray therapy should always follow, and this is the only hope in all but very early cases. Arsenical preparations and, if necessary, blood transfusion should be employed to combat the accompanying anæmia.

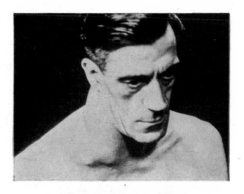

Fig. 224.—Advanced Hodgkin's disease of the cervical lymph nodes.

Prognosis.—The expectation of life of the average patient, who only seeks treatment comparatively late (fig. 224), is about eighteen months. A frequent terminal event is involvement of the mediastinum and lungs.

RETICULO-SARCOMA (See also p. 61)

Again the neck is a common site for this fortunately rare condition. It usually appears as a rapidly growing tumour. In

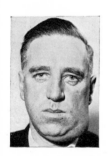

Fig. 225.— Reticulo-sarcoma, two months' duration. Proved histologically.

its early stages the affected lymph nodes are discrete and movable, but soon the neoplasm invades their capsules (fig. 225) and infiltrates surrounding structures. So rapid is the cellular activity that it is sometimes difficult to differentiate between subacute lymphadenitis and reticulo-sarcoma. In such cases the centre of the tumour softens, and ultimately the skin gives way, producing deep sloughing ulcers which bleed freely.

Treatment.—The prognosis is hopeless, although temporary regression occurs with deep X-ray therapy.

CAROTID-BODY TUMOUR

The carotid body, situated at the bifurcation (generally in the fork) of the carotid artery, is a moiety of the chromaffin system. Tumours thereof are usually classified as ganglio-neuromata, neuro-blastomata, or (less satisfactorily) as endotheliomata.

Practically always unilateral, they are rare and difficult to diagnose, for, contrary to expectation, many of these tumours exhibit less transmitted pulsation than the solid lumps from which they have to be differentiated. Clinically there are two types :

(*a*) In the larger proportion of cases the tumour increases in size very slowly ; indeed, it behaves very like a mixed parotid tumour (see p. 177). Unfortunately, as a rule, the lump is at least the size of a hen's egg before the patient seeks advice, and by this time the tumour is intimately blended with the carotid tree. This type is usually noticed first during adult life, although the youngest recorded case was at seven years (Bevan).

(*b*) The smaller proportion of carotid-body tumours occurs in patients of about sixty years of age. This variety gives rise to an irregular, hard lump, and it was called by Sir Jonathan Hutchinson " the potato tumour."

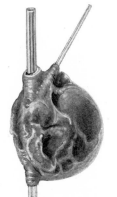

FIG. 226.—Carotid-body tumour successfully removed from a female patient, aged forty-five. Glass rods are in the carotid tree.

Treatment is even more difficult than the diagnosis. Very few of these tumours are radio-sensitive. By the time the patient seeks relief, so blended is the highly vascular tumour with the carotid tree (fig. 226) that its removal is impossible without ligation of the common carotid artery ; and in a few cases ligation of the common carotid is followed by hemiplegia or death.

Electro-encephalography has been employed to determine whether or not ligation of the common carotid artery will render the corresponding cerebral hemisphere dangerously anæmic. After having exposed the artery under local anæsthesia, a piece of tape is passed around the common carotid artery and it is temporarily occluded while the test is being carried out. (Lambert Rogers.)

In a small percentage of cases a patient with a carotid-body tumour complains of attacks of sudden faintness and collapse. This is the carotid sinus syndrome, and, with these warning signs, ligation of the common carotid artery is a perilous undertaking.

Arthur Dean Bevan, Contemporary. Professor of Surgery, Rush Medical College, Chicago.
Sir Jonathan Hutchinson, 1828–1913. Surgeon, London Hospital.
Lambert Rogers, Contemporary. Professor of Surgery, Welsh National School of Medicine, Cardiff.

CHAPTER XII

THE THYROID GLAND AND THE THYROGLOSSAL TRACK

THE thyroid gland is developed mainly from the median bud of the pharynx (the thyroglossal duct), which passes from the foramen cæcum at the base of the tongue to the isthmus of the thyroid. The major part of the lateral lobes also arises from this structure. Lateral buds from the fourth branchial cleft amalgamate with, and complete, the lateral lobes. The parathyroids and the thymus are derived from the third and fourth branchial clefts.

ECTOPIC AND ABERRANT THYROIDS

The whole thyroid gland may be situated in some part of the thyroglossal track, in which case the rings of the trachea are easily palpabel. **Lingual thyroid** (fig. 227A) is the commonest of these rare abnormalities. This variety of ectopic thyroid gland gives rise to a rounded swelling at the back of the tongue beneath the foramen cæcum (fig. 228). In about 10 per cent. of cases removal of a lingual thyroid is followed by myxœdema, for the abnormally situated gland is the only thyroid tissue present.

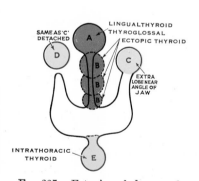

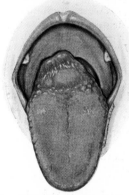

FIG. 227.—Ectopic and aberrant thyroids. A and B are ectopic thyroids, C, D, and E are aberrant thyroids.

FIG. 228.—Lingual thyroid.
(*H. Wapshaw.*) (*British Journal of Surgery.*)

Thyroglossal ectopic thyroid.—In the case of an ectopic thyroid situated in the upper two-thirds of the neck (fig. 227B), the swelling it causes is usually mistaken for a thyroglossal cyst (p. 222), which is much more common. When performing an operation for a supposed thyroglossal cyst, if the swelling is found to be solid, and composed of thyroid substance, some of the thyroid tissue should be spared, in order to prevent myxœdema, because, again, this type of ectopic thyroid may be the only thyroid tissue present.

Lateral aberrant thyroids (fig. 227 C and D) are exceedingly uncommon, and are liable to become malignant. Many authorities deny their existence, and state that supposed malignant aberrant thyroids are secondary deposits in lymph nodes from a primary growth in the thyroid gland.

Intrathoracic aberrant thyroid is a precursor of complete intrathoracic goitre (p. 217).

A goitre is an enlarged thyroid gland.

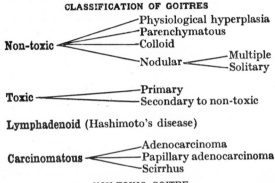

CLASSIFICATION OF GOITRES

Non-toxic — Physiological hyperplasia / Parenchymatous / Colloid / Nodular — Multiple / Solitary

Toxic — Primary / Secondary to non-toxic

Lymphadenoid (Hashimoto's disease)

Carcinomatous — Adenocarcinoma / Papillary adenocarcinoma / Scirrhus

NON-TOXIC GOITRE

Ætiology.—Non-toxic goitre may be endemic or sporadic. There is evidence to show that in some districts, e.g. North America and Switzerland, the goitre is caused by deficiency of iodine in the water-supply, and by the addition of a trace of iodine to the water-supply at regular intervals, or by supplying a table-salt containing one part of potassium iodide to 100,000 parts of sodium chloride, the number of cases has been reduced.

The principal regions in which endemic goitre occurs are the great watersheds—the valleys of the great mountain ranges.

In Europe.—The Alps and Pyrenees.

In India.—The Himalayas and the Punjab Plains.

In Africa.—The Sudan, Egypt, and Sierra Leone.

In North America.—The Rocky Mountains and the basins of the Great Lakes and the St. Lawrence River.

In South America.—The Andes.

In Australasia.—The great plains east of the Southern Alps of New Zealand.

In England there was formerly a " goitre belt " extending from Cornwall, northwards via the Cotswold Hills and the Chilterns, into Derbyshire (the Pennine Chain), with offshoots into Cheshire and North Wales.

In England the incidence of adeno-parenchymatous goitre has diminished considerably in comparison with years gone by ; a change that is usually attributed to the improved distribution of fish, with its high iodine content, and also to a better water supply.

Thus, it seems that iodine deficiency may be overcome by so simple a factor as a weekly call to an isolated village by a fishmonger's van (Young).

PHYSIOLOGICAL HYPERPLASIA (*Syn.* GOITRE OF PUBERTY)

Clinical Features.—The only symptom is a swelling in the neck (fig. 229). The condition is almost confined to females.

Matthew Young, 1884–1940. Lecturer in Anatomy, University College Hospital, London.

The thyroid is enlarged evenly and comparatively soft to the touch. Sometimes the deformity is considerable. Usually the enlargement subsides gradually, and has all but disappeared by the twentieth to twenty-second years.

Treatment.—The adoption of hygienic measures, the elimination of septic foci, and the administration of a harmless iodine preparation, such as syr. ferri iod. ʒj (4 ml.) t.d.s., is all that is necessary.

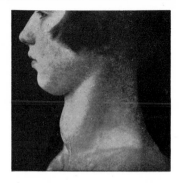

FIG. 229.— Physiological hyperplasia of the thyroid gland.

The use of thyroid extract and Lugol's solution (see p. 214) is discouraged, for not a few examples of thyrotoxicosis have been produced by their exhibition in these cases.

PARENCHYMATOUS GOITRE

Parenchymatous goitre is due to an increase in the epithelial elements of the gland without any appreciable colloid accumulation (Joll). This form of goitre occurs particularly as an endemic variety. It attacks both sexes, often, in goitrous districts, in very early life. When it appears at puberty it is indistinguishable from simple hyperplasia, except by the passage of time. Usually the deformity caused by the swelling is the only symptom. Parenchymatous goitre is a precursor of colloid goitre, and probably of nodular goitre as well.

Treatment.—Unless the swelling is extravagant, the patient is kept under observation until the possibility of the enlargement being a physiological hyperplasia has passed.

COLLOID GOITRE

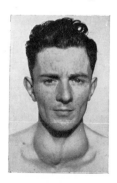

FIG. 230.—Colloid goitre.

The swelling feels fairly elastic and tolerably smooth to the palpating fingers, and usually the whole of the thyroid gland is affected. While clinically it resembles the last variety, microscopically the thyroid vesicles are greatly distended with colloid and lined by flattened cells. By the time the stage of colloid goitre has been reached, the deformity is very obvious (fig. 230). Patients between twenty and thirty years of age are usually affected. Symptoms of pressure upon the air-passages are infrequent. In a few cases this form of goitre becomes toxic.

Cecil Joll, 1885–1945.   Surgeon, Royal Free Hospital, London.

Treatment.—Partial thyroidectomy is advised, in order to reduce the size of the gland to more normal limits. If any toxic symptoms are present the thyroidectomy should be of the subtotal variety.

NODULAR GOITRE

Multiple nodular goitre (*syn.* adenoparenchymatous goitre) is usually encountered in patients over thirty years of age. The whole gland is studded with rounded swellings, some of which are of a considerable size. The nodes are encapsulated masses containing colloid (fig. 231). In long-standing cases calcification of the walls of the nodes occurs. The unsightly swelling, when it has reached a distressing size, is the most common symptom which brings the patient to seek relief.

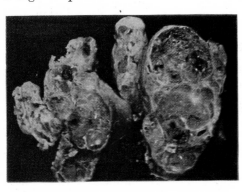

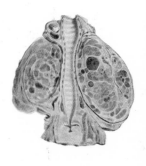

FIG. 232.—Scabbard trachea caused by a multiple nodular goitre.

FIG. 231.—Multiple nodular goitre. Specimen removed at operation. Showing the cut lateral lobes and the pyramidal lobe.

(*British Journal of Surgery.*)

Pressure upon the trachea may develop. When the goitre is mainly unilateral, the degree of tracheal displacement is sometimes fantastic. Nevertheless, it is not so much this type which produces dyspnœa as the bilateral, deep, but not obviously great, enlargement. Here the continuous compression of the sides of the trachea decreases its transverse diameter (fig. 232), and, if unrelieved, a time comes when this portion of the airway is but a mere antero-posterior slit ("scabbard trachea").

Treatment.—The only treatment is surgical, and partial thyroidectomy should be recommended, not only to rid the patient of the deformity and for the relief of pressure symptoms, but because of the possibility, though small, of secondary thyrotoxicosis. Moreover, in about 17 per cent. of cases a carcinomatous change eventually occurs.

Solitary Nodular Goitre.—A favourite site for this solitary localised swelling is at the junction of the isthmus with one lateral lobe of the thyroid gland (fig. 233). Formerly considered to be an adenoma, this frequently well-encapsulated lesion, in its earlier stages, is microscopically similar to parenchymatous goitre. Sooner or later colloid degeneration occurs (fig. 234),

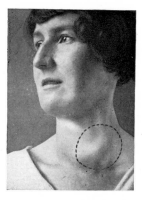

FIG. 233.—Solitary nodular goitre.

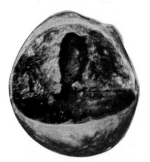

FIG. 234.—Large solitary nodule of the thyroid showing the interior. Colloid degeneration has occurred.

and between the masses of colloid the scanty stroma is richly supplied with thin-walled blood-vessels, from which hæmorrhage into the encapsulated swelling can occur. When the swelling is in juxtaposition to the trachea, hæmorrhage into the swelling can cause sudden death by asphyxia. In old-standing cases calcification in the walls of the swelling commonly occurs.

Treatment.—Surgical treatment should be strongly advised, not only for cosmetic reasons, but because in at least 25 per cent. of cases thyrotoxic symptoms develop about the age of forty; furthermore, this is the commonest form of goitre to become malignant. In addition, there is the danger of sudden hæmorrhage into the swelling.

Because of the high incidence of the development of carcinoma in solitary nodular goitre—as many as 24 per cent. are found to be malignant on histological examination—sub-total hemithyroidectomy, which ensures removal of the node intact within its capsule, is the correct form of treatment.

In cases where a hæmorrhage occurs into the swelling, causing symptoms of asphyxia, the patient sometimes succumbs before surgical aid is available. Relief of intracapsular tension by the insertion of a wide-bore needle has been successful, but in less favourable circumstances, or when this measure fails, an incision over the swelling, *dividing the pretracheal cervical fascia* which permits the goitre to bulge into the wound (instead of pressing upon the trachea), has proved a life-saving measure.

TOXIC GOITRE

Ætiology.—The cause of primary toxic goitre is unknown, but it is believed to be due to over-production of a thyrotrophic hormone of the pituitary. The onset is abrupt, and in a number of cases dates from a crisis in the patient's life in the form of a mental shock. The majority of patients also give a history of a severe or repeated infection of the nasopharynx.

Primary Toxic Goitre (*syn.* Exophthalmic Goitre, Graves' Disease, Basedow's Disease).—The symptoms often appear in the third and fourth decades of life, but may occur earlier or later. Eighty-five per cent. of patients are females. The disease

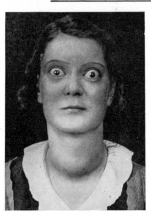

FIG. 235.—Primary toxic goitre.
(*Professor A. J. Wayne.*)

progresses by acute exacerbations and remissions. It is well to remember that the exophthalmos or the goitre may be absent, but seldom both. In a typical case, the protuberant eyeballs, giving a startled look, are unmistakable (fig. 235). Curiously, exophthalmos is sometimes mainly or entirely unilateral. The thyroid gland is enlarged uniformly, and feels smooth and firm. Because of its vascularity, a " thyroid thrill " is often obtained.

In the early stages of the disease the appetite is voracious, but in spite of this the patient loses weight. Due to increased metabolism, there is polyuria, and the patient often complains of having to get up two or three times during the night to micturate. In well-established cases attacks of diarrhœa add to the general wasting. Muscular weakness progresses as the disease advances, and this applies to the myocardium as well as to the skeletal musculature.

Cardiovascular Disturbance.—Tachycardia is a leading symptom. In an acute exacerbation the pulse is very rapid. Usually the blood-pressure is raised, and the slightest excitement accentuates the circulatory turmoil. Eventually the heart

Robert Graves, 1797–1853. Physician to the Meath Hospital, Dublin.
Karl Basedow, 1799–1854. General Practitioner, Mersburg, Germany.

weakens, and auricular fibrillation is a frequent accompaniment of advanced cases.

Nervous Symptoms.—Early cases are commonly diagnosed as neurasthenia. The patient is restless and highly strung. The extended hands shake, and the protruded tongue is tremulous.

Vaso-motor disturbances are in evidence. The patient sweats readily, and is subject to sudden flushing of the face and neck. She is intolerant of heat, and all the symptoms become accentuated in the warmer weather. Insomnia is the rule, and hysterical weeping without provocation is one of the least of many mental abnormalities which may complicate the situation.

Metabolic Activity is Elevated.—*The basal metabolic rate* (B.M.R.) is a valuable method of confirming the clinical diagnosis of thyrotoxicosis, and assessing the degree of metabolic upset. The patient, under strict resting conditions, breathes 50 per cent. oxygen from the Benedict-Roth apparatus, the exhaled carbon dioxide and water vapour being absorbed by a soda-lime tower in the apparatus. After corrections for room temperature and other factors, the oxygen absorbed by the patient over a given time is measured. Calculations are made against the normal for a patient of the same age, sex, and surface area. The resulting figure, if normal, falls between − 15 and + 15 of the normal average. Figures over + 15 are found in hyperthyroidism (thyrotoxicosis), below − 15 in hypothyroidism (myxœdema).

Medical treatment includes rest in bed, a light nutritious diet with copious fluids, and plenty of glucose. Sedatives such as luminal $\frac{1}{2}$ gr. (30 mg.) twice daily are prescribed.

Thiouracil.—A course of one of the preparations of thiouracil is given. Methylthiouracil is the preparation commonly employed in this country at the time of writing, but the more expensive preparation propylthiouracil is less liable to be accompanied by untoward reactions. Thiouracil by, it is believed, combining with the iodine in the thyroid gland, prevents the synthesis of thyroxin. This drug often exercises a strikingly beneficial effect, which is sometimes maintained for as long as small amounts of the drug are continued. The dose given is usually 0·2 gm. (3 gr.), rising to a maximum of 0·6 gm. (9 gr.) daily, until a definite response is obtained, the criteria being a fall in the pulse-rate, a loss of vaso-dilatation, an increase in weight, and a fall in the basal metabolic rate. After this response the dose is reduced to 0·2 or even 0·1 gm. (3 or even 1·5 gr.) daily. During the exhibition of this drug repeated leucocyte counts are necessary, especially during the initial stages of the treatment, because leucopenia, and sometimes the dangerous condition of agranulocytosis, is liable to

Francis Gano Benedict, Contemporary. Director, Nutrition Laboratory, Carnegie Institution, Washington, D.C.
Paul Roth, Contemporary. Director of Physical Therapy, Battle Creek Sanatarium, Michigan, U.S.A.

CARBIMAZOLE   10 - 50 mg.   p.d.

occur.   Watch should also be kept for pyrexia, sore throat, skin rashes, lymphadenopathy, jaundice, and nausea.   Any of these untoward signs and symptoms is a signal that the drug should be discontinued, or the dose of it reduced.

Treatment by thiouracil does not reduce the size of the goitre ; indeed, in many cases the thyroid gland becomes larger, hence it is contraindicated if the gland is retrosternal.   Furthermore, it renders the substance of the gland very vascular and friable, and consequently is inferior to Lugol's solution as an immediate pre-operative measure.   If the patient reacts favourably to thiour-acil, a maintenance dose can be continued for six months, or longer.   When the thiouracil is discontinued, relapses are fre-quent, and on this account, even if the patient reacts favourably, it is usual to advise operation if the goitre persists, or, after a relapse, as soon as the thyrotoxic symptoms have been counter-acted by a second course of the drug.

Radio-active iodine is a new means of controlling primary thyrotoxicosis. Radio-active iodine administered orally has its iodine absorbed rapidly by the secreting cells of the thyroid.   If a small dose of 100 millicuries is given to a normal individual, 30 to 60 per cent. is excreted in the urine within forty-eight hours.   In a thyrotoxic patient less than 20 per cent. is excreted.   This is made use of as a diagnostic test, and as a method of calculating the thera-peutic dose required.   One appropriate dose brings about a clinical im-provement within three weeks.   A second or a third dose can be adminis-tered in necessary cases.

Operative   Treatment.—Careful   pre-operative   preparation occupying at least fourteen days is essential.   The régime of rest in bed, a high fluid intake (including glucose), and sedation is the same as that outlined in medical treatment.   As soon as the patient's general condition warrants it, the date of operation should be fixed.   If the patient has been receiving thiouracil, this is discontinued.   In any case, pre-operative medication with Lugol's solution is commenced.   Lugol's solution is 5 per cent. of iodine dissolved in 10 per cent. potassium iodide.   Lugol's solu-tion is best given in milk or orange juice, either of which masks its taste and colour.   In an average case, 10 minims (0·6 ml.) is given three times a day for twelve to fourteen days, when its maximum effect is reached.   Lugol's solution controls thyrotoxicosis as effectively as thiouracil, but after fourteen days its beneficial effects commence to wane.   Its great advantage over thiouracil as a pre-operative drug is that it renders the gland less vascular and friable.

Jean Guillaume Auguste Lugol, 1786–1851.   Physician, Hôpital Saint-Louis, Paris.

Sub-total Thyroidectomy.—Due to better pre-operative preparation with thiouracil and Lugol's solution, local anæsthetic by infiltration or cervical nerve block is now considered less essential, and is being supplanted by general anæsthesia administered via an endotracheal tube. Kocher's well-known collar incision is made, and the flap is dissected up to the level of the hyoid. A vertical median incision is now made through the fascio-muscular planes from the hyoid bone to Burns's space. By suitable retraction it is possible to expose the lateral lobes. If the goitre is a large one, it is necessary to divide the pre-tracheal muscles. Commencing usually on the right side, the superior pole is freed and the superior thyroid vessels ligated. The middle and inferior thyroid veins are then secured and divided. After suitable dissection the lobe can be delivered into the wound. A special dissection for the inferior thyroid artery is now seldom employed, but if this ligation is undertaken, the artery should be tied well away from the gland, to avoid the recurrent laryngeal nerve. When all is in readiness, about nine-tenths of one lateral lobe

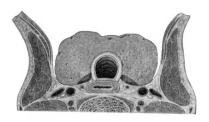

FIG. 236.—Diagram showing the relative amount of a lateral lobe which is removed in toxic goitre, and the portion which remains protecting the parathyroid glands and the recurrent laryngeal nerve.

are resected together with the isthmus (fig. 236). The slice which remains protects the parathyroids and recurrent laryngeal nerve. Provided the patient's condition remains good, which is the rule, sub-total lobectomy is repeated on the other side. The wound is closed, usually with drainage, but if hæmostasis is perfect it may be closed entirely.

In exceptional circumstances the second lobe may be left until the patient has had a further course of medical treatment.

Post-operative Treatment.—The patient is propped up in the sitting position and suitable doses of omnopon and luminal are prescribed. The pulse must be watched closely. While it is important that the patient should have a high fluid intake, she should not receive the fluid intravenously, for fear of embarrassing the heart. Only if the necessary amount of fluid cannot be administered by mouth, via a transnasal intragastric

Theodore Kocher, 1841–1917. Professor of Clinical Surgery, Berne.
Allan Burns, 1781–1813. Extramural lecturer in Surgery and Anatomy, Glasgow.

tube, or per rectum, should the intravenous route be chosen. One drachm of Lugol's solution in milk is given per rectum a few hours after operation. Minims 10 (0·6 ml.) of Lugol's solution are given t.d.s. in fruit juice for five or six days. It is then discontinued.

Post-operative Complications.—Hæmorrhage.—The nurse should be instructed to watch for excessive hæmorrhage, particularly at the back of the dressing, for the blood tends to trickle posteriorly. Reactionary venous hæmorrhage is the usual type, particularly if the patient vomits. Hæmorrhage may be concealed owing to clotting. Any undue bulging of the neck must be reported immediately.

Treatment.—The wound must be reopened as soon as possible. If the bleeding point cannot be found, the wound is packed for twenty-four hours and then resutured.

Dyspnœa.—Urgent dyspnœa may result from blood-clot pressing upon the trachea. In such circumstances it is necessary to reopen the wound immediately and proceed as outlined above. Dyspnœa may also be due to bilateral damage to the recurrent laryngeal nerves. If oxygen fails to relieve the dyspnœa, temporary tracheotomy or intratracheal catheterisation is required.

Alteration to the Voice.—After an extensive thyroidectomy, nearly all patients speak in a whisper for a few days, to spare undue movement in the region of the wound. If hoarseness or aphonia persists, it is probable that there has been damage to one or both recurrent laryngeal nerves (see p. 247).

Acute post-operative hyperthyroidism is much less common than formerly, owing to better pre-operative medical preparation of very toxic patients. It may come on suddenly immediately after operation, or may sometimes be delayed for several hours. The symptoms are increasing pulse-rate, restlessness, and vomiting.

Treatment.—Ten to 20 minims (0·6 to 1·2 ml.) of Lugol's solution should be injected intravenously as a first-aid measure. When the temperature is above 103° F. (39°C.), ice packs are applied. There should be no delay in administering efficient continuous oxygen therapy. As soon as possible the administration of continuous intravenous saline and glucose, to the first pint (600 ml.) of which is added 50 to 100 minims (3 to 6 ml.) of Lugol's solution, is commenced.

Tetany.—When this complication supervenes, it is usually about twenty-four hours after the operation. It is due to parathyroid insufficiency, and its frequency has been greatly diminished by modern operative technique. The patient complains of cramps, and characteristic signs are spasms of the muscles of the legs and arms, the hands assuming the "obstetrical position."

Treatment consists in giving large doses of calcium promptly. In the first instance, 20 per cent. calcium gluconate is injected intravenously in doses of 10 to 20 ml. (⅓ to ⅔ oz.), and repeated if necessary. When the spasms are controlled, calcium lactate may be given by mouth, 30 to 60 gr. (2 to 4 gm.) four-hourly, for several days. If the tetany is not controlled by calcium, the administration of parathormone is usually successful.

Exophthalmic ophthalmoplegia is a rare complication. It consists of a marked increase in the exophthalmos, followed by paralysis of all the voluntary muscles of the eyeball. Radiotherapy sometimes proves valuable. If this fails, orbital decompression must be carried out by transfrontal removal of the roof of the orbit (Naffziger's operation).

Howard C. Naffziger, Contemporary. Surgeon-in-Chief, University of California, San Francisco, U.S.A.

SECONDARY TOXIC GOITRE

Thyrotoxicosis may be secondary to some form of pre-existing simple goitre. It is more frequently encountered in women over forty who have had a solitary nodular goitre for years—often since their 'teens. Secondary thyrotoxicosis is also prone to occur in retrosternal goitres. Although symptoms of secondary toxic goitre are less severe than those of primary toxic goitre, the condition is steadily progressive, and remissions are absent. Cardiovascular symptoms (see p. 212) are most in evidence, and many of these patients have myocardial degeneration. Exophthalmos is nearly always absent. The basic metabolic rate is higher than normal, but not so high as it is in primary toxic goitre.

Treatment.—As secondary thyrotoxicosis seldom responds satisfactorily to thiouracil, the treatment is usually surgical. The same careful pre-operative treatment as detailed for primary toxic goitre is necessary.

INTRATHORACIC GOITRE (*Syn.* RETROSTERNAL GOITRE)

Depending upon whether all or a part is below the level of the sternal notch, an intrathoracic goitre is said to be complete or incomplete, the former being comparatively rare. With few exceptions, goitres wholly intrathoracic are left-sided. While all other types of goitre are far more common in women, intrathoracic goitre is commoner in men. A goitre wholly within the thorax is frequently overlooked, and because it is very liable to become toxic, the symptoms to which it gives rise are mistaken for asthma or heart disease.

An intrathoracic goitre usually displaces the trachea. Sometimes the patient complains that sleeping on one side (usually the right) produces such difficulty in breathing (fig. 237) that he always sleeps on his other side. Owing to years of delay in diagnosis calcification often occurs in the walls of intrathoracic goitres, rendering radiological diagnosis unquestionable.

As a submerged goitre enlarges, dilatation of the superficial thoracic veins over the upper part of the chest wall

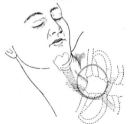

Fig. 237.—Intrathoracic goitre, showing the reason for the dyspnœa.
(*After Lahey.*)

(fig. 238), due to pressure upon one or both innominate veins, is liable to occur, and is characteristic.

Treatment.—As soon as the thyrotoxicosis, if any, is controlled, the first step in the operative removal of an intrathoracic goitre should be ligation and mobilisation of the superior pole of the lateral lobe concerned. The middle thyroid veins are

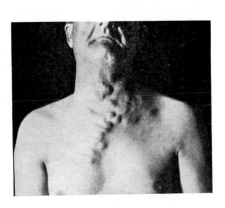

Fig. 238.—Engorgement of the superficial thoracic veins in a case of intrathoracic goitre. (*Professor Rendle Short.*)

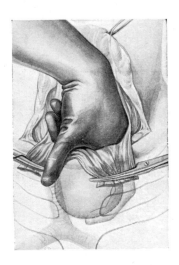

Fig. 239.—A stage in the delivery of an intrathoracic goitre.

next divided between ligatures. The finger is passed into the mediastinum *behind* the tumour (fig. 239). Pressure from below and gentle traction from above applied to the mobilised lateral lobe will, in most cases, permit of the mass being delivered. Oozing from the intrathoracic cavity which accommodated the tumour is controlled by packing. If the above technique is employed, splitting the sternum (see fig. 257, p. 228) in order to get access is rarely necessary.

LYMPHADENOID GOITRE

Lymphadenoid goitre (*syn.* Hashimoto's disease ; struma lymphomatosa) nearly always attacks women in the late forties. The patient is inclined to obesity and has the facies of early myxœdema. The gland is symmetrically enlarged, fairly hard, and somewhat lobulated (fig. 240). The condition has frequently been mistaken for malignant disease. Macro-

K. *Hashimoto*, Contemporary. Surgeon, Okayama, Japan.

scopically the colour of the gland tissue varies from palest pink to yellowish white (fig. 241).

The pathology of lymphadenoid goitre has been the subject of conflicting opinion. At the present time many regard it as a local form of lymphoid reticulosis.

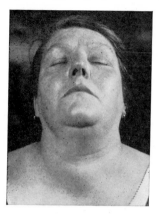

FIG. 240.—Hashimoto's disease.

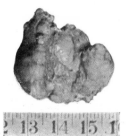

FIG. 241.—Complete thyroidectomy specimen removed from patient shown in Fig. 240.

Treatment.—Lymphadenoid goitre is, according to Sir Stanford Cade, usually radio-sensitive, and a rapid response to deep X-ray therapy serves to distinguish the condition from carcinoma —a differential diagnosis which otherwise is impossible clinically. Other workers have not found deep X-ray treatment permanently satisfactory, and thyroidectomy has been performed. With either form of treatment, a degree of myxœdema requiring the administration of thyroid extract usually follows.

CARCINOMA OF THE THYROID

Adenocarcinoma usually commences in a pre-existing solitary nodular goitre, which previously was thought to be a fœtal adenoma. In different series a varying percentage up to 4 per cent. of solitary nodular goitres removed by operation were found on histological examination to be adenocarcinomata still encapsulated. When the tumour breaks through its confines local growth is usually slow, but it tends to invade veins, and becomes disseminated by the blood-stream, especially to the lungs and bones (fig. 242).

Papillary Adenocarcinoma.—Although this is a slowly growing neoplasm, and the tumour often attains a large size before breaking its confines, in this instance spread to the regional lymph nodes is usual, distant metastases being rare. Lateral aberrant thyroids are particularly prone to this form of malignancy. All lateral aberrant thyroids should be considered potentially malignant (Cattell).

Scirrhous Carcinoma.—Unlike the other varieties of carcinoma of the thyroid, scirrhous carcinoma usually occurs in a normal gland. Its growth is more rapid than either of the foregoing varieties of carcinoma of the thyroid. Distant metastases occur early, as well as involvement of the regional

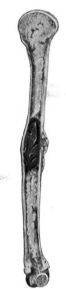

FIG. 242.— Secondary thyroid tumour in the humerus.(*Joll.*) (*British Journal of Surgery.*)

Sir Stanford Cade, Contemporary. Surgeon, Westminster Hospital, London.
Richard Bartley Cattell, Contemporary. Surgeon, Lahey Clinic, Boston, U.S.A.

lymph nodes. Very rarely a thyroid neoplasm is found to be squamous-celled, and possibly in a few instances the growth arises in a fœtal rest of the thyroglossal duct.

Clinical Features.—In the early stages it is impossible to diagnose carcinoma of the thyroid gland, particularly from its most frequent precursor—solitary nodular goitre. When, because of its hardness and irregularity, and even its macroscopical appearance at operation, carcinoma is suspected, it sometimes transpires that the patient is suffering from Hashimoto's disease. Again, unless metastases have occurred, it is impossible to distinguish scirrhous carcinoma from Riedel's thyroiditis until a microscopical examination has been undertaken. Hoarseness due to involvement of a recurrent laryngeal nerve is not infrequent. In advanced cases (fig. 243) the carotid vessels, being surrounded by the growth, cannot be felt. Pain referred to the ear (auricular branch of the vagus nerve) suggests that the main trunk of the vagus has become implicated.

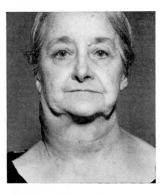

FIG. 243.—Advanced carcinoma of the thyroid.

Treatment.—Deep X-ray therapy, or the administration of radio-active iodine, can be tried, but most of these tumours are not radio-sensitive.

Total Thyroidectomy.—While, in reasonably early cases, complete thyroidectomy offers a good chance of cure, the prognosis is to a large extent dependent upon the type of growth revealed by histological examination of the specimen.

Palliative Operation.—When it is not feasible to perform total thyroidectomy, as much as possible of the tumour should be removed, together with the pretracheal muscles. It also may be advisable to perform tracheotomy.

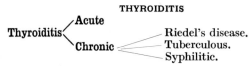

THYROIDITIS

Thyroiditis — Acute
            — Chronic — Riedel's disease.
                       — Tuberculous.
                       — Syphilitic.

Acute thyroiditis is exceedingly rare. It is sometimes primary, but more often secondary to such conditions as tonsillitis and pneumonia. Suppuration is rather infrequent. Treatment follows orthodox lines for local inflammation.

Bernhard Riedel, 1846–1916. Professor of Surgery, Jena, Germany.

Chronic Thyroiditis.—Riedel's thyroiditis (*syn.* ligneous thyroiditis) is also very rare. The condition occurs in males as well as in females. Many of the patients are young adults, a fact which may help to distinguish the condition from scirrhous carcinoma. Microscopically the thyroid is converted into a mass of fibrous tissue. At any rate in the early stages, the pathological process is mainly unilateral. The diseased thyroid becomes intimately adherent to surrounding structures, and infiltrates the pretracheal muscles ; compression of the trachea is the leading symptom. Riedel himself called the condition " iron-hard strumitis " ; certainly its hardness is so great that it may blunt the knife.

Treatment.—Deep X-ray therapy is seldom beneficial. Owing to the extreme density of the gland and its adherence to surrounding structures, thyroidectomy is an extremely arduous undertaking. When dyspnœa is in evidence, resection of the isthmus is the best treatment.

Tuberculosis of the thyroid is exceedingly uncommon. It is sometimes associated with thyrotoxicosis.

Syphilis of the thyroid is also very infrequent, and it is usually mistaken for a malignant tumour. Whenever malignancy is suspected, the possibility of syphilis should be eliminated (Crotti).

CONDITIONS DUE TO DEFICIENT THYROID SECRETION

CRETINISM (INFANTILE HYPOTHYROIDISM)

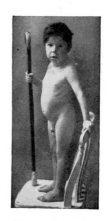

Fig. 244.—A cretin boy aged thirteen. With thyroid extract he soon became nearly normal.

In this country cretinism is sporadic. It appears in healthy families, the other children being normal and the mother presenting no thyroid aberration. The condition is due to absence of the thyroid gland, or to its complete, or almost complete, destruction *in utero.* Cretinism as exhibited in *adolescent and adult life* (fig. 244) can hardly be mistaken. The patient is a dwarf ; the skin is dry, redundant, and wrinkled ; pads of fat are often found in the supraclavicular region. The cretin's mentality is usually below normal, but not necessarily so. *In early infancy,* when it is so necessary to diagnose the condition if it is to be remedied, it is easily overlooked. The principal features at this time are a protuberant tongue and a listless infant who seldom cries and is disinclined to take nourishment. The face is pale, puffy, and somewhat wrinkled. The child snores when asleep. On examination the hands seem thick and short. The anterior fontanelle is open widely. The temperature is subnormal, and, what is most important, the rings of the trachea can be palpated easily.

Treatment consists in administering 1 to $2\frac{1}{2}$ gr. (60–150 mg.)

André Crotti, Contemporary. Surgeon, Mount Carmel Hospital, Columbus, Ohio, U.S.A.

of thyroid extract twice a week, increasing the dose as necessary. Throughout life medical supervision is necessary, for the patient must always take a correct amount of thyroid extract.

MYXŒDEMA (HYPOTHYROIDISM IN THE ADULT)

Myxœdema commonly arises idiopathically, but the same train of symptoms follows extirpation of too much of the thyroid gland. The idiopathic form usually affects women between thirty and forty-five. Its onset is slow, and the patient becomes mentally and physically inert. She feels cold weather intensely. There is an increase in her weight, but the fat has an abnormal distribution ; for instance, there is often a " hump " over the seventh cervical and first dorsal vertebræ. The breasts themselves do not enlarge, but there are deposits immediately below them. The facies coarsens (fig. 245) and the complexion becomes sallow. Much of the hair falls out, and that which remains is dry, lustreless, and prematurely grey.

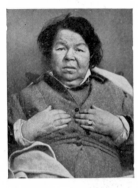

FIG. 245.—Myxœdema.
(Royal Infirmary, Newcastle upon Tyne, Clinical Collection.)

In well-established cases a diminished menstrual flow or amenorrhea is usual. On palpation the skeletal muscles seem hard, and the "mucin"[1]-laden subcutaneous tissues feel adherent to them. The symptoms can be completely cured by appropriate and continued doses of thyroid extract.

ANOMALIES OF THE THYROGLOSSAL TRACK

Thyroglossal cyst may be present in any part of the thyroglossal track (fig. 246). The common situations, in order of

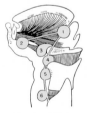

FIG. 246.—Possible sites of a thyroglossal cyst: (1) Beneath the foramen cæcum. (2) In the floor of the mouth. (3) Suprahyoid. (4) Subhyoid. (5) On the thyroid cartilage. (6) At the level of the cricoid cartilage.

frequency, are beneath the hyoid (fig. 248), in the region of the thyroid cartilage (fig. 249), and above the hyoid bone

[1] Mucin. This is not mucin, but a fluid containing about 13 per cent. of (stored) protein. (Best and Taylor's *Physiology*.)

Sir William Gull, 1816–1890. Physician to Guy's Hospital. First described myxœdema.

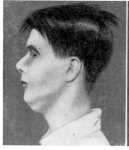
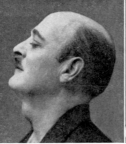
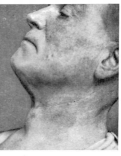

FIG. 247.—Suprahyoid thyroglossal cyst. FIG. 248.—Subhyoid thyroglossal cyst. The commonest variety. FIG. 249.—Thyroglossal cyst in relation to the thyroid cartilage.

(fig. 247).   Such a cyst occupies the middle line, except in the region of the thyroid cartilage, where the thyroglossal track is pushed to one side, usually to the left, viz. :——————————————————→

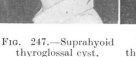

Thyroglossal cysts are the seat of recurrent attacks of inflammation (fig. 250), and when inflamed they are often mistaken for abscesses and incised. This is one way in which a thyroglossal fistula arises.

Thyroglossal fistula (fig. 251) is rarely congenital.   Most often it follows local extirpa-

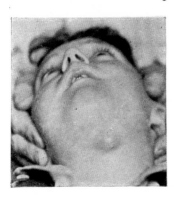

FIG. 250.—Inflamed thyroglossal cyst.

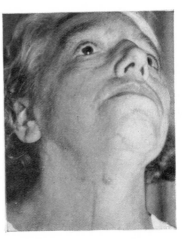

FIG. 251.—A thyroglossal fistula following incision of an inflamed thyroglossal cyst.

tion or incision of a thyroglossal cyst.   Long-standing fistulæ are inclined to be situated low down in the neck, and fig. 252

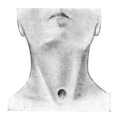

Fig. 252.—A long-standing thyroglossal fistula. The semilunar fold is characteristic.

shows an example that had been present for twenty years. The hood of skin with its concavity downwards (due to uneven rates of growth of the neck as a whole and of the thyroglossal track) is characteristic. A thyroglossal fistula is lined by columnar epithelium, discharges mucus, and is the seat of recurrent attacks of inflammation.

Treatment of a thyroglossal cyst and a thyroglossal fistula is essentially the same. Every vestige of the thyroglossal track must be removed right up to the foramen cæcum, otherwise a discharging fistula is almost inevitable. Because of difficulty in defining the track in the region of the hyoid bone, the centre

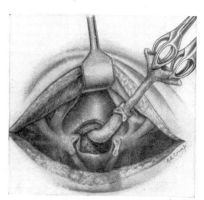

Fig. 253.—Complete extirpation of the thyroglossal track. Note that a portion of the body of the hyoid bone has been removed, and the dissection is proceeding towards the foramen cæcum.

of this bone is resected in the course of the dissection (Sistrunk's operation) (fig. 253). Before embarking upon the removal of a supposed thyroglossal cyst, it is well to make sure that there is a thyroid gland present in the normal position, for the swelling in question may be an ectopic thyroid (see p. 207).

Walter E. Sistrunk, 1880–1933. Surgeon, Mayo Clinic, Rochester, U.S.A.

CHAPTER XIII

THE PARATHYROID GLANDS, THE THYMUS AND THE ADRENAL GLANDS

THE PARATHYROID GLANDS

THESE small glands, reddish-brown in colour and usually four in number, are situated typically in two pairs. They are normally placed outside the thyroid capsule, but one or more of them may be embedded in the thyroid gland. Indeed, in 8 per cent. of subtotal thyroidectomies, a portion of parathyroid tissue is found in the extirpated material. The upper pair are situated behind the superior poles of the thyroid gland ; the inferior pair are inconstant in position (fig. 254). The parathyroid glands, by

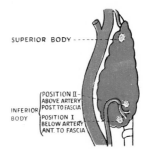

SUPERIOR BODY

FIG. 254.—The usual positions of the parathyroid glands. Coronal section.

(*After Sir James Walton.*)

POSITION II—
ABOVE ARTERY
POST TO FASCIA

INFERIOR
BODY

POSITION I
BELOW ARTERY
ANT. TO FASCIA

virtue of their hormone, parathormone, exercise a controlling influence upon the metabolism of calcium and phosphorus.

Hypoparathyroidism.—The accidental removal of two or more parathyroid glands in the course of thyroidectomy sometimes results in tetany (p. 217). Tetany also occurs occasionally, (*a*) in the new-born idiopathically, (*b*) in adults with long-continued vomiting due to pyloric obstruction, or (*c*) after operations upon the stomach. None of the groups (*a*), (*b*), (*c*) have been proved to be connected with parathyroid deficiency.

Hyperparathyroidism may be due to a tumour of one of the normally placed parathyroid glands, or to a tumour of an ectopic parathyroid gland situated in connective tissue surrounding the cervical œsophagus or in the region of the thymus gland. The tumour, usually an adenoma, is always relatively small (2 to 4 cm. ($\frac{3}{4}$–1$\frac{1}{2}$ in.) in diameter) and upon clinical examination of the neck, is most unlikely to be palpated. A parathyroid tumour cannot be demonstrated by radiography. Occasionally hyperparathyroidism is caused by simple hyperplasia of the parathyroids. The only method of confirming the possibility of hyperparathyroidism is by biochemical investigations. These show:

1. Increased excretion of calcium in the urine.
2. Increased excretion of phosphorus in the urine.
3. Elevation of serum calcium.
4. Decrease of inorganic phosphorus in the blood.

Hyperparathyroidism gives rise to two very different trains of symptoms:

1. Osteitis fibrosa cystica (von Recklinghausen's disease) (p. 1096).

2. Multiple or recurrent urinary calculi (p. 652).

Frequently the urinary (usually renal) calculi precede the bone disease by many years.

PARATHYROIDECTOMY

Parathyroidectomy is the only treatment of hyperparathyroidism. The thyroid gland is exposed as for thyroidectomy, and a parathyroid tumour (fig. 255) is sought by sight and touch in the position of the normal parathyroid glands. When such a tumour is found, it is resected, together with the lateral lobe of the thyroid concerned, if the tumour is embedded in thyroid tissue (fig. 256). When a parathyroid tumour is not found, and the normal parathyroids appear to be the seat of

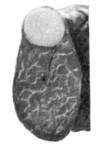

Fig. 256.—Tumour of the left superior parathyroid embedded in the superior pole of the thyroid gland. Case of osteitis fibrosa.
(Lucy and Hill.)
(British Journal of Surgery.)

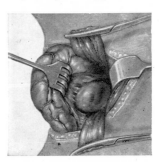

Fig. 255.—Parathyroid tumour exposed.

hyperplasia, two, or occasionally, when large, three of the glands should be removed. Should the parathyroids appear normal and an ectopic parathyroid tumour cannot be located by palpation and blunt dissection in the region of the cervical œsophagus or in the superior mediastinum, the wound is closed. If, during convalescence, the biochemical tests still

Friedrich Daniel von Recklinghausen, 1883–1910. Professor of Pathology, Strasburg.

indicate that the patient is harbouring a parathyroid tumour, a second operation is indicated.   This time the sternum is split and the tumour is sought in the anterior mediastinum, removing the thymus, if necessary. After parathyroidectomy calcium lactate by mouth, in large doses, should be prescribed for four or five days, to forestall the possibility of post-operative tetany.

When hyperparathyroidism can be cured, the diseased skeleton recalcifies, and it is improbable that urinary calculi, if entirely removed, will recur.

THE THYMUS

After puberty the normal thymus atrophies, so that in adults it is almost entirely replaced by fat.

Hypertrophy of the thymus occurs in cases of toxic goitre, Addison's disease, leukæmia, acromegaly and some cases of myasthenia gravis.

Thymic asthma occurs in babies and young children.   There are recurrent attacks of laryngeal spasm, and the larynx is usually poorly developed.   The diagnosis is made on X-ray examination, when a shadow in the region of the thymus is present.

If given in time deep X-ray therapy cures the condition.

Dubois " abscesses " sometimes occur in congenital syphilis.   The thymus becomes vacuolated.   The spaces are filled with turbid fluid, which is not true pus.

Thymic Cysts.—Simple cysts of the thymus have been reported in the literature.

Thymoma is a tumour of the thymus gland.   The term embraces a number of neoplasms which are difficult to classify owing to their varying histological appearances.

Some of these tumours are primarily malignant and, behaving as lymphosarcomata, they invade the mediastinum, causing compression of the air passages and the great veins.   Others are encapsulated, and contain polyhedral cells, suggesting an origin from Hassell's corpuscles.   This variety is at first benign, but later becomes malignant.   It is the latter variety which is sometimes associated with myasthenia gravis.   The diagnosis of a thymoma is largely made on an X-ray examination, a lateral radiograph being especially valuable.

Treatment.—Tumours still confined to the thymus should be removed by thymectomy.   The organ is approached by splitting the sternum (fig. 257).   When the tumour is widespread and non-encapsulated, deep X-ray therapy should be tried, but usually recurrences take place, and the condition is rapidly fatal.

Myasthenia gravis is essentially a disorder which has its seat in neuro-muscular junctions.   It usually commences in early adult life, and is more common in women.   The disease is some-

Paul Dubois, 1797–1871.   Profssor of Obstetrics, University of Paris.
Arthur Hill Hassall, 1817–1894.   Physician, Royal Free Hospital, London.

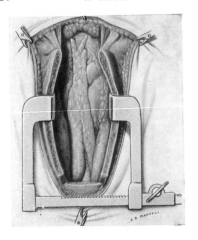

FIG. 257.—Exposure of a tumour of the thymus by splitting the sternum.

(*Geoffrey Keynes.*)
(*British Journal of Surgery.*)

times associated with primary toxic goitre. At first the muscles are easily tired, but recover with rest. Muscles supplied both by cranial and spinal nerves are affected. Ptosis (fig. 258), squints, diplopia, dropping of the jaw, difficulties in swallowing and extreme fatigue on the least exertion are the usual symptoms. The affected muscles may show the myasthenic reaction—fatigue

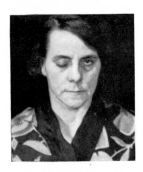

FIG. 258.—Myasthenia gravis. Before prostigmin.

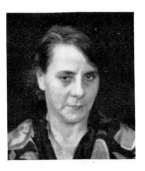

FIG. 259. — Myasthenia gravis. Ten minutes after an injection of prostigmin.

with faradic, but not with galvanic, stimulation. A lateral radiograph of the superior mediastinum may reveal a thymic tumour.

Treatment.—Prostigmin with ephedrine results in temporary improvement (fig. 259) in an otherwise progressive disease. A number of patients have been cured by complete thymectomy; in a minority relapses have occurred. The best results are obtained in the younger patients with long histories (Keynes).

Geoffrey Langdon Keynes, Contemporary. Emeritus Surgeon, St. Bartholemew's Hospital, London.

In 10 per cent. of cases the removed thymus contains a tumour. In the remainder the thymus is either normal or shows simple hyperplasia.

THE ADRENAL GLANDS

Calcification in an Adrenal Gland.—A calcified adrenal gland is difficult to interpret in an X-ray picture (fig. 260) ; it is liable

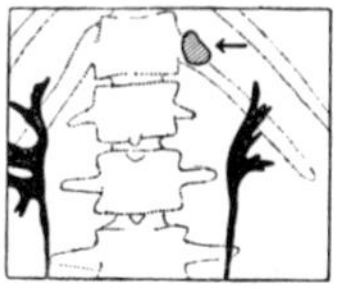

Fig. 260.—Tracing of a radiograph, showing calcification of the left adrenal gland.

to be confused with a renal calculus. Areas of calcification in the adrenal glands have been observed in Addison's disease.

ADRENAL APOPLEXY

Adrenal apoplexy occurs unilaterally or bilaterally, the latter being more common. Bilateral hæmorrhages are nearly always fatal. Adrenal apoplexy has been classified into six clinical groups:

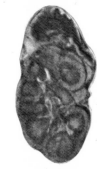

Type 1.—Is a cause of sudden death in infants (fig. 261). At necropsy the only finding is hæmorrhage into both adrenal glands.

Type 2.—Fulminating purpura with adrenal hæmorrhages, known as the Waterhouse-Friderichsen syndrome, occurs in children. The adrenal hæmorrhages are but a manifestation of the hæmorrhagic tendency.

Type 3.—Asthenic type. Asthenia progresses to a fatal termination.

Type 4.—Nervous type. Characterised by delirium, convulsions, and coma.

Type 5.—Peritoneal type. The symptoms simulate acute hæmorrhagic pancreatitis.

Fig. 261.—Adrenal of a newly born infant, s h o w i n g hæmorrhage into it.

Type 6.—Spontaneous perirenal hæmatoma. Except in a few cases due to bursting of an aneurism of the renal artery, spontaneous perirenal hæmatoma is possibly due to adrenal apoplexy. Following prompt operation, a few patients thus afflicted have recovered.

THE SURGICAL ASPECTS OF ADDISON'S DISEASE

Cases are recorded where an adrenal gland, removed with aseptic precautions shortly after death, has been transplanted into the sheath of the rectus abdominis or the breast of a patient suffering from Addison's disease (fig. 262). In a number of instances this has resulted in a dramatic

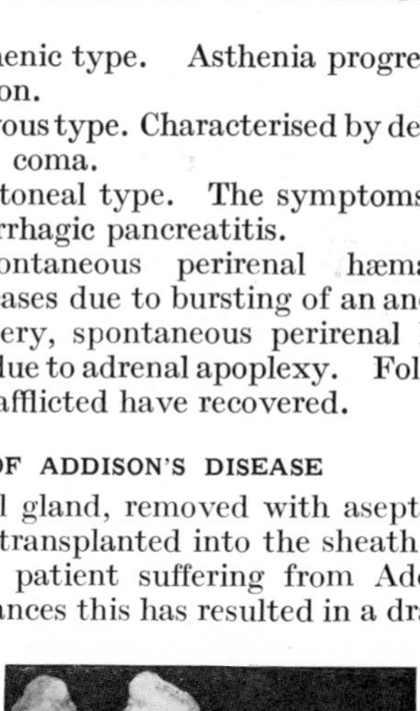

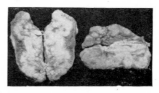

Fig. 262.—Addison's disease. Adrenal glands riddled with caseating tuberculosis.

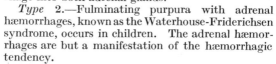

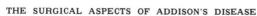

Rupert Waterhouse, Contemporary. Physician, Royal United Hospital, Bath, England.
Carl Friderichsen, Contemporary. Director of the Children's Department, Sundby Hospital, Copenhagen.
Thomas Addison, 1793–1860. *Physician, Guy's Hospital, London.*

improvement in the patient's condition, although it is usually only temporary. Such grafts, of course, are difficult to obtain. As a substitute three 50-mg. pellets of desoxycorticosterone acetate can be implanted in the same way. The good effects are also short-lived, but reimplantations of further pellets can be undertaken.

THE ADRENO-GENITAL SYNDROME

Pre-pubertal type occurs in infancy or early childhood, and as in these cases the adreno-genital syndrome is always due to a malignant growth of the adrenal cortex, it is described on p. 231.

Post-pubertal type may be caused by (*a*) hyperplasia, (*b*) adenoma, or (*c*) carcinoma of the adrenal cortex. It tends to produce a reversal of sex, i.e. signs of virilism appear in women and feminism in men, but feminism in men from this cause is extremely rare (Broster). Those most often affected are young women, and it is more prone to occur in Jewish and Spanish women than in those of other races. The commonest cause of the post-pubertal type of the syndrome is adrenal cortical hyperplasia. The leading symptoms and signs are amenorrhea, an excessive growth of hair on the face (fig. 263), atrophy of the breasts, alterations in bodily contour and muscular development, a tendency to adiposity, a deepening of the voice, and an enlargement of the clitoris.

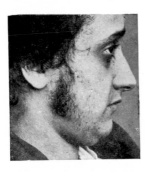

Fig. 263. — Adreno-genital syndrome in a woman of twenty-eight.
(*S. L. Simpson*)

Difficulty in diagnosis arises from the fact that symptoms of the adreno-genital syndrome resemble those of Cushing's syndrome (due to basophil adenoma of the pituitary gland) (p. 864). In both syndromes there is an increased excretion of androgens in the urine, but in the case of the adreno-genital syndrome, the 17-Ketosteroid excretion is usually over 200 mg. in twenty-four hours.

Treatment.—In the case of the adreno-genital syndrome it is most unusual to be able to palpate a tumour of the adrenal gland, a difficulty which is increased by the obesity of the patient. If the condition is strongly suspected, left laparotomy is performed. Should the left adrenal gland be obviously larger than the right, or when both are enlarged (bilateral hyperplasia) the left adrenal gland is removed. If the right adrenal gland is found to be the

Lennox Ross Broster, Contemporary. Surgeon, Charing Cross Hospital, London.
Harvey Cushing, 1869–1939. Professor of Neuro-Surgery, Yale University.

larger, the wound is closed and a fortnight later the right adrenal gland is removed by an incision in the loin, through the bed of the resected twelfth rib.   Removal of one adrenal gland in the case of bilateral hyperplasia improves the condition, but it is not curative.   When the lesion is unilateral the results of adrenalectomy are excellent.   In order to combat possible post-operative adrenal cortical insufficiency, 20 mg. of desoxycorticosterone is given intramuscularly during the first twenty-four hours after operation ; this is followed by daily decreasing doses of the drug.

ADRENAL TUMOURS

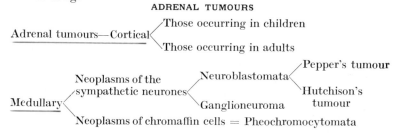

Adrenal tumours—Cortical — Those occurring in children / Those occurring in adults

Medullary — Neoplasms of the sympathetic neurones — Neuroblastomata — Pepper's tumour / Hutchison's tumour / Ganglioneuroma

Neoplasms of chromaffin cells = Pheochromocytomata

TUMOURS OF THE ADRENAL CORTEX

Tumours of the adrenal cortex arise in the zona fasciculata, and are divided into two varieties :

Those occurring in children.—Little girls are the usual victims. Puberty is precipitated ; the child of four or five presents a full growth of pubic hair and well-developed breasts.   In the case of a boy of seven, the child was bearded, and had to be shaved daily. Often this neoplasm is very malignant and secondaries soon appear in the liver, spleen, and in bones, notably the skull.

Treatment.—If the adrenal glands are explored soon after the appearance of the initial symptoms, it may be possible to remove a primary growth before metastases have occurred.

Those occurring in adults.—Both adenomata and carcinomata of the adrenal cortex occur, and these tumours are sometimes associated with the adreno-genital syndrome.   On the other hand, a patient without any signs of this syndrome with an adrenal cortical tumour may seek advice on account of an abdominal swelling.   Cortical adenomata tend to become carcinomatous, and it is this variety that attains considerable dimensions before metastases occur.   Metastasis takes place via the adrenal vein to the retroperitoneal and mesenteric lymph nodes, to the lungs, and in late cases the contralateral adrenal is often involved.   Bones are seldom the site of secondary deposits, but in other respects, including macroscopical appearance and behaviour, the tumour closely resembles a Grawitz' tumour of the kidney (p. 678).   When an adrenal tumour is large enough to be palpable, a depression of the upper portion of the renal pelvis can usually be demonstrated by pyelography.   The tumour can be differentiated from a Grawitz' tumour by the 17-Ketosteroid content of the urine, which is high in the case of an adrenal cortical tumour, and normal in the case of a Grawitz' tumour.

Treatment.—If adrenalectomy can be performed before metastasis has occurred, the prognosis is good.   The operation is best conducted through an incision in the bed of the resected twelfth rib.

TUMOURS OF THE ADRENAL MEDULLA

Tumours of the sympathetic neurones.   Neuroblastomata occur in two forms, both of which are very rare :

(*a*) *Pepper's tumour* occurs in very young children under two years of age.   It is rapidly fatal, giving rise to metastases in the liver, which becomes greatly enlarged.   The mesenteric lymph nodes and the lungs also become involved.   Formerly it was thought that the right adrenal gland was more often the seat of this primary tumour, but according to Boyd there is no substantiation for this statement.

(*b*) *Hutchison's tumour* occurs in older children.   It is slightly less malignant than the foregoing.   Metastases occur chiefly in bones, especially those of the orbit and skull.

Treatment.—Although these tumours are radio-sensitive, recurrence is almost inevitable.   An occasional case of survival after deep X-ray therapy has been reported.

Ganglioneuroma is relatively benign, and occurs in adults as well as children.   These grow to a large size and form one of the varieties of retroperitoneal sarcoma.

Treatment.—If completely removed at a comparatively early stage, a cure can be expected.

Tumours of the chromaffin cells.   Pheochromocytoma, which owes its name to the presence of chromaffin granules, is another very rare adrenal tumour.   Pheochromocytoma occurs in adults of both sexes.   The tumour is usually innocent, and it produces an excess of adrenalin, consequently the blood pressure is raised, and often there are paroxysmal attacks of extreme arterial hypertension.   The paroxysmal attacks, which last for a few minutes to several hours, are accompanied by cutaneous flushing and a sensation of suffocation.   The blood pressure may register as much as 300 mm. Hg.   The attacks are followed by great prostration and glycosuria.   In some cases the tumour is large enough to be palpated.   More usually it has to be demonstrated radiologically (*a*) by a depression of the renal pelvis in a pyelograph, or (*b*) by perirenal insufflation of air.

Treatment.—The tumour should be removed by operation.   The immediate post-operative mortality is considerable, but those who survive are cured.

Paul Grawitz, 1850–1932. *Professor of Pathology, Greifswald, Germany.*
William Pepper, Contemporary. *Physician, Dean of the Medical Faculty, University of Pennsylvania.*
William Boyd, Contemporary. *Professor of Pathology and Bacteriology. University of Toronto.*
Robert Hutchison, Contemporary. *Consulting Physician, London Hospital.*

CHAPTER XIV

THE PHARYNX AND THE LARYNX

TONSILS AND ADENOIDS

Surgical Anatomy.—The conception that the lymphadenoid tissue of the naso-pharynx is Nature's barrier to bacterial invasion can be fostered, and the ætiology of certain cervical inflammations can be visualised and better understood, if Waldeyer's inner and outer rings (fig. 264) are studied. The

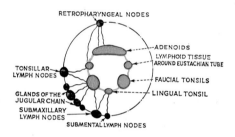

RETROPHARYNGEAL NODES

ADENOIDS
LYMPHOID TISSUE
AROUND EUSTACHIAN TUBE

TONSILLAR
LYMPH NODES

FAUCIAL TONSILS

GLANDS OF THE
JUGULAR CHAIN

LINGUAL TONSIL

SUBMAXILLARY
LYMPH NODES

SUBMENTAL LYMPH NODES

FIG. 264.—Waldeyer's rings.   Inner ring—first barrier to infection ; outer ring—second barrier.

faucial tonsils are the largest and most important moieties of the inner ring.   Tonsillar tissue normally contains crypts, usually tortuous, which extend right through the tonsillar substance to the external capsule.   These crypts can, and often do, harbour pus and micro-organisms.   The capsule is a definite structure composed of fibrous and elastic tissue, and muscle fibres.   It clothes the lateral two-thirds of the circumference of each tonsil, the median third of the circumference being that portion of the tonsil which lies between the pillars of the fauces and is readily accessible to clinical examination.

The tonsil has an exceptionally good blood supply (fig. 265). It is well to bear in mind the vulnerable but infrequent anomaly of the internal carotid artery forming a complete circular coil (fig. 266), but it is reassuring for those who enucleate tonsils with a guillotine to know that they drag the tonsil away from the danger zone (Brown Kelly).

Wilhelm von Waldeyer, 1836–1921.   Professor of Pathology, Berlin.
Adam Brown Kelly, 1865–1941.   Surgeon to Ear, Nose, and Throat Department, Victoria Infirmary, Glasgow.

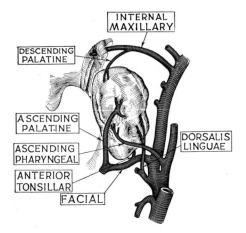

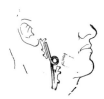

Fig. 266. — Internal carotid artery forming a complete circular coil.
(*After A. Brown Kelly.*)

Fig. 265.—The arterial supply of the tonsil.
(*After Fowler.*)

ENLARGEMENT OF THE TONSILS

Enlarged tonsils are not necessarily infected ; a certain amount of hypertrophy is common in early childhood. As adult life approaches the tonsils, together with other lymphoid tissues, tend to undergo a process of involution. Excessive hypertrophy is often bilateral. Occasionally the tonsils are so large that they almost meet in the middle line.

Considerable adenoid hypertrophy causes the patient to snore loudly at night and to breathe through the open mouth, giving that well-known vacant expression (fig. 267). Added to this, hearing is impaired by the hypertrophied lymphadenoid tissue obstructing the orifice of the Eustachian tubes.

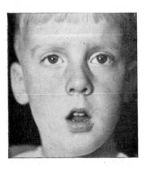

Fig. 267.—The adenoidal facies. Tonsillar hypertrophy is a usual accompaniment. (*Dr. Bauer.*)

Acute follicular tonsillitis is a common condition characterised by pyrexia associated with a sore throat, the most usual causal organism being a streptococcus. On examination the tonsils are swollen, and yellow spots due to pus in the crypts of the mucous membrane can often be discerned. The lymph nodes of the neck are usually enlarged and painful. The condition must be distinguished from diphtheria, and ulceration due to Vincent's spirillum, by a bacteriological examination. Mild cases

Bartolommeo Eustacchio, 1524–1574.   *Professor of Anatomy, Rome.*
Jean Hyacinthe Vincent, 1862–1950.   *Professor of Medicine, Val-de-Grâce (Military) Hospital, France.*

may resemble the small "snail track" ulcers of secondary syphilis.

Treatment.—Aspirin is administered to relieve pain, and penicillin lozenges are prescribed. When the infection has subsided, the question of the advisability of tonsillectomy, or removal of a portion of tonsillar tissue left behind at a previous tonsillectomy, will arise.

Chronic tonsillitis is often associated with hypertrophy. During early childhood chronically inflamed tonsils are usually soft, but as puberty is reached, they frequently become indurated, due to recurrent attacks of inflammation and subsequent fibrosis. The tonsillar lymph node of the jugular chain is usually palpable.

Sometimes pus and débris can be expressed from infected tonsillar crypts. In suitable instances suction of the tonsils enables a bacteriological examination to be made.

MALIGNANT TUMOURS OF THE TONSIL

Neoplasms of the tonsil are of three varieties :

	Approximately
Carcinoma, usually squamous-celled . .	85 per cent.
Reticulo-sarcoma	10 ,, ,,
Lymphoepithelioma	5 ,, ,,

All are extremely malignant, and all are difficult to diagnose in their early stages. In the case of **carcinoma of the tonsil**, the patient is commonly an elderly man, and pain is a leading symptom. The pain is severe and radiates to the ear, and, unlike that of tonsillitis, it is unilateral. Later, bleeding occurs, and as the ulcer deepens the loss of blood may be copious. **Reticulo-sarcomata** usually occur earlier in life, and the first complaint is of a lump in the throat with discomfort on swallowing. Later the growth spreads, and forms a swelling of the palate, which has been mistaken for a peritonsillar abscess. In all varieties the cervical lymph nodes soon become involved, and in reticulo-sarcoma distant metastases are not long delayed.

In order to confirm a diagnosis, a biopsy is necessary, and sufficient material must be removed to assist in what is often a difficult histological diagnosis. It is usually conceded that a biopsy of a tonsillar tumour stimulates the rapid growth of the neoplasm. It is therefore advised to carry out the biopsy with a diathermy knife only after the patient has been subjected to deep X-ray therapy.

Treatment should be by deep X-rays or by teleradium, when available. Except in early cases, the prognosis is poor.

TONSILLECTOMY

While indiscriminate extirpation of tonsils and adenoids is to be deprecated, there can be no question that removal of greatly hypertrophied and infected tonsils and adenoids confers enormous benefits upon the individual. In children particularly, when this source of recurrent infection and respiratory obstruction has been removed, the general condition improves remarkably.

Indications for Tonsillectomy.—1. Hypertrophy of such a degree as to cause respiratory obstruction. Such examples are usually associated with adenoids.

2. After an attack or repeated attacks of acute tonsillitis.

3. Chronic tonsillitis, accompanied by frequent sore throats or quinsy.

4. Tuberculous cervical adenitis where the tonsils are suspected of being the primary focus of infection.

Tonsillectomy.—Tonsils can be removed by dissection or by enucleation with a guillotine.

Dissection.—This method is more exact and bleeding is far less in evidence. Either local or general anæsthesia can be employed. The mouth is kept open and the tongue depressed with a Davis's gag (fig. 268). The

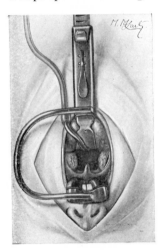

tonsil is seized with volsellum forceps. An incision is made through the mucous membrane, and the capsule of the tonsil is exposed. The tonsil is removed by dissection, starting at the upper (palatal) pole. When the pedicle is defined, it is severed by a wire snare.

By Enucleation with the Guillotine.—When the tonsils have been removed with the guillotine (fig. 269) considerable hæmorrhage occurs. This soon ceases when the pharynx has been cleared with swabs upon a holder, and ice-cold water, which should always be in readiness, is applied to the face.

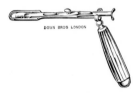

Fig. 268.—Removal of the tonsils by dissection. Exposing the tonsillar capsule.

Fig. 269.—A guillotine.

The patient is kept in the operating theatre until the bleeding has ceased and the air-way is clear.

After-treatment of Patients who have Undergone the Guillotine Operation.—Until the patient has recovered consciousness he should be kept with his head low and well over to one side (fig. 270). On no account should he be permitted to lie on his back or be left unattended.

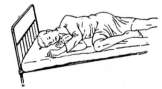

Fig. 270.—Position of patient after tonsillectomy.

The original Davis's gag was invented by Dr. Davis, of Boston, Mass. Edmund G. Boyle, Anæsthetist, St. Bartholomew's Hospital, perfected it.

Hæmorrhage after Tonsillectomy.—The main disadvantage of the guillotine operation is that occasionally serious renewed hæmorrhage occurs from the tonsillar bed. In such cases prompt measures are necessary. The most important of the immediate measures are : (1) removal of clot from the tonsillar bed (fig. 271), (2) the application of pressure and

FIG. 271.—Hæmorrhage from the tonsillar bed may be due to clot preventing the surrounding musculature from contracting. (*After Lee Macgregor.*)

styptics by means of a swab on a holder, (3) the administration of morphia. If bleeding persists in spite of these measures, the patient should be returned to the operating theatre, and under general anæsthesia the bleeding-point is sought and ligatured. When the bleeding-point cannot be found, coaptation of the pillars of the fauces with sutures will arrest the hæmorrhage. These stitches should be removed after twenty-four hours. The usual methods of replenishing the circulation after loss of blood must be invoked.

Removal of adenoids is usually undertaken at the conclusion of an operation for tonsils. Adenoids are removed with a curette (figs. 272, 273). If considerable hæmorrhage follows the removal of adenoids, the post-nasal space should be packed firmly with gauze, which is removed at the end of twenty-four hours.

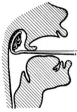

FIG. 272.— Curettage of adenoids.

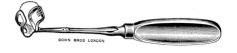

FIG. 273.—An adenoid curette.

PERITONSILLAR ABSCESS (*Syn.* QUINSY)

Peritonsillar abscess is nearly always an extension of acute suppurative tonsillitis. The general symptoms are often severe. Locally, in addition to the signs of the preceding tonsillitis, there is a diffuse swelling of the soft palate, most in evidence near the superior border of the affected tonsil. The swelling displaces the œdematous uvula to the contralateral side.

Treatment, in the early stages, is the same as that for acute follicular tonsillitis. In addition, penicillin should be administered intramuscularly. If suppuration occurs, evacuation of pus in the following manner should not be delayed.

A scalpel is prepared by winding a strip of strapping around the blade so that only

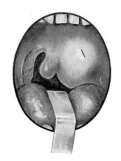

FIG. 274.—Peritonsillar abscess, showing site of incision.

1 cm. ($\frac{2}{5}$ in.) of the tip projects. An incision is made in the position shown in fig. 274, which is usually described as midway between the base of the uvula and the third upper molar tooth. Dressing forceps are now pushed firmly *directly backwards*. As soon as pus is encountered the forceps are widely opened and withdrawn.

Parapharyngeal abscess is similar to the above, but the maximum swelling is behind the posterior faucial pillar, and there is little or no œdema of the palate. The abscess is opened with a really blunt instrument, such as a tongue depressor. Often the gloved finger will suffice (Watson-Williams).

RETROPHARYNGEAL ABSCESS

Two forms occur :

Acute.—*Between* the prevertebral fascia and the pharynx.

Chronic.—*Behind* the prevertebral fascia.

Acute retropharyngeal abscess is most commonly seen in children under the age of four. It is the result of suppuration of the lymphatic nodes which occupy the space. In infants the condition is sometimes very acute, and accompanied by rigors, convulsions, and vomiting. The neck is held rigidly, usually on one side, and saliva dribbles from the child's mouth. Its feeds are regurgitated, and dyspnœa is an important feature. The posterior wall of the pharynx is swollen. This is sometimes only visible when the base of the tongue has been firmly depressed. A localised projection may be felt digitally. The only condition with which acute retropharyngeal abscess is likely to be confused is laryngeal diphtheria.

A less acute form is seen in older children as a complication of middle-ear disease.

Treatment.—The anæsthetised child is held upside-down, and a pair of dressing forceps guided by the finger is thrust into the abscess cavity, the contents of which are evacuated before the patient is laid prone. Suitable chemotherapy is prescribed.

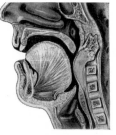

Fig. 275.—Chronic retropharyngeal abscess secondary to tuberculous disease of the cervical vertebræ.

Chronic retropharyngeal abscess is often due to an extension of tuberculosis of the cervical vertebræ (fig. 275), and this possibility should always be confirmed or eliminated by suitable radiographs of the cervical spine. Cases of chronic retropharyngeal abscess due to tuberculous retropharyngeal lymph nodes are not uncommon. When the collection of pus is large, in addition to

Eric Watson-Williams, Contemporary. Aural Surgeon, Bristol Royal Infirmary.

the retropharyngeal swelling, there is a fullness behind the sterno-mastoid on one side.   A chronic retropharyngeal abscess must never be opened into the mouth, for such a procedure will lead to secondary infection.   The pus should be evacuated by an incision behind the sternomastoid.   The dissection towards the retro-pharyngeal space is conducted carefully until the abscess is opened.   The cavity is then mopped dry and the wound closed. The treatment of the tuberculous process must then receive attention.

DIVERTICULUM OF THE PHARYNX

Congenital lateral diverticulum is really a blind internal branchial fistula (p. 185) opening into the fossa of Rosenmüller.   Occasionally such a fistula becomes greatly distended and food lodges within it.

Pharyngeal Pouch—Ætiology.—There is a weak area in the musculature of the pharynx in the middle line posteriorly, at its extreme lower end near its junction with the œsophagus.   This is Killian's dehiscence, which is bounded above and laterally by the inter-digitating fibres of each half of the inferior constrictor, and below by the sphincteric portion of the crico-pharyngeus muscle.   When the pharynx is viewed from within, a dimple can be seen in the mucous membrane at this point in the normal subject (fig. 276).   If the intrapharyngeal pressure

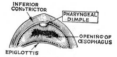

FIG. 276.—The pharyn-geal dimple.

is raised, the mucous membrane will tend to be forced through this weakness.   The probable cause of increased intrapharyngeal pressure is intermittent spasm of the crico-pharyngeus due to inco-ordination of the intricate neuro-muscular mechanism of the region.   This theory is sub-stantiated by an inquiry into the early history of the patients, some of whom state that they had ex-perienced attacks of slight difficulty in swallowing since adolescence.   So commences a pharyngeal pouch (fig. 277).

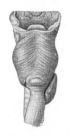

FIG. 277.—Early pro-trusion of the mucous mem-brane in the middle line posteriorly through Kil-lian's dehis-cence. *(Raven.)* *(British Journal of Surgery.)*

Clinical Features.—As time goes on, the sac becomes larger and fills with food at every meal. Unable to expand posteriorly because of the resist-ance of the vertebral column, the pouch turns out-wards, usually to the left (fig. 278), and obtrudes itself into the side wall of the neck.   In about

Justav Killian, 1860–1921.   Professor of Otolaryngology, Berlin.
Gohann Rosenmüller, 1771–1820.   Professor of Anatomy and Surgery, Leipzig.

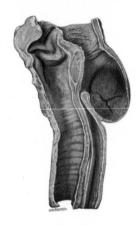

FIG. 278.—Museum specimen of a pharyngeal pouch, showing compression of the adjacent œsophagus. (*British Journal of Surgery.*)

one-third of cases a pharyngeal pouch is large enough to form a visible swelling. Sometimes the pouch can be seen to enlarge when the patient drinks. Patients presenting themselves with this condition are usually, but not necessarily, elderly, and it is twice as common in men as in women. The complaint is dysphagia, for when the sac becomes full, its lower part presses upon the œsophagus (fig. 279). Regurgitation of undigested food often occurs. An irritable cough and a gurgling noise in the neck

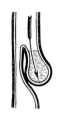

FIG. 279.—Showing how a pharyngeal pouch causes dysphagia.

may also be symptoms. Some intelligent patients acquire a knack of overcoming their disability. It is recorded that Lord Jeffrey, a Scottish nobleman, was in the habit of emptying his pouch with a large silver spoon after every meal. Other sufferers have found that they can swallow their food better if the pouch

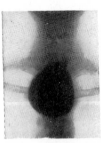

FIG. 280.—Radiograph of a pharyngeal pouch after a barium meal.
(*Capps and Dunhill.*)
(*British Journal of Surgery.*)

is full, and accordingly take porridge as a first course. Notwithstanding these ingenious devices, eventually there is progressive loss of weight due to semi-starvation, and cachexia is sometimes extreme.

The patient should be investigated by radiography after the ingestion of barium (fig. 280). Quite often the fundus of the pouch will be seen invading the mediastinum.

Treatment.—When the diverticulum is a small one, and the symptoms confined to slight difficulty in swallowing, the passage of an œsophageal bougie at intervals may keep more serious symptoms in abeyance. In these circumstances a conservative course should be followed, because a small pouch is much more difficult to remove than a large one.

In cases where the pouch is of a considerable size, operation is strongly advised, because progressive symptoms are inevitable. When there is extreme emaciation, a preliminary temporary gastrostomy is occasionally required.

The operation may be performed in two stages, or the whole procedure completed in one stage. The two-stage procedure was designed to prevent mediastinitis, but this danger appears to have been exaggerated. The operation can be conducted under local anæsthesia or endotracheal general anæsthesia.

The Two-stage Operation.—At the first stage a longitudinal incision is made along the anterior border of the sternomastoid in the lower half of the neck. The pouch is approached by mobilising the lateral lobe of the thyroid gland. It is necessary to ligate and divide the middle thyroid veins, and sometimes the inferior thyroid artery in addition. When this has been completed, the lateral lobe is retracted forwards, and the internal jugular vein is retracted backwards. At this stage a large stomach tube is passed by the anæsthetist and it enters the pouch ; the tube is guided by the surgeon from the pouch into the œsophagus, and there it remains during the operation as a helpful guide in determining the limits of the neck of the sac during the later stages of the dissection.

The walls of the sac vary in thickness ; in some cases they are so thin that great care must be taken not to tear them.

When the pouch is free, it is exteriorised by stitching the muscles to it in such a way that its opening into the pharynx inclines downwards rather than upwards.

The skin is then closed about the unopened sac.

The second stage is undertaken about fourteen days later. The pouch is cut off level with the skin. The mucosa is dissected up for a short distance and the wound closed in two layers.

The One-stage Operation.—The dissection of the pouch is precisely similar to that of the first stage of the two-stage procedure, except that most operators approach the pouch through a transverse incision at the level of the cricoid cartilage. Having freed the pouch completely, a cuff of the outer layer of the pouch is dissected from the mucous membrane. This permits of the closure of the neck of the sac, which must be very accurately performed in two layers, alternatively the neck of the sac is clamped, and after the pouch has been excised with the diathermy knife, the stump is closed in two layers in the same manner as a duodenal stump is closed after gastrectomy. The wound is closed with drainage.

After-treatment (one-stage operation).—The patient is fed through an indwelling transnasal gastric tube for three days. Fluids only are permitted for the next three days. After this, semi-solids are given, and the diet is then gradually increased.

Complications :

1. **Infection.**—As stated previously, severe infection of the wound is now infrequent. Infection can be prevented, or if it occurs can be combated with chemotherapy.

2. **Pharyngeal Fistula.**—The fistula usually closes spontaneously.

NEOPLASMS OF THE PHARYNX

Benign tumours are extremely rare, and include papilloma, lipoma, and angioma. The first two should be removed by excision, and an angioma, which is sometimes the source of hæmorrhage, should be destroyed with a diathermy knife.

Malignant tumours are relatively common. With the exception of nasopharyngeal tumour, which has been considered already on p. 136, they are carcinomatous.

Surgical Anatomy.—For purposes of description of the sites for carcinoma of the pharynx, the pharynx proper is divided into the oropharynx and the laryngopharynx. The laryngopharynx, which extends from the epiglottis above to the commencement of the œsophagus at the level of the sixth cervical vertebra below,

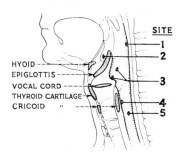

HYOID
EPIGLOTTIS
VOCAL CORD
THYROID CARTILAGE
CRICOID "

SITE
1
2
3
4
5

Fig. 281.—Sites of carcinoma of the oropharynx and laryngopharynx.

1. The posterior wall of the oropharynx.
2. The epilarynx.
3. The sinus pyriformis and the lateral wall of the epipharynx.
4. The postcricoid region.
5. The posterior wall of the hypopharynx.
(After Sir Stanford Cade.)

is further divided into an epipharynx above the upper border of the cricoid cartilage, and a hypopharynx below this line (fig. 281).

1. Carcinoma of the posterior wall of the oropharynx usually occurs in women over sixty-five years of age. The lesion is of the ulcerative type. Spread to the regional lymph nodes is comparatively late. The symptoms are not severe, and pain is a very late complaint. There is discomfort at the back of the throat, fœtor, and blood-stained sputum.

2. Epilayrngeal Carcinoma.—This group embraces growths which were formerly known as extrinsic carcinoma of the larynx. The lesion is situated on an ary-epiglottic fold, the epiglottis, or on the vallecula, and is either of the ulcerative or the papillary type. Epilaryngeal carcinoma is most often seen in men between fifty and sixty. The earliest symptom is hoarseness. Later there are attacks of dyspnœa associated with the expectoration of blood-stained sputum. The diagnosis is made by indirect laryngoscopy.

3. Carcinoma of the Sinus Pyriformis and the Lateral Wall of the Pharynx.—Again, this group occurs chiefly in men about fifty years of age but, unlike the foregoing, may be called the silent type, by which is meant that the neoplasm does not give rise to symptoms until an advanced stage has been reached. Tumours of the lateral wall are often papillary, while those of the pyriform fossa (fig. 282) are of the ulcerative type. In a number of instances the appearance of a mass of malignant lymph nodes below the angle of the jaw (fig. 283) is the only reason for the patient seeking advice. Exceptionally, the patient presents himself at an earlier stage,

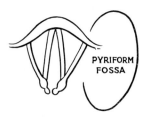

Fig. 282.—The pyriform fossa is the most frequent site of a silent laryngo-pharyngeal carcinoma.

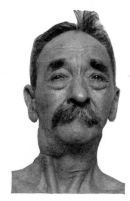

Fig. 283.—Malignant lymph nodes of the neck. Secondary to laryngo-pharyngeal carcinoma in the "silent" area. The patient presented himself on account of the lump in the neck.

because of slight difficulty in swallowing saliva, as opposed to food. Pain is absent. The presence of the growth can be shown with a laryngeal mirror, but sometimes its extent cannot be determined without the aid of direct laryngoscopy.

4. Post-cricoid carcinoma occurs on the anterior wall of the hypopharynx at the level of the cricoid cartilage. The patient is nearly always a woman of about forty years of age, who gives a history of increasing dysphagia. Many of these neoplasms are secondary to the Plummer-Vinson syndrome. Indirect laryngoscopy seldom reveals the growth, which lies hidden beneath a pool of mucus. Radiographic examination after a barium swallow is often helpful in determining the site of the lesion. Direct pharyngoscopy is the most informative, and allows a portion of the growth to be removed for biopsy.

5. Carcinoma of the posterior wall of the hypopharynx occurs at a lower level than the foregoing. The patient is usually an elderly man, and the symptoms are precisely those of carcinoma of the upper third of the œsophagus ; indeed, it is usually impossible to determine if the growth begins in the extreme end of the pharynx or in the commencement of the œsophagus.

Treatment.—Carcinoma of the oropharynx is best treated by deep X-ray therapy, or teleradium when available. In comparatively early cases this causes regression or disappearance of

Henry S. Plummer, 1874–1936. Physician, Mayo Clinic, Rochester, U.S.A.
Porter P. Vinson, Contemporary. Physician, Mayo Clinic, Rochester, U.S.A.

the growth, but the eventual prognosis is poor. **Carcinoma of the laryngopharynx** is also treated by deep X-ray therapy and teleradium. Many of these neoplasms are radio-sensitive, but the eventual prognosis is poor, particularly when the carcinoma is situated in the " silent " area.

In a few instances the tumour is radio-resistant, and when the patient's general condition is good and the lesion is tolerably circumscribed, Trotter's operation of transhyoid pharyngotomy, combined, if necessary, with excision of the involved larynx, is sometimes indicated.

Trotter's operation is usually performed in conjunction with a dissection of the lymph nodes of the neck. Preliminary tracheotomy is performed. After the lymphatic nodes have been extirpated, the cervical fascia, previously raised in the form of a flap, is stitched to the prevertebral muscles. In this way the posterior part of the wound and the carotid vessels are shut off from the area which will be exposed to infection from the pharynx. The lateral lobe of the thyroid is mobilised and displaced forwards. The inferior constrictor muscle is detached from the thyroid and cricoid cartilages. The great cornu of the hyoid bone and the posterior two-thirds of the ala of the thyroid cartilage are removed without opening the mucous lining. The pharynx is then incised longitudinally and packs are inserted into the œsophagus below and the glottis above. The tumour is then excised with a margin of healthy mucous membrane. If the resulting defect is small, the edges are reunited ; if it is large, a tube is passed into the stomach and the pharynx is packed. A plastic operation is performed later. When it is known beforehand that the defect in the

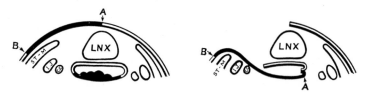

FIG. 284.—Trotter's method of reconstructing the pharynx from a flap of the skin (A–B) of the neck after excision of an extensive pharyngeal carcinoma.

pharyngeal wall is likely to be a large one, the operation is performed through a rectangular skin flap hinging at the level of the sternomastoid, and after the growth has been excised the first stage of the plastic procedure is carried out as shown in fig. 284. In the early post-operative period, the patient is fed by a tube through the fistula.

Wilfred Trotter, 1872–1939. Surgeon, University College Hospital, London.

THE LARYNX

ACUTE ŒDEMA OF THE GLOTTIS

Ætiology.— *Inflammatory*

1. Scalds, corrosives, insect stings.
2. Extension of acute inflammation, especially acute streptococcal tonsillitis, diphtheria, and Ludwig's angina (see p. 196).

Non-inflammatory

1. Local dropsy (renal or heart failure).
2. Extension of carcinoma of the base of the tongue, oropharynx, or laryngopharynx.
3. Pressure on great cervical veins.
4. After massive doses of potassium iodide (rare).
5. Angio-neurotic œdema, including serum sickness.

The œdema is an exudation into the submucosal tissue of the rima glottidis. The patient complains of pain as though he had a foreign body in the throat. The œdema is liable to spread to the ary-epiglottic folds and the sub-glottic region, and cause urgent dyspnœa. If laryngoscopic examination is possible, the entrance to the larynx can be seen presenting an appearance not unlike that of a cervix uteri. Digital examination will reveal swelling of the parts. In obscure and not very urgent cases, the urine should be examined for albumin and casts.

Treatment.—Inhalation of medicated steam and spraying with a dilute solution of cocaine and adrenalin afford relief in early and mild cases. When dyspnœa is urgent, tracheotomy or laryngotomy should be performed forthwith.

THE RELIEF OF URGENT OBSTRUCTIVE DYSPNŒA

The two emergency measures to be considered are tracheotomy and laryngotomy—tracheotomy for children, laryngotomy for adults (fig. 285).

Laryngotomy.—As a temporary measure for relieving sudden laryngeal

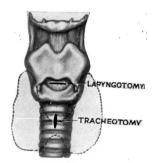

Fig. 285.—Emergency openings into the windpipe.

Wilhelm von Ludwig, 1790–1865. Professor of Surgery and Midwifery, University of Tübingen.

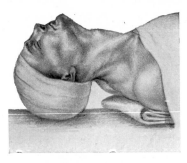

FIG. 286.—Position for laryngotomy and tracheotomy.

obstruction in adults, laryngotomy is unsurpassed.

Operation.—Local anæsthesia is employed. The patient's head is extended and held in the middle line (fig. 286). A transverse incision is made at the upper border of the cricoid cartilage. The cricothyroid membrane is opened and a laryngotomy tube (fig. 287) inserted.

Tracheotomy.—The usual indications are as follows :

1. Acute inflammation of the larynx, causing urgent dyspnœa. The most notable example in this category is diphtheria in children.

2. Laryngeal stenosis, following inflammation, leprosy, tuberculosis, or new-growth.

3. Bilateral abductor paralysis of the vocal cords.

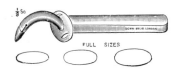

FIG. 287.—Butlin's laryngotomy tube.

4. Foreign bodies in the glottis threatening asphyxia, when facilities for direct peroral laryngoscopy are not available.

5. As a preliminary to certain operations, particularly extirpation of the larynx.

Tracheotomy for diphtheria is accomplished as follows : Local anæsthesia is employed, because any form of general anæsthetic is liable to cause spasm of the glottis, which, superadded to œdema, may result in complete obstruction. In all cases the child is pinned in a blanket so that a sudden movement of the arms may not embarrass the surgeon. When preparations are complete, a small sandbag is inserted beneath the shoulders, and an assistant keeps the head strictly in the midline.

The surgeon, standing at the right side of the patient,, places his left index finger on the upper border of the cricoid cartilage and makes an incision vertically downwards for 1 to 1½ inches (2·5 to 3·75 cm.), dividing skin, fascia, platysma, pretracheal fascia, and passing between the infrahyoid muscles. If seen, the isthmus of the thyroid gland is divided between hæmostats. In an emergency, hæmorrhage is ignored. A cricoid hook (fig. 288) is then inserted under the cricoid cartilage and grasped in the left hand. The hook steadies the trachea and brings it to the surface of the wound. The trachea is incised with a scalpel, the second and first rings being divided from below upwards : the lower the tracheotomy the less will be liability to laryngeal stenosis. A tracheal dilator is inserted through the wound, the cricoid hook removed, and the edges of the tracheal wound are gently separated, the surgeon placing a swab over the wound so that the violent expiratory efforts which follow do not spray membrane, infected mucus, and blood over himself and his assistants. When respira-

Sir Henry Butlin, 1845–1912. Surgeon, St. Bartholomew's Hospital, London.

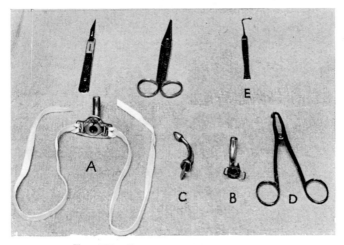

FIG. 288.—Instruments for tracheotomy.
A. Outer tube with tapes attached. B. Inner tube. C. Pilot.
D. Tracheal dilators. E. Cricoid hook.

tory efforts have become less violent, a tracheotomy tube on a pilot is inserted into the trachea, the dilator is removed, and the surgeon keeps his
finger on the tube while the assistant ties the attached tapes around the
patient's neck. The inner tube is then fixed in position, and one or two
silkworm-gut stitches are introduced if necessary. Anti-diphtheritic
serum is given and a nurse remains in constant attendance. The inner tube
is removed and washed in sodium bicarbonate solution every four hours,
or more often if necessary, and in four to seven days the tracheotomy tube
itself can usually be dispensed with.

In the case of a less urgent tracheotomy all bleeding is stopped before the
trachea is opened. The injection of a few drops of 2 per cent. cocaine
before the trachea is incised prevents the bout of coughing which follows
the insertion of the tube. If the operation is performed on an adult, a
small window may be cut in the trachea and the isthmus of the thyroid
gland divided if necessary.

Intratracheal catheterisation is a substitute for laryngotomy
and tracheotomy as a method of overcoming dyspnœa in certain
cases of temporary laryngeal obstruction.

RECURRENT LARYNGEAL NERVE INJURY : PARALYSIS OF THE VOCAL CORDS

Damage to one recurrent laryngeal nerve (figs. 289A and 289B),
which usually results from implication of the nerve by a goitre,

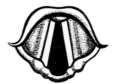

FIG. 289A.—Normal larynx on inspiration. Indirect laryngoscopy.

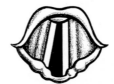

FIG. 289B.—Paralysis of the left
vocal cord. (Inspiration.)

or as a result of injury to the nerve during thyroidectomy, causes varying degrees of hoarseness, or even complete loss of voice. The condition, however, tends to improve if the contralateral vocal cord is fully active.

Damage to both recurrent laryngeal nerves causes abductor paralysis ; this is an occasional and very serious complication of thyroidectomy. In a number of instances one recurrent laryngeal nerve was probably implicated by the goitre before the operation. Bilateral abductor paralysis results in severe dyspnœa because the glottic chink cannot be opened sufficiently on inspiration.

Formerly permanent tracheotomy was often required. Modern treatment consists in Kelly's operation. After resecting

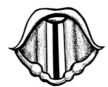

Fig. 289c.—Bilateral abductor paralysis of the vocal cords.

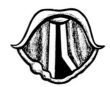

Fig. 289d.—Showing the result of Kelly's operation. Sufficient glottic space has been created to allow normal breathing.

a window in the thyroid cartilage, the crico-arytenoid joint is exposed and disarticulated. The freed arytenoid cartilage is directed to the window and anchored there. By displacing the vocal cord the glottic chink is widened posteriorly.

FOREIGN BODIES IN THE LARYNX

Various objects held in the mouth are inhaled accidentally. Occasionally the foreign body is arrested in the larynx.

The first symptoms are those of acute laryngeal obstruction ; they are usually transient, and very rarely does death from asphyxia result. These symptoms are succeeded by those of irritation. There is retrosternal pain, persistent cough, and often expectoration of blood-stained mucus. From time to time paroxysms of dyspnœa, with a terrifying sensation of impending death, occur.

Treatment.—Immediate laryngotomy or tracheotomy is the correct treatment in urgent cases with obstructive symptoms. In less urgent cases radiography is indispensable when the foreign

Joseph Dominic Kelly, Contemporary. Professor of Oto-rhino-laryngology, Belle Vue Hospital, New York.

body is opaque to X-rays. When possible, direct laryngoscopy should be performed, and by its aid the object can be seized and removed through the natural passages.

LARYNGEAL TUBERCULOSIS

The larynx is rarely the seat of primary tuberculosis. In the majority of cases the primary focus is in the lungs, and the laryngeal mucosa becomes infected by the sputum. The mucous membrane appears œdematous and semi-translucent. Tuberculosis affects the arytenoid region and the epiglottis, as well as the vocal cords. Ulceration follows, and in many instances necrosis of the cartilage occurs eventually. Treatment by streptomycin is often effective, but the resulting stenosis of the larynx may necessitate permanent tracheotomy.

LARYNGEAL SYPHILIS

Secondary syphilitic manifestations are sometimes noted in the larynx. The mucous membrane becomes congested and mucous patches form. The voice is husky. Syphilitic laryngitis clears up under anti-syphilitic treatment.

Tertiary Syphilis.—The usual lesion is a gummatous infiltration,which attacks the epiglottis, and may implicate all the structures of the larynx. Necrosis of cartilage is liable to follow. The pathological process is arrested by anti-syphilitic treatment, but subsequent cicatricial contracture is liable to cause laryngeal stenosis. For severe contractions permanent tracheotomy is the only remedy.

NEOPLASMS OF THE LARYNX

Innocent.—**Papilloma** is the commonest innocent tumour of the larynx, although, at times, an angioma or fibroma is found in this situation. A papilloma of the larynx, when it occurs in adult life, is usually single, and its pedicle is attached to one of the true or false vocal cords. The symptoms to which it gives rise are similar to those of carcinoma of the larynx, from which it must be distinguished. The diagnosis is made by laryngoscopic examination. Rarely, a papilloma becomes malignant. In doubtful cases the growth should be submitted to microscopical examination. In children the growth is usually more vascular, softer, and implantation growths soon appear in the vicinity and tend to obstruct the glottis (fig. 290). The first symptom of laryngeal papillomatosis in children is recurrent attacks of dyspnœa, which some-

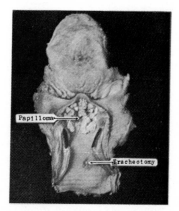

Fig. 290.—Papillomata of the vocal cords.

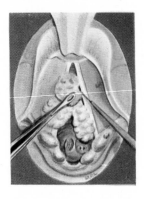

FIG. 291.—Papillomata of the vocal cords being removed by a diathermy needle via direct laryngo-scopy.   (*Water-colour painted from life by W. O. Lodge.*)

times become so urgent as to call for tracheotomy.

Treatment consists in removing the growths endoscopically with a snare or a diathermy needle (fig. 291). In recurrent cases laryngo-fissure is performed, and the growth is excised with a diathermy knife.

Malignant.—Carcinoma of the larynx, though rare, is more common than an innocent tumour of the larynx. It usually occurs between forty and sixty years of age, and men are ten times more often attacked than women. Carcinoma of the larynx was formerly designated intrinsic carcinoma of the larynx, to differentiate it from extrinsic carcinoma of the larynx, now classified as a variety of pharyngeal carcinoma. There are two varieties of laryngeal carcinoma—carcinoma of a vocal cord, which is relatively common, and subglottic carcinoma, which is rare.

Carcinoma of a vocal cord usually arises from the anterior half of one true vocal cord. It is most frequently of the papillary variety (fig. 292), but may be flattened or ulcerative, the last being uncommon. Due to the paucity or absence of lymphatic vessels of the vocal cords, carcinoma of the larynx remains locally malignant for a long period.

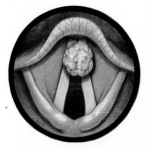

FIG. 292.—Carcinoma of a true vocal cord.

The first symptom is huskiness of the voice. The huskiness is progressive, and the patient can only speak in a low whisper, which finally gives place to aphonia. About this time the growth breaks through its cartilaginous confines, and secondary deposits occur in the cervical lymph nodes and elsewhere. Secondary involvement of the lymph nodes occurs very much later than in the case of epilaryngeal carcinoma.

The diagnosis is made by laryngoscopic examination, and

every patient with hoarseness persisting for more than three weeks should be submitted to this form of examination. According to the length of time the growth has been present, three stages of the disease are recognised :

1. The growth is confined to the vocal cord.
2. Subglottic extension with fixation of the cord.
3. Spread to the opposite cord.

Subglottic carcinoma is a less common variety which commences beneath the vocal cords. In this site the neoplasm grows steadily and silently, until dyspnœa develops. Unlike carcinoma of the vocal cord, metastasis is not so long delayed. The first lymph node to be involved is that on the crico-thyroid membrane.

Treatment of Carcinoma of the Larynx:

Stage 1.—Carcinoma of the larynx is nearly always radio-sensitive, and treatment by deep X-ray therapy and teleradium is tending to supplant surgical treatment. The results of treatment by laryngo-fissure with excision of the affected vocal cord is also extremely satisfactory in early cases.

Laryngo-fissure and Excision of the Growth.—Under local infiltration, a preliminary tracheotomy is performed. The thyroid cartilage is bisected in the middle line and the crico-thyroid membrane opened. The perichondrium in the region of the affected vocal cord is raised by blunt dissection, and the whole vocal cord, with a margin of healthy tissue, is removed. The larynx is repaired and the tracheotomy tube removed after a few days. The patient is left with a useful voice.

Stage 2.—**Fenestration with interstitial radium** is often employed with a high proportion of favourable results.

The larynx is exposed by a curved incision commencing above the level of the hyoid bone, and ending below the lower border of the cricoid cartilage. The flap is raised. The infrahyoid muscles are split, and a large window is cut in the ala of the thyroid cartilage, without opening the underlying mucosa. In cases of subglottic carcinoma a window is also cut in the cricoid cartilage. The object of removing the cartilage is to allow radium needles to come in closer proximity to the growth, and prevent radium necrosis. The radium needles are left in place seven to nine days.

Stage 3.—When this stage is reached, and deep X-rays have not proved effective, or when radium necrosis has occurred, total laryngectomy (fig. 293) may be indicated.

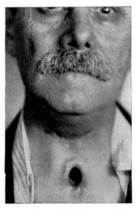

Fig. 293.—Patient after complete laryngectomy.
(Jackson and Babcock.)

Total Laryngectomy.—Of several incisions, one passing down the anterior border of the right sternomastoid muscle from the level of the hyoid bone to half an inch above the suprasternal notch, and then passing across the middle line to end near the base of the contralateral sternomastoid muscle, is most favoured. The large skin flap is raised. The operation is less difficult if it has not been necessary to perform tracheotomy. The sterno-hyoid muscles are split, and the sternothyroid muscles are divided near their insertion. The isthmus of the thyroid gland is clamped and divided and the lateral lobes of the thyroid gland are stripped from the larynx, a step which is facilitated by ligating and dividing the superior thyroid arteries. The larynx is separated from its muscular attachments on each side, and mobilised still further by cutting through the superior cornua of the thyroid cartilages. Attention is now directed to separating by blunt dissection the trachea and back of the cricoid cartilage from the œsophagus. The trachea is then divided between its first and second rings, the distal end of the trachea is brought out through a small stab incision in the supra-sternal notch, and fixed in this position, the anæsthetic being continued through a tube passed into the open trachea. The larynx is now hooked forwards, and after still further separating the back of the cricoid cartilage from the commencement of the œsophagus, the hypopharynx is opened. The inferior constrictor muscle and the pharyngeal mucosa is cut away from the thyroid cartilages on each side, care being taken to remove each pyri-form fossa. The thyrohyoid membrane is divided completely. The larynx is now free, except for the attachment of the epiglottis, which is excised with the larynx. There remains a wide gap in the pharynx, which can be wholly or partly closed by approximating the cut edge of the hypo-pharynx below to the severed thyrohyoid membrane and the base of the tongue, above. Any gap which remains is packed. The infra-hyoid muscles are approximated in the middle line. If it has been possible to close the pharynx, feeding can be accomplished through a tube passed from the nose into the stomach. If the pharynx has been left partially open, the feeding tube is passed through the wound which, in either case, is drained freely.

CHAPTER XV
THE ŒSOPHAGUS

As measured from the incisor teeth in the average adult :

At 7 inches (18 *cm.*)—the pharynx ends and the œsophagus commences.

At 11 inches (28 *cm.*)—the œsophagus is crossed by the left bronchus.

At 17 inches (43 *cm.*)—the cardiac orifice is situated and the œsophagus ends.

These figures, 7, 11, and 17, are of great importance in the surgery of the œsophagus. They represent the situations of anatomical narrowing, and consequently the points where ingested foreign bodies are likely to be arrested, and the situations where difficulty may be experienced during the passage of instruments. Furthermore, these points are the sites of election for innocent strictures and also for malignant disease, the commonest affection of the œsophagus.

INVESTIGATION OF THE DISEASES OF THE ŒSOPHAGUS

The œsophagus is very inaccessible, consequently clinical methods of examination are of little avail.

Until the twentieth century one of the chief methods of examining this organ was by inserting bougies blindly down the gullet. Aneurisms were frequent in those days, and it happened occasionally that an aortic aneurism escaped detection until a bougie was passed. The terrifying hæmorrhagic cascade through the victim's mouth clarified the diagnosis, but brought " blind " œsophageal instrumentation into disrepute. Another, and probably more frequent, accident of this nature was perforation of the œsophageal wall in the neighbourhood of a carcinomatous stricture. We have seen fatal cases of mediastinitis from this cause.

Radiography.—In the case of a swallowed foreign body impacted in the œsophagus, provided the object is opaque to X-rays, the diagnosis and site of arrest, as shown by X-ray examination, is absolute. Radiography after the ingestion of barium is of great value in detecting an œsophageal stricture or an ulcer, and in outlining an impacted foreign body non-opaque to X-rays.

s.p.—16

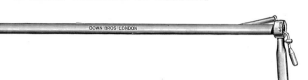

Fig. 294.—Chevalier Jackson's œsophagoscope.

Œsophagoscopy.—Examination with an œsophagoscope (fig. 294) enables the interior of the œsophagus to be examined visually, thereby aiding in arriving at an exact diagnosis which otherwise would be impossible. In addition, in the case of an impacted foreign body or of an œsophageal stricture, œsophagoscopy is an indispensable means of affording treatment.

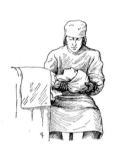

Fig. 295.—Chevalier Jackson's position for œsophagoscopy. The head of the patient is supported entirely by the hands of the seated assistant.

In performing œsophagoscopy it is essential to adopt Jackson's position (fig. 295). The instrument is passed entirely under vision, and once its beak has passed the cricoid cartilage, it can be moved down the œsophagus with comparative ease.

CONGENITAL ABNORMALITIES

It is estimated that one of the following anomalies occurs once in every 2,500 births :

1. Complete absence (so rare as to be a curiosity).

2. Atresia.

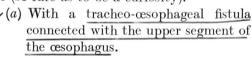

    (a) With a tracheo-œsophageal fistula connected with the upper segment of the œsophagus.

    (b) With a tracheo-œsophageal fistula connected with the lower segment of the œsophagus (80 per cent. of all cases).

    (c) With a tracheo-œsophageal fistula connected with both segments of the œsophagus.

3. Membranous stricture (very rare indeed).

4. Congenitally short œsophagus.

Congenital Atresia.—It is most important to be cognisant of the possibility of this anomaly, because its recognition within

Chevalier Jackson, Contemporary. Professor of Laryngology, Jefferson Medical College, Philadelphia.

forty-eight hours of birth, and subsequent surgical rectification, is the only hope of survival.

Clinical Features.—The new-born babe regurgitates all its first, and every feed. Saliva pours, almost continuously, from its mouth. Attacks of coughing and cyanosis are prone to occur (stomach contents regurgitating into the trachea). The abdomen becomes distended (dilatation of the stomach) due to swallowed air from the tracheal fistula (fig. 296).

Clinical Confirmation of the Diagnosis.—A catheter passed from the mouth becomes arrested in the œsophagus.

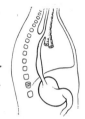

Radiological Confirmation.—Barium should never be used for these cases. Injection of 1 ml. of lipiodol down the catheter will demonstrate the septum. During this examination the prone position is advised, because in the rare event of the atresia belonging to categories (a) and (c) (see classification above), the medium is less likely to enter the trachea.

Fig. 296.— Tracheo - œso- phageal fistula, common variety.

Pre-operative Treatment.—Lam emphasises that the operation should not be an urgent, but a quasi-urgent, one, i.e. it should not be carried out in a matter of hours, but postponed for a day or two. Everything by mouth is forbidden and the saliva must be aspirated. The patient is supported by suitable parenteral fluid.

Operation.—Unless end-to-end anastomosis is impracticable (rare), a one-stage operation is the best, particularly when performed under local anæsthesia. During the operation 75 ml. of blood can be transfused with advantage. The vertebral ends of the second to the sixth ribs are divided, and short lengths of them are resected. The pleura is displaced from the bodies of the vertebræ. The upper segment of the œsophagus is located by a catheter within it, the lower segment is found, and its connection with the trachea is severed between ligatures as near to the trachea as possible. The two ends of the œsophagus are then anastomosed over a catheter, great care being taken to effect a leak-proof anastomosis. 30,000 units of penicillin are instilled into the mediastinum and the thorax closed with drainage.

Post-operative Care.—1. A special nurse, skilled in aspirating saliva, and an oxygen-tent-incubator are desirable.

Conrad C. Lam, Contemporary. Surgeon, Henry Ford Hospital, Detroit, U.S.A.

2. Nothing by mouth for five days.

3. Parenteral fluids, mostly 5 per cent. glucose, about 250 ml. (9 oz.) daily.

4. Feeding by mouth is started on the fifth day, commencing with ½ oz. (14 ml.) of 5 per cent. glucose every two hours. On the seventh day small milk feeds are begun.

Membranous Stricture.—A complete congenital membranous stricture has been treated successfully by division of the membrane through an œsophagoscope (Abel). The condition, which is very rare, is sometimes associated with hypertrophic pyloric stenosis.

Congenitally Short Œsophagus.—Because of the shortening, a portion of the cardiac end of the stomach lies above the diaphragm. The condition does not give rise to symptoms until adolescent or adult life, when peptic ulceration of the œsophagus (see p. 257) is prone to occur. It should be noted that most cases of short œsophagus seen in connexion with peptic ulceration are considered to be acquired, due to fibrosis consequent upon the inflammation.

INJURIES

Injuries of the œsophagus are uncommon. Perforation has occurred during the passage of instruments and from swallowing sharp-pointed objects. The site of the perforation is usually in the upper third of the œsophagus. The great danger is the development of mediastinitis. It is true that mediastinitis is a very lethal complication, but only if the involved closed fascial space is not drained soon enough. In the case of the retropharyngeal space and the superior mediastinum, an incision along the posterior border of the sternomastoid will enable the infected cellular tissues to be decompressed adequately. For the posterior mediastinum the posterior ends of two ribs should be resected over the site of the perforation (Phillips).

ŒSOPHAGEAL DIVERTICULUM

Traction diverticulum is of pathological interest only. The apex of the diverticulum is firmly attached to a tuberculous lymphatic node (fig. 297), the commonest site being the anterior wall of the œsophagus in the region of the bifurcation of the trachea. The diverticulum passes upwards. Food does not enter its open mouth, consequently it gives rise to no symptoms.

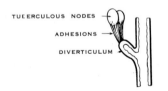

TUEERCULOUS NODES

ADHESIONS

DIVERTICULUM

Fig. 297.—
Traction diver-
ticulum.

Pressure diverticulum (*syn.* epiphrenic diverticulum) is rare, and occurs at the extreme lower end of the œsophagus. Such pouches cause dysphagia and restrosternal discomfort after food.

The diagnosis is made by radiography after a barium meal. Occasionally the symptoms are sufficiently troublesome to warrant excision of the diverticulum by an approach similar to that indicated in the surgical treatment of œsophageal peptic ulceration (see p. 257).

A. Lawrence Abel, Contemporary. Surgeon, Cancer Hospital, London.
Charles E. Phillips, Contemporary. Surgeon, Hospital of the Good Samaritan, Los Angeles, U.S.A.

PARALYSIS

The passage of food along the gullet is dependent entirely upon involuntary muscular peristalsis.   When the neuro-muscular mechanism of deglutition is paralysed, as occurs occasionally, notably as a complication of diphtheria, ingested material is regurgitated.   In established cases the difficulty has to be overcome by feeding through a stomach tube.

ŒSOPHAGEAL VARICES

The lower end of the œsophagus is one of the principal regions where the portal and systemic venous systems anastomose.   Dilatation of these anastomotic channels occurs in portal obstruction (p. 321).   They can often be visualised radiologically after a barium swallow.

PEPTIC ULCERATION OF THE ŒSOPHAGUS

Peptic ulceration of the œsophagus is a rare but important condition.   The ulcer or ulcers are nearly always situated in the terminal inch (2·5 cm.) of the œsophagus.   Œsophageal peptic ulceration is often associated with a sliding diaphragmatic hernia which permits intermittent prolapse of the first few inches of the cardiac end of the stomach into the thoracic cavity through the enlarged anatomical diaphragmatic hiatus.   The absence of an effective cardiac sphincter results in regurgitation of gastric juice into the œsophagus, and subjects its mucosa to the probability of peptic ulceration.

The condition is usually found in patients over fifty years of age, and men are slightly more often affected.   Unlike cardiospasm, pain is the leading symptom, and it generally occurs, not on swallowing, but at a varying time after meals, making the clinical history identical with that of a chronic gastric or duodenal peptic ulcer.   Dysphagia is sometimes an additional early symptom, which should direct attention to the lesion ; more often dysphagia is a late symptom and implies that some degree of stenosis of the ulcerated area has complicated the primary condition.   Formerly, the latter syndrome was considered to be due to " painful cardiospasm."   In rare instances perforation of the ulcer into the pleura, mediastinum or the pericardium occurs, and is usually fatal.   Congenitally short œsophagus, by allowing regurgitation of gastric juice, may produce peptic ulceration of the œsophagus in young subjects.

An X-ray following a barium meal often reveals a flake of barium in an ulcer crater situated in the extreme lower end of the œsophagus.   This, together with a widely open cardia, is a typical radiological finding.   It may be possible to visualise the ulcer by œsophagoscopy, but sometimes the ulcer is hidden by voluminous folds of mucosa.

Medical treatment is the same as that for gastric and duodenal peptic ulcers. In the early stages rest to the ulcerated area is afforded by drip feeding through a Ryle's tube. In order to minimise regurgitation of gastric juice into the œsophagus, the patient should sleep propped up with pillows. If there is any degree of stricture formation, the stricture should be dilated through an œsophagoscope. Recurrence is liable to follow the healing of the ulcer by conservative measures, because the cause (sliding hernia of the diaphragm) remains.

Surgical treatment.—When the symptoms recur rapidly and repeatedly after conservative measures, operation may be advisable. In comparatively early cases repair of the diaphragmatic hernia via the transthoracic route can be undertaken. When there is much stenosis, œsophagojejunostomy with exclusion of the stomach has proved successful (Allison).

ACUTE ŒSOPHAGEAL OBSTRUCTION

Foreign Bodies in the Œsophagus.—All sorts of swallowed foreign bodies have become arrested in the œsophagus : coins, pins, and dentures (fig. 298) head the list. When the object contains radio-opaque material, an urgent X-ray examination is called for. Moreover, whenever possible the patient should be screened immediately before œsophagoscopy is undertaken.

The foreign body having been seen (fig. 299), and if necessary, manipulated into a favourable position, it is grasped with suit-

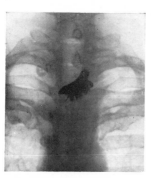

FIG. 298.—False teeth impacted in œsophagus.
(*James F. Brailsford.*)

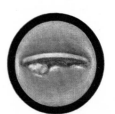

FIG. 299.—A penny in the œsophagus as seen through an œsophagoscope.

able forceps introduced through the œsophagoscope. The œsophagoscope, together with the forceps still grasping the foreign body, is then withdrawn steadily.

John Alfred Ryle, 1889–1950. Physician, Guy's Hospital.
Philip Rowland Allison, Contemporary. Thoracic Surgeon, General Infirmary, Leeds.

CHRONIC ŒSOPHAGEAL OBSTRUCTION

The causes of chronic œsophageal obstruction can be classified as follows :

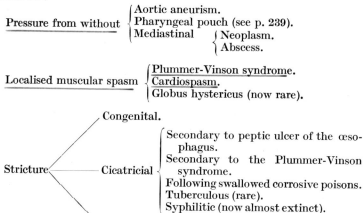

Pressure from without
- Aortic aneurism.
- Pharyngeal pouch (see p. 239).
- Mediastinal
  - Neoplasm.
  - Abscess.

Localised muscular spasm
- Plummer-Vinson syndrome.
- Cardiospasm.
- Globus hystericus (now rare).

Stricture
- Congenital.
- Cicatricial
  - Secondary to peptic ulcer of the œsophagus.
  - Secondary to the Plummer-Vinson syndrome.
  - Following swallowed corrosive poisons.
  - Tuberculous (rare).
  - Syphilitic (now almost extinct).
- Carcinomatous.

LOCALISED MUSCULAR SPASM

There are two important clinical entities associated with muscular conditions of the œsophagus. One affects the pharyngo-œsophageal junction and is known as the Plummer-Vinson syndrome. The other affects the extreme lower end of the œsophagus and is called cardiospasm, or achalasia.

The Plummer-Vinson Syndrome.—The patient is nearly always a middle-aged woman who comes complaining of difficulty or inability to swallow. Provided the clinician is aware of the existence of the syndrome, close examination nearly always provides clues to the diagnosis, but not all the following are necessarily in evidence in a given case.

The tongue shows evidence of glossitis. The changes in the mucous membrane vary from abnormal smoothness to advanced glossitis.

The lips and corners of the mouth are often cracked, giving the mouth a pursed appearance.

The finger-nails are brittle, and tend to be spoon-shaped (koilonychia) (fig. 300).

Fig. 300.—
Spoon - shaped
finger-nail.

The spleen is often somewhat enlarged.

The Blood.—Hypochromic anæmia is always present. Hypochromic anæmia is so called because the red corpuscles contain less hæmoglobin than normal. It seems probable that the

Henry S. Plummer, 1874–1936. Physician, Mayo Clinic, Rochester, U.S.A.
Porter P. Vinson, Contemporary. Physician, Mayo Clinic, Rochester, U.S.A.

dysphagia precedes the anæmia, which is due to lack of iron and other necessary ingredients of a balanced diet.

The dysphagia is due to spasm of the circular muscle fibres of the extreme upper portion of the œsophagus. In long-standing cases the orifice looks like a mere pin-hole. In comparatively early cases the mucous membrane of the neighbourhood shows inflammatory changes. Later the surface presents areas simulating leukoplakia. What is highly important to realise is that this lesion is definitely a pre-carcinomatous condition.

Treatment.—The dysphagia yields readily to dilatation of the stricture through an œsophagoscope. As always, gentleness must be used; even so, in cases of some standing bleeding will occur. The administration of tab. ferri. sulphate, gr. 3 (0·2 gm.) t.d.s., together with vitamins, is indicated. In refractory cases intravenous iron preparations can be employed. Sometimes blood transfusion is necessary. Once the anæmia is under control and the patient can swallow an adequate diet, rapid improvement occurs and is usually maintained.

CARDIOSPASM (Syn. ACHALASIA OF THE CARDIA)

Definition.—A condition of dilatation and hypertrophy of the whole length of the œsophagus in which, at post-mortem examination, no cause for the obstruction can be found.

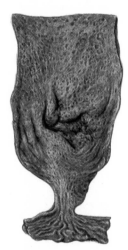

Pathology.—When slit up longitudinally it will be seen that not only is the œsophagus enormously dilated (fig. 301), but it is also lengthened. Its circumference at the distal end sometimes measures as much as 7 inches (18 cm.). As a rule there is no hypertrophy of the cardiac sphincter.

Ætiology. — The normal neuro-muscular mechanism of the cardiac sphincter is upset. Stokes found that the whole of Auerbach's plexus in the neighbourhood of the cardiac sphincter is destroyed and replaced by fibrous tissue. Mosher states that the cause of the fibrosis of the peri-œsophageal connective tissue and the musculature is infection, probably from œsophageal peptic ulceration.

Fig. 301.—Cardio-spasm. Necropsy specimen showing the typical flask-shaped dilatation. (*British Journal of Surgery.*)

Clinical Features.—Cardiospasm is usually found in women over forty years of

Adrian Stokes, 1887–1927. *Pathologist, Guy's Hospital, London.*
Leopold Auerbach, 1828–1897. *Frankfurt neurologist.*
Harry Peyton Mosher, Contemporary. *Professor Emeritus of Otolaryngology, Harvard University, Boston, U.S.A*

age.   The history is one of progressive dysphagia, but there are several special features.

The onset is insidious, and the patient sometimes only seeks relief after the symptoms have been present for many years. Curiously, not a few sufferers complain that the dysphagia is more in evidence when taking fluids.   Although the patient says she vomits, on closer interrogation it becomes apparent that there is regurgitation of food, often several hours after the meal. In advanced cases mucus and froth are brought up in considerable quantities.   There may be retrosternal discomfort, rarely amounting to pain.

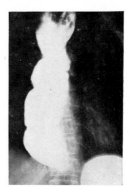

As a result of the obstruction the patient fails to obtain sufficient nourishment, and if unrelieved, death from starvation is a possible termination.

Radiography.—Radiological appearances are characteristic ; the enormous dilatation of the œsophagus is seen in no other condition (fig. 302).

Œsophagoscopy.—Once the instrument has passed the cricoid cartilage it appears to enter a gaping cave partially filled with dirty water, which laps to and fro with respiratory movement.   When the fluid has been aspirated the cardiac orifice is located with difficulty, owing to its contracted state.

FIG. 302. — Typical X-ray appearance after the ingestion of a barium meal in a case of cardiospasm.

Treatment.—

Dilatation with Mercury-loaded Tubes.—Rubber tubes, varying in size and each containing 1 lb. 5 oz. (600 gm.) of mercury, are employed.   On the first occasion the tube is passed under the vision afforded by the X-ray screen and a mark made at the level of the incisor teeth when the extremity of the tube is 2 inches (5 cm.) within the stomach.   The patient must learn to pass the tubes herself before meals. The treatment, which must be carried out conscientiously, is tedious for the patient.   Good results have accrued in comparatively early cases.

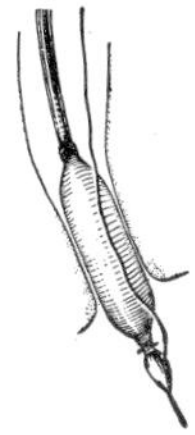

Plummer's Hydrostatic Bag.—A silk thread with a shot on the end is swallowed, and when the shot has entered the stomach, suitable bougies are passed by the " railroad " method. Once the sphincter is dilated sufficiently, the hydrostatic bag (fig. 303) is inserted.

FIG. 303. — Plummer's hydrostatic bag *in situ.*

Operative treatment :

1. Œsophagocardiomyotomy (Heller's operation).—The upper abdomen is opened. Having mobilised the liver by division of the left triangular ligament, and having enlarged the œsophageal hiatus of the diaphragm, a tape is passed around the œsophagus, allowing it to be withdrawn into the abdomen. While the operation is in progress the dilated œsophagus is kept empty by means of a suction apparatus passed through the mouth. A longitudinal incision is made at the junction of the œsophagus and the stomach, dividing the muscular coat of the œsophagus, so as to expose, but not open, the mucosa. The muscle fibres are gently separated in much the same way as in Rammstedt's operation for hypertrophic pyloric stenosis (see p. 271).

2. Cardioplasty.—The preliminary steps of the operation to afford exposure of the gastro-œsophageal junction are similar to the above. A plastic œsophagogastrostomy is then carried out.

3. Mikulicz's operation has been superseded by the above procedures. It consists of opening the stomach and gently dilating the constricted cardia digitally. Although this method gave good results in many instances, there is a danger of rupturing the œsophagus, and in a few instances the stricture recurred.

BENIGN STRICTURE

Compared with obstruction due to carcinoma, simple stricture is rare. A few cases are congenital in origin (see p. 254). As set out in the table on p. 259, the causes of benign stricture are various. When consequent upon swallowing corrosive poisons, the strictures are usually multiple, the densest being at the level of the crossing of the left bronchus. The diagnosis is established by X-ray examination and œsophagoscopy.

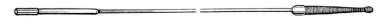

Fig. 304.—Chevalier Jackson's carrot-shaped œsophageal bougie.

Treatment consists of dilatation with bougies (fig. 304). In the first instance this should always be carried out under vision, and in some cases such treatment is continued at regular intervals. When the stricture has a very small lumen a special guide is passed, to the end of which a larger bougie is attached by a screw. By these means nearly all simple strictures can be kept patent, but " once a stricture always a stricture " is as true in this instance as in the case of the urethra.

In cases where a bougie cannot be passed from above or threaded along a swallowed string weighted by a small shot, retrograde bouginage can be attempted through a gastrotomy. If this measure is successful, after this bougies can be passed in the usual way. In extreme cases, where dilatation of a dense stricture is impossible, the choice lies between a permanent gastrostomy or excision of the œsophagus, similar to that used for malignant disease (p. 265).

Ernst Heller, Contemporary, Professor of Surgery, Leipzig.
Conrad Rammstedt, Contemporary. Chief Surgeon, Rafael Clinic, Münster.
Johannes von Mikulicz-Radecki, 1850–1905. Professor of Surgery, Breslau.

BENIGN TUMOURS

Simple tumours of the œsophagus are exceedingly rare. Papilloma of the œsophagus is usually solitary, and occurs in the upper third of the organ. Diathermy excision through an œsophagoscope is a satisfactory method of treatment. Myoma and a submucous lipoma causing symptoms of dysphagia have been removed successfully by the transthoracic approach.

MALIGNANT TUMOURS

Carcinoma of the œsophagus is by no means rare, but it is not as frequent as carcinoma of the stomach or the large bowel, including the rectum.

Ætiology.—As with carcinoma in other situations, our ignorance concerning its cause is abysmal. It has been suggested that post-cricoid carcinoma is favoured by swallowing hot fluids (see p. 46).

Pathology.—As pointed out already, the growth nearly always occurs at one of the sites of anatomical narrowing. The relative frequency of the situation of the growth is shown in fig. 305.

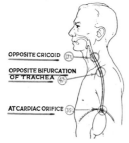

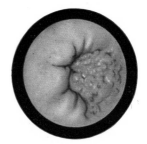

FIG. 305.—The relative frequency of œsophageal carcinoma.	FIG. 306.—Carcinoma of the œsophagus as seen through an œsophagoscope.
(*Lawrence Abel's statistics.*)	(*A. Lawrence Abel.*)

Macroscopically three types can be recognised :

1. An annular constriction.
2. A papilliferous mass (fig. 306).
3. A carcinomatous ulcer.

The first variety is usually found at the cardia.

Microscopically, when derived from the mucosa of the upper two-thirds of the organ, the growth is squamous-celled, while in the lower third it is often of the columnar type.

Modes of Spread.—Direct extension is the most usual form of spread. When the muscular coat has become invaded, periœsophagitis fixes the œsophagus to neighbouring structures, which eventually become involved in the neoplastic process. Spread by the lymphatics occurs comparatively late in the disease. From a growth in the cervical œsophagus cervical lymph nodes, usually those of the left supraclavicular fossa, frequently become implicated. Growths in the mid-œsophagus sometimes metastasise in the mediastinal lymph nodes, and in cases of carcinoma of both the mid-œsophagus and the cardiac end, the nodes around the lesser curvature of the stomach and the cœliac axis become the seat of secondary deposits.

Terminal Complications.—Untreated, the growth causes death in one of the following ways :

1. Progressive cachexia and dehydration.

2. Pneumonia from perforation into some part of the bronchial tree.

3. Mediastinitis from perforation into the posterior mediastinum.

4. Erosion of the aorta (very rare).

At necropsy one often marvels at the comparative absence of metastatic deposits.

Clinical Features.—Men between forty-five and seventy are the usual victims. The disease is comparatively rare in women ; when it occurs it is usually situated at the commencement of the organ. The first symptom is a feeling of " weight," " heaviness," or " oppression " behind the sternum. Later, the leading symptom is dysphagia. In surgical out-patient practice the patient often presents himself when he can no longer swallow milk puddings and such-like semi-solids. By this time the growth must have involved at least three-quarters of the lumen of the œsophagus. Regurgitation of food (œsophageal pseudovomiting) is also a common symptom. The regurgitated material is alkaline, mixed with mucus and saliva, and possibly streaked with blood. Pain is conspicuous by its absence until complications have arisen.

Diagnosis.—In this instance clinical methods of examination are peculiarly impotent. The patient can, however, usually indicate fairly accurately where he feels the food is obstructed. Early cases can be diagnosed with certainty only by œsophagoscopy. When the disease is more advanced, the growth fig. 307), or more usually the stenosis produced by it, can be demonstrated by X-rays after barium emulsion has been swallowed.

Treatment is divided into palliative—to avert starvation—and curative. Unfortunately, the condition is usually diagnosed so late that only the former can be contemplated.

Palliative treatment consists in either performing gastrostomy or intubating the neoplastic stricture with a Symond's or a Souttar's tube introduced through an œsophagoscope.

X-ray Treatment.—Deep X-ray therapy is sometimes curative in cases of carcinoma of the cervical œsophagus. It also causes temporary regression of the growth in the middle third of the œsophagus, but it has no effect on growths situated at the cardiac end.

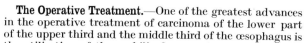

Fig. 307.—Comparatively early carcinoma of the œsophagus.

(Radiograph by G. R. Mather Cordiner.)

The Operative Treatment.—One of the greatest advances in the operative treatment of carcinoma of the lower part of the upper third and the middle third of the œsophagus is the utilisation of the mobilised stomach to restore the continuity of the alimentary canal after the tumour-bearing area and the œsophagus distal to it have been excised. The stomach, usually approached from the thorax through the diaphragm, is freed from all its omenta, leaving a fringe of omentum attached to the greater and lesser curvatures. In this fringe are arterial arcades which receive their blood supply from the right. It is most important that the left gastric artery be ligated and divided near its origin from the cœliac axis (fig. 308), so as to ensure the integrity of one of the main components of this collateral circulation.

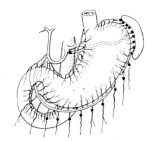

Fig. 308.—Mobilisation of the stomach with preservation of a vascular supply.

1. *The Upper Third. (a) In the Neck.*—The treatment is precisely similar to that of carcinoma of the hypopharynx, which has been dealt with on p. 243.

(b) *In the Thorax above the Arch of the Aorta.*—The neck, thorax, and abdomen are prepared for operation, and the patient lies on his back.

Step 1.—An incision is made along the anterior border of the sternomastoid muscle. The middle thyroid vein is divided between ligatures. The inferior thyroid artery, which supplies the upper portion of the œsophagus, must be preserved. The thyroid gland is retracted anteriorly, and the sternomastoid posteriorly. The commencement of the œsophagus is exposed, and the tumour is sought with the finger. If it is found that the tumour can be separated from the trachea and from the arch of the aorta, the cervical wound is packed temporarily.

Step 2.—The patient is placed on his right side, with the left arm

Charters J. Symonds, 1852–1932. Surgeon, Guy's Hospital, London.
Sir Henry Souttar, Contemporary. Consulting Surgeon, London Hospital.
Franz Torek, Contemporary. Surgeon, Lenox Hill Hospital, New York. Performed the first successful excision of the œsophagus in 1914.

rotated forwards and upwards. Thoracotomy is undertaken through the bed of the excised sixth rib. The pleural cavity is opened, and the lung is retracted anteriorly. The pleura overlying the œsophagus is incised and the œsophagus dissected from its bed, the arteries supplying it from the aorta being divided and ligated. That part of the œsophagus containing the tumour is freed from surrounding structures, particular care being taken not to injure the thoracic duct and the left vagus nerve, which is divided below its left recurrent branch. Once the tumour-bearing area of the œsophagus has been entirely mobilised, the phrenic nerve is crushed and the diaphragm is incised from the œsophageal hiatus to the lateral thoracic wall.

Step 3.—The cardia is divided between two strong sutures. The distal end is invaginated into the stomach by means of a purse-string suture. The ligated free end of the œsophagus is carbolised and encased in a piece of rubber glove, and a second strong ligature tied tightly over the rubber, leaving the ends of the ligature long. The stomach is mobilised as described above. The uppermost part of the fundus is transfixed with two strong stay sutures.

Step 4.—A long hæmostat is passed from the cervical incision behind the arch of the aorta, and is made to grasp the long ends of the ligature surrounding the cut end of the œsophagus. The ligature, followed by the thoracic œsophagus, is pulled through the cervical incision. The forceps are again introduced into the thorax from the neck, this time in front of the aorta and behind the hilum of the lung. They grasp the two stay sutures attached to the fundus of the stomach, which is drawn up into the neck (Garlock). After applying penicillin to the mediastinum, the edges of the mediastinal pleura are attached to the stomach. The diaphragm is repaired about the stomach. The lung is re-expanded and the incision in the thoracic wall closed in layers with dependent stab drainage.

Step 5.—The patient is turned on to his back, and end-to-side anastomosis is performed between the cervical œsophagus above the growth and the fundus of the stomach, the œsophagus and the growth being detached in the process. Penicillin is applied to the anastomosis, and the wound is closed with drainage.

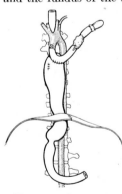

2. *The Middle Third* may be approached via the left pleural cavity in a similar way to the incision employed for the second stage above. Because of the danger of hæmorrhage from branches of the thoracic aorta, Allison frees the aorta as a first step by dividing between ligatures the upper six left, and then the corresponding right, intercostal arteries. The thoracic aorta can then be lifted up with tapes while the mobilisation of the œsophagus from its bed is carried out. The remainder of the operation, which includes incising the diaphragm and mobilising the stomach, dividing the œsophagus at the cardia and invaginating its distal end, is then performed. The fundus of the stomach is brought up into the thorax and joined to the œsophagus above the growth by end-to-side anastomosis (fig. 309), that part of the œsophagus containing the growth and the whole of the distal œsophagus being excised. Some surgeons prefer

Fig. 309.—Resection of the œsophagus for a growth in its middle third, utilising the mobilised stomach for restoring the continuity of the alimentary track (semi-diagrammatic).

John Henry Garlock, Contemporary. Surgeon, Mount Sinai Hospital, New York.

an approach to the mid-œsophagus through the right pleural cavity. The advantages claimed for this route are that after the vena azygos has been divided, the œsophagus is immediately available (fig. 310) and the aorta does

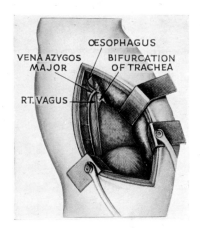

FIG. 310.—The surgical anatomy involved in œsophagectomy via the right pleural cavity. (*O'Shaugnessy and Raven.*) (*British Journal of Surgery.*)

not hamper the dissection. The disadvantage of this route is that the stomach is far less accessible through the right crura of the diaphragm. Ivor Lewis performs the operation in two stages. At the first stage the blood-vessels of the stomach are divided and ligated in the manner shown in fig. 308, and a temporary jejunostomy is performed. At the second stage, a week or ten days later, the right sixth rib is resected, the vena azygos divided and ligated, and the stomach brought up for anastomosis.

3. *The Lower Third.*—The thoraco-abdominal approach (p. 306) is employed. The left lung is retracted and the lower third of the œsophagus is freed from surrounding structures, a rubber-covered clamp being placed on the œsophagus towards the upper limit of this mobilisation. If necessary, portions of adherent pleura are left attached to the growth. The anterior layer of the lieno-renal ligament is divided, and the spleen is drawn forwards and to the right, and with it the fundus of the stomach. Exerting traction

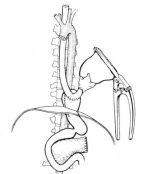

FIG. 311.—Resection of a growth at the cardiac end of the œsophagus through an abdomino-thoracic incision. The rubber-covered clamp above the growth referred to in the text has been omitted for purposes of clarity.

upon the stomach and the spleen, the left crus of the diaphragm is dissected free from the stomach. By dividing the sustentaculum lieni, the lesser sac is opened and the posterior surface of the tail and the body of the pancreas

Ivor Lewis, Contemporary. Medical Director and Surgeon, North Middlesex Hospital, London.

are displayed.   The splenic vein and artery are divided and ligated, the tail of the pancreas resected with a diathermy knife, and the cut surface of the body is sutured.   The stomach is now held to the posterior abdominal wall only by the left gastric artery, which is divided.   The great omentum is detached from the left half of the greater curvature and a similar portion of the gastro-hepatic omentum is detached from the lesser curvature: crushing clamps are applied across the stomach at this point.   The distal end of the stomach is closed and invaginated.   The whole mass, which comprises the cardiac end of the stomach, the spleen, and the tail of the pancreas, together with that part of the œsophagus containing the growth, can now be withdrawn.   The portion of the stomach which remains is brought up into the mediastinum for anastomosis with the œsophagus (fig. 311) above the rubber-covered clamp referred to at the commencement of the dissection.   The repair of the diaphragm and of the chest wall is similar to that of the preceding operations.

CHAPTER XVI

THE STOMACH AND DUODENUM

HYPERTROPHIC PYLORIC STENOSIS OF INFANTS
(*Syn.* CONGENITAL PYLORIC STENOSIS)

Ætiology.—The cause of the condition is unknown. Several theories have been put forward, the most acceptable being that the condition arises from an inco-ordination of the neuro-muscular mechanism of the stomach, or that there is an achalasia (primary failure of the sphincter to relax).

Pathology.—The muscle coats of the stomach are hypertrophied, especially the circular fibres in the region of the pylorus. This hypertrophy terminates abruptly, the duodenum being normal. When observed from the duodenal side, the pylorus has the appearance of a cervix uteri (fig. 312). The mucosa in the pyloric antrum is thrown into folds ; on transverse section two main longitudinal folds can often be distinguished. At necropsy the stomach shows mucous catarrh and petechial hæmorrhages, which are no doubt secondary to the stasis and vomiting. The muscular hypertrophy persists after all symptoms have been cured by Rammstedt's operation.

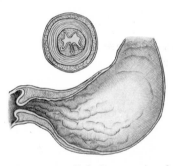

FIG. 312.—Pyloric stenosis of infants. Longitudinal and transverse sections of the stomach to show the enormous muscular hypertrophy. Note the abrupt termination.

Clinical Features.—In 48 per cent. of cases the child is the first-born (Still), and boys are six times more commonly affected than girls. The infant shows no tendency to vomit until it is *two or three weeks of age*. The vomits are large, and evidently consist of more than the last feed. Within two or three days the vomiting becomes projectile. The motions tend to become like those of a rabbit—small and dry. Naturally, loss of weight follows, and it is not long before the infant begins to look emaciated. On abdominal examination soon after the child has been fed peristalsis can be seen in the epigastrium passing from left to right, and there is an acorn-like swelling (the thickened

Conrad Rammstedt, Contemporary. Chief Surgeon, Rafael Clinic, Münster. Introduced his operation in 1913.
Sir Frederick Still, 1868–1941. Physician, Hospital for Sick Children, Great Ormond Street, London.

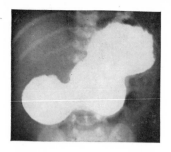

FIG. 313.—Radiograph six hours after the ingestion of a barium meal in a case of hypertrophic pyloric stenosis in an infant.

pylorus) in the right hypochondrium. If any doubt exists as to the diagnosis, a barium meal reveals pyloric obstruction (fig. 313), but the passage of a gastric tube, and aspiration of a large residue two hours after a feed, is equally informative.

Treatment.—*Medical.*—From time to time medical treatment is recommended as a principal measure for combating this condition. In most centres at the present time, for the majority of patients, medical treatment is employed for only two or three days, to prepare the patient for operation. In breast-fed babies in fair condition the time devoted to medical measures is reduced to forty-eight hours. Patients who, on account of complete pyloric obstruction, are admitted in a dehydrated condition should receive sufficient saline and glucose solution, given intravenously or into the bone marrow of the tibia, to restore the fluid balance. This results in a remarkable improvement in the general condition ; the sunken eyes and cheeks and depressed fontanelle fill out ; the dry skin and mucous membrane become moist, and the output of urine increases. A gastric tube is passed, and after aspirating and measuring the amount of retained gastric contents, the stomach is washed out with normal saline. Eumydrin (atropine methyl-nitrate) 1 : 10,000 of water, freshly made, is given half an hour before each feed, beginning with 0·5 to 1 ml. and increasing to 2·5 to 3 ml.

Alternatively, lamellæ of pylostropin can be placed under the tongue. Toxic symptoms (erythema and hyperpyrexia), though less common than when atropine is used, do arise, and are signs that the dose of the drug should be decreased or discontinued. Small, frequent feeds of milk (if possible the mother's milk), diluted with 5 per cent. glucose, are given. Medical treatment is used exclusively in subacute cases. In this type of case the patient has often reached the age of about two months before the symptoms become obvious. In such patients if, as a result of medical treatment, the gastric residue decreases in amount, a cure by non-operative means can be

Elisabeth Svensgaard, Contemporary. Physician, Rigshospitalet, Copenhagen. Introduced eumydrin as a therapeutic improvement on atropine in 1935.

anticipated. In patients who are admitted with signs of infection, especially of the mouth, a continuance of medical treatment is advisable until the infection is controlled, even if surgery would otherwise be indicated, because of the increased risk of post-operative gastro-enteritis.

Surgical.—When operation is advised comparatively early, the recovery rate in breast-fed babies approaches 100 per cent. Among bottle-fed babies the mortality is appreciably higher, owing to their greater susceptibility to gastro-enteritis (Levi).

Rammstedt's Operation.—*Preliminary Preparation.*—The stomach is washed out several times ; finally, one hour before operation. The prevention of chilling is of great importance. To this end the temperature of the operating theatre should be high (80° F.) and the infant's body is encased in wool, the upper abdomen alone being accessible.

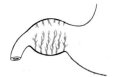

Fig. 314. — The upper part of the hypertrophied pylorus is comparatively bloodless. (*After Weeks.*)

Operation.—Local anæsthesia is usually advisable. The abdomen is opened by a right rectus-splitting incision. The hypertrophied pylorus is delivered and rotated so that its superior surface comes into view ; thus the most avascular portion (fig. 314) can be selected for the incision (fig. 315), which divides the hypertrophied muscle completely. Because the hypertrophied pylorus is often of the consistency of an unripe pear, it should be split by using a blunt dissector. On separating the edges with artery forceps, the pyloric mucosa bulges into the cleft which has been made in the muscle (fig. 316). Great care is taken not to penetrate the mucosa, an accident which is liable to occur at the duodenal " fornix " (see fig. 312). In order to be sure that there is no perforation, some air is squeezed from the stomach into the

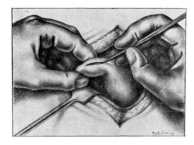

Fig. 315.—Rammstedt's operation.

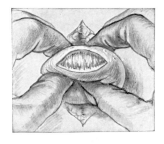

Fig. 316.—Showing the hypertrophied muscle divided and the mucous membrane bulging into the incision.

duodenum. If a perforation has occurred, it must be repaired carefully with interrupted sutures. The free entry of air into the duodenum also indicates adequate division of the muscle.

After-treatment.—To minimise the risk of cross-infection, and consequent gastro-enteritis, the patient must be segregated. Further infusions of

David Levi, Contemporary. Surgeon, Infants' Hospital, London.

glucose and saline, and, in patients in poor condition, plasma or blood transfusion should be given. The feeds must be very small and well-diluted, not more than ʒi being given at a time ; they are commenced eight hours after the operation.

Complications :

(i) *Hæmorrhage.*—It must be realised that in an attenuated infant the loss of even a drachm of blood is considerable. Bleeding from the incised muscle must receive meticulous attention.

(ii) *Persistent diarrhœa is* a troublesome and often fatal complication. It is minimised by thorough medical preparation, very careful after-feeding, and the administration of sulphasuccidine.

(iii) *Post-operation pyrexia* is rather common and is not necessarily of serious consequence. If excessive, tepid sponging is advisable.

(iv) *Burst abdomen is* a rare complication, and is more liable to occur in emaciated subjects.

CONGENITAL OCCLUSION OF THE DUODENUM

There is a septum, usually complete, across the duodenum (fig. 317). This occurs at the point of fusion of the fore- and mid-gut, and consequently

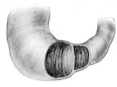

lies in the neighbourhood of the ampulla of Vater. The infant vomits *from birth*, and daily rapidly loses weight. In contradistinction to congenital pyloric stenosis the vomit contains bile. Laparotomy should be undertaken without delay. Duodeno-jejunostomy is the best procedure when, as is usually the case, the obstruction is in the second or third part of the duodenum (Ladd).

Fig. 317.—Congenital septal duodenal obstruction at the commencement of the third part of the duodenum. The gut above is enormously dilated.

(*After Ladd.*)

FOREIGN BODIES IN THE STOMACH

A variety of ingested foreign bodies reaches the stomach. Fortunately, for the most part they are opaque to X-rays. Sharply pointed or large objects are best removed promptly by gastrotomy. Rounded, smaller foreign bodies may be left to pass along the natural passages. Suitable doses of " Normacol " form a gelatinous pabulum, in which the article becomes embedded during its transit along the alimentary tract. That the journey is being accomplished can be verified by periodic examinations under the fluorescent screen (fig. 318).

Hair-ball of the stomach is accorded a prominent place among museum exhibits. The condition has always been rare, and now that most women wear their hair shorter than formerly, gastric hair-ball is exceptional, even among the feeble-minded. The treatment is removal of the mass by gastrotomy.

ACUTE DILATATION OF THE STOMACH

Acute dilatation of the stomach is a fairly com-

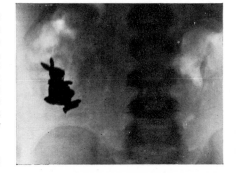

Fig. 318.—Embedded in " Normacol," this foreign body was passed naturally in three days.

Abraham Vater, 1684–1751. Professor of Anatomy and Botany, Wittenberg.
William E. Ladd, Contemporary. Emeritus Professor of Child Surgery, Harvard University, Boston, U.S.A.

mon post-operative complication. It can occur after any operation, or after the application (under an anæsthetic) of a plaster-of-Paris jacket, but the greatest incidence is after operations on the biliary passages and pelvic organs. More rarely, the condition complicates the state of shock, such as might be occasioned by a fractured femur.

Pathology.—In fatal cases the stomach is found enormously dilated ; it occupies the whole abdomen and the greater curvature may extend into the pelvis (fig. 319). The organ is filled with air and dark, watery fluid. Sometimes the dilatation ends at the pylorus ; more often it extends into the duodenum, and in a few instances the dilatation involves the extreme upper end of the jejunum. The gastric mucosa is scattered with petechial hæmorrhages.

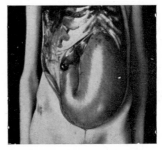

FIG. 319.—Acute dilatation of the stomach seen at necropsy.

Ætiology.—It has been suggested that the cause of the dilatation is compression of the third part of the duodenum by the superior mesenteric vessels, but as the dilatation does not regularly end in the middle of the third part of the duodenum, this hypothesis must be abandoned. Another explanation is that acute dilatation of the stomach is a local form of paralytic ileus. The swallowing of air (aerophagy) during the operation and in the immediate post-operative period, and the inability of a hypotonic stomach to expel the air, may play a part in starting the dilatation by inducing hyperæmia of the gastric mucous membrane, which in turn causes an excessive outpouring of secretion (succorrhœa).

Clinical Features.—The symptoms, which may come on with dramatic suddenness two or three days after operation, are those of profound shock accompanied by enormous, effortless vomits. In a fully-established case gallons of dark, watery fluid are brought up.

The vomitus consists mainly of water, a considerable quantity of mucus, occasionally pancreatic ferments have been found in it, but little or no hydrochloric acid. If some of the vomitus is placed in a test-tube and diluted with water, it will be seen to contain black particles (altered blood), which account for its characteristic colour.

So great is the quantity of fluid produced by a dilated stomach that in a matter of hours the patient becomes severely dehydrated. On abdominal examination a fullness in the epigastrium can often be seen, and splashing sometimes can be elicited, but in obese patients this may not be evident.

Prevention and Early Diagnosis of the Condition.—In a number of instances fully-established acute dilatation of the stomach can be prevented :

(*a*) By treating all patients with excessive post-anæsthetic vomiting by gastric aspiration and lavage, and retaining an indwelling gastric tube until it can be proved that fluid imbibed is passing down the alimentary canal.

(*b*) By passing a gastric aspiration tube when attention is drawn to a patient who has recently undergone an operation (particularly an abdominal or pelvic operation) by a rising pulse-rate, otherwise unexplained, epigastric discomfort, belching, slight hiccough and, on examination, some fullness in the epigastrium. These are the signs of impending acute dilatation of the stomach, and if the stomach can be emptied by aspiration before the patient commences to vomit, the dangerous stage of indubitable acute dilatation of the stomach is prevented.

Treatment.—In a fully established case, prompt action is imperative. The two principles are :

1. To empty the stomach and keep it empty.

2. To combat dehydration by administering continuous intravenous saline and glucose solution.

In the first instance it is best to employ a large stomach tube, and to empty the stomach by syphonage. In milder cases, and in fully established cases after the stomach has once been emptied, the stomach should be kept empty by aspiration or, preferably, by continuous suction through an indwelling Ryle's

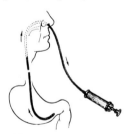

FIG. 320. — Aspirating the contents of the stomach via the nose.

or other small gastric tube passed, when possible, by way of the nose (fig. 320). The patient may drink as he pleases, and the ingested fluid is aspirated promptly. In this way the stomach is washed out. The amount of fluid given and the amount aspirated is measured and charted. When the amount withdrawn is unquestionably less than the amount given, the tube is removed and the continuous intravenous saline is discontinued.

By these measures, unless effective treatment has been delayed unduly, the stomach soon regains its tone.

PEPTIC ULCER

Peptic ulcers may be acute or chronic. Chronic ulcers are much the more common.

ACUTE PEPTIC ULCERS

Ætiology.—It is possible that these ulcers arise as toxic mucosal erosions, as is seen experimentally in animals after the injection of histamine and other poisons. They can arise as an inflammation of lymph follicles (follicular ulcers) or as submucosal hæmatomata (hæmorrhagic ulcers). Acute peptic ulcers have been found at post-mortem in hæmorrhagic diseases, uræmia, food poisoning, bacteræmia, and burns (see Curling's ulcer below).

Pathology.—Acute peptic ulcers are frequently multiple and can occur in any part of the stomach, but in the duodenum they are almost confined to the first part. These ulcers are oval or circular in shape, and vary in size from 1 to 2 mm. in diameter (when they are called erosions) to one or more cm. in diameter. They are shallow, punched out, and do not invade the muscular coats. When healing occurs they seldom leave a scar.

Clinical Features.—Acute peptic ulcers probably occur with great frequency. They give rise to short-lived attacks of dyspepsia which are not diagnosed, and the ulcer heals. Usually they are recognised only when they cause hæmatemesis. Occasionally an acute ulcer, particularly when it is situated on the anterior wall of the duodenum, perforates. By gastroscopy, it has been ascertained that acute peptic ulcers can be the cause of hæmatemesis at all ages and in both sexes. Such lesions have been seen to progress to chronic ulceration (Tanner).

Treatment.—If possible, the cause must be removed. Under medical treatment acute peptic ulcers tend to heal rapidly. Blood transfusion may be required for hæmatemesis. As improvement sets in, attention must be directed to the elimination of infected foci, particularly of dental origin. Dietetic irregularities must be corrected in order to prevent recurrence or chronicity.

Curling's ulcer (*syn.* duodenal ulcer following burns) is an acute ulcer in the second part of the duodenum, opposite the ampulla of Vater, and follows extensive cutaneous burns or scalds. The ulcer is small, clean cut, and deep. The cause is probably an infected embolus from the burnt area, or possibly it is the result of toxic products from the burned tissue being excreted in the bile. It is a very rare phenomenon.

CHRONIC PEPTIC ULCER

Ætiology.—The cause of chronic peptic ulcer is bound up with that of acute peptic ulceration, and has long been a matter for controversy. The following are the main theories which have been put forward. None is a satisfactory explanation for all the various forms of the lesion.

(a) *The Infective Theory.*—Bacteria, especially streptococci, from a distant focus are arrested in the gastric lymphoid follicles, which break down, forming an acute ulcer, which in turn becomes chronic.

(b) *Vascular Theory.*—Local embolism or thrombosis causes a devitalisation of an area of mucosa which is subsequently digested by gastric juice.

(c) *Chemical Theory.*—An abrasion or a lesion, caused by one of the above processes, fails to heal because of hyperchlorhydria.

(d) *Neurogenic Theory.*—That the ulcer is due to undue stimulation of the vagus nerves, which in turn results in hypersecretion and hypermobility of the stomach.

Thomas Curling, 1811–1888. Surgeon, London Hospital.
Norman Cecil Tanner, Contemporary. Senior Surgeon, St. James's Hospital, London.

(e) *Accessory Causes.*—Faulty diet, inadequate mastication, irregular hours of work, mental or physical strain, excessive smoking, and vitamin deficiency have at one time or another been blamed, and unquestionably are, to some extent, predisposing factors to the formation of a chronic peptic ulcer.

Pathology.—The ulcer-bearing area is shown in fig. 321. Outside this area ulcers are comparatively rare. A chronic peptic ulcer invades the muscular coats, which it tends to penetrate. Alternatively, the ulcer tends to heal, only to break down again, with further loss of tissue. Repetition of this cycle produces deformities, including pyloric stenosis and hour-glass contracture.

Fig. 321. — The ulcer-bearing area of the stomach and duodenum.

Chronic gastric ulcer is usually larger than a chronic duodenal ulcer. It varies in size, but in a well-established case it will admit the tip of a finger (fig. 322). The floor of a chronic gastric ulcer is situated in the muscular coats of the stomach,

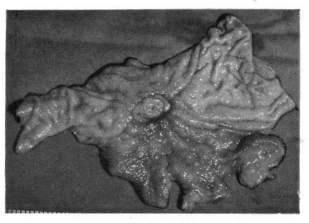

Fig. 322.—Chronic gastric ulcer on the lesser curvature of the stomach. Specimen removed by partial gastrectomy.

and as time goes on the ulcer occupying the posterior wall becomes adherent to, and later invades, the pancreas or the liver.

Chronic Duodenal Ulcer.—The ulcer is <u>always situated</u> in the <u>supra-ampullary portion of the duodenum</u>, and sometimes two ulcers are present : one on the anterior surface and one on the posterior surface of the first inch of the duodenum. The anterior ulcer tends to perforate, the posterior one is prone to penetrate into the pancreas and in so doing it often erodes an artery.

Microscopical Examination.—There is nearly always greater destruction of the muscular coat than of the mucosa. The base of the ulcer is filled with necrotic granulation tissue ; around this there is a zone of living granulation tissue. The arteries in the neighbourhood show evidence of endarteritis obliterans. At the margin of the ulcer there may be epithelial proliferation, and downgrowths of glandular tissue are apt to be found beneath the muscularis mucosæ. These downgrowths are sometimes wrongly interpreted as indicating a carcinomatous change (Boyd).

A chronic duodenal ulcer rarely, if ever, becomes carcinomatous. On the other hand, there is ample proof that a longstanding chronic gastric ulcer sometimes becomes malignant, but how frequently this change takes place is a matter of great difference of opinion. While a much higher figure has been given in many series, it would seem probable that it does not exceed 5 per cent., and, in the opinion of many, this estimate is too high. There is a consensus of opinion that an ulcer with a crater of more than 1 inch (2·5 cm.) in diameter is almost certainly malignant.

Pathology of the Living.—At operation the presence of a chronic peptic ulcer may be evident as a white scar under the peritoneal coat. Delicate vascular adhesions, salmon pink and fluffy in appearance, can often be observed in the immediate neighbourhood of the peritoneal aspect of the ulcer. At other times the ulcer must be sought for by palpation ; induration, frequently extensive in the case of a gastric ulcer, is centred over the mucosal lesion. When the ulcer is situated in the duodenum, the surrounding induration is not so evident, but if the ulcer is situated on the posterior wall it may be possible to feel the crater with the tip of the finger. A useful method of confirming the presence of a peptic ulcer, particularly one situated on the anterior wall of the duodenum, is to rub the peritoneal surface gently with a swab ; the peritoneum overlying the ulcer becomes speckled, as though sprinkled with cayenne pepper, a characteristic phenomenon due to minute petechial hæmorrhages (fig. 323). It is sometimes difficult to be certain whether a given

William Boyd, Contemporary. Professor of Pathology and Bacteriology, University of Toronto.

ulcer is gastric or duodenal.   The veins of Mayo (fig. 324) are a helpful landmark ; an ulcer situated to the right of these veins must be a duodenal ulcer.

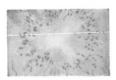

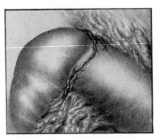

FIG. 323.—Petechial hæmorrhages around the peritoneal aspect of a chronic peptic ulcer.   These become very noticeable after gently rubbing the surface with gauze.

FIG. 324.—The veins of Mayo.

Incidence.—In men, chronic duodenal ulcer is considerably more common than gastric ulcer, the proportion being about 7 : 1.   In women the incidence of the two types of ulcer is about equal.   Gastric and duodenal ulcers can exist concomitantly.   From the years 1911–1941 there was a great increase in the number of deaths from chronic peptic ulcer, males over forty years of age being largely responsible for the rise. Since 1941 the death-rate from this cause has fallen (fig. 325). The frequency with which the duodenum is attacked, as opposed to the stomach, varies enormously in differ-

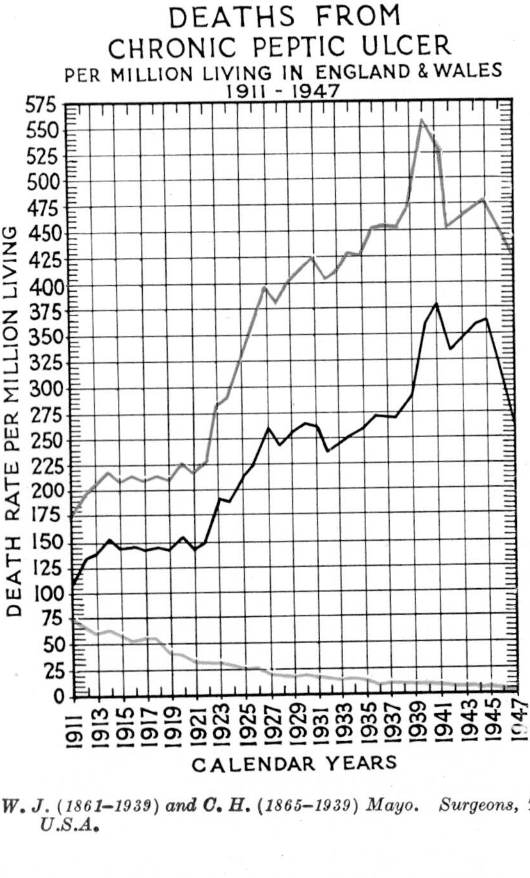

DEATHS FROM CHRONIC PEPTIC ULCER
PER MILLION LIVING IN ENGLAND & WALES
1911 - 1947

DEATH RATE PER MILLION LIVING

CALENDAR YEARS

FIG. 325.—*Red.* The incidence of deaths from chronic peptic ulcer in males over forty years of age.

Black. The incidence of deaths from chronic peptic ulcer in males between twenty and forty years of age.

Green. The incidence of deaths from chronic peptic ulcer in females aged twenty to forty.

(*Graph compiled by Denis Dooley and Allan Clain.*)

W. J. (*1861–1939*) *and* C. H. (*1865–1939*) *Mayo.   Surgeons, The Mayo Clinic, Rochester, U.S.A.*

ent localities. Even in Great Britain there is an almost unbelievable geographical variation. Thus, the relative incidence of duodenal to gastric ulcers in London is 1·2 : 1, in Leeds 4·4 : 1, and in Scotland 11·6 : 1 (Nicol).

THE CLINICAL FEATURES OF GASTRIC AND DUODENAL ULCERS CONTRASTED

It is an excellent practice to record the patient's history under seven headings, preferably in tabular form (see p. 280).

Chronic Gastric Ulcer.—The patient is usually beyond middle age, and by reason of a restricted diet, is often thin. In many instances the patient appears anæmic, and this is often confirmed by a hæmoglobin estimation. On careful enquiry certain features of the dyspepsia become manifest. Typically there is :

1. *Periodicity.*—The attacks last from two to six weeks, and are followed by intervals of freedom from two to six months. The attacks are more in evidence in the spring and autumn.

2. *Pain* is epigastric, and occurs half to one and a half or two hours after food. This variation often bears a direct relation to the position of the ulcer, viz. :——→ The longer the ulcer has existed the more does the pain radiate.

3. *Vomiting.*—In over 50 per cent. of cases vomiting is a notable symptom. It relieves the pain, and may be self-induced.

4. *Hæmatemesis and Melæna.*—Approximately 30 per cent. of cases have had hæmatemesis some time during the course of the disease, and half that number have had melæna.

5. *Appetite* is good, but the sufferer is afraid to eat.

6. *Diet.*—The patient avoids meat and certain other foods, which vary with the individual. Milk, eggs, and fish are the staple diet.

7. *Weight.*—Usually by the time the surgeon is consulted there has been some loss of weight.

On examination there is frequently deep tenderness in the epigastrium, especially during one of the periodic attacks.

Chronic duodenal ulcer can occur at any time during adult life, but is commonest between the ages of twenty-five and fifty. As has been pointed out already, it is more common in men. The usual history is as follows :

1. *Periodicity* is usually well marked, and classically the attacks come on in the spring and in the autumn. These

Bruce Millian Nicol, Contemporary. Surgeon, Colonial Medical Service, Nigeria.

attacks usually last from two to six weeks, with intervals of freedom from one to six months.

2. *Pain* is severe, and may double the patient up. It usually occurs two to two and a half hours after food. As it is often relieved by food, the pain is known as " hunger pain," and, classically, the patient carries biscuits, which he eats at frequent intervals to prevent this gastric torment. The pain, which is also relieved by alkalis, often awakens the patient in the early hours of the morning.

3. *Vomiting is very rare* in duodenal ulceration unless it is self-induced or stenosis has occurred. Regurgitation of burning fluid into the mouth (" water-brash " ; " heart-burn ") is an extremely common complaint.

4. *Hæmorrhage,* which manifests itself as hæmatemesis or melæna, or both, forms one of the most dangerous complications.

5. *Appetite* is exceptionally good, but the patient often refrains from eating during the attacks.

6. *Diet.*—In contradistinction to patients with a chronic gastric ulcer, those suffering from duodenal ulcer who have not been ordered a special diet seldom display much dietetic discrimination, although some of the more intelligent find it advisable to avoid butcher's meat and fried food.

7. *Weight.*—Usually there is no loss of weight ; indeed, the patient often tends to become plump.

On examination it is not unusual to find localised deep tenderness in the right hypochondrium.

SUMMARY

	Gastric Ulcer	Duodenal Ulcer
Periodicity .	Present	Well marked
Pain .	Half an hour after food	Two hours after food
Vomiting .	Considerable vomiting	No vomiting – water brush – heartburn
Hæmorrhage .	Hæmatemesis	Melæna
Appetite .	Afraid to eat	Good
Diet .	Lives on milk and fish	Eats almost anything
Weight .	Loses weight	No loss in weight

SPECIAL METHODS OF INVESTIGATION

Barium Meal.—In the case of a chronic *gastric* ulcer the radiological findings are often conclusive. When a penetrating ulcer of the lesser curvature is present, the characteristic finding

Lord Moynihan, 1865–1936. Surgeon, General Infirmary at Leeds. First described " hunger pain."

is a niche or crater filled with barium (fig. 326), with spasm of the circular fibres of the stomach causing a notch in the greater curvature opposite the ulcer, i.e. there is " a niche and a notch." The notch must be distinguished from hour-glass stomach. In other portions of the stomach the radiological findings may not be conclusive, but when a deep ulcer is present, there will be a niche seen throughout the examination, and a flake of barium persisting in the crater after the stomach is emptied. Unless there is pyloro-spasm,

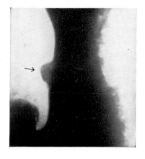

FIG. 326.—Large penetrating ulcer on the lesser curvature.
(*G. Mather Cordiner.*)

the rate of emptying in the case of an uncomplicated gastric ulcer is usually rapid, and there is no residue after six hours.

The radiological findings in the case of a chronic *duodenal* ulcer include hypermobility, i.e. several contractile waves present simultaneously. In an uncomplicated chronic duodenal ulcer the usual characteristic finding is initial rapid emptying of the major part of the meal, followed by delay of the remainder. In cases of longer standing, a deformity of the duodenal cap is often found, and sometimes an ulcer niche can be demonstrated (fig. 327) with persistence of a flake of barium in the ulcer crater after the stomach and duodenum have emptied.

The X-ray appearances of chronic peptic ulcer complicated by pyloric stenosis or hour-glass stomach are extremely characteristic (see pp. 293 and 294).

A hæmoglobin estimation is performed, and the stool and the vomitus, if any, are examined for occult blood.

Fractional Test Meal (fig. 328).—In the case of a chronic *gastric* ulcer the acid curve is not characteristic; it may

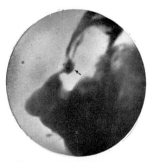

FIG. 327. — Ulcer niche localised on the posterior wall of the duodenal cap.
(*G. Mather Cordiner.*)

be slightly raised, but often it is normal. Of more diagnostic value is the presence of excess of mucus and perhaps a trace of blood in the gastric juice. In the case of an uncomplicated chronic *duodenal* ulcer, the acid curve rises precipitously (fig. 329),

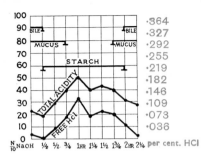

			per cent. HCl
		·364	
		·327	
		·292	
		·255	
		·219	
		·182	
		·146	
		·109	
		·073	
		·036	

FIG. 328.—Normal fractional test meal.

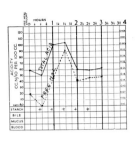

FIG. 329.—Typical steep curve of duodenal ulcer. (*Norman Tanner.*)

reaching a maximum about two hours after a meal. This is caused by spasm of the pylorus preventing reflux of alkaline duodenal content.

The following tests are also indicated when vagotomy is contemplated as a method of treatment for a chronic *duodenal* or an *anastomotic* ulcer :

Insulin Test Meal.—Insulin produces hypoglycæmia, a state which induces vagal stimulation, which in turn causes an increased secretion of gastric juice. Ten units or more of insulin are given intravenously, in order to produce a state of hypoglycæmia, which is measured by a blood-sugar reading about an hour later. A test meal taken during the state of hypoglycæmia shows an increase in the total and free acidity over and above that of the usual fractional test meal of that patient.

The Amount of Night Secretion of Gastric Juice.—If the night secretion of gastric juice, collected by suction via a Ryle's tube, exceeds 500 c.c. in twelve hours, it is confirmatory evidence of over-stimulation of the vagus nerves.

Gastroscopy (fig. 330) gives useful, but limited, information. After at least twelve hours' starvation, a suitable injection of morphia is administered. The patient is then given a 25-mg. tablet of amethocaine (a surface anæsthetic) to suck. Soon after this has dissolved a gastric aspiration tube is passed, and the contents of the stomach are aspirated. The patient is sent

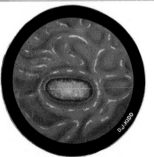

FIG. 330.—Chronic gastric ulcer; posterior wall of the stomach. Greyish colour due to penetration into the pancreas. (*J. Howell Hughes.*) (*British Journal of Surgery.*)

to the operating theatre with the tube in place.   After further aspiration, the tube is removed.   The gastroscope is passed and the stomach inflated with air.   The flexible extremity of Hermon Taylor's instrument (fig. 331) can be moved into different parts

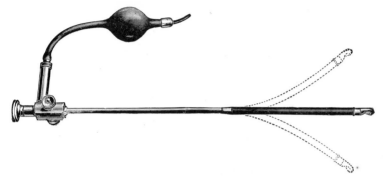

Fig. 331.—Hermon Taylor's flexible gastroscope.

of the stomach by means of a controlling wheel near the eye-piece, and with this instrument nearly all parts of the stomach can be examined, but positive X-ray evidence is more valuable than negative gastroscopic findings.   Gastroscopy is valuable in the diagnosis of shallow gastric ulcers, particularly acute ulcers, which do not show on radiography, in checking the results of medical treatment, and in the differential diagnosis between simple ulcer and carcinoma.   Gastroscopic examination is con-traindicated in the presence of inflammatory lesions of the mouth, pharynx, or œsophagus, and in patients with an aortic aneurism or spinal deformity.

TREATMENT OF CHRONIC PEPTIC ULCER

All are agreed that in the first instance treatment should be medical.   When necessary, dental attention should be insisted upon, and any source of focal infection must be eliminated as far as possible.   Whatever course is adopted, rest in bed is essential, and irregularities of diet must be avoided when the patient resumes his occupation.   Cannabis indica is an excellent drug for promoting restfulness and mental tranquillity, especially in highly strung patients (Douthwaite).

Apart   from   acute   complications,   the   indications   for

Georg Wolf, Contemporary, *Optical-instrument Maker, Berlin*, and *Rudolph Schindler*, Contemporary, *Associate Professor of Medicine, University of Chicago (formerly of Munich), invented the gastroscope in 1932.*
Hermon Taylor, Contemporary.   *Surgeon, London Hospital.*
A. H. Douthwaite, Contemporary.   *Physician, Guy's Hospital, London.*

operation in cases of chronic peptic ulcer may be summarised as follows :

1. Frequent relapses after efficient medical treatment.
2. A suspicion of malignancy.
3. Stenosis causing delay in emptying.
4. Large penetrating ulcer.
5. Hæmatemesis occurring more than once.
6. Economic reasons—adequate medical treatment impracticable.

OPERATIVE TREATMENT

Partial Gastrectomy.—Partial gastrectomy (fig. 332) (with, in the case of duodenal ulcer, resection of the first part of the

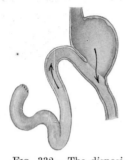

Fig. 332.—The disposition of the parts concerned after standard partial gastrectomy.

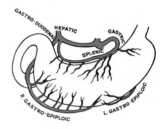

Fig. 333.—The arterial supply of the stomach.
(*After T. H. Somervell.*)

duodenum) is the most reliable and, in many cases, the only operation which will cure the condition permanently. There are several methods of performing partial gastrectomy, the most usual being the anterior or posterior Polya method. In all methods of partial gastrectomy, ligation of the arteries which supply the stomach (fig. 333) at the points indicated in fig. 334 is an inherent part of the procedure.

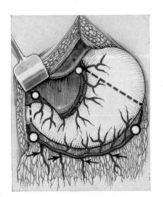

Fig. 334.—Points at which ligatures are applied to arteries in the operation of partial gastrectomy.

The upper abdomen is opened by a right paramedian incision. Having verified the diagnosis, the first step is to open the lesser sac between the stomach and the transverse colon. The gastro-colic omentum is freed from the greater curvature and the first part of the duodenum by clamping and

Eugers Polya, Contemporary. Surgeon, St. Stephen's Hospital, Budapest.

dividing this omental attachment and its contained blood-vessels close
to the stomach. The process is continued as far as the junction of the upper
third with the lower two-thirds of the greater curvature. In a similar
manner, the gastro-hepatic omentum is cleared from the superior surface of
the first part of the duodenum and lesser curvature. The duodenum is
then divided between clamps, and the duodenal stump is closed and invaginated, the suture line being reinforced by a covering of omentum.

The stomach is turned over to the left (fig. 335),
and is further cleared of omental attachment, as
necessary. A loop of jejunum is then brought up,
either in front of the transverse colon (anterior
Polya operation) or through an opening in the
transverse mesocolon (posterior Polya operation),
and is attached to the posterior stomach wall by
continuous or interrupted sero-muscular stitches
just proximal to the proposed line of division. The
stomach is divided between crushing clamps just
distal to this suture line. The lower two-thirds
of the stomach is now freed, and removed. A
rubber-covered stomach clamp grasps the stump
of the stomach, and the remaining crushing
clamp is removed. The jejunum is incised along
the length of its attachment to the stomach, and
end-to-side anastomosis is completed between the
cut end of the stomach and the jejunum. Stitching
the proximal loop of the jejunum to the lesser
curvature beyond the stump prevents kinking of
the loop, and is shown in fig. 332. The abdomen
is closed in layers.

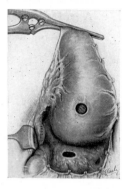

Fig. 335.—Partial gas-
trectomy in progress.
An ulcer penetrating
the pancreas has been
separated.

Gastro-jejunostomy is practised much less frequently than
formerly. The operation is not curative in the case of a chronic
gastric ulcer, and in the case of a chronic duodenal ulcer, particularly when the patient is young and the ulcer is associated with
a high acidity and hypermotility, gastro-
jejunostomy is, after a varying period of benefit,
too frequently followed by the development of
a gastro-jejunal ulcer. Gastro-jejunostomy
is now performed only in cases of simple pyloric
stenosis, and in cases of duodenal ulcer occurring in patients over forty-five who can be
shown to have a relatively low acidity, and slow
emptying of the stomach. A short-loop
posterior operation with a vertical stoma, and
the efferent loop nearer the greater curvature
(fig. 336), is the type of operation which gives
the best results.

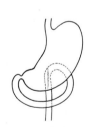

Fig. 336.—The
posterior, vertical,
short-loop gastro-
jejunostomy of
Mayo.

Vagotomy (vagus nerve section).—It has been proved that both hypermotility and hypersecretion of the stomach are diminished by complete
section of the vagus nerves. Dragstedt applied this knowledge to patients

*On September 27th, 1881, Wölfler, of Vienna, first performed gastro-jejunostomy, the operation
being suggested by Nicoladoni, his assistant.*
Lester Reynold Dragstedt, Contemporary. Professor of Surgery, University of Chicago.

suffering from peptic ulcer. Originally, the operation was undertaken by the thoracic route. The trans-abdominal approach is now generally favoured, and besides carrying a lower mortality, it has the advantage of enabling the lesion to be examined.

Indications.—1. An uncomplicated chronic duodenal ulcer occurring in a young subject, and where there is (*a*) hypermotility, as shown in the barium meal, (*b*) excessive secretion, as shown by the collection of the night secretion of gastric juice, and (*c*) a raised curve of the insulin test meal.

2. A gastro-jejunal ulcer occurring at the site of anastomosis after a gastro-jejunostomy or a partial gastrectomy.

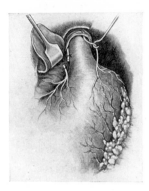

FIG. 337.—Bilateral vagotomy. Abdominal approach. (*After Dragstedt.*)

It is for the latter conditions that this operation has received the greatest approbation.

Surgical Anatomy.—Both vagi reach the stomach through the lesser omentum, and there divide into branches. The left vagus nerve supplies the anterior wall of the stomach and sends branches to the liver. The right vagus supplies the posterior wall and a large branch passes to the cœliac plexus. There is a constant intermediate branch which connects the two vagi (Thorek).

Operation.—The peritoneal cavity having been entered through a left paramedian incision, the left triangular ligament of the liver is exposed and made taut. This is divided and the left lobe is retracted to the right. The peritoneum covering the lower end of the œsophagus is incised and a finger is placed in the posterior mediastinum to mobilise the œsophagus so that its lower 3 inches can be delivered into the abdomen. The vagus nerves feel like taut cords, and they can be thus differentiated from the more yielding muscle of the œsophagus. A short length of each nerve is resected between ligatures—the objective being to ensure permanent loss of continuity (fig. 337).

COMPLICATIONS OF CHRONIC PEPTIC ULCER

Acute. { **Perforation.**
{ **Severe hæmatemesis** and/or **melæna.**

Intermediate. **Perigastric abscess.**

Chronic. { **Stenosis** { Pyloric stenosis.
{ Hour-glass contracture.
{ **Penetration** into neighbouring viscera, notably the pancreas.
{ **Neoplastic change.**

PERFORATED PEPTIC ULCER

Sex.—The ratio is 19 men to 1 woman (Illingworth).

Age.—The highest incidence is between forty-five and fifty-five years of age (fig. 338).

Location.—At the commencement of the present century the ulcer that perforated most frequently was situated in the stomach. During the past

Phil Thorek, Contemporary. Attending Surgeon, Cook County Hospital, Chicago.
Charles Frederick William Illingworth, Contemporary. Regius Professor of Surgery, University of Glasgow.

thirty years perforation of a duodenal ulcer has become much more common, and is now at least four times more frequent than perforation of a gastric ulcer.

Seasonal Variations.—The highest incidence is in December ; the lowest in the early autumn. The December peak, which increases steadily through that month, cannot be attributed to seasonal festivity.

Daily Variations.—Perforation of peptic ulcers is relatively uncommon on Sunday and Monday. Tuesday, Wednesday, and Thursday may be taken as average days ; Friday and Saturday vie with each other for pride of place for the maximum incidence. Rest from the week's labours on Saturday afternoon and Sunday may account for fewer perforations on Sunday and Monday.

Hourly Variations.—Uncommon during the night, the incidence rises sharply, (*a*) at the end of the morning ; (*b*) during the late afternoon. These peak periods coincide with those of physical fatigue (Jamieson).

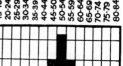

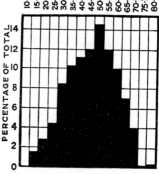

Fig. 338.—Age incidence of perforated peptic ulcer compiled from 1,055 cases of perforation collected from sixteen London hospitals. (*Stewart and Winser.*)

Ætiology.—Extra-large meals and extra pints of liquor typify what is implied by the " Christmas dinner " theory. This theory, so long a popular one, has no foundation in fact. It has been proved conclusively that the principal determining cause of perforation is physical fatigue and mental stress. The seasonal, daily, and hourly variations of incidence strongly support the latter hypothesis. In keeping with this theory are the facts that perforation became at least ten times as common during a famine period in Russia, and there was an abrupt rise in the incidence during the intensive air bombardment of London (Stewart and Winser).[1]

In the majority of cases the ulcer which perforates is situated on the anterior surface of the duodenum ; much less frequently it is situated on the anterior surface of the stomach, usually the lesser curvature. Very rarely an ulcer on the posterior wall of the stomach perforates into the lesser sac. In 80 per cent. of cases there is a history—often a long history—of peptic ulceration. In 20 per cent. there is no such history ; it is a " silent " chronic ulcer which perforates. Usually the symptoms of perforation come on with dramatic suddenness.

The gastric or duodenal contents escape through the perforation into the general peritoneal cavity, provoking widespread peritoneal irritation (peritonism). At that moment the victim cries out in agony, and, at any rate if the perforation is a large one and the stomach is full, he is riveted temporarily to the spot where

[1] Dr. D. N. Stewart and the late D. M. de R. Winser wrote their paper while they were medical students at Charing Cross Hospital, London.

Robert Ainslie Jamieson, Contemporary. Lecturer in Surgery, University of Glasgow.

the perforation felled him. The peritoneum reacts to this chemical irritation by secreting peritoneal fluid copiously. For a short time this outpouring relieves the pain, and the stage of reaction is at hand. This stage of reaction lasts but an hour or so, and is followed by diffuse bacterial peritonitis.

Clinical Features.—1. *Stage of Peritonism.*—Examination reveals a pale, anxious individual obviously in great pain. The temperature is usually subnormal, and *the pulse-rate frequently in the neighbourhood of 80 or 90* ; in a large majority of instances, during the first six hours, the pulse-rate is comparatively unaltered. The upper abdomen of a thin subject will be seen to be scaphoid, and it moves little or not at all with respiration (fig. 339). The

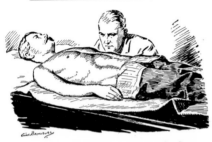

FIG. 339.—Watching for abdominal movement on respiration. In cases of perforated peptic ulcer abdominal movement is restricted or absent.

palpating hand at once recognises an abdominal rigidity which is general and board-like. The whole abdomen is tender and inclined to be dull to percussion. In a small percentage of cases, sufficient gas escapes to cause a diminution of the normal liver dullness in the mid-axillary line. A rectal examination sometimes reveals tenderness in the recto-vesical pouch. When a comparatively small perforation is situated in the duodenum, the escaping fluid is sometimes directed down the right paracolic gutter to the right iliac fossa. The symptoms then simulate closely those of acute perforated appendicitis.

2. *The Stage of Reaction.*—The severe abdominal pain lessens, and the patient says he feels better. The temperature becomes normal or elevated one degree, but the pulse-rate is usually still in the neighbourhood of 90. This temporary improvement in the general condition has been termed the " period of illusion," and it occurs between the fourth and sixth hours after the perforation. On examination there is a varying amount of rigidity, but it is not board-like ; there is tenderness, and because of the considerable quantity of free fluid present, shifting dullness can often be elicited.

Confirmation of a Doubtful Diagnosis.—When a perforation is present, in about 70 per cent. of cases a plain radiograph will reveal a crescent-shaped translucent area beneath the right cupola of the diaphragm (fig. 340). In cases of clinical doubt (for instance if the patient has been given morphine) when the gastric contents have been aspirated, 20 to 30 ml. of air are injected into the stomach. After the patient has lain on his left side for a few minutes a radiograph is taken in the sitting posture, and if a perforation is present the crescent-shaped translucent area will be seen in every case.

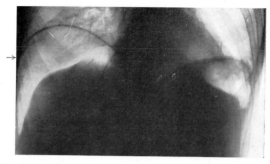

FIG. 340.—Showing gas beneath the diaphragm. Plain X-ray of a patient with a perforated duodenal ulcer.

3. *The Stage of Diffuse Peritonitis.*—After six or eight hours the signs gradually change to those of diffuse peritonitis. The abdomen slowly becomes distended and the intense rigidity tends to pass off. By this time enough free fluid has collected in the peritoneal cavity for shifting dullness to be elicited.

After the sixth hour the pulse-rate gradually increases, and with each passing hour the chances of recovery grow more slender.

Treatment.—Morphia should not be given until written permission for operation has been obtained. Operation, as soon as the general condition permits, is usually the best course. Laparotomy is performed (fig. 341) and the perforation is closed

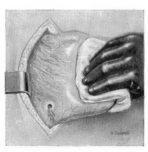

FIG. 341.—Perforated gastric ulcer exposed by laparotomy.

with interrupted sutures. In large perforations it is well to reinforce the suture line with a patch of omentum. With a mechanical sucker or swabs, free fluid in the peritoneal cavity is removed. Suprapubic drainage of the peritoneal cavity is employed in late cases, or when the leaking contents are foul, e.g. pyloric stenosis is present. Sulphonamide suspension having been introduced into the peritoneal cavity, the laparotomy incision is closed. The immediate after-treatment consists in saline infusions, and as soon as the patient awakens from anæsthesia he should be placed gradually in modified Fowler's position. Penicillin and

George R. Fowler, 1848–1906. Surgeon, Brooklyn Hospital, New York.
Ludwig Heusner, 1846–1916. Surgeon, Barmen, Germany. Performed the first successful operation for perforated peptic ulcer in 1892.

sulphonamide therapy have contributed to the improvement of results.

Non-operative Treatment.—Hermon Taylor advises non-operative treatment in *early* cases of perforated peptic ulcer. His instructions are as follows :

First twenty-four hours : Aspiration every half-hour. Three pints of fluid parenterally plus the amount of fluid aspirated.

Second twenty-four hours : Aspiration every hour, followed by drinks of 1 ounce water.

Third twenty-four hours : The same as the second twenty-four hours, but a mixture of milk and water instead of water only.

On the fourth day the tube is removed if the fluid chart proves that all the fluid taken by mouth is indubitably passing onwards.

In most clinics this form of treatment is not attempted, particularly in early cases, because the results of operative treatment carried out soon after the perforation has occurred are so good. For subjects in poor condition, for instance, those afflicted with chronic bronchitis or heart disease, the risks entailed are probably smaller than the risks that accompany operation.

Late Results of Perforated Peptic Ulcers.—As might be expected, there is a transient remission of symptoms due to the rest in bed and the careful dietetic supervision during convalescence. Elderly patients and those of any age with a very short dyspeptic history are the ones who are likely to remain symptom-free after successful treatment of a perforation (Illingworth). Nevertheless, within one year 40 per cent. of patients relapse, and within five years 70 per cent. On this account, those who have been fortunate enough to survive perforation should be warned to report, so that, if necessary, they may receive timely treatment for an active ulcer.

PERIGASTRIC ABSCESS

is an uncommon condition which can arise in one of two ways : (1) the amount of fluid escaping from a leaking duodenal ulcer due to a minute perforation may be small enough to be confined to Morison's right kidney pouch, and there become shut off from the rest of the peritoneal cavity by adhesions ; (2) an ulcer on the posterior wall of the stomach perforates into the lesser sac, the foramen of Winslow being occluded by adhesions.

Some days after an acute attack of upper abdominal pain a tender swelling appears in the epigastrium or right hypochondrium. Usually the temperature is elevated.

Treatment.—If on laparotomy an abscess of the first variety is found, it is best drained by a counter-incision in the flank. An abscess of the lesser sac can usually be most conveniently drained through the gastro-hepatic omentum. A gastric or duodenal fistula may follow drainage of a perigastric abscess.

SUBPHRENIC ABSCESS, see p. 386.

Rutherford Morison, 1853–1939. Professor of Surgery, University of Durham.
Jacob Winslow, 1669–1760. A Dane who migrated to Paris, and there established a school of anatomy.

HÆMATEMESIS AND MELÆNA

Ætiology.—Chronic peptic ulcer for which the
patient has received treatment . . . 85% of cases.

Acute peptic ulcer (p. 275)
" Silent " chronic ulcer } . . . . 10% ,, ,,

Œsophageal varices due to
  portal hypertension (p. 321)
Carcinoma of the stomach (p. 302)
Purpura (p. 315) } . . 5% ,, ,,
Hæmophilia
Pernicious and other anæmias

Pathology.—Slight bleeding due to the trauma of passing food
is a frequent accompaniment of all chronic peptic ulcers ; such
bleeding is demonstrated only by finding traces of blood in a
fractional test meal and occult blood in the stools. In about
20 per cent. of cases of chronic peptic ulcer, sooner or later a
sudden and serious hæmorrhage occurs, due to erosion of an
artery in the floor of the ulcer. Occasionally the artery thus
implicated is of considerable size, such as the splenic or the gastro-
duodenal artery ; more usually it is a branch of one of these
vessels. Even when a large vessel is eroded, death from
hæmorrhage (fig. 342) seldom results from the initial hæmorrhage. Far more frequently a large hæmorrhage is heralded by
two or three smaller ones on consecutive days, as in other cases
of secondary hæmor-
rhage.

Clinical Features.
— In the case of
serious hæmorrhage
from a *gastric* ulcer,
collapse and pallor
are followed by
hæmatemesis, which
is effortless vomiting
of coffee-ground
material, sometimes
followed by bright
red blood. When
severe hæmorrhage

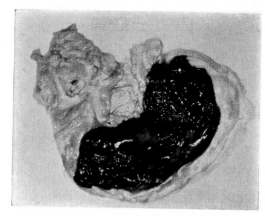

Fig. 342.—Fatal hæmatemesis from erosion of an
artery in the floor of a gastric ulcer.

takes place in a *duodenal* ulcer, the patient says he feels faint. This is followed by the passage of a melæna stool. So great may be the bleeding that bright red clotted blood is passed per rectum.

The patient looks pale, the pulse is rapid, and the blood pressure low. Quite often the bleeding comes on during a quiescent period of the ulcer, the patient having been free from symptoms of peptic ulcer for weeks or months.

Treatment.—*On admission* the collapsed patient is laid flat, and the foot of the bed is raised. Morphia, gr. $\frac{1}{6}$th (10 mgm.), is given four-hourly, and while arrangements (including cross-matching) are being made for blood transfusion, if the blood pressure is very low a plasma infusion is given. The important consideration is to replenish the circulation without overloading it, and a drip blood transfusion proportional to the estimated blood loss should be given. A pulse chart, if necessary half-hourly, is compiled, and a careful watch is kept on the blood pressure. A hæmoglobin estimation is unchanged at first, but commences to fall some hours after a severe hæmorrhage. As a result of these measures improvement usually occurs. The patient can now gradually be propped up in low Fowler's position.

Medical Treatment.—Feeding according to Witts' régime is commenced. This consists of a bland, semi-solid diet, providing about 3,000 calories a day, with a fluid intake of about 2,750 ml. ($4\frac{3}{4}$ pints) daily. Frequent pulse and blood-pressure readings are continued for at least three days after apparent cessation of the hæmorrhage. The drip transfusion is also continued at a rate of 30 drops a minute until the hæmoglobin estimation is satisfactory.

In patients under forty-five years of age the initial improvement is usually maintained. This permits a continuance of medical treatment, but, when possible, although it entails the risk of washing out the stomach, gastroscopy should be performed, and if the ulcer is visualised, it can be decided whether or not to rely upon medical treatment.

Surgical Treatment.—In patients over forty-five years of age continuance of medical measures for more than two, or at the most three, days is usually unsafe, for even if the bleeding has apparently ceased, or at any rate diminished, owing, perhaps, to the more sclerotic arteries, renewed bleeding frequently

Leslie John Witts, Contemporary. Nuffield Professor of Clinical Medicine, Oxford.

recurs more violently within a week.   The tendency, therefore, is to advise operation as soon as the patient has rallied from the initial hæmorrhage and he or she is deemed fit for operation.

Unfortunately, gastroscopy in these circumstances is seldom of any avail, owing to blood-clot in the stomach.   As a rule laparotomy, with the drip transfusion still running, must be undertaken to verify the diagnosis, and usually the only effective operation is partial gastrectomy with, if necessary, partial duodenectomy.   Extra-gastric ligation of individual arteries is unreliable, but when the condition of the patient is poor and the ulcer is situated in the stomach, gastrotomy with cauterisation of the ulcer and direct suture has proved effective.

Failure of repeated transfusions in recurrent Hæmorrhages. —If operative treatment is withheld, especially in patients of the older age groups, in spite of, or because of, the numerous transfusions, a uræmic state supervenes, accompanied by high blood urea and a low output of urine.   The cause of this condition is not known, but it is believed to be due to liver failure. When such a state supervenes it is too late for surgical treatment, and the patient usually succumbs.

PYLORIC STENOSIS

is usually the result of cicatrisation of a duodenal ulcer.   Occasionally it follows a prepyloric ulcer.

There is a history of a long-standing peptic ulcer, with the following modifications :

Periodicity is lost, and pain becomes constant.

Pain comes on immediately after food, and remains as a constant heavy discomfort, with attacks of colic due to excessive peristalsis.

Vomiting.—Very large foul and frothy vomits are characteristic. They usually occur once a day, commonly in the evening.   Classically, the patient recognises undigested food eaten one or more days previously.   Vomiting does not entirely relieve the discomfort.

On Examination.—In thin subjects with considerable stenosis of the duodenum or the pylorus, the outline of the full, dilated stomach can sometimes be observed.   Visible peristaltic waves passing from left to right are characteristic.   These patients may be mentally confused as a result of vitamin B deficiency or of alkalosis.

Barium Meal.—The stomach is large and low (fig. 343), and often takes more than six hours to empty.

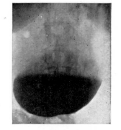

FIG. 343.—Typical X-ray appearance of pyloric stenosis. The barium meal lies as at the bottom of a bowl.
(Carl Krebs, Aarhus, Denmark.)

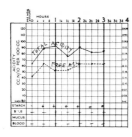

Fig. 344.—Plateau curve
of pyloric stenosis.
(*Norman Tanner*.)

Fractional Test Meal.—Registers a high *total* acidity, partly due to fermentation and partly due to union of free acid with food débris and mucus. The latter may result in lowering of the free HCl. The contour of the fractional test-meal curve tends to be raised, but flat—the so-called plateau curve (fig. 344).

Treatment. — Preliminary treatment with gastric lavage, a high-protein diet, and correction of chloride and vitamin (particularly B and C) deficiencies is necessary. In cases with a persistently low free HCl content, gastrojejunostomy gives satisfactory results. If, however, the ulcer is active, partial gastrectomy should be carried out.

HOUR-GLASS STOMACH

only occurs in women, and is due to cicatricial contracture around a saddle-shaped lesser-curve ulcer. In extreme cases the stomach is divided into two compartments, united by a channel which barely admits a pencil (fig. 345). The condition is sometimes associated with pyloric stenosis.

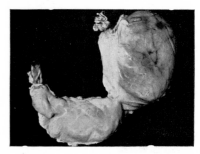

Fig. 345.—Hour-glass stomach.

History.—*Periodicity* is lost. The symptoms have become practically constant.

Vomiting is more frequent, and gives no relief to the discomfort.

The *appetite* becomes poor.

Weight.—Loss may be so great that carcinoma is suspected.

Barium meal is often very characteristic. We have known cases of hour-glass stomach reported as pyloric stenosis, owing to failure of the second pouch to fill. True hour-glass stomach (fig. 346) must be distinguished from gastric spasm of the hour-glass type, which is sometimes associated with an uncomplicated ulcer on the lesser curvature.

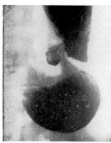

Fig. 346.—Hour-glass
contracture of the
stomach.
(*G. Mather Cordiner*.)

Fractional test meal shows a very low acidity.

Gastroscopy.—The gastroscope enters the upper compartment of the stomach, and the narrow, scarred channel leading to the lower compartment and the causative ulcer are usually seen.

Treatment.—Partial gastrectomy, with removal of the second pouch and the isthmus, is usually the best treatment. When the ulcer is defunct and the stenosed area consists entirely of scar tissue, union of the pouches by gastro-gastrostomy with a wide stoma is followed by complete amelioration of all symptoms.

ADHERENCE OF THE ULCER TO THE PANCREAS AND PENETRATION INTO IT (CHRONIC PERFORATION)

is a common complication of chronic gastric and duodenal ulcers situated on the posterior wall of the duodenum and the body of the stomach. It appears to be more common in England than in America.

History is one of chronic gastric ulcer with the following modifications:

Periodicity tends to be less definite, in that the intervals of freedom are short or absent.

Pain becomes more severe, constant, and passes to the back or the left shoulder.

Barium Meal.—If there is a definite crater in this region, the diagnosis is certain.

Gastroscopy may be needed to confirm the diagnosis of an early ulcer.

Treatment.—In deep, penetrating ulcers, and when medical treatment has failed, partial gastrectomy is indicated.

NEOPLASTIC CHANGE IN THE ULCER

The possibility of a malignant change occurring in a peptic ulcer is limited to a gastric ulcer. It is generally conceded that an ulcer with a crater more than 1 inch (2·5 cm.) in diameter is almost certainly malignant. A prepyloric ulcer is more prone to become carcinomatous than a lesser-curve ulcer.

History.—*Periodicity.*—The last attack continued much longer than usual, and there was no remission.

Pain is constant, but not as severe as formerly, and it is usually unrelieved by medical treatment.

Vomiting does not relieve the pain, and sometimes takes the form of regurgitation of foul material, or " coffee grounds."

Appetite is lost; in the early stages, especially for meat.

Weight.—The patient tends to lose weight rapidly.

Barium meal may show nothing characteristic in the early stages, but an ulcer crater which exceeds one inch in diameter should be assumed to be malignant until it has been proved otherwise.

Fractional test meal tends to have a low free hydrochloric acid content. Absence of free hydrochloric acid is a frequent finding in advanced cases. Owing to fermentation the total acidity may be increased.

Gastroscopy is the most certain method of making an early diagnosis. Nodular changes

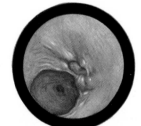

Fig. 347.—Early carcinomatous change in a chronic gastric ulcer seen by gastroscopy in a patient undergoing medical treatment for gastric ulcer. (*Hermon Taylor.*)

of one part of the ulcer edge and infiltration of the adjacent stomach wall may be seen (fig. 347).

Carcinoma of the stomach and its treatment are discussed on p. 302.

COMPLICATIONS AFTER GASTRIC OPERATIONS

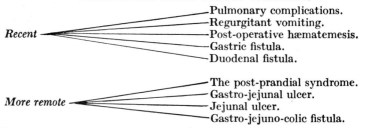

Recent — Pulmonary complications.
Regurgitant vomiting.
Post-operative hæmatemesis.
Gastric fistula.
Duodenal fistula.

More remote — The post-prandial syndrome.
Gastro-jejunal ulcer.
Jejunal ulcer.
Gastro-jejuno-colic fistula.

Pulmonary complications are liable to occur after gastric operations, but the frequency and gravity of post-operative pneumonia has diminished very considerably since the advent of penicillin therapy and modern anæsthesia.

Regurgitant vomiting is more prone to occur after gastro-jejunostomy than gastrectomy. During the first forty-eight hours after a gastric operation there is often a certain amount of regurgitation of bile, no doubt due, in part, to the local paresis set up by the operative trauma. If the stomach is kept empty by a gastric aspiration tube, the regurgitation usually subsides. Should it persist to the third day, it may be due to œdema of the stoma, or to mechanical obstruction. Œdema of the stoma is particularly liable to occur in patients with a low plasma protein ; a plasma infusion is therefore indicated in any case. If the amount of fluid aspirated indicates that there is obstruction at the site of anastomosis, the abdomen must be reopened, and usually the best procedure is anastomosis between the afferent and efferent loops.

Post-operative Hæmatemesis.—The bleeding usually comes from a vessel in the posterior line of suture. This complication has been almost completely circumvented by loosening the clamp, and observing the posterior suture line before completing the anastomosis.

The treatment closely follows that of severe hæmatemesis of the usual variety. It is sometimes necessary to reopen the abdomen to suture the bleeding vessel.

Gastric fistula can occur as the result of a leak in the suture line after partial or total gastrectomy. This serious complication is more liable to occur when the operation was performed for an ulcer which had extensively penetrated the pancreas, or the subject is debilitated. It can also occur after suture of a large perforated peptic ulcer. Jejunostomy under local anæsthesia, combined with suction and drainage of the fistula, sometimes proves effective.

Duodenal fistula is a more frequent, and also a very dangerous, complication. Leakage from the duodenal stump may give rise to diffuse peritonitis, which is often fatal. At other times the leak finds its way to the surface, and leads to the establishment of a duodenal fistula. Leakage from the duodenal stump sometimes follows cases where there has been difficulty in closing the duodenum satisfactorily. More often it is due to obstruction of the afferent jejunal loop by œdema of the gastro-jejunal stoma, or local paresis of the jejunum, and it can be prevented by a trans-nasal intragastric tube passed into the duodenum just before completing the anastomosis, thus keeping the duodenum empty by suction drainage, which is continued for forty-eight hours, or for such a time as it can be shown by the gastric intake and output chart that the stoma is functioning. Once a duodenal fistula has occurred, if the fistula is kept dry by suction drainage applied to the wound, and the skin protected by aluminium paste, or other protective coating, provided the general condition of the patient remains good, the fistula often heals. When the discharge from the fistula is profuse, temporary jejunostomy, by allowing nourishment to be given below the level of the fistula, if performed early will prevent general deterioration and aid in natural closing of the fistula.

The post-prandial syndrome (*syn.* the " dumping " syndrome) is not infrequent, and probably occurs in about 15 per cent. of patients who have been subjected to partial gastrectomy, particularly those in whom a very radical gastrectomy has been performed. The symptoms come on about a month after the operation, and may last for many months. There is a feeling of great distension, sweating, giddiness, and rapid action of the heart after each meal. The attacks last about half an hour, and in many instances are severe enough to necessitate recumbency. The symptoms terminate abruptly after vomiting of a considerable quantity of bile. Owing to the similarity of the attacks to those produced by an overdose of insulin, it was thought that the post-prandial syndrome was due to hypoglycæmia. This has been disproved, because although after gastrectomy there may be periods of hypoglycæmia, as tested by frequent blood-sugar estimations, these periods do not coincide with the post-prandial attacks, nor are they in any way related to the carbohydrate content of the meal. The attacks are almost certainly due to the too early passage of food into the jejunum—hence the term " dumping " syndrome.

The patients with this syndrome are often severely anæmic, and to remedy the anæmia and insist on small, very frequent meals, is all that can be done. It would appear that the condition can be minimised or prevented by reducing the size of the stoma at the time of the gastrectomy or, better, by constructing an inferior valve in addition to the superior valve shown in fig. 332 in the opening between the stomach and the jejunum.

Gastro-jejunal ulcer (*syn.* anastomotic ulcer).—A new ulcer at the site of the anastomosis is the bugbear of gastro-jejunostomy. Gastro-jejunal ulcer is not entirely limited to patients who have had gastro-jejunostomy performed, for it occurs occasionally after partial gastrectomy, and it implies that the operation has not been sufficiently radical.

Anastomotic ulcer occurs most frequently after operations upon cases of duodenal ulcer (fig. 348) with a very high free hydrochloric acid content.

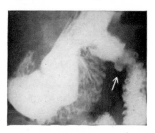

Fig. 348.—Gastro-jejunal ulcer. (*K. J. Yeo.*)

The symptoms, which appear months or sometimes years after the operation, are almost identical with those of duodenal ulcer, except that the patient frequently vomits and pain is referred to the left side. These ulcers sometimes perforate, and indeed are liable to all the complications of a primary peptic ulcer, except carcinoma. When hæmatemesis occurs it is likely to be most serious, for the middle colic artery is liable to be involved.

Treatment of Gastro-jejunal Ulcer.—Relapses are usual after medical treatment. Vagotomy is often successful in this condition. If it fails, and the original operation was a gastro-jejunostomy, the anastomosis can be undone, the ulcer excised, and the anatomy of the parts concerned reconstituted, or a partial gastrectomy can be performed. If the previous operation was partial gastrectomy, a more radical gastrectomy is the only curative measure. When severe hæmatemesis is the reason for the necessity for further operation, and it is found that the hæmorrhage is coming from the middle colic artery, in addition to measures to remedy the gastro-jejunal ulcer, ligation of the middle colic artery may so endanger the vascular supply of the transverse colon that this, too, must be resected.

Jejunal ulcer is another complication of partial gastrectomy performed on patients with a very high acidity. Vagotomy nearly always cures the condition.

Gastro-jejuno-colic fistula is a complication of gastro-jejunal ulcer. The ulcer penetrates and erodes the transverse colon. In addition to the symptoms of anastomotic ulcer, the unfortunate patient is troubled with diarrhœa after every meal, eructates foul gas, and may even vomit fæces. Loss of weight and strength, dehydration, and anæmia complete the picture. The treatment is first to perform colostomy at the hepatic flexure to prevent fæces entering the stomach. After further suitable preparation a second operation to repair the colon and undo the gastro-jejunostomy, combined, in some cases, with partial gastrectomy, has to be undertaken. This is one of the most difficult operations in surgery.

CONDITIONS WHICH MIMIC CHRONIC PEPTIC ULCER

Appendicular dyspepsia is a great imitator of chronic *duodenal* ulcer. Many of the symptoms of appendicular dyspepsia are clearly due to an associated duodenitis, and bleeding from the duodenal mucosa sometimes occurs in these cases. The patient is often cured entirely by the removal of the appendix, which in genuine cases is demonstrably diseased, and often contains pus.

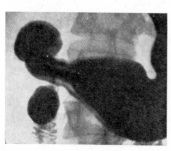

FIG. 349.—Typical duodenal diverticulum.

Duodenal Diverticulum.—The majority of duodenal diverticula occur in the second part of the duodenum and are found in the course of a barium meal (fig. 349). This variety of diverticulum is probably congenital. The sac consists of mucous membrane with a covering of fibrous tissue, the muscular layers of the gut being absent. In more than half the cases the diverticulum is without clinical significance. On the other hand, symptoms closely resembling those of chronic duodenal ulcer or more rarely those of chronic cholecystitis are produced by duodenal diverticula that fail to empty after six hours, or are inflamed. Tenderness to palpation during the radiological examination is therefore of importance. From time to time cases of perforation of a duodenal diverticulum have been reported. A diverticulum of the first part of the duodenum is always acquired as the result of scarring of a duodenal ulcer.

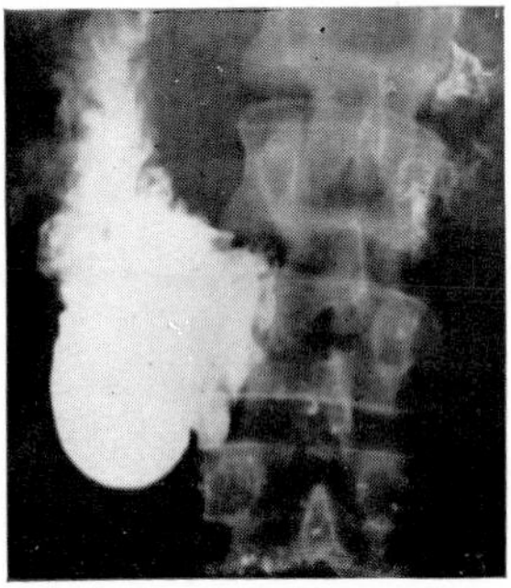

Treatment.—When the diverticulum is producing symptoms, and other relevant lesions have been excluded, excision of the diverticulum (or invagination of it, should it be close to the ampulla of Vater) is indicated.

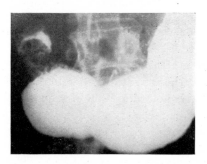

Fig. 350.—Duodenal ileus. Note the abrupt obstruction to the second part of the duodenum.

Chronic duodenal ileus is a rare condition, and the symptoms are akin to those of pyloric stenosis. Women are the usual sufferers. The duodenum is found considerably dilated up to the point where the superior mesenteric vessels cross it (fig. 350).

When the symptoms are persistent, anastomosis of the lowest part of the dilated duodenum to an adjacent loop of jejunum (duodeno-jejunostomy) is the best course (Wilkie), but the results are often disappointing.

Prolapsing Gastric Mucosa.—Hypertrophied gastric mucosa prolapses through the pylorus (fig. 351), thereby causing partial pyloric obstruction. This condition does not give rise to pathognomonic symptoms, but a long history of dyspepsia comparable with that of a pyloric ulcer is usual.

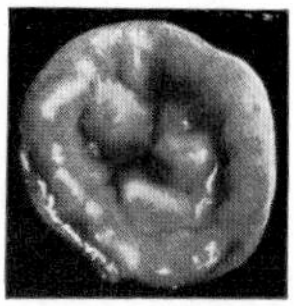

Fig. 351.—Prolapsing gastric mucosa viewed from the duodenal aspect of the pylorus. (*L. H. Appleby.*)

Fig. 352.—Showing the "jockey-cap" deformity. (*L. H. Appleby.*)

Prolapsing gastric mucosa should be suspected when the barium meal displays considerable delay (six hours) in emptying, combined with a "jockey-cap" residue in the duodenal cap (fig. 352), and a display of traceable mucosal patterns as the stomach eventually empties. Partial gastrectomy gives excellent results (Appleby).

Syphilis of the stomach produces thickening of the wall and mucosal ulceration with symptoms and X-ray findings identical with those of peptic ulcer or cancer. The differential diagnosis is particularly difficult because ulcer or cancer of the stomach may be present in a patient with a positive Wassermann reaction (Meyer).

Sir David Wilkie, 1882–1938. Professor of Clinical Surgery, University of Edinburgh.
Lyon H. Appleby, Contemporary. Chief Surgeon, St. Paul's Hospital, Vancouver, British Columbia.
Karl A. Meyer, Contemporary. Senior Surgeon and Medical Superintendent, Cook County Hospital, Chicago.

Gastroptosis often produces symptoms which simulate those of a gastric ulcer. The leading difference in the symptoms of the two conditions is that in gastroptosis periodicity of attacks is usually lacking. The symptoms tend to be present constantly week in and week out ; also the appetite is prone to be poor. The symptoms are inclined to be improved by recumbency and pregnancy. In spite of these differences, it must be admitted that in some cases the symptoms which gastroptosis produces are identical with those of chronic gastric ulcer.

Fig. 353.— Narrow sub-costal angle as found in cases of gas-troptosis.

On Examination.—Gastroptosis should be suspected if the patient has a narrow subcostal angle (fig. 353). In such circumstances Rovsing's sign should be sought. The epigastrium is viewed tangentially. If the beating aorta can be seen to cause epigastric pulsation, the sign is positive. Visible pulsation signifies that the cushion-like structure, the stomach, has slipped down, and has left bare the aorta beneath the abdominal wall.

Fractional test meal usually shows hypochlorhydria. Especially in gastroptotic females, there is sometimes complete absence of free hydrochloric acid.

Barium meal reveals the ptosed state of the stomach. It is not unusual for the lesser curvature to be well below the level of the umbilicus (fig. 354).

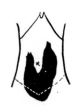

Fig. 354.— Profound gas-troptosis. (*From an X-ray.*)

Treatment.—Physiotherapy and exercises to increase the tone of the abdominal muscles are sometimes beneficial. In older patients a well-fitting abdominal belt is helpful. Fluids should not be taken with meals—small, dry meals, with fluids at least half an hour before, should be the rule. In a few cases, in order to eliminate definitely the possibility of a gastric ulcer or carcinoma, gastroscopy, or even laparotomy must be undertaken.

ACUTE PHLEGMONOUS GASTRITIS (*Syn.* ACUTE SUPPURATIVE CELLULITIS OF THE STOMACH)

Acute phlegmonous gastritis is due to a streptococcal infection of the submucosa of the stomach. This is an extremely rare condition which, as a rule, involves the whole stomach. There is a still rarer variety which is limited to the pyloric region. Most of these cases are diagnosed as perforated peptic ulcer, or acute pancreatitis, and are revealed only when laparotomy has been performed. In the past, acute phlegmonous gastritis

Thorkild Rovsing, 1862–1927. Professor of Surgery, University of Copenhagen

was usually fatal.   The best procedure is to incise the serosal coat, provide drainage, and treat the patient with massive doses of penicillin.

VOLVULUS OF THE STOMACH

Axial rotation of the whole stomach is an exceptional emergency occurring in patients with profound gastroptosis.   The greater curvature is rotated upwards, and both the pyloric and the œsophageal orifices become occluded.   There is acute upper abdominal pain, and regurgitation of everything taken by mouth.   Great abdominal distension is present and a gastric aspiration tube cannot be passed.   On laparotomy the distension is often so great that the organ must be emptied by a trocar and cannula before untwisting can be accomplished.   Before closing the abdomen, the anterior wall of the stomach should be fixed by sutures to the abdominal wall, to prevent recurrence of the volvulus.

GASTRIC TETANY

Gastric tetany, due to alkalæmia, sometimes complicates simple or malignant pyloric obstruction, particularly when there has been long-continued vomiting, or much alkaline medicine has been ingested.   The spasms, which are usually confined to the extremities, are accompanied by dyspnœa and cyanosis.   If the stomach is dilated, it should be emptied and kept empty by aspiration.   Continuous intravenous saline and glucose should be administered without delay.   The blood calcium level must be raised by the administration of calcium (see parathyroid tetany, p. 216).   An acidifying mixture, e.g. ammonium chloride by mouth, is prescribed in addition.

RUPTURE OF THE DUODENUM

TRAUMATIC RUPTURE OF THE DUODENUM is a rare accident, usually the result of a blow on the right flank.   The rupture may be intra- or extra-peritoneal, or both.

Intraperitoneal Rupture.—The tear can usually be sutured.

Extraperitoneal Rupture.—The initial symptoms are often slight, and the condition is overlooked until an abscess forms.   When such an abscess is opened, a duodenal fistula results.

Duodenal Fistula.—The most usual causes are as follows :
1. As a complication of partial gastrectomy.
2. Opening an abscess connected with a perforated duodenal ulcer.
3. Traumatic rupture of the duodenum.
4. As a complication of transduodenal choledochotomy.
5. As a complication of right nephrectomy.

The duodenal contents well up on to the surface, and pancreatic enzymes soon digest and excoriate the skin.   When the fistula discharges copiously, unless measures are taken to prevent it, dehydration will take place rapidly.

Treatment.—Continuous suction is sometimes very successful, for it removes the digestive ferments, and permits the wound to heal.   Especially in traumatic cases, where the deficiency in the wall of the duodenum is considerable, pyloric occlusion combined with gastro-jejunostomy prevents starvation and puts the fistula at rest.

GASTRIC NEOPLASMS

Benign tumours are rare and unimportant.   Myomata, fibromata, and adenomata are found from time to time.   The last particularly sometimes gives rise to intussusception of the stomach.   Diffuse polyposis of the gastric mucosa sometimes occurs ; it is usually mistaken for carcinoma until a histological examination has been made.   Angiomata and lipomata of the stomach are pathological curiosities.

CARCINOMA OF THE STOMACH

Carcinoma of the first part of the duodenum is almost unknown : carcinoma of the stomach is one of the captains of the men of death. Twelve thousand persons die annually from this disease in England and Wales, and 38,000 in the United States of America (Payne). While from youth to senility no age is exempt, it will be seen from the graph (fig. 355) that the highest incidence is between forty and sixty. Males are somewhat more frequently attacked than females.

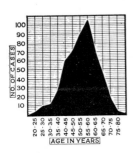

FIG. 355.—Age-incidence of cancer of the stomach. Compiled by Payne from 506 cases occurring at St. Bartholomew's Hospital.

Ætiology.—Certain clinical facts throw some light upon the frequency with which the stomach is attacked. As gastric cancer does not occur in animals, and as negroes are almost exempt, it is reasonable to argue that highly civilised man, by pouring hot, semi-solid, and fluid nourishment into the stomach, is subjecting his gastric mucosa to a form of repeated irritation which predisposes to malignancy. There is some evidence to support the belief that carcinoma ventriculi occurs more frequently in patients suffering from pernicious anæmia, a condition in which atrophic gastritis is nearly always found.

PATHOLOGY.—The growth originates much more frequently in the distal third of the stomach ; least often in the proximal third (fig. 356).

Microscopically.—The growth is usually columnar-celled, but cubical, and even squamous-

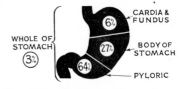

FIG. 356.—Incidence of carcinoma in various portions of the stomach.

celled neoplasms arise near the œsophageal orifice, although the last type probably arise in the œsophagus.

Macroscopically. — The following is Borrmann's classification :

Type 1.—A cauliflower-like growth with sharply defined edges. Its surface is nodular (fig. 357), later it ulcerates.

Type 2.—An ulcer with an irregular base and an in-

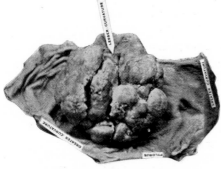

FIG. 357.—Carcinoma of the stomach ; type 1. Specimen removed by partial gastrectomy.

Reginald Theodore Payne, Contemporary. Surgical Assistant, British Post-graduate Medical School, London.
Robert Borrmann, Contemporary. Director of the Krakenanstadt Pathological Institute, Bremen.

durated edge. Small irregular superficial ulcers are sometimes present on the edge.

Type 3.—Also an ulcer, but one edge of the ulcer is shallow. Diffuse nodular infiltration extends outwards from this shallow area.

Type 4.—Diffuse infiltrating carcinoma. It has no definite edge. The infiltrated area may or may not have ulcers on its surface. This is the commonest type. When the whole stomach is involved it is known as the leather-bottle stomach (see p. 307).

The Spread of Gastric Cancer.— No better illustration of the various modes by which carcinoma spreads can be taken than the case of the stomach.

(*a*) *Direct Spread.* — As the growth enlarges, it tends to invade neighbouring viscera. The pancreas, transverse colon, mesocolon, œsophagus, or liver may be involved.

(*b*) *Lymphatic Spread* (fig. 358) :

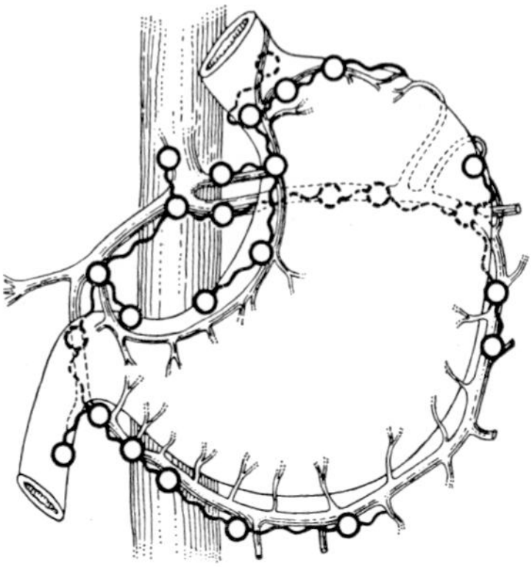

1. *By Emboli.*—Small clumps of carcinoma cells are swept along the lymphatic vessels, to become arrested in the neighbouring lymph nodes.

Fig. 358.—The distribution of the regional lymph nodes of the stomach. Note their relationship to the arteries. (*After Taylor and Nathanson.*)

2. *By Permeation.*—Carcinoma cells grow along the lumina of the lymphatic vessels. At operation lymphatic vessels, enlarged and white from contained neoplasm, can sometimes be demonstrated.

(*c*) *Spread by the Blood-stream.*—Minute portions of the growth are carried by the venous system to the liver and other more distant organs.

(*d*) *Transcolomic Implantation.*—Carcinoma cells sometimes fall from the stomach into the peritoneal cavity. They gravitate to the pelvis, where secondary tumours palpable on rectal examination may develop. On occasions, in the female, they alight upon the ovaries, giving rise to **Krukenberg's tumours** (fig. 359), which are sometimes an occasion for diagnostic confusion. These tumours are premenopausal, as after the climacteric the ovaries atrophy. It may well be that in the case of Krukenberg's tumours the spread of carcinoma from the stomach is not

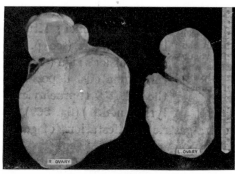

Fig. 359.—Krukenberg's tumours from a woman of thirty-seven.

by transcolomic implantation, but by lymphatic spread. Indeed, this is the view of most gynæcologists at the present time.

Friedrich Krukenberg, Contemporary. Ophthalmologist, of Halle. Wrote a classical thesis on malignant tumours of the ovary at the age of twenty-four.

CLINICAL FEATURES

Six clinical types are met with in practice :

(1) *Acute Onset.*—In 10 per cent. of cases the onset of symptoms is abrupt, being ushered in with a short history of acute indigestion, sometimes complicated by hæmatemesis, or even perforation. A wise clinician assumes that every patient over the age of forty-five complaining of rapidly oncoming dyspepsia is suffering from carcinoma of the stomach, until it has been definitely proved otherwise.

(2) *Insidious Onset.*—The patient feels tired and weak. There is probably some epigastric discomfort, but pain is not a leading symptom. Anorexia, especially for meat, is a cardinal symptom in these cases. This type simulates closely (*a*) pernicious anæmia : carcinoma of the stomach is frequently mistaken for pernicious anæmia, and vice versa. (*b*) On-coming uræmia, such as may be occasioned in cases of prostatic ob-struction.

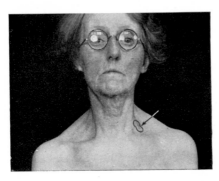

FIG. 360.—Troisier's sign found in the course of a routine examination for vague dyspepsia of recent origin. In this case there was a visible as well as a palpable mass of lymph nodes in the left supra-clavicular fossa.

(3) *Latent Type.* — The symptoms and signs are extra-gastric, i.e. they are not at first sight referable to the stomach. Such mani-festations as painless jaundice due to secondary deposits at the hilum of the liver ; ascites from carcino-matosis peritonei ; Kruken-berg's tumours (see p. 303) and Troisier's sign (enlarged carcinomatous deposits in the left supraclavicular lymph nodes) (fig. 360), are examples of the diverse extra-gastric manifestations of gastric carcinoma.

(4) *Secondary to a Chronic Gastric Ulcer.*—After years of typical attacks of symptoms of chronic gastric ulcer the symptoms change. The clinical features of this variety have been discussed on p. 295.

(5) *Carcinoma of the cardiac end of the stomach* often closely

Charles E. Troisier, 1844–1919. Professor of Pathology, Paris.

simulates œsophageal obstruction, from which it must be differentiated.

(6) *Carcinoma of the Pylorus.*—The symptoms are identical with those of simple pyloric stenosis. The features favouring a malignant origin of the stenosis are a comparatively short history in a patient past the meridian of life.

INVESTIGATION OF A SUSPECTED CASE

In the more universal adoption of all the following methods of examination lies the hope of earlier diagnosis.

X-ray frequently reveals a character- istic deformity of the stomach (fig. 362). Only advanced cases give typical radiographic appearances.

Test Meal.—Blood is often present in the aspirated gastric contents. Achlorhydria is the rule in advanced

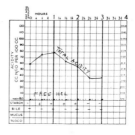

Fig. 361. — Fractional test meal in a case of carci- noma of the stomach.

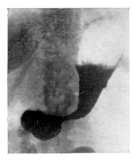

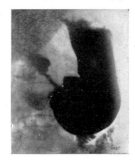

A   B

Fig. 362.—Typical radiographic appearances in carcinoma of the stomach, (A) of the body of the stomach, (B) of the pyloric antrum.
(*Carl Krebs, Aarhus, Denmark.*)

cases (fig. 361). A low acidity is suggestive but not confirmatory evidence of a gastric neoplasm.

Gastroscopy.—If the tumour can be visualised, its character- istics are usually obvious. Its nodularity, the presence of several irregular superficial ulcers, the irregular multicoloured ulcer base, the " frozen " appearance of the adjacent mucosa all point to its nature. In cases of doubt a second examination after two weeks' medical treatment will show it has failed to respond (Tanner).

TREATMENT

There is no curative treatment except subtotal or total gastrectomy, and this is possibly curative only when the growth has not grossly infiltrated neighbouring organs and there are no obvious secondary deposits beyond those in the immediate vicinity of the gastric wall.

Subtotal gastrectomy for cancer differs from subtotal gastrectomy for peptic ulcer in the following particulars: the greater and lesser omenta are removed entirely. The lymph nodes round the cardiac orifice and all the nodes round the upper lesser curvature of the stomach are stripped downwards and removed with the growth. The transection of stomach must be at least $1\frac{1}{2}$ inches (3·75 cm.) above the palpable limit of the growth. When neighbouring organs, e.g. the liver, colon, pancreas, are invaded locally, the involved part must be resected with the stomach.

Total gastrectomy is obviously a formidable undertaking, but clearly, when successful, it offers a greater prospect of a cure, particularly when the growth is situated in the upper half of the stomach. Technical difficulties are being surmounted, and the thoraco-abdominal approach (see fig. 363), which gives good

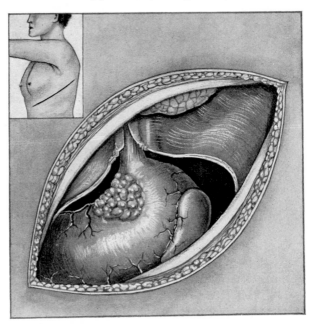

FIG. 363.—The thoraco-abdominal approach to the stomach gives good access to the organ for total gastrectomy. (*After F. R. Harper.*)

access to the lower end of the œsophagus as well as to the stomach, is gaining in popularity as the best route for total gastrectomy.

The results of treatment of carcinoma of the stomach are depressing. Even in cases apparently suitable for radical gastrectomy, recurrence after several months or years is common. The occasional patient who is alive and well five years after subtotal or total gastrectomy makes perseverance with total gastrectomy the only form of curative treatment worth while.

Experience shows that in cases of mobile (as opposed to fixed) but inoperable carcinoma of the stomach partial gastrectomy often brings relief, and life in comparative comfort may be appreciably prolonged.

THORACO-ABDOMINAL APPROACH TO THE STOMACH AND LOWER ŒSOPHAGUS

Intratracheal anæsthesia is employed. The patient is placed on the operating table with the left side of the thorax uppermost in the true lateral position. The incision follows the ninth rib, and extends from the angle of that rib to the lateral border of the left rectus abdominis. The ninth rib is excised within the limits of the incision, and the thorax entered through the bed of the rib. The pulmonary ligament is divided and the lung falls away from the diaphragm. The incision is then carried farther forward for about 2 inches (5 cm.), and the peritoneal cavity is opened. Starting anteriorly, the diaphragm is completely split to the œsophageal hiatus. Rib spreaders having been inserted, remarkable exposure and access is obtained (fig. 363).

LEATHER-BOTTLE STOMACH (*Syn.* LINITIS PLASTICA : GASTRIC FIBROMATOSIS)

There is a generalised and localised form of leather-bottle stomach.

When localised, it is the pyloric antrum which is mainly involved. The stomach wall is enormously thickened (fig. 364),

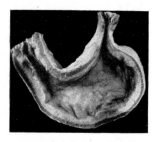

FIG. 364. — Leather-bottle stomach, showing the enormous thickening of the stomach wall.

and feels, as its name implies, like leather. The mucosa in specimens we have examined appears quite normal. Microscopically there is an enormous overgrowth of fibrous tissue in the subserosa and submucosa, which sometimes spreads between the muscle fibres and strangulates them. The blood-vessels show evidence of endarteritis. It is usually difficult or impossible to find any evidence of carcinoma, even in serial sections, but secondaries are sometimes to be found in the regional lymph nodes. While the consensus of opinion favours the view that leather-bottle stomach is always an atrophic scirrhus carcinoma, some consider that the condition is due to syphilis, or other chronic inflammations.

The symptoms are those of pyloric obstruction, but the small capacity of the stomach on X-ray examination makes the diagnosis tolerably certain.

Treatment.—In the localised variety, partial gastrectomy, and in the diffuse, total gastrectomy, offer hope of prolonging life, and even of a cure, but recurrence is unfortunately only too common.

SARCOMA OF THE STOMACH

Sarcoma of the stomach is very rare, and is usually mistaken for carcinoma until a histological examination has been made.

There are three main varieties :

1. Round or spindle-celled, from the submucosa.
2. Fibro-sarcoma, from the subserosa.
3. Lympho-sarcoma.

The prognosis is not always as hopeless as one might expect. Indeed, there are several reported cases of cures after partial gastrectomy. Type 2 is a comparatively benign growth, and sometimes gives rise to a tumour of immense size, which is mistaken for an ovarian cyst.

DUODENAL NEOPLASMS

are exceedingly uncommon. Adenomatous polyps and adenomyomata have been reported from time to time as a cause of severe melæna. Carcinoma of the first part of the duodenum, where ulceration is so common, never occurs. Carcinoma of the second part of the duodenum has been described, but most of these cases appear to arise in the ampulla of Vater (see p. 374).

CHAPTER XVII
THE SPLEEN AND THE LIVER
THE SPLEEN

MOVABLE SPLEEN (*Syn.* WANDERING SPLEEN)

Curiously, in general visceroptosis the spleen is the one abdominal organ which maintains its correct anatomical position. Movable spleen is a congenital abnormality which occurs more often in women. The condition is of great rarity, and the diagnosis is seldom made correctly in the first instance. Movable spleen does not become grossly ptosed because the organ is supported by the phrenico-colic ligament (*syn.* sustentaculum lienis). Movable spleen is sometimes associated with postural albuminuria owing to pressure on the left renal vein and temporary congestion of the kidney.

Torsion of the splenic pedicle sometimes occurs in the wandering organ. The torsion may be acute or chronic, acute cases presenting the symptoms of an intra-abdominal catastrophe. Chronic torsion may result in atrophy of the spleen, and after a period of indefinite abdominal discomfort all symptoms abate.

Treatment.—A movable spleen giving rise to symptoms should be removed.

RUPTURE OF THE SPLEEN

usually occurs as the result of a traffic or industrial accident of the "crushing" or "run-over" type. Blows on the abdomen and falls on to a projecting object are other sources of the violence. Much more rarely, the rupture is due to a direct wound, viz. a stab or bullet wound, or to a fractured rib driven inwards and penetrating the diaphragm. Several cases of spontaneous rupture of a normal spleen have been reported, but in all probability in these there has been an accident which has been forgotten or suppressed by the patient.

Cases of ruptured spleen may be divided into three groups :

1. **The Patient Succumbs Rapidly, Never Rallying from the Initial Shock.**—This type is very rare in temperate climates ; only complete avulsion of the spleen from its pedicle gives rise to the symptoms which characterise this group. In countries where malaria is rife, splenic rupture is often rapidly fatal, and advantage has been taken of this knowledge by murderers in

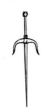

FIG. 365.
—A larang,
which, being
interpreted,
means " for-
bidden."

China, who achieve their end by digging the victim beneath the left ribs with an implement known as a larang (fig. 365).

2. **Initial Shock ;   Recovery from Shock ;   Signs of a Ruptured Spleen.**—This is the usual type seen in surgical practice. After the initial shock has passed off, there are signs which point to an intra-abdominal disaster, and by correlating these signs it is often possible to arrive at a correct pre-operative diagnosis.

General signs of internal hæmorrhage are incon-stant.   Perhaps the most helpful is increasing pallor and a rising pulse-rate.

Local Signs.—(*a*) Abdominal rigidity is present in more than 50 per cent. of cases ; it is most pronounced in the left upper quadrant.

(*b*) Local tenderness is found constantly.

(*c*) Shifting dullness in the flanks is often present.

Ballance's sign is said to be pathognomonic of splenic rupture.   There is a dull note in both flanks, but on the right side it can be made to shift, whereas on the left it is constant.   The interpretation is that there is blood in the peritoneal cavity, but the blood in the neighbourhood of the lacerated spleen has coagulated.

(*d*) Abdominal distension commences about three hours after the accident, and is due to paralytic ileus.

(*e*) Kehr's sign is pain referred to the left shoulder.   There may be hyperæsthesia in this area.   This sign is present very often if especially sought.

3. **The Delayed Type of Case.**—After the initial shock has passed off, the symptoms of a *serious* intra-abdominal catas-trophe are postponed for a variable period up to fifteen days, or even more.

Delay of serious intraperitoneal bleeding is explained in one of the following ways :
(*a*) The great omentum, performing its well-known constabulary duties, shuts off that portion of the general peritoneal cavity in the immediate vicinity of the bleeding.
(*b*) A subcapsular hæmatoma forms and later bursts.
(*c*) Blood-clot temporarily sealing the rent becomes digested by escaping ferments due to injury to the tail of the pancreas.

Treatment of Rupture of the Spleen.—Immediate laparotomy and splenectomy is the only reliable course.   Blood is mopped up and the abdomen closed completely.   When circumstances

Sir Charles Ballance, 1856–1936.   Surgeon, St. Thomas's Hospital, London.
Hans Kehr, 1862–1916.   Surgeon, Halberstädt, later Berlin.   He died of septicæmia con-tracted during his work.

permit, blood transfusions should be given before, during, and after the operation. In the absence of stored blood, auto-transfusion at the time of the operation is indicated.

Auto-transfusion.—Extravasated blood is collected from the peritoneal cavity by means of a suction apparatus. After mixing it with 3·8 per cent. sodium citrate solution, 2 ounces (60 ml.) in 1 pint of blood (570 ml.), it is strained through several layers of sterile gauze and gravitated into a vein.

The results of timely operation for traumatic rupture of the spleen are excellent.

When the organ is damaged by a stab wound or missile penetrating the left plural cavity, access to the spleen is best obtained by excising the thoracic and diaphragmatic wounds, and enlarging the opening in the diaphragm.

Post-operative Complications.—From time to time the following complications occur after splenectomy for rupture of the spleen.

Acute dilatation of the stomach.

Left pleural effusion is due, no doubt, to bruising of the diaphragm at the time of the accident or to trauma during splenectomy.

Peritoneal effusion is due to a wound of the tail of the pancreas. The effusion lasts three or four weeks, and usually lessens gradually in amount. It is accompanied by slight pyrexia.

Persistent hiccough is the result of irritation of branches of the left phrenic nerve upon the under-surface of the left side of the diaphragm.

"Burst" abdomen is liable to occur where the tail of the pancreas has been wounded, for escaping ferments digest the catgut in the abdominal wound. In order to forestall this complication, wire sutures should be employed.

Hæmatemesis from temporary congestion of the fundus of the stomach, due to ligation of the vasa brevia.

RUPTURE OF A MALARIAL SPLEEN

As has been mentioned, in tropical countries this is a frequent catastrophe. The delayed type of rupture (following a trivial injury) is also very common, and the patient is admitted with a perisplenic hæmatoma (fig. 366). If splenectomy can be per-formed before the hæmatoma bursts into the general peritoneal cavity, the prognosis is less grave.

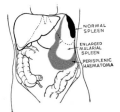

The operation is considerably more difficult than in the case of a ruptured normal spleen. Surgeons with tropical experience have surmounted these difficulties by ligating the splenic vessels as they run along the superior border of the body of the pancreas, before disturbing the hæmatoma (Andreasen).

Fig. 366.—Normal spleen, malarial spleen, perisplenic hæmatoma. Note that the splenic contour is lost when the capsule has ruptured.

Anthony Turner Andreasen, Contemporary. Formerly Professor of Surgery, University of Calcutta.

ENLARGEMENTS OF THE SPLEEN

The spleen is a meeting-place of medicine and surgery. The following is a useful table of the causes of enlargement of the organ. Those conditions of particular surgical importance will be considered in detail.

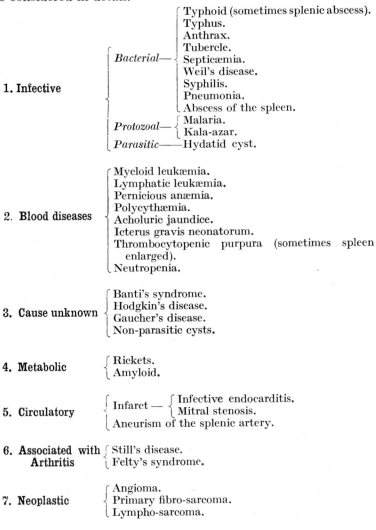

1. Infective
- *Bacterial*—
  - Typhoid (sometimes splenic abscess).
  - Typhus.
  - Anthrax.
  - Tubercle.
  - Septicæmia.
  - Weil's disease.
  - Syphilis.
  - Pneumonia.
  - Abscess of the spleen.
- *Protozoal*—
  - Malaria.
  - Kala-azar.
- *Parasitic*——Hydatid cyst.

2. Blood diseases
- Myeloid leukæmia.
- Lymphatic leukæmia.
- Pernicious anæmia.
- Polycythæmia.
- Acholuric jaundice.
- Icterus gravis neonatorum.
- Thrombocytopenic purpura (sometimes spleen enlarged).
- Neutropenia.

3. Cause unknown
- Banti's syndrome.
- Hodgkin's disease.
- Gaucher's disease.
- Non-parasitic cysts.

4. Metabolic
- Rickets.
- Amyloid.

5. Circulatory
- Infarct —
  - Infective endocarditis.
  - Mitral stenosis.
- Aneurism of the splenic artery.

6. Associated with Arthritis
- Still's disease.
- Felty's syndrome.

7. Neoplastic
- Angioma.
- Primary fibro-sarcoma.
- Lympho-sarcoma.

ANEURISM OF THE SPLENIC ARTERY

Of 183 consecutive aneurisms found in the course of necropsies at the Jena Pathological Institute, nine were of the splenic artery. The symptoms

Adolph Weil, 1848–1916.   Director of the Medical Clinic, Dorpat, Esthonia.   Developed laryngeal tuberculosis and subsequently practised at various spas.
Thomas Hodgkin, 1798–1866.   Curator of the Museum to Guy's Hospital, London
Sir Frederick Still, 1865–1941.   Physician, Hospital for Sick Children, London
A. R. Felty, Contemporary.   American Physician.

of the condition are vague. In reported cases the spleen has been found more or less enlarged. Rupture of a splenic aneurism usually presents symptoms similar to those of spontaneous rupture of the spleen. In such a case St. Leger Brockman heard a bruit over the left hypochondrium, and was thereby enabled to make a correct pre-operative diagnosis. Splenectomy, together with excision of that part of the artery containing the aneurismal sac, has been performed successfully.

INFARCTION OF THE SPLEEN (Fig. 367)

The patient, who is often suffering from subacute infective endocarditis or auricular fibrillation, is seized with agonising pain in the left hypochondrium. In a case seen by us, symptoms mimicked those of a perforated gastric ulcer, but the heart lesion helps the clinician to elucidate the diagnosis. When the embolus is aseptic the symptoms pass off in a few days.

ABSCESS OF THE SPLEEN

If a splenic embolus is infected, and the primary condition does not prove fatal, a splenic abscess may be expected to follow. Other sources of metastatic abscesses of the spleen are typhoid fever, osteomyelitis, otitis media, and puerperal fever. An abscess of the spleen can also occur by direct extension of infection from a diverticulitis or carcinoma of the splenic flexure of the colon. An abscess in the upper pole of the spleen may rupture and form a subdiaphragmatic abscess. If the abscess is in the lower pole, rupture of it results in diffuse peritonitis.

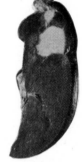

Fig. 367.— Infarct of the spleen.

Treatment.—As a rule, owing to dense adhesions, drainage of the abscess is the only course. Very rarely, it is possible to perform splenectomy with the abscess *in situ*.

CYSTS

Cysts of the spleen are very rare. There are several varieties.

1. *Single, usually unilocular, non-parasitic cysts* are of two varieties : (a) *True cysts*, including dermoids and those lined by epithelium. (b) *False cysts*, which often reach a large size and contain blood-stained fluid and often cholesterol crystals. They tend to be situated at one or other pole of the spleen. They are supposed to be due to ancient subcapsular hæmorrhage or degeneration of an infarcted area.

2. *Small multiple cysts* are sometimes encountered at necropsy, and occasionally at operation. They have no clinical significance.

3. *Polycystic Spleen.*—Polycystic disease is sometimes confined to the spleen, but is more often associated with congenital cystic kidneys and liver. Occasionally the pancreas is similarly affected.

4. *Hydatid Cyst of the Spleen.*—A number of cases of hydatid cyst of the spleen have been reported, and in this situation hydatid cysts are readily removed with the whole spleen.

ACHOLURIC JAUNDICE (Syn. SPHEROCYTOSIS)

Acholuric jaundice is jaundice without bile in the urine. Spherocytosis is a term which gives a clue to the underlying pathology. The erythrocytes, instead of being biconcave, are

R. St. Leger Brockman, Contemporary. Professor of Surgery, University of Sheffield.

s.p.—20

biconvex. Not all of them are so shaped, but a proportion are, according to the severity of the condition. Biconvex (spheroidal) red cells burst more easily than normal red cells ; indeed, the biconvexity may be said to be the first stage of hæmolysis. There are two pathognomonic laboratory tests for this condition :

The Fragility Test.—There is an increased fragility of the red cells. Normally, erythrocytes begin to hæmolyse in 0·47 per cent. of saline. In this condition hæmolysis occurs in 0·6 per cent., or even in solutions which more nearly approximate physiological saline.

The Reticulocyte Count.—To compensate for the loss of erythrocytes by hæmolysis, the bone marrow discharges into the circulation immature red cells, which differ from the adult cells by possessing a reticulum. This cannot be seen in the usual blood films, but can be demonstrated readily by vital stains. After a hæmolytic crisis of acholuric jaundice (see below), the reticulocyte count is very much increased from the normal, very low, figure to as much as 85 per cent.

There are two forms of the disease—congenital and acquired.

Congenital acholuric jaundice can appear in either sex, and either the father or the mother can transmit it, there being a familial history of similar jaundice in the parent concerned. Sometimes the patient is born jaundiced, or becomes so early in life. In some families the disease is accompanied by severe crises of red blood-cell destruction ; thus, with the onset of a crisis, an erythrocyte count may fall from 4½ millions to 1½ millions in less than a week. These crises may be so severe as to cause death in infancy. More usually the jaundice, although variable, is very mild, and may not appear until adolescent or even adult life. In adult cases there is often a history of attacks of gall-stone colic ; indeed, in 50 per cent. of cases the patient has pigment stones in the gall-bladder.

On Examination.—The spleen is large, weighing 2 to 3 lb., and is therefore easily palpable in thin subjects. The blood examination shows secondary anæmia, and the characteristic fragility test and the increased reticulocyte count given above.

Treatment.—If the patient is so anæmic as to render blood transfusion advisable, this must be carried out with great caution, because patients with acholuric jaundice tend to hæmolyse donor blood. Therefore, after careful cross-matching, a small transfusion (not more than half a pint) is given, and if there is no untoward reaction, a similar transfusion is repeated on the following day. Provided that gall-stones, if present, receive appropriate treatment, splenectomy will render the patient symptom-free. Splenectomy and cholecystectomy performed at the same time is a big undertaking, and in frail subjects it is sometimes advisable to remove the spleen and the diseased gall-bladder separately, with an interval of a few weeks between the operations.

After splenectomy the jaundice disappears, but the tendency to spontaneous hæmolysis persists ; it has been demonstrated twenty-five years after removal of the spleen.

From time to time cases are encountered when a patient suffering from acholuric jaundice is admitted with obstructive jaundice due to pigment stones in the bile duct. In such cases the stones in the common bile duct must be removed by chole-dochotomy, and the treatment of the acholuric jaundice deferred until some time later, when full recovery from the obstructive jaundice has occurred.

Acquired acholuric jaundice is less common than the foregoing. The onset is usually in the third decade. Females are six times more often affected than males. The hæmolytic crises are very severe, and the result-ing anæmia profound. In the acquired form of this disease hæmolysis of donor blood occurs, however carefully cross-matching is performed. Blood transfusion, therefore, is contraindicated in these cases, but of course plasma can be administered, if necessary, during and after splenectomy. Because of the impossibility of utilizing blood transfusion, the results of treatment are not so satisfactory as those of the congenital form of the disease.

PURPURA

Purpura is a condition of great importance to the surgeon. It forcibly intrudes into his diagnostic arena ; on rare occasions it is the cause of an intussusception, but more frequently sub-serosal hæmorrhages produce signs similar to those of acute intestinal obstruction ; it may give rise to profound hæmaturia or alarming hæmorrhage from a mucous lining of the body, e.g. epistaxis, hæmatemesis, melæna or, in the case of young females (in whom the condition is particularly common), menorrhagia so severe as to render the patient in danger of exsanguination. It is, therefore, a condition which frequently calls for blood trans-fusion, and certain carefully selected cases are benefited by splenectomy.

During the attacks there are small petechial hæmorrhages into the skin. Sometimes these are numerous, and form ecchymoses (fig. 368).

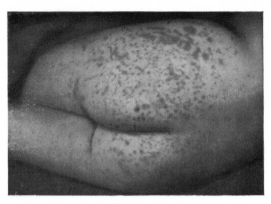

FIG. 368.—Purpura. *Dr. W. H. Cant.*)

Thrombocytopenic Purpura.—Before the age of puberty this disease is divided evenly between the sexes, but over that age there is a preponderance of five females to one male (Evans). In less than 50 per cent. of cases the spleen is palpably enlarged. In addition to hæmorrhages into the skin and from mucous membranes, there is a greatly reduced blood-platelet count (the normal blood-platelet count is 250,000 to 400,000 per cu. mm.). In some cases the platelet count is reduced to zero. The coagulation time of the blood is normal, but the clot fails to contract, and, consequently, the bleeding time is lengthened. When cutaneous hæmorrhages are not much in evidence, the fragility of cutaneous capillaries may be rendered apparent by the tourniquet test. The cuff of a sphygmomanometer is applied to the upper arm, and inflated to just below the systolic blood-pressure, thus causing venous congestion. Within a quarter of an hour petechial hæmorrhages occur in the skin both under and distal to the constricting agent.

Treatment.—While due attention should be directed to eradicating demonstrable foci of infection and, in necessary cases, to maintaining a safe hæmoglobin level in patients who are losing blood, in spite of the fact that the spleen is not necessarily enlarged, splenectomy is the only measure which offers some prospect of a cure. At operation the spleen is found

Sir Horace Evans, Contemporary. Physician, London Hospital.
Paul Kaznelson, Contemporary, of Prague. Performed the first successful splenectomy for thrombocytopenic purpura in 1916.

to be free from adhesions, and therefore easy to remove. Even in cases where hæmorrhage is otherwise uncontrollable, splenectomy sometimes has a dramatic effect. The procedure is empirical. A number of permanently successful cases following splenectomy have been reported. Late relapses are fairly numerous, and are more common in females. While this sex disparity remains unexplained, it has been suggested that the hypertrophy of an accessory spleen accounts for the purely temporary nature of the benefit which accrues in some cases.

NEUTROPENIA

Primary neutropenia is a rare condition occurring most often in women between the ages of thirty and sixty. It is associated with chronic ill-health, including recurrent oral and skin infections. The spleen is usually moderately, sometimes greatly, enlarged. The blood-count shows persistent leukopenia, varying between 1,000 and 2,000 per cu. mm., with less than 20 per cent. of neutrophils. Bone-marrow biopsy reveals increased cellularity and granular cells predominate. Splenectomy is often curative, and after its performance the white-cell count becomes normal.

Secondary neutropenia is sometimes associated with Felty's syndrome, and, if so, splenectomy may improve the general health, but it has no effect on the arthritis.

LYMPHATIC LEUKÆMIA

is of surgical importance in the differential diagnosis of enlarged lymph nodes and splenic enlargement. The diagnosis is made by an examination of the blood. The only treatment (and this is palliative) is deep X-ray therapy. In the past, splenectomy was tried for this condition, and was found to be useless. Recently it has been suggested that splenectomy is helpful to those undergoing deep X-ray therapy, because after splenectomy the patient is able to retain red-blood cells given by transfusion, which otherwise would be destroyed in the spleen. In this condition both the liver and the spleen are greatly enlarged (fig. 369).

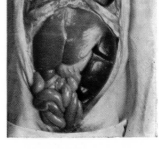

Fig. 369.—Leukæmia. Showing the enlarged liver and spleen as displayed at necropsy.

GAUCHER'S DISEASE

is characterised by enormous enlargement of the spleen, which may weigh 8 or 9 lb. The pathogenesis of the disease is uncertain. The hypothesis that it is a primary tumour of the spleen has been abandoned. It is generally classed as a disorder of lipoid storage. In the majority of cases the splenic enlargement begins in early childhood, usually before the age of twelve, although the patient rarely seeks advice before adult life. Until the splenic enlargement becomes massive the symptoms are few. There is slight anæmia of the chlorotic type, and the patient usually presents a brownish-yellow discoloration of the skin of the hands and face ; this discoloration is due to a deposit of hæmosiderin. A curious conjunctival thickening is a characteristic feature which helps to clinch the clinical

Phillipe Charles Ernst Gaucher, 1854–1918. Physician to St. Louis Hospital, Paris.

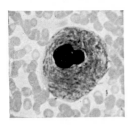

Fig. 370. — Typical Gaucher's cell from bone marrow obtained by sternal puncture.

(*M. L. Thomson.*)

diagnosis. Jewesses appear to be more prone to this disease than the rest of humanity. The diagnosis can be confirmed by sternal puncture (fig. 370). When the disease appears early in life, extensive skeletal changes, including coxa vara, kyphosis, pathological fractures, and dwarfism, are liable to occur.

Treatment.—Splenectomy rids the patient of a large abdominal swelling, but the operation is difficult because of perisplenitis and friability of the splenic pulp. The end results of this, the only treatment, are not encouraging, for the patients seldom survive more than two years. The cause of death is usually intercurrent infection, often tuberculosis.

NEOPLASMS

New-growths of the spleen are strikingly uncommon. Of the benign tumours, cavernous hæmangiomata and lymphangiomata have been encountered. Of the malignant, a few examples of primary fibro-sarcoma have been described. Lymphosarcoma is somewhat more common. Metastases of carcinoma in the spleen are extremely rare.

PORTAL HYPERTENSION

Largely due to the work of Whipple, Banti's disease (splenic anæmia), Egyptian splenomegaly, and the common condition of atrophic cirrhosis of the liver are now included under one heading —portal hypertension.

The normal pressure in the portal vein and its main tributaries is never more than 10 mm. of water ; in portal hypertension it rises to as much as 500 mm. of water. The portal venous pressure is measured by inserting a needle into the vein at operation.

Portal hypertension may be intra- or extrahepatic.

Intrahepatic hypertension is caused by cirrhosis of the liver. Due to the fibrosis around the intrahepatic portal vessels, less and less of the portal blood can traverse the liver substance ; consequently intravenous portal pressure rises, and the collateral circulation between the portal and the systemic venous systems opens up.

Extrahepatic Hypertension.—The obstruction occurs in various parts of the portal tree. This may be due to :

1. (*a*) Congenital stricture of the portal fissure, consequent upon the over-active closure of the ductus venosus and the umbilical vein.

(*b*) Congenital malformations of the portal vein.

Allen Oldfather Whipple, Contemporary. Professor of Surgery, Columbia University. New York City.
Guido Banti, 1852–1925. Professor of Pathology, University of Florence.

ANASTOMOSES BETWEEN THE PORTAL AND SYSTEMIC VENOUS SYSTEMS

	Site of Anastomosis	Portal Vessels	Systemic Vessels	Signs and Symptoms
1	Plexus around lower end of œsophagus.	Œsophageal branches of left gastric vein.	Lower systemic œsophageal veins.	Hæmatemesis.
2	Plexuses around lower third of rectum and anal canal.	Superior hæmorrhoidal vein.	Middle and inferior hæmorrhoidal veins.	Bleeding internal hæmorrhoids.
3	Around umbilicus.	Para-umbilical veins (run along the round ligament of the liver).	Superficial veins of the anterior abdominal wall.	Caput Medusæ.
4	At the upper pole of an enlarged spleen (becoming adherent to the diaphragm).	New accessory blood-vessels.	Diaphragmatic veins.	None.
5	Between bare area of liver and diaphragm.	Veins in liver substance.	Diaphragmatic veins.	None.
6	Extraperitoneal fat.	Veins of ascending and descending colon.	Inferior phrenic, renal, and lumbar veins.	None.
7	Liver—fissure for ligamentum venosum.	(Very rarely.) Patent ductus venosus joining left branch of portal vein with inferior vena cava.		None.

2. Thrombosis of the splenic vein, one of the other large tributaries of the portal vein, or the portal vein itself. Sometimes thrombosis of the splenic vein is due to fibrosis following chronic pancreatitis, and bilharzial infestation of the head of the pancreas, and consequent fibrosis, probably accounts for Egyptian splenomegaly.

3. Compression of the portal trunk by enlarged lymph nodes, neoplasms, or a cyst (rare).

In congenital extrahepatic hypertension small veins in the lesser omentum dilate, and carry the blood to the portal fissure. This may be so exaggerated as to appear at operation as a cavernous hæmangioma. In other varieties of Banti's syndrome, as time goes on, the anastomotic channels set out in the above table become increasingly involved.

Clinical Features.—Atrophic Cirrhosis of the Liver.—It is a mistake to regard the condition as necessarily confined to alcoholic subjects. The disease progresses through three stages :

First Stage.—The liver hypertrophies. The spleen may be slightly enlarged.

Second Stage.—The liver contracts and becomes lobulated (hob-nail). The spleen usually does not greatly enlarge.

Third Stage.—Progressive ascites occurs (fig. 371). There

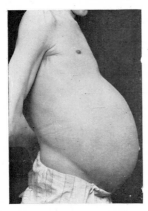

may be hæmatemesis from œsophageal varices and bleeding from associated hæmorrhoids. Sometimes, in advanced cases, the veins surrounding the umbilicus enlarge, forming a caput Medusæ.

The Banti Syndrome.—When the condition is due to congenital obstruction of the portal fissure, the symptoms come on in infancy. In other cases (the majority) they appear in adolescent or adult life. The Banti syndrome is also divided into three stages :

First stage sometimes lasts a long time, even for five to ten years. The patient feels run down and his friends tell him he looks pale. On examination the spleen is found to be enlarged. The blood-count shows a secondary anæmia with leukopenia. During the latter part of the first stage hæmatemesis may occur.

Fig. 371.—Cirrhosis of the liver with ascites.

Second stage is characterised by enlargement of the liver. The edge of the organ feels hard and slightly irregular. This stage is a comparatively short one, lasting from six to eighteen months. Recurrent hæmatemesis is usual.

Third Stage.—Fluid begins to collect in the peritoneal cavity; this is due to increasing portal hypertension. As the disease progresses the patient becomes more and more anæmic, and finally jaundiced. The liver decreases in size, due to increasing cirrhosis. Sometimes there is bleeding from the associated hæmorrhoids. Throughout this stage repeated hæmatemeses occur, which often determine the fatal issue (fig. 372).

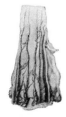

Fig. 372.—Œsophageal varices in a case of fatal "hæmatemesis" occurring in a patient suffering from Banti's disease. (*G. F. Walker.*) (*British Journal of Surgery.*)

Necropsy reveals a large adherent spleen, with a sclerotic splenic artery. The splenic vein is much enlarged and is often as large as a thumb. The liver is cirrhotic, the peritoneum opaque and spattered with milk-white patches.

INVESTIGATION OF A PATIENT WITH SIGNS OF PORTAL HYPERTENSION

The physical examination includes palpation of the spleen and the liver, and inspection of the anal canal for hæmorrhoids.

Examination of the Blood.—In cases of the Banti syndrome there is a secondary anæmia with leukopenia. Any case of portal hypertension may be complicated by a low hæmoglobin estimation due to loss of blood. In necessary cases cross-matching is undertaken, with a view to subsequent blood transfusion.

Tests for Liver Insufficiency.—Among the most helpful in this respect are the first five listed on p. 330.

Aspiration liver biopsy is a method of confirming the presence or absence of hepatic cirrhosis. The procedure is not without danger of internal hæmorrhage. When performed under vision during peritoneoscopy, this danger is reduced. Failure to aspirate a cylinder of liver occurs in from 5 to 10 per cent. of cases.

Excretion urography is valuable by showing the presence and state of each kidney. If both kidneys are functioning normally, the left kidney may be sacrificed in order to provide an artificial collateral circulation via the renal vein.

A barium meal sometimes displays œsophageal varices.

Œsophagoscopy is occasionally necessary to confirm the presence of the varices, and exclude peptic ulceration of the œsophagus as the cause of the bleeding.

SURGICAL MEASURES TO RELIEVE PORTAL HYPERTENSION

Laparotomy is performed, and ascitic fluid, if present, is evacuated. The liver and spleen are examined. The site of the obstruction is ascertained by measuring the portal pressure in the portal vein itself and its main branches, and, if facilities exist, by performing venography of the portal system on the operating table. According to the site of the portal obstruction, and taking into consideration the results of the pre-operative investigations, the operator is presented with a choice of procedures :

1. **The Talma-Morison Operation.**—The surfaces of the liver and spleen are scrubbed with gauze to encourage subsequent adhesion between these organs and the parietal peritoneum. The omentum is then fixed to the parietes at several points, particularly to the peritoneal edges of the incision. After the operation, several further tappings are necessary, but in successful cases the ascites abates, and large veins coursing over the abdominal wall bespeak the establishment of an efficient collateral circulation between the portal and systemic circulations.

While this operation has been performed for many years, the number of successful outcomes are few, and have been limited to patients in whom the operation was performed early in the course of hepatic cirrhosis. It is now comparatively rarely performed.

2. **Splenectomy** should still have pride of place in comparatively early cases of the Banti syndrome, and in the following circumstances :

(*a*) When the pressure in the portal vein is not more than 150 mm. of water. Splenectomy reduces the amount of portal blood by about 40 per cent. This enables a cirrhotic liver to cope with the lesser amount of portal blood without causing back-pressure effects. In addition, it removes the vasa brevia, which may be a source of serious gastric hæmorrhage.

(*b*) When there is thrombosis limited to the splenic vein, provided the left gastric (coronary) vein does not open anomalously into the splenic vein, instead of directly into the portal vein.

3. **Ligation and Division of the Splenic Artery.**—In cases of thrombosis of the splenic vein, the splenic artery goes on pumping into the spleen blood which can only escape with difficulty through the collateral circulation. Therefore, if, as is sometimes the case, the enlarged spleen is densely adherent, division of the splenic artery between ligatures will cause " physiological " splenectomy with the same beneficial effects as extirpation of the organ. This operation has an additional advantage in leaving intact the adventitious collateral circulation between the upper pole of the spleen and the diaphragm (Digby Chamberlain).

A. Sape Talma, 1847–1918. Professor of Medicine, Utrecht.
Rutherford Morison, 1857–1939. Professor of Surgery, University of Durham.
Digby Chamberlain, Contemporary. Professor of Surgery, University of Leeds.

Following splenec-
tomy (fig. **373**), the
patient may be cured.
In other cases he or
she may remain
symptom-free for
years. Should symp-
toms return, some
form of porto-caval
anastomosis is often
still possible.

**4. Porto-caval
Anastomosis.**—Many
years ago Eck showed

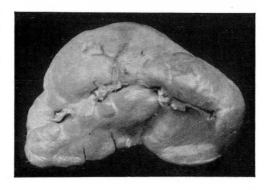

FIG. 373.—Specimen of a spleen removed for
Banti's syndrome.

experimentally that after the portal vein had been by-passed
into the inferior vena cava, the liver continued to perform
its manifold functions via the hepatic artery and vein. The
operation, which has undergone a number of modifications, was
first performed by Whipple and his associates, using a vitallium
tube to aid the implantation of the distal end of the severed
portal vein into the inferior vena cava. Subsequently direct
anastomosis by suture, after irrigating the lumina of the vessels
concerned with heparin, was found to give more lasting results.
In all the operations to be described, heparinisation of the
patient for forty-eight hours post-operatively helps to prevent
the occurrence of thrombosis at the site of the anastomosis.
Should oozing from the wound occur, the exhibition of heparin
must be discontinued forthwith.

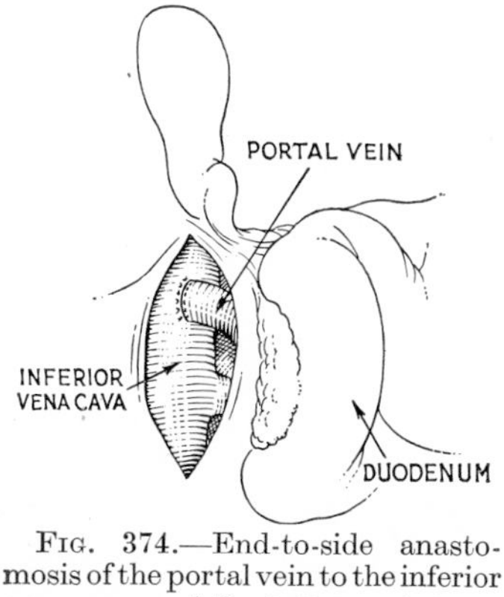

End-to-side Porto-caval Anasto-

mosis.—The portal vein is dissected
from the common bile duct, and
divided close to the portal fissure.
The proximal end is ligated. The
distal end is lightly clamped, and
after temporarily occluding the
inferior vena cava with rubber-
covered clamps, or better still the
special clamp illustrated in fig.
376, end-to-side anastomosis is
performed (fig. **374**).

PORTAL VEIN

INFERIOR
VENA CAVA

DUODENUM

FIG. 374.—End-to-side anastomosis of the portal vein to the inferior
vena cava. (*After L. M. Rousselot.*)

*Nicolai Vladimirovitch Eck. Russian Physiologist. Successfully performed lateral anasto-
mosis between the portal vein and inferior vena cava of dogs in 1877.*

Spleno-renal vein anastomosis is an alternative procedure, and when the spleen is relatively free from adhesions and the splenic vein is unquestionably patent throughout its course, it is both effective and rather less difficult to perform than the foregoing. It is especially indicated in cases of congenital extrahepatic hypertension when the portal vein is surrounded by engorged veins, making porto-caval anastomosis impracticable. The spleen is mobilised and the splenic artery is ligated. The radicles of the splenic vein are dissected, and the longest is selected for the anastomosis, and temporarily occluded by a rubber-covered bulldog clamp. The remaining veins are tied close to the spleen, which is removed. Left nephrectomy is performed, conserving as much as possible of the renal vein, which is similarly clamped, and end-to-end anastomosis carried out between the splenic vein and the renal vein. If the splenic vein is long enough to be approximated to the renal vein without tension, the end of the splenic vein can be anastomosed to the side of the renal vein without sacrificing the kidney (fig. 375).

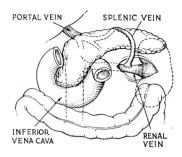

Fig. 375.—End-to-side anastomosis of the splenic vein to the left renal vein. (*After L. M. Rousselot.*)

When there is thrombosis of the main portal vein the possibility of effecting a cure is slender. Anastomosis of the distal cut end of the superior mesenteric vein and the inferior vena cava is very difficult, and the amount of blood that it carries from the portal to the systemic circulation is insufficient for a lasting improvement. Anastomosis of the distal end of the inferior mesenteric vein to the left renal vein has given more promising results.

Transthoracic side-to-side porto-caval anastomosis is the most recent development of the surgical treatment of portal hypertension. This operation is more time-consuming, but in patients who are fit to undergo it, the results are encouraging. With the patient in the lateral position, right side uppermost, the ninth rib is resected. The pleura and then the diaphragm are opened. This approach allows side-to-side anastomosis between the portal vein and the inferior vena cava. No dissec-

tion of the portal vein from the
common bile duct is necessary. A
special clamp (which permits opening
the vena cava without occluding the
entire blood-supply through it) is
placed on the inferior vena cava.
With very little dissection the portal
vein can be approximated to the
inferior vena cava, and after clamps
have been applied to the portal
vein, side-to-side anastomosis is performed (fig. 376).

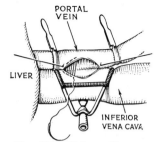

FIG. 376.—Side-to-side porto-
caval anastomosis being performed via the transthoracic
route with the aid of a special
clamp on the inferior vena cava.
(*After A. H. Blakemore.*)

SPLENECTOMY

The indications for splenectomy are :
1. Rupture.
2. Aneurism of the splenic artery.
3. Movable spleen with symptoms.
4. Acholuric jaundice.
5. Thrombocytopenic purpura.
6. Neutropenia.
7. Certain cases of portal hypertension, as described on p. 322.
8. Cysts.
9. Chronic abscess.
10. Gaucher's disease.
11. New-growths.

From the surgical standpoint the spleen may be said to have
two pedicles—the gastro-splenic omentum and the lieno-renal
ligament ; the splenic artery and vein lie in the latter (fig. 377).

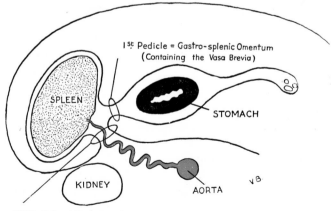

FIG. 377.—The spleen has two pedicles. The splenic vessels lie in the lieno-
renal ligament.

A left paramedian incision is made and the organ is palpated with special reference to adhesions. Division of adhesions on its convex aspect is effected at the expense of the diaphragm rather than of the splenic capsule. Once the organ is free, its pedicle is identified. The gastro-splenic omentum is divided, between ligatures. The main pedicle (the lieno-renal ligament), having been grasped between the fingers, it is divided little by little, clamping, then cutting as close to the spleen as possible, until the organ is free. This technique does away with the necessity for mass ligation where, so to speak, all the eggs are placed in one basket, and it minimises considerably the possibility of wounding the tail of the pancreas.

PHYSIOLOGICAL EFFECTS OF SPLENECTOMY

1. Spleniculi (Miniature Spleens) Hypertrophy.—It is not uncommon to find in the gastro-splenic omentum of a normal subject one, two, or even three spleniculi. After the spleen has been removed these tiny spleens enlarge. A case is on record where, some years after splenectomy, the dimensions of a hypertrophied spleniculus rivalled those of a normal spleen.

2. Bone Marrow Changes its Character.—Within six months red marrow replaces yellow marrow in many of the long bones (Rendle Short). This accounts for fleeting bone pains " like rheumatism," which are sometimes a matter of serious concern to the patient.

3. Changes in the Blood.—*Initial Changes :*

(*a*) Leucocytosis.

(*b*) Decreased red blood-corpuscles.

(*c*) Diminution in hæmoglobin.

These changes are maximal between two weeks and two months.

(*d*) Increased coagulability.

(*e*) Increased platelet count.

After two months lymphocytosis is invariable, and is independent of the cause for which the spleen was removed.

After many months there is moderate eosinophilia, and the mast cells increase in number.

Experimentally, in splenectomised animals, it has been shown that there are alternating periods of hæmatogenesis and hæmatogenous jaundice, hinting that there may be an interaction between the liver and spleen in the construction and destruction of red blood-corpuscles.

A. *Rendle Short, Contemporary. Emeritus Professor of Surgery, University of Bristol.*

4. There is more iron in the tissues.

5. Increased susceptibility to the effects of sunlight. At the Veterinary Research Laboratory at Onderstepoort, Transvaal, it has been shown that splenectomised sheep are very sensitive to strong sunlight. The practical outcome of this research is that a patient on whom splenectomy has been performed should not reside in the tropics.

THE LIVER
CONGENITAL ABNORMALITIES

Riedel's Lobe.—There is a tongue of liver projecting from the right lobe, which forms a palpable mass beneath the right costal margin. This accessory lobe (fig. 378) must be distinguished from an enlarged right kidney.

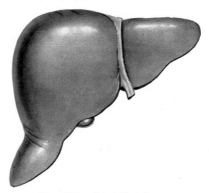

FIG. 378.—Riedel's lobe.

HEPATOPTOSIS (*Syn.* MOVABLE LIVER)

Hepatoptosis is usually part of a general visceroptosis. There is a congenital form which is due to the absence of certain ligamentous supports of the liver. Almost without exception the patient is a female, and in extreme cases the liver descends below the umbilicus. When it is impossible to control this displacement by a belt, operation has been advised and practised successfully. After scarification of its dome, so as to invite adhesion to the diaphragm, the liver is slung to the abdominal wall and lower costal cartilages.

INJURIES

Rupture of the liver is a frequent and, when extensive, an extremely grave accident. The violence which produces this injury is usually of a crushing type. A considerable proportion of cases of rupture of the liver are associated with other severe injuries, and the mortality is high. Tears in the liver are sometimes found at necropsy in subjects who have died from other causes ; small tears, therefore, probably occur frequently, but do not give rise to serious symptoms. Rupture of the right lobe is six times more common than of the left, and the tear is usually on the anterior or the superior surface of the organ. Very often a rib or ribs on the right side is fractured. Four clinical types are encountered :

Bernhard Riedel, 1846–1916. Professor of Surgery, Jena, Germany.

1. There are neither special symptoms nor signs of a ruptured liver. They are those of a hæmoperitoneum, and cannot be distinguished from a ruptured spleen.

2. Occasionally, but less commonly than in the case of a ruptured spleen, the symptoms and signs of serious intra-abdominal hæmorrhage are delayed for hours, or even days.

3. There are signs of a hæmoperitoneum with localising signs of pain, tenderness, and rigidity in the right upper quadrant.

4. A large subcapsular hæmatoma gives rise to a palpable, tender, enlarged liver.

Treatment.—In the first three types a blood transfusion is of primary importance. If it were not usually impossible to eliminate rupture of the spleen, or other intra-abdominal organ, it might be best to treat many of these cases conservatively. In the fourth type conservative measures should be employed, and often the patient recovers without operation, although he may become slightly jaundiced during convalescence or peri-umbilical jaundice may be noticed. In other cases, laparotomy must be undertaken. As soon as the peritoneum is opened, owing to the decrease in intra-abdominal pressure, hæmorrhage from the liver becomes violent. It can be controlled by passing a finger into the foramen of Winslow and compressing the hepatic artery and portal vein between the finger and thumb. When the tear is accessible and moderate in size, it is repaired by mattress sutures which, if introduced in the manner shown in figs. 379 and 380, accomplish their mission in a surprisingly effective manner. If the tear is on the superior surface of the liver, it can be rendered more accessible by dividing the round and falciform ligaments and, when necessary, resect-

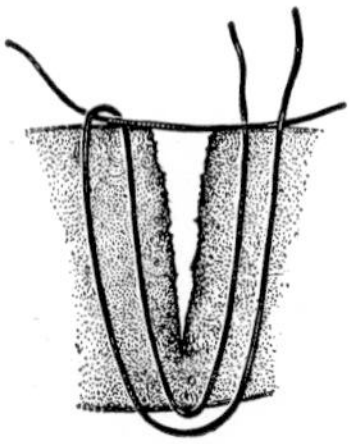

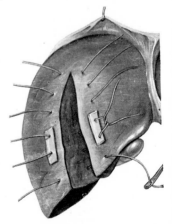

FIG. 379.—After the mattress suture has been tied not too tightly (to prevent cutting through), the ends of the loose strand which has been laid beneath are tied together.

FIG. 380.—Alternative method of liver suture. A piece of costal cartilage is removed, split into two, and used as shown to prevent the sutures cutting out.

Jacob Winslow, 1669–1760. A Dane who migrated to Paris, and there established a school of anatomy.

ing the costal margin. Suture is much to be preferred, but if the tear is not accessible, or very extensive, recourse must be had to packing with absorbable gauze or a length of gauze roll, the end of which is left protruding from the abdominal wound. Unabsorbable packing should remain *in situ* for five days, and then be removed gradually.

Wounds of the liver occur as the result of gunshot injuries and stab wounds. When, as is commonly the case, the wound of entrance is in the right lower thorax, the thoraco-abdominal approach, excising the wound of entrance, is the best. In some cases the wound of the liver is comparatively small, and no serious bleeding occurs. If the wound is a large one, the same principles of arresting hæmorrhage given above are employed. As one would expect, the mortality is highest when the wound has to be packed.

Traumatised liver produces a toxic substance which gives rise to pathological changes in the kidneys. This leads to a rise in non-protein nitrogen of the blood, a reduction of urinary output, and the appearance of albumin and casts in the urine.

ENLARGEMENTS OF THE LIVER

General enlargement

With jaundice

Regular
- Infective hepatitis.[1]
- Cholangitis (secondary to common duct stone impaction).
- Pylephlebitis.[1]
- Carcinoma of head of pancreas.
- Novarsenobillon poisoning (look for vein puncture at elbow).

Irregular—Late secondary carcinoma.

Without jaundice

Regular
- Portal cirrhosis, 1st stage.
- Failing heart.
- Leukæmia.
- Rickets.
- Amyloid (examine spleen and urine).

Irregular
- Secondary carcinoma.
- Gummata.
- Banti's syndrome, 2nd stage.

Localised lump
- Is it the gall bladder ?
- Hydatid.
- Amœbic abscess.[1]
- Hepatoma.
- Riedel's lobe.

Massive irregular enlargement
- Polycystic disease (examine kidneys).
- Cystadenoma.
- Secondary melanoma.

[1] Pyrexia or rigors are a feature.

LIVER FUNCTION TESTS

Owing to its manifold functions, there is no single test by which the liver can be stated to be functioning normally. Therefore several tests are usually undertaken in each patient, and in some instances the individual test must be repeated. Some of these tests attempt to demonstrate the presence or absence of liver insufficiency, while others are designed to help in the differential diagnosis of a case of jaundice. Among a large number of tests available are the following :

1. **Estimation of serum albumin** is a good general test of the state of liver function. A level below 2·5 mgm. per cent. indicates that liver function is greatly impaired, and the patient is unfit for operation. A level above 4 mgm. per cent. is satisfactory.

2. **Bromsulphalein test** is a sensitive test for the identification of early impairment of liver function. After an intravenous injection of the dye, not more than 30 per cent. of it should be present in the serum at the end of an hour. An increase in this amount suggests liver damage. The test is of no value in the presence of jaundice, as bile pigments interfere with the colorimetry.

3. **Serum Alkaline Phosphatase.**—The concentration of this enzyme is increased particularly in cases of biliary obstruction. It is apparently secreted into the circulation from the damaged liver cells or bile capillaries. The test is invalid during the period of skeletal growth or in bone diseases.

4. **Quick's Test.**—This test is only of value if it has been proved that renal function is unimpaired. The principle of the test depends on the administration of sodium benzoate and the collection of urine over a stated period. The hippuric acid which has been formed from the glycine of the patient in this period is precipitated from the urine and its amount determined by weighing.

5. **Galactose Tolerance Test.**—The liver is capable of converting galactose into glycogen. The patient is given 40 gm. of galactose by mouth. Normally the galactose in the blood should not rise above 40 mgm. per 100 ml. If it does, or if any is retained in the blood at the end of two hours, the carbohydrate metabolism of the liver is impaired.

6. **Urine Urobilinogen Estimation.**—Normally the liver oxidises nearly all the urobilinogen reabsorbed from the intestine, and only very small amounts (below 3 mgm.) are excreted in twenty-four hours. Liver damage interferes with this oxidisation ; consequently large amounts (from 5 to 300 mgm.) of urobilinogen are excreted in the urine, the amount depending on the severity of the liver damage.

7. **Thymol Turbidity and Flocculation Tests.**—A saturated solution of thymol buffered at pH 7·8 (3 ml.) is added to serum (0·05 ml.). A turbidity or flocculation usually develops in cases of hepatitis, but results are mainly negative in biliary obstruction (Maclagan).

ABSCESSES OF THE LIVER

A liver abscess can be due to many causes, and the infection reaches the liver in one of several ways, viz. :

Via the Portal Vein
- Suppurative appendicitis.
- Actinomycosis of the right iliac fossa.
- Inflamed hæmorrhoids.
- Diverticulitis.
- Amœbic abscess.
- Infected carcinoma of the colon.
- Typhoid (rare).

Armand J. Quick, Contemporary. Associate Professor of Pharmacology, Marquette University, U.S.A.
Noel Francis Maclagan, Contemporary. Chemical Pathologist, Westminster Hospital, London.

Along the Bile Ducts—Stone impacted in common duct.

Via the Hepatic Artery ⟨ General pyæmia.
Actinomycosis of the neck.
Infection of a hydatid cyst.

From the Umbilicus ⟨ Along the umbilical vein of the new-born.
Along the veins of Sappey.

By Direct Extension ⟨ From a subphrenic abscess.
From an empyema thoracis.
From a penetrating wound.

PYLEPHLEBITIS Syn. PORTAL PYÆMIA)

Pathology.—Particularly when occurring secondarily to appendicitis, the commonest cause, the liver is often riddled with abscesses (fig. 381). These abscesses are connected together, forming a " canal and cavity " system (H. M. Turnbull). In rare instances there is localisation of the infection.

Clinical Features. — Repeated rigors as a rule usher in this frequently fatal condition. The patient soon becomes slightly jaundiced, and the liver is found to be somewhat enlarged and tender. When there is no known focus of infection, the rectum should be examined for inflamed hæmorrhoids.

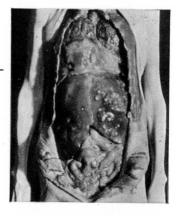

FIG. 381.—Pylephlebitis. Liver riddled with small abscesses.

If a swinging temperature and rigors occur in the course of acute appendicitis, pylephlebitis is one of the first conditions to be considered. In the early stages pylephlebitis is often difficult to differentiate from subdiaphragmatic abscess.

Prophylaxis.—(*a*) Hæmorrhoids should never be removed in an acutely inflamed state. (*b*) Ligation of the ileocolic vein in addition to appendicectomy is to be recommended in those rare cases of early acute appendicitis where rigors are in evidence or when a gangrenous appendix lies in the retro-ileal position.

Treatment.—In early cases penicillin and sulphonamide therapy may possibly abort the infection. When pylephlebitis is fully established, the outlook is practically hopeless, but it is more than justifiable to perform laparotomy. If the ileocolic or superior mesenteric vein is thrombosed, ligation is performed, and any obvious localised abscess is drained. A specimen from one of these abscesses is collected. After the organism responsible has been cultured, it may be found to be sensitive to streptomycin, and if so, this should be given.

CHOLANGITIS

By cholangitis is meant a state of inflammation of the bile ducts, but it is the radicles of the biliary tree lying within the liver, as opposed to the extrahepatic ducts, that should be visualised as being the seat of the infection. This is a rare complication of impacted stone in the common bile duct (see p. 351).

Infective hepatitis (*syn.* catarrhal jaundice) occurs in both sporadic and epidemic forms, and is probably due to a filterable virus. Young adults are usually affected. Most commonly the condition commences abruptly with nausea, and perhaps vomiting, together with general malaise and mild pyrexia. The pre-icteric phase lasts a few days, and is followed by mild jaundice. The liver becomes palpable and tender, and the jaundice lasts for two or three weeks. Occasionally the disease occurs in a more severe form, and the jaundice is so profound that it renders the differential diagnosis between this condition and jaundice due to a stone in the common bile duct or carcinoma of the head of the pancreas extremely difficult. When such is the case, liver function tests 5, 6, and 7, listed on p. 330, are particularly helpful.

Syringe jaundice is a variety of infective hepatitis. The interior of the syringe becomes contaminated by blood drawn into the syringe from a person suffering from infective hepatitis. Therefore, all syringes should be boiled or autoclaved afresh for each patient, and not sterilised in spirit. The same condition may occur after plasma infusion. Plasma should not be " pooled " in large quantities, and the ideal is to treat all plasma with ultra-violet irradiations, which are lethal to the virus.

ICTERUS GRAVIS NEONATORUM (*Syn.* ERYTHROBLASTOSIS INFANTUM)

Icterus neonatorum is noticed in more than half of all newly born infants. It appears from the second to the fifth day after birth, and then fades gradually. It requires no treatment.

Icterus *gravis* neonatorum, as its name implies, is a serious malady. The baby is born jaundiced. The condition is due to immunisation of the mother to a dominant antigen factor present in the red blood-cells of the fœtus inherited from the father. In 90 per cent. of cases the antigen is the rhesus factor. The mother is sensitised by the fœtal erythrocytes passing through the placenta or, less frequently, by a blood transfusion with Rh.-positive blood. The antibodies of the mother passing through the placenta violently hæmolyse the infant's blood. The first-born rarely suffers. A golden-coloured vernix caseosa and a hypertrophied placenta should arouse the obstetrician's suspicion. The condition must be distinguished from congenital obstruction of the bile ducts and syphilitic hepatitis, but an enlarged spleen and, more particularly, the finding of a greatly increased number of erythroblasts on several blood examinations, should make the diagnosis of icterus gravis neonatorum clear. Until a few years ago the condition was looked upon as almost hopeless. Great success has followed transfusion with Rh.-negative blood of the correct ABO group ; particularly successful is exsanguination-transfusion.

ACTINOMYCOSIS OF THE LIVER

produces the well-known " honeycomb " liver. The ray fungus reaches the organ in one of the following ways :

1. Secondary to actinomycosis of the right iliac fossa, 50 per cent.
2. Direct continuity .   .   .   .   .   . 20 ,, ,,
3. Metastasis, particularly from the neck   .   . 30 ,, ,,

For the treatment of the original actinomycotic lesion intensive iodine and penicillin therapy will doubtless have been tried. Usually by the time the liver is involved the prognosis is hopeless, but at least one patient with hepatic actinomycosis has recovered (Chitty).

TUBERCULOSIS OF THE LIVER

is exceedingly uncommon. When present it is usually secondary to ileo-cæcal tuberculosis.

AMŒBIC LIVER ABSCESS (SYN. DYSENTERIC ABSCESS)

is one of the terminations of amœbic hepatitis, which in turn is a complication of amœbic dysentery.

Pathology.—*Entamœbæ histolyticæ* (fig. 382) pass from the colon along the portal vein and enter the liver. Here they colonise and live at the expense of the liver cells, causing them to liquefy. The amount of liver destruction is proportionate to the size of the colony and the resistance of the host. In 70 per cent. of cases the abscess is solitary ; in 30 per cent. more than one abscess is present. Except in long-standing cases, amœbæ can be isolated from a scraping of the abscess wall. The content of the abscess cavity seldom contains the parasite ; indeed, the

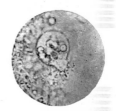

FIG. 382. — Enta-mœba histolytica.

pus is usually sterile. Characteristic pus from an amœbic liver abscess is chocolate-coloured, and consists of broken-down liver cells, leucocytes, and red blood-cells. When the abscess is solitary it is usually situated in the postero-superior surface of the right lobe. The right lobe of the liver is so frequently the seat of an amœbic abscess because blood from the intestine goes mainly to the right lobe of the liver, while blood from the spleen goes mainly to the left lobe (Bernard Shaw). Nearly always the perihepatitis causes the liver to become fixed to the diaphragm and the abdominal wall ; consequently the liver may be prevented from enlarging in a downward direction.

An amœbic abscess of the liver runs a variable course :

1. In early stages of amœbic hepatitis with abscess threatening, resolution often occurs under emetine treatment.

Hubert Chitty, Contemporary. Consulting Surgeon, Bristol Royal Infirmary.
Arthur Frederick Bernard Shaw, Contemporary. Professor of Pathology, University of Durham.

2. When an abscess forms the liver enlarges, most often in an upward direction. It is at this stage that surgical intervention is called for.

3. It may become encapsulated and remain dormant for long periods.

4. Unrecognised and untreated, it often bursts into neighbouring viscera (fig. 383), or, less frequently, points beneath the skin overlying the liver.

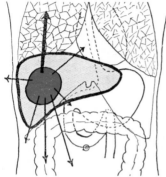

FIG. 383.—Directions in which a tropical liver abscess may burst.
(*After Cope.*)

The bursting of a liver abscess into the lung and the expectoration of a quantity of chocolate-coloured sputum occasionally results in a natural cure.

Bacterial infection is a rather frequent and serious complication of amœbic liver abscess. While solitary amœbic abscess is most amenable to combined emetine and surgical treatment, the prognosis in cases of multiple amœbic liver abscesses is extremely poor.

Clinical Features.—White males between twenty and forty years of age are usually affected ; women rarely suffer from this disease. As a rule, the condition develops soon after an attack of amœbic dysentery while the patient is resident in a tropical or sub-tropical country. Less frequently its appearance is delayed, sometimes for many years. Occasionally it occurs in a carrier who has not had dysentery ; indeed, it frequently appears in persons who have had mild diarrhœa not diagnosed as dysentery, and consequently have not had treatment for that condition.

Early Symptoms.—Anæmia, loss of weight, and an earthy complexion are often the first symptoms.

Pyrexia rising to 101° F. (38°C.) at night, with profuse sweating, is nearly always present. Rigors occasionally occur, especially in the early stages.

Pain is constantly present in the liver area, and is occasionally referred to the right shoulder.

Tenderness and *rigidity* in acute cases are comparable to that of acute cholecystitis. In old-standing chronic cases tenderness is often absent.

Enlargement of the liver can often be demonstrated by clinical methods (fig. 384), but it is not unusual for an abscess to be present in a liver which is fixed by perihepatitis, and therefore the liver cannot enlarge in a downward direction.

Basal lung signs on the corresponding side are always present in acute cases of hepatic abscess.

Leucocytosis is present in nearly all cases. Polymorphonuclear cells constitute, at the most, only 75 per cent. of the total count.

Examination of the stools for amœbæ should be undertaken, but their absence does not exclude the diagnosis of amœbic abscess of the liver.

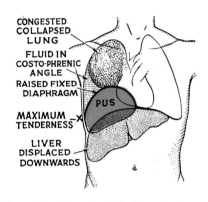

CONGESTED
COLLAPSED
LUNG
FLUID IN
COSTO-PHRENIC
ANGLE
RAISED FIXED
DIAPHRAGM
PUS
MAXIMUM
TENDERNESS
LIVER
DISPLACED
DOWNWARDS

FIG. 384.—The physical signs of a tropical liver abscess (commonest site). *(After Andreasen.)*

Sigmoidoscopy sometimes reveals the characteristic ulcers (p. 425).

Radiography (antero-posterior and lateral positions) often reveals an elevation and fixation of the right cupola of the diaphragm.

Treatment.—When amœbic hepatitis is even suspected, intramuscular injections of emetine hydrochloride (1 grain daily for ten days) are commenced, and are continued for three or more weeks if the diagnosis of an amœbic infection is confirmed.

Aspiration.—When, in spite of emetine treatment, the temperature does not settle, if the pain persists, and particularly if the presence of a suspected abscess is confirmed radiologically, aspiration should be undertaken in the operating theatre. Secondarily infected abscesses should be treated by aspiration in the first instance ; secondary infection can only be discovered by examining the pus. Indeed, when secondary infection is present, it can often be overcome by aspiration and, if the organism present be sensitive, by the instillation of 50,000 units of penicillin into the cavity, together with appropriate sulphonamide therapy (Andreasen). Even if this plan does not succeed, as a result of the conservative measures, the patient's general condition usually improves. Aspiration must be conducted in the operating theatre. The important technique of introducing a wide-bore hollow needle into the abscess cavity in various locations is shown in fig. 385. In some cases the abscess

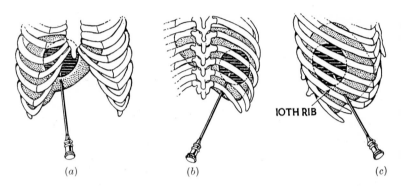

IOTH RIB

(a)   (b)   (c)

Fig. 385.—Aspiration of an amœbic hepatic abscess. (a) in the anterior part of the liver ; (b) in the posterior part of the liver ; (c) located near the dome of the diaphragm.

eludes the aspirating needle, in which event laparotomy should be performed, thus allowing the liver to be explored by the aspirating needle more thoroughly. At the same time laparotomy permits the exclusion of a primary carcinoma of the liver, which closely resembles an amœbic liver abscess in its onset and physical signs, and at times is even accompanied by a low pyrexia.

After-treatment.—A full course of emetine hydrochloride (gr. 1 (64 mgm.) daily for ten days) with an interval of fourteen days, followed by a second course of ten days, must be given.

Open operation should be avoided if possible, the only indications being when secondary infection is not controlled by chemotherapy, or when the abscess threatens to invade the skin. For the former, an approach similar to that used for a subphrenic abscess (see p. 386) is employed.

HEPATIC SYPHILIS

As far as the liver is concerned, syphilis, always an accomplished actor, can, and often does, deceive the clinician, and even the operator. Gummata give rise to rounded masses in the liver. These swellings sometimes simulate closely a liver abscess. Multiple gummata of the liver give signs not unlike secondary carcinoma when examined clinically, although, when displayed to the light of day, they lack the characteristic umbilicated appearance of the latter. Syphilitic cirrhosis is sometimes accompanied by ascites.

HYDATID DISEASE OF THE LIVER

Although the parasite may develop in many parts of the body, in 70 per cent. of cases it does so in the liver. It enters this organ through radicles of the portal vein.

Source of Infection.—Dogs are the chief cause of hydatid disease in human beings. Dogs become infected by feeding on the offal of infested sheep and, to a lesser extent, cattle (Fontana) (fig. 386). As would be expected, the disease is

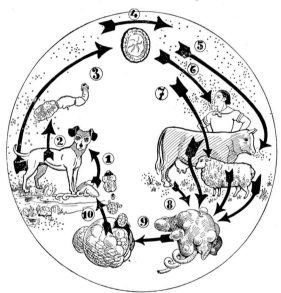

Fig. 386.—The life-cycle of the tænia echinococcus. Offal (1) infected with hydatid cysts is eaten by a dog (2). The tænia echinococcus (3) develops in the dog's intestine. This parasite is made up of a head and three segments, the last of which contains about 500 eggs (4), which are expelled from the dog's intestine on to grass, vegetables, etc. Cattle (5), human beings (6), or sheep (7) ingest the eggs. The liver (8) is the organ most frequently infested with hydatid cysts, a larval form of tænia echinococcus. Such cysts (9) harbour thousands of heads of the echinococcus (scolices) (10). (*Fontana.*)

relatively common in the sheep-rearing districts of Australasia and South America, while for the same reason, in the British Isles, Wales shows the highest incidence.

Pathology.—A hydatid cyst consists of two distinct layers. There is the adventitia made up of fibrous tissue, the result of the liver's reaction to the parasite, and the laminated membrane

Velarde P. Fontana, Contemporary. Professor of Surgical Pathology, the University of Montevideo.

formed of the parasite itself.   The adventitia is grey in colour, and intimately blended with the liver. The laminated membrane is whitish and elastic, and contains the hydatid fluid.   The laminated membrane closely resembles a child's uncoloured balloon filled with water.   Hydatid fluid registers a specific gravity of 1,005 to 1,009, contains no albumin, occasionally a trace of sugar, and, when not too old, hooklets and scolices.

The only living part of a hydatid cyst is a single layer of cells (germinal epithelium) lining the cyst. This secretes : (a) internally : the hydatid fluid ; (b) externally : the laminated membrane (fig. 387a).   The laminated membrane is of

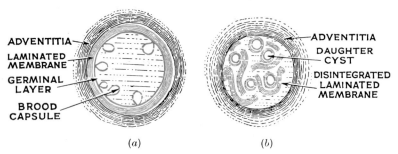

ADVENTITIA

LAMINATED
MEMBRANE

GERMINAL
LAYER

BROOD
CAPSULE

ADVENTITIA

DAUGHTER
CYST

DISINTEGRATED
LAMINATED
MEMBRANE

(a)   (b)

FIG. 387.—(a) Typical hydatid cyst.
(b) Development of daughter cysts (not common).

variable thickness, according to the age of the cyst, and is composed of white hyaline material.   The surrounding tissues of the host react to the presence of the parasite by entombing it in fibrous tissue—the adventitia.   Referring again to the germinal epithelium : here develop brood capsules within the cyst, attached by pedicles to its innermost wall.   Within the brood capsules, scolices (heads of future worms) develop. Should damage to the laminated membrane occur, this membrane disintegrates (Dew), and the brood capsules, becoming free, grow into daughter cysts (fig. 387b).   In this event the mother cyst no longer exists as such, but the hydatid fluid and its content are confined only by the adventitia.

Hydatid cysts grow slowly.   It is most unusual for them to give rise to symptoms and signs until many years after the original infestation.

Clinical Features.—In their early stages hydatid cysts are symptomless.   In the course of time, owing to the prepon-

Harold Dew, Contemporary.   Professor of Surgery, Sydney.

derance of cysts in the lower part of the liver, a visible and palpable swelling in the upper segment of the abdomen is discovered. The size which a hydatid may attain without causing much disturbance of health would seem to be limited only by the volume of the peritoneal cavity.

In academic circles undue prominence is accorded to the hydatid thrill, a sign which is rarely present, even in advanced cases. Percussion reveals dullness over the swelling continuous with the liver dullness. When the liver is enlarged upwards by the cyst the diagnosis is much more difficult, and among other conditions a differential diagnosis must be made between hydatid cyst and tropical liver abscess.

Naturally, when a patient hails from a locality where hydatid disease is rife, the diagnosis is simplified. In obscure cases radiography and immunological tests are of great diagnostic assistance.

The Intradermal Test (Casoni's test) is comparable to the tuberculin reaction, and is positive (fig. 388) in 75 per cent. of cases of hydatid disease.

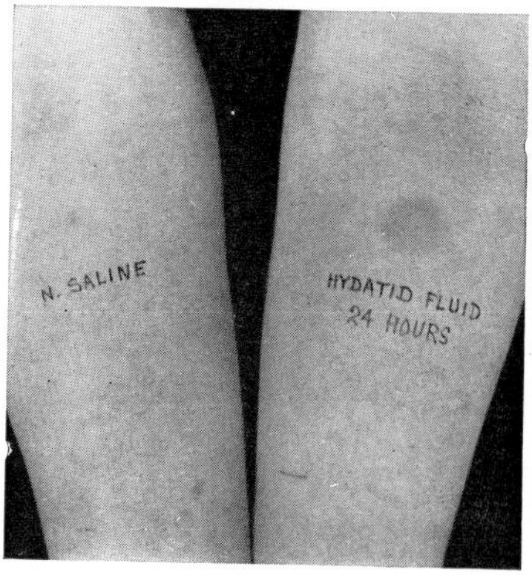

FIG. 388.—Casoni's test. Positive reaction.

The Complement Fixation Test, although more complicated, is of greater accuracy.

A blood-count often, but not invariably, shows an eosinophilia (6 per cent. or more).

Course of the Disease.— 1. Occasionally the parasite dies. The fluid is absorbed, and all that remains is an encapsuled, laminated, bile-stained membrane, such as is occasionally found at necropsy (fig. 390). In very old-standing cases the walls of the dead parasite calcify.

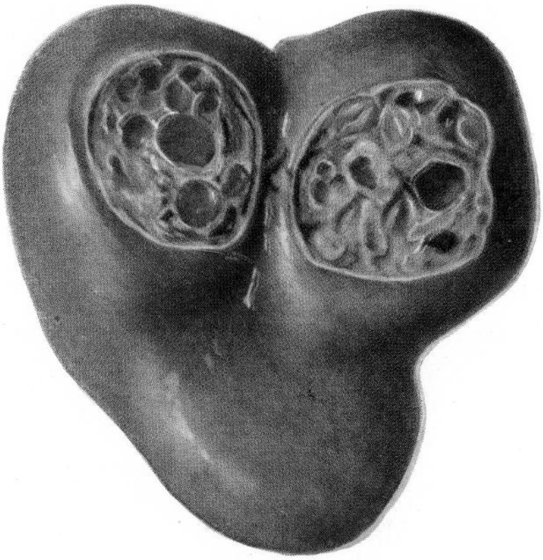

FIG. 389.—Multiple hydatid cysts in the liver. The patient, who had never left England, died after a street accident.

Tomasso Casoni, Contemporary. Physician, Ospedale Coloniale, Vittorio Emanuele III, Tripoli.

2. Usually the cyst enlarges gradually, and becomes manifest by its size. It is at this juncture that surgical intervention is indicated.

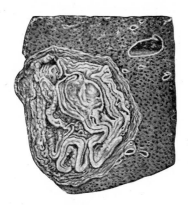

Fig. 390.—An encapsuled hydatid found at necropsy. (*Aschoff.*)

3. Complications arise. " It is the onset of complications that makes the morbidity not much inferior to that of malignant disease " (Fortacin).

Complications {
  Rupture {
    into the peritoneal cavity.
    into the alimentary canal.
    into the biliary channels.
    into a pleural cavity.
  }
  Suppuration.
}

Rupture into the peritoneum is accompanied by profound shock, and all the signs of general peritonitis. A green discoloration about the umbilicus has been noted in rare instances. As with any case of rupture of a hydatid cyst, anaphylactic phenomena, notably urticaria, are prone to occur. The treatment of intraperitoneal rupture must be immediate, and directed to combating shock and cleaning the peritoneal cavity. Even in those who survive, the ultimate prognosis is poor, for the disease must tend to become disseminated in the peritoneum.

TREATMENT OF HYDATID CYST OF THE LIVER

The only treatment is surgical, for there is no drug which has the slightest effect upon the course of the disease.

The cyst is exposed by an incision which gives the best access. The peritoneal cavity is packed off ; finally, a black pack, wrung out in 2 per cent. formalin, is tucked around the exposed liver—*black* so that daughter cysts and scolices will show up against the background ; *formalin* because this antiseptic kills the parasites. The cyst is aspirated, and a quantity of formalin solution is introduced so as to render the cyst about three-quarters full. An incision is made through the liver overlying the cyst, and the adventitia is opened. This brings the rubbery laminated membrane into view. Very gently the laminated membrane is grasped with ovum forceps, and separated from the adventitia. The aim in view should be to separate the laminated membrane and deliver it intact. This is possible in

José Blanc y Fortacin, Contemporary. Professor of Surgery, Madrid.

uncomplicated cases. In complicated cases it is sometimes necessary to remove the laminated membrane piecemeal. When the cyst can be cleanly enucleated, the resulting cavity in the liver can be closed completely. In less favourable circumstances it is advisable to drain the cavity, particularly when infection is present, when there is bile in the cyst cavity, or uncertainty of its complete removal. No attempt should be made to remove the adventitia. We have seen the liver irreparably split during an ineffectual attempt to excise an adventitia in the belief that it was the laminated membrane. In all cases full precautions should be taken to prevent spilling the contents of the cyst into the peritoneal cavity or the layers of the abdominal wall. Such precautions minimise the possibility of dissemination of the disease. A calcified hydatid cyst should not be interfered with unless it is infected.

NEOPLASMS OF THE LIVER

Benign.—**Angiomata.**—Cavernous angioma is the commonest primary neoplasm of the liver. It is usually small, and causes no symptoms. Large angiomata occasionally arise ; they are frequently in the left lobe, and may attain enormous dimensions.

Congenital cystic liver occasionally accompanies congenital cystic kidney.

Malignant.—**Primary carcinoma of the liver** is very uncommon in European races, but is relatively common in African natives, Malayans, and Chinese. Two pathological varieties are described :

1. **Hepatoma** arises in the liver cells. There are great variations in the malignancy of this tumour, which nearly always commences in the right lobe. At one end of the scale is a relatively benign, firm, slowly growing tumour, and at the other a rapidly growing, soft neoplasm prone to undergo necrosis, which soon metastasises within the liver, but rarely outside the organ. Primary carcinoma of the liver sometimes occurs in areas of regeneration which accompany portal cirrhosis (Turnbull).

2. **Cholangioma** arises in the intrahepatic bile ducts and is columnar-celled. It grows to a large size, and metastasising within the liver, is rapidly fatal.

Clinical Features of Primary Carcinoma of the Liver.—The patient sometimes presents on account of a palpable swelling, which may or may not be painful. The latter variety is sometimes accompanied by a low pyrexia, in which event it may be difficult to distinguish from an amœbic abscess. More often there is rapid loss of weight, anorexia, and, on examination, a large, irregular liver is found, and it is impossible to differentiate by clinical methods such a swelling from a secondary carcinoma of the liver, which, in white races, is very much more common.

Treatment.—Laparotomy should be performed when the patient's general condition is good and the swelling is solitary. If, at operation, the tumour is found to be firm in consistency,

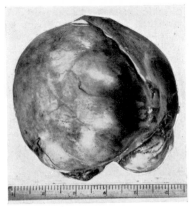

FIG. 391.—Hepatoma resected from the liver successfully.

indicating that it is a relatively benign hepatoma, even if it is of considerable dimensions (fig. 391), excision should be carried out. In this connection the tumour may be found on laparotomy to be a primary carcinoma of the gall-bladder invading the liver ; this, too, is often remediable by resection. When resecting a tumour of the liver, the best method of arresting hæmorrhage is to pass and tie deep interrupted sutures ½ inch (1·25 cm.) beyond the proposed line of section. The resection itself usually takes the form of a wedge, which should include ½ inch (1·25 cm.) of healthy liver on all sides of the tumour. The resulting raw surfaces of the cut liver are approximated by mattress sutures of the type depicted in fig. 379.

SECONDARY NEOPLASMS OF THE LIVER

Secondary Carcinoma.—As is well known, the liver is a favourite site for carcinomatous metastases (fig. 392). Characteristically secondary growths in the liver, owing to degeneration of cells in the centre, are umbilicated.

Secondary Sarcoma.—The liver is not an uncommon site for secondary deposits in cases of sarcoma, but the lungs show a higher incidence.

Secondary melanoma occurs in the liver with unfailing regularity unless the primary growth, re-

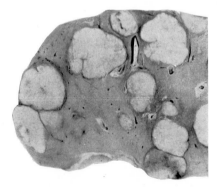

FIG. 392.—Secondary carcinoma of the liver.
(*University of Liverpool Pathological Museum.*)

gional lymph nodes, and intervening lymphatic vessels can be excised satisfactorily. As long as fifteen years have elapsed between the removal of the primary growth and the appearance of the secondary (see also p. 139).

CHAPTER ⌐XVIII

THE GALL-BLADDER AND BILE DUCTS

CONGENITAL ABNORMALITIES

VARIATION in the anatomical arrangement of the bile passages is not unusual. For instance, the gall-bladder may enter the common duct directly (fig. 393a), the cystic duct being absent.

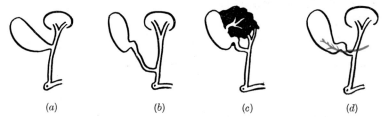

(a)   (b)   (c)   (d)

FIG. 393.—Some anatomical anomalies of the bile passages.

Conversely, sometimes the cystic duct is of considerable length, and opens into the common duct near the pancreas (fig. 393b). An accessory cholecysto-hepatic duct may open into the gall-bladder (fig. 393c). The cystic artery, and right hepatic artery from which it springs, at times lie anteriorly to the ducts (fig. 393d). These are the more important of the possible variations in this region. They are of great importance in operative surgery.

Congenital atresia of the bile ducts occurs more commonly in male than in female infants. Jaundice is apparent, not at, but soon after, birth, is steadily progressive, and accompanied by enlargement of the liver. Without treatment the infant survives about three weeks. The condition is distinguished from icterus gravis neonatorum (p. 332) by a blood examination, the absence of enlargement of the spleen, and the presence of clay-coloured stools.

Treatment.—After a transfusion of blood and injections of vitamin K, laparotomy should be performed during the first week of life. In about 30 per cent. of cases a remediable condition will be found (fig. 394).

Cystic dilatation of the common bile duct (*syn.* choledochus cyst) can be explained by partial congenital atresia of the supra-duodenal portion of the common bile duct. While the bile ducts

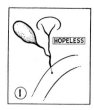 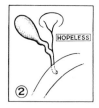 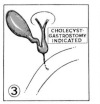 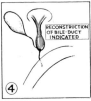

FIG. 394.—Symposium of the various types of congenital obstruction to the bile ducts, irremediable and remediable.

become dilated, the chief abnormality is a narrow-necked diverticulum arising from the common bile duct. During childhood or adolescence a palpable cystic swelling develops in the right hypochondrium, and sometimes becomes immense. Females are four times more commonly affected than males. There are attacks of pain, often associated with transient jaundice. Infection of the cyst is a frequent complication, and may prove fatal by extension of the infection along the dilated bile ducts to the liver (cholangitis).

Treatment.—Anastomosis of the cyst with the duodenum is a most successful form of treatment. When this is impracticable, anastomosis with the jejunum should be carried out.

Duplication of the Gall-bladder.—Cases have been reported of patients with two gall-bladders. Sometimes one of them alone contains calculi.

The Gall-bladder may have a Mesentery.—It is in these cases that the rare abdominal emergency, **torsion** of the gall-bladder, occurs. Cholecystectomy is the treatment, and because of the laxity of the parts it is seldom difficult.

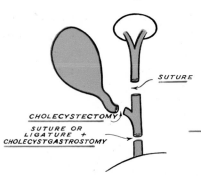

FIG. 395.—A symposium of methods of treating early complete tears of the biliary tract.

TRAUMATIC RUPTURE OF THE BILE PASSAGES

Rupture of the gall-bladder or the bile passages is a rare abdominal injury, usually the result of a run-over accident. It is unlikely that a correct preoperative diagnosis will be made, for the signs are identical with those of rupture of the small intestine. When the abdomen is opened, bile is found within the peritoneal cavity.

The best methods of treating these injuries are represented in fig. 395.

ACUTE CHOLECYSTITIS

There are two forms of acute cholecystitis—non-obstructive and obstructive.

Acute Non-obstructive Cholecystitis.—All grades of acute inflammation, from catarrhal to gangrenous cholecystitis, occur. The infecting organism is usually the colon bacillus or a streptococcus, or both. Especially in fulminating cases, Cl. welchii and other anaerobic organisms may be implicated. Typhoid and paratyphoid cholecystitis can occur as a complication of these fevers. Perforation is exceptional, save in the case of acute typhoid cholecystitis.

Acute obstructive cholecystitis is very much more common than the foregoing. It is due to a gall-stone becoming impacted in the cystic duct, or in Hartmann's pouch (fig. 396). When

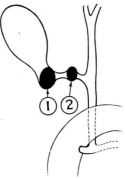

Fig. 396.—The sites of impaction of a gall-stone in acute obstructive cholecystitis.
1. In Hartmann's pouch.
2. In the cystic duct.

the contents of the gall-bladder are sterile, the imprisoned bile is absorbed, and mucus is excreted, giving rise to a thin-walled, transparent mucocele of the gall-bladder. Untreated, the mucocele becomes infected, and an empyema of the gall-bladder follows. In most instances, when impaction occurs the gall-bladder is already the seat of long-standing chronic infection, and the ensuing virulent acute cholecystitis causes the thickened gall-bladder to become intensely inflamed, with its mucous membrane swollen and perhaps gangrenous in places. The subsequent events are variable. Usually, perhaps on account of muscular contraction during vomiting, or more certainly because of conservative treatment, some degree of disimpaction of the stone occurs, and the muco-purulent contents of the gall-bladder escape by way of the cystic duct. Less frequently the impaction persists, and an empyema of the gall-bladder results. On

*William H. Welch, 1850–1934. Pathologist, Johns Hopkins University, Baltimore, U.S.A.
Robert Hartmann, 1831–1893. Professor of Anatomy, Berlin.*

account of the present, and probably previous, attacks of cholecystitis, there are adhesions between the gall-bladder and the omentum. These protective barriers are responsible for the fact that even when an infected obstructed gall-bladder perforates, a local abscess usually ensues. The site of perforation is at the fundus, which is farthest away from the blood supply, or somewhat more rarely, at the neck, from pressure necrosis by the impacted stone. Occasionally perforation into a neighbouring hollow viscus takes place (p. 353). Only in 0·5 per cent. of cases does perforation into the general peritoneal cavity supervene.

Clinical Features of Acute Cholecystitis.—The onset is sudden and agonising in the obstructive variety—more gradual in the non-obstructive. The pain is located in the right hypochondrium, and there is pyrexia, sometimes to 101° F. (38° C.) or more. Occasionally fulminating cases are ushered in by rigors. Rarely is there jaundice. On examination tenderness and rigidity are found in the right hypochondrium. If the patient can be persuaded to relax, particularly in obstructive cases, a mass consisting of the inflamed gall-bladder with attached omental adhesions can be felt. In cases of mucocele of the gall-bladder before infection has occurred, pyrexia is absent, and following the acute attack of pain, a large pyriform swelling can be palpated.

Treatment.—Experience shows that in more than 90 per cent. of cases the symptoms of acute cholecystitis subside with conservative measures and penicillin therapy. The patient is placed in Fowler's position, and for the first twenty-four hours continuous intravenous saline and glucose solution is administered. Nothing is given by mouth during this period. If vomiting is in evidence, the stomach is kept empty by aspiration through an indwelling Ryle's tube. Hot applications to the right hypochondrium and Pethidine (B.P.C.), 2 ml. (100 mg.), intravenously three times a day help to relieve the pain. After twenty-four hours glucose drinks are allowed, and if the temperature, pulse, and other physical signs show that the inflammation is subsiding, after the bowels have been emptied by an enema, the diet is increased gradually. About a fortnight after the acute symptoms have subsided cholecystectomy is carried out. When there is uncertainty about the diagnosis, e.g. high retrocæcal appendicitis or a leaking duodenal ulcer cannot be excluded, or, after a

George Ryerson Fowler, 1848–1906. Professor of Surgery, New York Polyclinic School.

period of twenty-four to thirty-six hours, the pulse and temperature are not falling, the pain persists and the physical signs point
to an empyema of the gall-bladder, urgent laparotomy must be
performed.   In such circumstances it is usually advisable to
limit the operation to cholecystostomy with removal of the impacted stone, although, in the opinion of some surgeons, even in
these circumstances cholecystectomy is often the operation of
choice.   When, on account of the absence of pyrexia and the
presence of a large pyriform swelling in the right hypochondrium,
the diagnosis of mucocele of the gall-bladder is probable,
after excretory pyelography has been performed to exclude a
right hydronephrosis, operation is best carried out in a matter
of hours.   In these circumstances most operators would favour
cholecystectomy.

Typhoid fever is now comparatively rare.   Because of the
danger of perforation in acute typhoid cholecystitis, immediate
laparotomy must be advised.

Should an infected gall-bladder perforate into the general
peritoneal cavity, diffuse peritonitis supervenes readily and
rapidly.   In such circumstances the only hope lies in immediate
drainage of the peritoneal cavity and the gall-bladder.   It is
extremely unusual for perforation to occur while the patient is
undergoing conservative treatment for cholecystitis.

CHRONIC CHOLECYSTITIS AND GALL-STONES

are best considered together, because chronic cholecystitis
often leads to gall-stones.   Furthermore, a sterile metabolic gall-
stone, particularly the solitary cholesterol stone, by temporarily
occluding the cystic duct, favours the development of both
acute and chronic cholecystitis.

Metabolic gall-stones are rare in comparison to infected stones,
and are produced by an error of metabolism causing an over-
production of cholesterol or pigment in the bile.   There are two
varieties, to which may be added a third, so rare as to be
a pathological curiosity, and the exact ætiology of which is
unknown.

1. *The cholesterol stone* sometimes attains a considerable size,
and is usually solitary.   It is rounded or oval in shape, and is sometimes composed of pure cholesterol when, like tallow, it is feebly
translucent.   More often bile pigments become deposited on

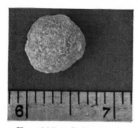

Fig. 397.—Solitary gall-stone from a gall-bladder. It is unfaceted.

its surface (fig. 397). This type of stone is not uncommon. It tends to occupy Hartmann's pouch, and its presence favours infection of the gall-bladder, when it may be accompanied by infected stones. On section the interior of a cholesterol stone will be found to radiate ─────────→

2. *Pigment stones* are rare, and are composed of bile pigments. Deposits of bile pigment usually take the form of dark biliary mud, which is largely composed of biliverdin. Biliary mud is more often found and formed in the bile ducts than in the gall-bladder. Pigment calculi, which are sometimes associated with acholuric jaundice and are found in the gall-bladder as well as the bile ducts, are small, black, and numerous, and on analysis are found to be composed of calcium biliverdinate. Owing to their metallic hardness they are difficult to section, and they are amorphous ─────────────→

3. *Calcium carbonate stone* is solitary and round. It is the rarest of all biliary calculi, and cuts like chalk.

Infected stones, which are much more common than other varieties, are produced by infection of the gall-bladder. They are multiple and by mutual pressure they become faceted. The stones are frequently all of much the same size, which suggests that they were formed at one and the same time. Often the gall-bladder is packed with stones (fig. 398). " Every gall-stone is a tombstone erected to the memory of the organisms dead within it " (Moynihan). These stones are composed of cholesterol, biliverdin, and calcium, and consequently are some-times designated " mixed calculi." On section they are found to consist of alter-nating layers of cholesterol and bile pig-ments ─────────────→

Cholesterosis of the Gall-bladder.— On slitting up a gall-bladder removed because of supposed chronic cholecystitis,

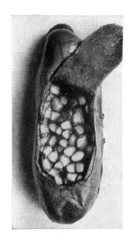

Fig. 398.—Gall-bladder packed with calculi.

Lord Moynihan, 1865–1936. Professor of Surgery, University of Leeds.

it is sometimes found to be the seat of cholesterosis, and is known as the "strawberry" gall-bladder (fig. 399). The pin-head yellowish deposits are composed of cholesterol esters, and although it was thought that this condition was due to infected cholecystitis, nearly always the gall-bladder and its contents are sterile. The condition is due to an error in cholesterol metabolism, and may be the first stage of the formation of a cholesterol stone.

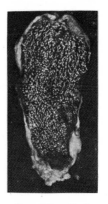

Fig. 399.—Cholesterosis of the gall-bladder.

CHRONIC CHOLECYSTITIS

can occur apart from gall-stones, although, if it is present long enough, gall-stones will almost certainly form in the infected gall-bladder. The infection may reach the gall-bladder by the blood-stream (hæmatogenous infection), or from the liver by means of the bile (hepatogenous infection), but according to Evarts Graham, because of the greater ease of culturing organisms from the cystic lymph node than from the gall-bladder, and the frequency of concomitant chronic hepatitis with subcapsular scarring, the most usual path of infection from the liver to the gall-bladder is lymphatic. Retrograde infection along the bile ducts from the duodenum is improbable. When the gall-bladder is chronically infected it loses its normal bluish translucency and elasticity, and becomes thickened and opaque ; its mucous membrane shows evidence of chronic inflammation. Variable adhesions are found about the gall-bladder ; sometimes these are exceedingly dense.

Clinical Features.—A fat, fertile, flatulent female of forty or fifty is the classical sufferer from gall-stones. Useful as is this clinical memorandum in emphasising that 75 per cent. of all cases occur in women, it must be stressed that both chronic cholecystitis and gall-stones may appear at a much earlier age, even in childhood, and long after the age of fifty.

Silent Gall-stones.—It is possible for calculi to be present in the gall-bladder and give rise to no symptoms during a long lifetime. They are sometimes found in the course of an operation for another condition. About 5 per cent. of necropsy subjects over fifty years of age have stones in the gall-bladder which have not contributed to the cause of death.

Inaugural symptoms of stones in the gall-bladder and chronic cholecystitis are synonymous. There is reflex dyspepsia, which

Evarts A. Graham, Contemporary. Professor of Surgery, Washington University, U.S.A.

in some respects simulates that of chronic peptic ulcer, but in typical cases differs from it in the following particulars. Period-icity, so frequently present in cases of chronic peptic ulcer, is lack-ing. The patient feels distended soon after meals, and women find it necessary to loosen their corsets. Flatulence is a regular accompaniment. Sometimes there is heart-burn in addition. This is made worse by fried or fatty foods, which the patients tend to avoid. These symptoms often continue for years. In cases where gall-stones are present in the gall-bladder, due to the passage of a small stone down the cystic duct, or to a large one temporarily occluding the mouth of the cystic duct, gall-stone colic may supervene.

Gall-stone Colic.—Suddenly the patient experiences ex-cruciating pain in the epigastrium and right hypochondrium. The pain shoots to the back or between the shoulder-blades. In severe cases it " doubles her up," and she rolls in agony on the floor. The attack, which lasts for upwards of two hours and is usually accompanied by vomiting and retching, often passes off as suddenly as it came. In most cases, heat somewhat relieves the pain, and in old-standing cases a brown pigmentation of the skin over the right hypochondrium bespeaks frequent hot applications.

Physical Signs.—When examined soon after an attack of gall-stone colic, a tender enlarged gall-bladder may be palpated. Deep tenderness in the right hypochondrium can often be elicited during the stage of the inaugural symptoms.

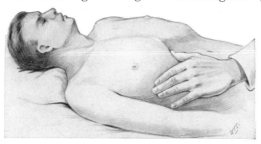

FIG. 400.—Murphy's sign.   (Moynihan's method.)

Murphy's Sign.—If continuous gentle pres-sure is exerted over the right hypochondrium (fig. 400) while the patient takes a deep breath, there is a "catch in the breath " just before the zenith of the inspiration.

Boas's Sign.—There is an area of hyperæs-thesia posteriorly be-tween the ninth and eleventh dorsal segments on the right side.

Sometimes the symptoms, especially in non-calculous chronic chole-cystitis, are anomalous and are easily overlooked; for instance, pseudo-anginal attacks sometimes have their origin in a gas-laden stomach secondary to a diseased gall-bladder (Miller).

Stones in the Common Hepatic and Common Bile Ducts.—

Transient jaundice, preceded by biliary colic, are the leading

John B. Murphy, 1857–1916.   Professor of Surgery, North-western University, Chicago.
Ismar Boas, 1858–1938.   Gastro-enterologist, Berlin.
Charles Miller, 1875–1939.   Physician, University College Hospital, London.

features of a stone in the common bile duct. The attack usually lasts for a few hours or, at the most, for a few days. After the attack has passed off bile can be demonstrated in the urine for several days after the yellow tinge of the skin and conjunctivæ is no longer perceptible. Tenderness in the right hypochondrium can usually be elicited soon after the attack.

If the stone was small enough, it may have been swept into the duodenum by a flow of bile during a period of relaxation of Oddi's sphincter, for the bile ducts, having no musculature in their walls, are unable to help to expel the stone. How often a stone is passed along the natural passages into the duodenum no one knows. If a further similar attack occurs at a later period, this is sometimes presumed to be due to another gall-stone, but this is not by any means necessarily the case. A stone (in two-thirds of all cases it is single) or stones arrested in the common bile duct have nearly always migrated from the gall-bladder. Pigment stones alone are formed in the bile ducts. Whatever the composition of a stone arrested in the common bile duct, during its sojourn there it receives an additional coating of calcium bilirubinate, and becomes larger and, even if previously faceted, ovoid in shape. Because the presence of a stone impedes the flow of bile, the common bile duct dilates above and at the site of the obstruction. Above the stone other stones may form or, what is more usual, biliary mud or gravel accumulates. A stone in the common hepatic duct is usually accompanied by one or more stones at a lower level. A stone or stones may be present in the common bile duct for months or even years without giving rise to serious symptoms. Conversely, impaction is liable to supervene.

Impaction of a stone (fig. 401) can occur in the supraduodenal

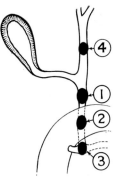

Fig. 401.—1. Stone impacted in the supraduodenal portion of the common bile duct (commonest site).

2. Stone impacted in the retroduodenal portion of the common bile duct (second most common site).

3. Stone impacted in the ampulla of Vater (10 per cent. of cases).

4. Stone impacted in the common hepatic duct (very rare).

Note that the gall-bladder is usually contracted because of chronic cholecystitis.

Ruggiero Oddi, 1845–1906. Surgeon and Anatomist, Rome.

or retroduodenal portions of the common duct (which are the usual sites), or at the ampulla of Vater or, very rarely, in the common hepatic duct. When impaction takes place severe biliary colic occurs, and the colic continues at varying intervals. With each episode of pain the jaundice deepens. Gradually the pain lessens, and usually passes off completely, but the jaundice persists. Nevertheless, unlike other types of jaundice, from which it must be distinguished, it varies in intensity from day to day. This variation is due to exacerbations of the concomitant cholangitis rather than to a ball-valve action of the impacted calculus. Similarly, the stools are seldom clay-coloured for more than two or three days at a time. As bile salts accumulate in the blood the skin commences to itch, sometimes intolerably. The patient loses weight. There is mild pyrexia. From the viewpoint of differential diagnosis, perhaps the most important sign is that in cases of calculus impaction the depth of the jaundice varies. Another, less reliable, sign is the absence of palpable enlargement of the gall-bladder (see Courvoisier's Law, p. 374). If the obstruction is not relieved, one of the following dangerous complications ensues :

(*a*) *Liver Function becomes Increasingly Impaired.*—When liver function becomes seriously depressed, pigment excretion ceases ; resorption of pigment from the stagnant bile in the dilated obstructed ducts occurs, but the mucous membrane of the ducts continues to secrete mucus, thus the ducts above the impacted calculi become distended with " white bile." The finding at operation of " white bile " is of grave, but not necessarily fatal, significance.

(*b*) *Suppurative Cholangitis Supervenes.*—When there is stagnation of bile, infection is prone to occur. Suppurative cholangitis is ushered in by a rigor, and later the temperature chart reveals those sudden elevations, precipitate descents, and complete intermissions, known colloquially as the " steeple chart." There is malaise and loss of appetite. Pain is not a marked feature, but it may be referred to the right shoulder. The jaundice deepens, and an enlarged tender liver can often be detected. Unless the bile passages are drained and the patient receives appropriate chemotherapy, the condition is nearly always fatal. At necropsy an engorged, bile-stained liver riddled with multiple pin-head abscesses is found.

Abraham Vater, 1684–1751. Professor of Anatomy and Botany, Wittenberg.

(*c*) The gall-stone ulcerates through the wall of the common duct, and diffuse general peritonitis supervenes. This form of bile peritonitis occurring in a subject with a grossly impaired liver function is rarely amenable to operative, or any kind of, treatment, although operation should be attempted. At operation the perforation in the common bile duct may be minute and difficult to find. If possible the common bile duct should be drained, and also the general peritoneal cavity.

(*d*) On rare occasions the stone ulcerates into the duodenum or jejunum, and a natural cure follows.

SPECIAL METHODS OF INVESTIGATION

Radiography.—When gall-stones are present in the gall-bladder they can be demonstrated by a plain X-ray in 30 per cent. of cases.

Cholecystography should never be performed in the presence of jaundice, because of the danger of increasing liver damage by the dye. For the same reason it should not be performed in the presence of acute cholecystitis.

The test depends upon the excretion in the bile of tetrahalogen compounds of phenolphthalein. The evening meal, consisting of an egg, bread and butter, and stewed fruit, is taken at 6 p.m. Soon after the meal the patient takes 6 capsules of tetraiodophenolphthalein (Opacol) at half-hourly intervals with water. No food of any kind is allowed until the radiological examination has been made, but the patient is permitted and urged to drink water. Films are taken at 9 a.m., 11 a.m., and 12 noon the following day. Then a glass of milk with cream is given (to empty the gall-bladder), and a final film is taken.

Normally, the gall-bladder is visualised by this method (fig. 402). A reliable sign of obstructive cholecystitis is failure of the

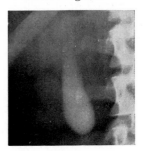

Fig. 402.—A normal cholecystogram.

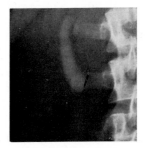

Fig. 403.—Same after a fatty meal.

gall-bladder to cast a shadow in any of the serial radiographs. It is, of course, essential to be certain that the patient has ingested the dye. If there is any question of the dye having been vomited, or if the patient is suffering from diarrhœa at the time of the examination, the examination should be repeated. Distortion of the gall-bladder or the presence of gall-stones are frequently demonstrated by cholecystography. Failure of the gall-bladder to contract after a fatty meal suggests chronic cholecystitis.

A negative cholecystogram does not exclude gall-stones, for small calculi may be present which cast no shadow or filling defect in the dye-filled gall-bladder.

Liver function tests are often valuable in determining the extent of liver damage. Some of these tests set out on p. 330 are designed to help in the differential diagnosis of jaundice.

The icteric index is a colorimetric estimation of an acetone extract of the blood serum. The normal icteric index is 5. This laboratory test is useful in estimating the degree of jaundice, and repeated estimations are valuable in determining the degree of progressive and intermittent jaundice with more precision than clinical observation.

THE TREATMENT OF CHRONIC CHOLECYSTITIS AND CHOLELITHIASIS

Morphine and its derivatives, so long the standard treatment of gall-stone colic, do not relieve the pain as often as would be expected. What should be given is a drug which relaxes spasm of involuntary muscle (morphine causes such musculature to contract). A drug falling into this category is pethidine (B.P.C.) 2 ml. intravenously four-hourly, or 50 mgm. orally.

Following an attack of gall-stone colic there is considerable depression of liver function, and operation should never be contemplated until at least a week after such an attack. Should jaundice follow, the diagnosis of impacted stone in the common bile duct is made, and the preparation for operation, the indications for operation, and the nature of the operation are described later. In other circumstances, unless there is some definite contraindication, the correct treatment for chronic cholecystitis, with or without stones, is cholecystectomy. Cholecystostomy is now comparatively rarely employed, except in the aged, or when operation has to be undertaken urgently for empyema of the gall-bladder, or when adhesions are so dense as to render the identification of the junction of the cystic and common ducts impossible.

LAPAROTOMY FOR CHRONIC CHOLECYSTITIS AND GALL-STONES

It is important to have the patient in the " gall-bladder position," that is with the lower dorsal and upper lumbar vertebræ arched over the bridge with which most operating tables are provided or, failing this, over a pneumatic cushion or a sandbag. The incision may be a right paramedian, or a transverse one, according to preference. When the peritoneum has been opened the gall-bladder is located and examined. The field is isolated with packs. After examining the gall-bladder, particularly when the patient gave a history of a previous attack with jaundice, the common bile duct is palpated for a stone. If this examination is negative, so great is the danger of overlooking a stone in the common bile duct that, when facilities exist, a cholangiogram should be taken on the operating table.

Cholangiography.—Traction by forceps is applied to the neck of the gall-bladder so as to render the cystic duct taut. The duct is nicked with sharp-pointed scissors half an inch from its junction with the hepatic duct. By means of a malleable cannula, or a portion of a ureteric catheter, attached to a syringe, lipiodol or neohydreol is injected into the common duct. When the cannula is within the lumen of the cystic duct, instruments which would obscure the field are removed, and 5 to 10 ml. of the fluid is injected. An X-ray exposure is made as the last of the fluid is injected, and the film is ready for inspection in about five minutes.

A normal cholangiogram is sufficient evidence that exploration of the common bile duct is unnecessary (fig. 404), and cholecystectomy can be proceeded with. A positive cholangiogram (fig. 405) provides information regarding the presence of a stone

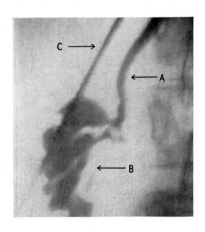

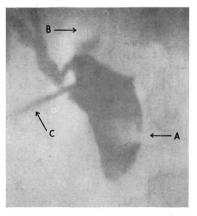

Fig. 404.—Normal cholangiogram, showing A, common bile duct, B, opaque medium in duodenum. C is the cannula used for injection.

Fig. 405.—Cholangiogram showing stone in common duct, A. Owing to spasm of sphincter no medium has entered the duodenum. B indicates dilated hepatic ducts. C is the cannula used for injection.

in the common bile duct, and is an indication that choledocho-lithotomy is the first consideration. Obstruction from other causes, such as carcinoma of the ampulla, may also be visualised.

Cholecystectomy.—By dissection the junction of the cystic, the common hepatic, and the common bile ducts is displayed (fig. 406). Removal of the gall-bladder should never be com-

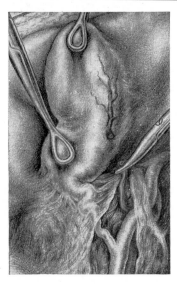

menced until all three ducts have been clearly exposed. The cystic duct is then divided between liga-tures. The cystic artery is ligated and severed. The peritoneal coat of the gall-bladder is incised

Fig. 406. — Cholecystectomy. The junction of the cystic, com-mon hepatic, and common bile ducts has been displayed and the cystic artery has been clamped and divided.

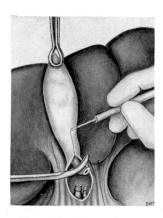

Fig. 407.—The peritoneum over the gall-bladder is in-cised with a diathermy knife.

(fig. 407) and dissected off the gall-bladder with a diathermy knife, so as to form a flap on either side of the bared gall-bladder. Gentle traction on the neck of the gall-bladder facili-tates diathermy dissection of the organ from its bed. Careful watch must be kept for an abnormal cholecysto-hepatic duct (see fig. 393c) which, if seen, is ligated. Persistent oozing of bile from one spot in the liver bed is indicative of division of this duct, and calls for thorough coagulation of the adjacent liver by means of diathermy. In this circumstance drainage of the wound is advisable. Proceeding towards the fundus, the gall-bladder is removed about an inch at a time, and at each stage the gall-bladder bed is coagulated with the diathermy button and the peritoneal flaps approximated over it before proceeding to the next stage, until the gall-bladder has been removed (fig. 408). The abdomen is closed. Provided hæmostasis is perfect and an abnormal cholecysto-hepatic duct has not been divided, drainage of the area of operation is unnecessary.

Choledocholithotomy. *The supra-duodenal route.*—Most stones in the common bile duct can be removed by this route. After the free edge of the gastro-hepatic omentum has been

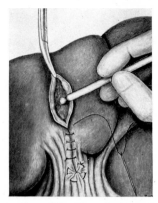

Fig. 408.—Coagulation of the gall-bladder bed with a diathermy button.

palpated upwards and downwards as far as possible, if a stone can be felt, an attempt is made to manœuvre it into a position midway between the entrance of the cystic duct and the superior border of the duodenum. If this can be accomplished, the stone having been steadied between the finger and thumb, the peritoneum overlying the duct is incised and dissected from the duct, which is opened longitudinally directly on to the stone, enabling it to be removed by a scoop. The interior of the duct is then explored upwards and downwards with the scoop for further stones. When the stone cannot be felt, or cannot be manipulated into the optimum position just described, after incising the peritoneum overlying the supraduodenal portion of the common bile duct, a length of the underlying structure is displayed. When there are numerous adhesions, and especially when the gall-bladder has been removed at a previous operation, it is sometimes difficult to be certain whether the structure in question is the common bile duct or the portal vein. Aspiration through a fine hypodermic needle connected to a syringe will settle this point. As soon as about ¾ inch (2 cm.) of the common bile duct has been exposed, the duct is transfixed by two stay sutures and a longitudinal incision into the duct is made between them. Escaping bile is mopped up, or removed by suction. Through this opening it may be possible to identify the stone and remove it with a scoop or forceps (fig. 409). After removal of the stone or stones by either of the above methods the common bile duct is cleared of any mud

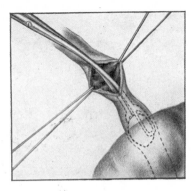

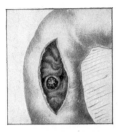

Fig. 410. — The trans-duodenal approach to a stone impacted in the ampulla of Vater.

Fig. 409.—Choledochotomy. The stone has been seized with Desjardins' forceps.

or grit by introducing and removing strips of ribbon gauze, followed by irrigation with saline solution. Finally, a bougie or blunt probe is passed through the ampulla of Vater into the duodenum. Drainage of the common bile duct should always follow ; it is best carried out by means of a T-tube (fig. 411).

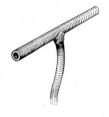

The horizontal limbs are passed into the duct, which is closed about the vertical limb.

The transduodenal route is indicated when a stone is found to be wedged near the ampulla of Vater and it cannot be retrieved from above. The duodenum is mobilised and its anterior wall incised. The contents of the duodenum, if any, are evacuated, preferably by suction. Sometimes the stone can be seen in the mouth of the ampulla of Vater, and is easily removed by a scoop. At others the wall of the ampulla must be divided in order to reach the stone. After removal of the stone the incision in the duodenum is repaired by closing it transversely with two layers of sutures. The supraduodenal portion of the common bile duct is drained, as in the previous operation, and dependent drainage of the peritoneal cavity in the region of the duodenum is provided.

Fig. 411.—T-tube for draining the common bile duct.

In the majority of cases, when a stone or stones can be removed with comparative ease by the supraduodenal route, cholecystectomy can be carried out in addition. In other circumstances additional cholecystostomy can be performed, or

Abel Desjardins, Contemporary. Surgeon, Dispensaire Henri de Rothschild, Paris.

the diseased gall-bladder can be left for removal on a future occasion.

TREATMENT WHEN JAUNDICE COMPLICATES CHOLELITHIASIS

To commence with, conservative treatment, which includes a high glucose intake to build up the store of liver glycogen, and so protect the liver, together with the exhibition of pethidine, if there are further attacks of pain, is instituted. With these measures the depth of the jaundice may diminish, the amount of bile in the urine lessen, and the stools become increasingly coloured. Such a train of events sometimes culminates in complete disappearance of the jaundice, and implies disimpaction of the stone, or possibly passage of a small stone into the duodenum. In such circumstances cholecystography can be safely undertaken, and if the liver function tests are satisfactory, it will be possible to undertake laparotomy under the same conditions as have been described already.

At any time during conservative treatment if, over a period of days, the jaundice is found to be increasing rather than decreasing, and particularly when any degree of jaundice is accompanied by pyrexia, operation should be planned to take place within two or three days. Jaundiced patients tend to ooze from a cut surface. This tendency to bleed is due to a diminution of prothrombin in the blood, which results from failure of absorption of vitamin K from the alimentary canal, which in turn is consequent upon diminution of bile salts in the alimentary canal. To raise the prothrombin level of the blood, injections of vitamin K 10 mg. are given intramuscularly twice or three times a day for two or three days. In patients with pyrexia chemotherapy is also given. In a jaundiced patient, the length of the operation should vary inversely with the depth of the jaundice. In patients who are deeply jaundiced, or who show signs of suppurative cholangitis, operation should be limited to draining the common bile duct (choledochostomy), removing a stone or stones only if they are readily accessible. If it is impracticable to remove an impacted calculus, a biliary fistula will probably result, and further operation will have to be undertaken later, when the jaundice abates.

After-treatment of Cases when the Common Bile Duct has been Drained.—In jaundiced patients vitamin K is continued for a week after the operation. A high carbohydrate fluid diet is given, and Felamine (a preparation of urotropin and cholic acid) is prescribed as a biliary antiseptic. The drainage from the tube in the common bile duct is watched closely. In a deeply jaundiced patient, if white bile is succeeded by yellow, and then green bile, the prognosis becomes increasingly good. In jaundiced patients no attempt should be made to remove the tube until the jaundice has disappeared. In other patients, on the eighth day after operation the vertical limb of the T-tube is occluded by a hæmostat for ten minutes ; if pain is not experienced, it remains occluded for another ten minutes. The absence of pain at the end of this time is a sign that the common bile duct is patent and the bile is passing through the horizontal limb of the tube into the lower end of the common bile duct, and entering the duodenum. If pain is experienced, it may be due to spasm of Oddi's sphincter associated with pancreatitis, but it is more likely that the lower end of the duct is occluded by a stone. If, a few days later, the vertical limb of the tube is occluded with the same result, a post-operative cholangiogram is taken by injecting lipiodol down the tube. This gives information regarding obstruction to the common bile duct. When there is no pain after clipping the tube, the tube is removed in non-jaundiced patients or as soon as the jaundice has disappeared and the temperature is normal. When, by intention or oversight, a stone has been left in the lower end of the common bile duct, instillations of solution G (see p. 651) via the T-tube can be tried in the hope of dissolving the stone, but, as a rule, further operation will be required.

BILIARY FISTULÆ

(a) Due to a Stone Ulcerating through the Wall of the Gall-bladder

1. *Into the Stomach.*—The patient may vomit the stones.

2. *Into the Duodenum.*—A gall-stone in the neck of the gall-bladder may ulcerate through into the duodenum. This is the commonest internal biliary fistula. If the stone is over one inch (2·5 cm.) in diameter, intestinal obstruction follows, the stone becoming impacted in the ileum about two feet above the ileo-cæcal valve (p. 471).

3. *Into the Colon.*—No untoward complication follows, as a rule, but a large stone may become impacted in the rectum.

4. *Through the Skin of the Umbilicus.*—The gall-stones are extruded on to the surface.

5. *Into the Peritoneum.*—Diffuse peritonitis quickly supervenes.

(b) Post-operative Fistula

1. *After Cholecystostomy.*—Occasionally a cholecystostomy opening fails to close naturally. When the cystic duct is occluded, the discharge is mucus. If there is partial or complete obstruction to the common duct, the fistula discharges bile.

2. *After Cholecystectomy.*—(i) Due to a severed accessory cholecysto-hepatic duct. In this instance the amount of bile is comparatively small, and the fistula heals spontaneously.

(ii) Due to injury of the common bile duct during cholecystectomy. This accident will never occur if the operation is performed in the manner that has been described. It is more liable to occur when the gall-bladder is removed from the fundus towards the cystic duct, instead of in the reverse direction, and a way in which this happens is depicted in fig. 412.

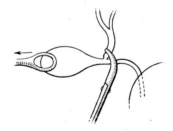

FIG. 412.—One method by which the common bile duct may be severed in cholecystectomy. The accident is more common when the gall-bladder is removed from its fundus towards the cystic duct.

(iii) Due to accidentally or intentionally leaving a stone in the lower end of the common bile duct after choledocholithotomy or choledochostomy.

(iv) Due to a fibrous stricture developing after choledocholithotomy at the site where the stone was impacted or to pre-existing chronic pancreatitis (p. 370).

Reconstruction of the Common Bile Duct.—This difficult operation is indicated in cases of a biliary fistula following injury of the common bile duct during cholecystectomy (see p. 356), and in cases of stricture of the common bile duct. Painstaking efforts must be made to identify and approximate the two ends of the common duct. If necessary the duodenum is displaced inwards and the duct is dissected from the pancreas in order to facilitate approximation (fig. 413). The ends of the duct are united, and a T-tube is introduced below the anastomosis. Should the tube be inserted through the junction the scar which remains after removal will predispose to a stricture at the already narrowed site of union of the duct.

CARCINOMA OF THE GALL-BLADDER

Carcinoma of the gall-bladder is more frequent than is generally supposed ; 5 per cent. of cases of stones in the gall-bladder are associated with carcinoma (Rolleston). This is convincing support for the theory that carcinoma is often inaugurated by chronic irritation. Microscopically carcinoma of the gall-bladder is commonly spheroidal-celled, but owing to

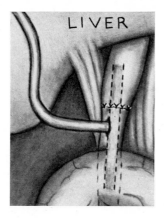

FIG. 413.—Reconstruction of the common bile duct.

prolonged irritation and metaplasia it may become squamous-celled. There are no characteristic symptoms or signs ; by the time there is an [unmistakable palpable tumour the case is inoperable. When the neoplasm is confined to the gall-bladder cholecystectomy offers considerable hope of a cure. Even when the growth has involved the liver locally, cholecystectomy, together with extirpation of a wedge of liver substance, may occasionally cure the patient.

Sir Humphrey Rolleston, 1862–1944. Physician, St. George's Hospital.

CHAPTER XIX

THE PANCREAS

INJURIES

INJURIES to the pancreas are uncommon on account of its deeply placed, protected position. In many instances when the pancreas is damaged, other organs are involved simultaneously.

Type 1.—The patient, who has had a severe injury to the upper abdomen, presents signs of a serious lesion of some intra-abdominal organ, and it is thought wise to explore. When the pancreas is the injured organ, there is often blood-stained fluid in the lesser sac, and fat necroses are sometimes present.

Type 2 (Milder Injuries).—The first intimation that the pancreas has been lacerated is often the development of a pseudo-pancreatic cyst (p. 369).

Treatment.—When the abdomen has been opened soon after the injury, a ruptured pancreas has many times been sutured successfully. The sutures should be of unabsorbable material, such as cotton. In other cases recovery has ensued after packing the rent and draining the lesser sac. Drainage is essential in all cases.

ACUTE PANCREATITIS (*Syn.* ACUTE NECROSIS OF THE PANCREAS)

Pathology.—The following outstanding features can be seen at necropsy. The great omentum and subperitoneal fat are studded with opaque areas termed fat necroses. If these are dabbed with a solution of cupric acetate they will be seen to stain an intense blue (Benda's test).

Fat necroses are not always limited to the abdominal cavity. They can sometimes be demonstrated beneath the pleura and pericardium, and even in the subsynovial fat of the knee joint.

The peritoneal cavity, especially the lesser sac, contains a blood-stained exudate, which, in very acute cases, seems to be almost pure blood. The retroperitoneal tissues in the vicinity are infiltrated with blood-stained fluid, or, more rarely, with pure blood, giving the appearance of a retroperitoneal hæmatoma. The pancreas is swollen, and in some cases all or part of it is necrotic. Sometimes the gall-bladder is thin-walled and normal in appearance ; more often it is thickened and fibrotic from previous chronic cholecystitis. In over 50 per cent. of cases the gall-bladder contains stones. The stones are nearly always small, and occasionally a stone or stones is found in the common bile duct. On culture the bile may be found to be infected, most often with B. coli or streptococci.

Carl Benda, 1857–1933. Professor of Anatomy, Berlin.

When the lesser sac has been drained and the patient survives, portions of the peripancreatic tissue and even of the pancreas may be discharged through the wound as putty-like material. Upon analysis this material has been shown to be composed largely of calcium stearate.

In a few cases of historic interest some demonstrable cause for the necrosis of the pancreas has been discovered ; for instance, a gall-stone, a pancreatic stone, or a round worm has been found blocking the ampulla of Vater.

Ætiology.—The cause of acute pancreatitis has not been fully elucidated. An older theory was that cholecystitis (perhaps with gall-stones) causes a reflex spasm of the muscle of Oddi, and consequent regurgitation of infected bile along the pancreatic ducts. Newer experimental work proves that Oddi's sphincter is too weak to effect this regurgitation. Rich and Duff found metaplasia of the epithelium of the pancreatic duct in a high percentage of cases of acute pancreatitis. Obstruction to a pancreatic duct would favour stasis of secretion, and infection.

The following theory (Eve's hypothesis) is a rational explanation of the widespread distribution of the fat necroses :

1. Bacteria can convert trypsinogen into trypsin.

2. In acute pancreatitis there is a *Bacillus coli* or other bacterial infection of the pancreatic ducts.

3. The bacteria activate free trypsinogen in the inflamed pancreas.

4. This trypsin erodes the pancreatic tissue.

5. Thus all the pancreatic enzymes are set free, including :

6. Steapsin (lipase), which splits fat into glycerine and fatty acid.

7. The free fatty acid combines with calcium to form soaps=*fat necrosis* (fig. 414).

Clinical and Clinico-pathological Features.— The patient is classically a robust fat man about forty years of age, but there are many sufferers who do not conform to this type ; indeed, in about 50 per cent. of cases the patient is a woman. In its most severe forms, acute pancreatitis

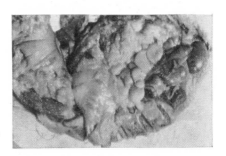

Fig. 414.—Necropsy on an obese subject. Death from acute pancreatitis. The colour photograph shows the hæmorrhage into the lesser sac in the upper part of the picture, and fat necroses on the great omentum. These can be seen particularly in the centre of the lower part of the illustration.

comes on very suddenly, and in this respect it simulates a perforated peptic ulcer. There is often a history of previous attacks of upper abdominal pain, and it is probable that fulminating cases are a culmination of a series of attacks of subacute pancreatitis. The salient features of acute pancreatitis are as follows :

Abraham Vater, 1684–1751. Professor of Anatomy and Botany, Wittenberg.
Ruggiero Oddi, 1845–1906. Surgeon and Anatomist, Rome.
Arnold Rice Rich, Contemporary. Professor of Pathology, Johns Hopkins University, Baltimore, U.S.A.
George Lyman Duff, Contemporary. Professor of Pathology, McGill University, Montreal.
Sir Frederick Eve, 1853–1916. Surgeon, London Hospital.

Pain is agonising, mainly epigastric, and passes through to the back.

Vomiting is repeated, and retching is in evidence.

The temperature is at first subnormal, and later it rises to 99° F. (37·4° C.), or more.

The pulse is nearly always rapid from the commencement of the attack (cf. Perforated Peptic Ulcer, p. 288).

Rigidity is not board-like, and in severe cases is absent because the patient is collapsed. This helps very considerably in the differential diagnosis between acute pancreatitis and perforated peptic ulcer. However, considerable rigidity is to be expected after three or four hours, by which time pancreatic ferments have escaped into the general peritoneal cavity.

Tenderness is pronounced in the epigastrium, and may be present in the loins, particularly the left.

Cyanosis.—Cyanosis is a fairly common accompaniment of the most acute forms of acute pancreatitis. It is due to the profundity of the toxæmia, though, perhaps, anoxæmia, due to the inflamed pancreas preventing full excursions of the diaphragm, plays a part.

The serum amylase is raised from the normal 4 to 50 units to 200 units or more in about 80 per cent. of cases.

Unfortunately this biochemical test has serious disadvantages. It is occasionally absent in cases of acute pancreatitis, and is sometimes positive in cases of perforated duodenal ulcer, probably because pancreatic enzymes in the duodenal contents are absorbed from the peritoneal cavity. The serum amylase has also been found to be raised in some cases of inflammatory lesions of the small intestine such as Crohn's disease, and in pneumococcal peritonitis. The reason for the elevation in the last two conditions is not clear.

Diastatic index of the urine is raised to 200 units or more in a large percentage of cases of acute pancreatitis. This test is as fallible as the serum amylase test.

Loewi's mydriatic test is a confirmatory sign which is applied easily. The pupils are examined : into one conjunctival sac 4 drops of fresh 1 in 1,000 adrenalin solution are instilled ; after five minutes 4 more drops are instilled, and the pupils examined again after half an hour. While adrenalin has no effect upon the pupil of a healthy individual, in acute pancreatitis a positive reaction—namely, dilatation of the pupil—is frequently obtained. The test is not uniformly reliable but is worth taking into consideration.

Serum Calcium.—Owing to the free fatty acids combining with the serum calcium to form soaps in the areas of fat necrosis, the amount of calcium in the blood is reduced. This reduction is not appreciable until about forty-eight hours after the commencement of the attack. Calcium gluconate should be administered to overcome the deficiency.

Glycosuria is present in only about 15 per cent. of cases of acute pancrea-

Otto Loewi, Contemporary. *Professor of Pharmacology (retd.), Graz.*

titis. It is of little diagnostic significance unless it is known that glycosuria was not present previously.

Discoloration of the skin is a rare manifestation of acute pancreatitis seen in cases of two or three days' standing. Grey Turner first described it in the loins, and likened it in appearance to that of late extravasation of urine. Other observers have described a similar discoloration around the umbilicus. The cause of the phenomenon is the action on the subcutaneous fat of pancreatic ferments that have escaped from the retroperitoneal tissues, either directly or via the round ligament of the liver.

TREATMENT

Delayed Treatment.—When the diagnosis of acute pancreatitis can be made with confidence, delayed treatment similar to that detailed in the chapter on peritonitis is becoming increasingly employed. Because of the difficulties in diagnosis, it is true that patients with milder symptoms than those of the ultra-acute type (acute pancreatitis varies considerably in intensity) tend to be selected for delayed treatment, but in centres where the delayed treatment is strongly advocated, a substantial proportion of ultra-acute cases are also treated expectantly. After a few hours of the treatment the condition of the patient must be re-assessed. If, as a result of gastric aspiration, intravenous saline and glucose and the administration of pethidine and atropine, the general condition improves and the pulse-rate falls, conservative measures are continued. When the intense pain does not abate, Alton Ochsner advocates splanchnic block. Penicillin is given to prevent infection of necrotic material and the exudate. If an abscess develops it is opened preferably, but not necessarily, by the posterior route, i.e. an incision is made beneath the right 12th rib and the finger burrows towards the head of the pancreas. Operation is subsequently required if, as sometimes happens, a pseudo-cyst of the pancreas becomes evident, in which case drainage of the lesser sac by the anterior route is employed. In most instances resolution occurs without these complications. During convalescence cholecystography is undertaken, and pre-operative and operative treatment similar to that of subacute pancreatitis is carried out three weeks after all symptoms have subsided. In cases where an abscess or a pseudo-cyst had to be drained, further operative measures should not be undertaken for at least three months.

Early Operative Treatment.—Some surgeons consider that, after saline infusion to correct the depleted fluid loss by vomiting, together with plasma infusion, if necessary, early laparotomy

G. Grey Turner, Contemporary. Emeritus Professor of Surgery, Post-graduate Medical School, London.
Alton Ochsner, Contemporary. Professor of Surgery, University of Tulane, New Orleans.

should be carried out. Laparotomy will also be required when doubt exists as to the diagnosis, i.e. when perforation of a peptic ulcer or high intestinal obstruction cannot be ruled out. When the abdomen is opened the diagnosis is clinched at once by the blood-stained exudate and fat necrosis. The pancreas is explored most readily by opening the lesser sac between the stomach and transverse colon (fig. 415). In a few cases, where there is ptosis of the stomach, the pancreas can be more conveniently exposed through the gastro-hepatic omentum.

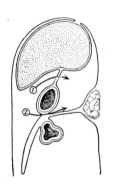

FIG. 415.—Routes of approach to the pancreas.
1. Through the gastro-hepatic omentum. (Rarely used.)
2. Between the stomach and the colon.

In most cases the operation should be limited to drainage of the lesser sac and of the general peritoneal cavity, and unless the condition of the patient is desperate, it is advisable to perform cholecystostomy or choledochostomy in addition. The abdominal wall should be closed with unabsorbable, preferably wire, sutures, which resist digestion by pancreatic ferments.

Post-operative Treatment.—As soon as the patient has been returned to bed, continuous intravenous saline or plasma infusion is continued as necessary. Continuous oxygen therapy is of value. The skin of the abdominal wall must be protected from excoriation by pancreatic ferments, as described on p. 427. Drainage should be maintained as long as the discharge continues.

SUBACUTE PANCREATITIS

gives rise to symptoms similar to those of acute cholecystitis ; indeed, in many instances the diagnosis is not made until laparotomy has been performed after the attack has subsided. So satisfactory is delayed treatment in these cases that it is generally conceded that this course should be followed. When the symptoms have abated the relevant investigations and the pre-operative treatment are identical with those of cholecystitis.

Laparotomy after Acute or Subacute Pancreatitis has Subsided.—On opening the abdomen it is likely that some evidence of fat necrosis will still be present, and the pancreas will feel enlarged.

Attention is directed to the gall-bladder. The course to be followed will vary according to whether the gall-bladder is thin-walled and comparatively normal, or thick-walled, fibrotic, and full of stones. Cholangiography is helpful in determining the presence of a stone in the common bile duct, and stricture or spasm of the ampulla of Vater. One method of treatment, only applicable when the gall-bladder is not thickened or fibrotic, is to perform cholecyst-duodenostomy or cholecyst-jejunostomy, with the object of by-passing the bile in the event of the ampulla being stenosed, or becoming so from fibrosis following the pancreatitis. When the gall-bladder is small, fibrotic, and full of calculi, cholecystectomy must be performed. This, together with removal of stones (if any) from the common bile duct, dilatation of the ampulla (if possible), followed by choledochostomy, is the usual method of treatment. More recently division of the mouth of the ampulla and its contained circular muscle fibres has been carried out. If a small bougie can be passed through the ampulla, a sphincterotome is then passed into the duodenum. The blade is opened, and the instrument retracted until it engages the papilla. The knife is closed, and the sphincterotome is withdrawn. In the absence of this special instrument, or when it cannot be passed into the duodenum, the ampulla is approached by the transduodenal route, and divided with sharp-pointed scissors. The duodenum is closed as described on p. 358 and the common bile duct is drained with a T-tube.

Chronic pancreatitis is a condition quite apart, and will be considered later.

PANCREATIC CALCULI

Stones in the pancreatic ducts are very infrequent. The symptoms are similar to those of chronic pancreatitis or of gall-stones. Pancreatic calculi have been demonstrated radiologically.

Treatment.—The stone, or stones, should be removed by an incision into the duct of Wirsung through the substance of the pancreas, or by slitting up Oddi's sphincter, according to circumstances. As the duct of Wirsung lies nearer the posterior than the anterior aspect of the gland, it is generally advised that the pancreas, together with the duodenum, should be mobilised and the duct approached from behind. After removal of the stone, the pancreas is sutured. After the pancreas has been incised, drainage is essential.

PANCREATIC CYSTS

True Pancreatic Cyst (fig. 416).—In 40 per cent. of cases a cyst of the pancreas is a true cyst, and falls into one of the following categories :

(a) *Retention cysts*, due to impaction of pancreatic calculi or fibrosis around the duct of Wirsung.

(b) *Cyst-adenomata.*—Most true cysts belong to this group.

Johann Wirsung. Prosector at Padua ; was murdered when entering his house at night in 1643.

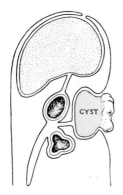

FIG. 416.—True pancreatic cyst.

(c) *Congenital Cystic Disease.*—Very rare indeed.

(d) *Fibro-cystic disease of the pancreas.*

(e) *Hydatid Cyst.*—The ubiquitous hydatid completes the list.

The cyst commences in the body or, less frequently, in the tail of the pancreas. Only in occasional cases is the head the seat of origin. The cyst, which is filled with watery brown fluid or mucoid material, is generally unilocular. It is lined by columnar or cubical epithelium, which tends to degenerate, and many of these cysts have a wall consisting mainly, if not entirely, of fibrous tissue. Most often the swelling comes to the surface between the stomach and the colon. Sometimes it protrudes between the stomach and the liver.

Clinical Features.—Epigastric discomfort and the presence of a swelling are the usual reasons that cause the patient to seek advice. On examination there is a swelling, sometimes a very large swelling, centrally placed above the umbilicus. The swelling is fixed, and in many instances it is so tense that fluctuation cannot be elicited. As a rule transmitted pulsation from the abdominal aorta is very noticeable, but the pulsation becomes less pronounced or ceases when the patient is examined in the knee-elbow position. In this way the possibility of the swelling being an aneurism of the abdominal aorta is eliminated. Its fixity distinguishes it from a mesenteric cyst, and the fact that it rarely, if ever, invades the pelvis usually rules out the possibility of the swelling being an ovarian cyst. A barium meal shows displacement of hollow viscera ; usually the stomach is displaced upwards and the transverse colon downwards (fig. 417). When the swelling arises in the tail of the pancreas it may be impossible to differentiate it from a hydronephrosis until pyelography has been performed. In those exceptional cases where the cyst arises in the head of the pancreas, the symptoms are identical with those of a choledochus cyst.

Treatment.—In exceptional circumstances the cyst can be removed by dissection. In most of the cases

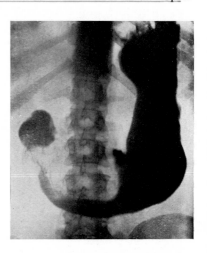

FIG. 417.—Pancreatic cyst causing gastric deformity.

when this has been possible the swelling proves to be a cystadenoma connected to the pancreas by a comparatively narrow neck, or it arises from the tail of the organ. The majority of very large thin-walled cysts are treated by marsupialisation of the peritoneum and parietes to the cyst wall (fig. 418) before opening the cyst. When the contents are evacuated the cavity is drained or packed with gauze. A sinus results which closes after a variable period. In some cases the contents of the cyst are rich in proteolytic ferment, and the skin around the resulting fistula requires constant attention to prevent excoriation. It is not possible to predict in a given case whether a pancreatic fistula and its attending evils will occur or not. On this account most authorities now recommend anastomosis of a thick-walled cyst to the jejunum in the following way : the contents of the cyst are evacuated. About 18 inches from its commencement the jejunum is divided. The distal end is closed and invaginated, and side-to-side anastomosis is carried out between it and the cyst wall. The proximal end of the divided jejunum is then implanted into the side of the distal jejunum below the anastomosis. This type of internal drainage prevents food entering the cyst.

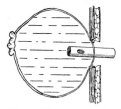

Fig. 418.—Marsupialisation of a pancreatic cyst.

Pseudo-pancreatic cyst (fig. 419), although rare, is more common than the foregoing, and accounts for 60 per cent. of all cases. In the majority of pseudo-pancreatic cysts the collection of fluid in the lesser sac is the result of an injury to the pancreas. More rarely it follows acute or subacute pancreatitis, and exceptionally it is the result of a minute perforation of a peptic ulcer situated on the posterior wall of the stomach. The condition commences as peritonitis limited to the lesser sac, the foramen of Winslow becoming occluded in the process, thus preventing involvement of the general peritoneal cavity.

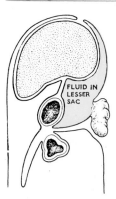

FLUID IN LESSER SAC

Fig. 419.—Pseudo-pancreatic cyst.

Clinical Features.—A supra-umbilical cystic swelling follows three or four days up to two or three weeks, and even longer, after an abdominal injury ; this is the typical history. As a rule, in traumatic cases, abdominal pain, frequent vomiting, and tenderness are in evidence when the patient comes under observation, although an interval of freedom from symptoms, sometimes lasting many days, has occurred since the blow. In other cases the swelling develops during the conservative treatment of acute or sub-acute pancreatitis. Exceptionally the patient is admitted with a pseudo-pancreatic cyst and gives a history of an attack of severe abdominal pain occurring a week or more previously.

Treatment.—The lesser sac should be drained, usually by an opening between the stomach and the colon. The skin around the wound requires protection from digestion by pancreatic ferments. This can be accomplished by painting it with aluminium paint or by applying kaolin in lanoline ointment. In the early post-operative period the discharge is best removed by suction. In favourable cases the wound heals in about six weeks, and remains healed. In a few the pancreatic fistula continues to discharge, or healing is followed by a further pseudo-pancreatic cyst, which has to be opened.

Congenital cystic disease of the pancreas sometimes accompanies congenital cystic disease of the kidney and liver.

Fibro-cystic disease of the pancreas is a rare disease of early childhood, and is characterised by cystic dilatation of the pancreatic ducts with increasing fibrosis of the acinar tissues. Concomitantly the bronchi and

Jacob Winslow, 1669–1760. A Dane who migrated to Paris, and there established a school of anatomy.

bronchioles are obstructed by thick tenacious mucus, which eventuates in bronchiectasis. The disease, which appears to be due to an autonomic imbalance of the nervous control of the secretory mechanism of the pancreas and of the pulmonary mucous glands, gives rise to symptoms of respiratory distress, the passage of bulky, pale, offensive stools, and severe nutritional deficiency. The condition is ultimately fatal. Remarkable, if temporary, improvement has followed right splanchnectomy. The indication for this operation is as follows : in fibro-cystic disease of the pancreas the duodenal contents aspirated through a duodenal tube show an absence of trypsin. A splanchnic block is performed, and duodenal aspiration again carried out. Should trypsin be found in the aspirated material, it is indicative that splanchnectomy will prove of benefit.

PANCREATIC FISTULA

The quantity and composition of the discharge varies very considerably. As to quantity, in many cases the amount is only a few ounces daily ; in others it is as much as two litres in the twenty-four hours. Such a loss of fluid and electrolytes, unless counterbalanced, is a menace to life. As a rule the fluid is charged with active ferments, and full precautions must be taken to prevent auto-digestion of the abdominal wall. The exception is the discharge following marsupialisation of a true pancreatic cyst, when a thin mucoid fluid, which is no doubt derived from epithelial remnants lining the walls of the cyst, drains without excoriating the skin or without any detriment to nutrition.

Treatment.—When the leakage is watery and profuse, the juice should be removed by continuous suction through a catheter attached to an electric pump, and methods to protect the skin of the abdominal wall, as have been described already in the section on Pseudo-Pancreatic Cyst, are instituted. Returning the fluid aspirated from the fistula to the patient via a transnasal intragastric tube should be tried. If this method causes nausea and vomiting, the fluid imbalance must be maintained by intravenous saline and glucose. Plasma infusion or blood transfusion may be necessary. In most cases there is a gradual lessening of the amount of leakage. Among the methods recommended for hastening closure are a protein-free diet ; conversely other authorities advise a high protein and fat diet. Still others have had success by affording complete alimentary rest, nutrition being maintained parenterally with intravenous saline and glucose, together with the administration of protein hydrolysate intravenously, for as long as seventeen days. Conservative treatment is usually successful, although it is sometimes protracted.

In a few instances a long-standing fistula with a fibrous wall has been cured by dissecting it, together with a margin of skin from the abdominal wall past the level of the peritoneum, and implanting the mouth of the fistula into a loop of jejunum.

CHRONIC PANCREATITIS

Chronic pancreatitis is not an uncommon disease, but the symptoms are obscure, and the diagnosis is always fraught with considerable difficulty. The inflammation is sometimes limited to the head of the pancreas. At others the whole organ is involved. There are three clinical types of chronic pancreatitis :

Type 1. *Associated with Cholecystitis.*—This is the commonest type, and sometimes attention is first drawn to it after the gall-bladder has been removed and the symptoms still persist.

Type 2. *Associated with Obstruction of the Common Bile Duct.*—A chronically inflamed and probably fibrotic head of the pancreas causes constriction of the common bile duct near its termination. Jaundice is a leading symptom.

Type 3. *Chronic relapsing* (syn. *calcareous*) *pancreatitis* may be an end result of Type 1. The whole of the excretory mechanism tends to be replaced by fibrous tissue. Occasionally the islets of Langerhans are also implicated, and diabetes results. Calcification occurs in fibrous replacement, and the whole of the organ may become calcareous.

Clinical Features.—There are no pathognomonic symptoms or signs of chronic pancreatitis. Because of its inaccessible situation, it is exceedingly unlikely that the chronically inflamed pancreas will be felt on palpation.

In the first type the symptoms are often overshadowed by those of the concomitant cholecystitis, but laboratory tests for pancreatic insufficiency may be positive. These include :

1. *An excess of free starch in the stool.*
2. *Azotorrhœa.*—There are many unaltered striated muscle fibres in the fæces. When positive, this is the most reliable of these tests.
3. *Steatorrhœa.*—The normal fat content of the fæces is about 20 per cent., but in chronic pancreatitis it may rise to between 50 per cent. and 90 per cent. This is present only in late cases.
4. *The diastatic index of the urine* may be increased.
5. *The serum amylase* may be increased. If the blood amylase rises during attacks of pain, it is said to be very suggestive that the attacks are due to chronic pancreatitis rather than to biliary colic.
6. *The absence of pancreatic ferments in the duodenal test meal* is confirmatory evidence of obstruction of the pancreatic duct or to dysfunction of the gland.
7. *Glycosuria and a lessened sugar tolerance* occurs only late in the course of that type of the disease which affects the whole organ.

In the second type, laparotomy must be performed in order to differentiate this condition from carcinoma of the head of the pancreas. Even then the differentiation of the two conditions is often extremely difficult. Methods which are employed to establish this all-important differential diagnosis are described later.

In the third type, at first the pain is severe and recurring. As the disease progresses the pain often becomes constant and intolerable. Although by the time this stage has been reached wasting, anæmia, and signs of pancreatic insufficiency will be in evidence, pain is the dominant feature. An X-ray may show that the gland is calcareous.

Treatment : *Type* 1.—When chronic pancreatitis is diagnosed preoperatively, or if it is strongly suspected at laparotomy for chronic cholecystitis, provided the gall-bladder is even moderately

Ernst Langerhans, 1847–1888. Professor of Pathology, Freiburg.

healthy, it should be preserved.   Cholangiography, by showing
constriction of the intrapancreatic portion of the common bile
duct and poor discharge of the medium into the duodenum, helps
to confirm the diagnosis.   After emptying the gall-bladder and
removing the stones (if any), the common bile duct should be
opened, and if there are any stones within it, they are removed.
The common bile duct is drained by a T-tube and cholecyst-
duodenostomy or cholecyst-jejunostomy is carried out.   Many
favour the last procedure if it is performed in the manner
described for the internal drainage of a pancreatic cyst (p. 369).

When the gall-bladder is small and fibrotic, which is unusual
in cases of chronic pancreatitis, cholecystectomy with drainage
of the common bile duct is usually performed.   Prolonged drainage of the common bile duct sometimes results in resolution of
chronic pancreatitis, but relapses are liable to occur.   Most
often the abdomen is reopened because of attacks of pain similar to those produced by a stone in the common bile duct.   In
such circumstances further drainage of the common bile duct
affords relief of the pain, but to prevent repetition of this train of
events more radical measures are necessary.   In this type of
case reconstruction of the common bile duct (p. 360) will probably remedy the condition.

Type 2.—On laparotomy in a jaundiced patient the difficult
differential diagnosis between an operable carcinoma of the head
of the pancreas and chronic pancreatitis can sometimes be settled
by cholangiography ; an abrupt complete blockage of the end
of the common bile duct supports the diagnosis of carcinoma.
In other circumstances mobilising the duodenum and the head
of the pancreas permits the latter to be palpated thoroughly, and
a pancreatic calculus or a growth in the neighbourhood of the
ampulla of Vater may be felt.   A frozen section of a small wedge
of the head of the pancreas, if it is positive for carcinoma, settles
the diagnosis.   If the section shows chronic pancreatitis, this
does not rule out an early growth in the periampullary region.
Removal of a small piece of the head of the pancreas for biopsy
is followed by considerable hæmorrhage, which can be controlled
by sutures.   In cases where a diagnosis of chronic pancreatitis
can be made with assurance, some form of internal drainage of
the gall-bladder is followed by a long survival and freedom from
symptoms.

Type 3.—Thoraco-lumbar sympathectomy for the relief of pain has been carried out with success. The only alternative measure is total pancreatectomy.

NEOPLASMS

Islet-celled tumours are most often adenomata arising in the islets of Langerhans. Rarely are they carcinomata. Islet-celled tumours are usually single, although in 10 per cent. of cases two or more of them are present. They are greyish-white or pink in colour, and rarely exceed more than a few millimetres in diameter. They are smoother and firmer than normal pancreatic tissue, and are commonly situated towards the tail of the pancreas, but the head of the organ is not exempt. Consequently, when the pancreas is explored for a suspected adenoma, not only should the tail and body of the organ be palpated thoroughly, but the duodenum should be mobilised so that the head of the pancreas can be palpated between the finger and thumb.

Clinical Features.—The patient, usually a woman over forty years of age, suddenly complains of dizziness, often faints, and sometimes becomes maniacal. The attacks become increasingly frequent, and occur most often in the early morning or when the patient has been without food for some time. These symptoms are analogous with those found in insulin overdosage (hyperinsulinism) and are due to hypoglycæmia. Attacks can be provoked by a very small dose of insulin, or by exercising after fasting. Glucose alleviates the symptoms quickly. The patient is usually found to have a persistently low blood-sugar, 50 mg. per cent. or less. In all cases the blood-sugar is very low during and immediately after the attacks. Attacks of " insulin shock," the finding of a blood-sugar of 50 mg. per cent. or less, and the prompt relief of symptoms by the ingestion of glucose, constitute what is known as Whipple's triad.

Treatment.—If other causes of hypoglycæmia can be excluded, exploration of the pancreas should be undertaken. A transverse upper abdominal incision gives good access to the whole pancreas, which must be palpated systematically in the manner described already. The organ is approached through the gastrocolic omentum. When a tumour has been found, it is enucleated. The bed is closed by sutures. In cases where a tumour cannot be felt, the tail and the body of the pancreas as far as the crossing of the superior mesenteric vessels is resected, in the hope that the tumour will be found in the excised portion of the gland. Resection of the body of the pancreas is facilitated by splenectomy. When the splenic vessels which supply the body and tail of the pancreas are ligated, hæmorrhage from the pancreas is more readily controlled. Sometimes the adenoma is only found on serial section of the excised specimen. At others no tumour is found, but the patient is relieved of the symptoms. It is possible, therefore, that hyperplasia of the islets of Langerhans gives rise to these symptoms. Persistence of blood-sugar below 50 mg. per cent. after operation is very suggestive that an adenoma has been overlooked, and it has sometimes been discovered at a second operation.

CARCINOMA OF THE PANCREAS

Clinically, carcinoma of the pancreas can be divided into two varieties—carcinoma of the body and tail, and carcinoma of the head.

Carcinoma of the Body and Tail.—When the growth commences

Allen Oldfather Whipple, Contemporary. Professor of Surgery, Columbia University, New York City.

in the body, as it does in about 3 per cent. of cases, or in the tail, which is very rare, the carcinoma is spheroidal-celled, often of the scirrhous variety, but sometimes encephaloid. In these situations symptoms are insidious, and generally resemble those of carcinoma of the stomach. Often by the time the patient seeks relief, metastases have occurred in the retroperitoneal lymph nodes and the liver. In the minority of patients violent pain passing through to the back, due to involvement of the cœliac plexus, is the leading feature. When laparotomy is performed early, and the growth is situated towards the tail of the organ, it can be resected with comparative ease and some lasting cures have been reported.

Carcinoma of the Head of the Pancreas.—In two-thirds of all cases of carcinoma of the pancreas the growth is situated in the head of the organ, and it never attains the size of a fist ; rarely is it more than a quarter of this size. The leading features of a neoplasm in this situation are due to obstruction to the common bile duct by the growth. Most often the carcinoma arises in the acini and is spheroidal-celled. Typically it gives rise to the following symptoms and signs :

Previous History.—Often there is no previous history of indigestion or attacks of biliary colic.

Jaundice, steadily progressing, is the leading symptom. The icteric tinge becomes deeper and deeper until, at last, the skin and conjunctivæ assume an almost mahogany shade. It should be noted that in over 50 per cent. of cases of carcinoma of the head of the pancreas jaundice precedes the pain.

Pain is variable and is often of a dull, boring character.

The temperature is normal.

The stools become clay-coloured, and often remain so.

Wasting occurs, but this is not diagnostic, for patients with a stone impacted in the common bile duct also waste rapidly.

Courvoisier's law states that if in a jaundiced patient the gall-bladder is enlarged, it is *not* a case of stone impacted in the common bile duct, for previous cholecystitis must have rendered the gall-bladder fibrotic. There are several exceptions to this law, notably (*a*) double impaction, when there is one stone in the cystic and another in the common bile duct, (*b*) transmitted pressure of a stone in the cystic duct compressing the common hepatic duct, and (*c*) a pancreatic calculus causing obturation at the ampulla of Vater.

Periampullary Carcinoma.—In about one-third of the cases the neoplasm is columnar-celled and arises in the ampulla of Vater,

Ludwig T. Courvoisier, 1843–1918. Professor of Surgery, Basle.

in the termination of the pancreatic ducts, or in the duodenal mucosa adjacent to the ampulla. Even when an operation specimen is examined, or at necropsy, it is often impossible to decide which of these structures was the seat of origin. They are, therefore, conveniently grouped together under the term " periampullary carcinoma." While at the commencement of the disease the symptoms conform to type, in a matter of about a month, due, it is believed, to necrosis of a portion of the growth, the pent-up bile escapes into the duodenum. Consequently the jaundice becomes variable, the stools become coloured, and there may be melæna from the bleeding growth. Moreover, pyrexia from infection of the necrotic growth and consequent cholangitis heightens the similarity of the symptoms of this form of neoplasm to obstruction of the common bile duct by a gall-stone. In periampullary carcinoma a barium meal may reveal a filling defect in the second part of the duodenum, and blood is likely to be present in a duodenal test meal. Cases of periampullary carcinoma of the pancreas submitted to radical operation offer a better prognosis than the more usual variety of carcinoma of the head of the pancreas.

When any case of carcinoma of the head of the pancreas becomes advanced, obstruction to the portal vein, with accompanying ascites, is liable to occur. Obstruction of the inferior vena cava, followed by cyanotic œdema of the lower extremities, may complicate the terminal phase of the disease.

Differential Diagnosis.—As may be inferred from the foregoing description, the differential diagnosis between stone impacted in the common bile duct, carcinoma of the head of the pancreas, and infective hepatitis is extremely difficult in atypical cases. Laboratory tests which are designed to help in the differential diagnosis are numerous, and most of them, while providing assistance in early cases, fail to do so in late cases because by that time hepatitis is often superimposed on obstructive jaundice due either to carcinoma of the head of the pancreas or a stone impacted in the common bile duct.

The Van den Bergh Reaction.—Bilirubin which has been resorbed from the bile passages after being excreted by the liver differs from that which has not passed through the liver. The former gives immediate violet coloration with Erlich's diazo reagent. This constitutes a positive direct reaction. Bilirubin which has not passed through the liver gives the reaction only after a considerable delay, or after the addition of alcohol. This is

A. A. Hymans van den Bergh, Contemporary. Professor of Medicine, University of Utrecht.
Paul Ehrlich, 1854–1915. Bacteriologist, Director of the Institute for Experimental Therapy,
    Frankfurt on Main.

an indirect reaction. In early cases of obstructive jaundice the positive direct reaction is helpful in distinguishing the jaundice from that produced by infective hepatitis.

Urobilinogen in the Urine.—If the liver function is damaged, the amount of urobilinogen in the urine rises greatly. In early cases of obstructive jaundice it is normal or raised very little, but in infective hepatitis it is present in excessive amounts.

Serum alkaline phosphatase and thymol tests are also of value in distinguishing obstructive from non-obstructive jaundice (see p. 330). Thus obstructive cases usually have high phosphatase values and negative thymol tests, whereas in hepatitis the findings are exactly opposite.

There remain cases in which the diagnosis cannot be settled unless laparotomy is performed. If the liver function tests are adequate and the patient is prepared with a high glucose intake and vitamin K injections, laparotomy may prove that the condition is remediable.

Treatment.—When the patient is deeply jaundiced and the liver function is poor, preliminary cholecystostomy is performed through a small incision, with a view to improving the patient's general condition. In other circumstances laparotomy is performed, a blood transfusion being given and continued throughout the operation.

When the growth is inoperable as shown by secondary deposits, cholecyst-duodenostomy or cholecyst-jejunostomy, according to preference, is carried out. Either of these measures afford relief to the obstructed common bile duct. The jaundice disappears gradually, but within a few days there is complete relief of the accompanying pruritus.

When the pathological process is limited to the head of the pancreas doubt may arise as to whether the condition is due to carcinoma or to chronic pancreatitis. A fibrotic mass in the head of the pancreas, due to chronic pancreatitis, may simulate exactly a scirrhous carcinoma. Methods available for determining this differential diagnosis have been discussed on p. 372.

Excision of the Head of the Pancreas.—The whole of the duodenum is mobilised as far as the crossing of the superior mesenteric vessels. The pylorus is freed and the right gastro-epiploic and superior pancreatico-duodenal vessels are ligated. The stomach is divided between clamps just proximal to the pylorus. The third part of the duodenum is divided between clamps close to the crossing of the superior mesenteric vessels. The distal end of the duodenum is closed and invaginated. Attention is directed to the common bile duct, which is freed by dissection from the portal vein, and the dissection is carried as far as possible behind the first part of the duodenum, where the common bile duct is temporarily clamped and divided above the growth. Dissection of the head of the pancreas from the retroperitoneal tissues permits access to the posterior surface of the head of the pancreas. The most exacting part of the operation—freeing the superior mesenteric vessels from the uncinate process and from the groove in the back of the neck of the pancreas in which they lie—is commenced from below. The inferior pancreatico-duodenal artery is ligated and a number of veins issuing from the pancreas to join the superior mesenteric vein must be ligated and divided. Once the superior mesenteric vein is freed from the pancreas and followed to its termination in the portal vein, there remains only to dissect the uncinate process of the pancreas from its connective tissue attachment to the inferior vena cava, and the head of the pancreas is ready for resection through its neck. Reconstruction of the parts left by this ablation is now undertaken. A loop of the commencement of the jejunum is drawn up in front of the transverse colon. Into the apex of the loop the common bile duct, previously temporarily clamped, is implanted with fine sutures. The cut surface of the pancreas is treated in one of two ways: (*a*) the dilated main duct is ligated and the raw surface is oversewn; (*b*) the whole thickness of the cut surface of the neck of the pancreas is implanted into the jejunum.

Controversy is centred around the better method of dealing with the stump of the pancreas. Implantation of it into the jejunum is difficult because the capsule of the pancreas is thin and does not hold sutures well, but advocates of the method state that the incidence of serious pancreatic fistula is less than when the duct of Wirsung is ligated and the raw surface is oversewn. Finally, the cut edge of the stomach is anastomosed to the side wall of the jejunum (fig. 420). The abdominal wall is closed with wire

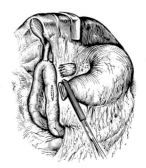

Fig. 420.—Reconstruction after a one-stage operation for excision of the head of the pancreas. The neck of the pancreas is oversewn. Alternatively, the neck of the pancreas is implanted into the side of the jejunum.

sutures, and drainage is provided. Transfusion of blood should be continued after the operation, as necessary, and vitamin-K injections continued for several days.

The operation of excision of the head of the pancreas has been undertaken in stages. Among other procedures cholecyst-jejunostomy and gastro-jejunostomy have constituted the first stage, but most surgeons now favour the one-stage operation described above.

The mortality of this extensive operation is probably about 15 per cent. The complications are principally those of leakage from the pancreas or the common bile duct anastomosis.

CHAPTER XX

THE PERITONEUM, OMENTUM, MESENTERY, AND RETROPERITONEAL SPACE

ACUTE PERITONITIS

NEARLY all varieties of peritonitis are due to an invasion of the peritoneal cavity by bacteria. To such an extent is this true, that when the term " peritonitis " is used without qualification, bacterial peritonitis is implied.

Paths of Bacterial Invasion.—1. Via perforation of some part of the gastro-intestinal track.

2. Extension of the inflammation from an inflamed intra-peritoneal organ, e.g. appendicitis, cholecystitis.

3. By transmigration through damaged gut wall, e.g. un-relieved intestinal obstruction.

4. From or via the Fallopian tubes.

5. Through a penetrating wound of the abdominal wall.

6. Hæmatogenous infection.

7. Post-operative.

Even in non-bacterial peritonitis (e.g. intraperitoneal rupture of the bladder or a hæmoperitoneum) the peritoneum becomes infected by trans-migration of organisms from the bowel, and so what may be termed mechanical or chemical peritonitis becomes a peritonitis in the usual sense of the term.

Bacteriology is very variable, and accounts to a large extent for the mildness or virulence of the peritonitis. Aerobes (B. coli, streptococci, B. proteus, and B. pyocyaneus) and anaerobes (Cl. welchii) are among the main causative organisms. The infection is frequently mixed, and the B. coli is the predominating organism. The most virulent forms of peritonitis are due to hæmolytic streptococci and Cl. welchii. Gonococcal and pneumococcal peritonitis constitute distinct clinical entities.

Factors which favour localisation of peritonitis are anatomical and pathological.

Anatomical.—Excluding the subphrenic spaces, which will be considered later, the greater sac of the peritoneum is divided into (*a*) the pelvis and (*b*) the peritoneal cavity proper. The latter is re-divided into a supracolic and an infracolic compart-

Gabriello Fallopio, 1523–1562. Anatomist and Professor of Surgery, University of Pisa.

ment by the transverse colon and transverse mesocolon, which deters the spread of infection from the former to the latter. The lower abdomen is divided into a right and a left compartment by the mesentery and the bodies of the vertebræ, which hinders the passage of infection from one side to the other, but both compartments communicate freely with the pelvis. When the supracolic compartment overflows, as is often the case when a peptic ulcer perforates, it does so over the colon into the right supracolic compartment, and so, by way of the right paracolic gutter, to the right iliac fossa, and thence to the pelvis.

Pathological.—Inflamed peritoneum loses its glistening appearance and becomes reddened and velvety. Flakes of fibrin appear and cause coils of intestine to become adherent with one another and to the parietes. There is an outpouring of serous fluid rich in leucocytes and antibodies, which soon becomes turbid, and if localisation occurs the fluid becomes frank pus. Peristalsis is retarded in affected coils, and this helps in preventing distribution of the infection to other coils. The greater omentum, by enveloping and becoming adherent to inflamed structures, often forms a substantial barrier to the spread of infection.

Factors which tend to cause diffusion of peritonitis are as follows :

(*a*) The virulence of the infecting organism may be so great as to make the localisation of the infection difficult or impossible.

(*b*) An inflamed appendix, or other hollow viscus, perforates before the natural defences set out above have had time to come into action.

(*c*) A considerable area of chemical peritonitis (due to the escape of gastric or duodenal contents) upon which a bacterial infection is superadded, is unlikely to remain localised unless the perforation is a small one and has become sealed—a relatively infrequent happening.

(*d*) Violent peristalsis occasioned by the administration of a purgative or an enema often causes a widespread distribution of a previously localised infection. The ingestion of food, or even water, by stimulating peristaltic action, hinders localisation.

CLINICAL FEATURES

Localised peritonitis is intimately bound up with the causative lesion, e.g. acute appendicitis, acute cholecystitis, acute diverticulitis, and the initial symptoms and signs are those of the lesion. When infection spreads from an inflamed viscus to the neighbouring peritoneum, provided conditions are favourable, the process of walling-off from the general peritoneal cavity by adhesions occurs. On this account localisation is unlikely until at least twenty-four hours have elapsed since the commencement of the attack. When the peritoneum becomes inflamed the temperature, and especially the pulse-rate, rise. The pain increases and usually there is repeated vomiting. The most important sign is rigidity of the abdominal wall over the quadrants of the abdomen which is involved. In cases of pelvic peritonitis arising from an inflamed appendix in the pelvic position, the abdominal signs are often slight, deep tenderness of one or both lower quadrant alone being present, but a rectal or vaginal examination reveals tenderness of the pelvic peritoneum. With appropriate treatment localised peritonitis usually resolves. In about 20 per cent. of cases an abscess follows. Infrequently, localised peritonitis becomes diffuse. Conversely, in favourable circumstances diffuse peritonitis can become localised, most frequently in the pelvis.

Diffuse (syn. Generalised) Peritonitis.—The most obvious example is that caused by perforation of a peptic ulcer. In this instance the onset of symptoms is followed in a matter of minutes by widespread board-like abdominal rigidity. The commonest cause of diffuse peritonitis is gangrene or perforation of an inflamed appendix occurring within twenty-four hours of the attack, that is before there has been time for the infection to become walled-off from the general peritoneal cavity. Diffuse peritonitis from any cause may be divided into three stages :

1. *Early.*—This is the stage of diffusing or spreading peritonitis. Pain, which was limited to one quadrant of the abdomen, becomes more widespread ; the exception to this rule is post-operative peritonitis, in which pain is almost absent. Vomiting becomes very frequent, bile-stained, and often effortless. The patient lies supine, with his knees flexed. The temperature is usually raised, but in fulminating cases it may be subnormal. The pulse-rate is elevated. A rising pulse-rate, as shown by a two-hourly or, in very acute cases, a one-hourly pulse-chart, is an indication that the peritonitis is failing to resolve. On examination the tongue is moist and the face some-

what flushed. Inspection of the abdomen shows that there is little or no respiratory movement of the abdominal wall. Palpation reveals widespread abdominal rigidity. On auscultation of the abdomen no sound of peristalsis can be heard.

2. *Intermediate.*—The third day is the critical one in diffuse peritonitis. In cases where a favourable outcome can be confidently expected, the pulse-rate ceases to rise, or commences to fall. The temperature, which may have been normal or subnormal, rises and less fluid is withdrawn on gastric aspiration. If the inflammation is not subsiding, the pulse-rate continues to rise. The rigidity to some extent passes off, and gives place to distension. The whole abdomen is acutely tender. The amount of fluid removed by gastric aspiration increases, and becomes fæculent. Even after an enema, little or no flatus is passed.

3. *Late Stage.*—On the fourth or fifth day the patient's condition becomes extremely grave. The whole abdomen is grossly distended. The pulse becomes thready and rapid. The eyes are sunken but bright, the nose is pinched, the lips are dry, the forehead is clammy, and the facies drawn and anxious (Hippocratic facies).

TREATMENT

Early Operative Treatment.—After adequate preparation by measures detailed under conservative treatment, early operation is indicated in cases of perforation of any hollow viscus and in peritonitis due to an inflamed appendix of under forty-eight hours' duration. If it is decided that operation is necessary, an injection of morphia or one of its derivatives is administered intravenously while the preoperative measures are carried out. In this group of cases early operation, by preventing further extravasation of infected material or by extirpating the focus of infection, usually results in rapid resolution of the inflammation. Post-operative treatment includes chemotherapy and many of the measures included under conservative treatment.

Drainage is not required in many cases of early infection of the peritoneum. After dealing with the primary focus, purulent exudate is removed by aspiration or by gentle mopping and the abdomen is closed. Apart from drainage of residual abscesses, which will be considered later, drainage of the peritoneal cavity is recommended in the following circumstances :

Suprapubic drainage by a tube passed into the pelvis through

Hippocrates, by common consent the Father of Medicine, was born in the Island of Cos about 460 B.C.

a stab incision in the middle line above the pubis is advised :

1. After suture of a perforated peptic ulcer when there is considerable extravasation of fluid and more than six hours has elapsed from the time of perforation.

2. After appendicectomy in cases of peritonitis due to perforated obstructive appendicitis.

3. In the uncommon cases of diffuse peritonitis due to perforation of the small or large intestine, or to perforation of an infected gall-bladder or bile duct.

Drainage through the flank is especially called for when retroperitoneal tissues are infected, as is often the case in gangrenous retrocæcal appendicitis.

A suprapubic drainage tube is usually turned on the second day, and removed on the third day. A drainage tube in the flank, if a considerable amount of pus is being discharged, should be left in place for upwards of five days.

Conservative treatment is indicated :

1. In any case of diffuse peritonitis where the general condition is poor.

2. In localised peritonitis due to cholecystitis.

3. In most cases of peritonitis due to appendicitis of over forty-eight hours' duration.

4. In peritonitis due to salpingitis.

5. In pneumococcal peritonitis.

In cases where conservative measures are employed, there is usually a decided improvement within six hours, which is maintained. Patients undergoing this form of treatment require careful watching and repeated examination. Operation is required when the response to the treatment is not wholly satisfactory, or in cases of non-resolution of a local abscess.

Posture.—High Fowler's position is not now considered advisable. Most surgeons, however, favour a modified Fowler's position, whereby the patient is propped up with pillows, with a soft pillow under the knees and with the head of the bed raised on six-inch blocks (fig. 421). Frequent changes of posture are advisable, the patient being encouraged to adopt the position of greatest ease. These modifications discourage the development of phlebothrombosis decubiti, and they also facilitate respiration.

Albert John Ochsner, 1858–1925. Surgeon, Augustana Hospital, Chicago, formulated the conservative treatment of late cases of diffuse peritonitis.
George Ryerson Fowler, 1848–1906. Professor of Surgery, New York Polyclinic School.

FIG. 421.—The bulwarks of the conservative and post-operative treatment of peritonitis : (1) Modified Fowler's position. (2) Intranasal gastric aspiration. (3) Continuous intravenous saline. (4) Charts : (a) Two-hourly pulse and temperature chart. (b) Fluid intake and output chart. (c) Sulphonamide or penicillin chart.

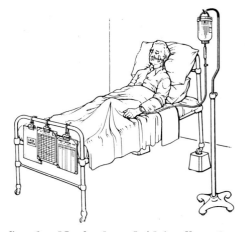

Rest to the Alimentary Canal.—No food or fluid is allowed to be ingested until the inflammation has subsided, as indicated by a fall of the pulse-rate to the eighties and a corresponding fall in the temperature. The bowels are left confined, unless they are opened naturally ; enemata are not given until the acute stage is over, but a flatus tube is passed. There should be no vomiting or potential vomiting (i.e. material withdrawn by the intranasal gastric tube) for forty-eight hours before fluids are allowed by mouth, and the bowels should have acted before even milky foods are commenced. Usually these criteria are reached by the fourth day, but in severe cases it may be the fifth or sixth day.

Gastric aspiration by a Ryle's tube, preferably passed transnasally, is commenced and continued as long as bile or intestinal contents is withdrawn. With the tube in place the patient is allowed to drink, provided the fluid is aspirated promptly. In this way the stomach is washed out. If, after the tube has been withdrawn, vomiting recommences, or the patient hiccups, the tube must be reinserted. Especially when the tube is not in place, frequent mouth-washes are given.

Intravenous saline and glucose is administered by the drip method at the rate of forty drops a minute. In cases of severe peritonitis associated with paralytic ileus, when the intravenous route is the only one by which the patient can receive nourishment for several days, the addition of a preparation of amino acids for intravenous administration is valuable in maintaining the patient's strength.

Chloride depletion is apt to occur as a result of vomiting,

John Alfred Ryle, 1889–1950. Professor of Social Medicine, University of Oxford.

gastric suction, sweating, or discharges, and correction of excessive loss is necessary for efficient metabolism.

The Fantus test is easily performed and indicates the amount of chloride
which is being excreted. Ten drops of acidified urine are placed in a test
tube and mixed with one drop of 20 per cent. potassium chromate. Silver
nitrate solution (2·9 per cent.) is added drop by drop until a permanent red
colour is obtained. The number of drops of silver nitrate represents the
amount in grammes of sodium chloride in a litre of urine (normally 3 gm.).

Charts.—A two-hourly pulse-rate chart is recorded graphic-
ally. In anxious cases, when the advisability of operation is un-
decided, a one-hourly chart is compiled. The temperature is
recorded every four hours. No less important is an intake and
output chart, which must be kept for as long as the patient is
receiving fluids intravenously.

Sedative Drugs.—While the patient is being watched to determine if there is a favourable response to conservative measures,
morphia and its derivatives should be withheld. Once it has
been decided to treat the case conservatively, morphia grain
$\frac{1}{4}$ (16 mg.) or omnopon grain $\frac{1}{3}$ (20 mg.) is given subcutaneously,
or half that dose intravenously.

Chemotherapy is given via the intravenous drip, or intramuscularly when the intravenous drip has been discontinued.

1. **Penicillin,** 50,000 units, three-hourly.

2. **Sulphonamide** in a soluble form is given, 2 gm. initially
followed by 1 gm. four-hourly until a total of 30 gm. has been
given. This dosage maintains the blood-level of the sulphonamide at 6 to 8 mg. per 100 ml., which is the most effective
concentration without being dangerous.

3. **Streptomycin** or other antibiotics can be given in addition
to the above.

In severe cases all three bactericides should be given. The
most generally used is a combination of the first two.

Local heat is applied to the abdomen, if the patient finds it
comforting. The best means is by an electrically heated pad ;
failing this, a hot-water bottle is employed.

The conservative treatment is considered at some length in
relation to late cases of appendicitis (p. 498).

COMPLICATIONS OF PERITONITIS

All the complications of a severe bacterial infection are possible,
but the special complications of peritonitis are as follows :

1. Intestinal obstruction (see p. 468).

Bernard Fantus, Contemporary. Director of Therapeutics, Cook County Hospital, Chicago.

2. Paralytic ileus (see p. 475).

3. Residual abscesses.

Abscess formation following local or diffuse peritonitis usually occupies one of the situations shown in fig. 422. When palpable, an intraperitoneal abscess should be treated by marking out its limitations on the abdominal wall, and careful daily examination. If the abscess is getting larger or fails to resolve, it should be opened, when possible by an extraperitoneal incision. The incision is made on the lateral side of the swelling. The layers of the abdominal wall are divided until the peritoneum is

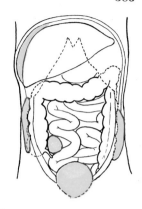

FIG. 422. — Common situations for residual abscesses.

reached. With the finger, the extraperitoneal tissues are separated gently from the peritoneum, until the abscess is opened. In the case of an abscess in either paracolic gutter, a counter incision in the loin is made to accommodate a drainage tube. The layers of the original incision are approximated and corrugated drainage to the wound is provided.

PELVIC ABSCESS

is common, because the vermiform appendix is commonly pelvic in position and also because the Fallopian tubes are a frequent focus of infection. A pelvic abscess can also occur as a sequel to any case of diffuse peritonitis. Pus can accumulate in this area without serious constitutional disturbance, and unless the patient has been carefully examined from day to day, such abscesses may attain considerable proportions before being recognised. The most characteristic symptoms of a pelvic abscess are diarrhœa and the passage of mucus in the stools. It is no exaggeration to say that the *passage of mucus, occurring for the first time in a patient who*

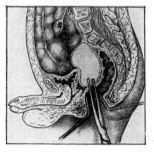

has, or is recovering from, peritonitis, is pathognomonic of pelvic abscess. Rectal examination reveals a bulging of the anterior rectal wall which, when the abscess is ripe, becomes softly cystic. It is inaccurate to say that it fluctuates, unless fluctuation can be elicited between it and the abdominal wall. Fluctuation cannot be tested with one finger. Left to Nature, a proportion of these abscesses burst into the rectum, after which the patient nearly always recovers rapidly. It is too hazardous to wait for this possible happy termination. A pelvic abscess should be drained deliberately. In certain cases, notably those where the primary focus is

FIG. 423.—Opening a pelvic abscess into the rectum.

in the Fallopian tubes, vaginal drainage through the posterior fornix is chosen. In other cases, where the abscess is definitely pointing into the rectum, rectal drainage (fig. 423) is employed. If any uncertainty exists as to the presence of pus, an aspirating needle introduced through the rectal wall into the bulging swelling will settle the question. Drainage of a pelvic abscess into the rectum is exceedingly efficacious in selected cases, but occasionally, in the case of a large abscess which can be palpated above the pubes, lower laparotomy should be undertaken in order to be quite certain of the diagnosis. Provided the abscess is shut off from the general peritoneal cavity, a point which can be ascertained undeniably when the abdomen has been opened, rectal drainage of a pelvic abscess is preferable to suprapubic drainage, which in many cases unavoidably breaks down Nature's barriers, and exposes the general peritoneal cavity to the dangers of spreading infection.

SUBPHRENIC ABSCESS

Anatomy.—The complicated arrangement of the peritoneum results in the formation of seven spaces in which pus may collect. Three of these spaces are on either side of the body, and one approximately in the midline (fig. 424).

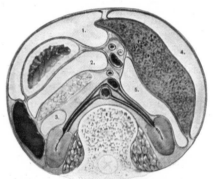

FIG. 424.—Anatomical relationships of five types of subphrenic abscess. 1. Left anterior intraperitoneal; 2. Left posterior intraperitoneal; 3. Left extraperitoneal; 4. Right anterior intraperitoneal; 5. Right posterior intraperitoneal.

Left Side.—*Anterior intraperitoneal,* bounded above by the diaphragm, behind by the left lateral ligament and left lobe of the liver, the gastro-hepatic omentum and anterior surface of the stomach. To the right is the falciform ligament, and to the left the spleen, gastro-splenic omentum, and diaphragm.

Posterior intraperitoneal, which is the upper part of the lesser sac (or omental bursa). Consequently, it is bounded behind by the diaphragm, pancreas, mesocolon, and transverse colon, in front by the Spiegelian lobe, gastro-hepatic omentum, and stomach, and to the left by the lieno-renal ligament, spleen, and gastro-splenic omentum. On the right side is the duodenum, above which is the foramen of Winslow.

Extraperitoneal, which is normally only a potential space. When an abscess forms, pus collects near the upper pole of the left kidney, and strips the peritoneum off the diaphragm.

Right Side.—*Anterior intraperitoneal,* which lies between the right lobe of the liver and the diaphragm. It is limited posteriorly by the anterior layer of the coronary and the right lateral ligaments, and to the left by the falciform ligament.

Posterior intraperitoneal (*syn.* Rutherford Morison's kidney pouch) lies transversely beneath the right lobe of the liver. It is bounded on the right by the right lobe of the liver and the diaphragm. To the left is situated the foramen of Winslow, and below this lies the duodenum. In front are the liver and gall-bladder, and, behind, the upper part of the right kidney and diaphragm. The space is bounded above by the liver, and below by the transverse colon and hepatic flexure.

Adrian van den Spiegel, 1578–1625. Professor of Anatomy and Surgery, Padua.
Jacob Winslow, 1669–1760. A Dane who migrated to Paris, and there established a school of anatomy.
Rutherford Morison, 1853–1939. Professor of Surgery, University of Durham.

Extraperitoneal, which is the " bare area " of the liver.

Falciform Ligament.—The two layers are occasionally separated by a collection of pus, which either tracks forwards from the bare area of the liver, or arises from infection around the umbilicus.

Ætiology.—The commonest causes of subphrenic abscess are appendicitis, and gastric or duodenal ulcers, especially following perforation or operation. In a series of seventy-eight cases of subphrenic abscess, we found that appendicitis was the cause in no less than thirty. However, owing to the growing tendency to select the time for operation with discretion, subphrenic abscess is a less common complication of appendicitis than formerly. Although an empyema is frequently associated with a subphrenic abscess, infection of the subphrenic spaces rarely if ever follows an empyema.

Clinical Features.—The symptoms and signs of subphrenic infection are frequently obscure, and it is well to remember the aphorism, " Pus somewhere, pus nowhere else, pus under diaphragm " (Barnard).

Symptoms.—A common history is that when some infective focus in the abdominal cavity has been dealt with, the condition of the patient improves temporarily, but after an interval of a few days or weeks, symptoms of toxæmia reappear. Owing to rapid absorption of toxins, the patient steadily, and often rapidly, loses ground. Sweating, wasting, and anorexia are present. The patient sometimes complains of epigastric fullness, abdominal discomfort or pain in the shoulder on the affected side, owing to irritation of sensory fibres in the phrenic nerve, and referred pain along the descending branches of the cervical plexus.

Signs.—General signs are those of toxæmia, with increasing listlessness, wasting, and anæmia.

If the abscess is anterior, abdominal examination will reveal some tenderness, rigidity, or even a palpable swelling. Sometimes the liver is displaced downwards, but more often it is fixed by adhesions. Examination of the chest is of extreme importance, and in the majority of cases pressure signs at the base of the lung or evidence of effusion or empyema are to be found. Anaerobic organisms in the pus sometimes form gas in sufficient quantities to be recognised clinically. In these cases percussion demonstrates four zones (fig. 425).

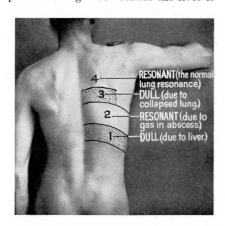

Accessory Investigations.—(i) *Blood Count.*—A relative and absolute leucocytosis is the rule.

(ii) *X-ray.*—A simple radiograph sometimes demonstrates the presence of gas, or of a pleural effusion. On screening, the diaphragm is often seen to be elevated and its movements impaired.

FIG. 425.—Subphrenic abscess with gas. The four areas of differential percussion.

(iii) *Needling.*—Which is the final court of appeal.

If the needle has penetrated a subphrenic abscess, the movements of the diaphragm are transmitted to the needle, which consequently oscillates during respiration. In the case of an empyema these movements are

Harold Leslie Barnard, 1868–1908. Surgeon, London Hospital.

absent. Needling should always be performed in the operating theatre, and if pus is discovered the needle is left *in situ* as a guide to the abscess, and the operation performed forthwith.

Differential Diagnosis.—Pylephlebitis, tropical abscess, and empyema give rise to most of the diagnostic difficulties.

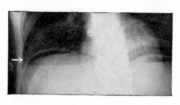

FIG. 426.—Radiograph showing subphrenic abscess containing gas. (*K. J. Yeo.*)

Other conditions which have been confused with a subphrenic abscess include perinephric abscess, splenic infarct following ulcerative endocarditis, pancreatic cysts, and renal tumours.

Treatment.—Many cases of subphrenic infection do not proceed to suppuration, and resolution is encouraged by chemotherapy. The clinical course of suspected cases is watched, and blood and radiological examinations are made at suitable intervals. If suppuration seems probable, surgical intervention is indicated.

If a swelling can be detected in the subcostal region or in the loin, an incision is made over the site of maximum tenderness, or over any area where softening, œdema, or redness is discovered. The parietes usually form part of the abscess wall, so that contamination of the general peritoneal cavity is unlikely.

If no swelling is apparent the subphrenic spaces should be explored from behind after removal of the twelfth (and possibly eleventh) rib. The diaphragm is incised below the pleural reflection, and a finger is inserted beneath the diaphragm so as to explore the adjacent area. Most abscesses can be discovered by this method, which obviates opening either the pleura or peritoneal cavity.

Transpleural drainage is rarely necessary. Unless well-marked adhesions are present in the pleural cavity, or urgent drainage is required on account of toxæmia, a two-stage operation should be performed as for an abscess of the lung (p. 982).

SPECIAL FORMS OF ACUTE PERITONITIS NOT CONSIDERED ELSEWHERE

Pneumococcal Peritonitis.—There are two forms of this disease :

1. Primary.
2. Secondary to pneumonia.

Primary pneumococcal peritonitis is the more common. The patient is very often an undernourished girl between five and ten years of age, and infection is believed to occur via the vagina and Fallopian tubes. After the age of ten pneumococcal peritonitis becomes comparatively rare. A possible explanation is that about this time the vaginal secretion becomes acid. When primary pneumococcal peritonitis occurs in a male child the explanation is difficult. A blood-borne infection seems probable.

Pneumococcal peritonitis is seen less frequently than formerly;

perhaps this is due to the greater cleanliness and the higher standard of living of the hospital patient (Barrington-Ward). Pneumococcus type I is the most usual offender.

Clinical Features.—The onset is sudden, and the earliest symptom is pain localised to the lower half of the abdomen. The temperature is raised to 103° F. (39·8° C.) or more, and there is usually frequent vomiting. After twenty-four to forty-eight hours a characteristic symptom is profuse diarrhœa, sometimes blood-stained. There is usually increased frequency of micturition. The last two symptoms are due to severe pelvic peritonitis. Herpes on the lip or nostril is often present. In acute forms of the disease, even in cases where there is no involvement of a lung, there is a tinge of cyanosis of the lips and cheeks. On examination rigidity is usually bilateral, and is less than that due to appendicitis.

Differential Diagnosis.—In some cases, especially in males, it is sometimes impossible to exclude a perforated appendix. A leucocytosis of 30,000 or more with approximately 90 per cent. polymorphs speaks more for pneumococcal peritonitis than appendicitis. Even so, it is sometimes impossible to exclude with complete certainty a perforated appendix. The risk of treating expectantly a gangrenous appendix with spreading peritonitis outweighs the risk of a small incision in pneumococcal peritonitis (Sir John Fraser).

Treatment.—In typical cases where the diagnosis can be made with assurance, the patient should be placed in the modified Fowler's position and nepenthe is prescribed in suitable doses, according to age. Heat is applied to the abdomen. Intravenous saline and glucose infusion is administered by the drip method. Penicillin and sulphonamide preparations are given, the former in doses of 200,000 units daily. Under such treatment resolution often occurs or, after at least fourteen days, a localised abscess forms, which will require drainage. Operative treatment is necessary when the condition cannot be distinguished from acute appendicitis with peritonitis. If, on opening the abdomen, odourless fibrinous and sticky exudate is found, and the appendix is not more inflamed than the rest of the intestine, the pus should be aspirated or removed with swabs, and the abdomen closed. Chemotherapy is commenced, or continued. In all cases oxygen therapy is advisable. In severe

Sir Lancelot Barrington-Ward, Contemporary. Consulting Surgeon, Hospital for Sick Children, Great Ormond Street, London.
Sir John Fraser, 1885–1947. Surgeon, Royal Edinburgh Hospital for Sick Children.

cases repeated small blood transfusions are beneficial in the later stages of the illness.

Gonococcal Peritonitis.—Pelvic peritonitis is a common complication of gonococcal salpingitis. Usually the disease is localised to the pelvis, but diffuse peritonitis of gonococcal origin is not uncommon. In gonococcal peritonitis the abdominal rigidity is not marked and tenderness is bilateral, but sometimes one side is more tender than the other. A vaginal examination shows tenderness in the pouch of Douglas. The finding of gonococci in a smear taken from the cervix uteri is helpful confirmatory evidence in suspected cases. When gonococcal peritonitis can be diagnosed with irrefutable accuracy, conservative treatment is extremely satisfactory, and in the majority of cases resolution occurs. In the minority a localised pelvic abscess forms, and such an abscess is drained effectively through the posterior fornix. In cases where difficulty in diagnosis arises and pelvic appendicitis cannot be excluded, laparotomy must be performed. If the appendix is normal and the Fallopian tubes are found to be intensely inflamed, and there is a thin, purulent, odourless peritoneal exudate, the pus is mopped up or aspirated, and the abdomen closed without drainage. Penicillin is extremely effective in these cases. After the acute phase has subsided, salpingectomy is often required.

Streptococcal peritonitis is sometimes due to puerperal infection, and if so, is a notifiable disease. It is more common after first deliveries. Rigidity is seldom much in evidence ; this, at any rate in part, is due to the stretched condition of the abdominal musculature. The lochia may be offensive but not necessarily so. Diarrhœa is common.

The sheet anchors in treatment of post-partum streptococcal peritonitis are modified Fowler's position, intravenous saline given in accordance with the patient's needs, and chemotherapy. Primary streptococcal peritonitis occasionally occurs idiopathically, no primary focus being demonstrable. Rightly, the abdomen is opened, usually on a diagnosis of acute appendicitis. In streptococcal peritonitis the peritoneal exudate is odourless, thin, contains small flecks of fibrin, and may be blood-stained. In these circumstances the pus is aspirated, the abdomen closed, and the measures detailed in the conservative treatment of peritonitis carried out. Even so, the mortality of this condition is high.

Acute Tuberculous Peritonitis.—It is doubtful if tuberculous peritonitis is ever acute. However, patients with tuberculous peritonitis sometimes have acute exacerbations which resemble so closely acute peritonitis that the abdomen is opened. Straw-coloured fluid escapes, and tubercles are seen scattered over the peritoneum and great omentum. Tubercles occasionally simulate fat necroses (see p. 362) or the nodules of peritoneal carcinomatosis. The latter feel hard when rolled between the finger and thumb, making their differentiation tolerably simple. On opening the abdomen and finding tuberculous peritonitis, the fluid is evacuated, a portion of the diseased omentum is removed for histological confirmation of the diagnosis, and the wound closed without drainage.

CHRONIC TUBERCULOUS PERITONITIS

Usually children are affected, but it is not rare for the disease to make its first appearance in early adult life, when females outnumber males by two to one. Exceptionally the disease becomes manifest in patients over forty years of age.

Origin of the infection :

1. From tuberculous mesenteric lymph nodes.
2. From tuberculosis of the ileo-cæcal region.
3. From a tuberculous pyosalpinx.
4. Very occasionally it is due to a blood-borne infection from pulmonary tuberculosis.

There are four varieties of tuberculous peritonitis :

Ascitic Form.—The peritoneum is studded with tubercles, and the peritoneal cavity becomes filled with pale, straw-coloured fluid. The onset is insidious. There is loss of energy, some loss of weight, and the child becomes pale. The patient is usually brought for advice because of abdominal enlargement (fig. 427). Pain is often completely absent ; in other cases there is considerable abdominal discomfort which may be associated with constipation or diarrhœa. On inspection dilated veins can be seen coursing beneath the skin of the abdominal wall. Shifting dullness is readily elicited. In the male child congenital hydroceles sometimes appear, due to the ascitic fluid being forced from the peritoneal cavity into patent tunicæ vaginales. Because of the increased intra-abdominal pressure, an umbilical hernia commonly occurs. On palpation a transverse solid mass can often be made out (fig. 428). This is rolled-up great omentum infiltrated with tubercles.

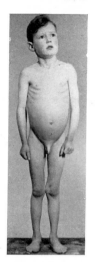

Fig. 427. — Abdominal tuberculosis. Ascitic form.

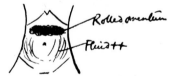

Fig. 428.—Physical signs recorded in a case of the ascitic form of tuberculous peritonitis.

The diagnosis is seldom difficult, except when it occurs in an acute form or when it first appears in an adult, in which case it has to be differentiated from other forms of ascites.

Treatment.—Sanatorium treatment, which includes heliotherapy, is usually effective. Laparotomy with evacuation of ascitic fluid is often followed by considerable improvement, probably due to an outpouring of fresh ascitic fluid more plentiful in antibodies. In favourable cases with general treatment, including heliotherapy, this fluid is gradually absorbed, there is a steady gain in weight, and eventual recovery. Streptomycin is valuable in all forms of tuberculous peritonitis not responding to heliotherapy.

Encysted (*syn.* loculated) form is similar to the above, but one part of the abdominal cavity alone is involved. So is produced a localised intra-abdominal swelling which gives rise to difficulty in diagnosis. In a female above the age of puberty, when the swelling is in the pelvis, an ovarian cyst will probably be diagnosed. In the case of a child it is sometimes difficult to distinguish the swelling from a mesenteric cyst. For these reasons laparotomy is often performed, and if an encapsulated collection of fluid is found, it is evacuated and the abdomen is closed. The general treatment already detailed is required, but the response to this treatment is more rapid. Late intestinal obstruction is a possible complication.

Fibrous (*syn.* plastic) form is characterised by the production of wide-spread adhesions, which cause coils of intestine, especially the ileum, to become matted together and often adherent to the parietal peritoneum. Typically the condition is accompanied by wasting and attacks of abdominal pain. On examination the adherent intestine with omentum attached, together with the thickened mesentery, may give rise to a palpable swelling or swellings. The first intimation of the disease may be subacute or acute intestinal obstruction. Sometimes the cause of the obstruction can be remedied easily by the division of bands ; more often it can only be overcome by lateral anastomosis between an obviously dilated loop and a collapsed loop of small intestine, or by ileo-colostomy. If the obstruction does not occur, or can be overcome, the prognosis, considering the intraperitoneal chaos, is fairly good.

Purulent form is rare. Amidst a mass of adherent intestine and omentum tuberculous pus is present. Intraperitoneal cold abscesses form, and point on the surface, commonly near the umbilicus, or burst into the bowel. In this type, which is a frequent complication of tuberculous pyosalpinx, a fæcal fistula is a common and serious development. In addition to prolonged general treatment, operative treatment may be necessary for the evacuation of cold abscesses and possibly for intestinal obstruction. If the patient survives long enough to overcome the infection, it may be possible to close a fæcal fistula, which usually persists because of obstruction distal to it. Closure must therefore be combined with some form of anastomosis between the segment of intestine above the fistula and an unobstructed area below. The prognosis in the purulent variety of tuberculous peritonitis is poor.

PERITONEAL ADHESIONS

Congenital bands and membranes, which are never a cause of acute intestinal obstruction, must be distinguished from inflammatory peritoneal adhesions. The following are encountered from time to time :

1. *The cystico-duodenal band* runs from the gall-bladder to the pylorus.

2. *The mesocolic band of Pringle* passes from the mesocolon to the duodenojejunal flexure.

3. A congenital band attaching the ileum 4 inches from the ileo-cæcal junction to the right ovary or the posterior abdominal wall.

4. *Jackson's membrane,* which is comparatively common, runs from the great omentum, enveloping like a shroud an unusually lax, capacious cæcum and ascending colon. When this veil is gently pulled so as to make

Seton Pringle, Contemporary. Consulting Surgeon, Royal City of Dublin Hospital, Ireland.
Jabez N. Jackson, 1868–1935. Surgeon, Kansas City, U.S.A.

it move upon the cæcum, its contained blood-vessels become the more apparent (fig. 429).

5. *Payr's membrane* is a similar structure over the splenic flexure.

6. *Toldt's membrane* is found over the pelvic colon.

Inflammatory peritoneal adhesions may follow any form of peritonitis or any abdominal operation. While complete resolution without any sign of adhesions may result after widespread peritonitis or an intraperitoneal abscess, e.g. appendix abscess, on other occasions adhesions are dense and bind together the abdominal viscera. Especially after laparotomy, hollow viscera and the omentum often become adherent to the abdominal wall. Peritoneal adhesions are a frequent cause of intestinal obstruction. Recent adhesions are separated easily. Old-standing adhesions, tough and sometimes vascular, require scissors or scalpel for their division. Often the cause of intestinal obstruction is found to be a single adhesion, sometimes surprisingly thin, which can be divided between hæmostats. Peritoneal adhesions tend to reform, and to avoid recurrence an extensive area of adherent intestine which has been freed should be covered with a free omental graft to prevent it again becoming adherent.

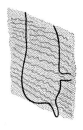

Fig. 429.—Jackson's membrane.

Talc Granuloma.—Talc (silicate of magnesium) which is still used as a lubricant for rubber gloves, is the cause of peritoneal adhesions, and granulomata in the Fallopian tubes have been reported. Potassium bitartrate, which is completely soluble, should be used for this purpose.

Lycopodium spores in glove dusting-powder are also a cause of peritoneal adhesions, and sometimes the spores produce multiple nodules on the peritoneal surface which simulate those occurring in carcinoma peritonei or tuberculous peritonitis.

ASCITES

A large collection of serous fluid within the peritoneal cavity occurs in a number of divergent conditions, and although ascites is a symptom and not a disease, it is convenient to consider the common causes of the condition together. The abdomen is distended evenly, with fullness of the flanks, which are dull to percussion. Usually shifting dullness is present, but when there is a very large accumulation of fluid, this sign is absent. In such cases, on flicking the abdominal wall, a characteristic fluid thrill is transmitted from one side to the other. In the female, ascites must be differentiated from an enormous ovarian cyst (fig. 430).

Edwin Payr, Contemporary. Emeritus Professor of Surgery, Leipzig.
Carl Toldt, 1840–1920. Professor of Anatomy, University of Vienna.

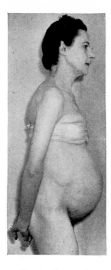

FIG. 430. — The absence of any cause for ascites made the diagnosis of ovarian cyst probable in this case. Diagnosis confirmed by operation.

Type 1.   *A Failing Heart or Chronic Nephritis.*—The ascitic fluid is part of a general dropsy. The fluid is a light yellow serum of low specific gravity, about 1,010.

Type 2.   *Portal Hypertension.*—Ascites may occur from hepatic cirrhosis or in late cases of the Banti syndrome, when enlargement of the spleen will be evident. The serum is darker in colour than the foregoing, and the specific gravity is about 1,015.

Type 3.   *Tuberculous Peritonitis.*—The fluid is pale yellow and usually clear. The specific gravity is comparatively high, often 1,020 or over. The fluid is rich in lymphocytes. Even after centrifugalisation tubercle bacilli can rarely be found, but their presence can be demonstrated by culture or guinea-pig inoculation.

Type 4.   *Secondary Carcinoma of the Peritoneum.*—The fluid is dark yellow and frequently blood-stained. The specific gravity is high, 1,020 or over. Microscopic examination often reveals cancer cells.

Type 5.   *Chronic Constrictive Pericarditis (syn.* Pick's Disease). In addition to the peritoneal effusion, effusions occur into the pleural cavities. The specific gravity is about 1,015.

The differential diagnosis between tuberculous peritonitis occurring in an adult and carcinoma peritonei is sometimes impossible by clinical methods. Those skilled in the use of the peritoneoscope employ this instrument to view the peritoneal cavity and by this means distinguish tubercles from secondary malignant deposits. More usually laparotomy is performed for this purpose.

Treatment.—When the ascites accompanying a failing heart or chronic nephritis does not respond to medical treatment, paracentesis (tapping) is necessary. The surgical measures adopted to relieve portal hypertension have been described on p. 322, but even when, as a result of one of the operations described, hæmatemesis from œsophageal varices ceases, repeated tapping of accumulations of peritoneal fluid is usually necessary.

Friedel Pick, 1867–1926. Physician, of Prague.

Although tapping the peritoneal cavity and aspirating the fluid from the pleural cavity gives temporary relief in Pick's disease, treatment should be directed to the cause—obliterative pericarditis (see p. 995).

Paracentesis Abdominis.—The bladder having been emptied by a catheter, under local anæsthesia puncture of the peritoneum is carried out with a moderate-sized trocar and cannula at one of the points shown in fig. 431. In cases where the effusion is due to cardiac failure the fluid must be evacuated slowly. In other circumstances this precaution is unnecessary. If the cannula becomes blocked with fibrin, it is cleared with a probe. After the fluid has been evacuated the puncture is sealed, and a tight binder is applied to the abdomen.

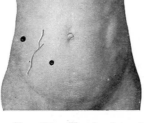

Fig. 431.—Usual points of puncture for tapping ascites. The bladder must be emptied by a catheter before the puncture is made. Note the relationship of the sites of puncture to the deep epigastric artery.

NEOPLASMS OF THE PERITONEUM

Carcinoma peritonei is a common terminal event in many cases of carcinoma of the stomach, colon, ovary, or other intraperitoneal organs and also of the breast. The peritoneum, both parietal and visceral, is studded with secondary growths, and the peritoneal cavity becomes filled with ascitic fluid. It is remarkable how often a patient riddled with intraperitoneal carcinoma preserves her nutrition, and looks and feels comparatively well until the last. Withdrawal of the fluid by tapping renders the patient more comfortable.

Pseudo-myxoma Peritonei.—This rare condition occurs more frequently in females. The abdomen is filled with a yellow jelly, large quantities of which are often more or less encysted. The condition arises in one of two ways. Most often from rupture of a pseudo-mucinous cyst of the ovary not otherwise malignant ; less often from rupture of a mucocele or diverticulum of the appendix. The condition is painless, and there is no impairment of general health for a long time. When the condition arises from the appendix the mass is often more localised, but in cases of ovarian origin the whole peritoneal cavity is involved. It is highly improbable that a correct preoperative diagnosis will be made. At laparotomy masses of jelly are scooped out, and the primary focus, if it can be found, is removed. Unfortunately, recurrence is usual. In one of our patients laparotomy and evacuation of quarts of jelly was undertaken on four occasions in a little over a year. When pseudo-myxoma peritonei arises from a mucocele of the appendix, repeated recurrence is less common. Pseudo-myxoma peritonei is locally malignant, but does not give rise to metastases. Deep

X-rays may be tried in order to prevent re-formation of the myxomatous material.

THE GREAT OMENTUM

Rutherford Morison called the great omentum the " abdominal policeman." Relatively larger and structurally more

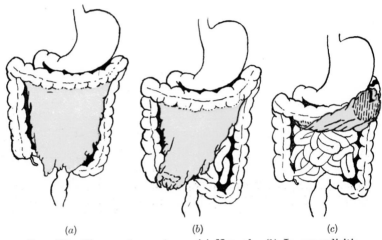

(a)   (b)   (c)

FIG. 432.—The great omentum. (a) Normal. (b) In appendicitis.
(c) In a (comparatively small) laceration of the spleen.

substantial in the adult than in the child, the discharge of its life-saving constabulary duties becomes more effective after puberty, and they remain unabated throughout life. The great omentum attempts, often successfully, to limit intraperitoneal infective processes (fig. 432). For instance, an acutely inflamed appendix is often found wrapped in omentum, and this saves many a patient from developing diffuse peritonitis. Sufferers from herniæ are also greatly indebted to this structure, for it often plugs the neck of a hernial sac and prevents a coil of intestine from becoming strangulated.

Torsion of the Omentum.—Torsion of the omentum (fig. 433) is a rare emergency, and consequently is seldom diagnosed correctly. It is usually mistaken for appendicitis with somewhat abnormal signs. A tender lump

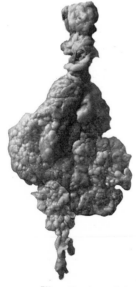

FIG. 433.—Torsion of the great omentum. Specimen removed by operation.
(*Archibald Ronald.*)

may be present in the abdomen. The blood-supply having been cut off, the twisted mass sometimes becomes gangrenous, and peritonitis may follow.

Treatment.—The abdomen having been opened, the pedicle above the twist is ligated securely and the mass removed.

THE MESENTERY

A wound of the mesentery can follow a severe abdominal contusion, and is a cause of hæmo-peritoneum. In about 60 per cent. of cases the mesenteric laceration is associated with a rupture of the intestine. If the tear is a large one, and

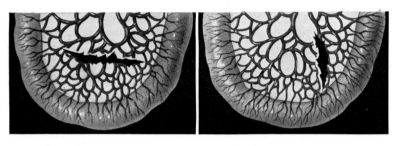

| FIG. 434. | FIG. 435. |

Laceration of the mesentery. A transverse tear (fig. 434) often imperils the blood-supply of a segment of intestine, making resection necessary. A longitudinal tear (fig. 435) can be closed by suture.

especially if it is transverse (fig. 434), the blood-supply to the neighbouring intestine is cut off, and a limited resection of gut is imperative. Small wounds and wounds in the long axis (fig. 435) should be sutured.

Torsion of the Mesentery (see Volvulus Neonatorum, p. 458, and Volvulus of the Small Intestine, p. 467).

Embolism and Thrombosis of the Mesenteric Vessels (see p. 472).

Acute Non-specific Mesenteric Lymphadenitis.—The mesenteric lymph nodes, particularly those in relationship to the lowest two or three feet of the ileum, become inflamed and considerably enlarged. There is a small quantity of sterile free fluid in the peritoneal cavity. Histologically a node removed at operation shows hyperplasia, but no organisms can be found on culture of the peritoneal fluid or from the substance of the node.

Clinical Features and Differential Diagnosis.—The patient is most often a male between three and ten years of age, but the condition is sometimes found in adolescents and adults. The attacks are usually recurrent, the patient giving a history of previous similar attacks. There are spasms of general abdominal colic with intervals of freedom in which the patient moves about without pain. This feature should lead the clinician to suspect the condition. Nausea, and sometimes vomiting, accompanies the attack. The temperature is raised, and there is a leucocytosis of 15,000 or more on the first day of the attack, but this falls on the second day. The initial reading is higher and falls more rapidly than in acute appendicitis. In many cases the condition is indistinguishable from acute appendicitis, but the following features help to differentiate acute non-specific lymphadenitis from acute appendicitis. Sometimes the condition is mildly epidemic, and is preceded by upper respiratory infection. The rigidity, although present, is not as great as that in acute appendicitis. The point of maximum tenderness is higher and more medial than in that condition. The most valuable differentiating sign is shifting tenderness ; after lying the patient on the left side for a few minutes, the site of maximum tenderness referred to changes to the level of the umbilicus or to the left of that point (Ian Aird). The differential diagnosis between non-specific lymphadenitis and tuberculous mesenteric lymphadenitis is considered in the section which follows immediately.

Treatment.—There is no treatment of acute non-specific lymphadenitis, which is a self-limiting disease. Appendicectomy must sometimes be performed because of difficulty in diagnosis, but the removal of the appendix does not confer any immunity from further attacks.

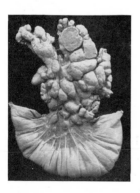

FIG. 436.—Massive tuberculosis of the lymph nodes of the mesentery.

Tuberculosis of the Mesenteric Lymph Nodes (fig. 436).—Although still fairly common, tuberculous mesenteric lymphadenitis is considerably less common than acute non-specific lymphadenitis, and it has become increasingly less frequent in Britain during the past twenty-five years. Tubercle bacilli, usually but not necessarily bovine, are ingested, and enter the mesenteric lymph nodes by way of Peyer's patches. Sometimes only one lymph node is infected ; usually there are a number, those connected with the lower

Ian Aird, Contemporary. Director of Surgical Unit, Post-Graduate Medical School, London.
Johann Peyer, 1653–1712. Anatomist, Schaffhausen, Switzerland.

ileum being especially involved. The infection probably always occurs during childhood. In many instances the condition causes no symptoms, and the affected node or nodes become calcified, their presence being apparent only at an X-ray examination, during the course of an abdominal operation for another condition, or at necropsy. Less frequently the tuberculous process is more active, and gives rise to general symptoms. The patient, usually a child under ten years of age, loses appetite, looks pale, and there is some loss of weight. Sometimes abdominal pain is the cause of the patient being brought for advice ; usually this pain is not severe, but rather a discomfort, and is often constant. On examination the abdomen is somewhat protuberant and there is tenderness on deep pressure to the right of the umbilicus. In these circumstances the condition has to be distinguished from acute non-specific mesenteric lymphadenitis. If, on deep palpation, the nodes are palpable as round, tender masses most frequently to the right of and near the umbilicus, the condition is almost certainly tuberculous. A normal leucocyte count favours tuberculosis, and in a child a positive patch test is confirmatory evidence. On occasions the abdominal pain is acute and may be accompanied by vomiting. This, combined with tenderness and some rigidity in the right iliac fossa, makes the diagnosis from sub-acute appendicitis almost impossible. When, as is sometimes the case, the tuberculous infection of the mesenteric lymph nodes becomes reactivated in adolescent or adult life, the diagnostic difficulties are even greater.

A plain X-ray may show calcified lymph nodes, but as such a condition can co-exist with appendicitis, in some cases laparotomy for appendicectomy and visualisation of the lymph nodes is necessary. If the mesentery is found to be in an inflamed state with caseation of some of the lymph nodes, the diagnosis of active tuberculosis of the nodes is confirmed.

Treatment.—In all active cases of tuberculous mesenteric lymphadenitis general treatment as for tuberculous peritonitis must be carried out. The prognosis with this treatment is excellent. In a few instances a local abscess forms, usually in the right iliac fossa, when the tuberculous pus should be evacuated and the abdomen closed without drainage.

Tuberculous Mesenteric Lymph Nodes as a cause of Intestinal

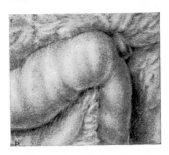

FIG. 437.—Obstruction by angulation. The gut had become adherent to a tuberculous lymph node.

Obstruction.—Remote rather than recent tuberculous mesenteric adenitis can be the cause of intestinal obstruction. For instance, a coil of small intestine becomes adherent to a caseating node, and is thereby angulated (fig. 437), or a free coil may become imprisoned by passing beneath the site of adherence and the mesentery.

As a cause of Pseudo-mesenteric Cyst.—When tuberculous mesenteric lymph nodes break down, the tuberculous pus may remain confined between the leaves of the mesentery, and a cystic swelling having the characteristics of a mesenteric cyst is found. When such a condition is confirmed at operation the tuberculous pus should be evacuated without soiling the peritoneal cavity, the wound closed, and general treatment continued until the infection has been overcome.

Calcifying Mesenteric Lymph Nodes as a Confusing X-ray Shadow.—Sometimes the shadow cast by a calcified mesenteric lymph node or nodes may simulate that of a ureteric calculus or renal calculi. A change of posture often causes lymph-node shadows to alter in position. Pyelography clarifies the diagnosis in doubtful cases.

Cysts.—The following varieties of mesenteric cysts exist:

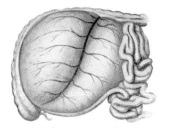

FIG. 438.—A large mesenteric cyst.
(*Higgins and Lloyd.*) (*British Journal of Surgery.*)

Chylous cysts are thin walled, lined by endothelium and filled with lymph or chyle. They may be situated anywhere in the mesentery, and often attain a great size (fig. 438).

Enterogenous cysts are usually situated in the mesentery of the lower ileum. They have a thick fibro-muscular wall, are lined by columnar or flattened epithelium, and filled with mucinous fluid. This form of mesenteric cyst is believed to be derived from an intestinal diverticulum which has become sequestrated from the intestinal canal during embryonic life.

Teratomatous cysts are filled with sebaceous material.

The following, while not being mesenteric cysts in the academic meaning of the term, give rise to the same physical signs, and are treated in the same manner. From the practical point of view they *are* mesenteric cysts:

Serosanguineous cyst is probably traumatic in origin, but a history of an accident is seldom obtained.

Tuberculous Abscess of the Mesentery.

Hydatid Cyst of the Mesentery.

Clinical Features.—The patient is nearly always a child, and may be brought because of an abdominal swelling, or on account of one of the complications of the cyst. A cyst of the mesentery presents characteristic physical signs. These have been well summarised by Tillaux, and are known as Tillaux's triad.

1. There is a fluctuating swelling in the abdomen near the umbilicus.

2. The swelling moves freely in a plane at right angles to the attachment of the mesentery (fig. 439).

3. There is a zone of resonance around and a belt of resonance across the cyst.

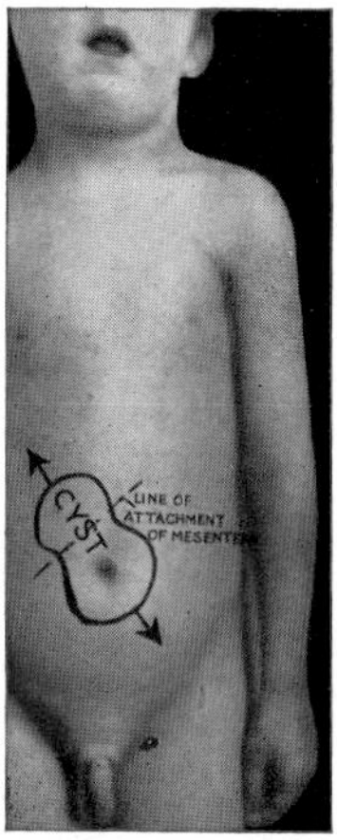

If the diagnosis is in any doubt, a barium meal will show the hollow viscera displaced around the cyst.

Complications.

1. Intestinal obstruction.
2. Rupture.
3. Infection.
4. Torsion of that portion of the mesentery containing the cyst.
5. Hæmorrhage into the cyst.

Treatment.—*Enucleation* is the ideal treatment, but it is seldom possible, except in the case of small cysts.

FIG. 439. — A mesenteric cyst moves freely in the direction of the arrows, i.e. at right angles to the attachment of the mesentery.

Resection, which of necessity must include the involved segment of intestine, is generally required in the case of an enterogenous cyst. If the cyst occupies the extreme lower end of the mesentery, the continuity of the alimentary canal is restored by ileo-cæcostomy. In other situations end-to-end anastomosis of the small intestine is performed. In the chylous variety resection is often a severe undertaking, owing to the large amount of the small intestine that is implicated.

Marsupialisation.[1]—In the chylous variety marsupialisation is a less drastic procedure which often gives satisfactory results. When torsion of the mesentery containing the cyst has occurred

---

[1] Marsupialisation. Marsupials are animals which carry their young in an open pouch.

Paul Tillaux, 1834–1904. Professor of Surgery, University of Paris.

and obstruction is present, it may be necessary to resect because of gangrene or impending gangrene of the intestine.

The peritoneum is closed above and below the cyst, leaving a small area uncovered. The cut edge of the peritoneum is sewn to the cyst wall around the bare area, through which the cyst is drained (fig. 440).

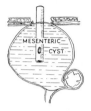

F I G .   4 4 0.— Method of treating a large mesenteric cyst by marsupial- isation.

NEOPLASMS

Tumours situated in the mesentery give rise to physical signs similar to those of a mesenteric cyst, the sole exception being that they sometimes feel solid.

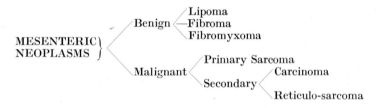

MESENTERIC NEOPLASMS

Benign — Lipoma, Fibroma, Fibromyxoma

Malignant — Primary Sarcoma; Secondary — Carcinoma, Reticulo-sarcoma

THE RETROPERITONEAL SPACE

Pus or blood in the retroperitoneal space tends to track to the corresponding iliac fossa. If a retroperitoneal hæmatoma or an abscess develops, it should be evacuated by an incision through the abdominal wall, meticulously avoiding opening the peritoneum.

Retroperitoneal Cyst.—A cyst developing in the retroperitoneal space often attains very large dimensions, and has at first to be distinguished from a hydronephrosis. After this condition has been eliminated by a pyelogram, because it presents the same clinical features, a retroperitoneal cyst can seldom be diagnosed with certainty from a retroperitoneal tumour, until displayed at operation. The cyst may be unilocular or multilocular. Many of these cysts are believed to be derived from a remnant of the Wolffian duct, in which case they are filled with clear fluid. Others are teratomatous, and are filled with sebaceous material.

Kaspar Wolff, 1733–1794.   German anatomist.

Excision of these and other retroperitoneal swellings is best performed through a transperitoneal incision.

Primary neoplasms of the retroperitoneal space are confined to lipomata, lipo-sarcomata, and sarcomata. Although neuro-blastomata and gangliomata of the adrenal gland are retro-peritoneal tumours, they have now been segregated as clinical entities, and have been dealt with on p. 232.

Retroperitoneal lipoma, in the first instance, is usually mistaken for a hydronephrosis, a diagnosis which is ruled out by pyelography. Women are more often affected. These swellings sometimes reach an immense size. We have removed such a tumour weighing $5\frac{1}{2}$ lb. (2·5 kgm.), and much larger specimens have been recorded. Retroperitoneal lipomata some-times undergo myxomatous degeneration, a complication which does not occur in fatty tumours elsewhere. Moreover, undoubt-edly they sometimes become malignant, and may be looked upon as liposarcomata (fig. 441). An example of this malig-nant change occurred in a middle-aged woman under our care.

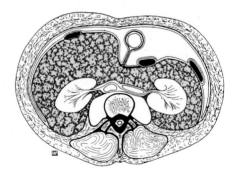

Fig. 441.—Rapidly growing retroperitoneal lipo-sarcoma.
After Reynolds.)

Retroperitoneal sarcoma presents signs similar to a retro-peritoneal lipoma. The patient may seek advice on account of a swelling, or because of indefinite abdominal pain. On other occasions the tumour, by pressure on the colon, causes symptoms of subacute intestinal obstruction. On examination a smooth fixed swelling, which is not tender, is palpated. The most prob-able original diagnosis is that of a neoplasm of the kidney. This is ruled out by pyelography. The ureter, however, may be displaced by the tumour. Exploratory laparotomy should be performed, and when operable the tumour is removed. Often it is found widely disseminated in the retroperitoneal space, rendering complete removal impossible, in which case a portion is excised for section. Even when removed at a comparatively early stage, recurrence always takes place, and these tumours must be looked upon as being necessarily fatal. Deep X-ray treatment should be tried.

CHAPTER XXI

THE INTESTINES

Some Points in Surgical Anatomy.—It is of great practical importance to be able :

1. To distinguish various portions of the intestinal canal at sight.

2. To know in which part of the abdomen the upper coils, as opposed to the lower coils, of the small intestine lie in relationship to the anterior abdominal wall.

3. To be able to tell which is the proximal and which the distal end of any loop under consideration.

4. To distinguish irrefutably large from small intestine.

For practical purposes these problems are settled as follows :

1. The mesentery of the jejunum has only two series of arches of blood-vessels, whereas the lower ileum has several series of arches.

2. Monks's method of intestinal localisation roughly indicates the disposition of the upper, middle, and lower thirds of the small intestine (fig. 442).

3. The mesentery, after being made taut, is examined. As the mesenteric attachment runs from

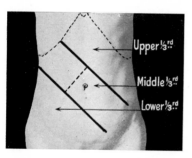

Fig. 442.—Monks's method of localising the small intestine upon the surface.

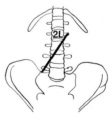

Fig. 443.—The attachment of the mesentery.

left to right (fig. 443), and palpation reveals the mesentery is not twisted, then the upper end of the bowel in the wound is the proximal end. Such a test is useful, but not as easy to perform in the living as in the dissecting-room subject.

4. As the " small " intestine is sometimes found enormously distended, and the " large " gut entirely collapsed, size is no criterion. The large gut is characterised by its tæniæ coli and appendices epiploicæ.

Embryology.—Beneath the notochord appears the primitive alimentary canal, which is continuous with the yolk sac (fig. 444). This canal becomes differentiated into :

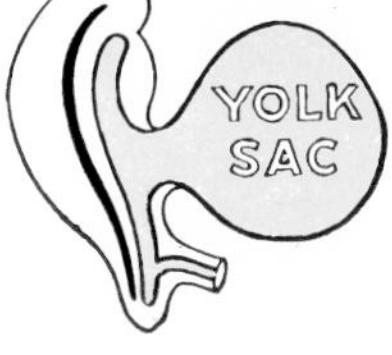

Fig. 444.—Embryo showing the primitive alimentary canal and the yolk sac.

George H. Monks, 1853–1933. Surgeon-in-Chief, City Hospital, Boston, U.S.A.

1. *The fore-gut,* from which are developed the pharynx, œsophagus, and stomach, together with the duodenum as far as the ampulla of Vater.

2. *The hind-gut,* which is the forerunner of the descending colon, pelvic colon, rectum, and the anal canal as far as the pectinate line.

3. *The mid-gut,* which gives origin to the remainder of the intestinal canal.

The mid-gut is continuous with the yolk sac, but as development proceeds, the communicating channel between these two structures dwindles into the *vitello-intestinal duct.* Later still the duct disappears entirely, except in 2 per cent. of individuals, where its inner extremity is represented by a pouch, so well known as Meckel's diverticulum. The mid-gut grows apace, and becomes differentiated into large and small intestine, the junction being indicated by an out-growth, which later forms the cæcum. As the gut, which now is suspended by a mesentery, elongates it also rotates, and the rotation of the various portions in relation to the middle line is depicted in fig. 445. At the fourth week of intrauterine life the greater part of the mid-gut is extruded, and comes to lie within the umbilical cord. This is a temporary physiological hernia, which sometimes persists (see Exomphalos). The normal process of rotation occurs during the act of reduction of the physiological hernia.

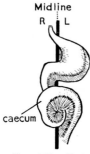

FIG. 445.—Rotation of portions of the alimentary canal on either side of the middle line.

CONGENITAL MALFORMATIONS OF THE GUT

Congenital atresia of the duodenum (see p. 272).
Congenital atresia of the small intestine (see p. 460).
Volvulus neonatorum (see p. 458).

Failure of Descent of the Cæcum.—The cæcum remains under the right lobe of the liver—a normal situation of the structure in the mangabey monkey. This anomaly, which is not infrequent, is of importance, because it leads to remarkable displacements of the vermiform appendix.

HIRSCHSPRUNG'S DISEASE AND MEGACOLON

Megacolon is characterised by enormous dilatation and hypertrophy of the pelvic colon, which sometimes extends into the descending colon but rarely involves the more proximal parts of the large intestine. The pelvic mesocolon is elongated and thickened, and its blood-vessels are enlarged. All coats of the dilated intestine show gross pathological changes. The serous coat is thickened, the circular fibres of the muscle coat are extensively hypertrophied, while the tæniæ coli are unaffected and appear inconspicuous. The mucous lining is chronically inflamed and frequently ulcerated. In congenital Hirsch-

Abraham Vater, 1684–1751. Professor of Anatomy and Botany, Wittenburg.
Harald Hirschsprung, 1830–1916. Physician, Queen Louise Hospital for Children, Copenhagen.

sprung's disease there is a terminal spastic segment of bowel
varying in length involving the anal canal, the rectum, and sometimes a portion of, or exceptionally all, the pelvic colon ; in
this segment there is no hypertrophy.   The hypertrophy and
dilatation of the colon above is secondary to an absence of
peristalsis in this terminal spastic segment.   On histological
examination of the spastic segment the cause of the immobility
is evident.   There is a complete absence of parasympathetic
ganglion cells, and this absence is continued for a distance of 1
to 5 cm. ($\frac{2}{5}$ths to 2 inches) into the transitional zone between the
terminal spastic segment and the hypertrophied portion
(Bodian).   Above this, parasympathetic ganglion cells are
present as in normal intestine (fig. 446).   In other varieties of

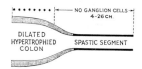

FIG. 446.—Showing the essential pathological histology in congenital Hirschsprung's
disease.   (*After M. Bodian.*)

megacolon the dilatation and hypertrophy extend to the anal
canal.   In some cases the condition is acquired ; in the
remainder the ætiology is obscure and the term idiopathic
dilatation of the colon cannot be bettered.

Clinical Features.—Males are six times more frequently
affected than females.   While the disease often originates from
birth, or soon afterwards, it varies in severity.   Obstinate constipation is the leading symptom ; many days, or even weeks,
elapse without evacuation.   Purgatives have little or no effect.
Enemata are of more assistance.   In its most severe forms
the infant suffers from attacks of acute-on-chronic intestinal
obstruction which are relieved by the passage of a rectal tube
and irrigations, but unless operative treatment is undertaken in
cases not responding to conservative measures, death results
from intestinal obstruction or from peritonitis following perforation of a stercoral ulcer.   In less severe cases the patient
survives infancy.   The abdomen remains enormously distended
(fig. 447) and the patient is often anæmic.   In a few instances,
in spite of the bowels acting only at intervals of a week or longer
and a distended abdomen, the patient reaches adult life and

Martin Bodian, Contemporary.   Morbid Anatomist, Hospital for Sick Children, London.

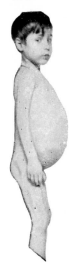

FIG. 447.
—Hirsch-
sprung's dis-
ease.
(*W. Mercer.*)

the general health remains unimpaired. Twistington Higgins divided cases of megacolon into three categories :

1. **Acquired megacolon** is encountered in older children. The condition is sometimes found to be the result of congenital stricture of the anal canal or a fissure-in-ano ; others are probably due to bad habits. A rectal examination reveals fæces immediately above the anal sphincter.

2. **Hirschsprung's Disease (mild type).**—The examining finger passes through the anal canal and a short segment of contracted rectum, and encounters a mass of fæces.

3. **Hirschsprung's Disease (severe type).**—The finger enters the rectum, which is empty.

Barium Enema.—Radiography after a barium enema provides considerable help in differentiating between the varieties of megacolon. In Hirschsprung's disease the barium enema shows the extent of the inactive segment with a greatly distended pelvic colon above (fig. 448). The appearance is in sharp contrast to acquired megacolon, which shows dilatation of the whole of the rectum and a varying amount of the pelvic colon.

Treatment of acquired megacolon is directed to the cause, if any is present. A stricture of the anal canal is dilated at intervals, or a fissure is treated by injection or operation. All cases require regular enemata and bowel education. In the less severe type of Hirschsprung's disease, in addition to these measures, the injection of spinal anæsthesia, which para-

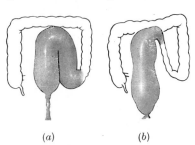

(*a*)   (*b*)

FIG. 448.—Radiological appearances : (*a*) Hirschsprung's disease ; (*b*) acquired megacolon. (*After B. C. H. Ward.*)

lyses the anterior roots at least as high as T5, has been found beneficial (Telford) although it may have to be repeated. For a number of years lumbar ganglionectomy or excision of the presacral nerve, together with division of the inferior mesenteric nerves, was practised and gave some excellent immediate results, but relapses were so common that these measures have been largely abandoned. Radical operation which aims at excision of the aganglionic spastic terminal segment has given better results. After a preliminary course of enemata, the operation is performed in stages.

Stage 1.—A transverse colostomy with a spur is constructed. This entirely defunctions the colon distal to it. Further colonic irrigations are given until the left half of the colon is completely emptied of fæcal accumulation.

Stage 2 is an abdomino-perineal resection of the rectum and the commencement of the funnel-shaped dilated colon, and anastomosis of the hypertrophied colon to the anal mucosa ¾ inch (2 cm.) above the ano-cutaneous margin, with preservation of the sphincters. Denis Browne achieves this in the following manner. Through a left lower paramedian incision the rectum and part of the colon, including the commencement of the hypertrophied colon, are freed from their attachment as far as the levator ani. A sigmoidoscope is passed from the anus into the commencement of the hypertrophied colon, and two needles 18 inches (45 cm.) long, each carrying a strand of braided silk which encircles the colon, are passed through the intestinal wall into the lumen of the sigmoidoscope at diametrically opposite points, and thence out of the anus. Traction is applied to these silk loops and the colon is intussuscepted into the rectum (fig. 449). Further traction causes prolapse of the rectum and the commencement of the hypertrophied colon outside the anus. The prolapsed portion is excised about ¾ inch (2 cm.) from the anal margin by dividing with a diathermy knife and uniting the resulting cut edges with sutures of linen thread; little by

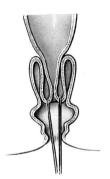

Fig. 449.—Method of intussuscepting the terminal part of the hypertrophied colon into the rectum and out of the anus. (*After Denis Browne.*)

little the circumference of the intussuscepted colon is joined to that of the anal canal, the intussuscepted aganglionic segment being thereby excised. The closely sutured colo-anal junction is then inverted into the anal canal. The pelvic floor having been reconstructed, the abdominal wall is closed.

Stages 3 *and* 4 are, respectively, crushing the spur of the transverse colostomy and closure of the colostomy.

GENERAL VISCEROPTOSIS (*Syn.* GLÉNARD'S DISEASE)

All the intra-abdominal organs are ptosed. The patient is nearly always a woman.

Rovsing recognised two types of general visceroptosis :

Maternal Visceroptosis.—As a result of repeated pregnancies the abdominal wall loses its tone and the intra-abdominal organs slide downwards.

Virginal Visceroptosis.—From childhood the patient shows signs of ptosis. She has a long, narrow, upper abdomen (see p. 300), and tends to stoop. She is of the " drooping lily " type, and, as she grows older, is constantly ailing. Although, no doubt, there are uncomfortable sensations

Denis John Browne, Contemporary. Surgeon, Hospital for Sick Children, London.
Franz Glénard, 1848–1920. Physician at Vichy. Ill health compelled him to leave Paris.
Thorkild Rovsing, 1862–1927. Professor of Surgery, University of Copenhagen.

from the ptosed organs, only too often the patient becomes hypochondriacal.

Treatment is unsatisfactory. A well-fitting abdominal belt, put on each morning before the patient arises, and worn all day, is of great service. Massage and exercises are helpful, especially in the maternal type.

TRAUMATIC RUPTURE OF THE INTESTINE

The intestine can be ruptured without any external wound. The most frequent cause of such an accident is a kick in the

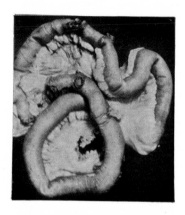

FIG. 450.—Traumatic rupture of the small intestine. Note the prolapse of the mucous membrane.

abdomen, the rupture probably being produced by a coil of intestine being crushed against the sacral promontory. Rupture of the intestine is said to be more frequent where a fixed part of the alimentary tract joins a free portion, such as the duodeno-jejunal flexure, but this has not been our experience. The latter type of lesion is sometimes met with after run-over accidents.

In small perforations the mucosa prolapses and tends partially to seal the rent (fig. 450); consequently the early signs are misleading. In general it may be stated that the signs simulate closely those of a perforated gastric ulcer.

In the type of injury under consideration, laceration of the mesentery is a frequent operative finding. The intestinal tube is not necessarily breached, but owing to devascularisation, its viability may be so imperilled as to render resection of the infarcted segment (fig. 451) imperative.

Traumatic rupture of the large intestine is very much less frequent. Compressed-air rupture of the colon is sometimes the result of a damnable form of practical joke, whereby a hose, carrying air under considerable pressure, is turned on near the victim's anus.

Blast injuries of the abdomen sustained during air-raids resulted in a number of cases of traumatic rupture of the intestine.

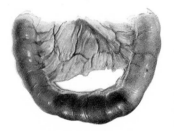

FIG. 451.—Laceration of the mesentery resulting in infarction of the associated portion of gut.

The pelvic colon was found to be injured more frequently than other segments of the intestine. Rupture of the upper reaches of the rectum is not unknown during sigmoidoscopy. In some cases of ulcerative lesions the air insufflation has been sufficient to perforate the intestinal wall.

Treatment.—In all cases of rupture of the intestine immediate laparotomy must be performed. In many instances simple closure of the perforation is all that is required. In others, e.g. where the mesentery is lacerated, resection may be required. In the case of the large intestine, exteriorisation, if possible, is often the procedure of choice. Except in early cases of high jejunal perforation, the general peritoneal cavity must be drained.

INTESTINAL DIVERTICULA

Literally, a diverticulum means a wayside house of ill-fame, and these wayside houses certainly live up to their evil reputation. When diverticulitis is spoken of, it is assumed that colonic diverticulitis is implied, otherwise the site of the diverticulum is defined, e.g. duodenal diverticulitis.

Diverticula occur in many parts of the alimentary canal from the duodenum to the rectum. Some of them are undoubtedly congenital in origin, for example Meckel's diverticulum, but the majority are thought to be acquired (Edwards). Evidence that acquired diverticula of the small intestine originate as a mucosal herniation through a point of entrance of blood-vessels into the wall of the intestine is found in the fact that most of these diverticula (Meckel's excluded) arise from the mesenteric side of the bowel (fig. 452).

Fig. 452.—Diverticulum at the *mesenteric* border of small intestine.

Meckel's diverticulum and the remainder of the vitello-intestinal duct give origin to many conditions of surgical interest and importance. Attention will first be directed to the vitello-intestinal duct and its remnants.

1. The vitello-intestinal duct occasionally remains patent (figs. 453 and 454), giving rise to an umbilical fistula, which discharges mucus and, rarely, fæces.

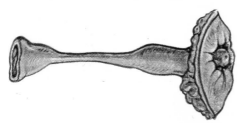

Fig. 453.—Patent vitello-intestinal duct opening into the umbilicus. (*A. L. Taylor.*)

Johann Meckel, 1781–1833. Professor of Anatomy, Botany, and Obstetrics in Berlin.
Harold Edwards, Contemporary. Surgeon, King's College Hospital, London.

2. Much more frequently only a small portion of the duct near the umbilicus remains unobliterated. This gives rise to a sinus which discharges mucus. The epithelial lining of the sinus often becomes everted to form an enteroteratoma (" raspberry " tumour).

3. Sometimes both the umbilical and the intestinal ends of the duct close, but the mucous membrane of the intervening portion remains and an intra-abdominal cyst develops (fig. 454).

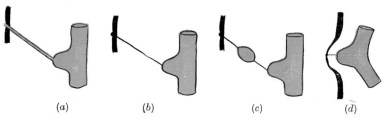

(a)   (b)   (c)   (d)

Fig. 454.—Varieties of anomalies connected with the vitello-intestinal apparatus. (a) Umbilical fistula. (b) Intraperitoneal band. (c) Intra-abdominal cyst. (d) Meckel's diverticulum adherent to the sac of a congenital umbilical hernia.

4. With its lumen obliterated or unobliterated, the vitello-intestinal duct provides an intraperitoneal band which is a potential danger, for intestinal obstruction is most prone to occur. The obstruction results from a loop of intestine passing under or over, or becoming twisted round the band (fig. 455).

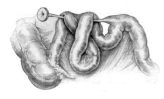

Fig. 455.—Meckel's diverticulum and its vitello-intestinal duct causing intestinal obstruction.

5. A vitello-intestinal cord connected to Meckel's diverticulum, but not attached to the umbilicus, becomes adherent to, or knotted around, another loop of intestine, and so causes intestinal obstruction.

6. Sometimes a band extending from the umbilicus is attached to the mesentery near its junction with a distal part of the ileum. In this case the band is probably an obliterated vitelline artery, and is not necessarily associated with a Meckel's diverticulum.

Coming now to Meckel's diverticulum itself, it will be recalled that the structure is present in 2 per cent. of the human race ; that it is situated upon the anti-mesenteric border of the small intestine, 2 feet (60 cm.) from the ileo-cæcal valve, and that it is usually 2 inches (5 cm.) long. One need not be acquainted with abdominal surgery for any length of time to realise that the diverticulum may be of much greater length, sometimes up to 2 feet (60 cm.) In 16 per cent. of cases Meckel's diverticulum contains in its mucosal lining gastric or pancreatic epithelium, or both (epithelium heterotopia).

The actual diverticulum, as opposed to its vitello-intestinal duct, can give rise to a number of pathological conditions :

Inversion of the diverticulum is a frequent cause of intus-susception, especially during adolescent life.

Meckelian Diverticulitis.—Acute inflammation of the diverticulum produces the symptoms, signs, and complications of acute appendicitis.

At an operation for acute appendicitis, if the appendix appears normal, an inflamed Meckel's diverticulum should be sought.

Peptic ulceration occurs at the junction of the heterotopic gastric epithelium and the intestinal epithelium. The ulcer is therefore usually situated towards the base of the diverticulum or in the intestinal wall immediately adjacent. Such ulcers are much more common in males than in females. The symptoms often occur in a child about eight years of age, but they may not appear until adolescent or adult life. Pain is similar to that of a duodenal ulcer, but it is not relieved by taking food or alkalis. The passage of blood, usually bright red per rectum, often follows the pain. In a child the occurrence of pain similar to that of duodenal peptic ulcer, associated with melæna and with a negative X-ray of the stomach and duodenum, should be suggestive of this condition. Not infrequently the condition remains unrecognised until the ulcer perforates (fig. 456). Severe recurrent melæna, sometimes unassociated with pain and otherwise unexplained, is another reason for finding an ulcer-bearing diverticulum at operation. Meckel's diverticulum is extremely difficult to demonstrate radiologically, and the absence of such a diverticulum cannot be assumed from the results of a barium-meal examination.

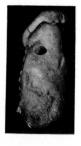

Fig. 456.—Per-forated ulcer in a Meckel's diverticulum.

Treatment.—It is unnecessary to remove a Meckel's diverticulum found in the course of an operation for another condition, because it is often a harmless structure. Excision is essential when it is inflamed, perforated, or if it is found to be the cause of an intussusception. When the diverticulum has a narrow neck it can be removed in the same way as a vermiform appendix. If its base is wide, crushing clamps are applied transversely to the long axis of the intestine and the diverticulum is excised between them. The base is closed with two layers of sutures ; the outer layer should be of unabsorbable material because occasionally ferments from a pancreatic heterotopia digest catgut sutures. In some instances, especially in cases where a peptic ulcer is situated in the mouth of the diverticulum, it is preferable to excise the segment of intestine bearing the diverticulum and restore the continuity of the intestine by end-to-end anastomosis. A patent vitello-intestinal duct should be excised together with the diverticulum when the child is about six months of age. When a vitello-intestinal band gives rise to acute intestinal obstruction it may be expedient to excise the band only, and to invaginate the cut end into the diverticulum.

ACQUIRED DIVERTICULA

The incidence in the various segments of the alimentary canal varies greatly (fig. 457).

Duodenal diverticulum (see p. 298).

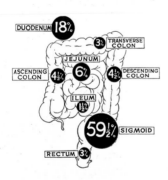

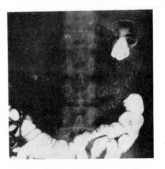

Fig. 457.—Incidence of diverticula in various portions of the intestine. Meckel's diverticulum and diverticulum of the cæcum, both definitely congenital conditions, are excluded.

(*After Dixon, Deuterman, and Weber.*)

Fig. 458.—Diverticulum of the jejunum three hours after ingestion of barium. The patient was a woman of fifty-six, with a fourteen-years' history. The symptoms were ameliorated by excision of the diverticulum.

Jejunal Diverticula.—These pouches vary in size, are sometimes single, but more often they are very numerous. Usually they are symptomless, but occasionally a solitary diverticulum (fig. 458) gives rise to two main symptoms : (*a*) vague abdominal discomfort and sometimes pain, particularly after meals ; (*b*) flatulence, sometimes very pronounced and associated with loud borborygmi. It is possible that the closure of the mouth of one of these diverticula is the explanation of the formation of a mesenteric cyst—a condition otherwise difficult to explain (see p. 400).

Diverticulum of the cæcum is almost certainly congenital, for it has a complete muscular coat. The diverticulum is solitary and is situated on the medial aspect of the intestine just above the ileo-cæcal valve. Its neck is narrow, and the diverticulum is subject to attacks of acute inflammation which are indistinguishable from acute appendicitis. When chronically inflamed it produces gross thickening of the ileo-cæcal region and dense adhesions. The cause of the chronic inflammation may not be evident until the cæcum has been resected.

Colonic diverticulosis—the presence of diverticula in the colon—can be demonstrated in at least 5 per cent. of persons over forty years of age subjected to radiological examination after a barium enema. Males are twice as often affected as females, and individuals with this condition are often stout. The pelvic colon is the usual seat of diverticulosis. The descending and transverse colons are sometimes involved. Diverticula of the ascending colon are most unusual.

Pathogenesis. — The diverticula contain no muscle in their walls. They are herniations of mucous membrane through the muscular coat of the large intestine, and occur most often nearer the mesenteric than the anti-mesenteric border of the colon, in close proximity to a tænia coli (fig. 459), and occur where the muscle coat is penetrated by an arteriole. Sometimes the diverticulum passes into an appendix epiploica. As a rule, appendices epiploicæ of a diverticula-bearing

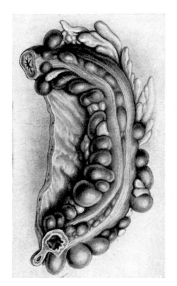

Fig. 459.—Pelvic colon with multiple diverticula.

pelvic colon are well developed and contain fat of a bright-yellow hue. The segment of colon bearing the diverticula is always spastic with a diminished lumen. The cause of the diverticulosis has been attributed to increased intra-colic pressure due to chronic constipation or purgation, and also to degeneration occurring in the parasympathetic ganglion cells of the affected large intestine.

Radiological Findings.—Colonic diverticula, as such, give rise to no symptoms. On radiographic examination by a barium meal, or better by a barium enema, the affected colon is shown to have lost its normal segmented appearance, is more contracted

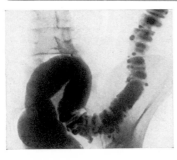

than normal, and globular shadows in relation to the colon are readily demonstrated. Sometimes only two or three are present; more often upwards of a score are visible (fig. 460). In early cases the diverticula are retractile and empty as the colon empties. In cases of longer standing the walls of the diverticula having become fibrous, the shadows persist for a considerable time after the enema has been evacuated.

Fig. 460.—Barium enema. Diverticulosis of pelvic colon.
(*R. Mather Cordiner.*)

Sometimes the diverticula are filled with fæcal concretions, in which case they may give a crescentic shadow, due to the interior of the diverticulum being only partially filled with barium. In a small percentage of cases the diverticula become the seat of inflammation.

Acute Diverticulitis.—In typical cases the pain commences at the umbilicus and passes to the left iliac fossa, and there is also maximal tenderness in the left iliac fossa, which makes the diagnosis from appendicitis simple. In other cases when the inflamed diverticulum is situated in a loop of the colon lying in the pelvis, and tenderness is only elicited by pelvic examination, the differentiation between the two conditions is not apparent until laparotomy has been performed. Usually perforation of a diverticulum does not occur suddenly because the neighbouring appendices epiploicæ tend to partially seal the perforation and an abscess in the left iliac fossa or in the pelvis results (fig. 461). In comparatively few cases the perforation into the general

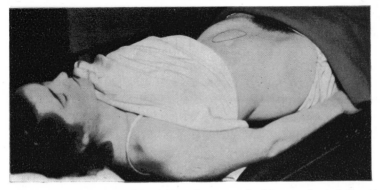

FIG. 461.—Abscess of the abdominal wall connected with a perforated diverticulum of the pelvic colon.

peritoneal cavity does occur suddenly, usually after the ingestion of a purgative during an attack of pain. The high bacterial content of the colon sets up an especially virulent peritonitis.

Chronic diverticulitis is more common than the foregoing and is accompanied by peridiverticulitis. In early cases flatulent dyspepsia and constipation are the main symptoms. Sufferers from chronic diverticulitis are liable to toxic phenomena such as lumbago, sciatica, and neuritis. As the condition progresses there are attacks of abdominal pain associated with diarrhœa and the passage of mucus, but rarely of blood. On palpation a thickened, tender pelvic colon may be felt in the left iliac fossa, or by bimanual examination, but as the patient is often obese, deep tenderness in the left iliac fossa is sometimes the only physical sign. Peridiverticulitis of long standing results in stenosis of the affected segment of bowel, and chronic or acute-on-chronic intestinal obstruction ensues. Intestinal obstruction can also arise from pericolonic adhesions implicating the small intestine. As a result of the inflamed colon becoming adherent to a loop of ileum, an entero-colic fistula sometimes ensues and is a cause of persistent diarrhœa. Vesico-colic fistula is the commonest internal fistula connected with diverticulitis. Usually it becomes manifest after the patient has had several attacks of diverticulitis, but it may occur without warning, the patient presenting entirely on account of symptoms of cystitis accompanied by pneumaturia. A fæcal fistula frequently follows incision of a paracolic abscess arising from diverticulitis.

Differential Diagnosis.—Many of the manifestations of chronic diverticulitis closely resemble those of a carcinoma of the colon. Colonic diverticula revealed by a barium enema can, of course, be concomitant with a carcinoma of the colon. If the growth takes the form of an ulcer or is of the papilliferous variety, radiological appearances are characteristic, as also are the sigmoidoscopy findings. The radiological appearances of an inflammatory and a malignant annular stricture are not always distinctive. Sigmoidoscopy shows a stricture in both peri-diverticulitis and annular carcinoma. The absence of bleeding when the walls of the strictured portion are swabbed favours diverticulitis. On laparotomy there is no distinguishing feature, and enlargement of the paracolic lymph nodes may be inflammatory. Even when the affected portion of the colon has been excised it is difficult to determine which of the two conditions is present, but should the mucous surface be ulcerated it usually proves to be a carcinoma. The final verdict in such cases rests on microscopical examination.

Similar difficulties occur when a vesico-colic fistula is found (see p. 419).

TREATMENT

Acute Diverticulitis.—When the diagnosis can be made with assurance, conservative treatment similar to that of the delayed treatment of appendicitis should be employed ; as a result either resolution or abscess formation occurs. A paracolic abscess should be drained. A fæcal fistula often results, and for this a waiting policy should be adopted, for after several months the fistula may close spontaneously. When diffuse peritonitis consequent upon perforated diverticulitis occurs early operation is imperative. If, owing to cicatrisation of the pelvic mesocolon exteriorisation of the leaking segment is impossible, the peritoneum may be stitched around the perforation so as to construct an external fæcal fistula ; in addition, suprapubic drainage of the peritoneal cavity is necessary. An alternative measure is to perform suprapubic drainage of the peritoneal cavity and transverse colostomy.

Chronic Diverticulitis.—In early cases medical treatment is sometimes effective. Purgatives are discarded and liquid paraffin substituted, and the diet should contain little residue. Courses of sulphaguanidine or sulphasuccidine are given. In cases with recurring attacks of pain in spite of this treatment, a defunctioning transverse colostomy should be undertaken. At the end of six months, if there is no stenosis of the affected segment as shown by a barium enema, the colostomy can be closed. When acute or chronic intestinal obstruction is present temporary transverse colostomy should be performed. After a sufficient interval (at least several weeks) this is followed by resection and end-to-end anastomosis of the diseased segment.

A **vesico-colic fistula** is treated by transverse colostomy, which is maintained for at least six months. In a few cases the fistula heals ; more often an operation to separate the two structures must be undertaken. The opening in the bladder is closed with sutures and an indwelling catheter is left in place for ten days. The perforation in the colon is closed and reinforced by an omental graft.

An Entero-colic Fistula.—It may be possible to separate the two hollow viscera and close the perforation in each. A large perforation usually entails resection of a segment of small intestine. Likewise, if the perforation in the large intestine cannot be closed with safety, the segment is either exteriorised or resected. If resection is necessary, a temporary transverse colostomy or cæcostomy must be performed to prevent distension and strain on the suture line.

TUBERCULOSIS OF THE INTESTINE

(*a*) **Tuberculous ulceration** affects particularly the ileum. These ulcers are usually multiple, and are placed transversely (see fig. 469) (cf. typhoid ulcer). Tubercles over their peritoneal surface allow of recognition at operation. Perforation is rare, but cicatricial contracture of the gut wall is a frequent and serious complication. Excision of the affected segment is sometimes possible. At other times the disease is widely distributed through the small intestine, and curative treatment is not possible.

(*b*) **Hyperplastic tuberculosis of the cæcum** simulates closely carcinoma of the cæcum, and is mimicked by actinomycosis of the right iliac fossa and chronic appendix abscess. There is a mass in the right iliac fossa. Radiography after a barium meal often reveals a filling defect (fig. 462), which at least tends to eliminate the possibility of an appendix abscess. Even on laparotomy, there is no certain means of telling if the mass is tuberculous or neoplastic. The treatment is excision of the cæcum and right third of the colon.

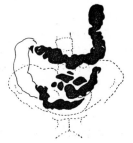

Fig. 462.—Stierlin's filling defect present in tuberculosis and carcinoma of the cæcum.
(*After Cawadias.*)

Eduard Stierlin, 1878–1919. Professor of Surgery, Munich.

(c) **Generalised tuberculosis of the colon** is rare outside sanatoria, a fact that makes it probable that it is secondary to tuberculosis elsewhere. Early cases may be mistaken for appendicitis, for the disease usually begins in the right half of the colon. Later, chronic blood-stained diarrhœa is the leading symptom, and the clinical picture simulates closely that of ulcerative colitis. Heliotherapy and general treatment are usually advised.

REGIONAL ILEITIS (*Syn.* CROHN'S DISEASE)

Regional ileitis is a localised affection of a granulomatous nature usually confined to the lower ileum, but it may extend to the cæcum and farther along the large intestine. In exceptional cases regional ileitis occurs in the jejunum. Occasionally several segments of intestine are affected at the same time or, as is more frequent, successively. It is essentially a cicatrising inflammation with ulceration of the mucosa.

Pathological Histology.—In the early stages there is œdema and infiltration by lymphocytes and leucocytes of the submucosa and, to a lesser extent, of the other coats, with a varying degree of ulceration of the mucosa. A characteristic finding is lymphadenoid hyperplasia of the submucosa with the presence of non-caseating giant-celled systems. In the later stages of the disease ulceration extends into, and obliterates, the submucosa, but giant-celled systems may be found in the neighbouring mesenteric lymph nodes. In many respects the condition resembles tuberculosis, but caseation in the wall of the diseased intestine or in the affected mesenteric lymph nodes never occurs, and tubercle bacilli cannot be demonstrated. Regional ileitis has been classified as a granuloma due to a non-specific virus. Hadfield and others are opposed to this view, and are of the opinion that it is a reticulosis.

Clinical Features.—Young adults are most often affected. The disease may be divided into four stages, in any of which a swelling may be palpable in the right iliac fossa or on pelvic examination.

First (or Acute) Stage.—A peritoneal reaction gives rise to symptoms indistinguishable from acute appendicitis, and it is at operation that the condition is first recognised. The affected portion of the intestine is bright red with a fibrinous exudate on its peritoneal surface. The corresponding mesenteric lymph nodes are enlarged and the mesentery is thickened. Occasionally, in acute-on-chronic cases, perforation of the intestine leading to local or diffuse peritonitis occurs.

Burrill B. Crohn, Contemporary. Physician, Mount Sinai Hospital, New York.
Geoffrey Hadfield, Contemporary. Sir William H. Collins Professor of Human and Comparative Pathology, Royal College of Surgeons, London.

Second Stage.—Mucosal ulceration predominates. Diarrhœa with the passage of blood and mucus is usual. There is progressive loss of weight, a varying degree of secondary anæmia, and sometimes evening pyrexia.

Third stage is characterised by symptoms of subacute or chronic intestinal obstruction. Cicatrisation of the ulcerated area has progressed to such an extent that the lumen of the intestine is narrowed (fig. 463).

Fourth stage is that of adhesion and fistula formation. The adhesions are dense, abscess formation is common, and fistulous

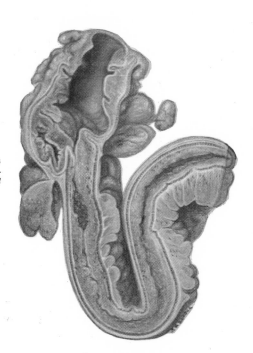

Fig. 463. — Crohn's disease. Third stage. *(Sir Lancelot Barrington-Ward and R. E. Norrish.)*

tracks develop on to the surface or into neighbouring hollow viscera. In such circumstances the possibility of actinomycosis must be suspected.

X-ray Diagnosis.—In the early stages X-ray after a barium meal often shows lack of segmentation and feeble or absent peristalsis in the affected portion of the intestine, the lumen of which remains constant in diameter. The third stage particularly gives a characteristic radiograph. The terminal ileum

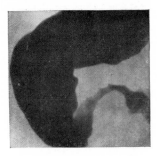

FIG. 464.—The "string" sign of Kantor.

is so constricted that what is known as the " string " sign of Kantor (fig. 464) is produced.

Treatment.—In the acute stage, when the abdomen has been opened in the belief that the symptoms are due to acute appendicitis, unless there is a long history of similar attacks, it is best to close the abdomen forthwith, for early acute regional ileitis sometimes terminates in complete resolution. In patients giving a long history, and particularly when some degree of intestinal obstruction is present, division of the healthy ileum 6 inches (15 cm.) above the diseased portion with closure of the distal end, followed by ileo-transverse colostomy, sometimes gives relief. Nevertheless, once regional ileitis is firmly established, so often does the disease persist and progress in spite of this short circuit that after an interval of about three weeks a second operation with resection of the diseased portion of the intestine is to be recommended. In the rare event of acute perforation the disease will certainly have progressed to the ulcerative stage. Closure of the perforation together with, in early cases, defunctioning ileo-transverse colostomy and drainage of the peritoneal cavity is the best course. In late cases suture of the perforation and drainage of the peritoneal cavity is all that should be attempted in the first instance.

In non-acute cases primary resection of the affected segment should be undertaken. In about 20 per cent. of cases, after an interval of freedom up to two years, the disease recurs in another segment of the intestine, usually that adjacent to the anastomosis, and further resection is required.

ACTINOMYCOSIS OF THE RIGHT ILIAC FOSSA

The commonest starting-point of abdominal actinomycosis is in the ileo-cæcal region, and the condition no doubt arises from swallowed streptothrices. A mass of granulation tissue forms in the submucosa, followed by ulceration of the mucous membrane. These changes are similar to those of hypertrophic tuberculosis. Unlike tuberculosis, cicatrisation and consequent narrowing of the lumen of the intestine does not occur, neither

J. L. Kantor, Contemporary. Gastro-enterologist, Vanderbilt Clinic, Presbyterian Hospital, New York.

are the mesenteric lymph nodes involved. Moreover, suppuration occurs and the disease spreads into the retroperitoneal tissues. Unchecked, the abdominal wall frequently becomes riddled with indurated discharging sinuses and eventually the liver, especially the right lobe, becomes involved by way of the portal vein, and a honeycomb liver results—a condition which is practically hopeless. In some cases the right lung becomes implicated by direct extension through the diaphragm.

Clinical Features.—The usual history is that appendicectomy has been performed for acute or subacute appendicitis. Possibly if the appendix was subjected to histological scrutiny the streptothrix actinomyces would be found. More usually this examination is omitted, or the fungus is not discovered, and about three weeks after the operation a mass forms in the right iliac fossa, and a little later still the wound commences to discharge. At first the purulent discharge is thin and watery ; later, because of secondary infection, it becomes thicker and odorous. Other sinuses form, and fæcal fistulæ are liable to develop. At any stage of the disease, if pus is collected and allowed to trickle down the side of a test-tube, sulphur granules may be discovered. The pus should be kept warm and sent for immediate bacteriological examination. Several examinations are frequently required before the streptothrix is found.

Another clinical type is that of a patient, most usually a young adult male, who presents with vague abdominal pain. On examination a hard, slightly tender mass is found in the right iliac fossa. Extension of the disease to the psoas muscle sometimes causes fixation of the hip in flexion. Such a finding is characteristic, but is only present when the condition is fairly advanced. No help is derived from radiology in distinguishing actinomycosis of the right iliac fossa from hypertrophic tuberculosis or carcinoma of the cæcum ; a deformity of the cæcum is found in all these conditions. Actinomycosis rarely gives rise to obstructive symptoms. When, as is sometimes the case, there is a history of a more or less sudden onset of pain some weeks previously, a subsiding appendix abscess is probably diagnosed, but the mass does not resolve. There is loss of weight, anæmia, and occasional pyrexia. A negative patch test helps to eliminate tuberculosis, but in most instances laparotomy is performed with one of the following findings : an abscess is encountered and drained ; the mass is found to be densely adherent to the posterior abdominal wall, and irremovable ; the mass is sufficiently mobile for right hemi-colectomy to be carried out. Unfortunately, the last procedure is often followed by actinomycotic fistula formation at the site of the anastomosis, but this is sometimes prevented by recognition of the condition from the pathological specimen and early intensive general treatment.

Treatment.—Iodine in milk should be given in the same way as that described for facio-cervical actinomycosis (see p. 201). Penicillin, 1,000,000 units daily for upwards of three to four months, is curative in some strains of actinomycosis ; in others it has little or no effect. Deep X-ray therapy is valuable in the case of multiple sinuses of the abdominal wall.

ULCERATIVE COLITIS

is characterised by the formation of multiple minute ulcers in the rectum and the pelvic colon, but sometimes involving the whole of the colon. Occasionally the pathological process spreads to the terminal part of the ileum. As time goes on the minute ulcers may coalesce to form larger ones. In long-standing cases there is always considerable intramural fibrosis of the colon. The cause of the condition is unknown. It has been attributed to special diplococci and to streptococci which are sometimes found on culture of the stools. It is now certain that these findings are incidental. As a rule the disease commences between the ages of twenty and forty, although occasionally it is encountered during childhood.

Fulminating type is ushered in with a temperature of 102° to 103° F. (38·9–39·4° C.) and incessant diarrhœa containing blood, mucus, and pus. In such circumstances the condition must be differentiated from bacillary or amœbic dysentery and typhoid. These infections are eliminated by bacteriological examinations of the stools, blood culture, and a Widal reaction. A scraping from the rectal wall obtained through a proctoscope may be necessary to rule out amœbic dysentery.

Chronic type is far more common. As a rule the initial attack is of moderate severity, but exacerbations at intervals of weeks, months, or, in mild cases, years occur. As the disease progresses the patient becomes wasted and severely anæmic from diarrhœa

Fernand Widal, 1862–1929. Pathologist. Physician to the hospitals of Paris.

and loss of blood. Often during the attacks there are 10 to 20 stools per day, accompanied by tenesmus.

Barium Enema.—In well-established cases the radiological appearance is characteristic. In the affected portion the colonic shadow is diminished in calibre. It appears as a rigid tube without haustrations. Occasionally craters of large ulcers may be outlined by the barium.

Sigmoidoscopy is valuable in the diagnosis of early cases and in mild cases when the pathological effects of the disease are insufficient to alter the barium shadow. The granular, reddened mucosa dotted with tiny ulcers (fig. 465) is very different from the picture seen in amœbic dysentery, where there are large deep ulcerations with the intervening mucosa comparatively healthy. As ulcerative colitis progresses, the ulceration may become so severe that practically no normal mucous membrane remains. In mild cases, when the passage of occasional blood and mucus per rectum is the only symptom,

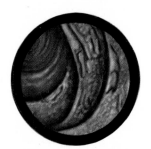

Fig. 465.—Ulcerative colitis. The granular inflamed appearance of the mucosa is characteristic. (*After Lockhart-Mummery.*)

sigmoidoscopy may be the means of differentiating the condition from a carcinoma of the pelvic colon.

Complications :

Pseudo-polyposis occurs in 19 per cent. of cases, and only in those of considerable standing.

Carcinoma.—An adeno-carcinoma supervenes in one of the pseudo-polyps in 5 per cent. of cases.

Stricture formation sometimes follows successful medical treatment and ileostomy. The stricture is most usually located at the recto-sigmoid junction.

Massive hæmorrhage is rare, but in half the cases in which it occurs the patient succumbs.

Perforation of an ulcer into the general peritoneal cavity occasionally occurs, especially in the fulminating type.

Recto-vaginal fistula, or a colo-vaginal fistula, sometimes complicates long-standing cases in females.

Perianal fistula, preceded by an ischio-rectal abscess, occurs in about 5 per cent. of late cases, and follows perforation of the rectal wall by an ulcer.

Polyarthritis often accompanies long-standing severe cases.

Treatment.—To correct dehydration copious fluids are administered. Intravenous saline and glucose is required in severe cases. There must be a high caloric intake (at least 3,000 calories per day). The aim is to provide a large amount of protein and carbohydrates with a minimum of fat and a low residue. Fluids thickened with skimmed milk powder provide increased protein. Dextrinised starch, malt, lactose, and chocolate are valuable. In cases of extreme wasting casein hydrolysate, 100 grammes (3½ oz.) daily, is given, preferably by mouth but, if necessary, intravenously so that amino acids can be absorbed without the necessity of previously being digested. Animal charcoal in 2-drachm (8 ml.) doses, or kaolin ½ ounce (15 gm.) helps to relieve the discomfort from flatulence. Vitamins are given to supplement those contained in the diet. Of great value are vitamins A, B, C, D, and K. Vitamin D is especially required because of the low content of fat in the diet. Vitamin K may help in controlling the bleeding. To combat anæmia, which is often serious, multiple small transfusions are more effective than large, less frequent ones. Blood transfusion should be continued until the hæmoglobin has reached a level of about 80 per cent. Liver extract, given parenterally, is also indicated. Phthalylsulphathiazole is administered in large doses, 1 gramme (15 gr.) four-hourly for six weeks. Some recommend that the sulphonamide should be given per rectum 6 grammes (90 gr.) in 6 ounces (180 ml.) of mucilage of starch run in slowly, with the foot of the bed raised, and retained as long as possible. Chloromycetin is helpful in some cases because of its bactericidal effect on streptococci and coli groups of organisms. Penicillin has also been given with a view to reducing infection by penicillin-sensitive organisms without, as a rule, any lasting beneficial effect. Morphia is necessary in early severe cases. Later, a combination of phenobarbitone, codeine, and belladonna is useful.

Operative Treatment.—*Indications :* (1) When perforation of an ulcer has occurred ; (2) in acute fulminating cases ; (3) after serious hæmorrhage ; (4) when the condition is not cured or controlled after some months of medical treatment.

In the case of a perforation into the general peritoneal cavity, ileostomy should be performed in addition to closure of the perforation and suprapubic drainage. In all other instances when surgical treatment is advised, about six days' intensive pre-operative preparation by the methods already enumerated is carried out. During this time the skin of the abdominal wall is hardened by the application of tannic acid jelly.

Ileostomy.—All are agreed that the ileum must be completely divided, so as to put the colon at rest. Opinion is not unanimous as to the best way of dealing with the distal end of the ileum. Some close the distal end and return it to the abdomen. The advantage of this method is that the single opening is easier to fit with a bag. The danger of the procedure is that if healing is followed by a stricture of the colon, the blind end may burst open. Others bring the distal end out of a stab incision (fig. 466).

FIG. 466.—Ileostomy as described in the text. Showing the distal end brought out through a stab incision.

A McBurney muscle-splitting incision is made mid-way between the umbilicus and the anterior superior iliac spine. The terminal portion of the ileum is examined, and if it is quite healthy a point about 1 foot (30 cm.) above the ileo-cæcal valve is chosen for the bisection ; otherwise an indubitably healthy area is selected higher up. The mesentery is ligated and divided at right angles to the intestine for a distance of 1 to 1½ inches (2·5 to 4 cm.). A stab incision is made 2 inches (5 cm.) above the original incision and through this is inserted a small crushing intestinal clamp, which is made to grasp the lower end of the devascularised intestine. Another similar clamp is placed, through the original incision, on the intestine immediately adjacent. After carefully packing off the area the ileum is divided between these crushing clamps with a diathermy knife. The distal end of the ileum is brought through the stab incision and there anchored by a single stitch transfixing the skin edge and the mesentery. The proximal end is brought into the grid-iron incision so that about 2 inches (5 cm.) of it projects above skin level. A purse-string suture is inserted, passing through an avascular part of the mesentery, picking up the peritoneum of the iliac fossa below the cæcum, next the lateral edge of the paracolic gutter, and lastly through the lateral leaf of the peritoneum of the grid-iron incision. When this suture has been tied it obliterates a tunnel which is a potent cause of strangulation of a loop of intestine passing upwards through the otherwise unobliterated para-ileal gutter. The peritoneum is closed, including the mesentery in the stitch, and the muscles are approximated around the loop, but no stitch passes through the intestinal wall. The extremities of the skin incision are closed. The clamps can be removed at once and a temporary bag applied, or the exteriorised intestine and the surrounding abdominal wall is covered with vaseline-gauze and a catheter connected to a suction apparatus removes the fluid fæces from the proximal limb.

The skin of the abdominal wall requires great attention to prevent excoriation, some degree of which is inevitable. A paste of aluminium 10 parts and zinc oxide 90 parts is perhaps the best of many applications. The stools thicken in a few weeks, and are usually semi-solid in a few months.

The Koenig-Rutzin bag, which is fixed to the skin by latex-

Charles McBurney, 1845–1913. Surgeon, Roosevelt Hospital, New York.

rubber adhesive, simplifies the management of an ileostomy. The bag is fitted two months after the operation, in order to give time for the ileostomy opening to contract, as each bag is made to measure. With a view to overcoming the difficulties of fitting an apparatus and preventing skin excoriation, a prehensile ileostomy is sometimes preferred. This consists in enveloping the projecting proximal wall of the exteriorised intestine with split skin grafts.

The Results of Ileostomy.—In a number of cases when the colon is completely rested, only a little mucus is expelled per anum from time to time. The patient gains in weight and the bleeding and tenesmus cease. When ileostomy is performed early in the course of ulcerative colitis, it may be possible to close the artificial anus and restore the continuity of the intestine by uniting the ileum to the ascending colon. Such a measure should not be undertaken under two years, and the indications for it are when a barium enema shows an absence of stricture formation and a return of normal haustration. If there is a distal ileostomy opening, fæces from the artificial anus can be collected, mixed with water and gravitated into the distal stoma. Provided this causes no symptoms on several occasions, cure of the colitis can be presumed, but in spite of these precautions in some instances the condition re-awakens and a new ileostomy must be performed. As yet the number of cases of ileostomy successfully closed without recurrence of symptoms is very small.

In about 50 per cent. of well-established cases of ulcerative colitis, ileostomy, while causing improvement in the patient's general condition, does not quieten the ulcerative process, and partial colectomy must be carried out. In the first instance a right hemi-colectomy is undertaken and the distal end of the transverse colon is brought out as a colostomy. Often this is insufficient because the main disease lies in the left half of the colon, which after an interval of several weeks is excised, the recto-sigmoidal junction being inverted and closed. In a few instances where the rectum is involved a perineal or a radical excision must be performed before the disease is eradicated.

THE SURGICAL ASPECTS OF INTESTINAL AMŒBIASIS

Pathology.—Entamœbæ histolyticæ pass through the mucous membrane of the large intestine into the submucosa, and there produce an inflammatory reaction. The centre of the congested area so formed undergoes necrosis, the mucous membrane in the centre gives way, and an ulcer results. The ulcer, which has been described as " bottle-necked," because of its considerably undermined edges, has a yellow necrotic floor (fig. 467) from which blood and pus exude. While such ulcers may be scattered through the large bowel, they are frequently confined to the cæcal or recto-sigmoidal areas (Nevin).

Clinical Features.—Dysentery is only one manifestation of the disease. In various guises amœbiasis obtrudes itself into the surgeon's diagnostic arena :

Appendicitis or Amœbiasis?—In tropical countries where amœbiasis is endemic this is a constantly recurring problem requiring considerable surgical judgment. To operate upon a patient with amœbic dysentery is to invite an exacerbation of amœbiasis that may prove fatal. Especially in cases where a palpable mass is present, the bowel is

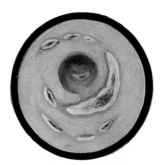

Fig. 467. — Sigmoidoscopic findings in amœbic dysentery.

(M. A. Arafa.)

friable and satisfactory closure of the appendix stump becomes difficult, or impossible. The death-rate from peritonitis and wound infection in the notorious Chicago epidemic of 1933 was appalling, which emphasises that surgeons in temperate climates should be familiar with the condition. In the case of amœbiasis of the right iliac fossa there is rarely rigidity, and pain commences in the right iliac fossa. Routine sigmoidoscopy is of great value. If real doubt exists as to the differential diagnosis, 1 grain (60 mg.) of emetine hydrochloride in 20 ml. (5 drachms) of normal saline given intravenously very slowly is likely to produce substantial amelioration of symptoms within two hours (Andreasen).

Perforation.—The most common sites are the cæcal and recto-sigmoidal regions. Usually perforation occurs into a confined space where adhesions have previously formed, and a pericolic abscess results, which eventually needs draining. When there is sudden fæcal flooding of the general peritoneal cavity, usually life must be despaired of, although Andreasen and others have had success by sewing the peritoneum down to the site of perforation and then performing terminal ileostomy, together with drainage of the peritoneal cavity.

Intestinal obstruction is a common complication of amœbiasis, and the obstruction is due to the adhesions associated with pericolitis.

Alarming rectal hæmorrhage due to the separation of slough is liable to occur.

Fibrous stricture may follow the healing of amœbic ulceration.

Hæmorrhoids frequently become acutely inflamed during an exacerbation of dysentery. The amœbiasis should be treated before the hæmorrhoids.

Granuloma.—Progressive amœbic invasion of the wall of the rectum or colon, with secondary inflammation, may produce a granulomatous mass indistinguishable from a carcinoma. Biopsy or the exhibition of emetine as a therapeutic test will prevent mistakes in diagnosis. Amœbiasis and carcinoma occasionally co-exist (Naunton Morgan).

THE SURGICAL COMPLICATIONS OF TYPHOID AND PARATYPHOID

Chloromycetin exerts a rapidly curative effect on typhoid and paratyphoid infections ; consequently complications are less frequently

Robert Wallace Nevin, Contemporary. Surgeon, St. Thomas's Hospital, London.
Anthony Turner Andreasen, Contemporary. Formerly Professor of Surgery, University of Calcutta.
Clifford Naunton Morgan, Contemporary. Surgeon, St. Mark's Hospital, London.

encountered than formerly. When any of the surgical complications of typhoid arise, chloromycetin should be given in addition to other necessary treatment.

1. *Intestinal hæmorrhage* may be the leading symptom. In three cases in our practice torrential rectal hæmorrhage has been the first indication of a typhoid infection. The condition must be distinguished from purpura with intestinal symptoms, and intussusception. A Widal reaction should be employed, and if negative, repeated in suspected cases. Blood transfusion may be necessary.

2. *Perforation.*—Perforation of a typhoid ulcer usually occurs during the third week; occasionally it is the first intimation of the disease (ambulatory typhoid). The ulcer is longitudinal to the long axis of the gut (fig. 468), and in the case of typhoid, it is situated in the lower ileum.

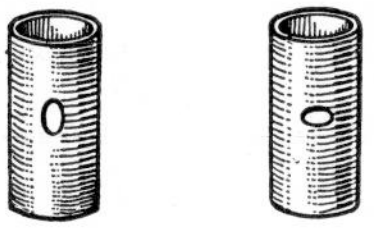

FIG. 468.   FIG. 469.

FIG. 468.—A typhoid ulcer is longitudinal to the long axis of the gut. (Peyer's patch necrosis.)

FIG. 469.—A tuberculous ulcer is transverse (because it follows the lymphatics).

In paratyphoid B, perforation of the large gut sometimes occurs. Treatment is to perform laparotomy under local anæsthesia as soon as the diagnosis is probable, and to close the perforation with sutures. The prognosis is very poor.

3. Spontaneous rupture of the enlarged *spleen* has been recorded.

4. *Liver abscess* is more often a complication of paratyphoid.

5. *Gall Bladder.*—Acute typhoid cholecystitis sometimes occurs (p. 347). Gallstones occasionally contain typhoid bacilli. Chronic typhoid cholecystitis can result in the patient becoming a typhoid carrier.

6. *Phlebitis.*—Venous thrombosis, particularly of the left common iliac vein, is a not very infrequent complication of typhoid fever.

7. *Genito-urinary Complications.*—Typhoid cystitis, pyelitis, bacilluria, and epididymo-orchitis all occur.

8. *Parotitis.*—Typhoid is a common cause of suppurative parotitis. In this instance the onset of parotitis is usually of grave significance (see p. 172).

9. *Joints.*—All degrees of arthritis, from a mild effusion to suppuration, have occurred as a complication of this disease.

10. *Bone.*—Typhoid osteomyelitis and typhoid spine are discussed in Chapter xli.

11. *Larynx.*—Typhoid perichondritis is met with occasionally, and typhoid laryngitis has been known to obstruct the airway.

TUMOURS OF THE SMALL INTESTINE

Compared with the large intestine, the small intestine is rarely the seat of a neoplasm.

Benign.—Submucous lipoma, leiomyoma, and adenoma occur from time to time, and usually reveal themselves by causing an intussusception.

Malignant *carcinoma* most often occurs between forty and fifty years of age. The jejunum is affected three times more often than the ileum. The most frequent symptoms are those of intestinal obstruction, and in about 40 per cent. of cases a palpable tumour is present. Because the content of the small intestine is fluid, by the time intestinal obstruction has ensued metastasis has occurred. In cases where a lump cannot be felt a correct pre-operative diagnosis has sometimes been made by injecting barium emulsion through a Miller-Abbott, or similar, tube. Another train of symptoms is dyspepsia associated with increasing anæmia, in which case a tumour, often of the papilliferous variety, may be revealed radiologically after a barium meal. Infrequently, a carcinomatous ulcer perforates into the general peritoneal cavity.

Sarcoma is very rare indeed, and of several varieties lymphosarcoma and myosarcoma are the least uncommon. Young persons, often children, are the usual sufferers. The neoplasm tends to convert the affected intestine into a rigid tube without much interference with the size of its lumen. Loss of weight and anæmia are the chief symptoms, and as a rule the tumour gives rise to a palpable swelling.

Argentaffin tumour is similar to a carcinoid tumour of the appendix. It occurs in the lower ileum, and is a cause of intestinal obstruction. It may become malignant and metastasise to the regional lymph nodes. At operation the tumour can be recognised by its yellow colour.

Treatment.—Usually wide resection of that portion of the intestine bearing the growth, together with its mesentery, followed by end-to-end anastomosis is indicated. The prognosis in the case of carcinoma of the jejunum is very poor, but in the ileum it is fair. An argentaffin tumour, being of low-grade malignancy, if widely resected has an excellent prognosis. Pedunculated innocent tumours can sometimes be removed by opening the intestine after applying light clamps above and below the tumour-bearing area. It is wise to defer such a procedure for a week or ten days if the tumour formed the apex of an intussusception.

TUMOURS OF THE LARGE INTESTINE

Benign

Lipoma is less frequently encountered in the large than in the small intestine, or in the rectum. Lipomata of the large intestine are almost confined to the cæcum. The tumour is submucous and in more than half the cases it is the cause of an intussusception. Other symptoms to which it gives rise are almost impossible to distinguish from those of a carcinoma of this region ; even macroscopical or microscopical blood is found in the stools. A barium meal may suggest a lipoma because of its smooth contour.

Multiple polyposis of the colon is a rare disease usually manifesting itself between puberty and the age of thirty. It is an inherited condition and is transmitted from both sexes to both sexes, though males are more frequently affected than females. The polypi are most often situated in the sigmoid and rectum, but they frequently extend into the descending colon and transverse colon, though rarely into the ascending colon. Often hundreds of tumours are present. The patient complains of attacks of lower abdominal pain associated with loss of weight, diarrhœa, and tenesmus, and the passage of blood and mucus, and sometimes pus—all symptoms very like those of ulcerative colitis. A rectal examination may reveal one or more of these polyps. Sigmoidoscopy shows a variety of neoplasms ranging from small sessile pink elevations to pedunculated tumours. A barium enema, especially a contrast barium enema, which is a radiograph following an injection of air after the barium has been partially evacuated, outlines the larger polypi.

Treatment.—In early cases when the polypi are limited to the rectosigmoid, fulguration through a sigmoidoscope, followed by sigmoidoscopic examination at regular intervals, may prove curative. Much more often a malignant change takes place in one or several of the tumours, and a radical excision of the rectum, together with, if necessary, staged resection of the affected colon, is the only curative treatment. Occasionally complete colectomy is necessary.

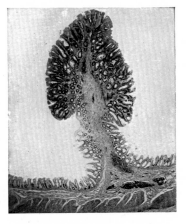

Fig. 470.—Pedunculated adeno-matous polyp of the intestine. Longitudinal section.   (*J. H. Saint.*)

Acquired adenomatous polyp (fig. 470) occurs in patients over forty years of age, and is often the precursor of papilli-ferous carcinoma. In specimens of carcinoma of the colon papillomata are often found adjacent to the malignant tumour.

Malignant
CARCINOMA OF THE COLON

Pathology. — Microscopically, the neoplasm is a columnar-celled carcinoma originating in cells which line the bowel, or in the crypts of Lieberkühn. Macro-scopically the growth takes the form of :

1. An annular constricting ring (fig. 471).

2. A tubular carcinomatous mass (fig. 472).

3. A carcinomatous ulcer (fig. 473).

4. A cauliflower proliferation, projecting into the lumen (fig. 474).

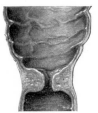 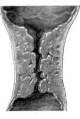 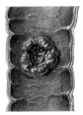 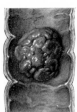

| Fig. 471. | Fig. 472. | Fig. 473. | Fig. 474. |
| Annular. | Tubular. | Ulcer. | Cauliflower. |

It is said that the annular form is the most malignant, in that it gives rise to secondary deposits comparatively early.   Type 4 is the least malignant form, and it is now certain that these papilliferous masses commence as simple adenomata.

Site.—The most frequent site is the pelvic colon, next the ascending colon, the splenic flexure, and the hepatic flexure, in that order, while the descending colon is the least common site for the neoplasm (fig. 475).

The Spread of Carcinoma of the Colon.—Generally speaking,

Johann Lieberkühn, 1711–1756.   Anatomist, Berlin.

carcinoma coli is a comparatively slowly growing neoplasm, and if extirpated thoroughly at a reasonably early period a cure can be hopefully anticipated.

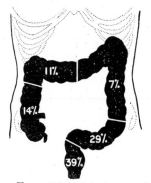

Fig. 475.—Relative frequency of carcinoma in various portions of the large intestine including the rectum.

Local Spread.—The growth is limited to the bowel for a considerable time. It spreads round the gut wall, and to a certain extent longitudinally, but it usually causes intestinal obstruction before it has penetrated surrounding structures. Particularly in cases of the ulcerative variety penetration of the serous coat occurs and, according to the segment involved, the abdominal wall, stomach, small intestine, spleen, the bladder, or uterus may become invaded by the growth. When a hollow viscus is thus implicated an internal fistula results; in other instances the perforation may lead to the formation of a local abscess and an external fæcal fistula.

Lymphatic Spread.—The groups of lymph nodes which drain the colon are as follows :

1. *The epicolic lymph nodes,* situated in the immediate vicinity of the bowel wall.

2. *The paracolic lymph nodes,* which lie in relationship to the leash of blood-vessels proceeding to the colonic walls.

3. *The intermediate lymph nodes,* which lie along the ileo-colic, right-colic, mid-colic, left colic, and the sigmoid arteries. In the last instance the paracolic nodes are often absent.

4. *The main lymph nodes,* which are aggregated around the superior and inferior mesenteric vessels, where they take origin from the abdominal aorta.

Spread by the blood-stream occurs late. Metastases are carried to the liver.

Clinical Features.—Carcinoma of the colon usually occurs in patients over fifty years of age, but it is not rare earlier in adult life. Exceptionally it appears in childhood.

Taking all sites into consideration, men are more frequently attacked than women, although carcinoma of the ascending colon is encountered more often in women.

A change in bowel habit is the most common early symptom. An adult who has had regular bowel habit all his life in a short space of time develops irregularity. The patient often states that he has *increasing* difficulty in getting the bowels to move and that he has to take *increasing* doses of purgatives. Because of the drastic purgation, attacks of constipation may be followed by diarrhœa.

Growths of the papilliferous type situated low in the colon

are inclined to give rise to a feeling of incomplete evacuation, which may result in tenesmus accompanied by the passage of mucus and blood, especially in the early morning. Often when the growth is of the annular type, chronic intestinal obstruction is the cause of the patient presenting himself. Increasing abdominal distension, attacks of colic, and borborygmi are then frequent symptoms. It is not unusual for a patient to be admitted suffering from acute-on-chronic intestinal obstruction due to a carcinoma of the colon, but giving only a short history of constipation. When the growth is situated in the cæcum or ascending colon the symptoms are often elusive. Anæmia, severe and unyielding to treatment, may be the predominating feature. If a palpable tumour is present the diagnosis is simplified. Growths in the ascending colon, and particularly those in the transverse colon, are often palpable at an early stage in thin subjects. A tumour present at one time and not at another, associated with attacks of pain, is characteristic of an intussusception. Sometimes patients with early carcinoma of the colon complain only of flatulent dyspepsia, a reflex feeling of fullness after food relieved by the passage of flatus or defæcation. It is in these cases particularly that radiological diagnosis is all-important.

Bimanual rectal examination occasionally reveals a hard, movable swelling in the recto-vesical pouch when the carcinoma is situated in a pendulous pelvic colon.

Sigmoidoscopy should be performed in cases where blood and mucus have been passed (fig. 476) and also in suspected cases when a barium enema is negative, because early growths in the lower part of the pelvic colon are not always visualised by radiography.

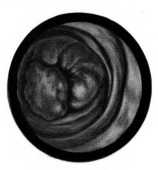

Fig. 476.—An example of the inestimable value of sigmoidoscopy. The patient had been diagnosed and treated for some weeks for " Ulcerative Colitis." A barium enema was negative. Sigmoidoscopy showed a small bun-shaped carcinoma giving rise to an intussusception.

Radiography after a barium enema often shows the growth as a constant, irregular filling defect. In cases of a growth involving only the mucous membrane, a contrast enema is very valuable. The barium emulsion is partly evacuated and air is injected into the colon. By this means the walls of the colon become delineated and a growth which fails to alter the contour of the barium-filled colon may be demonstrated. A tumour of the cæcum is more likely to be discovered by a barium meal than a barium enema. As a rule, in suspected cases of carcinoma of the colon, a barium meal is inadvisable because inspissated barium can precipitate intestinal obstruction when the lumen of the bowel is narrowed by a growth.

TREATMENT

The Test of Operability.—The abdomen having been opened, (1) the liver is palpated for secondary deposits; (2) the peritoneum, particularly the pelvic peritoneum, is palpated for implantations of the growth; (3) the various groups of lymphatic nodes which drain the particular segment are palpated. Their enlargement does not necessarily mean that these are invaded by metastases, for it may be inflammatory enlargement, as we have noted in diverticulitis; (4) the growth is examined with a view to ascertaining if it is fixed or free. So long as it can be mobilised sufficiently to be delivered into the wound it is operable.

Pre-operative Treatment.—When there is no intestinal obstruction, blood transfusion to correct anæmia, if present, enemata to cleanse the bowel, a high caloric and low residue diet, together with succinylsulphathiazole, 2 grammes (30 gr.) four-hourly for five days, are required. This sulphonamide has a slightly aperient action and it effectively reduces the number of virulent organisms ordinarily present in the colon. Streptomycin, 8 grains ($\frac{1}{2}$ gm.) twice daily by mouth can also be given with this object in view for forty-eight hours before the operation. These pre-operative bactericides have rendered resection and anastomosis of the colon far less dangerous than formerly. When intestinal obstruction is present, preliminary drainage of the intestine proximal to the obstruction must usually be performed (see p. 455).

Carcinoma of the cæcum, ascending colon, or hepatic flexure is treated, when operable, by hemi-colectomy (fig. 477). The abdomen is opened through a long paramedian incision.

The peritoneum just lateral to the ascending colon is incised and the incision is carried around the hepatic flexure. The right colon is elevated, with the leaf of peritoneum containing its

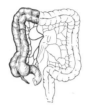

Fig. 477.—Showing the area to be removed when the growth is situated in the cæcum, ascending colon, or hepatic flexure.
(*After Arthur W. Allen.*)

vessels and lymph nodes, from the posterior abdominal wall, care being taken not to injure the ureter or the duodenum. The process of elevating the peritoneum is continued medially to near the origin of the ileo-colic artery, which is divided between ligatures, as also is the right colic artery when that vessel has a separate origin from the aorta. The mesentery of the last foot (30 cm.) of ileum and the leaf of raised peritoneum attached to the cæcum and ascending colon and hepatic flexure is, after ligation of the blood-vessels contained therein, divided as far as the junction of the right and middle thirds of the transverse colon. Many surgeons forthwith clamp and divide the ileum and the transverse colon at the level of their respective severed mesenteries, and excise the freed intestine (fig. 478). The divided ends of the large and small intestines can be closed, and a lateral anastomosis between the ileum and the transverse colon performed. Alternatively, an end-to-end ileo-transverse colostomy may be preferred. The defect in the posterior parietal peritoneum is repaired and the abdomen is closed.

Devine advises an exteriorisation method. The operation is carried out as above as far as ligature of the ileo-colic vessels and dividing the mesentery. Four inches (10 cm.) of the extreme end of that part of the ileum with its mesentery intact is

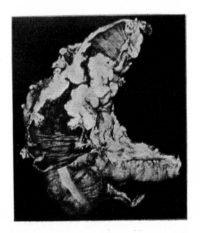

Fig. 478.—Adeno-carcinoma of the ascending colon. Specimen obtained by right hemi-colectomy.

Sir Hugh Devine, Contemporary. Senior Surgeon, St. Vincent's Hospital, Melbourne.

sutured to the transverse colon, and after repairing the defect in the posterior parietal peritoneum, the whole of the right colon and terminal ileum is brought out of the wound. The peritoneum of the anterior abdominal wall is closed around the neck of the ileo-colic approximation, and the abdominal wound is closed so as to leave 1 inch (2·5 cm.) of the coapted neck above skin level. Crushing clamps are then applied to the colon and to the ileum (fig. 479) and the whole mass, containing the growth and its lymphatic field, is excised with a diathermy knife. Devine employs this operation even in the presence of some degree of intestinal obstruction, in which event the proximal clamp is removed in six hours, but the clamp is partially reapplied in order that the intestine may be decompressed slowly. The continuity of the bowel is restored and the artificial anus is closed in a manner similar to that described and illustrated in the Paul-Mikulicz procedure.

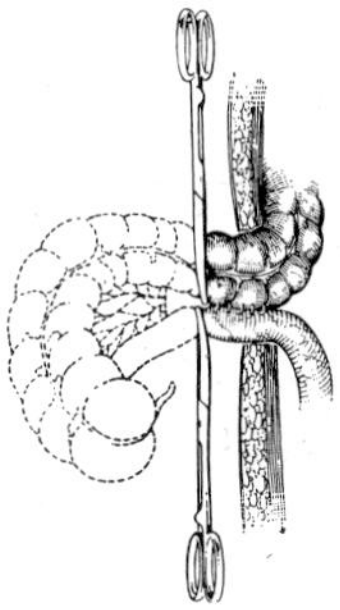

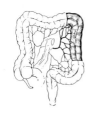

Fig. 479. — Right hemi-colectomy by the exteriorisation-resection method of Devine.

Carcinoma of the Transverse Colon.—

When there is no obstruction, ligation of the middle colic artery near its origin and excision of a V-shaped portion of the transverse mesocolon and the transverse colon with its attached great omentum, followed by end-to-end

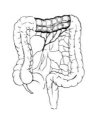

Fig. 480.—Showing the area to be removed when the growth is situated in the transverse colon. (*After Arthur W. Allen.*)

anastomosis, is a satisfactory procedure (fig. 480). If some degree of obstruction exists, after ligation and division of the blood-supply to the mesocolon, exteriorisation by the Paul-Mikulicz operation gives good results in this situation.

Carcinoma of the Splenic Flexure and Descending Colon.—

The phrenicocolic ligament is divided, and after incising the parietal peritoneum from the splenic flexure to the pelvic colon, the splenic flexure, descending colon, and pelvic colon are raised from the posterior abdominal wall in the same way as the ascending colon was raised on the right side. When this has been achieved, the left branch of the middle colic and the left colic arteries are ligated near their origin, and the peritoneal leaf with its contained lymph nodes is divided. The pelvic colon can be approximated to the transverse

Fig. 481.—Showing the area to be removed when the growth is situated at the splenic flexure or in the descending colon. (*After Arthur W. Allen.*)

Frank T. Paul, 1851–1941. Surgeon, Royal Infirmary, Liverpool.
Johannes von Mikulicz-Radecki, 1850–1905. Professor of Surgery, Breslau.

colon and the exteriorisation operation of Devine accomplished in a manner similar to that described in connection with right hemi-colectomy. Alternatively, excision with immediate intraperitoneal end-to-end anastomosis can be carried out (fig. 481).

Carcinoma of the Pelvic Colon.—For many years this was considered to be the ideal site for the Paul-Mikulicz operation. In this operation the pelvic colon is mobilised by incising the parietal peritoneum in the paracolic gutter, the sigmoid arteries are ligated, the peritoneal leaf divided, and the two limbs of the colon are approximated and the loop exteriorised (fig. 482).

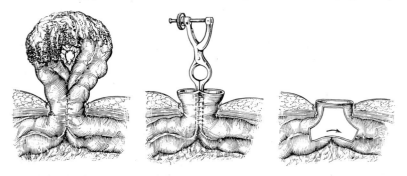

FIG. 482.—Stages in the Paul-Mikulicz operation.

The loop bearing the tumour is excised and an enterotome is placed on the intervening spur. If intestinal obstruction is present the last step is deferred and a Paul's tube is tied into the proximal limb of the colon. In these circumstances the application of the enterotome is postponed until the Paul's tube becomes loose and is removed—a matter of four or five days. An enterotome applied to the spur brings about restoration of the continuity of the colon by pressure necrosis, and the enterotome falls out in five or six days. Finally the colostomy is closed. When the pelvic colon is voluminous and the patient is thin, the Paul-Mikulicz is a satisfactory operation. If the abdominal wall is obese and the pelvic mesocolon short, the operation is difficult and a sufficient lymphatic area may not be removed. Because of these disadvantages other measures have largely superseded the operation. Devine recommends the construction of a defunctioning transverse colostomy as a first step. A similar operation to the Paul-Mikulicz is performed on the normal transverse colon to the right of the middle line, 4 inches

(10 cm.) of the transverse colon being united so as to form an effective spur. Devine divides the exteriorised loop between crushing clamps and brings the ends, via stab incision, through the skin and subcutaneous tissues, the original incision being closed. This puts the left colon at rest, relieves obstruction, if present, and permits thorough mechanical cleansing of the bowel (fig. 483). A few days before the second stage of the

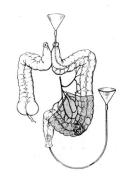

FIG. 483.—Defunctioning transverse colostomy employed as a preliminary measure to excision of the pelvic colon. The shaded portion shows the area to be removed. (*After Sir Hugh Devine.*)

operation sulphonamide wash-outs are given. At the second stage that part of the colon containing the growth is resected and an end-to-end anastomosis performed. Two or three weeks later, after healing of the anastomosis has taken place, the spur is crushed and the defunctioned segment allowed to function once more. Finally, the stomata of the colostomy are closed.

After-treatment.—Post-operative treatment includes the administration of penicillin to guard against chest complications and possible infection of the anastomotic area by cl. welchii. Phthalylsulphathiazole is usually given by mouth after anastomotic operations, 1·5 grammes (23 gr.) four-hourly. Its action is slightly constipating, and in this respect it is superior to succinylsulphathiazole, the purgative action of which, although slight, might endanger the suture line.

When the Growth is Found to be Inoperable.—If the growth is in the left colon, transverse colostomy is performed. If it is in the pelvic colon, left iliac colostomy is preferable. When there is an inoperable growth in the ascending colon, ileo-colostomy is the best procedure.

FÆCAL FISTULÆ

An external fistula communicating with the cæcum sometimes follows an operation for gangrenous appendicitis or the opening of an appendix abscess. A fæcal fistula can occur from necrosis of a gangrenous patch of intestine after the relief of a strangulated hernia, or from a leak after an intestinal anastomosis. The opening of an abscess connected with chronic diverticulitis or carcinoma of the colon frequently results in a fæcal fistula. Tuberculous peritonitis and ileo-cæcal actinomycosis are also causes of fæcal fistulæ, and they may be multiple.

External fæcal fistulæ can be divided into three varieties :

1. A direct track lined by granulation tissue communicating with the exterior.

2. A track lined by mucous membrane which protrudes above skin level.

3. A long, tortuous track lined by fibrous tissue and partly epithelialised, leading to some distant viscus.

A fistula connected with the duodenum or jejunum is bile-stained and contains undigested food. When the ileum or cæcum are concerned the discharge is fluid fæcal matter ; when the distal colon is involved it is solid or semi-solid fæcal matter. In some cases, when the leak from the small intestine or cæcum is small, it may be difficult to discern a fæcal discharge from pus. If charcoal is administered by mouth and a fæcal leak is present, the black granules will be easily distinguished in the discharge a few hours later. The site and length of a fæcal fistula can be determined by radiography after a barium meal or barium enema.

Treatment.—Fæcal fistulæ, especially those in connection with the small intestine, tend to heal spontaneously, if there is no obstruction beyond the fistulous opening. The abdominal wall must be protected from erosion by escaping intestinal juices as has been described in the section dealing with ileostomy (see p. 427).

The higher the fistula in the intestinal canal the more skin excoriation must be expected. This reaches its zenith in the case of a duodenal fistula (see p. 296). Some form of suction apparatus to remove the enzyme-laden discharge is a fundamental procedure.

Ferrum reductum, grains 5 (0·3 gm.) in capsules taken orally three times a day renders the intestinal contents less irritating to the skin. Phthalylsulphathiazole, by reducing the bacterial content of the discharge, assists in controlling the concomitant wound infection and favours healing. Fistulæ high in the alimentary track can result in dehydration and hypoproteinæmia. Intravenous saline and glucose, together with plasma infusions, may be required. In the case of a simple fistula where there is no protrusion of mucous membrane and the fistula fails to heal after a month, closure may be expedited by inserting an obturator in the following way : a disc of rubber, cut from the inner tube of a car, of suitable size, e.g. about 1 inch (2·5 cm.) in diameter, is transfixed by a mattress suture. The disc is rolled up and the resulting scroll is grasped with dressing forceps and inserted through the fistula into the intestine. When the forceps are removed the scroll opens in the lumen of the intestine. Traction on the suture approximates the disc to the wall of the intestine and occludes the internal opening of the fistula. The ends of the suture can be tied around a roll of gauze to keep it in place. When the healing of the fistula is almost complete one end of the suture is cut so that the remainder can be withdrawn, and the rubber disc passes along the bowel and is evacuated.

A fistula with mucosa visibly continuous with the skin edge will never close spontaneously. In some of these cases, where the opening is a large one, the intestine tends to prolapse upon the surface (fig. 484).

The operative treatment for

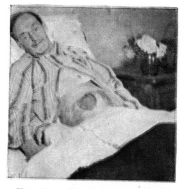

Fig. 484.—Fæcal fistula following acute appendicitis with gangrene of the cæcum. Aluminium paint is protecting the skin from excoriation.

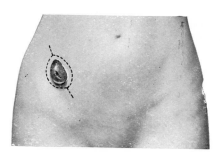

Fig. 485.—Incision for closure of a fæcal fistula of the cæcum.

closure of a fæcal fistula consists in making an incision as shown in fig. 485, and dissecting up the track through the abdominal wall and the peritoneum. The base of the fistula, now free, is crushed, ligated, and oversewn. The abdominal wall is then closed in layers. In the case of a fistula connected with colonic diverticulitis, if the fistula fails to heal after several months a defunctioning colostomy should be performed at a higher level. This step is always necessary in carcinoma as soon as the diagnosis is established. When there is no obvious cause for the fistula, the discharge must be examined on several occasions for the streptothrix or tubercle bacilli. The demonstration in a plain X-ray of many calcified tuberculous mesenteric lymph nodes favours tuberculosis as the cause. In complicated fistulæ operation is difficult, but in the case of the cæcum it is usually straightforward (fig. 485).

CHAPTER XXII
INTESTINAL OBSTRUCTION

INTESTINAL obstruction may be acute, subacute, chronic, or acute-on-chronic. The causes of intestinal obstruction are very numerous. In most instances the obstructing agent comes under one of four categories :

1. **Obturation.**—The lumen of the intestine becomes blocked by a foreign body, a gall-stone, a fæcolith, or inspissation of fæces or meconium.

2. **Intramural.**—The lumen becomes so narrowed by cicatrisation of its walls that the intestinal contents cannot pass. This occurs in inflammatory and malignant strictures. Also included under this heading are intussusception, volvulus, and kinking by adhesions.

3. **Extramural.**—The intestine is compressed from without. Herniæ, congenital or inflammatory bands, and pressure by an extrinsic tumour are the conditions that cause this type of obstruction. The last is rare.

4. **Loss of Propulsive Power.**—One segment fails to transmit peristaltic waves. Paralytic ileus and mesenteric vascular occlusion both come under this category.

The commonest causes of intestinal obstruction are an external hernia, carcinoma of the large intestine (including the rectum), inflammatory bands and adhesions, and paralytic ileus—in that order.

PATHOLOGY

There are four chief varieties of intestinal obstruction :

1. **Simple obstruction** in which the lumen of the intestine is occluded.

2. **Strangulation** where the blood supply to a segment of the intestine is seriously impaired or completely cut off.

3. **Closed-loop obstruction** in which a segment of intestine is shut off from above and below.

4. **Neurogenic obstruction** which arises from paralysis of the nervous mechanism controlling peristalsis.

Frequently more than one of these factors are present at the same time.

SIMPLE INTESTINAL OBSTRUCTION

The onset of acute mechanical obstruction causes increased peristaltic activity in the bowel above the obstruction. As a result of this activity the obstructed intestine and its mesentery become increasingly hyperæmic. When the obstruction is situated in the small intestine the following changes are noticed in the intestine below the obstruction. Peristalsis continues normally until the contents of the intestine have been absorbed and the residue has been passed onwards into the large intestine. The unobstructed small intestine then becomes immotile, contracted, and pale. Increased peristalsis continues in the proximal segment for a period of from forty-eight hours to several days. The lower the obstruction the longer does it last. If the obstruction is not relieved, a time is reached when increasing distension causes peristalsis to become less and less ; finally it ceases, and by this time the obstructed intestine is flaccid and paralysed.

Effects of Simple Intestinal Obstruction.—Loss of Fluids and Electrolytes.—The seriousness and rapidity of the loss is dependent on the level of the obstruction. Obstruction high in the small intestine, by preventing absorption from the ileum and leading to early and profuse vomiting, produces dehydration in a matter of twelve hours. The urine becomes scanty and chlorides disappear from it, and the blood chlorides, normally 500 mg. per cent., become progressively reduced. In the case of the lower ileum, which is a frequent site of intestinal obstruction, the loss is much slower, because for upwards of forty-eight hours absorption still takes place from the ileal mucous membrane above the obstruction. Nevertheless, as time goes on, for reasons stated below, the absorptive power of the ileum decreases. In colonic obstruction the amount of fluid loss is small.

Distension.—The intestine above the obstruction commences to distend as soon as the obstruction occurs, but before it can be recognised clinically, distension must be considerable. Distension is partly gaseous and partly fluid :

Gas.—At first the distension is mainly gaseous. In simple obstruction 68 per cent. of the gas is due to swallowed air, 22 per cent. to diffusion into the bowel lumen of gases from the blood-stream, and 10 per cent.

to bacterial decomposition of the intestinal contents (Hibbard). In closed-loop obstructions the gas must be derived entirely from the latter two sources. Whatever its original composition, the oxygen is quickly absorbed into the blood-stream and the gas becomes composed of about 90 per cent. nitrogen, the remainder being carbon-dioxide and hydrogen sulphide.

Fluid is mainly composed of intestinal juices. Each twenty-four hours there are secreted :

Saliva	approximately 1,500 ml. (2½ pints)
Gastric juice . . .	„ 2,500 ml. (4 „)
Bile and pancreatic juice .	„ 500 ml. (1 pint)
Succus entericus . . .	„ 3,000 ml. (5 pints)

7,500 ml. (12½ pints)

In obstruction of the ileum, these secretions are at first absorbed, but as the distension progresses the veins at the mesenteric border of the intestine become increasingly compressed ; consequently absorption of fluid by them becomes correspondingly diminished. The unabsorbed fluid accumulates in the obstructed intestine, and is further augmented by increased secretion of the œdematous, congested mucous membrane, which in turn still further distends the intestine. The diminution of the absorptive power of the ileal mucosa, which deprives the patient of water and salts, may prevent toxic substances due to the break-down of proteins, such as histamine, from entering the circulation.

Intestinal Toxins.—Prevailing opinion is that toxic absorption is not a lethal factor in simple obstruction as long as the intestine is viable. In late intestinal obstruction owing to breaking-down of the protein content of the intestinal juices, toxins *are* present in the obstructed intestine, but they do not enter the portal circulation for the reason given. In experimental animals a lethal dose of strychnine can be introduced into obstructed intestine, but it is not absorbed unless the obstruction is relieved and the contents of the obstructed segment pass into the healthy intestine below. Sudden release of obstruction of some standing therefore should, if possible, be postponed until the distended intestine has been decompressed by suction.

STRANGULATION

Primary strangulation resulting from herniæ, bands, intus-susception, and volvulus occurs concomitantly with intestinal obstruction, but the effects of the strangulation overshadow those of the obstruction. The dual lesion is the result of compression of the bowel *and its mesentery.* Mesenteric vascular occlusion alone gives rise to strangulation without mechanical obstruction.

Effects of Strangulation.—At first the venous return only is

James Sutherland Hibbard, Contemporary. Surgeon, Wichita, Kansas, U.S.A.

impaired, which causes the strangulated intestine, together with its involved mesentery, to become blue and congested.

Loss of blood volume into the congested loop depends on the length of the loop. When only several inches are involved, as is the case in a strangulated external hernia, it is not a matter of serious moment. If, however, a long loop of intestine (necessarily intraperitoneal) becomes strangulated, the loss of blood to the circulation is considerable. So great may be the amount of blood imprisoned in the loop that from a clinical standpoint it amounts to a serious internal hæmorrhage (Aird).

Distension.—At first the strangulated loop alone distends. The greatest distension is seen in cases where the venous return is completely occluded but the arterial supply is unimpaired. Unlike simple obstruction, the intestine above the strangulation does not distend ; indeed, it contracts for a time, varying from a few minutes to several hours. After this interval vigorous peristalsis occurs in the proximal intestine, but this is not accompanied by distension until there is retrograde thrombosis of its mesentery. Distension then appears both on the proximal and the distal sides of the strangulation (Chesterman). By this time gangrene of the strangulated loop is imminent.

The Onset of Gangrene.—Much depends on the tightness of the constricting agent. When the venous return is completely occluded, the colour of the intestine turns from purple to black. About this time, in many instances, owing to increased œdema at the point of obstruction, the arterial supply is jeopardised. Then the peritoneal coat loses its glistening appearance, the mucous membrane becomes ulcerated, and finally moist gangrene sets in.

Release of Toxins and Bacteria.—When the wall of the intestine becomes partly devitalised, both bacterial toxins and the products of tissue autolysis pass into the peritoneal cavity, there to be absorbed into the circulation. This is followed by the migration of bacteria, and peritonitis sets in. So it comes about that strangulation in an _external_ hernia is far less dangerous than intraperitoneal strangulation, for in the former the transudate containing lethal toxins and bacteria is limited to the small absorptive area of the hernial sac.

CLOSED-LOOP OBSTRUCTION

is present in the majority of cases of intestinal strangulation. In its pure form it is seen in carcinomatous stricture of the colon.

Ian Aird, Contemporary. Professor of Surgery, British Post-Graduate Medical School, London.
Judson T. Chesterman, Contemporary. Surgeon, City General Hospital, Sheffield.

Distally the colon is occluded by the neoplasm, while in one-third of cases the ileo-cæcal valve prevents regurgitation of the contents of the large intestine into the small intestine. Thus that part of the colon above the neoplasm is closed at both ends, and as a result of anti-peristalsis the pressure within the cæcum becomes so high as to compress the blood-vessels within its walls. Gangrene and perforation of the cæcum sometimes occurs from this cause. This is referred to as intramural, or secondary strangulation. In two-thirds of cases the ileo-cæcal valve permits regurgitation and the obstruction is of the simple variety.

Paralytic Ileus and **Mesenteric Vascular Occlusion** will be discussed under special forms of intestinal obstruction.

CLINICAL FEATURES OF ACUTE INTESTINAL OBSTRUCTION

Simple Obstruction.—The symptoms and signs vary with the nature and site of the obstruction, so much so that it should be possible to differentiate obstruction of the small intestine from obstruction of the large intestine.

When the Obstruction lies in the Small Intestine.—The first symptom is sudden, severe abdominal pain, which often comes without warning. The pain becomes increasingly intense and then passes off gradually, only to return at intervals of a few minutes to a quarter of an hour. These attacks of intestinal colic, which last from three to five minutes, spread all over the abdomen, but are localised chiefly at the umbilicus. In between attacks the patient is often quite free from pain. Recurring attacks of severe pain are a leading feature of all varieties of acute intestinal obstruction, with the exception of paralytic ileus, in which condition pain is slight, or absent.

When the jejunum is obstructed vomiting occurs with the first and each succeeding attack of pain. In the much more common obstruction of the ileum the patient may vomit once, following which there is an interval of several hours during which time the attacks of pain occur without vomiting. Ultimately copious, forcible, oft-repeated vomiting sets in. As acute intestinal obstruction progresses the character of the vomitus alters. Initially it contains partly digested food; next it consists entirely of mucoid fluid; thereafter the vomitus becomes yellow or green from regurgitation of bile; finally it is fæculent. This brown, evil-smelling fluid is jejunal contents ; the colour and smell are due to altered blood.

The pulse-rate and the temperature are normal in early cases, but in advanced intestinal obstruction the temperature becomes subnormal and the pulse-rate rises slowly. In early cases of obstruction of the small intestine abdominal distension is often slight or absent. Centrally placed distension is present in fully established cases of obstruction to the ileum.

Repeated vomiting leads to dehydration, and when the patient is first examined signs of dehydration—a dry skin, dry, brown tongue, and sunken eyes—may be present. The output of urine is small ; it is concentrated and contains little or no chlorides.

In view of the fact that external hernia is the commonest cause of intestinal obstruction, an examination of the hernial orifices should be undertaken early in the course of the clinical examination. In the absence of an irreducible hernia the abdomen is again inspected. Visible peristalsis may be present (fig. 486). In order to observe it the abdomen must be watched

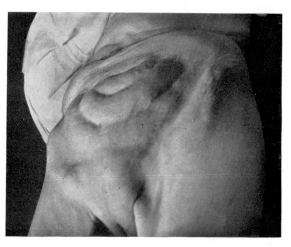

Fig. 486.—Visible peristalsis.   Intestinal obstruction due to the strangulated right femoral hernia, which can be seen.

for several minutes. If waves of peristalsis are seen and their appearance synchronises with an attack of intestinal colic, the information gained strongly supports a diagnosis of intestinal obstruction. In very thin subjects normal peristalsis is some-times visible, but in this instance the undulations are gentle and more constant; they do not come in waves and then depart, and their appearance does not coincide with an attack of pain. In the case of obstruction of the ileum, an obstructed coil may be felt to harden and soften intermittently when the hand is laid lightly upon the abdomen.

Borborygmi are sometimes loud enough to be heard by the unaided ear. More often auscultation is necessary. The sound of turbulent peristalsis coinciding with an attack of colic is valuable evidence of intestinal obstruction. In complete intestinal obstruction, after the contents of the bowel below the obstruction has been evacuated, there is absolute constipation— neither fæces nor flatus are passed. So it comes about that there may be a natural action of the bowels after the onset of the attack. Furthermore, it is commonplace for an enema to yield a small fæcal result. Of more diagnostic assistance is a second enema given half an hour later. If the obstruction is complete it is either returned without force, fæces, or flatus, or is retained and has to be siphoned back. In either of these circumstances the diagnostic significance is great, but if, as is sometimes the case, the enema is returned with a little flatus, or slightly coloured result, its diagnostic value is small.

When the Obstruction lies in the Large Intestine.—While many of the symptoms and signs are the same as those of obstruction of the small intestine, the commonly encountered acute-on-chronic obstruction of the large intestine, due in the majority of cases to carcinoma, has several distinctive features which help in distinguishing it from acute obstruction of the small intestine. In this instance intestinal colic does not come unheralded ; it is preceded by days or weeks of increasing constipation, which finally becomes complete. It is when flatus can no longer be passed that the acute symptoms arise. When the distal end of the large intestine is obstructed, distension is pronounced, especially in the flanks. No matter where the obstruction lies, whether in the ascending, transverse, or descending portions of the colon or in the rectum, the brunt of the obstruction is borne by the cæcum. This has been likened to a gun back-firing into its breech, and the cæcum becomes ballooned (fig. 487). Soon after the onset of intestinal colic, if the abdomen is watched, the cæcum can sometimes be seen to rise with each attack of colic, and fall as the colic passes off. It is not uncommon for vomiting

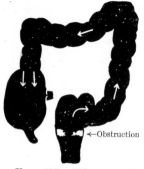

←Obstruction

Fig. 487.—Wherever the large intestine is obstructed the cæcum bears the brunt.

to be delayed for two or three days. On this account signs of dehydration are exceptional. On abdominal palpation a growth may be felt in the line of the colon, but it is usually obscured by the distension. A rectal examination will enable a carcinoma of the rectum or a mass of impacted fæces to be felt, and it may be possible to feel a growth in the pelvic colon which has prolapsed into the recto-vesical pouch. The diagnostic enemata referred to already are more likely to give conclusive evidence than is the case in obstruction of the small intestine.

Strangulation.—It is of the highest importance to distinguish strangulation from simple intestinal obstruction, because if the former is not relieved by an urgent operation, gangrene quickly follows. The diagnosis is made entirely by clinical methods. In some instances the differentiation is not difficult, for when the strangulation is a tight one, unlike simple obstruction, pain is never completely absent and spasms of intestinal colic recur three or four times a minute. Generalised tenderness and sometimes rigidity due to the extravasation of blood-stained fluid into the peritoneal cavity is also indicative that an early laparotomy should be performed. When a long loop of intestine is strangulated, there is an early rise in the pulse-rate, a fall in the systolic blood-pressure, and pallor. Much more difficulty is encountered when, as is often the case, the strangulation commences as a mild venous occlusion. In such circumstances the presence and character of local tenderness is of great significance, and frequently two or more clinical examinations at half-hourly intervals are required to detect signs of strangulation. In simple obstruction there may be an area of localised tenderness at the site of obstruction ; in strangulation there is always tenderness over an intra-abdominal strangulated loop, but the pain occasioned by pressure of the palpating hand is not relieved directly the hand is removed, as is the case in simple obstruction. This rebound tenderness is a distinctive sign of strangulation. Cases of intestinal obstruction in which pain persists in spite of one, or at the most two, hours of treatment by gastro-duodenal aspiration, even in the absence of any of the above signs, should be diagnosed as intestinal strangulation.

Radiography in the Diagnosis of Acute Intestinal Obstruction.—Plain X-ray films of the abdomen often give valuable information concerning the presence and site of intestinal obstruction. Frequently intestinal distension can be revealed by radiography before it is apparent clinically. Gas casts a shadow on the X-ray film and is present normally only in the stomach and colon.

In Obstruction of the Small Intestine.—Gas-filled coils of jejunum and upper ileum show as shadows one above another. The numerous valvulæ conniventes cause fine indentations of

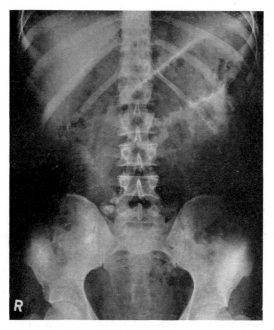

Fig. 488.—A plain X-ray in a case of acute obstruction to the small intestine by an inflammatory band.

the shadows (fig. 488). Although more centrally placed, these shadows are sometimes difficult to distinguish from the haustrations of the colon. The presence or absence of colonic obstruction can be shown readily by a radiograph after a barium enema. Loops of distended ileum appear as cylindrical shadows free from valvulæ conniventes. A radiograph taken in the erect position,

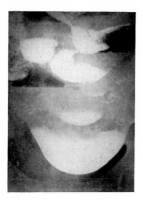

FIG. 489.—Fluid levels; subacute intestinal obstruction by bands. (*K. J. Yeo.*)

if the patient is well enough, or otherwise in the lateral horizontal position, may show multiple fluid levels (fig. 489).

In obstruction of the large intestine, plain X-ray films always show a large amount of gas in the cæcum. A barium enema gives concrete evidence of the presence and site of colonic obstruction.

TREATMENT OF ACUTE INTESTINAL OBSTRUCTION

There are three measures for overcoming and combating the effects of intestinal obstruction. They are: (1) gastro-duodenal or, when possible, gastro-intestinal suction drainage ; (2) replacement and maintenance of fluid and electrolytic balance ; (3) relief of the obstruction by operation.

The first two are always necessary preliminaries to the relief of obstruction by operation, and they are the mainstays of postoperative treatment. In some cases, as will be shown, they are used exclusively.

In every case of acute intestinal obstruction the first step is to empty the stomach by a transnasal aspirating tube and to keep the stomach empty by withdrawing the contents with a syringe or, preferably, by some form of continuous suction. The second step is to administer normal saline solution intravenously in proportion to the patient's needs. If signs of dehydration are present, the rate of flow should be 100 drops a minute until chlorides appear in the urine. The rate is then reduced to 60 drops a minute and saline-and-glucose solution substituted for the normal saline. The amount of saline solution and saline-and-glucose solution given intravenously, and the amount of fluid aspirated, is recorded, as also is the amount of urine passed. This enables an accurate fluid intake and output chart to be compiled later. During the first hour after admission the two enemata referred to in the section on diagnosis are given. When, on clinical examination, the cause of the obstruction is not obvious, radiographs of the abdomen are taken and the films examined. The clinical and radiographic data are correlated. The main indications for early operation, i.e. as soon as the fluid and electrolytic depletion has been corrected, are :

1. Obstructed or strangulated hernia (Chapter xxv).
2. Internal intestinal strangulation.
3. Acute or acute-on-chronic obstruction of the large intestine.

The most urgent of these is any form of intestinal strangulation. Gastro-duodenal aspiration should be continued throughout the operation, and also in most instances the intravenous infusion, which, in cases of strangulation, is supplemented by blood transfusion.

Relief of Obstruction by Operation.—When the cause of the obstruction lies within the abdomen but its site is doubtful, a right lower paramedian incision is employed.

When the Obstruction lies in the Small Intestine.—The hand is passed to the cæcum. In obstruction of the small intestine the cæcum is collapsed. The site of obstruction may be obscured by dilated coils of intestine, in which event an unobstructed contracted coil of ileum

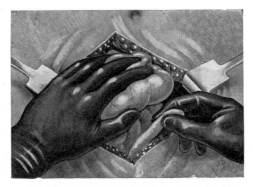

Fig. 490.—Acute intestinal obstruction : tracing a collapsed coil to the site of obstruction.

is sought (fig. 490) and followed upwards. This will guide the fingers to the site of obstruction which, if deeply placed, is exposed by displacing distended coils away from the site with warm, moist abdominal packs. Occasionally it is necessary to withdraw several coils of distended intestine before the site of obstruction can be displayed satisfactorily. Eviscerated coils must be kept covered by abdominal packs. The obstruction is relieved or short-circuited by one of the various methods described under special forms of intestinal obstruction.

Measures to be taken when the Intestine is Strangulated.—If, as is frequently the case in intra-abdominal strangulation, blood-stained fluid is present in the peritoneal cavity, the fluid should be aspirated or mopped up as completely as possible, for it is very toxic. After the relief of strangulation a decision must be reached as to whether the loop that was strangulated is viable. When it is black and the peritoneal coat has lost its sheen, when the mesentery shows a lack of arterial pulsation, or thrombosis of its veins, it is non-viable, if not already gangrenous, and resection followed by anastomosis must be carried out. In doubtful cases when the intestine is blue, purple, or dark red, it should be wrapped in a moist warm towel, while the anæsthetist administers pure oxygen. With the object of releasing arterio-spasm, which in part may account for the ischæmia, it is sound practice to inject about 10 ml. of a 1 per cent. solution of novocain into the base of the mesentery (Herrlin). A very fine hypodermic needle should be employed, and care taken not to prick a blood-vessel. If by these means the colour returns to pink, and especially if peristaltic contractions occur, viability is assured. Special attention should always be paid to the sites of previous constriction at each end of the loop. The proximal site of constriction, which has borne the brunt of the obstruction, sometimes alone is of doubtful viability, in which case it may be enfolded by passing sutures through the sero-muscular coats and covering the area with a patch of omentum. When the patient's general condition is too poor to withstand resection, doubtfully viable intestine should be returned to the peritoneal cavity, but obviously gangrenous intestine must be exteriorised and excised forthwith. If it is not excised, thrombophlebitis spreads from the veins of the extraperitonealised mesentery to the intraperitoneal mesentery, and so previously viable intraperitoneal intestine becomes gangrenous. Following this procedure a total fæcal fistula will result. Especially if the fistula is low in the small intestine, the patient may survive, and as soon as the general condition permits, the continuity of the intestine is restored by anastomosis.

When the obstruction lies in the large intestine it is usually due to a carcinoma or occasionally, in the case of the pelvic colon, to its imitator, diverticulitis, and the obstruction is of the acute-on-chronic variety. Acute-on-chronic obstruction of the large intestine should always be treated by early operation. If the patient's condition is good, laparotomy is performed through a right or left paramedian incision, according to the

John Samuel Herrlin, Jr., Contemporary. Surgeon, Fifth Avenue Hospital, New York City, U.S.A.

site of the obstruction. If the site is unknown, a right lower paramedian incision is employed. Distension of the cæcum at once confirms that the obstruction lies in the large intestine. Palpation of the pelvic colon and, if that be collapsed, the transverse colon, will readily lead to the obstruction. When removable obstruction is present in the ascending colon, at the hepatic flexure, or in the transverse colon, cæcostomy through a separate grid-iron incision is the best means of relieving the obstruction. If the obstruction lies in the pelvic colon, descending colon, or at the splenic flexure, transverse colostomy is performed. When the obstruction lies in the rectum or the lower part of the pelvic colon, left iliac colostomy is usually performed. For irremovable obstruction of the right colon ileo-transverse colostomy is employed. This measure is also used in cases of removable obstruction of the cæcum or ascending colon, although if the obstruction is not advanced, Devine's exteriorisation-resection (p. 436) is usually preferable in this instance.

When the distension is great and the condition of the patient is poor, blind cæcostomy is sometimes the best procedure. Under local anæsthesia, a McBurney's incision is made and, if possible, the cæcum is carefully brought to the surface. While a portion of it is held between the finger and thumb, it is punctured with a hollow needle connected to a suction apparatus. Deflation causes the thin, friable cæcal wall to become more substantial and permits more of the organ to be withdrawn, so that a rubber-covered clamp can be applied to it. Centred on the puncture, which is sealed by delicately grasping the immediate vicinity in the tip of a hæmostat, a purse-string suture is inserted. The cæcal wall is picked up by another hæmostat very near the first, and an incision is made into the cæcum between them. Through this a ½-inch (1·25-cm.) drainage tube is inserted and the purse-string suture is tied. The tube is anchored to the cæcal wall by a transfixing suture, and another purse-string suture is inserted and tied so as to invaginate the cæcal wall about the tube. If possible, a third purse-string suture is inserted and the process is repeated. The intestinal clamp is then removed. When the cæcum is mobile, all of it and the commencement of the ascending colon is brought out of the incision, and a glass rod is passed through the mesocæcum. In other circumstances the wall of the cæcum is fixed to the

Sir Hugh Devine, Contemporary. Senior Surgeon, St. Vincent's Hospital, Melbourne, Australia.
Charles McBurney, 1845–1913. Surgeon, Roosevelt Hospital, New York.

peritoneum at two points and the edges of the incision are lightly approximated above and below the protruding cæcum.

The disadvantages of blind cæcostomy are : (1) occasionally the cæcum is fixed to the posterior abdominal wall and it may be impossible to withdraw it ; (2) in closed-loop obstruction the cæcal wall may be on the point of perforating, in which case even the most gentle manœuvre is liable to result in perforation.

When the obstruction has been proved radiologically to be on the left side, *blind transverse colostomy* is to be preferred. The abdomen is opened through a short transverse incision over the right rectus muscle 2 inches (5 cm.) above the umbilicus. A portion of the transverse colon is delivered. After detaching the greater omentum from the loop, a glass rod is passed through the transverse mesocolon and the peritoneum is closed on either side, incorporating an appendix epiploica in each stitch. Vaseline-gauze is applied to the skin about the exteriorised loop, which is emptied by a hollow needle attached to a suction apparatus. The apex of the loop is then opened and a Paul's tube tied into it.

Gastro-intestinal Suction Drainage.—When intestinal strangulation can be ruled out, and the obstruction lies in the small intestine, gastro-intestinal suction drainage is the best form of treatment. This treatment should also be employed almost exclusively in paralytic ileus. In mechanical obstruction the combined effects of relieving distension by suction drainage and the administration of fluid intravenously greatly improves the general condition of the patient for operation, if that is necessary. Locally, diminution in size of the distended coils of intestine facilitates the operation, and closure of the incision. Another most important consideration is that if all or most of the highly toxic material is aspirated before operation, it spares the patient the danger of absorbing this material after the obstruction has been relieved.

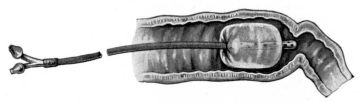

FIG. 491.—Showing the Miller-Abbott tube in position.

Frank T. Paul, 1851–1941. Surgeon, Royal Infirmary, Liverpool.

The gastro-intestinal tube, propelled by peristalsis, decompresses loop after loop (fig. 491) until it reaches the site of mechanical obstruction. Even in mechanical obstruction due to kinking of a coil or coils of intestine by adhesions, gastro-intestinal suction drainage alone sometimes brings about complete rectification.

There are two main types of gastro-intestinal tube :

The Miller-Abbott Double Lumen Tube.—One-third of the lumen is used for inflation of the balloon which is attached to the extremity of the tube ; two-thirds of the lumen are devoted to suction drainage. . . . . ⬤

The Cantor gastro-intestinal tube is a $\frac{3}{16}$-inch (0·5 cm.) single lumen tube to the end of which is attached a balloon containing 5 ml. (1½ drachms) of mercury. The first 20 inches (50 cm.) of the tube above the balloon is provided with multiple side holes of a length of ⅛ inch (0·3 cm.) in groups of four at intervals of 1 inch (2·5 cm.) with 4 inches (10 cm.) between each group.

The Miller-Abbott tube is 10 feet 8 inches (3·2 metres) in length, while the Cantor tube is 10 feet (3 metres) in length. The Miller-Abbott tube is calibrated in centimetres and the Cantor tube is calibrated in inches by its holes.

The Passage of a Miller-Abbott Gastro-intestinal Tube.—After preliminary cocainisation of the wider naris, the bag, folded round the end of the tube and well lubricated with liquid paraffin, is passed into the naso-pharynx and thence, while the patient sips water, into the stomach. When 2 feet (60 cm.) has been passed, the contents of the stomach are aspirated by a suction apparatus or a syringe. The tube is supported by allowing it to hang in a loop of tape fastened to the cheek with adhesive strapping. After the contents of the stomach have been aspirated the tube is advanced inch by inch at intervals of five minutes, while the patient sips water, until 2 feet 6 inches (75 cm.) has been paid out. The patient then lies on his right side for half an hour, continuous suction drainage being maintained. A radiograph is taken and this should show the tube lying along the greater curvature with its tip directed to the pylorus, in which case the patient sips more water and the tube is advanced another 2 inches (5 cm.). In favourable cases the tip of the tube should now have passed beyond the pylorus. If the tube is shown to be curled up in the stomach, it is withdrawn to the 60-cm. (2 feet) mark, and the process repeated. It may take many hours to negotiate the pylorus ; in some instances the method fails. Once the pylorus has been passed the balloon is inflated with 30 ml. of air and about 6 inches (15 cm.) of freshly lubricated tube is inserted every twenty minutes. Sometimes the tube is carried onwards spontaneously, therefore a loop is always left in readiness between the nostril and the tape. Cantor's tube is advanced in much the same way, the mercury-filled bag being the impetus for propulsion along the intestine once the pylorus has been negotiated.

Suction.—Wangensteen showed that in order to remove gas as well as fluid from the intestine a sub-atmospheric pressure of 75 cm. (30 inches) of water applied to the tube is the optimum negative pressure. Continuous suction is effected by an electric pump or by water-operated suction, as in Wangensteen's apparatus or one of its modifications. More commonly intermittent aspiration by a syringe is employed.

Thomas G. Miller, Contemporary. Professor of Clinical Medicine, University of Pennsylvania.
William O. Abbott, Contemporary. Associate in Medicine, University of Pennsylvania.
Meyer O. Cantor, Contemporary. Assistant Surgeon, Grace Hospital, Detroit, Michigan, U.S.A.
Owen Harding Wangensteen, Contemporary. Professor of Surgery, University of Minnesota, Minneapolis, U.S.A.

Maintenance of Fluid and Electrolytic Balance.—Once the fluid and salt loss have been restored, and commonly as much as 7 pints (4 litres) of normal saline are required if the patient shows signs of dehydration, and half that amount if such signs are absent, a fluid balance chart must be compiled and the daily fluid needs of the patient estimated. The fluid output comprises (a) the amount of urine passed—normally $2\frac{1}{2}$ pints (1,500 ml.) ; (b) the amount of gastro-intestinal contents withdrawn by suction—often as much as 5 pints (3,000 ml.) ; to which must be added (c) 1 pint (500 ml.) for invisible loss by the lungs and skin and (d) another 1 pint (500 ml.) if the patient is pyrexial for additional loss by perspiration. The total loss is therefore somewhere in the region of 8 pints (5,000 ml.). The total loss having been estimated, if it is reduced to litres and multiplied by eleven, it will give the rate at which the drip should be run (Aird).

There must be constant vigilance that the salt intake is adequate, but not excessive. The salt needs of a patient at rest are 3 grammes (45 gr.) per diem, to which must be added 5 grammes (75 gr.) for every litre removed by gastro-intestinal suction. A daily estimation of the urinary chlorides is a reliable check in this respect. If too much salt is given, especially in the elderly, œdema of the tissues and the lungs ensues.

During the first twenty-four hours after dehydration has been corrected by the administration of normal saline, a solution containing 5 per cent. glucose and 0·18 per cent. saline is given. A twenty-four-hour balance chart having been compiled, each day saline and glucose is given intravenously until the patient's requirement of salt for that day has been satisfied ; for the remainder of the twenty-four hours 5 per cent. glucose solution is substituted. The amount of fluid given by mouth is included in the intake ; most of this fluid is removed by suction in the early stages of decompression, but as more and more loops become decompressed an increasing amount of the fluid is absorbed by the decompressed intestine. Consequently the balance chart will show that less fluid is required intravenously.

Some special forms of intestinal obstruction will now be considered.

ACUTE INTESTINAL OBSTRUCTION OF THE NEW-BORN

Volvulus Neonatorum.—There are two types of volvulus neonatorum :

Type 1.—The cæcum lies in the upper right quadrant, and on laparotomy the ascending and transverse colons are readily visible. The duodenum is obstructed by the cæcum itself, or, more commonly, by a band connected thereto (fig. 492).

Type 2.—The small intestine presents, but the ascending colon, so readily visible in the previous variety, is hidden from view. This variety is a mid-gut volvulus (fig. 493). There are two, sometimes three, twists in

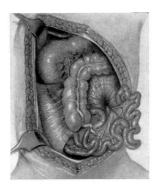

FIG. 492.—Volvulus neonatorum, Type 1. The incompletely rotated cæcum obstructs the third part of the duodenum. (*a*) The cæcum itself is the obstructing agent ; (*b*) A band connected to the cæcum is the obstructing agent.

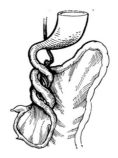

FIG. 493.—Volvulus neonatorum. Type 2.

a clockwise direction. The volvulus is not a tight one, so the mesenteric blood vessels are not, as a rule, compressed ; consequently there are no colour changes in the bowel.

Clinical Features.—The infant, apparently normal at birth, remains so for a few days. Vomiting then commences, persists and becomes bile-stained. There is very little abdominal distension, as the obstruction is a high one. A radiograph shows the stomach and duodenum filled with gas.

Treatment.—Unless laparotomy is performed and the volvulus untwisted, the condition is necessarily fatal. The abdomen should be opened through a long upper right paramedian incision. In Type 1 the peritoneal reflexion or any bands attached to the cæcum are divided so that the duodenum is completely freed, and the cæcum is placed in the left side of the abdomen. This converts the condition into one of complete non-rotation, with the large intestine on the left side and the small intestine on the right—a state that rarely gives rise to symptoms. In Type 2 it is best to eviscerate the small intestine and perform untwisting under vision, after which the duodenum is inspected to make sure that it is unobstructed. Again, it is usually best to place the cæcum on the left side of the abdomen.

Congenital intestinal occlusions always occur at the site of an embryological event (Bland-Sutton). Thus we may expect them particularly : (1) in the duodenum (liver and pancreatic buds) ; (2) at the lower end of the ileum (site of the obliterated vitello-intestinal duct) ; (3) in the rectum (junction of hind-gut and proctodæum). This expectation is borne out in practice. The commonest occlusion is imperforate anus.

Sir John Bland-Sutton, 1855–1936. Surgeon, Middlesex Hospital.

Congenital atresia of the ileum is due to a septum across the lumen of the gut (fig. 494), usually at the level of Meckel's diverticulum. Occasionally there is a complete gap in the continuity of the intestine, which may be associated with a corresponding mesenteric defect.

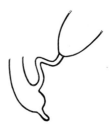

FIG. 494.—Congenital atresia of the ileum. The relative size of the gut above and below the septum is not exaggerated.

Clinical Features.—Unlike volvulus neonatorum, the infant commences to vomit on the day of birth, and the symptoms become progressively more severe as feeding is attempted. The amount of distension will vary with the duration of the obstruction. Radiography shows dilated small intestine with a lack of gas shadows in the large intestine.

Treatment.—After dehydration has been corrected the stomach is aspirated before, during, and after the operation. The extremely small diameter of the distal intestine makes the operation difficult. The contracted segment can be dilated by applying light clamps and then injecting air or saline solution into the intervening portion. Once dilated, and the clamps removed, the intestine does not contract so much as previously. Lateral anastomosis is performed between the dilated intestine above and the contracted intestine below. One layer of sutures only is used, as two layers would cause narrowing. Ladd employs a catheter in the contracted distal lumen, which is removed just before the anastomosis is completed. The mortality is over 75 per cent.

Congenital Duodenal Occlusion (see p. 272).

Imperforate Anus (see p. 509).

Meconium Ileus is an extremely rare form of intestinal obstruction in the new-born. The condition is usually, but not necessarily, associated with atresia of the main pancreatic duct. Like congenital intestinal atresia, the symptoms of intestinal obstruction come on during the first day of life. The X-ray appearances and the clinical features are the same as those of congenital intestinal atresia.

Operation should be undertaken as soon as dehydration and electrolytic balance have been corrected. The small intestine is grossly dilated and the terminal ileum is the usual site of the meconium impaction. After inserting a purse-string suture in the wall of the ileum, enterostomy is performed and a small catheter introduced into the lumen of the intestine, the purse-string being drawn tight, but not tied. Saline solution is injected into the intestine by a syringe, while the ileo-cæcal orifice is occluded by compressing it between finger and thumb. When the lower ileum has been thoroughly distended with fluid, the purse-string suture is loosened and the catheter removed, and the contents of the ileum allowed to escape into a sterile bowl, any solid portions being milked towards the enterostomy opening. The catheter is reinserted and the same procedure is performed in an upward direction until the intestine is freed from obstructing meconium. The purse-string suture is then tied, the suture-line reinforced, and the abdomen closed. Meconium ileus is sometimes associated with volvulus neonatorum.

ACUTE INTUSSUSCEPTION

One portion of the gut becomes invaginated into another immediately adjacent ; almost always it is the proximal into the distal. Occasionally the intussusception is retrograde.

Johann Meckel, 1781–1833. Professor of Anatomy, Botany, and Obstetrics, Berlin.
William E. Ladd, Contemporary. Emeritus Professor of Child Surgery, Harvard University, Boston, U.S.A.

Ætiology.—In a few cases there is some understandable cause, for, at the apex of the intussusception, a polyp, a papilliferous carcinoma, a submucous lipoma, or an inverted Meckel's diverticulum is found protruding. Obviously such a protrusion invites intussusception (fig. 495). In intussusception of infants there is no such demonstrable cause, and considerable ingenuity has been expended in accounting for this common form of intestinal obstruction.

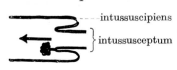

FIG. 495.—The mechanism of the production of an intussusception.

The following is a reasonable hypothesis for a condition that is otherwise difficult to explain.

Facts

1. Idiopathic intussusception occurs most often between the sixth and ninth months.
2. Between the sixth and ninth months there is a change in the infant's diet—it is weaned.
3. An idiopathic intussusception usually commences in some part of the last 2 feet (60 cm.) of the small intestine.
4. Peyer's patches are maximally aggregated in the lower ileum.

Theory

1. The alteration of diet brings about a change of intestinal bacteria.
2. This predisposes to inflammation of the intestinal tract.
3. Which in turn causes inflammation of Peyer's patches.
4. As a result Peyer's patches swell.
5. A swollen Peyer's patch produces an elevation protruding into the lumen of the gut comparable to one of the known causes of intussusception.

Other Theories :

The frequency with which enlarged lymph nodes at the ileocæcal angle accompany intussusception of infancy has led to the assumption that enlargement of these nodes favours intussusception.

Some consider that when the extreme terminal ileum is constricted by a spasm of intestinal colic, it is guided through the ileo-cæcal valve by the " bloodless " fold of Treves, which is well developed in infancy.

In hospital practice intussusceptions occur commonly at holiday time when children are taken out and given unsuitable food.

Pathology.—An intussusception is made up of three parts :

1. The entering, or inner, tube.
2. The returning, or middle, tube.
3. The sheath, or outer tube.

The outer tube is called the *intussuscipiens*. The inner and middle tubes together form the *intussusceptum*. The neck is the junction of the entering layer with the mass. That part which advances is the

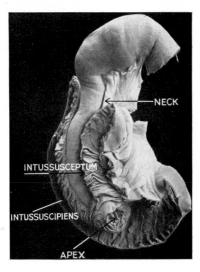

FIG. 496.—An intussusception dissected to show its constituent parts.

apex, and the mass which constitutes the intussusception (fig. 496) increases as it advances.

The blood-supply of the inner layers of the intussusception is liable to be cut off. It will be appreciated that the onset of gangrene is dependent upon the tightness of the invagination, and so it comes about that gangrene is especially liable to occur early in a small, tight intussusception, and it is the ileo-colic variety which produces this type because of the great pressure exerted on it by passing through the ileo-cæcal valve.

Varieties (fig. 497).—The following is a simple classification :
1. *Ileo-ileal.* Ileum is invaginated into ileum . Approx. 8 per cent.
2. *Ileo-colic.* An ileo-ileal intussusception which has passed through the ileo-cæcal valve into the colon . . . . . . ,, 36 ,,
3. *Ileo-cæcal.* The ileo-cæcal valve is the apex of the intussusception . . . . ,, 46 ,,
4. *Cæcal.* The caput cæci becomes invaginated ,, 2 ,,
5. *Colo-colic.* The colon is invaginated into the colon . . . . ,, 8 ,,

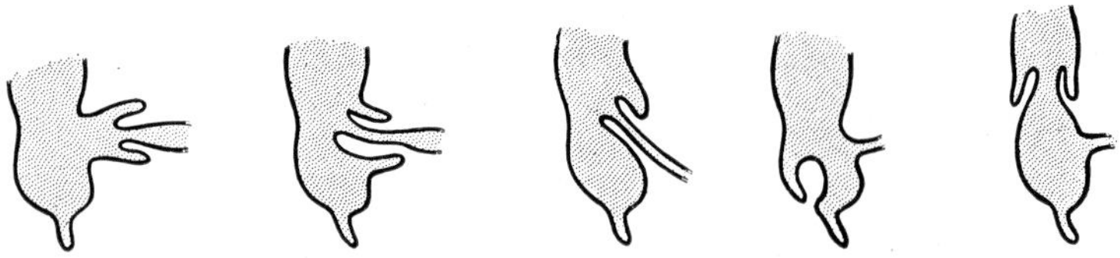

| ILEO-ILEAL | ILEO-COLIC | ILEO-CÆCAL | CÆCAL | COLO-COLIC |

FIG. 497.—Varieties of intussusception.

Clinical Features of Intussusception in Infants.—The patient is usually a fine, lusty male child between six and twelve months of age, and in perfect health when attacked. The onset is sudden. The child has a paroxysm of abdominal pain, draws up his legs, and screams. The patient may vomit shortly after the onset of the attack, but this is not a constant occurrence ; not until the intussusception has been present for about twenty-four hours is vomiting a conspicuous feature. The attacks, which last a few minutes and recur at about every fifteen minutes, are accompanied by facial pallor. They become progressively more severe. In between the attacks he lies listless and somewhat drawn. A normal stool may be passed in the early stages. Later, blood and mucus are evacuated, which together are very characteristic, and constitute the well-known " red-currant jelly " stool.

On Examination.—The abdomen is not distended. It is important to palpate with a warmed hand between the spasms, if possible while the baby is asleep. A lump, which hardens on palpation, may be felt in some part of the course of the colon

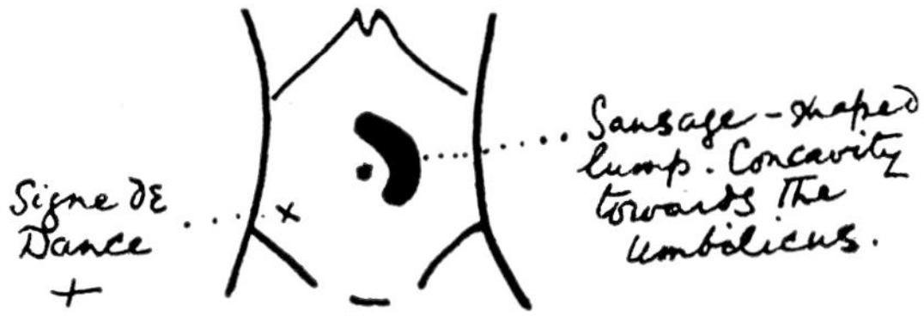

Fig. 498.—The physical signs recorded in a typical case of intussusception in an infant.

(fig. 498). If the lump is lying under the right or left costal margins it is sometimes not possible to feel it even under an anæsthetic. There is said to be a feeling of emptiness in the right iliac fossa (*signe de* Dance). On rectal examination, if the intussusception has travelled far enough, its apex, a conical mass which is aptly likened to the cervix uteri, will be felt. In the majority of cases the intussusception has not advanced far enough along the colon for the apex to be felt per rectum, but nearly always blood-stained mucus will be found on the examining finger. In a few instances the intussusception actually protrudes through the anus. This does not necessarily imply that the intussusception is of long standing, but rather that the patient is possessed of a long mesentery, rendering the small intestine unduly mobile.

Unrelieved, the pain becomes continuous. After twenty-four to thirty-six hours the abdomen commences to distend, and vomiting becomes copious. Absolute intestinal obstruction follows, and death from this cause, or from peritonitis secondary to the gangrene, is the rule. Once in a while a natural cure, due to sloughing of the intussusceptum, has been reported.

Jean Dance, 1797–1832. Physician, Hôpital Cochin, Paris.

Differential Diagnosis

1. *From Acute Entero-colitis.*—Unlike intussusception, diarrhœa is a leading symptom. As in intussusception, abdominal pain and vomiting often occur ; likewise blood and mucus may be passed, but in entero-colitis fæcal matter or bile is always present in the stools.

2. *From Purpura with Intestinal Symptoms (syn.* Henoch's purpura).— There is likely to be the characteristic rash, which is often mistaken for flea-bites. Intussusception is a not uncommon accompaniment of this form of purpura, consequently the differential diagnosis is not of vital importance, for exploratory laparotomy must be performed in suspicious cases.

3. *From Prolapse of the Rectum.*—This is readily eliminated. In prolapse the projecting mucosa can be felt continuous with the perianal skin. In intussusception protruding from the anus, the finger passes indefinitely into the depths of a sulcus.

Intussusception in adolescence is nearly always caused by an inverted Meckel's diverticulum (see p. 411).

Intussusception in adults is most often due to a papilliferous carcinoma ; consequently, the colo-colic type is frequent. Rarer causes are a papilloma or a submucous lipoma. Idiopathic intussusception is extremely uncommon except in Egypt, where a number of examples have been encountered immediately after the Mohammedan fasting seasons (Mooro).

TREATMENT OF INTUSSUSCEPTION

Preliminary Treatment.—Half an hour should be devoted to improving the general condition of the patient by the administration of saline and glucose. Especially in cases of over twenty-four hours' duration complicated by abdominal distension and vomiting, gastric aspiration should be carried out and continued during and after the operation. In all cases it is advantageous to empty the stomach as a part of the preliminary treatment.

In late cases operation without attempts at non-operative reduction is recommended, because the latter measures are unlikely to succeed.

Reduction by Hydrostatic Pressure.—Excellent results have been obtained from treatment by hydrostatic pressure, a form of therapy elaborated by Australian surgeons. The procedure should be undertaken in the operating theatre by the surgeon himself ; all must be in readiness to proceed with laparotomy. The patient is anæsthetised. A catheter, *not lubricated,* is inserted into the rectum for 3 inches (7·5 cm.). Lubrication makes the parts slippery and prevents proper compression of the buttocks. The catheter is connected by tubing to a glass reservoir filled with saline. The buttocks are pinched together and the reservoir is lifted to a height of 3½ feet (1 metre). Saline is allowed to run into the bowel for three or four minutes. The catheter is then removed and the fluid flows into a receptacle. The manœuvre is repeated two or three times.

If there is the slightest doubt as to whether the intussusception has been reduced completely, laparotomy is performed, but as in most instances the intussusception has been reduced as far as the cæcum, a grid-iron incision can be employed.

Edouard Henoch, 1820–1910. Professor of Diseases of Children, Berlin.
Abdel Mooro, Contemporary. Professor of Surgery, Cairo.

Reduction by barium enema is followed by good results in early cases (within twelve hours of the onset). Under a fluorescent screen, and without an anæsthetic, barium emulsion is permitted to run into the rectum through a catheter, from a height of 3 feet (90 cm.). An assistant must squeeze the buttocks together throughout the procedure. The apex of the intussusception can be seen outlined as a concave meniscus which, as a result of pressure exerted by the barium, gives ground, and the column of barium displays more and more of the colon, until the cæcum is reached. The chief difficulty is in deciding completeness of reduction at the cæcum, and unless barium can be seen to enter the small intestine, the success of the method is not assured, and operation through a grid-iron incision, as described under hydrostatic pressure, is carried out. In cases where successful reduction by barium enema is thought to have occurred, a suspension of powdered charcoal is instilled into the stomach through a gastric aspiration tube ; if the child remains without symptoms, and an enema given six hours later shows particles of charcoal in the resulting stool, there is no doubt that complete reduction has been effected.

Fig. 499.—Diagram showing the method of reducing an intussusception.

Operative Reduction.—In many centres treatment by operation is preferred to attempting reduction by one of the above methods. The abdomen is opened through a right lower paramedian incision. The first part of the reduction is accomplished by squeezing the lowest part of the sausage-like mass (fig. 499), and little by little the intussusception becomes unravelled. The last part of the intussusception is the most difficult to reduce and should be withdrawn and gently compressed in a warm, saline-soaked pack, to lessen the œdema. In the majority of instances reduction is completed easily by squeezing the apex of the intussusception, as shown in fig. 500. After reduction is completed, the terminal portion of small intestine, the caput cæci, and the appendix will be seen reddened and stiffened with œdema.

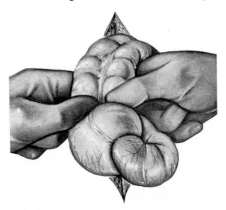

Fig. 500.—Method of reducing the terminal part of the intussusception. (*After R. E. Gross.*

Unless the diagnosis has been unduly delayed, the intussusception can be reduced. Thanks to earlier diagnosis, the number of irreducible intussusceptions in infants is getting smaller and the mortality is correspondingly lower.

If the intussusception cannot be reduced in the manner already described, the following methods are attempted, in sequence.

1. The little finger is inserted into the neck of the intussusception and an endeavour is made to separate adhesions between the intussuscipiens and intussusceptum, after which reduction is re-attempted (Cope's method).

2. Blunt-nosed forceps are used to stretch the intussuscipiens at the neck (fig. 501) (Daw's method).

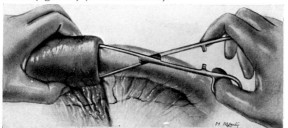

FIG. 501.—Daw's method of aiding the reduction of a tight intussusception.

Treatment of Irreducible and Gangrenous Intussusceptions.—If the above measures are not successful, rather than resort to forcible reduction or cutting the neck of the intussusception, resection followed by anastomosis should be carried out. Resection with anastomosis is also necessary when, after reduction of an intussusception, the involved intestine is of doubtful viability. The most expeditious, and probably the best method of carrying out resection and anastomosis is by Woodhall's ileo-transverse colostomy with exteriorisation of the divided ends of the ileum and transverse colon. This involves a wide resection. The ileum is doubly clamped and divided above the neck of the intussusception, and the cæcum, ascending colon and commencement of the transverse colon are resected, the transverse colon being then divided between clamps. An ileo-transverse colostomy is performed 2 inches (5 cm.) from the ends of the divided intestine and the abdominal wall is closed, leaving the clamps and about 1 inch (2·5 cm.) of the ends of the intestine protruding from the upper end of the incision (fig. 502). If distension arises, as it often does during the first three or four days, this procedure permits removal of the clamp on the small intestine for a short time, with escape of gas and fluid fæces. After seven days the anastomosis should be functioning satisfactorily, and the open ends of the bowel can be closed extraperitoneally.

An irreducible intussusception has been treated by inserting sutures so as to unite the intussuscipiens to the bowel entering the neck of the intussusception, special care being taken to close the space where the mesentery passes between the layers. By this measure peritonitis may be avoided, and occasionally the gangrenous detached intussusceptum is passed per rectum. Sloughing of the intussusception occurs and the continuity of the intestine is restored before the serious effects of intestinal obstruction arise (Montgomery). This method should only be employed in desperate cases.

After-treatment.—When reduction is effected easily, gastric aspiration should

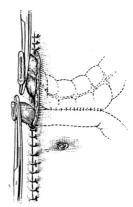

FIG. 502.—Woodhall's operation of ileo-transverse colostomy with exteriorisation of the divided ends of the small and large intestine.

Zachary Cope, Contemporary. Consulting Surgeon, St. Mary's Hospital, London.
Samuel Daw, Contemporary. Consulting Surgeon, The General Infirmary, Leeds.
Barnes Woodhall, Contemporary. Professor of Neurosurgery, Duke University, Durham, North Carolina.
Albert Horr Montgomery, 1882–1948. Chief Surgeon, Children's Memorial Hospital, Chicago.

be employed for twelve to twenty-four hours and saline and glucose administered intravenously, or by the intramedullary route. In infants, nepenthe minims 1 (0·06 ml.) is given by mouth every three or four hours. On the second day the gastric tube is removed and sips of water are given. A few hours later feeding is commenced, with the mother's milk if the infant is breast-fed or, if artificially fed, with citrated cow's milk. In cases where resection has been necessary, more vigorous methods of immediate after-treatment are required. Plasma infusions are valuable to combat shock. When the hæmoglobin estimation is reduced, as it often is, blood transfusion is necessary.

Recurrent Intussusception occurs in only 2 per cent. of cases of idiopathic intussusception. If a second operation is necessary to reduce an intussusception, in the endeavour to avoid still further recurrence, the last few inches of the ileum may be anchored to the ascending colon by sutures.

VOLVULUS

Compared with intussusception, volvulus is rare in this country. A volvulus is caused as a result of axial rotation of a portion of the alimentary track.

(*a*) **Volvulus Neonatorum** (see p. 458).

(*b*) **Volvulus of the small intestine,** other than the above, usually occurs in the lower ileum, and is favoured by the presence of an adhesion passing from the anti-mesenteric border of an intestinal loop (fig. 503) to the parietes or to the female pelvic organs.

Treatment is to untwist the loop, if possible. A causative adhesion should be divided and the stump of its intestinal attachment buried in the intestinal wall by a purse-string suture. When the intestine is gangrenous, resection followed by anastomosis is required.

FIG. 503.

(*c*) **Volvulus of the cæcum** occurs occasionally, especially when the right half of the colon is lax and mobile, and again it is favoured by a band of adhesions from the caput cæci to the peritoneum of the right iliac fossa, such as may follow appendicitis. The highest incidence is between twenty-five and thirty years of age. The symptoms are those of acute obstruction of the small intestine. In about 25 per cent. of cases there is a palpable tympanitic swelling not, as a rule, in the right iliac fossa, for in process of torsion the mobile cæcum moves out of the right iliac fossa into the mid-abdomen, or even to the left side. A plain radiograph shows loops of gas-filled ileum, and sometimes an especially large gas shadow which can be recognised as the cæcum. At first the obstruction is not absolute ; fæces and flatus may be expelled after an enema, but unless spontaneous untwisting occurs, the distension and attacks of intestinal colic continue.

Treatment.—Laparotomy should be performed. In early cases it is usually possible to untwist the organ. Sometimes before untwisting can be accomplished it is necessary to deflate the loop by the insertion of a hollow needle. The puncture is afterwards closed by a purse-string suture.

Untwisting should be followed by cæcostomy, which serves two purposes—
it relieves distension and it fixes the organ to the abdominal wall, thereby
preventing a recurrence.   If the volvulus cannot be untwisted in spite of
deflation, cæcostomy with ileo-transverse colostomy should be carried out.
If, however, the cæcum is gangrenous or its viability is not assured, Woodhall's method of excision with ileo-transverse colostomy is to be recommended.

(d) **Volvulus of the pelvic colon** is common in Eastern Europe.   The
predisposing causes are indicated in fig. 504.   The loop may rotate half a

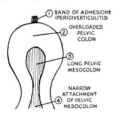

FIG. 504.—The pre-
disposing causes of
volvulus of the sig-
moid colon.

turn, in which event spontaneous rectification
sometimes occurs.   After the loop has rotated $1\frac{1}{2}$
turns the veins involved in the torsion are compressed, and the loop becomes greatly congested.
If, as is sometimes the case, it rotates more than
$1\frac{1}{2}$ turns, the blood-supply is entirely cut off, and
the loop becomes gangrenous. The rotation nearly
always occurs in an anti-clockwise direction.

Clinical Features.—Males are more commonly
affected than females, and the sufferers are usually
middle-aged or elderly.   There is often a history
of chronic constipation, and sometimes a history
of acute attacks of left-sided abdominal pain,
probably due to a partial volvulus, which
untwists itself and is followed by the passage of large quantities of flatus
and fæces.   As a rule the onset of volvulus of the pelvic colon is sudden
and is characterised by severe abdominal pain, usually coming on while the
patient is straining at stool.   Abdominal distension soon follows ; indeed,
in no other condition does extreme abdominal distension come on so
quickly.   If the patient is examined two or three hours after the commencement of the attack, the distension is mainly left-sided.   In a matter of six
hours the whole abdomen becomes distended.   Hiccough and retching occur
early ; vomiting is late.   Constipation is absolute, but an enema may be
returned blood-stained.   Occasionally the rectal wall is felt or seen by
sigmoidoscopy to be œdematous ; this is due to venous engorgement
consequent upon the superior hæmorrhoidal vein being caught up in the
torsion.

Treatment.—In early cases an attempt should be made to pass a rectal
tube with the patient in the knee-elbow position.   Sometimes the tube can
be passed with the aid of a sigmoidoscope when blind insertion fails.   If
this does not succeed, laparotomy must be performed.   An attempt is
made to untwist the gas-filled viscus.   If untwisting can be accomplished,
a rectal tube passed from the anus is manœuvred into the pelvic colon and
the loop is deflated.   To prevent recurrence, which so often follows
simple untwisting, a successful untwisting should be combined with a Paul-
Mikulicz operation which, on account of the long mesocolon, is especially
suitable in this instance.   If the volvulus cannot be untwisted, a Paul's tube
should be tied into it and the intestinal obstruction relieved by a cæcostomy
until the patient's condition improves sufficiently for resection to be carried
out.   When the volvulus is already gangrenous immediate resection is
imperative, after which a Paul's tube is tied into each end of the bowel.
The mortality in such cases is very high.

OBSTRUCTION BY BANDS AND ADHESIONS

By Bands.—Bands form an important group in the causes of
obstruction.   The band may be congenital, e.g. an obliterated

vitello-intestinal duct, or, more frequently, inflammatory, due to previous peritonitis. The band is often remarkably thin and fragile, as in fig. 505. Provided the gut is viable, division of the band or bands, and release of the obstructed loop, is the simplest and most satisfactory abdominal operation in surgery.

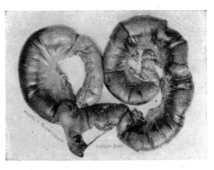

FIG. 505.—Strangulation by a band from Meckel's diverticulum, leading to gangrene.

By Adhesions

Type 1.—Post-operative fibrinous adhesions usually occurring between two days and three weeks after an abdominal operation.

Type 2.—Post-operative fibrous adhesions giving rise to symptoms at any time from months to many years after an abdominal operation.

Type 3.—Adherence of a loop or loops of intestine to inflamed intraperitoneal structures, e.g. a tuberculous mesenteric lymph node.

Type 4.—As a complication of the plastic form of tuberculous peritonitis.

Post-operative adhesions giving rise to intestinal obstruction usually involve the lower ileum. Operations for acute appendicitis necessitating drainage of the peritoneal cavity or drainage of an appendix abscess are the commonest precursors of this condition, while gynæcological operations closely follow as the second most common source of obstructing adhesions.

Treatment.—Gastro-intestinal suction drainage, combined with intravenous fluid therapy, is extremely beneficial (fig. 506) and sometimes curative in these cases. Nevertheless, constant vigilance is necessary, for strangulation, if not present initially, may develop during the course of such treatment. When operation is necessary, although many adhesions are often present, one only may be found to be causing the obstruction, in which case the condition is remedied easily by dividing this adhesion. At other times the intestine is angulated by adherence to the mesentery, the abdominal wall, another loop of intestine or, in the female, to the uterus or adnexæ. In these circum-

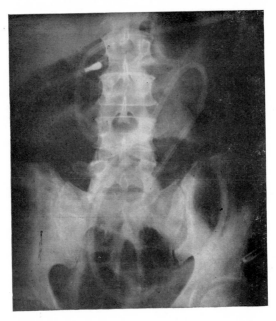

FIG. 506.—Tip of a Miller-Abbott tube arrested in the ileum. Case of obstruction to the small intestine due to adherence of the ileum to the transverse colon after resection of a carcinoma of the transverse colon. The condition of the patient was much improved by suction drainage, after which the coil was freed by operation.

stances it is sometimes possible to free the obstructed intestine by dissection. In order to prevent recurrence, the bare areas should be covered with omental grafts. In cases belonging to Type 1 (which are the ones most likely to be completely remedied by gastro-intestinal suction drainage) the obstructing adhesions of unorganised fibrin can often be broken with the finger, thereby relieving the obstruction. When adhesions are widespread and the small intestine so matted that a definite point of obstruction cannot be found, or it is inadvisable to attempt to free an adherent obstructed loop, anastomosis of an obviously distended loop to a collapsed loop has often resulted in the obstruction being overcome. When preliminary [gastro-intestinal suction drainage has been effective, the obstructed loops will be empty and the anastomosis should be performed between the collapsed loop containing the extremity of the tube and a collapsed loop not containing the tube.

OBSTRUCTION FROM STRICTURE OF THE SMALL INTESTINE

Cicatricial contracture is usually an aftermath of tuberculous ulceration. Multiple strictures are usually present, and the one with the smallest lumen becomes blocked with food residue or such object as a fruit stone. Malignant stricture is rare, although both carcinoma and sarcoma occur from time to time (p. 430).

Treatment.—Usually a simple stricture can be circumvented by lateral anastomosis. A malignant stricture should be excised and the continuity of the intestine restored by anastomosis.

OBSTRUCTION BY GALL-STONE (*Syn.* GALL-STONE ILEUS)

Obstruction by gall-stone usually occurs in old women. The gall-stone, which is 1 inch (2·5 cm.) or more in diameter, ulcerates through the neck of the gall-bladder into the duodenum. It passes down the small intestine, and becomes impacted about 2 feet (60 cm.) from the ileo-cæcal valve, because this is the narrowest part of the small gut. The symptoms are elusive. The patient experiences colic, accompanied by copious vomiting. As the obstruction is incomplete, there is often a fair result from an enema, and remissions of symptoms are frequent, but the vomiting returns, and by this time it is bilious. A radiograph occasionally demonstrates the calculus in the small intestine. In any event, the small intestine will be seen to be distended with gas. There is no abdominal distension until late, and late intestinal obstruction in an old person is an almost hopeless condition. On rare occasions a giant stone causes obstruction of the large intestine by ulcerating from the fundus of the gall-bladder into the transverse colon, and becoming impacted in the rectum.

Treatment.—A lower right paramedian incision is made. The loop containing the stone is delivered and packed off most carefully. After the application of rubber-covered clamps, the intestine is opened and the stone removed. It is an advantage to sew up the incision in the intestine transversely, to avoid constriction at this point. The gall-stone which causes intestinal obstruction is nearly always barrel-shaped

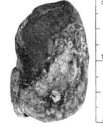

Fig. 507.—Gall-stone removed from the lower end of the ileum.

and unfaceted (fig. 507). If there is a facet it is advisable
to palpate the intestine above the obstruction for a possible
fellow-calculus.

OBSTRUCTION BY STERCOLITH

This gives rise to similar symptoms. It is much rarer, and usually
occurs in younger persons. The stercolith may contain as a nucleus a fruit
stone, or other foreign body.

Treatment is similar to the above.

OBSTRUCTION FOLLOWING THE INGESTION OF DRIED FRUIT

Obstruction of normal small intestine occurs occasionally after the
ingestion of large quantities of dried fruit, or unmasticated orange pulp.

At operation, if the obstructing mass cannot be milked along the small
intestine, it must be removed by making an incision into the intestine over
it, in the same way as described in the section on obstruction by a gall-
stone.

OBSTRUCTION DUE TO WORMS

An aggregation of ascaris lumbricoides may be the cause of low small
intestinal obstruction in children, usually under ten years of age. There is
debility out of proportion to that produced by the obstruction. The
obturation is inclined to follow the ingestion of an anti-helminthic. If it is
not known that the patient is suffering from ascaris infestation, a worm in
the vomitus or the presence of eosinophilia may be the means of making
a correct preoperative diagnosis. In this form of intestinal obstruction
laparotomy must be performed, but if possible the tangled mass should
be kneaded along the ileum into the cæcum. While opening the intestine
and removing worms has been followed by success, it has also been followed
by fatal post-operative peritonitis from a worm insinuating itself through
the suture line.

EMBOLISM AND THROMBOSIS OF THE SUPERIOR MESENTERIC VESSELS

Statistics differ as to whether arterial or venous mesenteric occlusion is
the more common. There is no question that the superior mesenteric
vessels are implicated much more often than the inferior mesenteric
vessels, but this may in part be due to the better collateral circulation of
the latter.

Embolism of the Superior Mesenteric Artery.—The embolus is derived
from a vegetation on the mitral valve, a left auricular appendage, an
atheromatous plaque arising from the aorta, or from a pyæmic infarct of
the lung which has led to thrombosis of the pulmonary vein.

Thrombosis of the superior mesenteric artery is less common than the
foregoing and is the result of arterio-sclerosis or thrombo-angiitis obliterans.

Thrombosis of the superior mesenteric veins occurs in portal hypertension and pylephlebitis.

No matter whether the occlusion is arterial or venous, hæmorrhagic
infarction occurs although, in the case of embolism, a short-lived pallor
has been observed at early laparotomy. The intestine and its mesentery
become swollen and œdematous, demarcation between infarcted and
healthy intestine being gradual. Blood-stained fluid is exuded into the
peritoneal cavity and the lumen of the infarcted intestine becomes filled
with blood. When the main trunk of the superior mesenteric artery
becomes occluded, so great is the area deprived of a blood-supply that

death nearly always results from peritonitis following gangrene (fig. 508). Frequently the embolus or thrombosis occludes a branch of the superior mesenteric vessels, when infarction of a few to many feet of the ileum occurs.

Clinical Features.—An embolus lodging in the superior mesenteric artery or thrombosis occurring in the corresponding vein gives rise to the same train of symptoms, but the former is likely to be more sudden in its onset. Repeated vomiting, with, it should be noted, sometimes blood-stained diarrhœa, ushers in this catastrophe. On examination an indefinite, movable, sub-umbilical, tumid lump can often be felt in thin subjects. The lump is the infarcted congested segment of small intestine. When blood is not passed per rectum, an enema may reveal its presence in the colon. The facial pallor and fall in systolic pressure closely resemble an internal hæmorrhage which, indeed, has taken place. Intestinal colic, a palpable lump, and the passage of blood per rectum are symptoms and signs similar to those of an intussusception, but mucus is not present with the blood. If it is known that the patient is suffering from one of the conditions which predispose to mesenteric thrombosis and embolus, the correct diagnosis is not difficult.

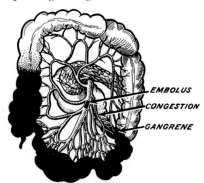

FIG. 508.—Embolus lodged in the superior mesenteric artery showing the widespread gangrene which results.
(*After Childe.*)

Treatment.—Some remarkable recoveries have followed solely from the administration of heparin or heparin and dicoumarol in their proper sequence (see p. 93). In many cases laparotomy has been performed, and when the infarction is limited to several feet of the small intestine, resection of the darkly congested or gangrenous intestine and its mesentery has been carried out. The post-operative administration of heparin and dicoumarol, by preventing extension of thrombosis, has improved the results of treatment by resection. In all cases, whether operation is undertaken or not, blood transfusion is required. In patients who recover with non-operative measures, obstruction may occur later from fibrosis of an area of the small intestine.

OBSTRUCTION DUE TO AN INTERNAL HERNIA

In certain parts of the abdomen peritoneal folds are found which bound recesses or fossæ into which pass a portion of small intestine, there to become obstructed or strangulated by the peritoneal fold guarding the recess. The recesses are as follows :

Fossæ about the Duodenum

(a) The Left Para-duodenal Fossa. The inferior mesenteric vein lies in its free border.

(b) The Right Duodeno-jejunal Fossa. The superior mesenteric artery runs in its free border.

(c) The Foramen of Winslow. The portal vein, common bile duct, and hepatic artery lie in its free border.

Fossæ about the Cæcum and Appendix

(a) *Superior Ileo-cæcal Fossa.* Between the general mesentery and a fold of peritoneum raised by the anterior single branch of the ileo-colic artery.

(b) *Inferior Ileo-cœcal Fossa.* Between the " bloodless " fold of Treves and the mesentery of the appendix.

(c) *The retro-cœcal fossa* behind the cæcum.

Intersigmoid Fossa is situated in the base of the pelvic mesocolon. Its mouth looks downwards.

*A Hole in the Mesentery.

A Hernia into the Broad Ligament.

The Supravesical Fossa** is bounded by the median and lateral umbilical folds (obliterated urachus and umbilical arteries). A loss of weight and a coincident loss of prevesical fat deepens the fossa.

A Congenital or acquired Diaphragmatic Hernia (see p. 599).

An internal hernia is an uncommon cause of intestinal obstruction. Often the patient gives a history extending over months or years of intermittent attacks of abdominal pain accompanied by vomiting. Many

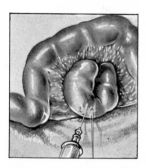

patients with obstruction due to an internal hernia are admitted in an advanced stage, the obstruction having been present for several days ; also strangulation is present in about one-third of the cases. Consequently the mortality in this variety of intestinal obstruction is high. There are no pathognomonic signs of obstruction due to an internal hernia ; in the majority of instances the obstruction is low in the small intestine, but para-duodenal herniæ are likely to give rise to obstruction to the jejunum. In the case of a hernia into the left para-duodenal fossa, intestinal obstruction is often associated with acute hæmorrhoids from compression of the inferior mesenteric vein. In many varieties of internal herniæ radiography not only confirms the diagnosis of intestinal obstruction, but often indicates the site. Particularly in high obstruction, even this aid to diagnosis sometimes fails.

Fig. 509.—Strangulation through a hole in the mesentery. Emptying the obstructed loop before attempting reduction.

Treatment.—Division of the constricting agent to release the imprisoned intestine can be carried out unreservedly in those herniæ *not* marked *. In the case of the foramen of Winslow, if the obstructed intestine cannot be withdrawn, the lesser sac is opened, and after the insertion of a purse-string suture, the distended intestine is emptied by means of an aspirating needle attached to a syringe or, better, to a suction apparatus. After deflation the purse-string suture is tied. This usually allows the intestine to be extricated, but if this is still impossible, mobilisation of the second part of the duodenum helps to enlarge the foramen. The principle of opening the fundus of the sac and emptying the intestine of its contents before attempting reduction should also be employed in cases of obstruction due to a hole in the mesentery (fig. 509), a left para-duodenal hernia, or duodeno-jejunal hernia. If this measure is unsuccessful in the case of a right duodeno-jejunal hernia, it is possible to divide the neck of the sac in a downward direction behind the superior mesenteric artery without injuring that vessel. When the left para-duodenal fossa is involved, the inferior mesenteric vein is so intimately blended with the para-duodenal fold that to divide any part of the latter must implicate the former. However, ligation of this vein in these circumstances is seldom followed by infarction of the left colon because pre-operative compression of the vessel has caused anastomotic channels to dilate.

Jacob Winslow, 1669–1760. A Dane who migrated to Paris, and there established a school of anatomy.

PARALYTIC ILEUS (*Syn.* ADYNAMIC ILEUS)

Neurogenic obstruction is due to failure of a segment of intestine to transmit peristaltic waves. In the majority of instances it is the ileum which is first and chiefly affected—hence the term paralytic ileus. The fault lies in the local neuro-muscular mechanism, probably in the nerve plexuses of Auerbach, situated between the circular and longitudinal muscle fibres of the intestine, and those of Meissner, in the submucous layer.

Following every abdominal operation, peristalsis ceases for about twenty-four hours. Often it returns in one segment, and is delayed in another. This is the cause of the common " gas pains " in the immediate post-operative period. Paralytic ileus often follows extensive abdominal operations. It is also frequently encountered after operations for diffuse or pelvic peritonitis. In the latter instance the primary condition is believed to be due to bacterial toxins diffusing from the peritoneum and causing direct damage to the intramural nerve plexuses. Plastic adhesions between loops of the ileum also play a part. These adhesions do not constrict the intestine or angulate it sufficiently to cause intestinal obstruction when peristalsis is normally vigorous, but when peristaltic waves have been enfeebled by toxic effects on the local nerve plexuses, such adhesions become formidable obstacles. Ileus following peritonitis is, therefore, mainly paralytic but partially mechanical.

Clinical Features.—Paralytic ileus should be suspected if the patient has neither passed flatus nor is there any result from an enema forty-eight hours after the operation. This suspicion becomes confirmed if there is no evidence of resumption of peristalsis after sixty hours. At first the distension is most apparent below the level of the umbilicus, but as the condition progresses the whole abdomen becomes involved. If gastric aspiration has not been commenced at an early stage, which is unlikely, the patient vomits repeatedly in an effortless manner. With gastric aspiration large quantities of bile-stained material continue to be withdrawn. In severe cases the abdomen becomes tense and drum-like, and the pulse-rate rises steadily. There is an absence of intestinal colic and no tenderness, except that to be expected in the region of the incision. On auscultation of the abdomen, in contradistinction to mechanical obstruction, there is complete silence.

Leopold Auerbach, 1828–1897. Anatomist, Breslau.
Georg Meissner, 1829–1903. Physiologist, Göttingen.

Reflex paralytic ileus presumably is due to interference with the extrinsic nervous control of intestinal musculature. It occurs in a number of heterogeneous conditions, which include fracture of the spine or ribs, a retroperitoneal hæmorrhage, or the application of a tight plaster jacket.

Paralytic Ileus in Uræmia.—Abdominal distension, vomiting, and hiccough are frequent accompaniments of advanced uræmia. Abdominal distension following prostatectomy may be uræmic in origin, although in some instances it occurs when the output of urine is satisfactory and the blood urea is normal or but little raised. In such cases the distension is probably reflex and it appears to affect the large more than the small intestine.

Management and Treatment.—Increase or decrease in the girth of the abdomen at the level of the umbilicus, measured with a tape-measure left in position, should be recorded four-hourly. Radiography shows many coils of small intestine filled with gas

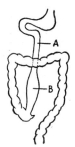

Fig. 510.—Showing how peristaltic stimulation by drugs often not only fails to relieve, but increases paralytic ileus.
(a) Comparatively healthy small intestine which responds to the stimulation, and thereby forces intestinal contents into (b) the paralysed segment which, unable to contract, becomes still further distended.

and often multiple fluid levels. Radiography, repeated daily, is valuable in assessing the effect of treatment on the distension. The general consensus of opinion is that all types of peristaltic stimulants have no place in the treatment of paralytic ileus. Too often they activate only the comparatively less affected jejunum and force more gas and some fluid into the paralysed ileum (fig. 510), with the result that the distension increases and a greater length of small intestine becomes totally paralysed. Morphia or one of its derivatives is the only drug which should be employed, and it is given in full doses every eight hours. The fluid balance must be adjusted daily by the administration of intravenous saline and glucose, the amount required being assessed by keeping a fluid intake and output chart. As hypoproteinæmia favours paralytic ileus, on the third or fourth day from the onset 1 pint (568 ml.) of the total fluid administered should be given as a plasma infusion. This can be repeated at intervals of forty-eight hours, as necessary. It is in cases of paralytic ileus that the Miller-Abbott or other type of intestinal tube with continuous suction drainage is especially valuable, and in this condition the tube can be made to negotiate the pylorus more easily than is the case in mechanical intestinal obstruction. If the measurements and radiograph show that distension is decreasing, the gastro-intestinal tube is clamped for a few hours, and if there is no vomiting or no increase in the distension, the tube may be removed and an enema given. If this is followed by even the passage of flatus, the paralysis has probably been overcome. In some instances the distension returns and the gastro-intestinal tube must be replaced. Throughout the treatment a rectal flatus tube is passed every six hours. When paralytic ileus persists in spite of these measures, the administration of a spinal anæsthetic sometimes is followed by immediate resumption of peristaltic activity.

In cases following peritonitis, when the symptoms persist after fourteen days of conservative treatment, especially if cessation of suction drainage is followed by abdominal pain and some intestinal sounds can be heard on abdominal auscultation, operative treatment is indicated, as the condition is partly mechanical. An upper left paramedian incision is made, and the first loop of jejunum to be encountered is anastomosed to the transverse colon. After this procedure the patient often passes flatus within twenty-four hours, and in forty-eight hours there is an action of the bowels.

At a much earlier stage, the fifth or sixth day, when the distension is very pronounced and a Miller-Abbott tube cannot be passed, or is not available, jejunostomy under local anæsthesia, with suction applied to the jejunostomy catheter, is a measure to be recommended.

CHRONIC INTESTINAL OBSTRUCTION

The various abnormalities and diseases giving rise to chronic intestinal obstruction are described in Chapters xxi and xxiv. There remains one condition to be considered here.

Fæcal impaction occurs principally in elderly, and often bed-ridden, patients. The mass of hardened fæces usually accumulates in the upper part of the rectum.

The symptoms are those of chronic intestinal obstruction, and attacks of spurious diarrhœa are a common accompaniment. A fæcal accumulation may form a palpable abdominal mass which can be indented.   When the mass is situated in the rectum, it can be indented by the palpating finger.

Treatment.—Enemata are usually insufficient.   The patient must be given an anæsthetic, and after the anal sphincter has been dilated, the mass is removed digitally or with a spoon.   In some instances fæcal impaction occurs above an innocent or malignant stricture of the rectum.   Especially in such cases, it may be necessary to resort to left iliac colostomy before the mass can be disimpacted.

CHAPTER XXIII
THE VERMIFORM APPENDIX

ACUTE APPENDICITIS

THE mortality from acute appendicitis in England and Wales has been more than halved during the decade 1938–1948 (fig. 511). Earlier diagnosis and appendicectomy while the inflammation is still confined to the appendix, the knowledge of the general public that it is dangerous to take or give to children a purgative in the presence of undiagnosed abdominal pain, more discrimination in performing immediate appendicectomy in late cases, and the control of infection by antibiotics and chemotherapy have all played a part in bringing about this remarkable improvement.

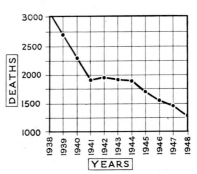

FIG. 511.—Deaths from appendicitis in England and Wales 1938–1948.

SURGICAL ANATOMY

The vermiform appendix is present only in man, certain anthropoid apes, and the wombat. Morphologically, it is the undeveloped distal end of the large cæcum found in many lower animals.

The appendix varies considerably in length and circumference. The average length is between 3 and 4 inches (7·5 to 10 cm.), but variations from ½ inch to 8 inches are not unusual. The lumen, which should admit a matchstalk, is irregular, being encroached upon by the multiple folds of mucous membrane lying parallel to its long axis. In infancy the orifice of the appendix is opened widely. As growth proceeds, the opening becomes narrow and partially occluded by a valve-like fold of mucous membrane—the valve of Gerlach.

From without inwards, the structure of the appendix is as follows. There is a peritoneal coat which completely invests it, except along the narrow line of attachment of the mesoappendix. The muscular coat resembles that of the small intestine, and is of uniform thickness. There is a well-developed submucous coat containing, especially in childhood

Joseph von Gerlach, 1820–1896. Professor of Anatomy and Physiology, Erlangen.

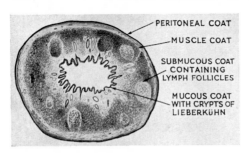

FIG. 512.—Cross-section of a vermiform
appendix.

and youth, a large number of lymphoid follicles which cause the mucous membrane to bulge into the lumen. The mucous membrane resembles that of the large intestine, but there are fewer crypts of Lieberkühn (fig. 512).

The **mesoappendix** springs from the lower surface of the mesentery, and when the appendix is free-lying, it is triangular in shape, but is subject to great variations. Often it does not extend to the tip of the organ. Sometimes as much as the distal one-third of the appendix is bereft of mesoappendix. Especially in childhood, the mesoappendix is so transparent that the contained blood-vessels can be seen. In many adult subjects it becomes laden with fat, which obscures these vessels.

The **appendicular artery,** a branch of the lower division of the ileo-colic artery, passes behind the terminal ileum to enter the mesoappendix a short distance from the base of the appendix. It then comes to lie in the free border of the mesoappendix; but for a variable distance from the tip, where the mesoappendix is lacking, the artery lies directly on the muscle wall beneath the peritoneal coat.

An accessory appendicular artery (fig. 513), a branch of the posterior cæcal artery, is present in nearly 50 per cent. of cases. When performing appendicectomy this vessel requires independent ligation.

The appendicular vein is a radicle of the ileo-colic vein, which drains into the portal system.

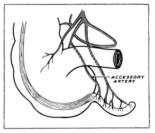

FIG. 513.—In nearly 50 per cent. of cases there is an accessory appendicular artery, a branch of the posterior cæcal.
(*After Seshachalam.*)

Lymphatic vessels draining the appendix follow the appendicular arteries between the layers of the mesoappendix. There are four or more of these channels, and they empty into the ileo-cæcal lymph nodes, situated between the layers of the mesentery of the small intestine at the ileo-cæcal angle.

McBurney's point was described by McBurney as lying between 1½ and 2 inches (3·75 and 5 cm.) from the right anterior superior iliac spine upon a line joining this spine and the umbilicus (fig. 514). It is now more generally taught as lying at the junction of the outer third with the

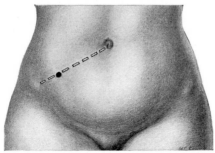

FIG. 514.—McBurney's point.

Charles McBurney, 1845–1913. Surgeon, Roosevelt Hospital, New York.

inner two-thirds of this line. McBurney's point is the classical site of greatest tenderness in appendicitis, and also a most useful point to have in mind when a grid-iron incision to expose the appendix is about to be made.

Inconstancy of Position.—The vermiform appendix is the only organ in the body which has no normal position. The relative frequency of the more usual positions occupied by the organ is depicted in fig. 515. In addition, the appendix must necessarily share in abnormalities in position of the cæcum. The most frequent of these is failure of the cæcum to descend, which results in the base of the appendix being situated in the right hypochondrium. Very occasionally the cæcum and appendix are situated in the left iliac fossa. This may be due to abnormal rotation of the gut during embryonic life, or to transposition of viscera.

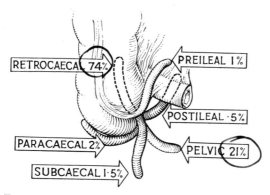

FIG. 515.—The various positions of the appendix.

Locating the Appendix.—Even when the cæcum is in full view it is not always an easy matter to find the appendix. In difficult cases the following method will be found to be of value in aiding the search. Trace any one of the tæniæ coli downwards : this must lead to the base of the appendix. If the organ is still not visible and it is certain that it has not been removed, it will probably be found buried in the posterior cæcal wall, and will be discovered by palpation and dissection.

ÆTIOLOGY

Until the close of the nineteenth century appendicitis remained un-recognised. Unquestionably, before this time it was a comparatively rare disease, but there can be no doubt that it existed even in remote times, for an acutely inflamed, perforated appendix was found preserved in the mummy of a young royal princess of Egypt (A. M. Spencer).

The riddle of appendicitis—its actual cause and its meteoric rise from an insignificant disease to the most common serious intra-abdominal inflammatory affection of Western civilised races—has been a matter for much divergent speculation. So far no satisfactory explanation has been forthcoming. The following ætiological factors are important, but for the most part they must be looked upon as purely contributory.

Fæcoliths and Strictures.—When an acutely inflamed appendix has been removed, some form of obstruction to its lumen can be demonstrated in a large percentage of cases. The obstructing agent is usually a fæcolith or a stricture ; exceptionally, a foreign body or threadworms are found.

Arthur M. Spencer, Contemporary. Deputy Superintendent, County Mental Hospital, Carmarthen, Wales.

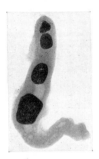

FIG. 516.—Fæcoliths. X-ray of an appendix after removal.

Fæcoliths (fig. 516) vary in size and have a laminated structure. They are composed of inspissated fæcal material, calcium and magnesium phosphates and carbonates, bacteria and epithelial débris ; rarely, a foreign body is incorporated in the mass.

The Abuse of Purgatives.—It is abundantly clear that the ingestion of purgatives, particularly castor oil, by patients with " stomach ache," and the violent peristaltic action which results, favours, and often determines, perforation of an inflamed appendix. " Purgation means perforation " is a wise adage.

Familial Susceptibility.—That there is sometimes a familial tendency to the disease cannot be disputed. This generally accepted fact can be accounted for by an hereditary malformation of the organ, which predisposes to infection. Thus the whole family may have a long retrocæcal appendix with a comparatively poor blood-supply, and many of its members fall victims to appendicitis in one form or another.

Race and Diet.—Appendicitis is particularly common in the highly civilised European, American, and Australasian countries, while it is rare in Asiatics, Africans, and Polynesians. Rendle Short has shown that if individuals from the latter races migrate to the countries where appendicitis is common, they soon acquire the local susceptibility to the disease. Even apes in captivity appear to acquire the human liability to appendicitis. These significant facts satisfy many that the rise of appendicitis amongst the highly civilised is due to an unbridled departure from a simple diet rich in cellulose. But this cannot be the whole explanation, for acute appendicitis occurs in lifelong vegetarians and even in babes at the breast.

Is Appendicitis an Endemic Disease ?—Many observers have noticed that cases of appendicitis occur in batches so regularly as to defy the vagaries of coincidence. It has been suggested that there is a relation between appendicitis and tonsillitis. Furthermore, like the tonsil, the lymphoid tissue of the appendix is scanty in infancy, becomes abundant during childhood, and commences to atrophy after the age of thirty. Appendicitis is more frequent during the years when the appendix is plentifully provided with lymphoid tissue.

BACTERIOLOGY

There is no one organism mainly responsible for appendicitis. Cultures from inflamed appendices usually reveal that the infection is mixed and there is hardly a pyogenic organism which has not been isolated from such specimens. The most common organisms present are the B. coli and streptococci, together with the Cl. welchii. In most instances the infecting organisms are normal inhabitants of the lumen of the appendix, although in the case of streptococci they may be blood-borne from a streptococcal infection of the throat.

PATHOLOGY

The menace of acute appendicitis lies in the frequency with which the peritoneal cavity is infected from this focus. Peritoneal infection takes place :

1. By perforation.

A. Rendle Short, Contemporary. *Emeritus Professor of Surgery, University of Bristol.*
William H. Welch, 1850–1934. *Pathologist, Johns Hopkins University, Baltimore, U.S.A.*

2. By transmigration of bacteria through the appendicular wall.

Attention has been directed to the value of the great omentum in attempting to limit the extent of the peritoneal invasion on the one hand, and on the other to the force-pump action of ingested purgatives in producing a widespread infection.

It is of great importance to recognise two types of acute appendicitis.

(a) *Non-obstructive Acute Appendicitis.*—The inflammation usually commences in the mucous membrane ; less often in the lymph follicles. Like any inflammatory process, it terminates in one of the following ways : (1) Resolution ; (2) Ulceration ; (3) Suppuration ; (4) Fibrosis ; (5) Gangrene. Non-obstructive acute appendicitis is less serious than the obstructive variety in that the mucopurulent products of inflammation have an opportunity of escaping along the lumen into the cæcum. Nevertheless, all grades of inflammation occur. One or more of the lymph follicles which early in the course of the inflammation become swollen, may break down and suppurate or, what is more common, suppuration occurring in the bottom of one of the crypts of Lieberkühn leads to a minute perforation of the mucous lining. In either event, once it reaches the loose submucous tissues, the infection progresses rapidly. The organ becomes turgid, bright red, and hæmorrhages occur into the mucous membrane. Swelling of the organ is restricted by its inelastic peritoneal coat, but expansion can occur into the leaves of the mesoappendix. Towards the tip this avenue is sometimes lacking; then the vascular supply of the distal part of the appendix is liable to become strangulated or the appendicular artery becomes thrombosed by extension of the infection to it. In these ways gangrene sets in. At other times the infection passes through one or more of the hiati where the blood-vessels pierce the muscularis to reach the subperitoneal coat. Here it spreads under tension, and a purulent blister is liable to form (fig. 517) and perforation results. As a rule, in non-obstructive appendicitis the inflammation progresses sufficiently slowly for protective

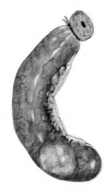

Fig. 517.—Acute appendicitis. Perforation imminent.

Johann Nathanael Lieberkühn, 1711–1756. Anatomist, Berlin.

adhesions to form, and the resulting peritonitis is localised. In many cases the infection never progresses beyond the mucous lining, and although the attack passes off, it is unlikely that a *status quo ante* ever takes place. Because the tip suffers most, fibrosis usually occurs therein. More rarely fibrosis following ulceration supervenes in the proximal end and the stricture thus formed predisposes to future acute appendicular obstruction.

(b) *Acute Appendicular Obstruction.*—About one-third of cases of acute appendicitis belong to this group. The obstruction can be by obturation (fæcolith, foreign body, or parasites) ; intramural (an inflammatory stricture) ; extramural (a congenital band. Rarely an appendix is strangulated in an external hernia). Of these, much the most common is a fæcolith.

Possibly œdema of Gerlach's valve or spasm of the circular musculature at the base of the appendix is sufficient to obstruct the lumen in some cases, but such obstruction cannot be proved. A kink is unlikely to cause complete obstruction.

When the lumen of an inflamed appendix is obstructed, the products of inflammation become pent up (fig. 518), and except in the rare event of the obstruction being overcome, the inflammation proceeds more rapidly and more certainly to gangrene or perforation than is the case when the appendix is unobstructed. Close examination of gangrenous appendices directly after their removal shows conclusively that they usually belong to the obstructive group (Wilkie).

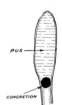

FIG. 518. —Acute obstructive appendicitis.

Often within twelve to eighteen hours the appendix distal to the obstruction becomes lifeless and green (fig. 519). When perforation occurs it does so suddenly, most often at the site of an impacted fæcolith, and before protective

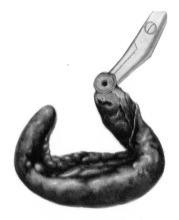

FIG. 519.—Acute obstructive appendicitis with gangrene. There is a large fæcal concretion impacted in the proximal end of the lumen of the organ.

Sir David Wilkie, 1882–1938. Professor of Surgery, University of Edinburgh.

adhesions have had time to form. The escaping purulent and gaseous contents being under high pressure, early widespread peritonitis is liable to ensue, especially if the appendix is free-lying.

CLINICAL FEATURES

Age Incidence.—Rare before the age of two, acute appendicitis becomes increasingly common during childhood and adolescence. The maximum incidence is between the ages of twenty and thirty; thereafter there is a gradual decline, but no age is exempt.

The patient often gives a history of similar slight attacks. The attack can commence at any time, but frequently it does so in the early hours of the morning, awakening the patient from sleep. Recent constipation is usual.

Non-obstructive Acute Appendicitis.—Typically, the first symptom is generalised abdominal pain, gradually becoming localised near the umbilicus or in the epigastrium. In severe cases this is followed in three or four hours by vomiting. Vomiting is reflex, and often as soon as the stomach is empty it ceases. In mild cases there is no vomiting, but nausea and anorexia are almost invariably present. During the first six hours there is rarely any alteration in the temperature or pulse-rate ; after that time slight pyrexia (99° to 100° F. (37·2–37·7° C.)), with a corresponding increase in the pulse-rate to 80 or 90, is usual. In severe cases, as time passes there is a further rise in the temperature to about 101° F. (38·3° C.) but seldom more, and the pulse-rate becomes correspondingly elevated. Only occasionally is the classical sequence of pain followed by nausea or vomiting reversed. In about twenty-four hours the pain becomes localised in the right iliac fossa.

In cases of under twelve hours' duration tenderness and some rigidity in the right iliac fossa is usually present. In spite of many exceptions, McBurney's point is the most usual site of maximum tenderness. Later, in progressive cases, the rigidity increases. Rovsing's sign is often helpful in strengthening the diagnosis ; even pressure is exerted over the pelvic colon. This forces gas into the cæcum. If pressure in the left iliac fossa causes pain in the right iliac fossa, the case is probably one of acute appendicitis. When the inflammation has implicated the walls of the appendix sufficiently to stretch its peritoneal

Reginald Fitz, 1843–1913. Physician, of Boston. Did much in first framing the clinical features of acute appendicitis.
Thorkild Rovsing, 1862–1927. Professor of Surgery, University of Copenhagen.

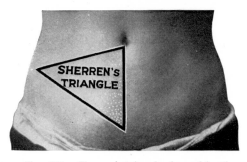

FIG. 520.—Sherren's triangle, formed by the umbilicus, the highest point of the iliac crest, and the right pubic spine.

coat, hyperæsthesia will be found in Sherren's triangle (fig. 520). When present, this is a most valuable sign.

Acute Appendicular Obstruction.—The onset is abrupt and the leading symptom is colic—severe generalised abdominal pain which comes and goes, and from the commencement of the attack is referred to the umbilicus. The temperature is usually normal and the pulse-rate in between the attacks is not necessarily accelerated. Vomiting occurs early and is usually repeated two or three times. After a few hours the pain passes to the right iliac fossa, but its spasmodic nature is maintained. The physical signs resemble those of non-obstructive acute appendicitis with the exception that when the appendix is free-lying the rigidity is more pronounced and comes on earlier. The presence of hyperæsthesia is of the utmost diagnostic value. Unlike non-obstructive appendicitis, it is present during the very early hours of the attack and remains until (1) the obstruction has been overcome ; (2) perforation occurs ; (3) gangrene supervenes.

Immediately after an obstructed appendix has perforated the violent abdominal pain disappears. The patient often says he feels better. Rigidity may be almost, if not entirely, absent, but soon the pulse-rate begins to rise steadily and other signs of diffusing peritonitis are not long delayed.

Every effort is made not only to diagnose acute appendicitis irrefutably, but also to diagnose the position of the appendix—whether it is retrocæcal, in the right iliac fossa, or pelvic. The special symptoms and signs likely to be encountered when the appendix occupies one of its more secluded positions are :

Retrocæcal.—Rigidity is often absent, and even on deep pressure tenderness may be lacking, the reason being that the cæcum, distended with gas, prevents the pressure exerted by the hand from reaching the inflamed structure. However, deep

James Sherren, 1872–1946. Surgeon, London Hospital.

tenderness is often present in the loin, and rigidity of the quadratus lumborum may be in evidence. Psoas spasm, due to the inflamed appendix being in contact with that muscle, may be sufficient to cause flexion of the hip joint, and to extend the joint brings on abdominal pain. Hyperextension of the hip joint may reveal abdominal pain in degrees of psoas spasm insufficient to cause flexion of the hip. An inflamed retrocæcal appendix occasionally is in contact with the ureter, in which event there may be slight hæmaturia and on microscopical examination pus cells are sometimes present in the urine.

Pelvic.—When the appendix lies entirely in the pelvis there is usually complete absence of abdominal rigidity, and often of tenderness. In some cases deep tenderness can be made out just above and to the right of the pubes. In either case a rectal examination reveals tenderness in the rectovesical pouch or the pouch of Douglas, especially in the right side of the pouch concerned. Psoas spasm may also be present when the appendix is in this position ; alternatively, spasm of the obturator internus is sometimes demonstrable when the hip is flexed and internally rotated. If an inflamed appendix is in contact with the obturator internus, this manœuvre will cause pain in the hypogastrium (Cope). An inflamed appendix in contact with the bladder causes increased frequency of micturition. Very occasionally early diarrhœa results from an inflamed appendix being in contact with the rectum.

Post-ileal.—The inflamed appendix lies against the mesentery, and if it is not removed early it may give rise to pylephlebitis. Coils of small intestine lie between the inflamed structure and the abdominal wall. Rigidity and deep tenderness are therefore liable to be slight or absent. Repeated vomiting is often much in evidence.

Maldescended.—The tenderness is in the subhepatic region. Hyperæsthesia, however, when present, occupies the usual area.

DIFFERENTIAL DIAGNOSIS

For purposes of differential diagnosis it is helpful to visualise the body as a house (fig. 521) and compare six parts of the house to the appropriate anatomical regions.

1. **The Attic** (i.e. *The Thorax*)

Pneumonia and pleurisy are associated with an increased respiratory rate. Pleurisy inhibits deep inspiration. Some

Zachary Cope, Contemporary. Consulting Surgeon, St. Mary's Hospital, London.

degree of cyanosis is usually present and the alæ nasi may move on respiration. Pleural friction or altered breath sounds should be detected by a stethoscope.

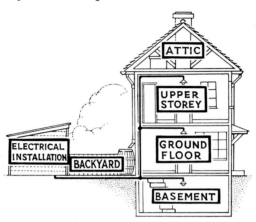

FIG. 521.

2. The Upper Storey (i.e. *Diaphragm to the Level of the Umbilicus*)

Perforated Peptic Ulcer.—Notably a perforated duodenal ulcer with duodenal contents passing along the paracolic gutter to the right iliac fossa. As a rule there is a history of dyspepsia and a very sudden onset. Rigidity and tenderness in the right iliac fossa is present in both conditions, but in a perforated duodenal ulcer it is most improbable that the rigidity is not as great or greater in the right hypochondrium.

Acute Cholecystitis.—Murphy's sign is often positive in cholecystitis and the pain radiates to the back. Early and repeated vomiting is usual. An enlarged gall-bladder may be felt. The unaltered area of hyperæsthesia when an inflamed or obstructed appendix lies in the right hypochondrium has been emphasised already.

Cyclical Vomiting.—There is a history of previous similar attacks. Rigidity is absent and acetone is found in the urine, but it should be remembered that acetonuria may accompany starvation.

3. The Ground Floor (i.e. *Umbilicus to the Brim of the Pelvis*)

Entero-colitis.—Diarrhœa is a prominent symptom, but there is also intestinal colic, slight pyrexia, and, not infrequently, vomiting. The difficulty of a differential diagnosis is increased

John B. Murphy, 1857–1916. *Professor of Surgery, North-Western University, Chicago.*

by the presence of tenderness in the right iliac fossa, which in the case of entero-colitis is due to inflamed mesenteric lymph nodes. There is no tenderness in the recto-vesical pouch, as is the case in pelvic appendicitis. In some cases the differentiation between appendicitis and entero-colitis is impossible, and it is safer to remove the appendix.

Non-specific Mesenteric Lymphadenitis.—The patient, usually a child, is completely free from pain in between attacks, which last a few minutes. Vomiting is usually absent. Shifting tenderness, when present, favours the diagnosis of non-specific mesenteric lymphadenitis, as also does a concomitant upper respiratory track infection.

Intestinal Obstruction.—The difficulty of differentiating severe early acute appendicular obstruction from obstruction to the small intestine may be very great. Vomiting is more persistent in the latter condition, and hyperæsthesia in Sherren's triangle greatly favours the former. In intestinal obstruction the pain remains localised to the umbilicus. If there is any doubt as to which of these two conditions is present, after the stomach contents have been aspirated and intravenous saline solution administered for an hour, the abdomen should be opened through a paramedian incision.

Regional ileitis in its acute form is indistinguishable from acute appendicitis unless a doughy mass of inflamed ileum can be felt. Often this is masked by overlying rigidity.

4. **The Basement** (i.e. *The Pelvis*)

Salpingitis.—Unlike early acute appendicitis, early salpingitis should be treated by non-operative measures. The history of a vaginal discharge, of menstrual irregularities and dysmenorrhœa, or burning pain on micturition are all helpful differential diagnostic points. The tenderness in salpingitis is more medial than that found in acute appendicitis, and is usually bilateral (fig. 522). On a rectal or vaginal examination the enlarged tender Fallopian tubes can be palpated. A smear from the cervix uteri examined microscopically sometimes clinches the diagnosis. In a few cases when the condition is mainly right-sided,

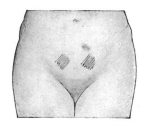

Fig. 522.—Typical distribution of abdominal tenderness in acute salpingitis.

the differential diagnosis is so difficult that it is wiser to explore the abdomen.

Ectopic Gestation.—It is unlikely that a *ruptured* ectopic pregnancy, with its well-defined signs of hæmoperitoneum, will be mistaken for acute appendicitis, but the same cannot be said for a right-sided tubal abortion, or more still for a right-sided unruptured tubal pregnancy (fig. 523). In the latter the

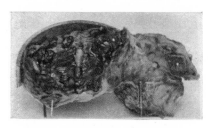

signs are very similar to those of acute appendicitis, except that the pain *begins* in the right side and there is often a history of a missed period. In tubal abortion signs of intraperitoneal hæmorrhage are likely to be manifest. When the internal bleeding has not been excessive the

FIG. 523.—Ectopic tubal gestation. Specimen removed by operation.

differential diagnosis between acute appendicitis and tubal abortion is not always simple, especially when the history of a missed period is lacking. The abdomen moves well on respiration, there is deep tenderness in the iliac fossa, but seldom rigidity. A vaginal examination reveals the cervix softer than usual, and the fornices are tender ; which is of considerable importance, since in inflammatory conditions the tenderness is only posterior and lateral.

(*b*) **Ruptured lutein cyst** (*syn.* apoplectic ovary) occurs particularly during the spring months, and in early womanhood. The patient is usually unmarried, or recently married and childless. The signs are similar to those of very early tubal abortion, but of course the history of a missed period is absent, as also is the sign of a soft cervix. In many of these cases it is practically impossible to rule out the possibility of a mild acute appendicitis.

5. **The Backyard** (i.e. *The Retroperitoneal Structures*)

Right Renal Colic.—In both renal and appendicular colic the right testis is often retracted. In typical renal colic pain commences in the loin and passes to the groin. This peculiar radiation, combined with the presence of urinary symptoms, serves to distinguish many cases from acute appendicitis. When renal colic is due to a stone in the right ureter there is often considerable rigidity in the right iliac fossa. An X-ray and an intravenous pyelogram, together with, if necessary, cystoscopy, will reveal the presence of a stone in the ureter or kidney, and also intermittent hydronephrosis, such as that occasioned by a Dietl's crisis. When these conditions have been excluded, it should be recollected that an inflamed retro-cæcal appendix adherent to the ureter can give rise to slight hæmaturia and a few pus cells in the urine from the right ureter. Therefore, if early acute retrocæcal appendicitis cannot be ruled out, it is safer to perform appendicectomy.

Right-sided acute pyelitis is accompanied and often preceded by increased frequency of micturition. The pain commences in the right side, and typically is higher and more posterior than that of appendicitis. The temperature is often 102° F. (38·9° C.) or more, and rigors are not infrequent. The enlarged tender kidney may be palpable.

Osteomyelitis of the iliac bone occasionally affects the crest of the ilium. The pain commences in the outer part of the right iliac fossa. Compression of the iliac crests causes acute pain. This sign is absent in appendicitis.

6. **The Electrical Installation** (i.e. *Central Nervous System*)

Tabetic crises are now rare. Severe abdominal pain and vomiting usher in the crisis. The absence of knee-jerks, and Argyll Robertson pupils readily confirm the diagnosis.

Pre-herpetic pain of the right tenth and eleventh dorsal nerves is localised over the same area as that of appendicitis. The absence of intestinal symptoms and rigidity should distinguish the condition. The herpetic eruption may be delayed for thirty-six to forty-eight hours.

Spinal conditions are sometimes associated with acute abdominal pain. Sudden irritation of a posterior nerve root in some phase of Pott's disease may give rise to acute pain in the right iliac fossa. Again, the absence of any intestinal symptoms and the probability of some degree of angular deformity with tenderness of the corresponding spinous process points to the probable diagnosis. A spinal tumour can also give rise to sudden right-sided abdominal pain, and in the absence of any interference with motor function such pain may be mistaken for that of appendicitis. The spinous process over the tumour is often acutely tender.

Joseph Dietl, 1804–1878. Professor of Pathology and Therapeutics, Cracow.
Douglas Argyll Robertson, 1837–1909. Ophthalmic Surgeon, Royal Infirmary, Edinburgh.
Percival Pott, 1714–1788. Surgeon, St. Bartholomew's Hospital, London.

PERFORATION AND GANGRENE

When perforation or gangrene occurs within twelve to twenty-four hours after the commencement of the attack, as is sometimes the case in acute appendicular obstruction, diffuse peritonitis is liable to result. In non-obstructive appendicitis particularly, and in obstructive appendicitis when perforation or gangrene develops after a period of twenty-four hours, especially when the appendix lies in a relatively secluded portion of the peritoneal cavity, the resulting peritonitis often becomes localised.

LOCAL AND DIFFUSE PERITONITIS are discussed in Chapter xx.

APPENDIX ABSCESS

On the third day (rarely sooner) after the commencement of an attack of acute appendicitis frequently a tender mass can be felt in the right iliac fossa beneath some rigidity of the overlying musculature. The other quadrants of the abdomen are free from rigidity or tenderness. The mass at this time is composed mainly of the great omentum, œdematous cæcal wall, and adherent œdematous portions of the small intestine. In the midst is a perforated or otherwise inflamed vermiform appendix.

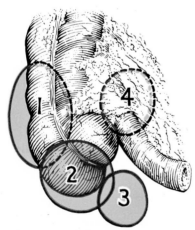

FIG. 524.—Positions of an appendix abscess palpable from the abdomen.
1. Retrocæcal.
2. Subcæcal.
3. Retrorectus.
4. Post-ileal (pre-ileal occupies the same position as 4, but lies in front of the ileum).

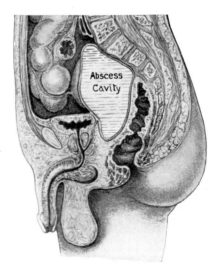

FIG. 525.—Appendix abscess invading the pelvis. Note the relationship to the rectum.

By the fourth or fifth day the mass becomes more circumscribed. As the rigidity passes off its periphery can be clearly defined. Accompanying the abscess there is variable pyrexia, but the pulse-rate is usually under 100. There is an increased leucocyte count with a relative increase of polynuclear cells. The site of the abscess varies with the position of the appendix. Although the commonest site of the abscess is in the lateral part of the iliac fossa (extension of retrocæcal suppuration) (fig. 524) and the second most common is in the pelvis (fig. 525), an abscess centred over McBurney's point is not so unusual as the percentages of the anatomical positions of the appendix would indicate. This is because perforation often implicates the proximal half of an inflamed appendix.

DIFFERENTIAL DIAGNOSIS

Twisted Ovarian Cyst.—If the patient is examined within twenty-four hours of the commencement of the attack, the diagnosis presents no difficulty, for it is so improbable that a definite mass will be found by this time in appendicitis. An appendix abscess is fixed in the iliac fossa ; a twisted ovarian cyst is more mobile.

Suppurative Iliac Lymphadenitis.—When right-sided, this condition sometimes simulates an appendix abscess. In the early stage psoas spasm is often in evidence. There is tenderness, some rigidity, and a palpable swelling above Poupart's ligament (fig. 526). Often the inguinal lymph nodes are unaffected. Suppuration of the iliac lymph nodes leads to an extraperitoneal abscess. There is usually a focus of infection due to such lesions as a scratch or a blister in the skin of the lower limb of the affected side.

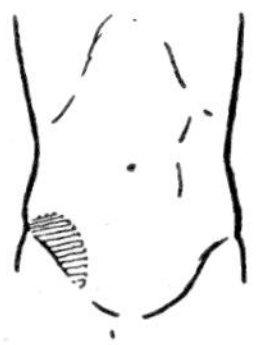

Fig. 526.—The usual situation of a lump connected with suppurating deep iliac lymph nodes.

Perinephric Abscess.—The point of maximum tenderness is in the angle between the last rib and the erector spinæ. In retrocæcal appendicitis or when there is an abscess following that condition, the tenderness is never present in this angle ; it is always below and more lateral.

TREATMENT OF ACUTE APPENDICITIS

The treatment of acute appendicitis is appendicectomy. If the diagnosis is made within forty-eight hours, all are agreed that the appendix should be removed urgently.

François Poupart, 1661–1708. Anatomist, Paris.
About 1888 Sir Frederick Treves, in London, and Thomas C. Morton, in Philadelphia, performed the first successful operations for acute appendicitis.

Appendicectomy.—A variety of incisions are practised. When the diagnosis is certain the grid-iron incision is the one most usually employed. When the diagnosis is in doubt the lower right paramedian incision is preferable because it gives good access to the pelvic organs in the female and, if necessary, it can be readily extended in an upward direction.

The Grid-iron Incision.—An incision from 2 to 4 inches (5 to 10 cm.) in length, according to the amount of subcutaneous fat, is made with its centre over McBurney's point, at right angles to a line joining the anterior superior iliac spine to the umbilicus. In the subcutaneous tissues an arterial twig from the superficial circumflex artery usually requires ligation. The external oblique is incised in the length of the incision. The fibres of the internal oblique and transversalis are separated, and after suitable retraction the peritoneum is opened. If it is found that more room is required, the sheath of the rectus muscle can be incised and the rectus muscle retracted medially.

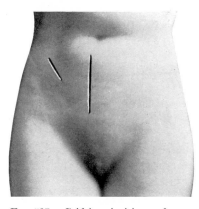

Fig. 527.—Grid-iron incision and para-median incision.

The paramedian incision is a vertical incision lying parallel to, and $\frac{1}{2}$ to 1 inch (1·25 to 2·5 cm.) to the right of the middle line. It commences 1 inch (2·5 cm.) below the level of the umbilicus and ends just above the pubes. The anterior rectus sheath is incised in the line of the incision and the rectus muscle is retracted laterally. Branches of the inferior epigastric vessels may require ligation. The transversalis fascia and the peritoneum are incised together, the peritoneal cavity being opened through the length of the incision. The advantages of the incision have been referred to already. Its disadvantages are (*a*) that it gives poor access to a retrocæcal appendix (it should be possible to diagnose retrocæcal appendicitis preoperatively) ; (*b*) if the incision becomes infected, its " trap-door " nature harbours infection.

The split right rectus incision lies in the same situation as the foregoing, the only difference being that the fibres of the rectus muscle are split in the line of the incision. Its advantages are more accessibility to the right iliac fossa and less susceptibility to prolonged infection, because pus deep to the rectus muscle can escape directly to the surface.

Removal of the Appendix.—It will be assumed that the abdomen has been opened by a grid-iron incision. A retractor is placed under the medial side of the peritoneum and the abdominal wall is lifted up. After removing purulent fluid with a mechanical sucker, packing is inserted into the wound on the medial side. Using an abdominal pack, the cæcum is withdrawn. A finger may be inserted into the wound to aid delivery of the appendix. Once the appendix has been delivered the cæcum is given to an assistant to hold. Morrant Baker forceps are applied around the appendix in such a way as to encircle the organ and yet not damage it (fig. 529). The mesoappendix is clamped in a hæmostat and severed. Sometimes only one such manœuvre frees the whole of the mesoappendix. When

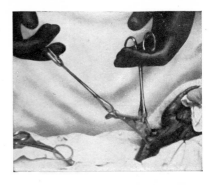

FIG. 528.—Showing the appendix delivered and the mesoappendix displayed.

the mesoappendix is broad, the procedure must be repeated with a second, or, rarely, a third, hæmostat. The appendix, now completely freed from its mesoappendix, is crushed near its junction with the cæcum in a hæmostat, which is removed and reapplied just distal to the crushed portion (fig. 529). Most operators tie a ligature around the crushed portion close to the cæcum.

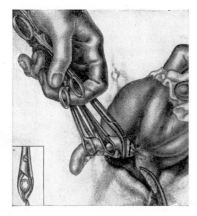

FIG. 529.—Appendicectomy. (Inset) Morrant Baker forceps in use.

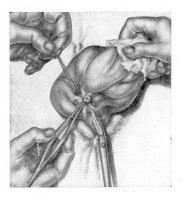

FIG. 530. — Appendicectomy. Inverting the stump of the appendix.

Others omit this ligature. In favour of ligation is that the appendicular artery may lie very close to the base of the appendix. A disadvantage of this ligature is that a small intramural abscess sometimes, if not always, forms between the ligature and the purse-string suture. Even if this is so, there is no evidence that it does harm.

A purse-string suture is inserted into the caput cæci about ½ inch (1·25 cm.) from the base. This stitch passes through

William Morrant Baker, 1839–1896. Surgeon, St. Bartholomew's Hospital, London.

the muscle coat, especially picking up the tæniæ coli. It is left untied until the appendix has been amputated with a scalpel close to the hæmostat, which is still applied to it. The stump is invaginated (fig. 530) while the purse-string suture is tied, thus burying the appendix stump.

Attention is now directed to ligating the mesoappendix. For this purpose transfixion sutures are safe and cannot slip.

Methods to be Adopted in Special Circumstances.—When the cæcal wall is œdematous, the purse-string suture is in danger of cutting out. If the œdema is of limited extent, this can be overcome by inserting the purse-string suture into more healthy cæcal wall at a greater distance from the base of the appendix. Occasions may arise when, because of extensive œdema of the cæcal wall, it is better not to attempt invagination, in which case the stump of the appendix should be ligated and the cut surface covered by stitching a near-by tag of fat or portion of greater omentum over it.

When the base of the appendix is inflamed, it should not be crushed, for fear of distributing infection by way of the lymphatics or blood-stream. It should be ligated close to the cæcal wall just tightly enough to occlude the lumen, after which the appendix is amputated and the stump invaginated.

When the base of the appendix is gangrenous, neither crushing nor ligation must be attempted. Two stitches are placed through the cæcal wall beneath the base of the gangrenous appendix, which is amputated flush with the cæcal wall, after which these stitches are tied. Further closure is effected by means of a purse-string suture, when possible, or by one of the methods described already.

Retrograde Appendicectomy.—In certain cases, especially when the appendix is retrocæcal and adherent, it is an advantage to commence by dividing the base of the organ between hæmostats. After the stump has been ligated and invaginated, the organ is removed from base to tip.

Drainage is unnecessary when the inflammation is confined to the walls of the appendix. If there is a purulent exudate limited to the immediate vicinity of the cæcum, this can be aspirated, and after appendicectomy the wound is closed. When there is a considerable collection of purulent fluid in the retro-cæcal space, drainage through a stab incision in the flank is required. When diffuse or pelvic peritonitis is present, drainage of the pelvis through a separate suprapubic mid-line incision is usually necessary. Local drainage of the abdominal wall, especially when there is considerable subcutaneous fat, with a narrow strip of corrugated rubber left in for forty-eight hours, is considered advisable by many in cases where purulent fluid has been in contact with the abdominal wound. The tubes are turned and shortened each day and are usually removed on the third or fourth day.

WHEN EARLY DIAGNOSIS HAS NOT BEEN MADE

If, for one reason or another, the diagnosis has been delayed until the third or fourth day of the disease, and there is local peritonitis or an appendix abscess, opinions differ as to the best course to adopt immediately. Surgeons are divided into two schools.

The *immediate school* advocate removal of the appendix, or drainage of an appendix abscess, under all conditions as soon as possible, irrespective of the time since the onset of the attack, although even disciples of this school often stipulate " unless the patient is recovering from the attack."

The *Ochsner-Sherren (delayed) school*, under certain conditions detailed below, institute a rigid non-operative régime, and while being *prepared* to operate immediately, they only do so if the signs point to failure of Nature to combat the infection.

The treatment is not merely a postponement of operation ; it is not a substitute for operation, but a preparation for it—essentially a surgeon's treatment, to be undertaken only in a surgical hospital, or a correspondingly equipped nursing home. But there are circumstances—for instance, in a small ship at sea—where conservative treatment would be less dangerous, by reason of these circumstances, than to attempt operation.

SELECTING CASES FOR THE " DELAYED " TREATMENT

The history is taken, and particular note is made of the number of hours since the onset. The history begins " ten, twenty-six, fifty-five *hours* ago," not " last Thursday," or " three days ago." The physical signs are then recorded in diagrammatic form. The extent of the rigidity is marked by shading ; the presence of a lump is drawn as near as possible to scale. The presence or absence of hyperæsthesia is always recorded, and the findings of a rectal examination are not omitted.

If the diagnosis of acute appendicitis is made and the history is of *under forty-eight hours' duration*, immediate operation is nearly always advised. If the diagnosis of acute appendicitis is made and the history is *over forty-eight hours' duration*, one should ask oneself the question, " Is there any reason why this appendix *should* be removed at once ? " The answer by one trained in the delayed treatment is, " It is safer to postpone operation for the time being, unless .. -

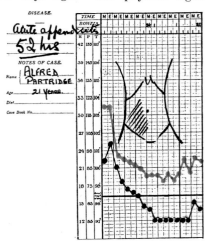

Fig. 531.—Chart of a case of acute appendicitis first seen fifty-two hours after the onset of the attack and treated by the Ochsner-Sherren method.

Albert J. Ochsner, 1858–1925. Professor of Surgery, University of Illinois, U.S.A
James Sherren, 1872–1946. Surgeon, London Hospital.

CONTRAINDICATIONS

1. The signs indicate that the inflammation is still confined to the appendix.

2. The patient's age is under ten years or over sixty-five.

3. The diagnosis cannot be made between acute appendicitis and some other intra-abdominal catastrophe normally requiring immediate operation.

4. The recent ingestion of a powerful purgative may be a justifiable indication for performing an operation which otherwise would be delayed.

TECHNIQUE OF THE "DELAYED" TREATMENT

Charts.—As a routine the pulse is recorded every two hours in graphic form on a special chart. In cases where anxiety is felt as to the advisability of continuing the treatment an hourly chart is employed. Temperature is

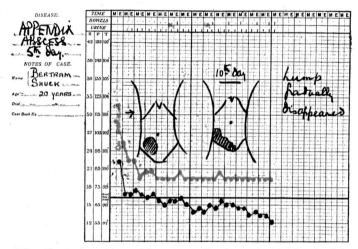

Fig. 532.—Chart of a patient with an appendix abscess treated by the Ochsner-Sherren method.

relatively unimportant, and it is recorded every four hours. Instructions are given to the nurse to record any vomiting on a separate piece of paper, known as a " vomit chart." On this is entered the time at which the vomitus was ejected, together with the quantity and character of the fluid.

Diet.—*Everything* is excluded by mouth, as even sips of water stimulate peristalsis. Mouth-washes are given frequently.

Intravenous saline and glucose solution is administered, care being taken to give the exact amount required for the individual patient. A fluid intake and output chart is compiled, and from this at the end of twenty-four hours the fluid needs of the patient for the next twenty-four hours are calculated.

On the fifth day of treatment, if the pulse and temperature are satisfactory, and the patient feels hungry, oral feeding is commenced. Small feeds of Benger's food, alternating with a cup of Bovril, are given. On the sixth day custard and jelly are allowed. After that the diet is gradually increased.

Application of Local Heat.—The best form is an electrically heated pad. Failing that, the patient is given a well-covered hot-water bottle to apply

Frederick Baden Benger, 1840–1903. Pharmaceutical Chemist, Manchester.

to the abdomen. Antiphlogistin, although often comforting to the patient, somewhat limits the finer perception of the palpating hand.

Drugs.—It should be particularly noted that no morphine or its derivatives are given in border-line cases (usually those between forty-eight and sixty hours after the onset of the attack) that are being watched closely for a few hours in order to observe whether the pulse-rate and other signs are tending to settle. Once it has been decided definitely to treat the patient by conservative measures, one dose of omnopon is given. Pain, as opposed to tenderness, is very seldom complained of after the first night of the treatment.

Antibiotics and Chemotherapy are, of course, employed by both schools, but it is convenient to include them here. Penicillin in doses of 100,000 units to 500,000 units, according to the severity of the case, six-hourly, is the most valuable of these agents, as it is inimical to Cl. welchii and many streptococci. If streptomycin, which is inimical to B. coli, is given in addition, many consider that chemotherapy can be omitted. In the absence of streptomycin, a water-soluble sulphonamide, 2 grammes (30 gr.) initially, followed by 1 gramme (15 gr.) four-hourly until 30 grammes (1 oz.) have been given, constitutes a course. All these agents can be added to the intravenous saline solution as long as it is running. Afterwards the antibiotics are given intramuscularly. Chemotherapeutic agents can be given by mouth in the latter stages of the delayed treatment of an appendix abscess. One advantage of antibiotics used alone is that there are no toxic effects. They do not induce nausea or vomiting, and are free from any danger of causing impairment of renal function.

Bowels.—The bowels are left confined if they are not opened naturally. On the fourth or fifth day a small glycerol enema is given. No purgatives of any kind are given until resolution is complete—that is, until the temperature and pulse have been normal for a week and pain and physical signs are absent—then liquid paraffin, 2 drachms (8 ml.) twice daily, is prescribed.

WATCHING FOR NATURE'S FAILURE TO COMBAT THE INFECTION

Instructions are given for the nurse in charge to watch the patient and report immediately (1) a rising pulse-rate, (2) vomiting, (3) pain, and, in the later stages of the treatment, (4) diarrhœa or the passage of mucus in the stools (pelvic abscess).

A rising pulse-rate in the early stages is the most reliable single sign that it is dangerous to proceed with the delayed method. If the pulse-rate has increased, or even if it is stationary towards the end of the first twenty-four hours of expectant treatment, operation is indicated.

Vomiting after the first few hours should always be regarded seriously, and this by itself may be a sufficient indication to abandon delayed treatment.

A patient undergoing delayed treatment should not complain of pain, as opposed to tenderness, after the first six hours of such treatment. If he does, there is usually something amiss, and there is a strong indication for operation.

THE OUTCOME

Under the delayed treatment about 90 per cent. of cases resolve without incident and the appendix is duly removed three months after the acute stage has abated, by which time usually the field of operation is singularly free from adhesions. In a few cases where the signs point to failure of the delayed treatment, urgent appendicectomy must be undertaken.

THE TREATMENT OF APPENDIX ABSCESS

The same controversy exists as in the case of acute appendicitis of more than forty-eight hours' duration. The immediate school proclaim an old and usually wise surgical axiom—" Where there is pus you must let it out." The delayed school state that the rule may be broken in the case of small and moderate-sized appendix abscesses, and the abscess should only be opened if it is getting larger or fails to resolve (fig. 533). They find that more than four-fifths of appendix abscesses resolve completely under the Ochsner-Sherren régime.

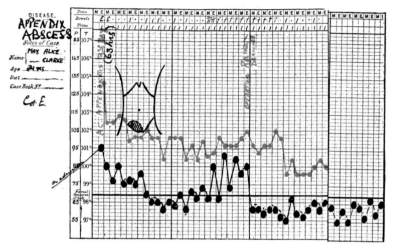

Fig. 533.—Chart of a patient with an appendix abscess treated by the Ochsner-Sherren method. In this case a pelvic abscess formed. The abscess was drained via the rectum.

Indications for Opening an Appendix Abscess.—(1) When the swelling is not getting smaller, or is increasing in size after the fifth day of treatment ; (2) when the temperature is swinging above 100° F. on several successive days ; (3) a pelvic abscess seldom resolves. Repeated rectal examinations are required to determine when it is ready for opening into the rectum (see p. 385).

Opening an Appendix Abscess.—The swelling is palpated under the anæsthetic.

A **retrocæcal appendix abscess** can be opened extraperitoneally. An incision from 1 to 2 inches (2·5 to 5 cm.) long, depending on the thickness of the abdominal wall, is made over the centre of the swelling, rather nearer the lateral than the medial aspect. The external oblique is incised and the fibres of the internal oblique are divided, instead of being separated, so as to give freer exit to the contents of the abscess. When the peritoneum has been reached the extraperitoneal tissues are separated in an outward and backward direction, until the abscess cavity is entered. The contents of the abscess are aspirated with a mechanical sucker, if available. In cases where the abscess cavity lies at some distance from the incision, more direct drainage is afforded by a counter-incision in the flank .in which case the original incision may be closed.

A subcæcal abscess can be opened in the same manner, the incision being placed nearer the anterior superior iliac spine.

A pre- or post-ileal abscess can only be reached through the peritoneal cavity. When the peritoneum has been opened, gauze packing is inserted so as to isolate the region from the general peritoneal cavity before opening the abscess.

A retro-rectus abscess that cannot be felt per rectum is best reached by a short rectus-splitting incision.

A pelvic abscess is opened into the rectum, as described on p. 385.

When it is necessary to drain an appendix abscess, no attempt should be made to perform appendicectomy, except in rare instances where the appendix is lying free in the abscess cavity. Usually the appendix is incorporated in the walls of the abscess.

COMPLICATIONS

The complications of appendicectomy for acute appendicitis with varying degrees of peritonitis, and to a lesser extent of an appendix abscess, include :

Recent

Residual abscess in the right iliac fossa.

Pelvic abscess (p. 385).

Residual abscess in the left paracolic gutter (p. 385).

Subphrenic abscess (p. 386).

Suppuration of the abdominal incision.

Pylephlebitis (p. 331).

Paralytic ileus (p. 475).

Intestinal obstruction from adhesions (p. 469).

Actinomycosis in the right iliac fossa (p. 422).

Thrombophlebitis of the femoral or ileo-colic vein (pp. 105 and 331).

Pulmonary complications (broncho-pneumonia ; empyema ; massive collapse of the lung).

Remote

Intestinal obstruction by bands and adhesions (p. 468).

Incisional hernia (p. 595).

Possibly right inguinal hernia if a low grid-iron incision has been employed (p. 578).

*　　　*　　　*　　　*　　　*

It is advisable to include the following practical problem :

After an operation for acute appendicitis the condition of the patient is unsatisfactory. The temperature is swinging and the pulse is elevated—signs which foretell of pocketing of pus. How would you investigate the case ?

1. *Examine the scar or wound and the abdominal wall* for an abscess of the abdominal wall.

2. *Consider the possibility of a pelvic abscess* (p. 385).

3. *Palpate the left iliac fossa* for an abscess in this situation.

4. *Examine the loin* for retrocæcal swelling and tenderness.

5. *Examine the legs*—to exclude the possibility of phlebitis.

6. *Examine the conjunctivæ for an icteric tinge and the liver for enlargement, and enquire if the patient has had rigors*—pylephlebitis.

7. *Examine the lungs*—pneumonia or empyema.

8. *Examine the urine for organisms* (pyelitis).

9. Lastly, *concentrate diagnostic endeavour upon the possibility of a subphrenic abscess.*

SUBACUTE APPENDICITIS

Subacute appendicitis is but a mild form of acute appendicitis, and requires no detailed consideration.

RECURRENT APPENDICITIS

Appendicitis is notoriously recurrent. This is perhaps the commonest form of appendicitis—mild subacute attacks which are so often attributed to " biliousness " or a " chill on the liver." The attacks vary in intensity, and the majority of cases ultimately culminate in severe acute appendicitis. If careful histories are taken from patients with acute appendicitis, over two-thirds remember having had milder but similar attacks of pain. This bespeaks the importance of recurrent appendicitis as a precursor of the more serious lesion.

CHRONIC APPENDICITIS

One should be careful to distinguish recurrent from chronic appendicitis. Many cases called " chronic appendicitis " are typical examples of the recurrent form of the disease. Chronic appendicitis is a comparatively rare affection ; it certainly exists, and its most typical symptoms are referred to the stomach and duodenum, and take the form of hyperchlorhydria and pylorospasm.

Pathology.—Appendices removed from patients suffering from true appendicular dyspepsia usually show a characteristic

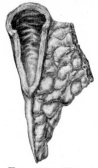

macroscopical change. There is obliteration of the lumen commencing at the tip and spreading along the organ for a variable distance. The walls of the obliterated portion can be seen to be composed almost entirely of white fibrous tissue (fig. 534). In long-standing cases the greater part of the organ is attenuated from fibrous contracture. In a few cases the fibrous changes are seen in the proximal end, but this is more characteristic of the recurrent type of the disease.

Fig. 534.—Chronic obliterative appendicitis.

Diagnosis is difficult. One should remember

constantly that in chronic appendicitis there are often no signs in the right iliac fossa—only referred symptoms elsewhere.

Radiology as an Aid to Diagnosis.—In the case of the vermiform appendix, radiology is not a great diagnostic aid. If the appendix cannot be visualised after an opaque meal, it suggests that its lumen is obstructed. If it fills and empties, it is indicative that at least part of the organ is healthy—but as nobody can tell the length of a given appendix until the organ has been displayed, there must always be uncertainty in the radiological diagnosis of appendicitis. Tenderness over the appendix during a radiological examination is contributory evidence of appendicitis, as also is delayed and irregular filling of the appendix. A barium meal followed by the ingestion of 2 drachms (8 ml.) of magnesium sulphate aids in the radiological diagnosis of a pathological appendix, the magnesium sulphate helping to fill the lumen of the organ with the ingested opaque material.

Treatment.—After thorough investigation, which includes a barium meal and cholecystography, if a diagnosis of reflex pylorospasm or appendicular dyspepsia has been made, the abdomen should be opened through a paramedian incision, so that other organs can be examined. Appendicectomy is carried out.

SPECIAL PATHOLOGICAL FORMS OF SUBACUTE AND CHRONIC APPENDICITIS

Mucocele of the appendix occurs when the proximal end of the lumen slowly becomes completely occluded, usually by a fibrous stricture, and the pent-up secretion remains sterile. The appendix is greatly enlarged ; sometimes it contains several ounces of mucus. The symptoms produced are those of mild subacute appendicitis unless infection supervenes, when the mucocele is converted into an empyema. Rupture of a mucocele of the appendix may result in pseudomyxoma peritonei.

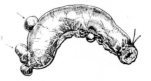

FIG. 535.—Appendicular diverticulosis.

Diverticula of the appendix can occur in conjunction with a mucocele. The intramural pressure rises sufficiently to cause herniation of the mucous membrane through the muscle coat at several points. More often diverticula (fig. 535) are found not in association with a mucocele, and often there is no demonstrable obstruction to the lumen. Usually the patient gives a history of previous recurrent attacks of appendicitis. It is probable that each diverticulum is the result of damage to the muscle coat by a previous intermural abscess which discharged into the lumen. Diverticula are present in 0·3 per cent. of appendices removed by operation.

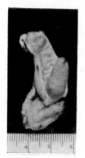

FIG. 536.—Intussusception of the appendix.

Intussusception of the appendix (fig. 536) is a very rare condition, and is most often seen in children. It can only be diagnosed at operation. The symptoms are usually not acute, and are often present for weeks or months. Untreated, the condition may pass on to an appendiculo-colic intussusception.

The treatment is appendicectomy, but if the intussusception cannot be reduced, the cæcum must be opened in order to effect this.

NEOPLASMS OF THE APPENDIX

Carcinoid tumour (*syn.* argentaffin tumour) is found once in about every 300 to 400 appendices subjected to microscopical examination, and occurs most usually in patients between twenty and thirty years of age. Females are more often affected than males. As a rule the appendix is removed because of symptoms of sub-acute or recurrent appendicitis. The tumour can occur

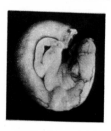

in any part of the appendix, but it frequently does so near the tip (fig. 537). Exceptionally, when it originates in the proximal part of the appendix, it gives rise to appendicular obstruction. The tumour is rarely more than $\frac{1}{2}$ inch (12 mm.) long and $\frac{1}{4}$ inch (6 mm.) in diameter. It feels moderately hard, and on slitting up the appendix the neoplasm is seen to occupy the walls of the appendix between the mucosa and the peritoneal coat. The tumour is of a bright yellow colour, due to contained lipoid,

FIG. 537.—Carcinoid tumour of the appendix. The solid bulbous tip is characteristic.

and probably arises in cells of the autonomic nervous system. Microscopically it is a spheroidal-celled carcinoma containing granules which stain readily with ammoniacal silver salts. In only 4 per cent. of cases does the tumour give rise to metastases.

Carcinoma is ten times less common than carcinoid tumour.

Adenocarcinoma is the least rare variety, and usually develops near the base and is intimately related to carcinoma of the cæcum (p. 435). When a carcinomatous mass has formed in the region of the caput cæci it is often impossible to state precisely where the growth originated, even after a careful pathological examination.

Colloid Carcinoma.—The whole appendix is involved and greatly enlarged. At first sight it may appear like a mucocele, but it is firm and solid.

Sarcoma is extremely uncommon.

Treatment of Neoplasms of the Appendix.—Appendicectomy suffices in carcinoid tumour. In colloid carcinoma removal of the appendix, together with 1 inch (2·5 cm.) of the related cæcal wall, has given satisfactory results. In other forms of neoplasm right hemicolectomy should be undertaken.

CHAPTER XXIV
THE RECTUM AND ANAL CANAL

EXAMINATION OF THE RECTUM

DIGITAL examination of the rectum is invaluable, and in cases where rectal disease is suspected it should be performed as a routine. Examination with a proctoscope (fig. 538) is also of paramount importance, but only the anal canal and a small part of the lower rectum can be inspected with this instrument. A sigmoidoscope is necessary for the visualisation of the upper reaches of the rectum. By its aid, provided the rectum has been emptied by suitable preparation, the valves of Houston are normally seen, and pathological conditions of the rectal wall are clearly apparent.

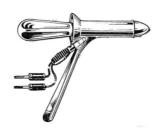

FIG. 538.—An illuminated proctoscope.

SURGICAL ANATOMY OF RECTUM AND ANAL CANAL

The rectum is 5 to 6 inches (12·5 to 15 cm.) long, and it extends from the third sacral vertebra to the apex of the prostate in the male, or $1\frac{1}{2}$ inches (3·75 cm.) below the tip of coccyx. It describes three lateral curves, two concave to left and one to right. The relative shortness of the longitudinal muscle coat forms the **valves of Houston** that are so much in evidence in sigmoidoscopy (fig. 539). Antero-posteriorly the rectum follows the curve of the sacrum and turns back at the level of the ano-rectal ring to become the anal canal.

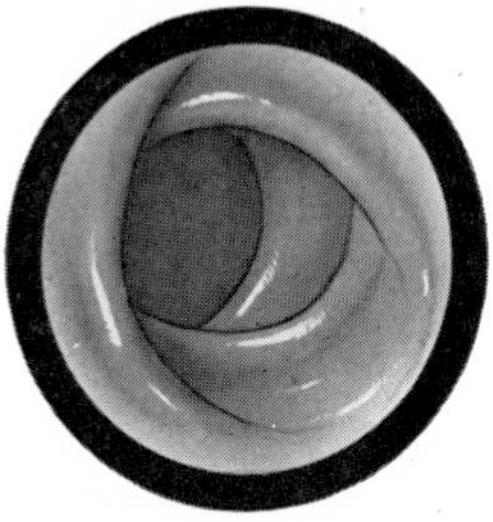

The rectal glands are tubular glands opening into the terminal part of the rectum, usually in the anal crypts. They are lined by transitional epithelium extending in the submucosa, and may pass between the fibres of the internal sphincter muscle. Infection of these glands is sometimes responsible for abscesses in this region.

The anal canal is $1\frac{1}{2}$ inches (3·75 cm.) long. In the upper part the lining epithelium is columnar. Three-quarters of an inch (2 cm.) above the anal verge the mucous membrane is thrown into a series of longitudinal folds—the columns of Morgagni (fig. 540), which are

FIG. 539. — Houston's valves as seen through a sigmoidoscope.

John Houston, 1802–1854. Physician, City of Dublin Hospital.
Giovanni Morgagni, 1682–1771. Professor of Surgery, Padua. He held the chair for fifty-six years.

joined below by transverse semilunar folds—the anal **valves of Ball** bounding crypts behind them (see fig. 540).

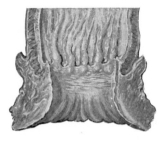

Fig. 540.—The anal canal showing the columns of Morgagni and the valves of Ball.

Just below the anal valves is the **pectinate line,** a most important region both morphologically and surgically. It represents (1) the site of fusion of the proctodæum and post-allantoic gut, and (2) the position of the anal membrane, remnants of which may frequently be seen as anal papillæ situated on the free margin of the anal valves. The pectinate line separates :

Above	*Below*
Columnar epithelium	from squamous epithelium
Autonomic nerves	from cerebrospinal nerves
Non-sensitivity	from extreme sensitivity
Pelvic lymph drainage	from superficial inguinal lymph drainage
Portal venous system	from systemic venous system

THE MUSCULATURE OF THE RECTUM AND THE ANAL CANAL

The longitudinal muscle, while clothing the whole of the circumference of the rectum, is more fully developed anteriorly and posteriorly than laterally. This muscle coat is continued on the wall of the anal canal to the level of the lower border of the **internal sphincter.** Here it terminates in two fibro-muscular septa. The outer septum divides the ischio-rectal space from the perianal space. The inner septum, called the intermuscular septum, separates the internal sphincter from the **subcutaneous external sphincter** and becomes firmly attached to the anal mucous membrane at the pectinate line. The intermuscular septum, becoming more muscular, continues downwards and outwards as the **corrugator cutis ani.**

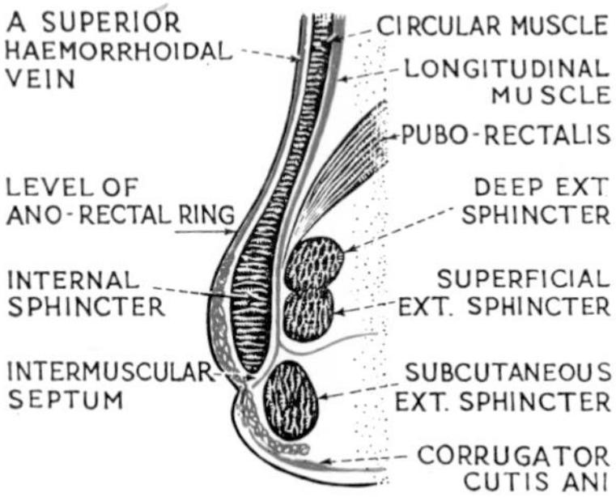

The Circular Muscle and Internal Sphincter.—The circular muscle forms a complete coat for the rectum. At the level of the ano-rectal ring it becomes thicker and forms the (unstriped) internal sphincter which terminates, in the adult, about ½ inch (1·25 cm.) above

A SUPERIOR HAEMORRHOIDAL VEIN

CIRCULAR MUSCLE

LONGITUDINAL MUSCLE

PUBO-RECTALIS

LEVEL OF ANO-RECTAL RING

DEEP EXT SPHINCTER

INTERNAL SPHINCTER

SUPERFICIAL EXT. SPHINCTER

INTERMUSCULAR SEPTUM

SUBCUTANEOUS EXT. SPHINCTER

CORRUGATOR CUTIS ANI

Fig. 541.—The musculature of the anal canal. (*After Naunton Morgan.*)

Sir Charles Ball, 1851–1916. Professor of Surgery, University of Dublin.

the anal margin. The external sphincters (striped) are three in number, from below upwards :

1. **The subcutaneous external sphincter** is situated beneath the skin at the anal margin. It is about ⅓ inch (1·25 cm.) thick.
2. **The superficial external sphincter** is attached to the coccyx.
3. **The deep external sphincter** is an annular muscle intimately blended with the pubo-rectalis portion of the levator ani.

The ano-rectal ring marks the junction between the rectum and the anal canal. It is formed by the fused parts of pubo-rectalis, deep external sphincter, longitudinal muscle, and internal sphincter. The ano-rectal ring can be clearly felt digitally, especially on its posterior and lateral aspects. Division of the ano-rectal ring results in permanent incontinence of fæces.

THE BLOOD-SUPPLY AND LYMPHATIC DRAINAGE OF THE RECTUM AND THE ANAL CANAL

The superior hæmorrhoidal artery is the direct continuation of the inferior mesenteric artery and constitutes the chief arterial supply to the rectum. Opposite the third sacral vertebra the artery divides into a right and a left branch, which descend on the postero-lateral wall. About half-way down the rectum each branch subdivides and pierces the rectal wall. The terminal branches run straight downwards, each in a column of Morgagni. The largest of these branches are situated in the left lateral, the right posterior, and the right anterior quadrants (Miles).

The middle hæmorrhoidal artery arises on each side from the internal iliac artery and supplies the muscle coat of the mid rectum. These arteries do not anastomose to any extent with the superior or inferior hæmorrhoidal arteries.

The inferior hæmorrhoidal artery arises on each side as a branch of the internal pudendal artery. Crossing the upper part of the ischio-rectal fossa, it breaks up into branches which supply the anal sphincters, anal canal, and the skin of the anal margin.

The internal hæmorrhoidal venous plexus lies in the submucosa of the anal canal and extends from the level of the pectinate line to that of the anal ring. The plexus drains into about six collecting veins which are situated in the submucosa of the rectum. About half-way up the rectum these branches pass through the rectal wall, and having reached the outside of the rectum, they unite to form the **superior hæmorrhoidal vein**, an important tributary of the portal vein. The **middle hæmorrhoidal veins** are small and comparatively unimportant. They drain into the internal iliac veins.

The external hæmorrhoidal venous plexus lies under the skin of the anal canal below the pectinate line and beneath the skin of the anal margin. It communicates above with the superior hæmorrhoidal plexus. The lower part of the inferior plexus drains into the internal pudendal veins and from thence into the internal iliac veins. By this plexus a free communication between the portal and systemic venous systems is established.

The lymphatic vessels commence above the pectinate line as a plexus in the submucosa. Collecting lymphatic vessels follow the superior hæmorrhoidal vessels and with them pass through the muscular coats of the rectum to reach the pararectal lymph nodes, which form a chain along the superior hæmorrhoidal artery. Efferent lymphatic vessels pass from the superior hæmorrhoidal nodes to the inferior mesenteric and aortic nodes, and thence to the cœliac nodes. There are also lymphatic vessels draining the ampulla of the rectum, which follow the middle hæmorrhoidal

W. Ernest Miles, 1869–1947. Surgeon, Cancer Hospital, London.

veins to the internal iliac lymph nodes. The lymphatic vessels below the pectinate line and those of the anal margin pass to the superficial inguinal lymph nodes.

THE FASCIAL SPACES

The perianal space is bounded below and on the inner side by the skin of the anal canal and the perianal skin, attached to which is the corrugator cutis ani muscle ; above by the intermuscular septum, which separates it from the submucous space and the ischio-rectal space. Externally it is unbounded, and communicates with the subcutaneous tissues of the buttocks. This space contains the subcutaneous external sphincter and the external hæmorrhoidal plexus.

The submucous space is situated in the upper two-thirds of the anal canal between the mucous membrane and the internal sphincter. Above it is continuous with the submucous space of the rectum. Below it is bounded by the intermuscular septum. This space contains the internal hæmorrhoidal venous plexus and lymphatic vessels.

The ischio-rectal space is bounded below by an outward extension of the intermuscular septum. The inner wall, from above downwards, is formed by the levator ani and the deep and superficial external sphincters. The outer wall has as its boundary the ischium and the obturator internus covered by the parietal layer of pelvic fascia. In this fascia lies a tunnel (Alcock's canal) containing the internal pudendal vessels and nerve. The inferior hæmorrhoidal artery and nerve pierce the inner wall of Alcock's canal and pass across the space to reach the external sphincter and the anal canal. Anteriorly the space is bounded by the triangular ligament and the transversus perinei muscles ; posteriorly by the great sacro-sciatic ligament, and the lower margin of the gluteus maximus. The space contains soft fat.

The pelvi-rectal space is situated beneath the pelvic peritoneum and above the levator ani.

EMBRYOLOGY

Early in embryonic life there is a common chamber—the cloaca—into

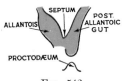

FIG. 542.

which open the hind gut and the allantois. The cloaca becomes separated into the bladder and post-allantoic gut (rectum) by the downgrowth of a septum (fig. 542). About this time an epiblastic bud, the proctodæum, grows in towards the rectum. Normally, fusion between these two structures occurs during the third month of intrauterine life.

CONGENITAL ABNORMALITIES

(a) **Imperfections in Development of the Anal Canal.**—The anal canal can be totally absent, represented by a dimple, or separated from the rectum by a membrane only (fig. 543). The degree of development of the anal canal is no criterion of the degree of development of the rectum. When the anal canal is entirely absent the sphincter muscles are likely to be absent also.

(b) **Imperfections in Development of the Rectum.**—The post-allantoic gut may be totally absent or incomplete when its

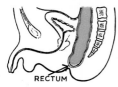

Fig. 543.—The anal canal separated from the rectum by a thin septum.

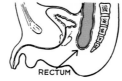

Fig. 544.—The anal canal separated from the rectum by a considerable interval.

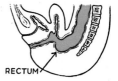

Fig. 545.—Congenital recto-vaginal fistula.

blind end terminates at the level of the prostate (fig. 544) or the cervix uteri.

(c) **Persistence of the Cloaca.**—*In the male* the communicating fistula is most often at the verumontanum, but it may occur anywhere from the base of the bladder to the membranous urethra. *In the female* the fistula usually opens into the vagina (fig. 545), and it is sometimes associated with a double vagina (failure of the Müllerian ducts to fuse).

IMPERFORATE ANUS

Clinical Features.—The abnormality may be noticed at birth, or detected only when the infant fails to pass meconium. Examination will show (1) a short anal canal ; (2) a dimple at the site of the anus (this is the commonest finding) ; (3) there is not even a dimple. In the last variety it is highly probable that the external sphincter muscle is absent.

If a recto-vaginal fistula is present, meconium will issue from the vulva. In males the presence of a recto-vesical fistula is manifest by meconium being passed per urethram with the urine, or as a constant dribble.

In any of these abnormalities the anal region should be inspected and palpated while the child cries. If this is accompanied by bulging, it is probable that the case is one of a simple septum.

X-ray Examination.—Six hours after birth sufficient air has collected in the large intestine to cast an X-ray shadow. With a metal button or a coin strapped to the site of the absent anus, or a metal bougie inserted into the blind anal canal, the infant is radiographed in the inverted position. The gas in the rectum will rise to the top and indicate the distance between the site of the metal indicator and the blind end of the rectum (fig. 546).

Fig. 546.—From an X-ray film.
(*After Wangensteen.*)

Johannes Müller, 1801–1858. Physiologist and embryologist, Bonn.

Treatment.—1. When it has been proved that the case is one of a simple septum, all that is necessary is to incise the septum crucially. Subsequent regular dilatations by the finger or a bougie are required.

2. More frequently the condition is not so simple, and if the distance between the blind end of the rectum and the anal dimple is not more than 2 inches (5 cm.), an incision is made in the middle line from the middle of the anal dimple to the coccyx, and a dissection is carried upwards in the hollow of the sacrum until the rectum is reached. The blind end is freed, drawn down, and having been opened and emptied, the edges of the opening are sutured to the skin in the anterior part of the incision. The divided sphincter is united and the posterior part of the skin incision is closed.

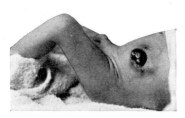

FIG. 547.—Left inguinal colostomy in an infant with imperforate anus (type 3). The child thrived.

3. When there is no anal dimple, and particularly when the distance from the blind end of the rectum to the surface is more than 2 inches (5 cm.), left inguinal colostomy is performed. Unless there is evidence of an external sphincter, a left inguinal colostomy (fig. 547) is preferable to an incontinent anal orifice in the natural situation.

4. In cases of imperforate anus with a recto-vesical fistula, the same operation as (2) should be carried out when possible. Sometimes, when the fistula is small, it closes spontaneously.

5. In cases with a vesico-vaginal fistula, operation can be delayed until the child is three or four years of age. It is sometimes possible to separate the rectum from the vagina, and establish a functioning anus in the normal position.

SACRO-COCCYGEAL SINUS (Syn. PILONIDAL SINUS)

There is a chronic or recurring sinus in the middle line about the level of the first piece of the coccyx (fig. 548). Typically a tuft of hairs projects from its mouth and loose hairs are a frequent content of the tract ; hence the term " pilonidal " (a nest of hairs).

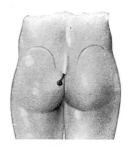

FIG. 548.—Probe in a pilonidal sinus.

Ætiology.—Three theories are held : (a) that the sinus arises from imperfect separation of the blind end of the neural canal from the ectoderm ; (b) that the sinus is a sequestration dermoid ; (c) that some cases are acquired by a hair puncturing the skin. The general consensus of opinion is that most cases are congenital in origin.

A dormant sinus is frequently awakened by local irritation or trauma ; for instance, riding in a hard-seated vehicle. During the 1939–45 war, so common was pilonidal sinus among jeep riders that it became known as " jeep disease."

Pathology.—In cases with a short history the primary sinus or sinuses are lined by squamous epithelium, leading to a cavity partly lined by squamous epithelium and partly by granulation tissue. In 50 per cent. of cases the blind sac contains hairs. In old-standing cases the hairs have been discharged and the wall of the cavity is mainly composed of granulation tissue. Secondary sinuses are always lined by granulation tissue.

Clinical Features.—Symptoms usually commence between eighteen and twenty-five years of age. Patients presenting later in life always give a history dating back to this period. Males are four times as commonly affected as females. The condition rarely occurs in blondes ; many of the patients are exceptionally hairy and are usually obese. In spite of the preponderance in dark-haired persons, the condition is practically confined to white races. The complaint is of a discharge, pain, or a tender swelling at the bottom of the spine. Even at the height of an attack of inflammation the constitutional symptoms are slight. Often there is a history of repeated attacks of abscesses in the region which have discharged spontaneously or have been incised. The primary sinus may have one, or as many as six, openings, all of which are strictly in the middle line between the level of the sacro-coccygeal joint and the tip of the coccyx. Unlike a fistula-in-ano, the sinus passes upwards and forwards towards the sacrum. It does not reach bone, but ends blindly near the bone. When an abscess forms, it may discharge through a primary sinus ; more frequently it points and bursts, or is incised to one side of the middle line, thus forming a secondary sinus. In at least 85 per cent. of cases the secondary sinus is on the left of the middle line (Oldham).

Treatment of an Acute Exacerbation.—Penicillin and sulphonamide therapy are given, and if an abscess points, it must be incised. In these circumstances a curative operation is postponed until the inflammation has become quiescent.

Jeep—U.S. Army reconnaissance motor vehicle.
J. B. Oldham, *Contemporary. Surgeon, United Hospital, Liverpool.*

Once a pilonidal sinus has become infected it will continue to discharge, or if the discharge ceases for a time, further attacks of inflammation follow.   While incision may become necessary, it is never curative, nor are X-rays or the application of caustics.

Pre-operative Treatment.—In hairy individuals pre-operative depilation of the skin of the area by X-rays is highly desirable.   Two or three days of preliminary treatment with penicillin is advisable.

Excision with marsupialisation is usually the operation of choice, because no guarantee can be given as to primary union after excision and suture. The theory underlying the marsupialisation operation is that in the primary track and the wall of the sac there are islets of squamous epithelium which help to epithelialise the wound. Using a probe, the sinus or sinuses and the sac are laid open, particular care being taken to open diverticula from the main channel. Overlying skin is cut away and the contents of the cyst are removed with a swab. Hæmostasis having been effected by forcipressure and hot packs, the skin edges are loosely sewn to the remaining deep part of the cyst wall. The cavity is packed with sulphonamide-petroleum jelly gauze and the bowels are kept confined for four or five days. After the bowels have been opened by an enema, the packing is removed. The patient then has baths twice a day ; following each bath the cavity is repacked. After a week the patient can attend as an out-patient for repacking of the wound, which heals in from three to six weeks.

Excision with primary suture may be successful, particularly in early cases, and especially in women. It should not be attempted when a secondary sinus is present or when the surrounding tissues feel indurated from long-standing chronic inflammation. An elliptical incision at least 2 inches (5 cm.) long and ¾ inch (2 cm.) wide is made. A solitary sinus should lie 1 cm. from the base of the ellipse ; if several sinuses are present, all are included in the ellipse with a margin of 1 cm. of skin. A block excision of the skin and fat containing the lesion is carried out down to the fascia overlying the coccyx. Hæmorrhage is controlled by forcipressure and hot packs. No ligatures are employed unless they are essential. When the bleeding has been controlled, a series of deep sutures is inserted ½ inch (1·25 cm.) from the skin edges, but not tied. The edges of the wound are then approximated with deep mattress sutures, after which the deeper sutures are tied over a roll of gauze. More gauze is applied, followed by firm, flexible adhesive plaster strapping.

OTHER CONGENITAL CONDITIONS

The Fovea Coccygea.—A little blind pit in the skin beneath the tip of the coccyx is occasionally noticed in the course of a clinical examination. The extremity of this corresponds to the attachment of the caudal ligament to the skin.

Sacro-coccygeal Teratoma.—It is a disputed point as to whether these neoplasms are derived from the neurenteric canal or from a parasitic twin.

Clinically, the tumour gives rise to a mass in the region of the sacrum (fig. 549), and is present at birth.

Treatment is excision, which is often possible. It may be necessary to resect a part of the sacrum.

Post-anal Dermoid.—The space in front of the lower part of the sacrum and coccyx is occupied by a soft, cystic swelling—a post-anal dermoid cyst (fig. 550).   These cysts are liable to become infected.   If a sinus is present, or the inflamed cyst bursts or is incised, a troublesome form of blind external fistula-in-ano results. Treatment is complete excision of the cyst and sinus, if present. In large cysts it is necessary to remove the coccyx in order to gain access.

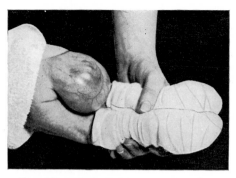

Fig. 549.—Congenital sacro-coccygeal tera-toma in an infant a week old. The tumour was excised successfully.

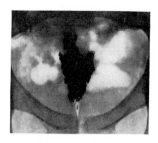

Fig. 550.—Post-anal der-moid cyst with sinus. In-jected with lipiodol. Sinus and cyst excised.

INJURIES

The rectum and anal canal may be injured in a number of ways, all of which are uncommon.

1. By falling in a sitting posture on to a spiked or blunt-pointed object, such as a broken shooting-stick or a broom-handle.

2. By the fœtal head during childbirth.

3. During the faulty administration of an enema by a syringe fitted with a bone, glass, or vulcanite nozzle.

4. During sigmoidoscopy, usually when examining a patient suffering from ulcerative procto-colitis or amœbic dysentery.

5. " Split Perinæum."—A lacerated wound of the perinæum, involving the anal canal, is an occasional pillion-riding accident.

6. Injuries due to warfare.

7. Compressed-air rupture (page 410).

Treatment.—If the rectum has been damaged the patient should be anæsthetised, and the rectum examined carefully with the finger and a speculum, special attention being directed to the anterior wall.

Extensive wounds of the rectum require prolonged rest and certain drainage. The former can be accomplished by performing left inguinal colostomy. The latter is aided by gaining access to the para-rectal tissues by removing the coccyx through a vertical incision and utilising this incision for the accommodation of corrugated rubber drainage.

When the peritoneum has been penetrated, laparotomy, with suture of the perforation and drainage, is called for urgently.

When the bladder has been penetrated, cystostomy and transvesical suture of the perforation is the best treatment.

FOREIGN BODIES IN THE RECTUM

The variety of foreign bodies which have found their way into the rectum is hardly less remarkable than the ingenuity displayed in their removal. A turnip has been delivered per anum by the use of obstetric forceps. A stick firmly impacted has been withdrawn by inserting a gimlet into its lower end. A tumbler, mouth looking downwards, has

several times been extracted by filling the interior with a wet plaster of
Paris bandage, leaving the end of the bandage protruding, and allowing the
plaster to set.

If difficulty is experienced in grasping any foreign body in the rectum,
recourse should be made early to a left lower laparotomy, which allows
that object to be pushed from above into the waiting assistant's fingers in
the rectum.   If there is considerable laceration of the mucosa a temporary
colostomy is advisable.

HÆMORRHOIDS (*Syn.* PILES)

Internal hæmorrhoids, which include intero-external hæmorrhoids, are exceedingly common.   Essentially the condition is
a varicosity of the internal hæmorrhoidal plexus, but because of
the communication of the internal with the external hæmorrhoidal plexus, if the former becomes varicose the latter, to
some degree, is involved also.   Whether seen externally when
prolapsed, or viewed through a proctoscope, hæmorrhoids are
arranged in three masses at 3, 7, and 11 o'clock with the patient
in the lithotomy position.   These are known as the left lateral
hæmorrhoid, the right posterior hæmorrhoid, and the right
anterior hæmorrhoid.   In between these three primary hæmorrhoids there may be secondary smaller hæmorrhoids, most often
in the left posterior quadrant, the next most frequent site being
in the left anterior quadrant.   Each primary hæmorrhoid can
be divided into three parts :

The pedicle lies in the rectum just above the ano-rectal ring.
As seen through a proctoscope, it is covered with pale-pink mucosa
through which large tributaries of the superior hæmorrhoidal
vein can be seen.   Occasionally a pulsating artery can be felt
in this situation.

The internal hæmorrhoid, which commences at the ano-rectal
ring and ends at the pectinate line.   It is bright red or purple,
and covered by mucous membrane.

The external hæmorrhoid lies between the pectinate line and
ends at the anal margin.   It is covered by skin, through which
blue veins can be seen, unless fibrosis has occurred.

Ætiology : *Hereditary.*—The condition is so frequently seen in members
of the same family that there must be a predisposing factor, such as a
congenital weakness of the vein walls or an abnormally large arterial
supply to the hæmorrhoidal plexus.

Anatomical.—(1) The collecting radicles of the superior hæmorrhoidal
vein lie unsupported in the very loose submucous connective tissue of the
rectum, where they are easily compressed by hard fæcal masses.   (2) These
veins pass through muscular tissue and are liable to be constricted by its
contraction during defæcation.   (3) The superior hæmorrhoidal veins and
the portal vein have no valves.

Exciting Causes.—Straining accompanying constipation, or that induced by over-purgation is considered to be a potent cause of hæmorrhoids. Less often the diarrhœa of enteritis, colitis, or the dysenteries aggravates latent hæmorrhoids.

Hæmorrhoids may be a symptom of some other condition or disease. During pregnancy hæmorrhoids commonly appear. " Pregnancy piles " are due to compression of the superior hæmorrhoidal vein by the pregnant uterus. The same effect can be produced by uterine fibroids, especially if the uterus is retroverted, or by a large ovarian cyst. Any form of portal hypertension is liable to be accompanied by hæmorrhoids. Straining on micturition consequent upon an enlarged prostate or a stricture of the urethra causes, or greatly aggravates, hæmorrhoids. Hæmorrhoids may be a symptom of inferior vena caval congestion caused by cardiac or pulmonary disease. Carcinoma of the rectum, by compressing or causing thrombosis of the superior hæmorrhoidal vein, gives rise to hæmorrhoids (fig. 551) sufficiently often to warrant it being a routine procedure to examine the rectum and the rectosigmoid junction for a neoplasm in every case of hæmorrhoids.

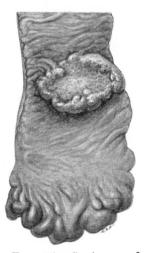

FIG. 551.—Carcinoma of the rectum associated with hæmorrhoids.

Symptoms : *Bleeding,* as the name hæmorrhoids implies, is the principal and earliest symptom. At first the bleeding is slight; it is bright red and occurs during defæcation, and it may continue thus for months or years. Hæmorrhoids that bleed at stool but do not prolapse are called *first-degree hœmorrhoids*.

Prolapse is a much later symptom. In the beginning the protrusion is slight and occurs only at stool, and reduction is spontaneous. As time goes on the hæmorrhoids do not reduce themselves, but have to be replaced digitally by the patient. Hæmorrhoids that prolapse only on defæcation are known as *second-degree hœmorrhoids*. Still later prolapse occurs during the day, apart from defæcation, when the patient is tired or exerts himself. Hæmorrhoids that prolapse apart from defæcation are called *third-degree hœmorrhoids*. By now the hæmorrhoids have become a source of great discomfort and a cause of a feeling of heaviness in the rectum.   Finally, in some cases, the hæmorrhoids become permanently prolapsed.

Discharge.—A mucoid discharge is a frequent accompaniment of prolapsed hæmorrhoids.   For the most part it is composed of mucus from the engorged mucous membrane, but it may be augmented by leakage of excessive ingestion of liquid paraffin.

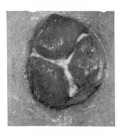

Fig. 552.—Typical third-degree hæmorrhoids.
(*E. T. C. Milligan.*)

Pain is absent unless complications supervene.

On inspection there may be no evidence of internal hæmorrhoids.   In more advanced cases redundant folds of skin or tags of skin can be seen in the position of the three primary hæmorrhoids.   When the patient strains, internal hæmorrhoids may come into view transiently, or if they are of the third degree they prolapse and remain prolapsed (fig. 552).

Palpation.—Internal hæmorrhoids, unless they are thrombosed, cannot be felt.

Proctoscopy.—A proctoscope is passed to its fullest extent and the obturator is removed.   The instrument is then slowly withdrawn.   Just below the ano-rectal ring internal hæmorrhoids, if present, will bulge into the lumen of the proctoscope.

Complications : *Profuse hæmorrhage* is not rare.   Most often it occurs in the early stages of the second degree.   The bleeding occurs mainly externally, but it may continue internally after the bleeding hæmorrhoid has retracted or has been returned.   In these circumstances the rectum is found to be full of blood.

Strangulation.—One or more of the internal hæmorrhoids prolapse and become gripped by the external sphincter.   Further congestion follows because the venous return is impeded.   Second-degree hæmorrhoids are most often complicated in this way.   Strangulation (fig. 553) is accom-

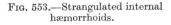

Fig. 553.—Strangulated internal hæmorrhoids.

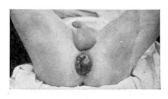

panied by considerable pain, and is often spoken of by the patient as an " acute attack of piles."   Unless the internal hæmorrhoids can be reduced within an hour or two, strangulation is followed by

Thrombosis.—The affected hæmorrhoid or hæmorrhoids become dark purple or black (fig. 554) and feel solid. Considerable œdema of the anal margin accompanies thrombosis. Once thrombosis has occurred the pain of strangulation largely passes off, but tenderness persists.

Ulceration.—Superficial ulceration of the exposed mucous membrane is a usual accompaniment of strangulation with thrombosis.

Gangrene occurs when strangulation is sufficiently tight to constrict the arterial supply of the hæmorrhoid. The resulting sloughing is usually superficial and localised. Occasionally a whole hæmorrhoid sloughs off, leaving an ulcer which heals gradually. Very exceptionally massive gangrene extends to the mucous membrane within the anal canal and rectum.

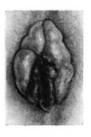

Fig. 554.— Strangulated internal hæmorrhoids with thrombosis.

Fibrosis.—After thrombosis, internal hæmorrhoids sometimes become converted into fibrous tissue. The fibrosed hæmorrhoid is at first sessile, but by repeated traction during prolapse at defæcation, it becomes pedunculated and constitutes a fibrous polyp that is readily distinguished by its white colour from an adenoma, which is bright red. Fibrosis following transient strangulation commonly occurs in the subcutaneous part of a primary hæmorrhoid. Fibrosis in an external hæmorrhoid favours prolapse of the corresponding internal hæmorrhoid.

Suppuration is uncommon. It occurs as a result of deep infection of the thrombosed hæmorrhoid. Throbbing pain is followed by perianal swelling, and a perianal or submucous abscess results.

TREATMENT OF INTERNAL HÆMORRHOIDS

Palliative treatment is recommended when the hæmorrhoids are a symptom of some other condition or disease. The bowels are regulated by liquid paraffin, ½ ounce (15 ml.) twice a day, and if necessary a small dose of cascara evacuant at night. A cream of equal parts zinc oxide and castor oil, inserted into the rectum from a collapsible tube fitted with a nozzle, at night and before defæcation, is of service.

In cases of strangulation, thrombosis, and gangrene, palliative treatment is to be strongly recommended. If the patient is seen soon after strangulation has occurred, treatment can be commenced by reducing the hæmorrhoids under a short pentothal anæsthetic. Once they are thrombosed, if the hæmorrhoids are replaced they prolapse almost immediately, so there is no point in attempting this manœuvre except in very early cases. In these circumstances the following measures will be found to give satisfactory results : the patient is put to bed and the foot of the bed is raised on blocks. One-quarter or ⅓ grain (16 or 20 mgm.) of morphia is administered, after which the anal region is shaved and the prolapsed mass is irrigated with a weak antiseptic solution. A quantity of gauze soaked in normal saline is applied to the anus, covered with jaconet, and kept in position by a four-tailed bandage. The dressing is changed every four hours. Liquid paraffin is given three times a day, and penicillin and sulphonamide are administered and continued for as long as necessary. If the bowels have not acted by the third day, a glycerine enema is given through a catheter. About the third or fourth day the œdema and inflammation will usually have subsided and the patient is permitted to have a daily bath. When the inflammation has abated, lead lotion is substituted for normal saline in the dressings. Under this treatment the mass gradually becomes smaller. By the end of a week or ten days the hæmorrhoids are barely visible. After a fortnight the case must be reviewed and treated on its merits. Most patients who have suffered from prolapsed thrombosed hæmorrhoids will require operation.

In cases where the patient has been admitted because of severe hæmorrhage, gentle irrigation of the rectum with warm saline solution, followed by compresses containing adrenaline solution if the bleeding hæmorrhoid is prolapsed, together with morphia, usually suffices to control the hæmorrhage. If the hæmorrhage continues in spite of these measures, it is controlled as described under Post-operative Hæmorrhage (p. 521). Often these patients are severely anæmic following the recent and more remote smaller hæmorrhages, and blood transfusion is required.

Cases suitable for injection treatment are those belonging to the first degree. Early cases of the second degree are sometimes cured by this method, but a proportion of them relapse.

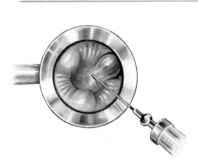

Fig. 555.—Injecting the pedicle above an internal hæmorrhoid.

Technique.—The patient should have an empty rectum, but no special preparation is necessary. A proctoscope is introduced, and the piles are displayed. The injection is made above the main mass of each hæmorrhoid (fig. 555) into the submucosa at or just above the ano-rectal ring. Using Gabriel's

W. B. Gabriel, Contemporary. Surgeon, St. Mark's Hospital, London.
In 1871, Mitchell of Clinton, Illinois, first used carbolic acid for injecting hæmorrhoids. Itinerant irregular practitioners exploited the method.

syringe (fig. 556) with the bevel of the needle directed towards the rectal wall, from 3 to 5 ml. of the following solution is injected :

> ℞   menthol gr. ii. (120 mgm.)
> 5 per cent. phenol in almond oil ad. ℨi. (30 ml.)

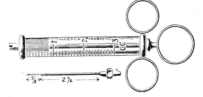

FIG. 556.—Gabriel's syringe for injecting hæmorrhoids.

The injection should produce elevation and pallor of the mucosa. The solution spreads in the submucosa upwards to the pedicle, and downwards to the internal hæmorrhoid and any secondary hæmorrhoids that may be present, but it is prevented by the intermuscular septum from reaching the external hæmorrhoid. There is a little bleeding from the point of puncture, which soon ceases. The injection is painless, and there is no special after-treatment. If there is only one hæmorrhoid present, it may be cured by one injection ; if all three hæmorrhoids are equally enlarged, each is injected at the same session. Often three sessions at fortnightly intervals are required. Care should be taken not to re-inject submucosa already sclerosed, otherwise sloughing may occur.

Cases unsuitable for injection treatment are : (1) third-degree hæmorrhoids ; (2) fibrosed hæmorrhoids ; (3) intero-external hæmorrhoids when the external hæmorrhoid is well defined and the groove between the external and the internal hæmorrhoids (the intermuscular septum) is poorly marked or absent ; (4) when the superior hæmorrhoidal artery can be felt pulsating in the pedicle. In these cases hæmorrhoidectomy should be performed.

HÆMORRHOIDECTOMY

Forty-eight hours' pre-operative treatment is necessary. An aperient, a little more than the patient usually takes, or, if none is habitually taken, ½ drachm (2 ml.) of cascara evacuant, is given on the evening forty-eight hours prior to the operation. On the following morning a small dose of effervescent saline is given before breakfast. On the evening before the operation a soap-and-water enema is administered, and the anal region is shaved. On the morning of the operation the rectum is washed out with water by means of a funnel and tube attached to a catheter.

Ligation and Excision.—With the patient in the lithotomy position the internal hæmorrhoids are prolapsed by traction on the skin tags related to the hæmorrhoids, or on the skin of the anal margin. Each primary internal hæmorrhoid is dealt with in turn, as follows : the internal hæmorrhoid is picked up with dissecting forceps and traction is exerted. This traction causes the pale-pink rectal mucous membrane to become thrown into a longitudinal fold (the pedicle) above the hæmorrhoid. Each pedicle is grasped in a hæmostat, as also is each external hæmorrhoid or skin tag connected with each primary hæmorrhoid. These pairs of hæmostats, when held out by the assistants, form a triangle. The operator takes the left lateral pair of hæmostats in the palm of his hand and places the extended forefinger in the anal canal to support the internal hæmorrhoid. In this way traction is applied to the skin of the anal margin. With scissors, a V-shaped cut is made, each limb of which is placed on either

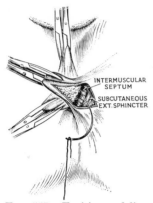

side of the skin-holding hæmostat. This cut traverses the skin and the corrugator cutis ani. Exerting further traction on the pair of hæmostats, the hæmorrhoid is dissected off the subcutaneous external sphincter by blunt dissection, and the fibrous intermuscular septum is seen at the upper edge of the muscle. The pedicle, including a portion of the intermuscular septum, is transfixed with a round-bodied needle (fig. 557) threaded with No. 4 chromic catgut, and the ligature is tied tightly behind and then in front of the tip of the pedicle-holding hæmostat, the double knot being situated beneath the tip of the hæmostat. Alternatively, a strong silk ligature can be used without transfixion, the pedicle-holding hæmostat being removed as the ligature is tied. Each hæmorrhoid having been dealt with in this manner and each pedicle having

Fig. 557.—Excision and ligation. Transfixion of the pedicle.

been firmly secured by one of the methods described, the hæmorrhoids are excised ½ inch (1·25 cm.) distal to the ligature, the ends of which are cut to within about ½ inch of the knot. Large secondary hæmorrhoids which cannot be included with the primary hæmorrhoids are treated by making a shallow cut into their inferior attachment and, after dissecting them up, they are ligated and excised separately. The stumps of the ligated hæmorrhoids are returned to the rectum by tucking a piece of gauze into the anal canal with closed scissors.

In making the V-shaped skin cuts, bridges about ¾ inch (2 cm.) wide were left between each cut. These are now trimmed so as not to leave any redundant overhanging skin edges (fig. 558). Bleeding subcutaneous

Fig. 558.—The black areas represent the trimmed skin cuts after removal of the three primary hæmorrhoids. (*After Milligan.*)

arteries having been secured, a rubber drainage tube with a diameter of ½ inch (1·25 cm.) is inserted into the rectum, and the corners of three pieces of petroleum-jelly gauze are tucked into the anus alongside the tube so as to cover the areas denuded of skin. A pad of gauze and wool, and a firmly applied T-bandage, complete the operation.

Post-operative Treatment.—The tube is removed after twenty-four hours, care being taken not to disturb the three pieces of petroleum-jelly gauze which by now have become adherent to the areas denuded of skin. A mild aperient is given on the evening of the second post-operative day and an olive-oil enema on the following morning, with which the dressings usually come away ; if not, they are removed. Baths and dressings are carried out twice a day after the first bowel movement. The wounds are irrigated with hydrogen-peroxide solution delivered by a tube from a douche can, and moist packing is tucked into the anal canal for ½ inch the aim being to lightly fill each of the skin wounds. On the seventh day a finger is passed into the rectum. On the eighth day, and until the wounds have healed, a St. Mark's dilator is passed daily. The patient can leave hospital on the fourteenth day. Dressing of the wound must continue. In the later stages a dry dressing is employed during the day and a zinc and castor-oil dressing at night. The wounds heal in three to six weeks.

Post-operative Complications :

Secondary hæmorrhage is rare, and when it occurs it does so about the seventh or eighth day after the operation. The hæmorrhage may be mainly or entirely concealed, but will become evident on examining the rectum.

Treatment.—The rectum should be washed out with saline solution after $\frac{1}{3}$ or $\frac{1}{2}$ grain (20 or 30 mgm.) of morphia has been given. Gauze is wound around one end of a rubber tube, $\frac{1}{2}$ inch (1·25 cm.) in diameter and 4 inches (10 cm.) long, to a thickness that it will just pass through a proctoscope. The proctoscope is passed and the tube with the dry gauze tampon is inserted into the rectum, and the proctoscope is removed. Some traction is applied to the tube and the gauze comes to lie against the ano-rectal ring. A large safety-pin is placed through the tube, and gauze is wound around the tube between the anal margin and the safety-pin. This maintains pressure on the bleeding area. The foot of the bed is raised on blocks and a blood transfusion is given, if necessary. Forty-eight hours later, after an injection of 5 ounces (150 ml.) of olive-oil into the rectum, the tube with the gauze is removed and a plain rubber tube is inserted for another twenty-four hours, in order to be sure that there is no further bleeding.

Retention of urine is not unusual after hæmorrhoidectomy in male patients. An injection of carbachol should be tried before resorting to catheterisation. Should the cause of the retention of urine be an enlarged prostate, treatment for this condition may be required.

ANAL PAPILLÆ

occur at the pectinate line, and are remnants of the ectodermal membrane which separated the proctodæum from the primitive rectum early in embryonic life. As these papillæ are present in fully 60 per cent. of patients examined proctologically, they should be regarded as normal structures. Anal papillæ can become elongated, as they frequently do in the presence of internal hæmorrhoids. Occasionally an elongated anal papilla or papillæ is found without hæmorrhoids, and is sometimes the cause of pruritus. An elongated papilla may become nipped in the external sphincter after defæcation, and by repeated traction on its pedicle may result in a fissure.

Treatment.—Using a slotted proctoscope, elongated papillæ without hæmorrhoids should be crushed and excised after injecting the base with local anæsthetic. When elongated papillæ complicate internal hæmorrhoids this is an indication for operative treatment of the hæmorrhoids.

EXTERNAL HÆMORRHOIDS

Acute perianal hæmatoma is loosely termed a " thrombotic pile." It is a small hæmatoma occurring in the perianal sub-cutaneous connective tissue, usually superficial to the corrugator

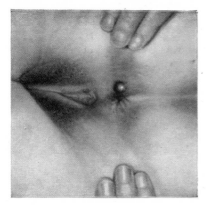

FIG. 559.—" Thrombotic " pile.

cutis ani muscle. The condition is due to the bursting of an anal venule consequent upon straining at stool, coughing, or lifting a heavy weight. The condition appears suddenly and is very painful, and on examination a tense, tender swelling which looks like an overripe cherry is seen (fig. 559). The hæmatoma is much more commonly situated in a lateral region of the anal margin than anteriorly or posteriorly. Untreated this hæmatoma may :

Resolve.
Suppurate.
Fibrose, and give rise to a cutaneous tag.
Burst and extrude the clot.

In the majority of cases resolution or fibrosis occurs. Indeed, this condition has been called " a five-day, painful, self-curing lesion " (Milligan).

Provided it is seen within thirty-six hours of the onset, a perianal hæmatoma is best treated as an emergency. Under local anæsthesia the hæmorrhoid is bisected and the two halves are excised together with ½ inch (1·25 cm.) of adjacent skin. This leaves a pear-shaped wound which is allowed to granulate. The relief of pain is immediate and a permanent cure is certain. On rare occasions in which a perianal hæmatoma is situated anteriorly or posteriorly it should be treated conservatively because of the liability of a skin wound in these regions to become an anal fissure.

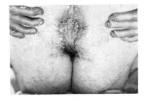

FIG. 560. — Condylomata ani.

Chronic external hæmorrhoids are often the external portions of intero-external hæmorrhoids. In the early stages they are varicosities of the external hæmorrhoidal plexus in positions corresponding to the three primary internal hæmorrhoids. Later, as a result of thrombosis, they are converted into skin

E. T. C. Milligan, Contemporary. Surgeon, St. Mark's Hospital, London.

tags. Skin tags without internal hæmorrhoids are often the result of one or more perianal hæmatomata. The sentinel skin tag associated with an anal fissure will be described presently.

Differential Diagnosis:

Anal warts are usually multiple and present the same characteristics as warts elsewhere. Occasionally they accompany gonococcal proctitis. Simple warts respond well to treatment by applications at weekly intervals of 25 per cent. podophyllin in liquid paraffin. After three or four applications, if there are any residual warts they should be excised.

Condylomata (fig. 560) have a smoother surface and are more pedunculated than the foregoing. Also they are usually moist, with a glairy discharge. There are likely to be other signs of secondary syphilis present, and the Wassermann reaction is positive.

Hypertrophic tuberculide of the anus is rare. These are multiple yellowish-brown papillomatous excrescences, and in some respects resemble a squamous-celled carcinoma. This is usually a primary form of tuberculosis, and the diagnosis is seldom established until microscopic examination of the excised specimen has been undertaken.

Treatment of Uncomplicated Skin Tags.—As they often result in pruritus, uncomplicated skin tags should be excised, after injecting local anæsthetic into the base of each tag.

ANAL FISSURE

Definition.—An elongated ulcer in the long axis of the anal canal.

Ætiology and Pathology.—A fissure is an aftermath of constipation, the mucosa being torn by a scybalous mass. At first there is an impalpable longitudinal abrasion of the mucous membrane. Later this becomes a small triangular ulcer, base downwards, and it is nearly always solitary.

ANTERIOR 11%

LATERAL 1%

POSTERIOR 88%

The fissure usually occupies the middle line posteriorly (fig. 561), and it rarely extends beyond the pectinate line. The floor of the

FISSURE

SENTINEL PILE

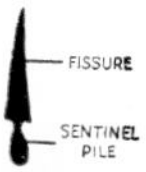

FIG. 561. — The usual locations of fissures.

ulcer is lined by granulation tissue and its base overlies the subcutaneous external sphincter. As chronicity is reached, the edges become indurated, the floor involves the subcutaneous external sphincter, and its base is the seat of a sentinel skin tag, due to œdema consequent upon inflammation and puckering of the skin by the contracted subcutaneous external sphincter. This tag is liable to become undermined and often gives rise to a subcutaneous abscess, the bursting or incision of which results in a dorsal fistula. Some cases of anal fissure are due to tearing down of a valve of Ball (fig. 562), but this fails to explain why the fissure is so frequently situated in the middle, or near the middle line posteriorly.

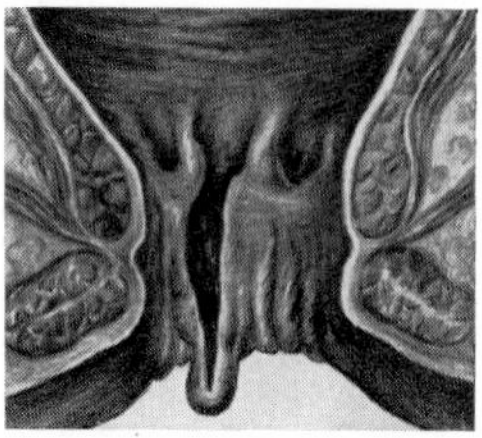

Blaisdell points out that a posterior anal fissure occurs over the unattached

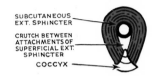

FIG. 562.—Anal fissure resulting from tearing of a valve of Ball.

FIG. 563.—"Blaisdell's Bar" theory.

subcutaneous external sphincter. When this muscle is stretched, it stands out like a bar (Blaisdell's bar) across the unsupported crutch between the coccygeal attachments of the superficial external sphincter (fig. 563). The overlying epithelium at this point is therefore not only greatly stretched, but placed in a most vulnerable position when a scybalous mass is being expelled.

Fibrosis of the submucosa due to chronic infection originating in an anal crypt or an anal gland, and fibrosis of the subcutaneous external sphincter muscle itself, and the narrowing of the anus that results from these causes, have each been held responsible for the liability of the mucosa to tear. An anterior fissure occurs almost exclusively in women, and may be explained by lack of support of the anal mucous membrane by a damaged pelvic floor.

Once an anal fissure is present, it seldom heals without surgical aid because :

1. The sphincter is always in action, and consequently the ulcer is never accorded that essential factor for spontaneous healing—rest.

2. It is constantly further aggravated by the patient postponing defæcation because of pain ; a vicious circle has set in.

Clinical Features.—The condition is more common in women, and generally occurs during the meridian of life. It is uncommon in the aged, because of muscular atony.

Pain is *the* symptom—sharp agonising pain during defæcation, and lasting an hour or more. The deeper the fissure the longer does the excruciating pain continue. As a rule it ceases suddenly, and the sufferer is comfortable until the next action of the bowel. Periods of remission for days or weeks occur. Exacerbations are due to renewed suppuration in the fissure. Reflex pain down the thighs simulating sciatica sometimes

Paul Carrier Blaisdell, Contemporary. Assistant Professor of Proctology, College of Medical Evangelists, Loma Linda, Los Angeles, California.

occurs. In extreme cases reflex frequency of micturition is not unusual.

Stools are frequently streaked with blood. In well-established cases of fissure they are narrow because the anus is narrowed, and are short, with a " nipped-off " appearance, caused by sudden muscular spasms.

Discharge.—A slight discharge of serum accompanies fully established cases. A purulent discharge follows if a subcutaneous abscess bursts into the anal canal or externally.

On Examination.—Frequently, in cases of some standing, a sentinel skin tag can be seen. This, together with a typical history and a tightly closed, puckered anus (fig. 564), is almost

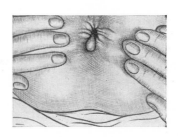

FIG. 564.—Sentinel " pile " associated with fissure. Puckering of the anus characteristic of fissure is also shown.

pathognomonic of the condition. By gently parting the margins of the anus, the lower end of the fissure can sometimes be displayed. Rectal examination causes great pain, but this can, to a large extent, be circumvented by inserting into the anal canal a pledget of cotton-wool previously moistened with water and then dipped into a bottle containing percaine crystals. The pledget should be left in place for about five minutes. In early cases the edges of the fissure are impalpable. In fully established cases a characteristic crater, which feels like a " button-hole," can be palpated. Multiple fissures raise a suspicion of syphilis, but they are also a complication of congenital stricture of the rectum. A fibrosed internal hæmorrhoid (fibrous polyp) is sometimes associated with a fissure below it. Palpation of the inner surface of the skin tag with a probe will reveal if it is undermined. Proctoscopy, on account of the great pain it produces, should not be attempted.

Treatment.—The pain of anal fissure is so great that usually the patient demands early relief.

Palliative Treatment.—Recent cases may respond to the

administration of liquid paraffin and lubrication of the anal
canal with an anæsthetic ointment before defæcation.

Injection Treatment is indicated in more advanced cases
without induration or a sentinel skin tag.

Five to 10 ml. of Proctocaine, Nupercaine-in-oil, or other oil-soluble
local anæsthetic is used, the dose varying according to the robustness or
otherwise of the patient. After shaving and sterilising the posterior
part of the skin of the anus, with the left forefinger in the rectum as a guide,
a hollow needle 2 inches (5 cm.) long and 20 standard wire gauge is inserted
into the subcutaneous tissues 1 inch (2·5 cm.) posterior to the anus. It is
then passed deeply into the external sphincter muscle to one side and a
little less than half the total dose of the previously warmed oil-soluble local
anæsthetic is injected into the muscle. The same procedure is adopted on
the contralateral side, leaving about ½ ml. to inject immediately beneath
the base of the fissure. The procedure often so relieves the pain and
muscular spasm that local treatment of the fissure can be undertaken. On

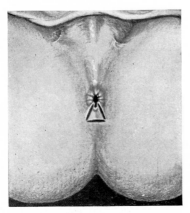

alternate days the fissure is cleansed
with pure Dettol on a pledget of cottonwool, after which Collosal ichthyol is
applied with a dressing of dry cottonwool over it (Gabriel). The anal canal
should be dilated at weekly intervals
with a St. Mark's dilator.

Fɪssuʀᴇᴄᴛᴏᴍʏ is the only permanently satisfactory treatment
for chronic cases. The fissure,
including a large triangular piece
of skin (fig. 565), and about ½
inch (1·25 cm.) of the subcutaneous external sphincter muscle in
the immediate vicinity of the fis-

Fɪɢ. 565.—Showing area of skin
excised in radical operation for
fissure-in-ano. *(After Gabriel.)*

sure, is excised. The object of
removing a large amount of skin
is to maintain drainage and to ensure that the anal part of the
wound is the last to heal.

Differential Diagnosis:

An anal chancre, which occurs in about 1 : 500 cases of primary chancre,
may simulate an anal fissure, especially when
the lesion is situated at the posterior margin of
the anus (fig. 566). Sometimes the lesion is dual
and symmetrical. Pain is not so much in evidence,
and there is more discharge and more induration
than in a case of recent anal fissure. As a history
of infection is usually lacking, it is advisable to
take a scraping from the base of any indurated
anal fissure of recent origin and examine the
exudate by dark-ground illumination for spirochætes.

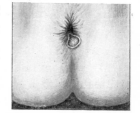

Fɪɢ. 566.—Anal chancre.

Tuberculous ulceration of the anus in its early stages is difficult to distinguish from an anal fissure. Undermining of the edges of the ulcer and the presence of active pulmonary tuberculosis usually determine the diagnosis.

Proctalgia fugax gives rise to attacks of severe ano-rectal pain at irregular intervals and not necessarily commencing during defæcation. The pain is due to spasm of the levator ani and sphincter muscles, and its cause is obscure. The administration of sedatives to relieve the pain is all that can be done.

Rectal crises of tabes are extremely uncommon. They are usually accompanied by diarrhœa and sometimes by rectal hæmorrhage. In every case of unexplained pain in the anal region the nervous system should be examined.

PRURITUS ANI

There is an intractable itching around the anus. The causes are very numerous and varied :

1. Lack of cleanliness, excessive sweating, and wearing woollen underclothing are common causes.

2. An anal or perianal discharge which renders the anus moist. The causative lesions include an anal fissure, fistula-in-ano, prolapsed hæmorrhoids, and an excessive ingestion of liquid paraffin.

3. A vaginal discharge, especially due to the trichomonas vaginalis, can cause irritation of the anus.

4. Parasitic causes. Threadworms should be excluded, especially in young subjects. Scabies and pediculosis pubis may infect the anal region. Mycotic diseases of the skin due to yeasts and fungi should be suspected when the anal skin shows some form of dermatitis which has a well-defined border. Microscopic and cultural examinations of muco-pus taken from the region is necessary to establish the diagnosis in this instance.

5. Allergy is sometimes the cause, in which case there is likely to be a history of other allergic manifestations, such as urticaria asthma, or hay-fever.

Treatment:

Hygienic Measures.—Washing the anus after defæcation, wearing cotton cellular underwear, and applications of calamine lotion are all that is necessary to cure some cases.

Removal of the Cause.—When a remediable cause is found, the appropriate medical or surgical treatment will frequently stop the itching.

Injection of Oil-soluble Anæsthetic.—Resistant cases from any cause are often greatly benefited by injections of an oil-soluble

anæsthetic. The preliminary injections are made posterolaterally, and between 15 to 20 ml. are injected into the deep
perianal tissues with a view to anæsthetising the inferior
hæmorrhoidal nerves. A week later a further injection of
5 ml. on each side antero-laterally is given. The injection of
oil-soluble local anæsthetic frequently renders the skin of the
anus partly anæsthetic, and results in cessation of scratching,
thus giving an opportunity for the dermatitis to be controlled or
cured by local measures. After a few weeks the injection may
be repeated, if necessary.

Tattooing.—Cantor tattoos the anus with cinnabar (mercuric
sulphide), using a tattooing machine with ten needles set to
penetrate to a depth of 2 mm.

Division of the Sensory Branches of the Internal Pudendal Nerve (Gabriel).
—In a small number of cases none of the measures described affords relief
for more than a week or two. For these the following operation is likely
to be curative. An incision about 3 inches (7·5 cm.) long is made in the
outer part of the ischio-rectal fossa parallel to the ischio-pubic ramus.
The incision is deepened until the ischial tuberosity and the outer edge of
the gluteus maximus are displayed. The anus is retracted to the opposite
side ; the inferior hæmorrhoidal nerves are found and traced to Alcock's
canal. The canal is opened and the internal pudendal nerve is identified,
and its fibres teased apart. Those fibres that do not respond to a mild
faradic current are divided. The operation is carried out on each side.

ANO-RECTAL ABSCESSES

The great majority of these abscesses arise from a focus within
the anal canal, and the infecting organisms are streptococci and
B. coli ; sometimes Cl. welchii is the predominating organism of
an ischio-rectal abscess. An indolent abscess, particularly an
ischio-rectal abscess without constitutional symptoms, may be
tuberculous in origin.

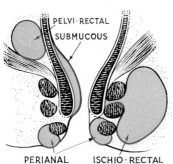

A **perianal abscess** is due to
infection of the perianal space,
and is the commonest variety of
ano-rectal abscess (50 per cent.
of cases). It can arise from an
anal fissure, as an infection of
a perianal hæmatoma, from infected prolapsed internal hæmorrhoids, or from extension of a
cutaneous boil. The abscess
may be entirely superficial to

Fig. 567.—Abscesses about the
rectum and anal canal.

Alfred Joseph Cantor, Contemporary. Proctologist, Flushing, New York.

the subcutaneous external sphincter (fig. 567) or arise deep to that muscle.

An ischio-rectal abscess occurs in 30 per cent. of cases of ano-rectal abscesses. The cause is often from infection of a torn valve of Ball, extension from an anal crypt, or from bursting of an infected intramuscular rectal gland. Perforation of the rectal wall by a sharp-pointed swallowed foreign body such as a fish-bone is sometimes found to be the cause. An ischio-rectal abscess is a rather frequent accompaniment of ulcerative procto-colitis. On rare occasions an ischio-rectal abscess complicates a carcinoma of the rectum. Occasionally an ischio-rectal abscess is bilateral, when the communicating canal is nearly always posterior.

A submucous abscess is comparatively rare, and occurs as a result of an abrasion of the mucous membrane above the pectin-ate line, from infected thrombosed internal hæmorrhoids or upward extension of infection from an anal crypt. The abscess lies between the mucosa and the internal sphincter. This type of abscess may be present concomitantly with an ischio-rectal abscess. The uncomplicated variety usually bursts spontane-ously into the rectum and gives rise to a submucous fistula.

A pelvi-rectal abscess is the rarest variety, and is situated above the levator ani and beneath the pelvic peritoneum. It arises as an extension of suppuration in the broad ligament in the female, or in the male from prostatitis, seminal vesiculitis, or a periurethral abscess. A pelvic appendix abscess or a pelvic abscess arising from colonic diverticulitis not infrequently results in a pelvi-rectal abscess. An abscess from any of these causes usually points in the rectum, and either bursts into the lumen or is opened into the rectum, but occasionally it bursts through the levator ani to infect the ischio-rectal fossa, as also may a psoas abscess.

Clinical Features.—There is throbbing pain, increased on defæcation.

A perianal abscess is readily recognised, and with a finger in the rectum and the thumb externally, usually it is possible to distinguish between the superficial and the deep variety of the abscess. The constitutional symptoms are slight.

An ischio-rectal abscess gives rise to a tender, brawny indura-tion in the corresponding side of the anal canal. Constitutional symptoms are more severe than those of perianal abscess, the temperature being 102° to 103° F. (38·9° to 39·4° C.). Men are more often affected than women. In the case of a *submucous abscess* the symptoms are more subacute than the foregoing. Rectal examination will reveal a tender oval swelling, usually on one lateral wall of the upper part of the anal canal and the lower part of the rectum. Sometimes this variety of abscess spreads downwards to invade the perianal space.

A pelvi-rectal abscess gives rise to considerable constitutional disturbance, and the symptoms and signs are obscure in the early stages. Rectal and (in the female) vaginal examination will reveal an indurated tender swelling in the recto-vesical pouch or the pouch of Douglas. If a pelvi-rectal abscess has invaded the ischio-rectal fossa, the signs of the ischio-rectal abscess may overshadow the deeper suppuration, which becomes apparent only when a greater amount of pus is evacuated than could be contained in the ischio-rectal fossa.

Treatment.—Only when the infection is clearly cutaneous (a boil) should penicillin be given and operation postponed unless pointing occurs. In all other cases early operation is imperative, and adequate drainage must be provided if a fistula is to be prevented. *A perianal abscess* should be incised in a cruciform manner and the four resulting triangular flaps cut away with scissors. If the subcutaneous external sphincter prevents free drainage, the muscle should be divided. *An ischio-rectal abscess* should be opened as soon as possible in the same manner, the floor of the ischio-rectal fossa being excised (fig. 568). If an opening into the anal canal above the subcutaneous external sphincter is found, this muscle is divided. When both ischio-rectal fossæ are involved, they are both treated in the manner described ; the connecting canal between the fossæ is laid open and over-hanging skin edges are cut away. If an extension is

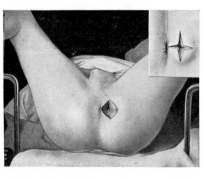

Fig. 568.—Excision of the skin forming the floor of the ischio-rectal fossa is an essential step in the efficient treatment of an ischio-rectal abscess.

present beneath the subcutaneous external sphincter, whether or not the extension opens into the anal canal, the subcutaneous external sphincter should be divided. If there is an opening into the anal canal between the superficial and deep external sphincter muscles, or between the deep external sphincter and the levator ani, a thick silk ligature is passed through the opening and knotted loosely below the muscle, and the ends of the ligature are left long. When the wound has filled in with granulation tissue the sphincter muscle will have had time to become fixed by fibrous tissue, and severing it will not endanger continence. *A submucous abscess* should be incised throughout its length through a proctoscope. *A pelvi-rectal abscess* involving the ischio-rectal fossa should be treated in the same way as an ischio-rectal abscess, except that the opening in the levator ani should be enlarged and a tube inserted into the abscess cavity above that muscle.

Both in the case of a perianal abscess and an ischio-rectal abscess, the wound is packed lightly, and subsequent treatment is similar to that detailed for internal hæmorrhoids. Penicillin and sulphonamide therapy are given in necessary cases.

FISTULA-IN-ANO

A fistula-in-ano is a track, lined by granulation tissue, resulting from a perianal abscess which has burst spontaneously or has been opened by a simple incision. The fistula continues to discharge, seldom if ever permanently healing without surgical aid, because of constant reinfection from the anal canal or the rectum, inadequate drainage, and repeated movement of the related musculature.

Classification.—The majority of fistulæ-in-ano are complete, i.e. they have an opening or openings on the skin around the anus and an internal opening in the anal canal or, rarely, the rectum. A few have no internal opening ; others have no external opening, and according to the old nomenclature incomplete fistulæ were designated as sinuses. A fistula which has no internal opening is now commonly called a blind external fistula, and a fistula with no external opening a blind internal fistula. Blind internal fistulæ are, as a rule, connected with undermining of the skin and subcutaneous tissues at the base of a fissure-in-ano, or as a sub-mucous extension of some other complete fistula. Blind external fistulæ include those originating in pelvi-rectal suppuration and from a chronic osteomyelitis of some part of the bony pelvis, or even a more remote origin in bone. For purposes of treatment fistulæ-in-ano are conveniently classified by Milligan and Morgan according to their relation to the ano-rectal musculature (fig. 569), with particular reference to the ano-rectal

Clifford Naunton Morgan, Contemporary.   Surgeon, St. Mark's Hospital, London.

ring, which must never be divided ; continence is dependent on the
integrity of the ano-rectal ring.

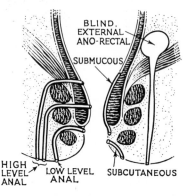

BLIND,
EXTERNAL
ANO-RECTAL
SUBMUCOUS

HIGH
LEVEL   LOW LEVEL   SUBCUTANEOUS
ANAL   ANAL

Fig. 569.—Varieties of fistulæ-
in-ano.

1. Subcutaneous and submucous fistulæ-in-ano   3·7 per cent.
2. Low-level fistulæ-in-ano .   .   .   .   76·2 per cent.
   (When complete, the internal opening lies in
   the anal canal between the subcutaneous
   external sphincter and the superficial external
   sphincter.)
3. High-level fistulæ-in-ano .   .   .   .   15 per cent.
   (When complete, the internal opening lies
   either between the superficial external and
   the deep external sphincters, or between the
   deep external sphincter and the levator ani.)
4. Ano-rectal fistulæ .   .   .   .   .   5·1 per cent.
   (Fortunately many of these fistulæ are blind
   internally.)

Clinical Features.—Commonly the principal symptom is a
persistent purulent discharge which irritates the skin in the
neighbourhood and causes discomfort.   Often the history dates
back for years.   Pain is not a usual symptom as long as the
opening is large enough for the pus to escape.   Frequently there
is a solitary external opening, usually situated within 1½ inches
(3·75 cm.) of the anus, presenting as a small elevation with
granulation tissue pouting from the mouth of the opening.
Sometimes superficial healing occurs ; pus accumulates and an
abscess again forms and discharges through the same opening,
or a new opening.   So there may be present two or more
external openings, usually grouped together on the right or left
of the middle line, but occasionally, when both ischio-rectal
fossæ are involved, a horse-shoe fistula (fig. 570) results.   As a
rule there is much induration of the skin and subcutaneous
tissues around the fistula.   On rectal examination occasionally

an internal opening can be felt as a nodule on the anterior or posterior wall of the anal canal at the level of the intermuscular septum. Irrespective of the number of external openings, there is almost invariably but one internal opening.

Probing.—The insertion of a probe affords valuable information as to the direction of the main channel, and with a finger in the anal canal it may be possible to feel the naked end of the probe protruding through the internal opening of the fistula (fig. 571). When an external opening is situated at a greater distance than 1½ inches (3·75 cm.) from the anus, a high internal connection can usually be anticipated.

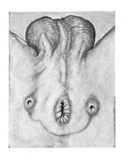

Fig. 570.—Horseshoe fistula - in - ano (tuberculous). Both ischio-rectal fossæ involved. There is often only one internal orifice.

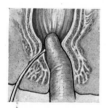

Fig. 571.—Method of demonstrating the internal opening of a fistula with a malleable probe.
(*After Bacon.*)

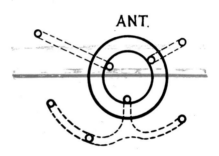

Fig. 572.—Illustrating Goodsall's rule.

Goodsall's Rule.—Fistulæ with an external opening in relation to the anterior half of the anus tend to be of the direct type (fig. 572). Those with an external opening or openings in relation to the posterior half of the anus usually have curving tracks, and may be of the horse-shoe variety.

Radiography.—Unless the course of the fistula can be clearly defined by probing, radiography after an injection into the external opening of a radio-opaque substance, such as lipiodol or bismuth paste, will give information concerning the extent and tortuosity of the main channel (fig. 573) and will often reveal side branches, if such be present.

David Henry Goodsall, 1843–1906. Surgeon, Metropolitan Hospital, London.

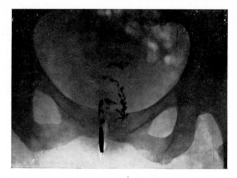

Fig. 573.—Fistula-in-ano visualised by an injection of lipiodol. (*W. B. Gabriel.*)

Special Clinical Types of Fistulæ-in-Ano :

1. **That Connected with an Anal Fissure.**—Unlike the usual fistula-in-ano, pain is a leading symptom. The fistula is very near the anal orifice, usually posterior, and the opening may be hidden by a skin tag.

2. **Tuberculous.**—If induration around a fistula is lacking, if the opening is ragged and flush with the surface, if the surrounding skin is discoloured and the discharge is watery, it strongly suggests that the fistula is due to a tuberculous infection. About 10 per cent. of fistulæ-in-ano are tuberculous.

3. **Fistulæ with many external openings** may arise from tuberculous proctitis, ulcerative procto-colitis, bilharziasis, and lympho-granuloma venereum with a fibrous rectal stricture. Mucoid carcinoma sometimes complicates long-standing fistulæ-in-ano.

Treatment.—The pre-operative preparation is similar to that described for hæmorrhoidectomy. *Subcutaneous and low-level anal fistulæ* are treated as follows : Using a probe director (fig. 574) the fistula is slit up from the external orifice A to the

Fig. 574.—A director with a probe-pointed malleable extremity is a useful instrument.

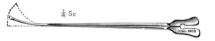

internal orifice B (fig. 575). A back cut is then made in the healthy tissue A–C. At this point an incision D–E is made at right angles to the main track. If multiple external openings are present, or if there are pockets from the main channel, they are all laid open. Overhanging skin and subcutaneous tissue between the lines B–D and B–E are cut away, leaving a triangular wound with shelving edges. In low anal fistulæ the subcutaneous external sphincter is divided. The objective is to leave a widely open triangular wound which is packed lightly and thereafter treated by

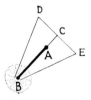

Fig. 575.—Diagram of the steps in laying open a fistula-in-ano.

For treating successfully Louis XIV's fistula-in-ano, Charles Félix, barber-surgeon to the Court, received a fee of a farm, 300,000 livres, and a title.

baths, syringing and moist flat packs, until the wound has healed
from the bottom.   *A submucous fistula* is laid open on a
director with a diathermy knife, to minimise hæmorrhage.
High anal fistulæ are dealt with by a two-stage operation
similar to that described for an ano-rectal abscess.

Tuberculous fistulæ-in-ano below the level of the deep external sphincter
respond to the surgical measures described for the corresponding non-
tuberculous fistulæ.   The operation should be performed under a low spinal
anæsthetic, and the excision, in this instance, is best carried out with a
diathermy knife.   Because of extensive ramifications and poor healing of
the tissues, tuberculous fistulæ-in-ano above the level of the superficial
external sphincter are usually inoperable.   In all cases of tuberculous
fistulæ-in-ano, whether or not surgical treatment is undertaken, sanatorium
treatment is advisable.

Fistulæ connecting the rectum with other organs are as
follows :

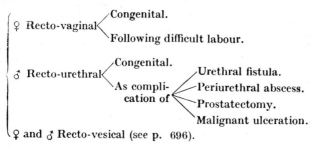

```
                    Congenital.
  ♀ Recto-vaginal
                    Following difficult labour.

                    Congenital.
  ♂ Recto-urethral                    Urethral fistula.
                    As compli-        Periurethral abscess.
                    cation of         Prostatectomy.
                                      Malignant ulceration.

  ♀ and ♂ Recto-vesical (see p. 696).
```

PROCTITIS

Inflammation of the rectal mucosa is sometimes limited to the
rectum ; at others it is associated with a similar condition in
the colon (procto-colitis).   The inflammation can be acute or
chronic.   The symptoms are tenesmus, the passage of blood
and mucus and, in severe cases, pus also.   In early cases of the
dysenteric group of procto-colitis diarrhœa is much in evidence,
but in other forms of proctitis the patient has an intense desire
to defæcate but the amount of fæces passed is small.   In acute
cases there are usually general symptoms of malaise and pyrexia
which are variable, and sometimes absent.   On rectal examination the mucosa feels swollen and is often exceedingly tender.
Proctoscopy is seldom sufficient and sigmoidoscopy is the more
valuable method of examination.   Skilled pathological assistance is required to establish or exclude the diagnosis of specific
infection by bacteriological examination and culture of the
stools, examination of scrapings or swabs from ulcers, and

serological tests. In chronic proctitis biopsy of a portion of the mucous membrane is occasionally necessary, especially when early carcinoma cannot be excluded.

Catarrhal proctitis can occur from very many causes, among which are irritation by scyballa, foreign bodies and intestinal parasites, repeated enemata, and over-purgation. The cause may be immediately apparent, or require much painstaking pathological investigation.

Acute granular proctitis is often an early manifestation of concomitant ulcerative colitis, although it occurs independently, when it may clear up completely after a few weeks of treatment. On proctoscopy and sigmoidoscopy the inflamed rectal mucosa is seen to have lost its shiny appearance. Usually small superficial ulcers are present.

Irradiation proctitis sometimes complicates deep X-ray and radium treatment of the pelvic organs, particularly for carcinoma of the cervix uteri. Usually the proctitis commences several months after the irradiation. Deep ulceration of the anterior wall of the rectum is a common finding and a recto-vaginal fistula may ensue. After prolonged local treatment and, if necessary, blood transfusion, the inflammation subsides with moderate stricture formation.

Proctitis Due to Specific Infections:

Bacillary Dysentery.—The proctological appearance is that of an acute purulent proctitis with multiple small shallow ulcers. Proctological examination is painful. The examination of a swab taken from the ulcerated mucous membrane is more certainly diagnostic than is a microscopical examination of the stools. Agglutination tests may render proctological examination unnecessary.

Amœbic Dysentery.—The infection is more liable to be chronic, and exacerbations after a long period of freedom from symptoms often occur. Proctoscopy and sigmoidoscopy are not painful. The appearance of an amœbic ulcer is described on p. 429. Scrapings from the ulcer should be transferred to a test-tube containing warm normal saline and sent to the laboratory for immediate microscopical examination.

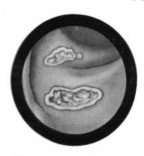

Fig. 576. — Tuberculous ulceration of the rectum. Sigmoidoscopic appearance.

Tuberculous proctitis is nearly always associated with active pulmonary tuberculosis, and is often complicated by a tuberculous fistula-in-ano or tuberculous ulceration of the anus. Submucous rectal abscesses burst and leave ulcers with an undermined edge (fig. 576). A hypertrophic type of tuberculous proctitis occurs in association with tuberculous peritonitis or tuberculous salpingitis. This type of tuberculous proctitis requires biopsy for confirmation of the diagnosis.

Gonococcal proctitis occurs in both sexes as the result of rectal coitus, and in the female from direct spread from the vulva. In the acute stage the mucous membrane is hyperæmic and thick pus can be expressed as the proctoscope is withdrawn. In the early stages the diagnosis can be readily established by bacteriological examination, but later, when the infection is mixed, it is more difficult to recognise. Specific treatment is so effective that local treatment is unnecessary.

Lympho-granuloma Venereum.—The modes of infection are similar to those of gonococcal proctitis, but in the female infection spreading from the cervix uteri via lymphatics to the pararectal lymph nodes is common. The proctological findings are similar to those of gonococcal proctitis. The diagnosis of lympho-granuloma venereum should be strongly suspected when the inguinal lymph nodes are greatly enlarged, although the enlargement may be subsiding by the time proctitis commences. Frei's intradermal test is positive in 95 per cent. of cases and the complement fixation test is even more accurate (see also p. 32).

Primary syphilis is very rare. A primary chancre situated on the anal or rectal mucosa is easily overlooked. The inguinal and iliac lymph nodes are greatly enlarged. By the time the symptoms of proctitis are manifest, the Wassermann reaction will be strongly positive. In venereal infections more than one infection may be present at the same time.

Bilharziasis is caused by the schistosoma mansoni, and gives rise to symptoms similar to those of dysentery. On examination in the later stages papillomata are frequently present. The

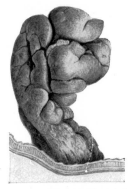

Fig. 577. — Bilharzial papilloma.

(*H. P. Keatinge, Cairo.*)

papillomata, which are sessile or pedunculated (fig. 577), contain the ova of the trematode, the mode of infection and life-cycle of which resembles that of schistosoma hæmatobium (see p. 710).

Untreated, the rectum becomes festooned, and prolapse of the diseased mucous membrane is usual. Multiple fistulæ-in-ano are prone to develop.

NON-MALIGNANT STRICTURE OF THE RECTUM AND ANAL CANAL

Congenital Stricture:

1. A stricture at the level of the pectinate line due to incomplete obliteration of the proctodeal membrane sometimes gives rise to symptoms during early childhood.

2. Patients who have had an operation for imperforate anus in infancy are often left with a stricture that requires periodic dilatation.

Spasmodic Stricture :

1. Chronic fissure results in spasm of the subcutaneous external sphincter, which may become fibrotic.

2. Rarely, a stricture of this variety is associated with some degree of megacolon, when it is due to over-activity of the sympathetic nerves and hypertrophy of the internal sphincter muscle.

Post-operative stricture, owing to the better operative treatment of hæmorrhoids, is now comparatively rare. It may

William Frei, Contemporary. Formerly Professor of Dermatology, Berlin.
August von Wassermann, 1866–1925. Director Institute for Experimental Therapy, Berlin.
Theodor Maximilian Bilharz, 1825–1862. German Physician.
Sir Patrick Manson, 1844–1922. Practised in Hong Kong. Later Physician to the Dreadnought Hospital, Greenwich.

follow removal of a large innocent growth or a conservative operation for carcinoma of the rectum.

Irradiation stricture can follow irradiation proctitis or the radium treatment of a squamous-celled carcinoma of the anal canal.

Inflammatory Stricture.—By far the most frequent, and possibly the only, cause of a tubular inflammatory stricture of the rectum is lympho-granuloma venereum. Stricture of the rectum also complicates ulcerative procto-colitis ; in this instance the stricture is annular, but often more than one is present.

Clinical Features.—Increasing difficulty in defæcation is the leading symptom. The patient finds that increasingly large doses of aperients are required, and if the stools are formed, they are " pipe-stem " in shape. In cases of inflammatory stricture, tenesmus, bleeding, and the passage of muco-pus are superadded. Sometimes the patient comes under observation only when subacute or acute intestinal obstruction has supervened.

Rectal Examination. — The finger encounters a sharply defined shelf-like interruption of the lumen at a varying distance

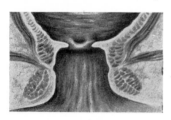

Fig. 578.—Simple annular stricture of the rectum.

from the anus. If the calibre of the stricture is large enough to admit the finger, it should be noted whether the stricture is annular (fig. 578) or tubular. Sometimes this point can only be determined after a stricture has been dilated. If free bleeding occurs after dilatation of a supposed inflammatory stricture, carcinoma should be suspected (Grey Turner), and a portion of the stricture should be removed for microscopical examination. Eighty per cent. of patients suffering from stricture of the rectum due to lympho-granuloma venereum are women. Frei's reaction is usually positive. This variety of rectal stricture is particularly common in negro races, and may be accompanied by elephantiasis of the labia majora.

Treatment:

Prophylactic.—The passage of an <u>anal dilator</u> during convalescence after hæmorrhoidectomy greatly reduces the inci-

G. *Grey Turner, Contemporary. Emeritus Professor of Surgery, Post-graduate Medical School, London.*

dence of post-operative stricture. Efficient treatment of lympho-granuloma venereum in its early stages should lessen the frequency of rectal stricture from this cause.

Dilatation by Bougies.—For anal and many rectal strictures dilatation by bougies at regular intervals, combined at first with lavage, is often satisfactory and occasionally curative. When the stricture is in the lower two-thirds of the rectum, Hegar's dilators are suitable for this purpose. Stricture of the upper third of the rectum should never be treated by dilatation because of the risk of extra- or intra-peritoneal perforation of the bowel. When the cause of the stricture is lympho-granuloma venereum, general treatment of the infection by sulphathiazole and aureomycin is a most important part of the treatment.

Internal proctotomy is necessary as a prelude to dilatation of a tight annular stricture. Guided by the finger, a blunt-pointed bistoury is inserted through the stricture and from four to six cuts are made in a posterior and postero-lateral direction.

Left iliac colostomy must be undertaken when a stricture is situated in the upper third of the rectum, when a stricture is causing intestinal obstruction, and in advanced cases of stricture complicated by fistulæ-in-ano.

Excision of the rectum is required if the stricture takes on a malignant change, and in some resistant cases of stricture due to lympho-granuloma venereum when the associated proctitis persists in spite of general treatment.

PROLAPSE OF THE RECTUM

Partial Prolapse.—The mucous membrane and submucosa of the rectum protrude outside the anus for not more than between $\frac{1}{2}$ to $1\frac{1}{2}$ inches (1·25 to 3·75 cm.). When the prolapsed mucosa is palpated between the finger and thumb, it is evident that it is composed of no more than a double layer of mucous membrane (cf. complete prolapse). The condition occurs most often at the extremes of life—in children between one and three years of age, and in elderly people. In children, partial prolapse often commences after an attack of diarrhœa, following severe whooping cough, or loss of weight and consequent diminution in the amount of fat in the ischio-rectal fossæ. In adults the condition is usually associated with third-degree hæmorrhoids. In the female a torn perineum predisposes to prolapse, and in

Alfred Hegar, 1830–1914. Professor of Obstetrics and Gynæcology, Freiburg.

the male straining from urethral obstruction.   In old age, both partial and complete prolapse are due to atony of the sphincter mechanism.

Complete prolapse is less common than the partial variety. The protrusion consists of all layers of the rectal wall.   It is more than 1½ inches (3·75 cm.) and commonly as much as 4 to 6 inches (10 to 15 cm.) in length.   On palpation with the finger inside the lumen and the thumb outside, the prolapse feels much thicker than a partial prolapse, and obviously consists of a double thickness of the entire wall of the rectum.   Any prolapse over 2 inches (5 cm.) in length contains anteriorly between its layers a pouch of peritoneum (fig. 579).   On this account Moschowitz

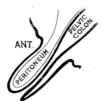

Fig. 579.—Complete prolapse, showing the pouch of peritoneum between the anterior layers.

considered that a complete prolapse is a sliding hernia occurring through the pelvic musculo-fascial diaphragm.   When large, the peritoneal pouch contains a loop or loops of small intestine which return to the general peritoneal cavity with a characteristic gurgle when the prolapse is reduced. The prolapsed mucous membrane is often arranged in a series of circular folds (fig. 580).   Complete prolapse is uncommon in children and in adults it can occur at any age.   Women are six times more often affected than men.   Many of the patients suffering from this condition are obese ;   the smaller number that are thin show signs of general visceroptosis.   In women

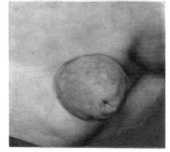

Fig. 580.—Complete rectal prolapse.   (*Professor Finch.*)

with extensive perineal tears, prolapse of the rectum may be associated with prolapse of the uterus.

Differential Diagnosis.—In the case of a child with abdominal pain, prolapse of the rectum must be distinguished from **ileo-cæcal intussuscep-**

Alexis Victor Moschowitz, 1865–1933.

tion protruding from the anus. Figs. 581 and 582 make the differential diagnosis clear. In **recto-sigmoid intussusception** in the adult there is a deep groove (2 inches (5 cm.) or more) between the emerging protruding mass and the margin of the anus.

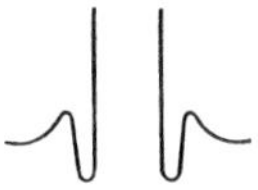

Treatment in Children.—Bowel training requires about a month in hospital. At first an enema is given after breakfast and the nurse supports the anus while the child defæcates in the left lateral position.

FIG. 581.— Partial prolapse of the rectum.

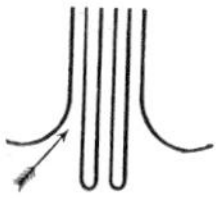

FIG. 582.— Ileo-cæcal intussusception protruding from the anus.

With a mild aperient at night, the child is taught to defæcate in this position at the same time each day ; after a month of this training together with, if necessary, a fattening diet, defæcation in the sitting position can often be resumed without return of the prolapse.

Submucous Injection.—When the above measure fails, injection of 5 per cent. phenol in almond oil is carried out under general anæsthesia. The submucosa at the apex of the prolapse is injected circularly, so as to form a raised ring, up to 10 ml. of the solution being injected. A similar injection is made at the base of the prolapse. Alternatively, if the prolapse cannot be drawn down the injections are given through a proctoscope. As a result of the aseptic inflammation following these injections, the mucous membrane becomes tethered to the muscle coat.

Perianal suture is used when the prolapse persists in spite of these measures. A stab incision with a tenotomy knife is made through the skin 1 inch (2·5 cm.) posterior to the anus in the middle line. A curved round-bodied needle carrying a No. 3 chromic catgut suture encircles half the anus, and emerges through a similar puncture at the anterior pole. The needle is reinserted and passed around the opposite side of the anus, to emerge at the original puncture. The suture is tied with the assistant's little finger in the anus, and each of the puncture wounds is closed by a single stitch.

Treatment in the Adult.—Submucous injections of phenol in almond oil is sometimes successful in cases of early partial prolapse.

Hæmorrhoidectomy may prove curative.

Excision of the Prolapsed Mucosa.—When the prolapse is unilateral the redundant mucosa can be excised after inserting and tying Goodsall's ligature (fig. 583) which, after the needles have been cut off, permits the base of the prolapsed mucous membrane to be ligated in three portions lying in juxtaposition. It should be noted that the foregoing measures are suited to partial prolapse only.

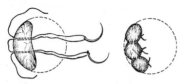

FIG. 583.—Goodsall's ligature.

Recto-sigmoidectomy is advised in relatively young patients when the prolapse is complete and remains outside the anus for long periods, causing the exposed mucous membrane to become ulcerated.

The pre-operative preparation is similar to that for hæmorrhoidectomy, but phthalylsulphathiazole, 5 grammes (75 grains) twice daily, is given for five days before the operation. With the patient in the lithotomy position, the prolapse is grasped in tissue forceps and drawn down as far as possible. A circular incision is made through the mucous membrane 1 inch (2·5 cm.) distal to the pectinate line (fig. 584). Numerous bleeding vessels in the submucosa are ligated. The lower cut edge of mucous membrane is dissected off the muscle coat, which is incised more distally throughout the circumference. The extraperitoneal fat is exposed and divided, and the underlying pouch of peritoneum is incised. This exposes the contained recto-sigmoid, which is grasped and drawn down as far as possible. The base of the peritoneal sac is sewn to the upper limit of the wall of the pelvic colon, special care being taken to close the lateral recesses. The edges of the pubo-

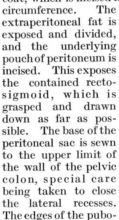

FIG. 584.—The mucous membrane of the prolapsed rectum is incised circumferentially 1 inch (2·5 cm.) below the pectinate line. (*After H. R. Thompson.*)

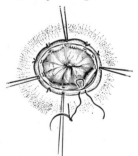

FIG. 585.—Suturing the cut edges of the pelvic colon to those of the rectum. Note the four stay sutures.

rectalis are sought and are approximated, so as to re-form the pelvic diaphragm. One inch (2·5 cm.) from the anal margin the pelvic colon is divided obliquely so that more of it projects posteriorly than anteriorly. When about three-quarters of the circumference has been divided, three stay sutures are inserted so as to unite the edges of the stump of the rectum to the edges of the pelvic colon, which lies within it. The mesocolon is secured in hæmostats and divided after ligating the superior hæmorrhoidal vessels contained therein. The remaining quarter of the pelvic colon is divided and a fourth stay suture is inserted. The cut edges of the pelvic colon are united to the cut edges of the rectum by interrupted mattress sutures (fig. 585). The anastomosis is then inverted into the anal canal.

Post-operative Treatment.—The bowels are kept confined for five days. On no account is an enema administered. Liquid paraffin and a small dose of cascara evacuant are given by mouth, and glycerine suppositories are inserted into the rectum on the fifth day. Sphincter exercises are commenced soon after the bowels have moved, and are carried out several times a day, if necessary aided by faradism. The success of the operation depends on the development of an efficient external sphincter.

Thiersch's operation consists in encircling the subcutaneous tissues of the anus with No. 20 gauge silver wire passed by means of a hollow curved needle, in the same way as that described for prolapse in children. The wire is tied while the proximal joint of an assistant's index finger is in the anal canal. This operation is preferable to the foregoing in elderly patients and in those in whom sphincter tone is lost.

ANAL INCONTINENCE
Aetiology :

Congenital.—(*a*) In cases of imperforate anus when a perineal anus has been established but the sphincter mechanism is partially or completely lacking ; (*b*) patulous anus associated with mental deficiency.

Traumatic.—By far the most frequent cause is as a complication of a complete perineal tear during parturition. Other injuries resulting in a torn anal sphincter are extremely rare.

Post-operative.—(*a*) After the ano-rectal ring has been severed during an operation for a high fistula-in-ano ; (*b*) following conservative resection of the rectum for carcinoma.

Associated with advanced complete prolapse with atony of the sphincter.

Interruption of the reflex arc responsible for sphincter control in diseases of the nervous system, notably tabes dorsalis.

Carcinoma of the Anus involving the Sphincter.

Treatment.—The only form that can often be completely remedied by operation is the postpartum variety. In these cases posterior perineorrhaphy with repair of the torn edges of the external sphincter often restores complete normality. Cases associated with complete prolapse may be benefited by Thiersch's operation. In cases where plastic operations fail, colostomy is often preferable to an incontinent natural anus.

BENIGN TUMOURS OF THE RECTUM

Adenoma is the commonest benign tumour of the rectum. Histologically it is composed of tubular glands similar to the glands of Lieberkühn, situated on a fibro-muscular stroma.

In children it occurs as a bright-red, slightly lobulated, pedunculated tumour in the lower rectum. Nearly always the patient is brought for advice because of the passage of bright-red blood. If the pedicle is long enough, the adenoma appears at the anus during defæcation, causing tenesmus and pain. On digital examination of the rectum a mobile, rounded lump is felt, the stalk of which can often be hooked beneath the

Michael Faraday, 1791–1867. English Physicist.
Karl Thiersch, 1822–1895. Professor of Surgery, Leipzig.
Johann Lieberkühn, 1711–1756. Anatomist, Berlin.

finger, permitting the bulbous end of the tumour to be withdrawn from the anus.

In adults an adenoma may give rise to similar symptoms, and it can occur at any age. Often adenomata are multiple, and are found on routine proctoscopy and sigmoidoscopy in cases of rectal hæmorrhage attributed to hæmorrhoids. The adenomata are often sessile and sometimes pedunculated (fig. 586). An adenoma of the pelvic colon not infrequently causes a local intussusception, and only on sigmoidoscopy is its true high origin discovered.

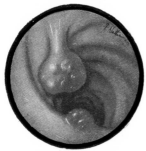

FIG. 586.—Rectal polypi seen through a sigmoidoscope.
(*W. R. Warner & Co., Ltd.*)

Differential Diagnosis. — Multiple adenomata of the rectum may be a part of multiple colonic polyposis, either hereditary or acquired (p. 431), and sigmoidoscopy, together with contrast radiography of the colon, is necessary to exclude this condition. Multiple adenomatous polypi must also be distinguished from inflammatory pseudo-polypi occurring as a complication of ulcerative colitis and those of hypertrophic tuberculosis. With the exception of those occurring in children, adenomata are prone to become malignant. The sign of malignancy, if the tumour can be felt, is induration of its base. Possibly its malignant nature may be detected microscopically after local excision. Recurrence after removal of an adenoma is proof that a malignant change in its base has occurred. Adult patients suffering from adenoma of the rectum must be examined sigmoidoscopically at intervals after the tumour has been excised, in order to detect possible recurrence.

Treatment.—A solitary pedunculated adenoma situated in the lower two-thirds of the rectum is easily removed by drawing it down, ligating its base by transfixion, and dividing the pedicle with a diathermy knife. Pedunculated adenomata too high to be delivered through the anus can be removed by a diathermy snare through a sigmoidoscope. Sessile adenomata can be destroyed by a stiff insulated electrode applied through a sigmoidoscope.

Papilloma occurs in middle-aged or elderly patients. It is a

villous tumour with finger-like projections consisting histologically of columnar epithelium on a fine connective tissue
stroma. It is usually sessile, but may become pedunculated.
When small, the sessile form is difficult to distinguish from an
adenoma, but it is more velvety in appearance and when
within reach of the finger it feels smoother. Untreated, the
tumour grows to a larger size than an adenoma, and it sometimes
completely encircles the rectum. While papillomata often
eventually become carcinomatous, they may remain innocent
for years. The most typical symptom is the passage of considerable amounts of clear mucus with bleeding occurring at
intervals. In 10 per cent. of specimens of carcinoma of the
rectum removed by excision the growth originates in a papilloma
(Dukes).

Differential Diagnosis.—In patients who have resided in
Egypt, bilharzial papilloma must be excluded.

Treatment.—*Local excision per anum* is satisfactory if the
upper limit of the tumour can be reached, in which case the
whole growth can be removed with a margin of healthy tissue.
When small, traction on the growth will elevate the mucous
membrane sufficiently to form a false pedicle, which can be
ligated by transfixion or, if too large for a single ligature, by
Goodsall's ligature. Still larger growths can be excised little
by little, commencing superiorly and drawing together the cut
mucous membrane as the growth is removed with a margin of
healthy tissue, inch by inch. *Excision of the rectum* is the only
treatment in growths situated high in the rectum and in those
involving all or most of the circumference.

Rare benign tumours of the rectum include submucous lipoma, leiomyoma, and hæmangioma. The last often causes serious, and if large sometimes fatal, hæmorrhage. When localised in the lower part of the
rectum or anal canal, a hæmangioma can be excised after applying
Goodsall's stitch. When the neoplasm is diffuse or lying in the upper part
of the rectum, colostomy and tying the inferior mesenteric artery has been
performed successfully.

Fibroma (*syn.* fibrous polyp) is not uncommon. It is not a neoplasm, but
is due to fibrosis of a thrombosed hæmorrhoid.

CARCINOMA OF THE RECTUM AND THE ANUS

THE RECTUM

Origin.—In about 30 per cent. of cases operation specimens
show that in some part of the length of bowel that has been

*Cuthbert Esquire Dukes, Contemporary. Director of Research Laboratories, St. Mark's
Hospital, London.*

removed, in addition to the carcinoma there are one or more
adenomata or papillomata. Undoubtedly adenoma and papilloma of the rectum are precarcinomatous conditions. In
approximately 3 per cent. of cases there is more than one
carcinoma present simultaneously. In 70 per cent. of cases the
growth is solitary. It begins as a nodule of atypical columnar
epithelium, the rapidly proliferating cells of which extend on
the surface by exuberant growth at its edges. At the same time
the submucosa is infiltrated. The less malignant varieties
continue to extend towards the lumen ; the more malignant
varieties soon become necrotic in their centre and give place to
an ulcer with indurated everted edges.

Local Spread.—The growth tends to spread circumferentially
around the lumen rather than in an upward and downward
direction. Usually a period of six months is required for
involvement of one-quarter of the circumference, and eighteen
months to two years for complete annular involvement. The
annular variety is common at the recto-sigmoid junction. After
the muscular coat has been penetrated the growth spreads into
the underlying fat, but is still limited by the fascia propria
(peri-rectal fascia). Eventually, rarely before eighteen months
from the commencement of the disease, the fascia propria
becomes penetrated. If penetration occurs anteriorly, the
prostate, seminal vesicles, or the bladder become involved in the
male ; in the female the vagina or the uterus are invaded. In
either sex, if the penetration is lateral, a ureter may become
implicated, while posterior penetration involves the sacrum and
the sacral plexus.

Lymphatic Spread.—Enlargement of lymph nodes from
bacterial infection is more frequent than enlargement from
metastasis, and microscopical examination is required to detect
carcinomatous involvement of the nodes. In early cases
lymphatic spread from a carcinoma of the rectum occurs almost
exclusively in an *upward* direction. After the muscular wall
of the rectum has been penetrated, the para-rectal nodes
situated within the fascia propria above the growth become
implicated. Thereafter the nodes related to the superior
hæmorrhoidal vessels become involved. Metastasis at a higher
level than the main trunk of the superior hæmorrhoidal artery
only occurs late in the disease. A radical operation should

ensure that the high-lying nodes are removed by ligating the inferior mesenteric artery and vein at the highest possible level, compatible with preserving the blood-supply to the descending and iliac colon. Only when the lymphatic vessels have become blocked by permeation of carcinoma cells does lymphatic spread occur in a downward direction. Lateral spread along the middle hæmorrhoidal lymphatic vessels to the iliac lymph nodes takes place mainly from deeply ulcerated growths situated in the rectal ampulla.

Venous Spread.—Involvement of the inferior hæmorrhoidal venous plexus by the growth does not necessarily imply that metastasis to the liver has taken place. As a rule this form of spread occurs late. Anaplastic and rapidly growing tumours in younger patients are much more liable to spread in this way than tumours of relatively low malignancy. Distant metastasis, other than to the liver, is unusual, that to the lungs being the least uncommon.

Peritoneal dissemination may follow penetration of the peritoneal coat by a high-lying rectal carcinoma.

As a rule carcinoma of the rectum does not metastasise early. From specimens removed at operation, Dukes classifies carcinoma of the rectum into three stages (fig. 587).

(A) The growth is limited to the rectal wall (15 per cent.).

(B) The growth is extended to the extra-rectal tissues, but metastasis to the regional lymph nodes has not yet occurred (35 per cent.).

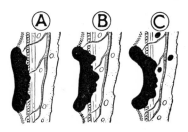

FIG. 587.—Cardinal varieties of carcinoma of the rectum from a practical standpoint.

(C) There are secondary deposits in the regional lymph nodes (50 per cent.).

This does not take into account cases that have metastasised beyond the regional lymph nodes or by way of the venous system.

Histological Grading.—In the great majority of cases carcinoma of the rectum is a columnar-celled adenocarcinoma. The more nearly the tumour cells approach normal shape and arrangement, the less malignant is the tumour. Conversely, the greater the percentage of cells of an embryonic or un-differentiated type, the more malignant is the tumour. Broders' histological classification into four grades has been simplified by Dukes into three grades :

Low grade = well-differentiated
tumours . . . . 11 per cent.   Prognosis good.
Average grade . . . 64 per cent.   „   fair.
High grade = anaplastic
tumours . . . . 25 per cent.   „   poor.

Mucoid (*syn.* **colloid**) **carcinoma** is present in 12 per cent. of cases. There are two forms ; much the more frequent is secondary mucoid degeneration of an adenocarcinoma. Histologically the glandular arrangement is preserved and mucus fills the acini. This type is of average malignancy. In a small number of cases the tumour is a primary mucoid carcinoma. The mucus lies within the cells, displacing the nucleus to the periphery, like the seal of a signet ring. Primary mucoid carcinoma gives rise to a rapidly growing bulky growth which metastasises very early and the prognosis of which is very bad. Occasionally secondary mucoid carcinoma arises in the mucous membrane surrounding the internal opening of a long-standing fistula-in-ano.

Clinical Features.—Carcinoma of the rectum occurs most frequently between forty and seventy years of age. It is not uncommon earlier in life, and of recent years more cases below the age of forty have been recorded than formerly. When the disease commences in youth, in spite of radical treatment death usually results within a year. Carcinoma of the rectum occurs nearly twice as commonly in men as in women. Carcinoma can attack any portion of the rectum or the adjoining sigmoid (fig. 588). Usually early symptoms are so slight that more often than not the patient does not seek advice for six months or more. The earliest and most constant symptom is bleeding. There is nothing characteristic about the colour, the amount, or the time at which the bleeding occurs. It is often slight and may occur during or immediately after defæcation, or be seen on the underclothing. It is usually bright red, but when the growth is situated in the recto-sigmoid it is often of a darker hue. Occasionally bleeding is serious and clots are passed. The next

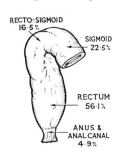

RECTO-SIGMOID
16·5 %
SIGMOID
22·5 %
RECTUM
56·1 %
ANUS &
ANAL CANAL
4·9 %

FIG. 588.—Sites of carcinoma of the rectum in 5,714 cases collected by H. E. Bacon.

Albert Compton Broders, Contemporary. Pathologist, Mayo Clinic, Rochester, U.S.A.

most frequent symptom is increasing constipation. The patient finds it necessary to take, or increase the usual dose of, aperients, and as a result a tendency towards diarrhœa ensues. A frequent symptom is a sensation that defæcation is incomplete ; consequently the patient endeavours to empty the rectum several times a day, often with the passage of flatus only. A patient who has to get up before the accustomed hour in order to defæcate, and one who passes blood and mucus in addition to fæces, is usually found to be suffering from carcinoma of the rectum. Pain of a colicky character accompanies advanced growths of the recto-sigmoid and is due to some degree of intestinal obstruction. When a deep carcinomatous ulcer of the rectum erodes the prostate or bladder, there is severe pain. Pain in the back, or sciatica, occurs when the growth presses upon or invades the sacral plexus.

Abdominal examination is negative in early cases.

In late cases metastases in the liver may be palpable. Perhaps a hydronephrosis from involvement of the ureter by the growth may be found. In late cases where the tumour is situated in the recto-sigmoid signs of obstruction to the large intestine are likely to be present. When the peritoneal cavity has been invaded there will be ascites.

Rectal Examination.—In about 90 per cent. of cases the growth can be felt digitally. The centre of the growth varies : in early proliferative cases it may be felt as a plateau or as a nodular friable protuberance with an indurated base. When the centre ulcerates, a shallow depression will be found, the edges of which are raised and everted ; this, combined with induration of the base of the ulcer, is the most frequent and an unmistakable finding. At a later stage the ulcer becomes crateriform, and its edges, although indurated and everted, are flatter than at an earlier stage. By this time the rectal wall is fixed to deeper structures. By bimanual examination it may be possible to feel the lower extremity of a carcinoma situated in the recto-sigmoid. Often a fold of mucous membrane separates the tip of the finger from actual contact with a growth within the sigmoid flexure. After the finger has been withdrawn, if it has been in direct contact with a carcinoma, it is covered with blood, or muco-purulent material tinged with blood. When a carcinomatous ulcer is situated in the lower third of the rectum, involved lymph nodes may be felt as one or more hard oval swellings in the extra-rectal tissues posteriorly or posterolaterally above the growth. In females a vaginal examination should be performed, and when the neoplasm is situated on the anterior wall of the rectum, with one finger in the vagina and another in the rectum, very accurate palpation can be carried out.

Proctoscopic examination will enable a growth in the lower third of the rectum to be seen.

Sigmoidoscopy is required in order to visualise a carcinoma in the middle or upper thirds of the rectum. This form of examination is of inestimable value when the growth is situated in the recto-sigmoid or the sigmoid. One or more enemata are necessary before a clear view can be obtained.

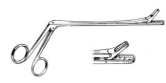

FIG. 589.—Yeomans' biopsy forceps.

Biopsy.—Employing biopsy forceps (fig. 589) by way of a proctoscope or sigmoidoscope, a portion of the edge of the tumour is removed. If possible another specimen from the more central part of the growth is obtained also. Expert histological examination will not only enable the diagnosis of carcinoma to be confirmed, but the tumour can be graded as to its relative malignancy.

Barium enema is usually unnecessary, except in cases of carcinoma of the pelvi-rectal junction or the sigmoid, when sigmoidoscopy fails to reveal the growth because of spasm of the bowel below it. A barium enema, especially an air contrast barium enema, is necessary when multiple adenomatous polyposis of the colon must be excluded.

Differential Diagnosis.—If an apparently benign growth shows evidence of induration or friability, it is certain that malignancy has occurred, even in spite of biopsy findings to the contrary. On the other hand, biopsy is invaluable in distinguishing carcinoma from inflammatory strictures and granulomata, including amœbic granuloma, which simulates a carcinoma very closely. Endometriosis produces a constricting lesion in the recto-sigmoid as well as a growth invading the rectum from the recto-vaginal septum. Growths invading the rectum from the recto-vaginal septum give rise to a very tender submucous elevation of the rectal wall. The condition occurs in females usually between twenty and forty years of age ; less often at the menopause. Dysmenorrhœa with rectal bleeding are the main symptoms. On sigmoidoscopy endometriosis involving the recto-sigmoid usually presents as a stricture with the mucosa intact. A barium enema may reveal a long filling defect in the recto-sigmoid. The final diagnosis is established by biopsy.

Frank C. Yeomans, Contemporary. Professor of Proctology, New York Polyclinic Medical School.

TREATMENT

The choice lies between a combined (abdominal and perineal) excision, a perineal excision, or a conservative operation with sphincter preservation. The first of these operative procedures is generally conceded to offer the best prospect of eradicating the disease.

Five days' pre-operative preparation similar to that for recto-sigmoidectomy (see p. 542) is necessary. Before commencing the operation in the male, a gum-elastic catheter is tied into the urethra.

The Abdomino-perineal Operation (Ernest Miles).—With the patient in high Trendelenburg's position, the abdomen is explored through a left paramedian incision. If the growth is deemed operable, after packing the small intestine away into the upper abdomen, the pelvic colon is withdrawn and examined. The inferior mesenteric vessels are divided and ligatured between their first and second sigmoid branches (fig. 590). The pelvic mesocolon is divided as far as its termination. The peritoneum on either side of the sigmoid and the rectum is incised, the incisions being carried down to the bottom of the pouch of Douglas or the recto-vesical pouch respectively. The retroperitoneal fat and connective tissue containing the regional lymph nodes are dissected forward, care being taken to avoid the left ureter (the right ureter is more laterally placed). By passing a hand into the hollow of the sacrum the retro-rectal fat and lymphatic tissues can be dissected forwards, aided by scissor cuts to divide fibrous bands, when necessary. Thus the dissection is carried to the level of the sacrococcygeal joint. The lower extremities of the para-rectal peritoneal incisions

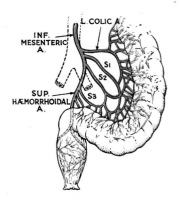

Fig. 590.—The usual disposition of the sigmoid branches (S1, S2, S3) of the inferior mesenteric artery.

are carried around the rectum to meet anteriorly, and separation of the rectum from the bladder and the seminal vesicles in the male, and from the upper part of the vagina in the female, is carried out, the ureters being avoided. After the anterior dissection has been completed, the rectum is tethered only by its lateral ligaments ; each is divided. After this complete mobilisation the pelvic colon is crushed at the junction of that part supplied by the sigmoid arteries and that which has been deprived of a blood-supply. The colon is divided with the diathermy knife and each end is ligated and invaginated. The distal end is encased in a rubber glove and pushed into the pelvis, and the peritoneal floor is united over it. The proximal end is brought through an incision in the left iliac fossa, and a terminal colostomy is constructed. The abdomen is closed. A catheter having been tied into the urethra, the patient is turned into the left lateral position and a perineal dissection is carried out through an incision similar to that described for the perineo-abdominal operation. Only the first few

W. Ernest Miles, 1869–1947. Surgeon, Cancer Hospital, London.
Friedrich Trendelenburg, 1844–1924. Professor of Surgery, Leipzig.
James Douglas, 1675–1742. Physician to Queen Caroline.

steps described for the perineal stage of that operation are necessary, after which the rectum with its lymphatic field intact is freed, and can be delivered from the wound. The perineal wound is treated in a manner similar to that described in the following operation.

Perineo-abdominal Operation (Gabriel).—Preliminary exploratory laparotomy through a right lower paramedian incision is performed. The liver and the peritoneum are examined for metastases. The degree of fixity of the growth is established from above, and it is often found to be less than was anticipated from a rectal examination. If the growth is operable the abdominal wound is closed by four or five silk-worm gut sutures tied over a roll of gauze. A sterile folded towel is placed over the gauze and retained in position by two pieces of adhesive strapping. The patient is turned into the left lateral position. After a small piece of gauze has been placed in the anal canal, the anus is firmly closed by two purse-string sutures of stout silk. An elliptical incision is made around the anus and the posterior end of the incision is inclined towards the right buttock so as to provide a slightly lateral scar subsequently. The posterior part of the incision is deepened and the coccyx is disarticulated and retracted forwards. The left forefinger is insinuated under the levator ani which is divided lateral to the finger, at first on one side and then on the other. The apex of skin anterior to the anus is grasped in a hæmostat, which serves as a retractor, and by scissors and gauze dissection the wound is deepened, when the catheter within the membranous urethra will be felt. Both in the male and the female a plane of cleavage will be found between the rectum and the prostate or the rectum and the vagina, respectively, if it is sought by the finger slightly lateral to the middle line. This plane having been determined, the strong median raphe of the perineum is divided, after which the rectum can be stripped from the prostate or the

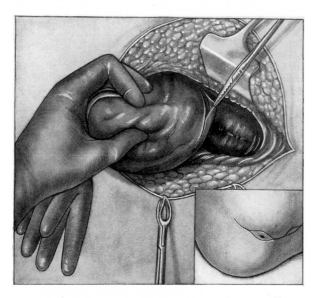

Fig. 591.—The rectum has been separated from the prostate and the recto-vesical peritoneal pouch is being opened. *Inset*: The skin incision. (*After Gabriel.*)

Richard von Volkmann (of Volkmann's contracture) was the first to excise the rectum for cancer in 1878.

William Bashall Gabriel, Contemporary. Surgeon, St. Mark's Hospital, London.

vagina. This accomplished, the posterior part of the wound is deepened. The strong fascia of Waldeyer, which arises from the lower sacral vertebræ and is inserted into the ano-rectal junction, is severed. The middle sacral artery will probably need ligation. The rectum can then be stripped off the sacrum by gauze dissection, aided here and there by dividing bands of fascia with scissors, until the level of the sacral promontory is almost reached. The mobilised rectum is enclosed in a sterile rubber glove which is secured by two strong silk sutures. By pulling the rectum downwards, and further dissection above the level of the prostate or vagina, the pouch of Douglas or the recto-vesical peritoneal pouch is seen. It is opened, keeping close to the bowel (fig. 591). The opening is enlarged on either side of the recto-sigmoid with long blunt-ended scissors, and the opening is extended upwards on each side of the recto-sigmoid as far as can be reached. The lateral ligaments of the rectum are now divided and the middle hæmorrhoidal vessels ligated if necessary (they are usually small, and ligation is not required). The rectum, with its superior hæmorrhoidal vessels intact, is now freed ; it is swabbed with flavine and pushed into the peritoneal cavity. Closure of the floor of the peritoneum is commenced anteriorly with a running suture of No. 1 chromic catgut. After three or four stitches have been placed, the last is locked. The needle is passed into a small swab and the excess of catgut is wound around the swab, and the swab with the needle and suture attached is pushed into the peritoneal cavity. After attending to hæmostasis of the perianal wound, it is closed anteriorly and posteriorly around a large drainage tube. If hæmostasis is unsatisfactory, or when the wound has been infected by perforation of the bowel during the dissection of an adherent growth, the posterior part of the wound is left open and a special rubber bag, which does not adhere to the wound, is inserted, followed by gauze packing. In either event a large dressing of gauze and wool is applied, and a triangular bandage and a many-tailed abdominal binder are left in place.

The patient is now turned on to his back and the table is tilted into a moderate Trendelenburg's position. Usually a drip blood transfusion is commenced at this stage. The abdominal wound is reopened and the small intestine is packed away from the pelvis. The rectum, covered by the rubber glove, is withdrawn. After further upward extension of the incisions in the peritoneum on either side of the bowel, the sigmoid and then the pelvic colon is withdrawn. By exerting traction on the bowel the mesocolon can be defined clearly and the inferior mesenteric vessels are ligated below the first sigmoid branch with strong silk passed on an aneurysm needle. A left iliac muscle-splitting incision 4 inches (10 cm.) long is made, the fibres of the internal oblique being divided at right angles in the lower half of the wound. The iliac colon is drawn out of this incision and the paracolic gutter is encircled with a running suture, which is not tied until the pelvic colon and the rectum have been passed through the incision up to the stitch ; the stitch is then tied, thereby closing the lateral space. The bowel is left lying on the abdominal towels. Closure of the pelvic floor (fig. 592), which was commenced from below, is completed, the tied inferior mesenteric pedicle being buried at the posterior extremity of the suture line. The paramedian incision is closed with stainless-steel sutures. The iliac colon is sutured to the peritoneum and the internal oblique. The pelvic mesocolon is ligated $1\frac{1}{2}$ inches (3·75 cm.) above the surface, and at this point the intestine is clamped and divided with a diathermy knife. The clamp having been removed, a No. 15 rubber catheter is sutured into the open mouth. After dressings have been placed on the abdominal wounds, the bandage and binder that were left in

Wilhelm von Waldeyer, 1836–1921. Professor of Pathology, Berlin.

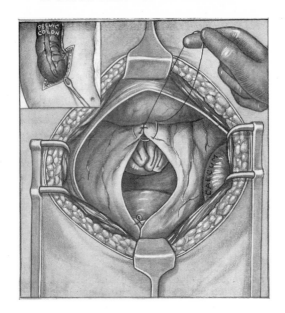

Fig. 592.—The cut edges of the pelvic peritoneum are being united over the space filled by packing left after excision of the rectum. *Inset*: The rectum and pelvic colon drawn through the left iliac incision to form a terminal colostomy. (*After Gabriel.*)

place are fastened in position. The patient is returned to bed and the foot of the bed is raised on blocks for six to twelve hours, the blood transfusion being continued as necessary. The catheter is removed from the colostomy after twenty-four hours, and the colostomy opening is trimmed on the tenth day.

Combined Simultaneous Excision of the Rectum.—With the patient in Trendelenburg-lithotomy position, the legs being supported in special crutches designed by Lloyd-Davies, access is afforded to the abdomen and the perineum at the same time. Two surgeons operate simultaneously, one performing the perineal dissection and the other the abdominal portion of the operation. This reduces considerably the time expended in performing the operation, and obviates turning the patient.

The Perineal Operation (Lockhart-Mummery).—This operation does not remove the lymphatic field in relationship to the inferior mesenteric artery, and it is now mainly reserved for poor-risk patients when the growth is in the ampulla or the anal canal. Laparotomy and left iliac colostomy are performed a fortnight before the excision. A perineal dissection is carried out exactly similar to that of the perineal stage of the perineo-abdominal operation. When the dissection is complete the vascular pedicle containing the superior hæmorrhoidal vessels is ligated and divided as high as possible. The rectum and the sigmoid can now be drawn down so that the latter is accessible. The sigmoid is divided between clamps with a diathermy knife, and the rectum is removed. A continuous mattress suture is applied over the clamp holding the sigmoid ; the clamp is removed as the stitch is tightened. Using the same needle, another layer of invaginating sutures is inserted. This is followed by reinforcing inter-

Oswald V. Lloyd-Davies, Contemporary. Surgeon, St. Mark's Hospital, London.
J. P. Lockhart-Mummery, Contemporary. Consulting Surgeon, St. Mark's Hospital, London.

rupted stitches. The ends of one of these is left long so as to prevent the closed stump from retracting into the pelvis. The edges of the parietal peritoneum are united to the seromuscular coat of the bowel stump. The long ends of the retractor stitch are then divided. Thus the closed end of the stump of bowel is left outside the peritoneal cavity. The dressing of the perineal wound is identical with that described in the perineo-abdominal operation.

Conservative Resection of the Rectum.—The majority of surgeons do not consider these operations to be sufficiently radical ; others have had good results with them.

The anterior operation is suited to growths of the sigmoid and recto-sigmoid junction. A preliminary defunctioning transverse colostomy is performed in cases where some degree of obstruction exists. The abdomen is opened in the left lower quadrant, and the inferior mesenteric artery and vein are ligated and divided between their first and second sigmoid branches. The remaining sigmoid vessels are divided and ligated immediately proximal to their bifurcation to form arcades, thus providing a greater length of viable pelvic colon. The recto-sigmoid is mobilised as in the abdominal stage of the abdomino-perineal operation, and the meso-rectum is divided 2 inches (5 cm.) below the growth. The bowel is then transected between right-angled clamps at this level. The pelvic colon is divided at a level of an unquestionably good blood-supply. An end-to-end anastomosis is carried out between the rectal stump and the pelvic colon. When the anastomosis lies low in the pelvis the peritoneum is united and sutured to the colon above the anastomosis ; the peri-rectal space is then drained by a tube passed into it through an incision over the coccyx, which is removed.

Procto-sigmoidectomy without Colostomy and with Preservation of the Sphincters (Bacon) is only applicable to growths situated in the upper two-thirds of the rectum or in the sigmoid. Through a left lower abdominal incision an extensive dissection of the sigmoid and the rectum is carried out, similar to the abdominal stage of the abdomino-perineal operation, up to the step of division of the pelvic colon, which is omitted. The abdomen is closed and the patient is placed in the lithotomy position. The rectum is lightly packed with gauze. The anus is everted by traction applied by forceps to the edges of the anal margin, and a circular incision is made through the anal epithelium just below the pectinate line. Grasping the upper cut edges in forceps, the dissection proceeds between the upper part of the anal canal and the superficial external sphincter, and then between the rectal wall medially and the internal sphincter laterally. Just above the internal sphincter the circular and longitudinal coats of the rectum are divided. The upper cut edges of the rectal wall are grasped in forceps and the preserved sphincters are retracted widely to permit removal of the fat in the ischio-rectal fossæ. Posteriorly the fascia of Waldeyer is divided ; anteriorly the detachment of the rectum from the prostate in the male or the vagina in the female is completed. Traction is now made on the bowel, and the levatores ani become taut. They are clamped and divided close to the ischium. Mobilisation of the rectum is now complete. The rectum and the sigmoid are withdrawn through the anus until at least 3½ inches (9 cm.) of viable colon above the ligated inferior mesenteric vessels protrudes outside the anal margin. The peritoneum is closed anteriorly and appendices epiploicæ of the colon are caught up in the posterior end of the suture line. The stumps of the levatores ani are approximated anteriorly. A mushroom-ended catheter is passed into the colon through a small anterior incision 3 inches (7·5 cm.) from the anal margin. A special clamp is applied, which permits the

Harry Ellicott Bacon, Contemporary. Professor of Proctology, Temple University, Philadelphia, U.S.A.

bowel to be clamped but avoids compressing the catheter. The colon distal to the clamp is excised. A drainage tube is placed in the presacral space for twenty-four hours. Eight days later the colonic mucosa is trimmed and united to the cut edges of the anal canal.

SARCOMA OF THE RECTUM

is very rare, and the symptoms are usually similar to those of a carcinoma· On examination a submucous tumour is found, the surface of which may be ulcerated.   Usually enlarged lymph nodes can be felt in the para-rectal tissues above the growth.   A biopsy will establish the diagnosis.   If a perineo-abdominal operation is performed before the growth has disseminated, there is a good prospect of a cure in cases of lympho-sarcoma and spindle-celled sarcoma. A reticular-celled sarcoma metastasises rapidly, and is fatal in spite of surgical or radio-therapeutic treatment.

CARCINOMA OF THE ANAL CANAL AND THE ANUS

Squamous-celled carcinoma occurs in the perianal skin or in the anal canal, the latter being more common in women.   Anal papillomata can become malignant (fig. 593).

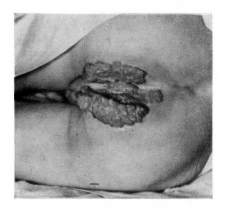

Fig. 593.—Neglected papillomata of the anus which have become malignant. The patient was a woman of forty-three years of age and symptoms had been present for eight years.

Columnar-celled carcinoma sometimes invades the anal canal from the lower part of the rectum.

Clinical Features.—Carcinoma of the anal canal and anus nearly always occurs in patients over sixty years of age.   In those cases commencing as papillomata there is but little pain or inconvenience in the early stages.   When ulceration occurs, there is often great pain on defæcation, tenesmus, and bleeding. The inguinal lymph nodes become enlarged, at first from the concomitant infection and later by metastatic deposits from the primary growth ; in the latter event they feel stony hard.

Treatment.—Radium or deep X-ray therapy is sometimes successful in squamous-celled tumours of low-grade malignancy situated outside the anal canal. When the tumour lies in the anal canal or if, by biopsy, it is graded of average or high malignancy, or when radiotherapy is not successful within a month, the perineo-abdominal operation should be performed, using the diathermy knife for the perineal stage of the operation. Inguinal lymph nodes are excised if they are the seat of secondary deposits.

Basal-celled carcinoma is very rare, and occurs at the anal margin. X-ray treatment should prove successful.

Melanoma is also very rare. It arises in the skin within the anus as a hard, dark, nodular mass, although when it becomes ulcerated the dark colour may be lost. It is usually highly malignant and metastasises by the lymphatic and venous systems. The inguinal lymph nodes are involved early, and are filled with cells containing melanin, even though the primary tumour is not dark in colour. Most cases are rapidly fatal in spite of surgical and radio-therapeutic treatment.

INOPERABLE CARCINOMA OF THE RECTUM, ANAL CANAL, AND ANUS

Only when the growth is absolutely fixed to the sacrum, or when extensive invasion has occurred to other organs anteriorly, or in the presence of widespread peritoneal involvement, is it inoperable. A palliative resection is now often undertaken in cases where metastasis to the para-aortic lymph nodes or to the liver has occurred but the rectum is removable. For inoperable growths left iliac colostomy is usually carried out, to relieve or prevent intestinal obstruction and to reduce infection by permitting lavage of the rectum from above as well as from below. When the secondary deposits cannot be completely removed, or when recurrence takes place, high-voltage deep X-ray therapy is sometimes of great benefit. The results of radium treatment of carcinoma of the rectum are poor. For the relief of pain an intrathecal injection of alcohol or cordotomy may be required.

CHAPTER XXV

HERNIA AND THE ABDOMINAL WALL

HERNIA

An external abdominal hernia is a protrusion of a viscus, usually within a peritoneal sac, through a weak area in the abdominal wall. The anatomical areas through which herniation is possible are shown in fig. 594.

At least twenty out of every thousand male inhabitants of

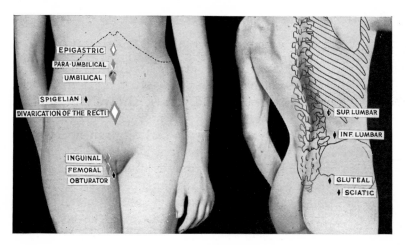

FIG. 594.—External herniæ.   Red = common.   White = not unusual.
Black = exceedingly rare.

Great Britain have a hernia (Sir Arthur Keith). The three varieties of external hernia commonly encountered are inguinal, femoral, and umbilical. Much the most frequent of these is inguinal, which occurs in 73 per cent. of cases ; then comes femoral, in about 17 per cent. of cases, and next umbilical, which occurs in about 8·5 per cent. This leaves 1·5 per cent. for the rarer forms. In this reckoning post-operative incisional hernia has not been included.

Ætiology.—In the great majority of cases no cause for the hernia can be found. In 4,780 cases of hernia in males over fifteen years of age the

Sir Arthur Keith, Contemporary. Master, Buckstone Browne Research Farm, Royal College of Surgeons.
The " saccular " theory of hernia was evolved by Hamilton Russell, 1860–1933. Surgeon, Alfred Hospital, Melbourne.

cause was unknown in 3,102 (Coley). It is highly probable, for reasons given later, that most oblique inguinal herniæ occur into a congenital pre-formed sac. Any condition that raises intra-abdominal pressure is liable to be followed by a hernia. Thus whooping cough is an exciting cause in childhood, and a chronic cough favours the development of a hernia in an adult. The stretching of the abdominal musculature during pregnancy is another factor in producing a hernia, particularly a femoral or an umbilical hernia. Straining on micturition consequent upon a stricture of the urethra or a fibrous prostate may precipitate a hernia, as also may straining on defæcation either from simple constipation or, in some instances, from an innocent or malignant stricture of the large intestine or rectum. Increasing obesity favours the development of an umbilical hernia in an adult. A powerful muscular effort or strain, such as that occasioned by lifting a heavy weight, often causes an inguinal hernia to descend into a pre-formed sac.

Accidental muscular strain as a cause of hernia is a question which is constantly being disputed in the law courts. Where there has been a proved undue muscular strain incurred during and because of the plaintiff's work, and the clinical features and/or operative findings are compatible with a recent origin of the hernia, compensation is usually allowed.

Pathological Anatomy.—As a rule, a hernia consists of three parts—the sac, the contents of the sac, and the coverings of the sac. In very exceptional cases of sliding inguinal hernia, the whole hernia consists of extraperitoneal large intestine, and perhaps a portion of the bladder.

The sac consists of a diverticulum of peritoneum which is divided into a mouth, neck, body, and fundus (fig. 595). In most cases the neck is well-defined, but in certain direct inguinal herniæ and in many incisional herniæ it is practically non-existent. The size of the body of the sac varies very greatly. The sac of a congenital hernia is not necessarily occupied. The sac resembles parietal peritoneum, but in many cases occurring in infancy and childhood it is more delicate than the parietal peritoneum with which it is continuous.

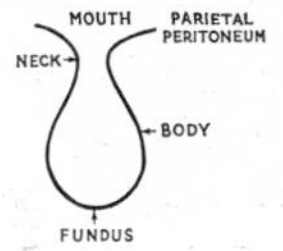

Fig. 595.—The various parts of a hernial sac.

In old-standing cases, especially after many years of pressure by a truss, the wall of the sac is comparatively thick and even (in places) of cartilaginous consistency.

Contents.—It has been said that every abdominal viscus except the liver[1] and the pancreas has been found at times among the contents of hernial sacs. The commonest are :

1. Omentum = omentocele (*syn.* epiplocele).

[1] Even a portion of the liver is present in the sac of a large exomphalos. (See p. 589.)

William B. Coley, 1862–1936. Surgeon, Hospital for the Ruptured and Crippled, New York.

2. Intestine = enterocele. Usually small intestine, but in some instances large intestine.

3. A portion of the circumference of the intestine = Richter's hernia.

4. A portion of the bladder, or a diverticulum of the bladder, is sometimes present in addition to other contents in direct inguinal, sliding inguinal, and in femoral herniæ.

5. Ovary and Fallopian tube, or testis.

6. A Meckel's diverticulum = Littré's hernia.

7. Fluid. As a part of ascites, or as a residuum thereof. Blood-stained fluid accompanies strangulation.

8. Loose bodies, such as detached small portions of greater omentum or appendices epiploicæ, which have undergone axial rotation.

Coverings are derived from the various layers of the abdominal wall through which the sac passes. In long-standing cases they become atrophied from stretching and so amalgamated that they are indistinguishable one from another.

A classification common to all herniæ is as follows :

1. *Reducible.*
2. *Irreducible.*
3. *Strangulated.*
4. *Obstructed* (syn. *incarcerated*).

} *Complications* of 1.

REDUCIBLE HERNIA

The hernia either reduces itself when the patient lies down, or can be reduced by the patient or by the surgeon.

The physical signs of reduction vary somewhat with the nature of the contents of the sac.

Intestine gurgles on reduction. The first portion is more difficult to reduce than the last.

Omentum is doughy, and the last portion is more difficult to reduce than the first.

Bladder.—There is often frequency of micturition, and possibly the hernia decreases in size after the bladder has been emptied.

IRREDUCIBLE HERNIA

A hernia is said to be irreducible when its contents cannot be returned to the abdomen, and there are no other serious symptoms. Such a condition is usually brought about by adhesions between the contents and the sac wall or from over-crowding in the sac. Irreducibility without other symptoms is almost diagnostic of an omentocele. Femoral and umbilical

August G. Richter, 1742–1812. Surgeon, Göttingen, Germany.
Johann Meckel, 1781–1833. Professor of Anatomy, Botany, and Obstetrics, Berlin.
Alexis Littré, 1658–1725. Teacher of Anatomy in Paris. Littré described " Meckel's "
    diverticulum in a hernial sac before Meckel was born.

herniæ are most often thus complicated. Inguinal herniæ are not often irreducible, but in long-standing cases they are frequently only partially reducible. Any degree of irreducibility predisposes to strangulation.

STRANGULATED HERNIA

A hernia becomes strangulated when the blood-supply of its contents is seriously impaired, rendering gangrene imminent. Gangrene may occur as early as five or six hours after the onset of the first symptoms of strangulation.

Although inguinal hernia is six times more common than femoral hernia, the greater liability of a femoral hernia to strangulate is brought out by referring to fig. 596. It should be noted that ventral herniæ, including umbilical, para-umbilical, and incisional herniæ, also frequently strangulate.

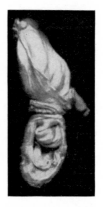

F I G . 5 9 7 .— Strangulation of a coil of small intestine in an inguinal hernia.

Strangulated Enterocele (fig. 597).

Pathology.—The intestine is obstructed, and in addition its blood-supply is constricted. At first only the venous return is impeded. The wall of the intestine becomes congested and bright red, and serous fluid is poured out into the sac. As the congestion increases the intestine becomes purple in colour.

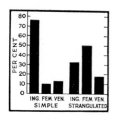

FIG. 596.—Hospital admissions of cases of simple and strangulated hernia ; inguinal, femoral, and ventral. (*D. M. Douglas.*)

As a result of increased intestinal pressure the strangulated loop becomes distended, often to twice its normal size. As venous stasis increases the arterial supply becomes more and more impaired. Ecchymoses appear under the serosa and spread until the whole wall of the imprisoned loop is involved. Blood is effused into the lumen of the loop, and also through the serosa, causing the fluid in the sac to become blood-stained. As the œdema increases the smooth shining serosa becomes dull and covered by a fibrinous, sticky exudate. By this time the walls of the intestine have lost their tone ; they feel flabby, and are very friable. The lowered vitality of the intestine favours migration of bacteria through the in-

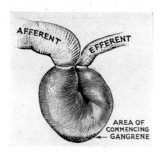

Fig. 598.—Gangrene usually first commences at the anti-mesenteric border of the intestine and next at the areas of constriction.

testinal wall, and the fluid in the sac becomes teeming with bacteria. Gangrene appears, first at the convexity of the loop and next at the rings of constriction (fig. 598), which become deeply furrowed and grey in colour. From the anti-mesenteric border the gangrene spreads upwards, and the colour changes, which vary from black to grey or green, are due to decomposition of blood in the sub-serosa. If the strangulation is un-relieved, perforation of the wall of the intestine occurs, most commonly on the convexity of the loop but nearly as often at the seat of constriction. The mesentery involved in the strangulation undergoes the following changes : it becomes congested and hæmorrhagic, and thrombosis of its vessels occurs. Finally it, too, becomes gangrenous. Peritonitis spreading from the sac to the peritoneal cavity is a usual terminal event.

Clinical Features.—Pain comes on suddenly, and is at first situated over the hernia. Generalised abdominal pain soon supervenes ; it is paroxysmal in character and is often located mainly at the umbilicus. Vomiting is forcible and usually oft-repeated. The hernia is tense, extremely tender, and there is no impulse on coughing. In cases of strangulation of the small intestine it is quite common to obtain a good fæcal result from an enema, and even from a second enema, but eventually complete constipation results. Unless the strangulation is relieved, the paroxysms of pain continue with increasing severity ; they do not stop until peristaltic contractions cease. With the onset of gangrene the pain ameliorates, and when paralytic ileus (often the result of peritonitis) develops, the pain ceases. Spontaneous cessation of pain is therefore of grave significance.

Strangulated Richter's Hernia (*syn.* **strangulated partial enterocele**).—The symptoms are not as severe as the foregoing, the patient may not vomit, and complete constipation does not develop for a long time. This form of hernia is particularly common in strangulated femoral hernia (p. 587).

Strangulated Omentocele.—The initial symptoms are similar to those of a strangulated enterocele, but the recurring attacks of generalised abdominal pain are not maintained. Vomiting may be absent and there need not be constipation. The findings on palpation of a strangulated omentocele are similar to those of strangulated enterocele. Unlike intestine, omentum can subsist on a very meagre blood-supply. The onset of gangrene is therefore correspondingly delayed, and it occurs first in the centre of the fatty mass. Unrelieved, a bacterial invasion of the dying contents of the sac will almost certainly occur. Infection is limited to the sac for days, and sometimes for weeks. This often terminates in extension of peritonitis from the sac to the general peritoneal cavity, and although deterioration of the patient's general condition takes place more slowly, ultimately the prognosis is nearly as grave as that of unrelieved strangulated enterocele.

OBSTRUCTED (*Syn.* INCARCERATED) HERNIA

An obstructed hernia is an irreducible hernia containing intestine whose lumen is obstructed from without or from within ; but the blood-supply to the obstructed loop is unimpaired. The symptoms are less severe and the onset more gradual than is the case in strangulation, but more often than not obstruction in a hernia terminates in strangulation. The term " incarceration " is usually employed when it is considered that the lumen of the intestine occupying the hernial sac is blocked with fæces. In rare instances when a segment of large intestine is situated in a large umbilical, an incisional, or a sliding inguinal hernia, this is, in fact, the cause of the obstruction. In such cases the scyballous contents of the hernia should be capable of being indented with the finger like putty. In these circumstances enemata may relieve the obstruction, but unless as the result of enemata the hernia becomes considerably smaller or wholly reducible and pain is completely relieved, early operation should be undertaken. As a rule no clear distinction can be made between obstruction and strangulation in herniæ ; consequently, as soon as gastro-intestinal suction-drainage and the administration of intravenous saline, as necessary, have improved the patient's general condition, operation should be undertaken.

INGUINAL HERNIA

SURGICAL ANATOMY

The external abdominal ring, a triangular aperture in the aponeurosis of the external oblique, lies $\frac{1}{2}$ inch (1·25 cm.) above and $\frac{1}{2}$ inch lateral to the spine of the pubis. Normally it will not admit the tip of the little finger.

The internal abdominal ring, which lies $\frac{1}{2}$ inch (1·25 cm.) above Poupart's ligament, midway between the symphysis pubis and the anterior superior iliac spine, is a ∪-shaped condensation of the transversalis fascia incomplete above. It is covered anteriorly by the transversus muscle, its base being situated below the free border of that muscle. The upper extremities of the ring are slung from the posterior surface of the transversus muscle and the ring moves upwards and outwards when the muscle contracts, thereby still further narrowing the aperture.

François Poupart, 1661–1708. Surgeon, Hôtel-Dieu, Paris.

The Inguinal Canal.—In infants the external and internal abdominal rings are almost superimposed, and the obliquity of this canal is slight. In adults the inguinal canal, which is about $1\frac{1}{2}$ inches (3·75 cm.) long, is directed downwards and medially between the internal and external abdominal rings. In the male the inguinal canal contains the spermatic cord, the ilio-inguinal and ilio-hypogastric nerves, and the genital branch of the genito-crural nerve. In the female the round ligament takes the place of the spermatic cord.

Fig. 599.

Boundaries of the Inguinal Canal.—Those fibres of the internal oblique which take origin from the outer two-thirds of Poupart's ligament arch over the spermatic cord (or round ligament), the superior fibres being inserted into the outer edge of the rectus abdominis. The inferior fibres, becoming tendinous, blend with the transversus muscle to become the conjoined tendon, which is inserted into the crest of the pubis. Thus the internal oblique forms part of the anterior wall (fig. 599) (a), the roof (b), and, as the conjoined tendon (c), part of the floor of the inguinal canal. Applying this knowledge, it is easy to remember the boundaries of the inguinal canal, viz. :

Anteriorly.—External oblique aponeurosis ; Poupart fibres of **internal oblique.**

Posteriorly.—**Internal oblique** (here conjoined tendon) ; deep epigastric artery ; fascia transversalis.

Superiorly.—**Internal oblique.**

Inferiorly.—Poupart's ligament.

Through the internal abdominal ring and down the inguinal canal passes an oblique inguinal hernia.

Hesselbach's triangle (fig. 600) is bounded medially by the outer margin of the rectus abdominis, laterally by the deep epigastric artery, and below by the medial half of Poupart's ligament. Through this triangle passes a direct inguinal hernia.

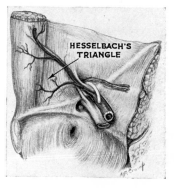

Fig. 600.—A direct hernia breaks through Hesselbach's triangle.

OBLIQUE (*Syn.* INDIRECT) INGUINAL HERNIA

This is the most common of all forms of hernia. It is generally agreed that an oblique inguinal hernia, at whatever age it appears, occurs into a preformed sac which is a partially or completely patent processus vaginalis. Normally the processus vaginalis becomes obliterated shortly before birth, at first at the internal abdominal ring, and a little later immediately above the upper pole of the epididymis ; the tunnel of peritoneum between these two points becomes a narrow fibrous cord. Failure to obliterate at either or both of these places results in an oblique inguinal hernial sac. The reasons for taking this

Franz Hesselbach, 1759–1816. Surgeon, Würzburg.

view are (*a*) the anatomical disposition of the sac is similar to that of the processus vaginalis ; (*b*) an empty sac in this position is often found at operation for other conditions, a hernia never having appeared ; (*c*) in post-mortem examinations in infants up to the age of four months the processus vaginalis is open in over 30 per cent. of cases ; (*d*) an oblique inguinal hernia commonly appears during infancy ; (*e*) in adults with an inguinal hernia of only a few days' duration the tissue binding the vas to the sac has been shown to consist of fibrous tissue without cellular elements.

In the first decade of life inguinal hernia is more common on the right side in the male. This is no doubt associated with the later descent of the right testis (see p. 788). After the second decade left inguinal herniæ are as frequent as right. The hernia is bilateral, or ultimately becomes so, in nearly 30 per cent. of cases.

There are various types of oblique inguinal hernia (fig. 601) :

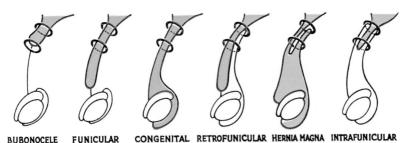

BUBONOCELE   FUNICULAR   CONGENITAL   RETROFUNICULAR   HERNIA MAGNA   INTRAFUNICULAR

Fig. 601.—Varieties of oblique inguinal hernia.

1. **Bubonocele.**—The hernia is limited to the inguinal canal, the processus vaginalis having been obliterated at the external abdominal ring. This type of hernia is seen commonly in young adults with a short history.

2. **Funicular.**—The processus vaginalis is closed only at its lower end, just above the epididymis. When the sac is occupied by hernial contents they are separated from the testis, which lies below the fundus of the sac. This type is frequent in adults with a history of some standing.

3. **Congenital** is rarely present at birth, but is commonly encountered in infancy. It may not appear until adolescent or adult life. There is a persistence of the prenatal condition

before the processus vaginalis becomes obliterated. The testis appears to lie within the lower part of the hernia.

4. **Retrofunicular.**—The processus vaginalis becomes obliterated above the epididymis, but the tunica vaginalis extends as a blind peritoneal pouch in front of the hernia. The only practical significance of this anomaly is that three serous membranes have to be opened before the contents of the sac are reached. Above, the space between the outer two serous membranes ends blindly in the region of the neck of the sac.

5. **Hernia Magna.**—This anomaly of the processus vaginalis provides an extremely large sac, even larger than the congenital. In contradistinction to the latter, it is loculated.

6. **Intrafunicular** (*syn.* encysted).—An empty tunica vaginalis gives rise to a serous coat around the sac. The condition has generally been noted as an extensive vaginal hydrocele surrounding the fundus and body of a hernial sac.

Clinical Features.—An oblique inguinal hernia can appear at any age, but it does so most frequently in infancy, childhood, or in early adult life. Males are at least twenty times more commonly affected than females ; in some series 99 per cent. of the patients are males.

In the early stages of the development of the hernia when the sac is still limited to the inguinal canal (bubonocele), the diagnosis

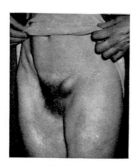

FIG. 602.—Left inguinal bubonocele.

presents some difficulty. Often the patient complains of pain in the groin or referred pain to the testicle when performing heavy work, or on exercise. The patient is asked to cough ; if a hernia is present there will be a transient bulging over the inguinal canal, which is better seen (fig. 602) than felt. In males the external abdominal ring can be palpated by invaginating the little finger into the scrotum. The presence of an enlarged external abdominal ring without a visible bulging and without an expansile impulse when the patient coughs is not evidence of the presence of a potential hernia.

When an oblique inguinal hernia has become large enough to reach the scrotum or labium majus, it produces a swelling which at first appears intermittently. In these circumstances the swelling can often be made to appear when the patient coughs, and it persists (fig. 603) until it is reduced. When the hernia cannot be made to come down at the time of the examination, an impulse can be seen and felt over the inguinal canal. On invagination of the scrotum the external abdominal ring will be found large enough to admit the little finger, which will pass along the inguinal canal in an upward and lateral direction. If

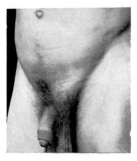

FIG. 603.—Oblique left inguinal hernia which became apparent when the patient coughed, and persisted until it was reduced.

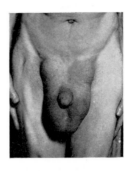

FIG. 604. — Bilateral oblique inguinal herniæ which have descended into the scrotum.

the individual constituents of the cord in the upper part of the scrotum are palpated between the finger and thumb, the vas will feel thicker on the affected side than on the contralateral side, because the empty hernial sac is intimately adherent to the vas. Local pain is unusual in a fully developed inguinal hernia unless complications have occurred.

As time goes on, unless it is supported by a truss, the hernia comes down as soon as the patient assumes the upright position (fig. 604). In large herniæ there is a sensation of weight, and dragging on the mesentery may produce epigastric pain. On palpation the swelling will be found to be issuing from the external abdominal ring. The spermatic cord lies posterior to the swelling, but in long-standing cases its constituent elements are so flattened that only the vas can be felt. If the contents of the sac are reducible, the inguinal canal will be found widely dilated.

The diagnosis of inguinal hernia in women is more difficult. In cases of bubonocele it is rarely possible to pass a finger into the inguinal canal, and reliance must be placed on a visible and palpable impulse over the inguinal canal on coughing. In those labial herniæ into which abdominal contents prolapse readily the diagnosis is much easier, and, unless the patient is stout, a finger can be introduced into the inguinal canal. In infants the swelling appears when the child cries. Sometimes an inguinal hernia is translucent in infancy and early childhood, but never in an adult.

Differential Diagnosis of Inguinal Herniæ.—An inguinal hernia must be distinguished from :

In the male.

(*a*) *A vaginal hydrocele* (see p. 804).

(*b*) *An encysted hydrocele of the cord* (see p. 804).

(*c*) *A femoral hernia* (see p. 581).

(*d*) *A maldescended testis occupying the inguinal canal* (see p. 788). An inguinal hernia is often associated with this condition.

(*e*) *A lipoma of the cord.* This is often an extremely difficult, but unimportant, diagnosis. It is usually not settled until the parts are displayed by operation.

In the female.

(*a*) *A femoral hernia.*

(*b*) *A hydrocele of the canal of Nück* (see p. 805) is the commonest differential diagnostic problem.

TREATMENT

A Truss.—Until the age of three months, or longer if the child is not thriving, a truss should be worn over an inguinal hernia. A skein of wool can be employed for this purpose, but its serious drawback is that it is liable to become saturated with urine. For this reason, and also because many cases are bilateral, a rubber-covered horse-shoe-shaped truss is preferable. In some instances the support of the truss may result in a cure of the hernia, but in nearly all cases the " cure " is only apparent and the hernia reappears later in life.

In adults, when operation is contraindicated because of cardiac, pulmonary, or other systemic disease, or when operation is refused, an adder-headed spring truss will control a moderate-sized inguinal hernia. For a larger hernia a rat-tailed truss with a perineal band will prevent the truss slipping. For an irreducible hernia a bag truss is sometimes employed, but as a rule operation should be urged in cases of irreducibility because of the danger of strangulation. A truss must be worn continuously during waking hours, kept clean and in proper repair, and

Anton Nück, 1650–1692. Anatomist, Leiden, Holland.

renewed when it shows signs of irreparable wear.   A good truss controls the hernia when the patient stands with his legs wide apart, stoops, and coughs violently.

Injection treatment is not often employed in Great Britain.   Those practised in the method obtain good results.   Treatment by injection is only attempted in small, completely reducible herniæ.   During the whole course of treatment a well-fitting truss must be worn both day and night, and for two months after the last injection.   A special truss must be worn for bathing and fitted immediately after the ordinary truss has been removed.   The truss is dispensed with gradually, at first during the night and about a month later is worn only during activities which entail muscular strain.   Finally it is discarded altogether.   Leigh Watson recommends the following solution :

Procaine (2 per cent. solution)	.	2 fl. dr.
Quinine urea hydrochloride .	.	1 dr.
Phenol	.	2 fl. dr.
Distilled water q.s. ad	.	4 fl. oz.

An average of ten to twelve injections at bi-weekly intervals are given. For the injection the patient is placed in semi-Trendelenburg's position. After sterilising and anæsthetising the skin over the inguinal canal, in an adult from 4 to 8 ml. 1 to 2 dr. of the solution is injected slowly into various parts of the tissues in the immediate vicinity of the hernia. A fibrous reaction follows, which in favourable cases obliterates the sac and narrows the inguinal canal.

OPERATIVE TREATMENT : INGUINAL HERNIOTOMY

Although the term " herniotomy " originally meant cutting the constriction of a strangulated hernia, it is now generally accepted as a term which indicates excision of a hernial sac.

Complete excision of the sac gives excellent results in infants, children, and in many young persons up to the age of twenty-five years suffering from oblique inguinal hernia.   Whether herniotomy alone is sufficient in young adults depends on the size of the internal abdominal ring.   If it is no larger than will admit the tip of a little finger, excision of the sac will suffice.   When the ring is enlarged, as it always is in those belonging to the older age groups, some form of repair of the posterior wall of the inguinal canal is required in addition.

An incision is made through the skin and subcutaneous tissues $\frac{1}{2}$ inch (1·25 cm.) above and parallel to the medial two-thirds of Poupart's ligament.   In large irreducible herniæ the incision is extended to the upper part of the scrotum.   After dividing the superficial fascia, the external oblique aponeurosis and the external abdominal ring are identified.   An incision is made through the external oblique aponeurosis in the line of its fibres so as to open the inguinal canal at the level of the internal abdominal ring.   The structures beneath the external oblique aponeurosis are separated from its deep surface before completing the incision into the external abdominal ring, which is divided.   In this way the ilio-inguinal nerve is

Leigh F. Watson, Contemporary.   Surgeon, Los Angeles, California, U.S.A.

safeguarded. The incision extends through the intercolumnar fascia, which is reflected from the pillars of the external abdominal ring on to the spermatic cord. A hæmostat is applied to each cut edge of the external oblique aponeurosis, and by blunt dissection the upper leaf is separated from the internal oblique aponeurosis, care being taken to avoid injuring the ilio-inguinal nerve. The lower leaf is likewise dissected until the inner aspect of Poupart's ligament is seen. The cremaster muscle is divided in the length of the inguinal canal and the spermatic cord is separated from it by blunt dissection. The cord is then hooked on the forefinger and the sac is usually easily apparent because it is whiter than the adjacent structures. If there is any difficulty in locating the sac, it should be sought near the internal abdominal ring. The infundibuliform fascia is incised. After separating this fascia from the sac, the latter is picked up with a hæmostat and separation of its entire circumference from surrounding structures is carried out with dissecting forceps. Thus the vas deferens and the spermatic vessels are separated from the sac. The dissection of these structures from the sac proceeds distally.

1. **If the hernia is a bubonocele,** the fundus is soon apparent, and it can be picked up in a hæmostat and completely freed distally.

2. **If the sac is of the funicular variety,** the fundus can be reached with a little more dissection, and the extremity must be separated from adhesions by sharp dissection.

3. **If the sac is of the congenital variety,** it becomes apparent at the upper pole of the testis that the sac is continuous with the tunica vaginalis. The sac is opened and any contents of it are reduced into the general peritoneal cavity. The sac is divided transversely between hæmostats about $\frac{1}{2}$ inch (1·25 cm.) above the testicle. The distal hæmostat is removed.

Isolating the Neck of the Sac.—Whatever type of sac is encountered attention is now directed to freeing the neck of the sac. This is accomplished by blunt and gauze dissection, which proceeds through the internal abdominal ring until the parietal peritoneum can be seen on all sides of the mouth of the sac. Only when the properitoneal fat is encountered on all sides and the deep epigastric vessels are seen on the medial side has the dissection reached the extremity of the neck. The fundus of the sac is opened, if this has not been performed already, into the peritoneal cavity, and any contents are reduced. In adults a finger is passed through the mouth of the sac and Hesselbach's triangle is palpated from within, thereby excluding or confirming the presence of a concomitant direct inguinal hernia. The neck of the sac is transfixed (fig. 605) and ligated as high as possible. The sac is excised $\frac{1}{2}$ inch (1·25 cm.) below the ligature. The incision in the cremaster muscle is approximated, the external oblique aponeurosis is sutured, and the subcutaneous tissues and the skin are closed.

In cases of congenital oblique hernia when the sac is veil-like, it should be opened at an early stage of the operation. At the upper margin of the inci-

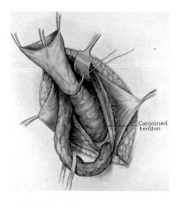

Conjoined tendon

FIG. 605.—Inguinal herniotomy. Transfixion of the neck of the sac for ligation and excision.

sion the lateral walls are divided transversely, the upper edges being
secured in hæmostats.   Exerting traction on each lateral wall, an incision
is made with a fine-pointed scalpel through the posterior wall of the sac.
The upper edge of the posterior wall, grasped in hæmostats, is dissected from
the constituents of the cord ; by this means a plane of cleavage is found
between these structures and the sac.   The lower margin is disregarded and
the body and the fundus of the sac remain (fig. 606), while the upper

FIG. 606.—In a very frail congenital inguinal hernia a
cuff of the sac near the neck is dissected as far as the
internal abdominal ring.   The cuff is transfixed and ligated.
The body of the sac is left *in situ*.

margin constitutes a complete ring of sac wall, which can be dissected like
a bubonocele until the junction of the neck with the parietal peritoneum is
reached.   Unless this method is adopted, the sac is liable to tear in a
vertical direction, especially in small children, and if this accident is not
recognised and remedied, a loop of intestine may be extruded into the
properitoneal tissues above the internal abdominal ring.

Inguinal Herniotomy in an Infant.—A short incision is made over the
external abdominal ring.   There is no need to open the inguinal canal.
The cord is lifted up and its coverings are incised.   According to circumstances, the sac is dealt with by one of the last two methods described
above.   If method two is practicable, it is not necessary to open the sac.
Once the neck of the sac has been freed, it is twisted two or three times
before transfixing and ligating it.

INGUINAL HERNIORRHAPHY

More than seventy methods of repairing the inguinal canal
after excision of the sac have been described.   One of these
procedures is required when the internal abdominal ring is
enlarged.   The more it is enlarged the greater the need for an
elaborate procedure designed to strengthen the posterior wall
of the inguinal canal.

Suture of the Transversalis Fascia.—This operation is mainly applicable
to young adults.   When the hernia is a large one and has been present for
a considerable time, the transversalis fascia is so stretched and atrophied
that its torn or stretched edges are unrecognisable.   When the edges of
the fascia at the internal abdominal ring can be felt, they can be picked up
with fine hæmostats and sutured together.   In other circumstances sutures
can be placed so as to approximate the transversalis fascia at the upper
margin of the internal abdominal ring to Poupart's ligament.   This step
is a usual preliminary in most of the methods of reinforcing the posterior
wall of the inguinal canal that follow.

Bassini's operation has been very widely practised for many years, and
is still employed with many permanently successful results.   Excision of
the hernial sac is performed in the manner described already.   The conjoined tendon is sutured to Poupart's ligament behind the spermatic cord.
The external oblique aponeurosis is reunited over the spermatic cord.   In
order to give good results, the conjoined tendon must be well developed

Edoardo Bassini, 1847–1924.   Professor of Surgery, University of Padua.

and the space between the tendon and Poupart's ligament must be small enough to allow the approximation of the latter to the former to be made without tension. Silk is the material most often employed for the sutures, but stainless steel wire and braided nylon are preferred by some. It should be noted that in a few cases the conjoined tendon is almost absent, the internal oblique aponeurosis being inserted entirely into the sheath of the rectus. It is agreed generally that suture of the internal oblique muscle, as opposed to tendon, to Poupart's ligament, is not efficient.

Reconstituting the posterior wall of the inguinal canal with floss silk (Maingot) is favoured by many surgeons. Meticulous asepsis is necessary. The instruments used are discarded and replaced by freshly sterilised ones after making the skin incision, after completing the dissection, and again when about to close the skin incision. Commencing medially and passing to the margins of the internal abdominal ring, the conjoined tendon and internal oblique aponeurosis are loosely darned to Poupart's ligament, the transversalis fascia being included in the stitches. Care is taken to avoid the ilio-inguinal and ilio-hypogastric nerves. The stitching is continued

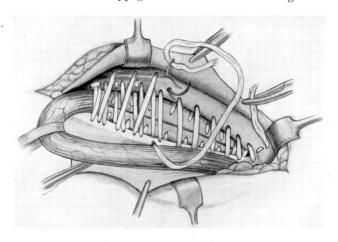

Fig. 607.—Reconstituting the posterior wall of the inguinal canal with floss silk. (*After Maingot.*)

from the internal abdominal ring to the starting-point, thus forming a lattice (fig. 607). The external oblique aponeurosis is approximated beneath the spermatic cord.

Hernioplasty with living fascia may be used to repair the inguinal canal :
(*a*) A strip of fascia $\frac{1}{2}$ inch (1·25 cm.) wide is cut from the upper leaf of the external oblique aponeurosis and, if necessary, a second strip from the lower leaf. The strip is left attached at its pubic end, the lateral end being divided where the aponeurosis becomes muscular. The free end of the strip is attached to a needle having an especially large eye (Gallie's needle) (fig. 608). The living suture is darned into the posterior wall of the inguinal canal. The external oblique aponeurosis is approximated over the cord.

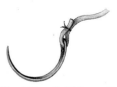

Fig. 608.—Gallie's needle. Showing the method of attaching a strip of fascia.

Rodney Maingot, Contemporary. Surgeon, Royal Free Hospital, London.
W. E. Gallie, Contemporary. Emeritus Professor of Surgery, Toronto.

This procedure is applicable in patients with a fairly good abdominal wall.

(*b*) When the external oblique aponeurosis is poorly developed and friable, a strip of fascia is obtained from the outer side of the thigh. This can be obtained through a long incision, or one of the various ingenious

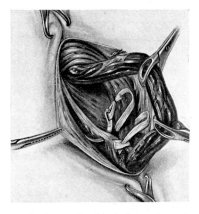

Fig. 609. — Hernioplasty. Strip of fascia lata being used to darn the walls of the inguinal canal.

patterns of fasciatomes which cut a strip from the fascia lata through a small skin incision can be employed. The fascial suture is used to darn the inguinal canal (fig. 609) in the same way as in (*a*).

(*c*) When the defect is large, and especially in recurrent cases, a fascia-patch transplant derived from fascia lata is sometimes the method of choice.

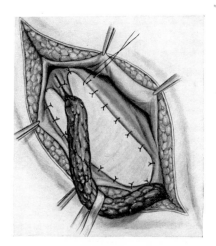

Fig. 610.—Reinforcing the posterior wall of the inguinal canal with a whole-thickness skin graft.

Hernioplasty with Whole-thickness Skin Graft (Mair).—At least forty-eight hours' preparation of the skin is necessary. The skin incision over the hernial site is so made as to include an ellipse of skin 2 inches (5 cm.) long and 1 inch (2·5 cm.) broad at its middle. The skin, with its subcutaneous tissues attached, is immersed in warm saline solution until it is

George B. Mair, Contemporary. Surgeon, Law Junction Hospital, Lanarkshire, Scotland.

required. The steps of the operation are the same as those for herniotomy, except that the external oblique aponeurosis is detached for a distance of ½ inch (1·25 cm.) from its pubic attachment in order to give better exposure of the structures to which the graft will be fastened medially. After excision of the sac the transversalis fascia is buttressed. The graft will be found to have contracted. It is divested of subcutaneous fat and its points are cut off. One of the ends is bifurcated for ½ inch (1·25 cm.). The unbifurcated end is sutured to the fascia over the symphysis pubis, and to the sheath of the rectus abdominis. The lower edge of the graft is attached to Poupart's ligament by interrupted sutures, its upper edge to the lower margin of the internal oblique aponeurosis and muscle (fig. 610). Finally the bifurcated ends which accommodate the spermatic cord issuing from the internal abdominal ring, are sutured together lateral to the cord. The external oblique aponeurosis is united over the spermatic cord and the skin is closed. In a few months a buried skin graft is converted into fibrous tissue.

STRANGULATED INGUINAL HERNIA

occurs at any time during life, and in both sexes. Males are more often affected than females, because inguinal hernia is so much more common in males. However, during infancy strangulated inguinal hernia is more common in females. In the presence of a patent hernial sac the hernia may descend for the first time and strangulate in three or four hours. More often strangulation occurs in patients who have worn a truss for a long time, and in those with a partially reducible or irreducible hernia. Because of the comparatively more yielding walls at the neck of an inguinal hernia, strangulation does not usually occur as quickly as is the case in strangulated femoral hernia, and in a number of cases strangulation is preceded by obstruction, but because the clinical demarcation between obstruction and strangulation is ill-defined, obstruction should be looked upon as an early stage of strangulation. Oblique inguinal herniæ commonly strangulate ; occasionally, when the sac is funicular, a direct inguinal hernia (p. 577) is the seat of strangulation.

The constricting agent is variable. In order of frequency it is :
1. The edge of the internal abdominal ring.
2. The edge of the external abdominal ring.
3. Fibres of the internal oblique in the inguinal canal.
4. Fibrosis of the neck of the sac itself.

In large herniæ :
5. Septa in the sac.
6. Adhesions within the sac.

Contents.—Usually small intestine is involved in the strangulation ; the next most frequent is omentum ; often both are implicated.   Occasionally large intestine is strangulated in a sliding hernia (p. 579) ; more often non-strangulated large intestine is present behind a sac containing strangulated small intestine.

Maydl's Hernia (*syn.* Hernia-in-W) (fig. 611) is a rare variety of strangulated inguinal hernia.   While the symptoms and signs resemble those of an ordinary strangulated enterocele, local tenderness over the hernia is not so great.   At operation two comparatively normal-looking loops of intestine are present in the sac.   After the obstruction has been relieved the strangulated loop will become apparent if traction is exerted on the medial limbs of the loops occupying the sac.

FIG. 611.—
Strangulation
in W.

Treatment of Strangulated Inguinal Hernia.—As a rule treatment by emergency operation is undertaken.   In early and previously reducible cases, taxis may be employed (p. 576).

Postural Treatment.—While arrangements are being made for the operation, provided not more than six hours have elapsed, it is a good practice to raise the foot of the bed, administer a full dose of morphia or omnopon (preferably intravenously), and lay a hot-water bottle over the hernia.   In a few instances the hernia reduces itself, rendering immediate operation unnecessary.

Operation.—The skin incision is the same as that described for inguinal herniotomy, but is somewhat longer.   The external oblique aponeurosis is exposed, and the sac, with its coverings, is seen issuing from the external abdominal ring.   In all but very large herniæ it is possible to deliver the body and fundus of the sac together with its coverings and (in the male) the testis on to the surface.   Each layer covering the anterior surface of the body of the sac near the fundus is incised, and if possible it is stripped off the sac.   In old-standing cases the coverings are very adherent one to another and to the sac, in which case it is better not to attempt to isolate the sac from its coverings.   When the sac has been incised, the fluid therein is mopped up or aspirated very thoroughly, for it is often highly infected. Attention is now directed to the inguinal canal.   The external oblique aponeurosis is incised and the external abdominal ring is divided.   Returning to the sac, a finger is passed into the opening, and employing the finger as a guide, the sac is slit up along its length.   If the constriction lies at the external abdominal ring or in the inguinal canal, it is readily divided by this procedure.   When the constricting agent is at the internal abdominal ring, by applying hæmostats to the cut edge of the neck of the sac and retracting them downwards, and at the same time retracting the internal oblique upwards, it may be possible to continue slitting up the sac over the finger beyond the point of constriction.   When the constriction is too tight to admit a finger, a grooved director is inserted and the constriction, as well as the neck of the sac, is divided with a scalpel under vision.   It is

Karl Maydl, 1853–1903. Surgeon, Prague.

very unlikely that the deep epigastric vessels will be wounded, but should this happen the vessels can be secured easily. In order to avoid these vessels as far as possible the constriction is divided in an upward and inward direction. It is usually advisable to make two or three nicks, rather than a bold incision. Once the constricting agent has been divided, the strangulated contents can be drawn down. Devitalised omentum is excised after being securely ligated in small sections. Viable intestine is returned to the peritoneal cavity. Doubtfully viable and gangrenous intestine is dealt with as described in Chapter xxii. If the hernial sac is of moderate size and can be separated easily from its coverings, it is excised, as hæmostats secure the rim of the peritoneum at its mouth, which is closed by a purse-string suture. When the sac is large and adherent, much time is saved by adopting the principle described for obviating excision of the body of a congenital hernia (see fig. 571). Having closed the mouth of the sac, if the condition of the patient is good, a simple form of herniorrhaphy can be carried out.

Treatment of Strangulated Inguinal Hernia in Infancy.— Performed within six hours of the onset of symptoms, taxis (fig. 612) is often possible and effective, because in infants gangrene does not occur early. Unless the patient is seen early in this period, it is best to administer a general anæsthetic, and if, after the abdominal muscles have become relaxed, the hernia cannot be reduced with very little pressure, open operation should follow immediately.

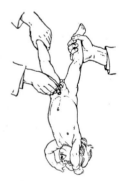

Fig. 612. — Taxis, using the " Judgment of Solomon " position.

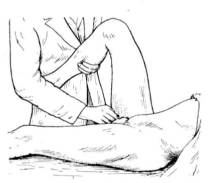

Fig. 613.—Applying taxis in the case of inguinal hernia. The thigh must be flexed and rotated internally.

Taxis as a method of treatment in other cases of strangulated inguinal hernia is useful in selected cases, but it should only be attempted in cases of strangulation (or obstruction) of under four hours, and when the hernia was previously completely reducible. The thigh must be flexed and internally rotated (fig. 613), which relaxes the pillars of the external abdominal ring. With the limb in this position, gentle even pressure is exerted with the finger and thumb upon the neck of the sac, while the other hand compresses the fundus.

The dangers of unskilled taxis are numerous. Among the most important are :

1. Reduction-en-masse (fig. 614). " The sac, together with its contents, is pushed forcibly back into the abdomen ; and as the bowel will still be strangulated by the neck of the sac, the symptoms are in no way relieved " (Sir Frederick Treves).

2. Reduction of gangrenous intestine.

3. Infected fluid may be expressed from the sac into the peritoneal cavity.

4. Contusion or rupture of the intestinal wall.

5. The sac may rupture at its neck and reduction of the contents is effected not into the peritoneal cavity, but extra-peritoneally.

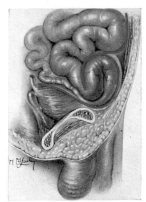

DIRECT INGUINAL HERNIA

A direct inguinal hernia is always acquired. The sac leaves the abdomen through Hesselbach's triangle. Some-times the sac passes through a defect in the conjoined tendon to enter the

Fig. 614. — Reduction-en-masse.

inguinal canal through its posterior wall ; at others it carries an atrophied conjoined tendon in front of it. In a few cases the conjoined tendon is congenitally absent, the internal oblique being inserted entirely into the sheath of the rectus abdominis. In these circumstances the integrity of Hesselbach's triangle is dependent on the fascia transversalis and a reflexion of Poupart's ligament on to the lateral edge of the rectus sheath. In the last two instances the sac is likely to be diffuse with a wide open mouth and little, if any, neck. In the former it may be funicular. Between 10 and 20 per cent. of inguinal

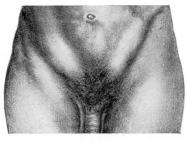

herniæ are direct. Often the patient is an elderly man with poor abdominal musculature, as shown by the presence of Malgaigne's bulgings (fig. 615). Predisposing factors are a chronic cough and straining on micturition. Exceptionally, a direct hernia appears in a young man with well-developed ab-

Fig. 615.—Malgaigne's bulgings.

Sir Frederick Treves, 1853–1923. Surgeon, London Hospital.
Joseph François Malgaigne, 1806–1865. Professor of Surgery, Paris.

dominal musculature ; its origin is then extremely probably traumatic.

Direct herniæ rarely attain a large size, and they do not descend into the scrotum because they are behind the transversalis fascia. Fifty-five per cent. are bilateral (Murray) (fig. 616). In contradistinction to an oblique inguinal hernia, a direct inguinal hernia lies behind the spermatic cord. A finger inserted into the external abdominal ring passes directly backwards into the abdomen. The deep epigastric artery lies lateral to the aperture, but because of its small size and the nature of its coverings, it cannot be felt. " Those who pretend to feel it surrender themselves to a flattering delusion " (Macready). At operation the distinguishing features are that the sac lies medially to the deep epigastric artery, and the spermatic cord is not attached to the wall of the sac. The sac is often smaller than the hernial mass would indicate, the protruding mass being composed, to a large extent, of extraperitoneal fat. A portion of the bladder is liable to be encountered in this tissue on the medial side. Direct inguinal herniæ that have stretched an intact conjoined tendon over them, or those in which the conjoined tendon is absent, never strangulate. Those that pass through the conjoined tendon rarely do so.

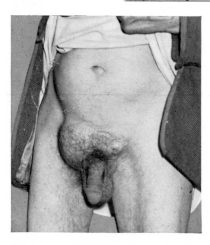

Fig. 616.— Bilateral direct inguinal herniæ.

Injury to the ilio-hypogastric or ilio-inguinal nerves during the gridiron operation for appendicitis appears to be associated with the development of a right inguinal hernia, usually, but not necessarily, of the direct variety (see also p. 928).

Treatment.—When there is no contraindication to operation, such as a chronic cough or poor abdominal musculature, operation is advised. In a diffuse variety there is no need to excise the sac ; it can be invaginated by a purse-string suture.

Robert W. Murray, Contemporary. Consulting Surgeon, David Lewis Northern Hospital, Liverpool.
J. F. C. H. Macready, 1850–1907. Surgeon to the Great Northern (now Royal Northern) Hospital, London.

The posterior wall of the inguinal canal is repaired by one of the more elaborate methods described already.

DUAL (Syn. SADDLE-BAG ; PANTALOON) HERNIA

There is a direct and an oblique hernia present on the same side. The deep epigastric vessels separate the two sacs. The condition is not a rarity, and is stated to be a rather common cause of recurrence, one of the sacs having been overlooked at the time of operation. By traction on the oblique sac, the direct sac can often be drawn lateral to the deep epigastric vessels, thus converting the two sacs into one.

SLIDING INGUINAL HERNIA (Syn. HERNIE-EN-GLISSADE)

Sliding herniæ are due to slipping of the posterior parietal peritoneum and the underlying cellular tissue, and it thus comes about that the posterior wall of the sac is not formed by the peritoneum, but by the cæcum on the right (fig. 617), and a portion of the pelvic colon and its mesocolon on the left.

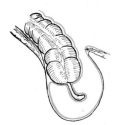

FIG. 617.—Hernie-en-glissade.

Sliding herniæ are nearly always found in middle-aged or elderly men. They are not uncommon, particularly on the right side. Any large globular inguinal hernia descending into the scrotum in a middle-aged or elderly man should be suspected of being a sliding hernia. The diagnosis cannot be made confidently before operation unless the patient has had a barium enema or a barium meal. These herniæ are subject to the same complications as other inguinal herniæ. It should be noted that the presence of the cæcum and appendix in the sac of a right inguinal hernia does not necessarily imply that the hernia is a sliding one. The cæcum with a complete investment of peritoneum, together with the appendix, is not infrequently found in large, oblique, right inguinal herniæ. The condition is a congenital abnormality due, it is believed, to the primitive cæcum becoming attached to the gubernaculum during intrauterine life.

The **operative treatment** is more difficult than in either of the foregoing forms of inguinal hernia. Great care must be taken to open the peritoneum lying over the middle or upper part of the anterior wall of the sac, and not to incise the fundus of the sac, which often consists of bowel wall. The possibility of a portion of the bladder being in the postero-medial part of the sac wall should be remembered. On the left side care must be taken to avoid damaging the sigmoid vessels. In most cases it is sufficient to excise the antero-medial portion of the sac and to close the opening in the peritoneum with a purse-string suture. The ptosed viscus is then reduced inside the abdominal wall. Herniorrhaphy by one of the methods which darn the posterior wall of the inguinal canal should be carried out, so as to form a floor upon which the ptosed viscus can rest. Some surgeons consider that orchidectomy is advisable so that the inguinal canal can be closed completely.

RECURRENT INGUINAL HERNIA

Recurrence after an operation for an inguinal hernia is more common in the case of a direct than an oblique hernia (fig. 618). In the former the recurrence rate is about 20 per cent. ; in the latter it is at least 10 per cent.

DIRECT.   INDIRECT.

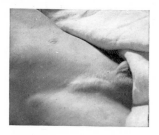

FIG. 618.—Recurrent oblique inguinal hernia.

In most instances the recurrence takes place within a year, but it may occur five years or more after the operation.

Many recurrent oblique herniæ are direct, but in a number of cases the recurrence is oblique, the new sac passing along the spermatic cord. In direct herniæ the recurrence occurs through Hesselbach's triangle, as did its predecessor. The following summarises the principal causes of recurrence :

Pre-operative.—Faulty selection of cases (e.g. those with Malgaigne's bulging, fig. 615)

Operative.—Faulty technique.

(a) Failure to ligate the neck as high as possible. A collar of extra-peritoneal fat is the guide for the correct site for the ligation.

(b) Tying stitches too tightly so that intervening tissues are devitalised.

(c) Imperfect hæmostasis, predisposing to infection.

Post-operative.—(a) Infection of the wound.

        (b) Constant cough.

        (c) Inadequate convalescence.

Treatment : Operative Treatment.—The skin scar is excised and the inguinal canal is opened. Dense adhesions are often encountered during the dissection of the inguinal canal. The sac is freed and excised, being ligated or sutured as high as possible. The inguinal canal is repaired by darning with floss silk or by one of the methods of hernioplasty. If Poupart's ligament is found to be weakened by the previous operation, Cooper's ligament can be used as the inferior point of attachment.

A truss is often advisable in cases of recurrent direct hernia when the patient has poor abdominal musculature. Injection treatment may be used in addition.

INTERSTITIAL INGUINAL HERNIA (*Syn.* INTERPARIETAL HERNIA)

Interstitial hernia is an uncommon condition usually occurring in males, and often associated with some degree of maldescent of the testis. An interstitial inguinal hernia is one in which the sac or a diverticulum thereof passes between two of the layers of the abdominal wall (fig. 619).

Inguino-superficial.—The sac emerges at the external ring and passes between the external oblique aponeurosis and the skin. Usually the testis is present in the swelling and the corresponding side of the scrotum is empty. The diagnosis presents no difficulty.

Intermuscular.—A diverticulum from an oblique inguinal hernia, or the whole sac, may insinuate itself between the muscle layers of the abdominal wall. In exceptional cases where there is a bilocular sac, it may be possible to feel the diverticulum fill as the contents of the sac are reduced. If strangulation occurs, it is often of the " en masse " variety (see p. 577).

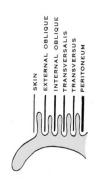

FIG. 619. — The positions that an interstitial diverticulum may occupy. The diverticulum alone may be present in any of the varieties, particularly the most superficial.

Sir Astley Cooper, 1768–1841. Surgeon, Guy's Hospital, London.

Properitoneal.—The hernia is usually bilocular, and is subject to the same danger of strangulation as the foregoing variety, from which it cannot be distinguished except at operation.

FEMORAL HERNIA

Surgical Anatomy.—The femoral canal is $\frac{1}{2}$ inch (1·25 cm.) long, and is conical, the base being directed upwards, where it is oval in shape, its transverse diameter measuring $\frac{1}{2}$ inch. The base is formed by the femoral ring, which is closed by a condensation of extraperitoneal tissue called the femoral septum. The latter is pierced by lymphatic vessels. The femoral canal contains areolar fat, lymphatic vessels, and the lymph node of Cloquet.

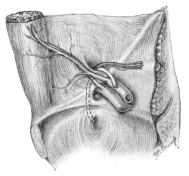

The femoral ring is bounded :

Anteriorly by Poupart's ligament.

Posteriorly by Astley Cooper's ligament, the pubic bone, and the fascia over the pectineus.

Medially by the concave knife-like edge of Gimbernat's ligament (fig. 620), which is also prolonged along the ileo-pectineal line as Astley Cooper's ligament.

Fig. 620.—The femoral ring and its immediate neighbourhood from within. The dotted structure is an abnormal obturator artery.

Laterally by a thin septum separating it from the femoral vein.

A hernia passing down the femoral canal descends vertically as far as the saphenous opening (fig. 621). Because of the narrowness of the canal at this point and the attachment of the superficial fascia to the lower part of the circumference of

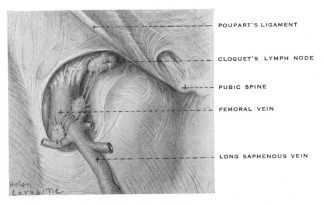

POUPART'S LIGAMENT

CLOQUET'S LYMPH NODE

PUBIC SPINE

FEMORAL VEIN

LONG SAPHENOUS VEIN

FIG. 621.—The relations of the saphenous opening.

Jules Germain Cloquet, 1790–1883. Professor of Clinical Surgery, Paris.
Antonio Gimbernat y Arbos, 1742–1790. Professor of Anatomy and Surgeon to the Santa Cruz Hospital, Barcelona.

the saphenous opening, the hernial sac is directed forwards,
pushing before it the cribriform fascia ; it then curves upwards
towards Poupart's ligament (fig. 622).   While it is confined to
the femoral canal the hernia is small, owing
to the inelastic walls of the femoral canal, but
once it escapes through the saphenous opening into the loose areolar tissue of the groin,
it enlarges, sometimes consider-
ably.   A fully distended femoral
hernia assumes the shape of a
retort (fig. 623), and its bulbous
extremity is often above
Poupart's ligament.   By the
time the contents have pursued so tortuous a path they are
usually irreducible, if not strangulated.

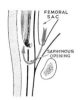

FIG.   622.—The
path taken by a
large femoral
hernia.

FIG. 623.

Throughout an operation for the repair of a femoral hernia, *on
the lateral side* the femoral vein, with the internal saphenous
vein emptying into it, must be protected.   *On the medial side*
of the neck of the sac the bladder must be identified and avoided.

Sometimes a diverticulum of the bladder finds its way down the femoral
canal, usually in association with a femoral hernia.   The condition should
be strongly suspected when two sacs are found.

An abnormal obturator artery arising from the deep epigastric
artery is present in fully 25 per cent. of cases ; some put it as
high as 40 per cent.   In its dangerous form (fig. 624) it was

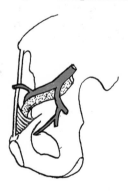
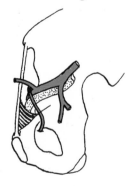
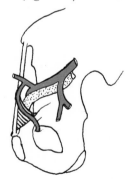

FIG. 624.

(a) Normal obturator
artery.

(b) Abnormal obturator
artery.   Non-dangerous
form.

(c) The same.   Danger-
ous form.   If Gimber-
nat's ligament is divided
from below, the artery
will be severed.

a source of great anxiety to a former generation of surgeons who practised the " lower " operation for strangulated femoral hernia. With the full exposure of the neck of the sac afforded by the inguinal route, this blood-vessel ceases to perturb the operator.

Ætiology.—Because a diverticulum of peritoneum passing into the femoral canal has never been found at necropsy on a new-born infant, and because femoral hernia is extremely rare in the early years of life, most consider that it is an acquired condition. Murray found an empty femoral peritoneal sac in 23 per cent. of 200 adult necropsies, and some believe that this lends support to the theory that a femoral hernia, like an oblique inguinal hernia, occurs into a preformed sac.

Clinical Features.—Femoral hernia is very rare before the age of fifteen, and extremely rare before the age of five. Between twenty and forty years of age the prevalence rises, and continues to old age. The condition is twice as common in females as in males. It is more common in women who have borne children than in nullipara ; consequently in many cases the increased intra-abdominal pressure of pregnancy must be responsible for the development of the hernia. Femoral hernia is twice as common on the right side (fig. 625) as it is on the left, and in 20 per cent. of cases it is bilateral. The symptoms to which a femoral hernia gives rise are less marked than those of an inguinal hernia. Adherence of omentum may cause a dragging pain, but the most usual complaint in an uncomplicated femoral hernia is the presence of a swelling. Oc-

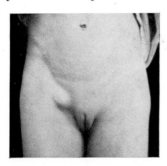

FIG. 625.—Right femoral hernia.

casionally numbness in the corresponding thigh is the principal symptom. Often a small femoral hernia gives rise to so little inconvenience that it is disregarded for years, until one day it strangulates. A small femoral hernia may be unnoticed by the patient. Although very large sacs are sometimes present, on the whole a femoral hernia is small and, especially in the obese, is difficult to find.

Differential Diagnosis
A reducible femoral hernia has to be distinguished :
(*a*) *From an Inguinal Hernia*
1. The swelling as seen when the patient stands is more laterally placed

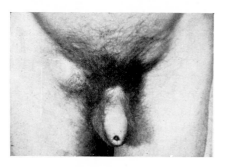

Fig. 626.—The patient has a left inguinal and a right femoral hernia.

than that of an inguinal hernia (fig. 626). In typical cases the swelling is manifestly below Poupart's ligament.

2. The neck of an inguinal hernia lies above and medial to the spine of the pubis, that of a femoral hernia below and lateral. If the spine of the pubis cannot be detected easily, the tendon of the adductor longus should be followed upwards.

3. When the tip of the little finger is insinuated into the external abdominal ring and the inguinal canal is found to be empty, or if the edges of the external abdominal ring are defined but will not admit the tip of the finger, then obviously the swelling cannot be an inguinal hernia.

(b) *From a Saphena Varix.*—An enlarged saphenous vein without obvious varicose veins in the neighbourhood is very liable to be mistaken for a reducible femoral hernia.

Both swellings appear when the patient stands and both disappear when she lies down. In both there is an impulse on coughing. A saphena varix (fig. 627) will, however, impart a fluid thrill to the examining fingers when the patient coughs, and usually a venous hum can be heard when a stethoscope is applied over the swelling.

(c) *From a Psoas Abscess.*—An examination of the back will usually clarify the diagnosis. In addition there is often a fluctuating swelling —an iliac abscess—which communicates with the swelling in question (fig. 628).

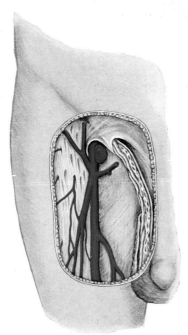

Fig. 627.—Saphena varix.

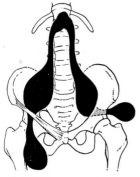

Fig. 628.—A psoas abscess appearing beneath Poupart's ligament may simulate a reducible femoral hernia. Likewise, when it points in the buttock, a gluteal hernia has been suspected. (*After Calot.*)

(*d*) *From a distended psoas bursa.*
The bursa disappears when the thigh is flexed.

(*e*) *From an obturator hernia* (see p. 596).

An **irreducible femoral hernia** (fig. 629) has to be distinguished :

(*a*) *From an Irreducible Inguinal Hernia.*—Even when it overlaps Poupart's ligament, a femoral hernia always lies to the lateral side of the pubic spine.

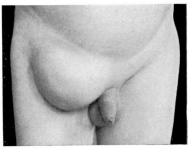

FIG. 629.—An irreducible femoral hernia with its fundus overlying Poupart's ligament.

(*b*) *From an Enlarged Femoral Lymph Node.*—If there are other enlarged nodes in the region the diagnosis is tolerably simple, but when one node only is enlarged, and that node is situated in or near the femoral canal, the diagnosis may be impossible unless there is a lead, such as an infected wound or abrasion on the corresponding limb or on the perineum.

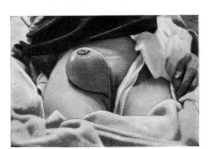

FIG. 630.—Hydrocele of a femoral hernial sac. The patient had previously had ascites, which abated under treatment with digitalin.

(*c*) *From a Hydrocele of a Femoral Hernial Sac.*—The neck of the sac becomes plugged with omentum or by adhesions, and a hydrocele results (fig. 630).

(*d*) *From Rupture of the Adductor Longus* (with hæmatoma).—If there is no superficial bruising, the diagnosis can be extremely difficult.

(*e*) *From a lipoma.*

(*f*) *From a femoral aneurism.*

TREATMENT OF FEMORAL HERNIA

Palliative Treatment.—A femoral truss is usually unsatisfactory. Furthermore, the great liability of femoral herniæ to strangulate is sufficient reason for urging the patient to have herniotomy performed. If necessary, the operation can be carried out under local anæsthesia.

Operative Treatment.—There are many methods of performing femoral herniotomy : the most generally accepted is the trans-inguinal operation.

TRANS-INGUINAL (LOTHEISSEN'S) OPERATION

The bladder is emptied by a catheter immediately before commencing the operation. An incision is made ½ inch (1·25 cm.) above and parallel to the inner two-thirds of Poupart's ligament, exposing the external oblique aponeurosis overlying the inguinal canal.

Georg Lotheissen, Contemporary. Surgeon, Kaiser Franz Josef Hospital, Vienna.

Femoral Stage.—The lower margin of skin and superficial fascia are dissected downwards below Poupart's ligament, and the lower margin of the wound is retracted to expose the deep fascia of the thigh and the related saphenous opening with the fat surrounding the body of the sac. The coverings of the sac are incised somewhat to the medial side, so as to be well away from the internal saphenous vein. The coverings, which are remarkably substantial compared with the contained sac, are peeled off by gauze dissection, each covering being incised before this procedure. When the sac is reached, if it is empty it will appear more opaque and whiter than its coverings ; when it is not empty the sac can be made to move over its contents. In either event the sac is cleared until its narrow neck can be seen disappearing beneath Poupart's ligament. If the sac is not empty, its fundus is opened. In the rare event of intestine being present in the sac, this is reduced into the peritoneal cavity by finger pressure. If thickened or adherent omentum is present, it is transfixed and ligated securely. The ligated stump or stumps of it are gently pushed through the neck of the sac into the abdomen. If the sac is a comparatively large one with omentum adherent to it, its neck is clamped about $\frac{1}{2}$ inch below Poupart's ligament and the body of the sac is excised. In other circumstances the sac is left alone for the time being.

Inguinal Stage.—The external oblique aponeurosis is incised in the line of its fibres in the length of the incision, the external abdominal ring being divided. The edges of the aponeurosis are dissected back to expose the conjoined tendon above and Poupart's ligament below. The cremaster muscle is reflected and the spermatic cord (or the round ligament) is elevated from its bed and retracted upwards and medially, so as to expose the posterior wall of the inguinal canal. The deep epigastric vessels are identified and an incision parallel to Poupart's ligament is made medially to these vessels through the fascia transversalis. If in the course of the dissection about to be made abnormal obturator vessels are encountered, they are divided between ligatures. The extraperitoneal fat is displaced in an upward direction, exposing the peritoneum. In this way the abdominal aspect of the neck of the sac passing through the femoral ring is displayed. If this peritoneal protrusion is cleared from fat and areolar tissue, first on the medial side exposing Gimbernat's ligament, and then very carefully on the lateral side, where it is in juxtaposition to the femoral vein, the sac (or the stump of it if the body has been excised from below) may be withdrawn by traction into the inguinal wound. If this manœuvre cannot be effected easily, the peritoneum above the neck of the sac is opened and a hæmostat is passed into the sac to grasp the fundus or, when the fundus has been excised, the stump that remains. The hæmostat is withdrawn, thus inverting the sac into the peritoneal wound. The sac having been delivered into the inguinal wound by one of these measures, the parietal peritoneum in relation to the neck is still further freed from the extraperitoneal tissue, particular care being taken to dissect away the bladder on the medial side. The sac is transfixed and ligated flush with the peritoneum, and excised. If the peritoneum has been opened, the opening is closed.

Repair of the Femoral Ring and the Inguinal Canal.—Three sutures are passed through the periosteum and Astley Cooper's ligament overlying the ilio-pectineal line, care being taken to protect the femoral vein (fig. 631). The free ends of these sutures are passed from the deep to the superficial surface of the conjoined tendon, which, when the stitches are tightened and knotted, is brought down and apposed to the ilio-pectineal line. If the conjoined tendon cannot be approximated to Cooper's ligament without tension, the anterior sheath of the rectus muscle may be incised. This mobilises the conjoined tendon considerably, but leaves a gaping defect in the rectus sheath. The edges of the defect are fastened to the rectus muscle by a running suture (Tanner's slide).

Alternative procedure. — The stitches traversing Cooper's ligament are passed through the inner third of Poupart's ligament, thus approximating these two structures. Recent statistics show that this method is followed by a higher recurrence rate than after approximating the conjoined tendon to Cooper's ligament.

Whichever of these expedients is employed, it is necessary to repair the lateral part of the opening in the transversalis fascia. The spermatic cord (or round ligament) is replaced, the cremaster muscle united, and the external oblique aponeurosis approximated by a running suture. The skin is closed.

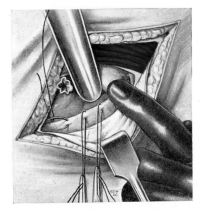

FIG. 631.—Method of placing the deep sutures referred to in the text. The finger is protecting the femoral vein.

Operation for a Recurrent Femoral Hernia.—Recurrence after operation is much less frequent than is the case in inguinal herniæ. After excision of the sac the femoral ring can be fortified by darning Cooper's ligament to the conjoined tendon with a strip of fascia taken from the external oblique, or by floss silk.

Strangulated Femoral Hernia.—It cannot be emphasised too strongly that femoral herniæ frequently strangulate, and gangrene often develops rapidly. This is because of the narrow unyielding nature of the femoral ring and the tortuous course taken by the sac. In 40 per cent. of cases of strangulated femoral hernia the obstructing agent (fig. 632) is not Gimbernat's ligament, but the neck of the femoral sac itself (Souttar).

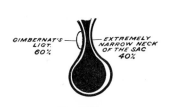

FIG. 632.

In extremely rare instances strangulation occurs at the saphenous opening, either by meshes of the cribriform fascia or the sharp upper edge of the saphenous opening.

A point upon which great emphasis should be placed is the frequent occurrence of a **Richter's hernia** (partial enterocele) (fig. 633). When only a portion of the lumen of the intestine is strangulated, the femoral swelling is sometimes no larger than a cherry. The patient may not vomit, or only vomits once or

Norman Cecil Tanner, Contemporary. Surgeon, St James' Hospital, London.
Sir Henry Souttar, Contemporary. Consulting Surgeon, London Hospital.

twice. Intestinal colic is present, but the patient, not having complete intestinal obstruction, may continue to have the bowels opened naturally, or at any rate respond to enemata. For these reasons gangrene of the knuckle of bowel has often occurred before operation is undertaken.

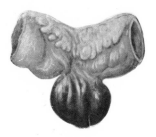

Fig. 633. — Gangrenous Richter's hernia from a case of strangulated femoral hernia.

Large irreducible femoral hernias of some standing often strangulate. Strangulated omentocele is a frequent occurrence in this situation.

Treatment.—Taxis should not be attempted. Immediate operation, if performed soon enough, is a life-saving and entirely satisfactory measure.

Operation for Strangulated Femoral Hernia.—The steps of the operation are similar to those described for non-strangulated femoral hernia, with the following important additions :

Femoral stage.—When the sac has been isolated from its coverings a dry pack should be placed beneath it. As soon as the sac is opened the blood-stained, highly infected fluid that escapes will be absorbed by the pack. A mechanical sucker is an advantage at this stage. When all the fluid has been mopped up the pack is changed for a warm moist one which envelops the sac beneath the lower margin of the wound during the inguinal stage of the operation.

Inguinal stage.—The peritoneum above the neck of the sac is opened as soon as it has been displayed clearly. Having inspected the abdominal aspect of Gimbernat's ligament, and if necessary having ligated and divided or retracted abnormal obturator vessels, a director is passed through the neck of the sac, and the neck of the sac on the medial side, together with Gimbernat's ligament, is nicked with a scalpel in two, or at the most three, places. This divides the obstructing agent, whether it be Gimbernat's ligament or a fibrotic neck of the sac. If necessary, Gimbernat's ligament can be partially avulsed from the pubic bone by a finger passed between it and the neck of the sac. By these means the very narrow femoral ring is widened considerably, so much so that, aided by gentle pressure from below, it is possible to withdraw strangulated intestine into the inguinal wound, and from thence to the surface. Strangulated intestine is dealt with according to circumstances, as described on p. 454. By reason of the free access to the mesentery afforded by the inguinal route, should resection of the intestine be necessary it can be undertaken much more readily than in the extremely narrow confines afforded by a purely femoral approach to the hernia. Strangulated omentum is best ligated and divided from below Poupart's ligament.

UMBILICAL HERNIA

Exomphalos is a rare condition occurring about once in every 6,000 births. Sometimes it is associated with other congenital abnormalities, such as spina bifida or a cleft palate. The condition is due to failure of all or part of the mid-gut to return to the abdominal cavity during early fœtal life. Sometimes a large sac ruptures during birth and the infant is born eviscerated (fig. 634). When the sac remains unruptured it is semi-translucent, and although very thin it consists of an amniotic membrane, a middle layer of Wharton's jelly, and an inner layer of extracœlomic peritoneum. In rare cases there is no peritoneal layer of the sac. The size of the sac varies very considerably. It may be only a finger-breadth expansion of the umbilical cord ; on the other hand, the pouch is sometimes as large as a fœtal

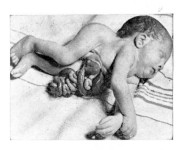

Fig. 634.—Exomphalos. The delicate amnionic covering burst during delivery.

head. Within the sac lies a varying amount of small and large intestine, and in 50 per cent. of cases a portion of the liver. In relatively small sacs the umbilical cord is attached to the summit of the protrusion and a possible accident is the inclusion of a loop of intestine or a Meckel's diverticulum in the ligature applied to the umbilical cord. In large sacs containing a portion of the liver the umbilical cord is attached to the inferior aspect of the swelling. The blood-supply to the outer walls of the sac was maternal, and within twelve to twenty-four hours they become dehydrated, and unless infection is prevented peritonitis supervenes.

Treatment.—(*a*) *Conservative.*—When the amount of extra-abdominal bowel is not great there is a good prospect of the sac becoming slowly epithelialised, provided infection can be prevented. To this end penicillin and sulphanilamide cream, together with a light gauze dressing, is applied at regular intervals. During conservative treatment a possible complication is intestinal obstruction, in which event as soon as gastric aspiration and the administration of fluid therapy have rendered the patient fit to undergo it, operation is carried out.

(*b*) *Operative.*—When the sac is large and contains part of the liver, which can be seen through the sac and is always present if the umbilical cord is attached to the lower margin of the sac, operation within the first few hours of life is necessary, for the sac is too large to epithelialise, and it often ruptures. The infant should not be fed in order to prevent further distension of the contents of the sac. A drip blood-transfusion is given and continued throughout the operation. A circular incision is made through the sac and its coverings at their junction with the abdominal wall. The umbilical arteries and vein are caught in hæmostats, trans-fixed, and ligated during this step. After separation of intestine from the sac wall by the finger, the sac is removed. If a portion of it is firmly attached to the liver, all but that part of the sac is cut away. The pro-lapsed viscera are reduced inside the abdomen, hollow viscera first and the liver last. It may be necessary to enlarge the opening in an upward direction before reduction is possible. If the defect in the abdominal wall is relatively small the peritoneum and posterior rectus sheath can be dissected and their edges united, after which the muscle and skin are closed by through-and-through sutures of silkworm gut or stainless steel wire. If the gap is so large that it is found impossible to approximate its edges, by undercutting the skin on either side, the edges of that elastic structure can be brought together, even if counter incisions towards the loin have to be made to permit closure. Three weeks later, when the wound is reopened, it will be found that the peritoneum and muscles can be closed in layers. In all cases the wound is dressed with penicillin and sulphanilamide powder, gauze, and a firm adhesive plaster. Ascorbic acid 100 mg. is given daily. For the first few days aspiration through an indwelling gastric tube may be necessary to relieve distension. The stitches are removed on the tenth day.

Umbilical Hernia in Infancy and Childhood.—On rare occasions a well-developed umbilical hernia is present at birth. The condition is believed to be due to intrauterine epithelialisation

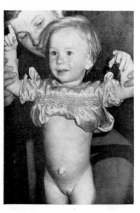

of a small exomphalos. In most cases of umbilical hernia appearing during infancy the hernia occurs into a congenital sac. Usually the first indication of an umbilical hernia is a small protrusion at the umbilicus which is noticed when the infant cries. Unsupported, the swelling becomes spherical and is present apart from crying. As it increases in size it tends to assume a conical shape (fig. 635). The diameter of an umbilical hernia appearing during infancy rarely measures more than 1 or at the most 2 inches (2·5 to 5 cm.).

FIG. 635.—Congenital umbilical hernia.

Such a hernia may be symptomless, but it sometimes gives rise to attacks of abdominal pain which are relieved by reducing the hernia. It is most unusual for obstruction or strangulation to occur in an umbilical hernia during infancy.

Conservative treatment is curative in about 75 per cent. of cases. The earlier it is commenced the better and quicker is the result, but at the best it will take six months. In early infancy the hernia can usually be controlled completely by the application of two strips of adhesive zinc oxide plaster 1 inch (2·5 cm.) in width applied in an X-shaped manner (fig. 636) so as to produce a ridge

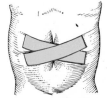

FIG. 636.—Method of strapping a small umbilical hernia in an infant.

of skin and subcutaneous tissue on either side of the umbilicus, which is kept enfolded. The strapping must be renewed when it shows evidence of becoming loose, and the mother should be instructed in the method of reapplication of the plaster in case it inadvertently becomes displaced while at home. The plaster must be worn continuously, and the child is washed, not bathed, during the whole period of treatment. For larger protrusions 1 inch (2·5 cm.) in diameter or more, a strip of 3-inch (7·5 cm.) strapping applied transversely so as to approximate the rectus muscles is satisfactory. Sometimes a year or more of such supportive treatment is necessary before the hernial opening becomes fibrosed.

Operative Treatment.—After the age of two years, if the appearance of the hernia cannot be accounted for by increased intra-abdominal pressure such as that produced by tuberculous peritonitis, portal hypertension, chronic cough, atresia meati or the pot-belly of rickets, or if conservative measures before the age of two have failed, operative treatment should be undertaken.

The apex of the hernia is grasped in tissue-holding forceps and retracted strongly towards the patient's head. A transverse incision about 1 inch long is made at the junction of the skin of the base of the hernia with that of the abdominal wall. When traction is released the incision will be found to be semi-circular around the lower half of the umbilicus. By dissection the fibrous wall of the hernia will be encountered beneath the subcutaneous tissue. The base of the fibrous wall is incised transversely, and the very thin peritoneal coat will come into view. Using fine, blunt-pointed scissors, the peritoneal sac is dissected from the fibrous wall throughout its circumference. At the apex the peritoneal sac is intimately adherent to the cutaneous umbilical cicatrix, and the peritoneum must be dissected from the skin with a scalpel. Not uncommonly the skin is nicked during this step ; the opening is closed easily with a single stitch. The peritoneal sac has now been separated completely from its attachments. In the rare event of a portion of omentum or vitello-intestinal duct being attached to the interior of the sac, it is opened. A tag of omentum is transfixed and divided near its attachment ; a vitello-intestinal band is excised and its intestinal attachment invaginated. The sac is ligated flush with the parietal peritoneum. The lower edge of the fibrous sac wall is stitched to the upper fibrous rim of the umbilical opening. What was the fibrous wall of the sac is imbricated over the first layer and attached to the rectus sheaths in the lower part of the wound. The skin may be closed by a subcuticular stitch or interrupted sutures.

In older children, and especially in youths, umbilical hernia is uncommon.

Umbilical Hernia in Adults.—It should be noted that umbilical hernia in adults often does not occur through the umbilicus.

It is a protrusion through the linea alba just above the umbilicus or, occasionally, just below that structure. These are, strictly speaking, para-umbilical herniæ. The hernia can occur through the umbilical cicatrix, when it may be a recurrence of the infantile form. As an umbilical hernia enlarges it becomes rounded or oval in shape, with a tendency to sag downwards

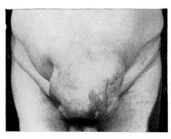

FIG. 637.—Large para-umbilical hernia.

(fig. 637). Umbilical herniæ in adults increase steadily in size and frequently attain very large dimensions. The neck of the sac is often remarkably narrow as compared with the size of the sac and the volume of its contents, which consist of omentum often accompanied by small intestine and, alternatively or in addition, a portion of the transverse colon. In old-standing cases the sac sometimes becomes loculated due to adherence of omentum to its fundus.

Clinical Features.—Women are affected five times more frequently than men. The patient is usually corpulent and between the ages of thirty-five and fifty. Increasing obesity with flabbiness of the abdominal muscles is an important factor in the production of umbilical hernia in an adult, and in women repeated pregnancy favours its occurrence. These herniæ soon become irreducible because of omental adhesions within the sac. A large umbilical hernia causes a local dragging pain by its weight. Gastro-intestinal symptoms are common and are sometimes due to traction on the stomach or transverse colon from greater omentum becoming adherent to the sac. Often there are transient attacks of intestinal colic due, almost certainly, to subacute intestinal obstruction. In old-standing cases intertrigo of the adjacent surfaces of the skin (fig. 638) is a troublesome complication.

FIG. 638.

Treatment.—Umbilical trusses are difficult to keep in position, and so far as controlling the hernia is concerned an abdominal belt is very little better. Untreated, the hernia increases in size, and more and more of its contents become irreducible. Eventually, in not a few instances, strangulation occurs. It is for these reasons that early operation should be advised in nearly all cases.

Mayo's Operation for Umbilical Hernia.—A transverse elliptical incision is made about the umbilicus (fig. 639). The neck of the sac is defined and opened. The contents passing through the neck are examined carefully piece by piece. Omentum is ligated and divided ; intestine is reduced into the abdomen. As soon as the contents have been dealt with,

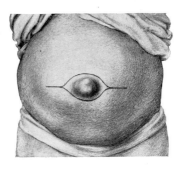

Fig. 639.—Para-umbilical hernia showing Mayo's incision.

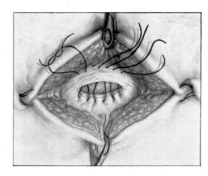

Fig. 640.—Mayo's operation for umbilical hernia.

the neck of the sac is amputated. The peritoneum and the aponeurosis on both sides of the umbilical ring are incised transversely for 1 inch (2·5 cm.) or more—sufficiently to allow an overlap of 2 or 3 inches (5 or 7·5 cm.). Three to five mattress sutures are then inserted as shown in fig. 640. When this row of mattress sutures has been tied the free upper margin is stitched to the sheath of the rectus abdominis and the aponeurosis in the middle line. It is important to denude this area of fat before stitching the flap in position. In order to prevent recurrence, or when recurrence has taken place, if the general condition of the patient will withstand a slightly more prolonged operation, a skin graft can be stitched over the imbricated portion of the abdominal wall in order to further support the area. The fat and skin are then approximated and the abdomen supported by a firm bandage. The patient should be confined to bed for at least fourteen days, and if she has a tendency to bronchitis, which is not unusual, it is wise to prescribe penicillin, and to order respiratory gymnastics.

Strangulation

Strangulation is a frequent complication of umbilical hernia in adults. Owing to the narrow neck and the fibrous edge of the linea alba, gangrene is liable to supervene unless early operation is carried out.

Operation.—In early cases the operation does not differ from that for non-strangulated cases, except reinforcement by a skin graft is never undertaken. Gangrenous contents are dealt with as in other situations. If the transverse colon is gangrenous, it should be exteriorised by the Paul-Mikulicz' method (see p. 438) and the gangrenous portion excised.

William J. Mayo, 1861–1939. Surgeon, Mayo Clinic, Rochester, U.S.A., described the operation in 1894.

If the ring is large enough to transmit the limbs of the colon unhampered, it is left alone ; otherwise it is enlarged.

Epigastric Hernia (*syn.* fatty hernia of the linea alba) commences as a protrusion of extraperitoneal fat through the linea alba along a point of penetration by a small blood-vessel. Swellings the size of a pea consist of extraperitoneal fat only. If the swelling enlarges it drags a pouch of peritoneum with it, when it becomes a true epigastric hernia. The mouth of the hernia is rarely large enough to permit a portion of a hollow viscus to enter it ; the sac is usually empty or contains a small portion of omentum. An epigastric hernia is usually situated midway between the umbilicus and the xiphisternum. Occasionally two or more herniæ are present one above the other in the middle line in this situation.

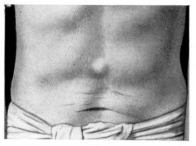

Fig. 641.—Epigastric hernia.

Clinical Features.—A small fatty hernia of the linea alba can be felt better than it can be seen, and may be symptomless, only being discovered in the course of a routine examination. On the other hand, an epigastric hernia consisting entirely of extraperitoneal fat may give rise to local pain and tenderness. When an epigastric hernia attains the size of a hazelnut it contains a pouch of peritoneum ; then it frequently gives rise to great pain which is sometimes associated with nausea and vomiting. An epigastric hernia (fig. 641) with symptoms occurs principally in male manual workers between thirty and forty-five years of age, and is probably a direct result of a sudden strain tearing the interlacing fibres of the aponeurosis. It is not uncommon to find that the patient has not noticed the hernia, but complains of symptoms suggestive of a peptic ulcer ; on the other hand, a patient suffering from a gastric or duodenal ulcer may attribute all his symptoms to the small epigastric hernia. When the symptoms are pain related to taking food, with nausea and vomiting, investigations which include radiography after a barium meal and a fractional test meal should be undertaken. It seems probable that severe gastric symptoms, which often occur without any lesion other than an epigastric hernia, are due to a portion of omentum near the greater curvature of the stomach being caught in the hernia and causing traction on the stomach. In these cases removal of the hernia and repair of the abdominal wall cures the patient. These herniæ sometimes become irreducible, but very rarely do they strangulate.

Treatment.—If the hernia is giving rise to symptoms operation should be undertaken.

A vertical incision is made over the swelling, exposing the linea alba, and the fat is cleared from the hernia by gauze dissection. This separation is possible because the fat of the hernia is covered by fascia transversalis. If the pedicle passing through the linea alba is very slender, it is separated on all sides of the opening by blunt dissection. After ligating the pedicle the small opening in the linea alba is closed by two or three unabsorbable sutures. When the opening is of such a size as to admit the tip of a little finger, after isolating the edges of the opening as described, it is enlarged for $\frac{1}{2}$ inch (1·25 cm.) above and below. The sac with its fatty coverings is dissected until its junction with the parietal peritoneum becomes apparent. The fundus of the sac is opened. Any contained omentum is returned to the peritoneal cavity ; if adherent it is ligated and divided near its attachment. The sac is ligated and excised. The abdominal wall can be repaired satisfactorily by overlapping the aponeurosis in a manner similar to that of the Mayo operation, but vertically instead of horizontally. In cases where the presence of a peptic ulcer cannot be excluded, the opening in the linea alba can be enlarged sufficiently to examine the stomach and duodenum.

Divarication of the recti abdominis is seen principally in elderly multiparæ. When the patient strains a gap can be seen between the recti abdominis below the umbilicus ; through this gap the abdominal contents bulge. When the abdomen is relaxed the fingers can be introduced between the recti.

Treatment.—An abdominal belt is all that is required.

A similar condition is occasionally met with in babies, only the divarication exists above the umbilicus. No treatment is necessary ; as the child develops a spontaneous cure usually results.

Incisional (syn. post-operative) hernia is not uncommon. It can occur after any variety of abdominal incision, but it is more frequent after lower than upper abdominal operations. Infection of the wound plays the largest part in the production of an incisional hernia, and the incidence is highest after operations for peritonitis, notably perforated appendicitis and appendix abscess. Other predisposing causes are severe post-operative cough, post-operative abdominal distension, and obesity. Post-operative hernia presents no difficulty in diagnosis. There are great variations in the degree of herniation.

The hernia may occur through a small portion of the scar, often the lower end, when the hernial sac has a neck.   More frequently there is a diffuse bulging of the whole length of the incision. A post-operative hernia, especially one through a lower abdominal scar, usually steadily increases in size, and more and more of its contents become irreducible.   Sometimes the skin overlying it is so thin and atrophic that normal peristalsis may be seen in the underlying coils of intestine.   Attacks of subacute intestinal obstruction are common, and strangulation may occur at the neck of a small sac or in a loculus of a large one.

Treatment.—*Palliative.*   An abdominal belt is sometimes satisfactory, especially in cases of a hernia through an upper abdominal incision.

Operation is usually advisable when the hernia is situated in the lower abdomen, but, particularly in large herniæ, it is a difficult undertaking.

An elliptical incision is made through normal skin so as to include the stretched scar.   The incision is deepened until normal aponeurosis can be seen on either side of the defect.   In the event of there being a comparatively narrow neck, the operation is conducted in a manner similar to that for an umbilical hernia up to the stage of closure of the abdominal wall.   In the more frequent diffuse hernia the skin must be dissected from the hernial sac.   Often the sac is deficient in places, and omentum or intestine is adherent to the undersurface of the skin, which must be dissected from intestine with great care.   Omentum can be ligated and divided, leaving a portion of it attached to the skin.   On completing this step there are often a number of holes in the peritoneal sac ; each of these is closed.   No attempt is made to remove the sac with its adherent contents.   Attention is then directed to excising scar tissue at the edges of the incision until the layers of the abdominal wall are apparent.   In some cases it is possible to approximate the fascia and muscles without tension ; if this is the case, interrupted sutures of silk or stainless steel wire are used for the approximation, together with deep through-and-through sutures to support the line of suture.   In a number of cases there is an actual loss of substance and some measure to bridge the defect must be employed.   After freeing the peritoneum from the abdominal musculature on either side, usually the peritoneum can be approximated.   A broad fascial patch with many tails can be inserted into the defect and beneath the abdominal wall, and the tails brought out through the muscle and aponeurosis, and sutured over the defect.   Even when the loss of tissue is too great to bring together the edges of the peritoneum, large defects in the abdominal wall have been treated successfully by interposition of tantalum wire mesh to bridge the defect.

OBTURATOR HERNIA

is a condition of great rarity.   The hernia passes through the obturator canal, which is below the femoral ring.   It occurs six times more frequently in women than in men, and most of the patients are over sixty years of age.

The swelling is liable to be overlooked because it is covered by the pectineus. It seldom causes a definite swelling in Scarpa's triangle, but if the limb is flexed, abducted, and rotated outwards, the hernia sometimes becomes more apparent. The leg is usually kept in a semi-flexed position and movement increases the pain. In more than 50 per cent. of cases of strangulated obturator hernia pain is referred to the knee along the course of the geniculate branch of the obturator nerve (fig. 642) (Howship-Romberg sign). On vaginal examination the hernia can sometimes be felt as a tender swelling at the obturator canal.

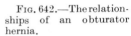

Fig. 642.—The relationships of an obturator hernia.

(*After Sir Cecil Wakeley.*)

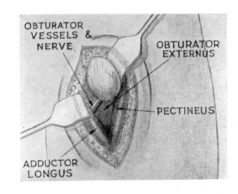

Cases of obturator hernia which have been reported have usually been cases of strangulation, and the diagnosis has not been made until the abdomen has been opened for intestinal obstruction. Having traced the site of obstruction to the obturator canal, the constricting ring can be stretched by inserting a hæmostat and gently opening the jaws, thus avoiding injury to the obturator vessels. Strangulation in this situation is often of the Richter type (see p. 588). The simplest and best method of dealing with the sac is to invert it, ligate the neck, and remove about half the sac. Stitches are passed through the stump and tied, thus forming a plug over the obturator canal, or the broad ligament can be sutured over the foramen.

GLUTEAL AND SCIATIC HERNIÆ

A *gluteal hernia* passes through the great sacro-sciatic notch, either above or below the pyriformis.

A *sciatic hernia* passes through the lesser sacro-sciatic notch.

Swellings under the gluteus maximus cause great difficulty in diagnosis because their individual character is masked by the overlying mass of muscle.

Differential diagnosis must be made between this condition and—

(*a*) A lipoma beneath the gluteus maximus.

(*b*) A cold abscess.

(*c*) A gluteal aneurism.

All doubtful swellings in this situation should be explored by operation.

Like an obturator hernia, these herniæ are only discovered in the course of laparotomy for intestinal obstruction. After the sac has been inverted, ligated, and excised, the opening may be closed by suturing to the edges of the opening a flap of fascia dissected from the pyriformis muscle. Even in non-strangulated cases, after exploring the site, the hernia is best dealt with from an abdominal approach.

Antonio Scarpa, 1747–1832. Anatomist and Surgeon, Venice.
John Howship, 1781–1841. English Surgeon.
M. H. Romberg, 1795–1841. German Neurologist.

Spiegelian hernia (*syn.* hernia through the linea semilunaris ; lateral ventral hernia) is exceedingly uncommon. It is so called because it occurs through the linea semilunaris (linea Spiegelii). As a rule, the hernia only apparently penetrates the abdominal wall, and does not give rise to an obvious swelling ; occasionally, as in Paul's case (fig. 643), there is a large protrusion.

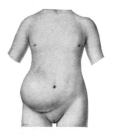

FIG. 643. — Spiegelian hernia.

(*From a photograph of a case under the care of Milroy Paul.*)

LUMBAR HERNIA

Apart from incisional herniæ following kidney operations, and the yielding of a scar of a lumbar abscess which has discharged externally, a hernia occasionally occurs (*a*) through the *superior lumbar triangle*, which is bounded by the 12th rib above, medially by the erector spinæ, and laterally by the posterior border of the internal oblique ; (*b*) through the *inferior lumbar triangle* (*syn.* triangle of Petit) which is bounded below by the crest of the ilium, laterally by the external oblique, and medially by the latissimus dorsi (fig. 644).

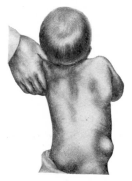

FIG. 644.—Inferior lumbar hernia. (*After Sultan.*)

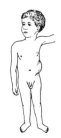

FIG. 645. — Phantom hernia following anterior poliomyelitis.

Differential Diagnosis.—A lumbar hernia must be distinguished from :

(*a*) A cold abscess pointing in this position.

(*b*) Phantom hernia due to local muscular paralysis (fig. 645). Lumbar phantom herniæ can result from many conditions which interfere with the nerve-supply of the affected muscles. We have seen a case follow herpes zoster.

HERNIA THROUGH THE PELVIC FLOOR

Several varieties are encountered :

(*a*) **Antero-lateral perineal hernia** occurs exclusively in women and passes through an opening anterior to the transversus perinei muscle to enter the labium majus. It is more frequent than

(*b*) **Postero-lateral perineal hernia,** which passes through the levator ani to enter the ischio-rectal fossa. This variety is more common in women, but occasionally occurs in men.

These herniæ are nearly always reducible and seldom strangulate. The anterior variety, which reduces backwards and upwards, must be

Adrian van der Spiegel, 1578–1625. Professor of Anatomy and Surgery, Padua.
Milroy Aserappa Paul, Contemporary. Professor of Surgery, University of Ceylon.
Jean Louis Petit 1674–1750. Director, Académie de Chirurgie, Paris.

distinguished from an inguinal hernia, which reduces from the labium majus into the inguinal canal. A lipoma in the labium majus or the ischio-rectal fossa is irreducible and painless.

Treatment.—A combined operation is generally the most satisfactory. The hernia is exposed by an incision directly over it. The sac is opened and its contents are reduced. The sac is cleared from surrounding structures and the wound is closed. With the patient in semi-Trendelenburg position, the abdomen is opened and the mouth of the sac is exposed. The sac is inverted, ligated, and excised, and the pelvic floor is repaired as well as possible.

(*c*) **Median sliding perineal hernia** is a complete prolapse of the rectum (see p. 540).

(*d*) **Post-operative hernia through a perineal scar** is not uncommon after excision of the rectum. It can be repaired by excising the scar, freeing and reducing the contents into the peritoneal cavity, closing the opening in the peritoneum, and approximating the edges of the levator ani. The wound is allowed to heal by granulation in the same way as after a perineal excision of the rectum.

DIAPHRAGMATIC HERNIA

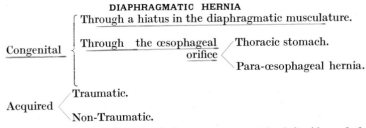

The majority of diaphragmatic herniæ occur on the left side and they are usually congenital. Following war wounds, a number of acquired cases have occurred, but in civil life traumatic cases are of the utmost rarity.

Diaphragmatic herniæ are difficult to diagnose clinically. By X-rays after a barium meal, hollow viscera, which often include the whole or part of the stomach, can be demonstrated occupying a part of the thoracic cavity. Strangulation sometimes occurs (p. 474).

Treatment.—Left phrenic avulsion, by paralysing the corresponding side of the diaphragm, sometimes brings relief. More often, an operation to close the defect should be undertaken. The best approach for this operation is the transthoracic. When the defect is a large one a patch of fascia lata can be utilised to occlude the abnormal opening.

Internal Herniæ, see p. 473.

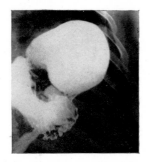

Fig. 646.—Radiograph showing the stomach in the thorax. Case of diaphragmatic hernia.

THE ABDOMINAL WALL

Ruptured rectus abdominis and torn deep epigastric vessels may occur in the following circumstances :

1. From a direct blow.

2. Following violent muscular effort.

3. During late pregnancy or delivery.

4. As a complication of tetanus.

5. Spontaneously during minor strains such as coughing or sneezing.

Except as a result of tetanus (see p. 26) it is probable that only a few fibres of the muscle are ruptured, and the main pathological event is tearing of the deep epigastric artery or, above the umbilicus, the superior epigastric artery.

Clinical Features.—The onset of the condition is accompanied by great pain. Muscular rigidity overlying the hæmorrhage is often extreme. Later, when the extreme rigidity has passed off, a firm mass (a hæmatoma) can be felt beneath the abdominal wall. The bleeding occurs into the extraperitoneal potential space. Occasionally in pregnant women the hæmorrhage from the deep epigastric artery may be so serious as to prove fatal (R. C. Thomas).

Differential Diagnosis.—When it occurs spontaneously or follows indirect violence, and the rigidity is situated in the right lower quadrant of the abdominal wall, the condition is extremely difficult to distinguish from acute appendicitis. When the condition follows direct violence it is impossible to differentiate a torn deep epigastric artery from an intraperitoneal lesion with certainty.

Treatment.—Usually, operation should be performed when the diagnosis is certain, or following direct violence when the condition cannot be distinguished from an intra-abdominal lesion. An incision is made over the affected portion of the rectus muscle, which is split. Blood and blood-clots are evacuated, and often a bleeding artery will need ligating. If the patient is seen twenty-four hours or more after the onset and a mass is palpable, a conservative course may be considered advisable. It will take some weeks before the blood-clot is absorbed, and penicillin should be administered to prevent infection.

Deep Lateral Hæmatoma of the Abdominal Wall.—A hæmatoma more laterally placed than the above following some days after an injury, and spreading beneath the fascia transversalis, is usually due to a rupture of the kidney on the corresponding side (see p. 628).

Rufus C. Thomas, Contemporary. Obstetric Consultant, County Borough of Croydon, England.

DISRUPTION OF AN ABDOMINAL WOUND

Occasionally a laparotomy wound bursts open and viscera are eventrated, usually between the fifth and fifteenth days after operation. The predisposing causes are hasty suture (from necessity), infection, persistent cough, abdominal distension, delayed healing in malignancy, and the too early removal of deep sutures, which should remain in place for ten days.

Prophylaxis.—When infection of the wound has supervened, or in other conditions in which it is thought that the stitches are liable to give way, the abdominal wall should be supported by " corsets " of adhesive plaster. In debilitated and aged subjects wound healing is retarded. The ingestion of vitamins, particularly vitamin C, and a high protein diet is indicated in such cases.

Treatment.—When the wound has disrupted, prompt action is imperative. Protruding intestine should be covered with a warm saline-soaked pack until the patient is anæsthetised, when, after carefully swabbing each coil with saline, it is returned to the abdomen and the abdominal wall is approximated by through-and-through sutures of braided nylon or strong silk. Contrary to what might be thought, peritonitis rarely supervenes.

INFECTIONS

Spreading cellulitis of the abdominal wall is a serious complication of a laparotomy, especially in cases of peritonitis. It presents the same clinical features as cellulitis in other situations.

Treatment.—Penicillin and sulphonamides are given. If after four or five days fluctuation can be elicited, incision into the lateral portions of the infected planes is usually necessary.

Abscess of the abdominal wall is seldom primary, but nearly always secondary to a focus within the abdomen, thorax, or the skeletal framework of the neighbourhood, e.g. ribs, spine, or crest of ilium.

NEOPLASMS OF THE ABDOMINAL WALL

Fibroma (*syn.* desmoid tumour).—Fibroma of the abdominal wall is a simple fibrous tissue tumour arising in the musculo-aponeurotic structures, especially those below the level of the umbilicus.

Ætiology.—Eighty per cent. of cases occur in women who have borne children, and the neoplasm occasionally occurs in scars of old hernial or other abdominal operation wounds. Consequently, trauma, e.g. the stretching of the muscle fibres during pregnancy, is a definite ætiological factor.

Pathology.—The tumour is composed of fibrous tissue containing multi-nucleated plasmodial masses resembling foreign-body giant-cells. It is usually of very slow growth, tending to infiltrate muscle in the immediate

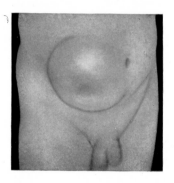

FIG. 647.—Giant-celled sarcoma of the abdominal wall.

neighbourhood, but eventually it undergoes a myxomatous change, when the tumour increases rapidly in size. Metastasis does not occur. Unlike fibromata elsewhere, no case has been recorded in which a sarcomatous change has taken place.

Treatment consists in excision of the neoplasm with a surrounding margin of at least ½ inch (1·25 cm.) of healthy tissue. Unless the tumour is excised widely, recurrence commonly takes place. After removal of a large desmoid tumour a plastic operation to fill the defect in the abdominal wall is required. These tumours are not radio-sensitive.

Sarcoma of the abdominal wall is rare, and is usually of the giant-cell variety (fig. 647). Radiotherapy is the best form of treatment.

THE UMBILICUS

The following table is a symposium of diseases of the umbilicus :

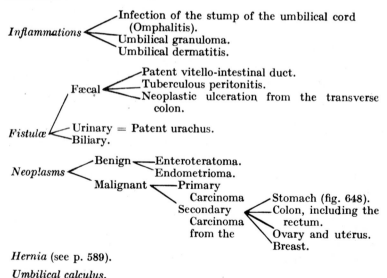

Inflammations — Infection of the stump of the umbilical cord (Omphalitis).
Umbilical granuloma.
Umbilical dermatitis.

Fistulæ — *Fæcal* — Patent vitello-intestinal duct.
Tuberculous peritonitis.
Neoplastic ulceration from the transverse colon.
Urinary = Patent urachus.
Biliary.

Neoplasms — Benign — Enteroteratoma.
Endometrioma.
Malignant — Primary Carcinoma
Secondary Carcinoma from the — Stomach (fig. 648).
Colon, including the rectum.
Ovary and uterus.
Breast.

Hernia (see p. 589).

Umbilical calculus.

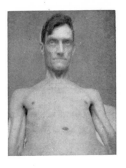

Fig. 648.—Secondary nodule at the umbilicus in a case of carcinoma of the stomach.

A few of these require special consideration.

Omphalitis (inflammation of the stump of the umbilicus) is usually due to a staphylococcal infection, and it may take one of several forms. A virulent infection passing along the umbilical vein before it is obliterated may give rise to liver abscesses and jaundice, which has to be distinguished from other forms of jaundice occurring in infancy (see p. 332). At other times the infection gives rise to a bacteræmia which results in osteomyelitis. If given early enough, penicillin often controls the latter variety of infection. Infection may take the form of a spreading cellulitis of the abdominal wall which usually resolves with treatment by penicillin. Extraperitoneal abscesses can occur (*a*) in the epigastrium from infection spreading from the umbilical vein, and (*b*) in either iliac fossa from infection passing along an umbilical artery. The former, when associated with vomiting, sometimes simulates hypertrophic pyloric stenosis, but the palpable lump is in the middle line and not to the right of it. When an extraperitoneal abscess forms in the right iliac fossa it is liable to be mistaken for an appendix abscess. Pressure over any of these swellings may cause pus to exude from the umbilicus. Aspiration and the instillation of penicillin sometimes cures the condition ; if this is not effective within a few days the abscess should be drained.

Mild local infection of the umbilicus is common after the cord has separated ; it usually quickly responds to applications of penicillin and sulphanilamide powder.

Granuloma.—Chronic infection of the umbilical cicatrix which continues for weeks causes granulation tissue to pout at the umbilicus. There is no means of distinguishing this condition from a commencing enteroteratoma, except biopsy, a procedure which is not justifiable. Usually an umbilical granuloma can be destroyed by cauterisation with a silver nitrate stick, keeping the umbilicus dry with antiseptic powder. An enteroteratoma continues to proliferate in spite of this measure.

Dermatitis of and around the umbilicus is common at all times in life. Fungus and parasitic infections are more difficult to eradicate from the umbilicus than from abdominal skin. Sometimes the dermatitis is consequent upon a discharge from the umbilicus, as is the case in enteroteratomata.

Fistulæ.—The umbilicus, being a scar, and a central abdominal scar, it is understandable that a slow leak from any viscus is liable to track to the surface at this point.

For instance, an enlarged inflamed gall bladder perforating at its fundus has been known to discharge its contents, including gall-stones, through the umbilicus. Again, we were confronted with a middle-aged woman in whom an unremitting flow of pus from a fistula at the umbilicus led to the discovery of a length of gauze left in the peritoneal cavity during hysterectomy five years previously.

Added to this, certain embryological remnants, to wit, the vitello-intestinal duct and the allantois (urachus), open here in early foetal life. Accordingly, it has been aptly remarked that the umbilicus is a creek into which many fistulous streams may open.

Patent Vitello-intestinal Duct has been discussed on p. 411.

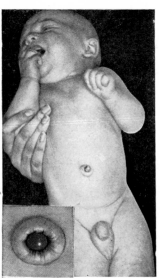

FIG. 649.—Enteroteratoma of the umbilicus.

Unlike the omphalo-mesenteric duct, usually a **Patent urachus** does not reveal its presence until maturity, or even old age. This is because contractions of the bladder commence at the apex of the organ and pass towards the base. A patent urachus, opening as it does at the extreme apex of the bladder, is temporarily closed during micturition, and so the potential urinary stream to the umbilicus is cut off. So it comes about that the fistula remains unobtrusive until a day when the organ is over-full, usually due to some form of obstruction, e.g. an enlarged prostate.

Treatment.—Usually no treatment is necessary other than that of removing the lower urinary obstruction. If the leak continues or a cyst develops in connection with the urachus, removal of the structure by dissection is indicated.

Enteroteratoma (*syn.* raspberry tumour) is commonly seen in infants (fig. 649), but occasionally later in

life.   The condition is due to a partially (occasionally a completely) unobliterated vitello-intestinal duct.   Mucosa prolapsing through the umbilicus gives rise to a raspberry-like tumour,
which is moist with mucus and tends to bleed.

Treatment.—If the tumour is pedunculated, a cotton ligature
can be tied around it, and in a few days the polypus drops off.
If the tumour reappears after this procedure, umbilectomy is
indicated.   Sometimes a patent vitello-intestinal duct, or more
often a vitello-intestinal band, will be found associated with a
Meckel's diverticulum.   The Meckel's diverticulum and the
attached cord or duct should be excised at the same time as the
umbilicus.   Histologically the tumour at the umbilicus consists
of columnar epithelium rich in goblet cells.

Endometrioma occurs in women between the ages of twenty and forty-
five.   A primary tumour may be situated in the umbilicus.   The umbilicus
becomes painful and bleeds at each menstruation, when the small fleshy
tumour between the folds of the umbilicus becomes more apparent.
Occasionally an umbilical endometrioma is accompanied by endometriomata in the uterus or ovary, but it is usually solitary.

Primary carcinoma of the umbilicus is very rare.   It is sometimes radio-
sensitive.   If it does not respond to radiotherapy it should be excised,
and also the lymph nodes of the groins if they are enlarged.   Even if the
primary tumour is radio-sensitive the lymph nodes must be extirpated.

Secondary Carcinoma at the umbilicus is much more common
than the foregoing, and is a late manifestation of the disease.

Umbilical calculus is composed of desquamated epithelium which
becomes inspissated and collects in a deep recess of the umbilicus.   A time
is reached when it gives rise to inflammation, and often a blood-stained
discharge.   The treatment is to dilate the orifice and extract the calculus.
In order to prevent recurrence, it may be better to excise the umbilicus
without attempting to remove the stone.

CHAPTER XXVI

URINARY SYMPTOMS. INVESTIGATION OF THE URINARY TRACT. ANURIA

URINARY SYMPTOMS

THREE symptoms, a veritable triple alliance, accompany most urinary affections. They are : pain, frequency, and hæmaturia.

Pain.—*Renal pain* is usually " fixed " in the loin. *Ureteric pain* is the well-known renal colic passing from the loin to the groin.. *Vesical pain* varies from a slight suprapubic discomfort to strangury, which is an intense pain during and after micturition referred to the tip of the penis or the labium majus. *Urethral pain* is a scalding pain during micturition. *Prostatic*

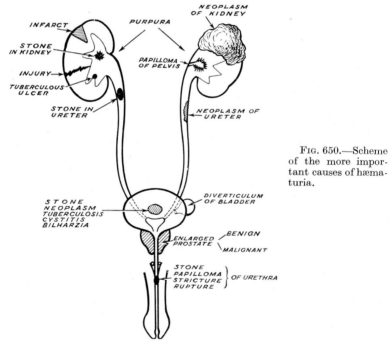

FIG. 650.—Scheme of the more important causes of hæmaturia.

pain is deep-seated in the rectum ; it is often referred to the suprapubic region and the iliac fossæ, or to the sacro-iliac joints.

Frequency.—The patient states that micturition is frequent. Of greater significance is the number of times he has to rise at night to empty his bladder.   In the clinical history the record of such an enquiry is usually entered thus $\dfrac{D}{N} = \dfrac{?}{3}$.

Hæmaturia.—Blood in the urine, however transient, is a symptom which should never be passed by lightly.   Painless hæmaturia is so often a symptom of new-growth in some part of the urinary tract that a complete renal investigation should be started at once, and the patient must not be discharged until the cause has been found.   If the hæmaturia is painful the patient demands relief, and the task of persuading him to undergo a thorough examination is less difficult.   The causes of hæmaturia are manifold.   The more common ones are depicted diagrammatically in fig. 650, and these conditions will receive appropriate attention in the text which follows.

INVESTIGATION OF THE URINARY ORGANS

The urine is examined chemically and bacteriologically.   For the former a twenty-four-hour specimen is collected under normal conditions.   For the latter a sterile specimen must be withdrawn with a catheter.   With a normal fluid intake, the amount of urine excreted by the kidneys is 50 ounces (1·5 litres) every twenty-four hours, and the average specific gravity of the urine varies from 1018 to 1020.

Tests of Renal Function

The Blood Urea is normally between 20 and 40 mg. per 100 ml. of blood.   A reading above 40 mg. is suspicious, and one more than 50 mg. is indicative that the kidney function is impaired.

Range of Specific Gravity.—The power of the kidneys to concentrate and dilute urine is a good test of their functional integrity.   Fluid is withheld for twelve hours overnight.   The specific gravity of the first two morning specimens should reach 1020.   Two pints (1·2 litres) of water are given by mouth.   Within four hours the specific gravity should reach as low as 1002.   A fixed specific gravity of 1010 under these varying circumstances is indicative of renal impairment.

Urea Concentration Test

All fluid is withheld for twelve hours.   The patient then receives 15 grammes of urea dissolved in 100 ml. of water.   Urea is a diuretic, and the excess of urea in the circulating blood should be eliminated in a few hours if the kidneys are healthy.   If the urine contains 2 to 2·5 per cent. of urea during the second and third hours after the intake, renal function may be regarded as satisfactory.   If there is under 2 per cent., there is deficient functional activity of the renal tissue.   The total output of urea per hour should be more than 1·5 gm. ; this is of more importance than the percentage (Swift Joly).   If the blood urea is high, the test is not reliable.

The Urea Clearance Test.—The test depends on the amount of urine passed in an hour, its urea content, and on an average blood urea.   It can

John Swift Joly, 1876–1943.   Surgeon, St. Peter's Hospital, London.

be performed in two ways : after witholding fluids for eight hours, 15 grammes of urea dissolved in 100 ml. of water is given by mouth, or the urea is omitted. Three-quarters of an hour later the bladder is emptied (by a catheter, if necessary) and this urine is discarded. A sample of blood is taken half an hour after the collection of urine has commenced. At the end of one hour the urine is passed or withdrawn. The average normal amount of blood cleared of urea in one minute has been found to be 54 ml. ; the result of the test is expressed as a percentage of this, and similar figures are obtained whether urea has been ingested or not. The normal limits of urea-clearance are from 70 to 120 per cent.

Excretory (*syn.* intravenous ; descending) pyelography.—The original German preparations Uroselectan-B and Perabrodil have been replaced by similar substances of British manufacture —Pyelectan (Glaxo) and Uropac (May & Baker). All these media contain about 50 per cent. of iodine, which renders them relatively radio-opaque. The preparations are supplied in 20-ml. ampoules of a sterile solution (adult dose). The contents of an ampoule, warmed to blood heat, is injected into the median basilic or median cephalic vein with the patient recumbent, the rate of injection being not greater than 10 ml. per minute. None of the solution must be permitted to escape into the tissues around the vein, for it is very irritating, and even when a small quantity is injected outside the vein, painful inflammation lasting for days follows, and may terminate in local necrosis. If the kidneys are functioning normally, the medium appears simultaneously in the calyces and pelvis of both kidneys in an X-ray film taken five minutes later. As a routine films are exposed at five, fifteen, thirty, forty-five, and sixty minutes. The concentration reaches its maximum in fifteen to thirty minutes (fig. 651), and nor-mally visible excretion is completed in one to one and a half hours. The later radiographs show the bladder filled with the medium. In order to display the termination of the ureters the patient should micturate immediately before the final radio-graph. The amount of residual urine in the bladder, if any, can also be demonstrated in this way. When the renal pelves and calyces fail to

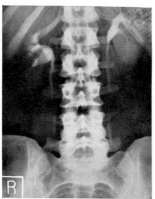

Fig. 651.—Normal excretory pyelogram.

A. von Lichtenberg, Contemporary. Late Professor of Urology, Berlin, now Budapest, announced the discovery of uroselectan in 1929.

empty within the normal limits, further radiographs are taken
at half-hourly intervals.

Anæsthesia.—For instrumental examination of the urinary organs local
anæsthesia of the urethra must be efficient.

In the Male.—The patient first empties his bladder. The glans penis is
washed with boric solution. The following anæsthetic is safe and effective,
but must be used within forty-eight hours of preparation, for after that
time it loses its potency.

Cocaine hydrochloride	. . .	gr. 3 (0·2 gm.).
Sodium bicarbonate	. . .	gr. 3 (0·2 gm.).
Aqua dist. ad	. . .	1¼ oz. (35 ml.).

Drachms 2 (8 ml.) of the solution is injected into the urethra and prevented
from escaping by the application of a penile clamp. Two minutes later,
without allowing any of the solution to escape, two further drachms are
injected, which forces the first injection into the posterior urethra. The
process is repeated on two further occasions at intervals of two minutes.
Thus a total of 8 drachms (32 ml.) is injected. By this time the posterior
and anterior urethræ are anæsthetised and instrumentation can proceed.

In the Female.—After cleansing the vulva, two injections of 2 drachms
(8 ml.) of the solution are given, followed by applying a small piece of
gauze soaked in the solution to the mouth of the urethra for five minutes.
After any form of instrumentation the patient should receive sulphathiazole, grammes 2 daily, together with an alkaline mixture for two days.
In special cases, when the likelihood of lighting up latent inflammation is
great, forty-eight hours' prophylactic treatment with streptomycin is
desirable.

Cystoscopy.—By cystoscopy, the interior of the bladder is
inspected and the ureteric orifices observed. If 7 ml. of a
0·4 per cent. solution (adult dose) of indigo-carmine are injected
intravenously, the excretion of the dye down the ureters can
be watched (fig. 652); normally it should appear within four
or five minutes. Delay of excretion of the dye on one side is
indicative of unilateral urinary obstruction or disease, while
delay on both sides suggests bilateral renal failure. By the
catheterising cystoscope ureteric catheters can be inserted into

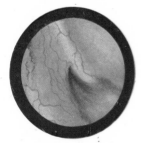

Fig. 652.—Discharge of
indigo-carmine down a right
normal ureter. Cystoscopic
appearance.

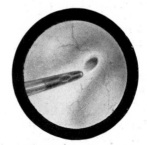

Fig. 653.—A ureteric
catheter about to enter
the left ureteric orifice.
Cystoscopic view.

*In 1877, Max Nitze, Professor of Urology, Berlin, in conjunction with Beneche, an optician
of Vienna, produced the first cystoscope.*

each ureter (fig. 653), and specimens of urine collected from each kidney. Such specimens are examined chemically and bacteriologically, and much information obtained.

Retrograde (syn. *instrumental*) *pyelography* is employed when a clearer definition of the calyces than that afforded by excretory pyelography is required. Such will be necessary principally (*a*) in cases of a non-functioning kidney ; (*b*) in cases where some part of the ureter fails to be visualised ; (*c*) in suspected cases of renal neoplasm or early tuberculosis. The ureters are catheterised, and the patient is conveyed to the radiological table. A sterile 12½ per cent. solution of sodium iodide is injected up the catheter until the patient experiences discomfort in the loin. A radiograph is then taken (fig. 654). For even better definition one of the organic iodine products used for excretory pyelography can be injected, instead of sodium iodide. They have the advantage of being entirely non-irritating.

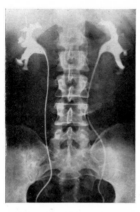

FIG. 654.—Normal retrograde pyelogram. The definition is much clearer, consequently this procedure is invaluable in confirming doubtful abnormalities visualised by the excretory method.

Normally, in an adult 7 or 8 ml. will be required to distend the pelvis of the kidney, but much larger quantities can be injected into hydronephroses. By this method it is possible to inject the pelves of both kidneys at the same sitting, but in cases of poor renal function it is advisable to make each examination independently. In either event, after the X-ray exposure has been made, as much of the medium as possible is aspirated from the renal pelvis.

Urethroscopy : (*a*) *Anterior urethroscopy* is employed when the presence of a urethral stricture or strictures is suspected, or in cases of chronic urethritis, in order to exclude or confirm the presence of an infected urethral crypt or a granuloma (a " soft " stricture). Anterior urethroscopy is conducted under air inflation of the urethra.

(*b*) *Posterior urethroscopy* permits inspection of the prostatic and membranous urethræ. Posterior urethroscopy is carried out under intermittent dilatation of the urethra with boric or oxycyanide solution. By posterior urethroscopy the internal urinary meatus can be seen as a crescentic fold forming the floor of the urethra. When the sphincter is relaxed, as it is in cases of congenital nocturnal incontinence, the whole periphery of the bladder neck is visible. When the prostate is enlarged, it can be seen as bulging of the floor and lateral walls of the urethra in the vicinity of the internal urinary meatus. The most notable normal spectacle of posterior urethroscopy is the verumontanum, which presents as an eminence on the floor of the prostatic urethra. On the summit of this projection is the sinus pocularis (fig. 655). Into the sinus pocularis open the ejaculatory ducts, the orifices of which can be seen but rarely. The verumontanum may be reddened and enlarged in cases of chronic vesiculitis. One or more of the numerous prostatic

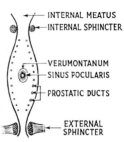

Fig. 655.—Structures on the floor of the posterior urethra.
(*After Ainsworth-Davis.*)

ducts which normally are difficult to visualise may be seen exuding pus in cases of chronic prostatitis.

Cystography: (*a*) *Excretory.*—The cystographs which accompany the later films of excretory pyelography usually are not dense enough to give a clear delineation of pathological conditions in the bladder.

(*b*) *Retrograde* is employed principally to confirm the presence and dimensions of a vesical diverticulum. A rubber catheter is passed and the contents of the bladder are evacuated. If a diverticulum is suspected, the patient lies on his face so as to favour drainage of urine from the diverticulum. A plain radiograph is taken to exclude a calculus in the diverticulum. The bladder is then filled with medium until the patient feels a desire to micturate. The solution can be $12\frac{1}{2}$ per cent. sodium iodide, but this often causes irritation and serious discomfort, and a 10 per cent. solution of an organic iodine compound casts as good a shadow without these objections. A radiograph is taken with the bladder full, and again after the bladder has been emptied. If there is a diverticulum present, it will remain full of medium after the medium has left the main cavity (see p. 693). The extent of a very large neoplasm of the bladder can sometimes be demonstrated better by cystography than by cystoscopy.

Urethrography is a means of visualising the outline of the urethra. It is of considerable value in cases of stricture, diverticulum, or fistula of the urethra, and for showing the relaxation of the internal sphincter associated with lesions of the spinal cord. In cases of stricture, it has an advantage over urethroscopy in that the length of the stricture can be demonstrated, whereas in urethroscopy the surface of the stricture only is seen. One of the media used for cystography is injected into the urethra by means of a urethral syringe. With the pelvis tilted at an angle of 45 degrees the film is exposed while the medium is flowing through the urethra into the bladder.

ANURIA (*Syn.* SUPPRESSION OF URINE)

Pre-renal Anuria.—The blood-pressure in the glomeruli is normally about 90 mm. of mercury ; when the systolic blood-pressure falls below 70 mm., filtration from glomeruli ceases. If the glomeruli are diseased, a higher pressure (up to 100 mm. of mercury) may be inadequate to maintain filtration. The causes of pre-renal anuria are traumatic shock, severe hæmorrhage, spinal anæsthesia, extensive burns, and dehydration from vomiting, diarrhœa, or excessive sweating.

Treatment.—Blood transfusion in the case of hæmorrhage, the treatment of shock (see p. 16) if that be the cause of the fall in the blood-pressure, or the administration of intravenous saline and glucose solution in cases of dehydration often restores urinary excretion. If hypotension is long maintained, damage to the renal epithelium results, and the condition passes on to renal anuria.

Renal anuria results from damage or destruction of the renal epithelium. The principal causes are :

Acute or chronic nephritis.

Acute pyelonephritis.

Incompatible blood transfusion (see p. 87).

The crush syndrome (see p. 19).

Cortical necrosis occurring in the toxæmia of pregnancy.

Poisoning by phosphorus, corrosive sublimate, phenol, lead, oxalic acid, or turpentine.

Reflexly, from too rapid emptying of the bladder in cases of retention of urine with overflow due to an enlarged prostate (p. 726).

Congenital cystic kidneys.

Bilateral renal tuberculosis.

Owing to destruction of renal epithelium, the last two are eventually necessarily fatal.

Clinical Features.—The onset of renal anuria is usually preceded by increasing oliguria. Anorexia is an early symptom which is followed by hiccough. Within a few days copious effortless vomiting is usual. By this time the blood urea is likely to be in the neighbourhood of 200 mg. per cent. The systolic blood-pressure is usually high—200 mm. of mercury, or more.

Unrelieved, about the sixth day increasing drowsiness, thirst, a dry skin, and a dry brown tongue are characteristic findings. The respiratory and pulse rates become slower and irregular, and Cheyne-Stokes' respirations are often in evidence. There may be muttering delirium, and coma. In spite of many new forms of treatment, the mortality of renal anuria remains considerably more than 50 per cent.

Treatment.—*The chief cause of death is pulmonary œdema due to excessive oral or parenteral fluid intake.*

Restrict Fluids.—This is a cardinal principle. The anuric patient requires only enough water (about 1 litre (1¾ pints) a day) to replace loss by sweating. If even a small excretion of urine is obtained, the intake is increased ; gently the kidneys are coaxed to excrete more.

Diuretics.—A good diuretic is an isotonic (4·285 per cent.) solution of sodium sulphate given intravenously by the continuous drip method. Alternatively one-fifth normal saline with 4 per cent. glucose can be used. These solutions should be given at the rate of 50 drops a minute. A diuretic should only be given early in the course of renal anuria, and if after the administration of 10 ounces (280 ml.) a flow of urine is not thereby promoted, the diuretic should be discontinued. If, as a result of administering a diuretic, urine is excreted, a total of 1 to 1½ pints (0·6–0·8 litre) can be given, and repeated on the following day.

A high fat diet helps to prevent the formation of urea and other toxic products. If, as is usual, the patient finds this diet distasteful, it can be given in fluid form through a gastric tube.

Venesection.—In advanced cases of uræmia, to venesect 1 pint and replace the blood loss by plasma sometimes tides the patient over a crisis.

Splanchnic Block Anæsthesia.—Twenty-five ml. of a 1 per cent. solution of procaine is injected successively on each side in the region of the renal pedicle, care being taken not to penetrate a blood-vessel. A number of successful cases, especially those of anuria associated with toxæmia of pregnancy and crush injuries, have followed bilateral splanchnic block.

Renal decapsulation, preferably bilateral, has been performed in a large number of cases of renal anuria with success. To be of value, it must be performed early in the condition.

Intestinal Perfusion.—A special triple-lumen intestinal tube is passed. One lumen is used to inflate a rubber balloon at the end of the tube ; the other two lumina are for the intake and output of the perfusion fluid.

John Cheyne, 1777–1836. Scottish Physician.
William Stokes, 1804–1878. Irish Physician.

The terminal orifice of the intake lumen is situated higher than that of the output lumen. In the absence of a special tube two Miller-Abbott tubes have been employed. The perfusion fluid is of the same composition as that described in connection with the artificial kidney. The perfusion fluid is gravitated at the rate of about 1 litre (1¾ pints) an hour, and with the diluted intestinal contents a considerable amount of urea is removed by aspiration or continuous suction. Late in uræmia repeated vomiting makes the passage of the tube through the pylorus impracticable ; indeed, even when used in early cases it often takes two or three days to negotiate the pylorus. The amount of urea that can be removed from the blood by this method is not sufficient to warrant its use in any but mild cases.

Peritoneal dialysis can be performed intermittently or continuously. The danger of the method is peritonitis, and to avoid this as far as possible 1,000 units of penicillin are added to each litre of the dialysing fluid, and penicillin is also administered directly to the patient. To prevent clotting in the tube or tubes, 10 mg. of heparin is added to each litre of dialysing fluid.

Intermittent Dialysis.—Under local anæsthesia, a tube of plastic ⅓ inch (1 cm.) in diameter is introduced into the peritoneal cavity through a muscle-splitting incision in the right iliac fossa. Two litres (3½ pints) of the dialysing fluid are gravitated into the peritoneal cavity and the tube is clamped for two hours. The clamp is then released and the fluid escapes from the peritoneal cavity. The majority of the fluid flows out spontaneously, but the remainder must be removed by suction. Another 2 litres are run into the peritoneal cavity, and the process is repeated for several days if necessary.

Continuous Dialysis.—A plastic tube is introduced into the peritoneal cavity above the umbilicus and a second perforated metal tube is inserted into the pelvis through a suprapubic incision. The dialysing fluid introduced through the upper tube is removed by suction through the lower tube.

The Artificial Kidney (Kolff).—Two glass cannulæ, to each of which is attached a piece of rubber tubing 10 cm. (4 inches) in length and filled with heparin and saline solution, are introduced one into the radial artery and the other into a superficial vein. The tubes are connected to a machine which consists of cellophane tubing 1 inch (2·5 cm.) in diameter and 40 metres (45 yards) long wound around a rotary horizontal cylinder immersed in a fluid of 6 gm. sodium chloride, 0·4 gm. of potassium chloride, 2 gm. of sodium bicarbonate, and 2 gm. of glucose to the litre. The blood moves through the cellophane tubing by gravity and is returned to the patient's veins by the pumping action of the rotating drum. By these means urea and other toxic products are removed from the blood by dialysis through the cellaphone tubing into the bath of rinsing fluid.

POST-RENAL (*Syn.* OBSTRUCTIVE) ANURIA

Calculous anuria arises in one of the following ways :

1. A calculus becomes impacted in the ureter of the only functioning kidney, the other kidney being congenitally absent, previously removed, or destroyed by disease.

2. Both ureters become obstructed by stones.

3. A calculus blocks one ureter, and the contralateral organ, seldom completely normal, also ceases to function. Whatever

---

W. J. Kolff, Contemporary. Physician, Municipal Hospital, Kampen, Holland.
Thomas G. Miller, Contemporary. Professor of Clinical Medicine, University of Pennsylvania.
William O. Abbott, Contemporary. Associate in Medicine, University of Pennsylvania.

the explanation of the phenomenon—it has been attributed to low blood-pressure caused by pain, and to a reno-renal reflex—the unobstructed side ceases to function until the obstruction on the obstructed side has been relieved.

In two-thirds of cases the obstruction lies at the uretero-pelvic junction or in the upper third of the ureter.

Clinical Features.—The condition commonly occurs in men between forty and sixty years of age. Usually there is a long history of urinary lithiasis and the patient may have undergone several operations for stone, but in 20 per cent. of cases anuria arises without previous symptoms.

Onset.—Typically an attack of renal colic precedes the anuria, the onset of which is sudden. In a few cases there is little, if any, pain, and the anuria is preceded by several days of increasing oliguria. The latter variety is usually due to a superimposition of pyelonephritis on kidneys (or a sole existing kidney) that have been functioning poorly on account of partial calculous obstruction.

Stage of tolerance usually lasts from three to six days. Exceptionally it is prolonged to as much as twelve days. The patient feels comparatively well and may continue his work for a few days. During this time the blood urea mounts steadily, and as it does so headache, sleeplessness, constipation, and lassitude supervene. By the end of this stage the blood urea is very high, often over 200 mg. per cent.

Stage of Uræmia follows, and is characterised by the same clinical features described in late renal anuria.

Diagnosis and Treatment.—Retention of urine is excluded by the passage of a urethral catheter. In anuria the bladder will be found to be empty, or it contains but a few ounces of blood-stained urine. If rigidity is present in one loin, the corresponding kidney is the one likely to be the last obstructed. A large palpable kidney is probably functionless and the seat of a hydronephrosis or pyonephrosis ; a recently obstructed kidney is never grossly enlarged. A plain X-ray film occasionally reveals the obstructing calculus. More often, because the obstructing calculus is small (it is seldom larger than an orange pip) and the film is obscured by intestinal gas shadows, the obstructing calculus is seldom visualised at this stage. Large branched calculi may be displayed in the kidney on the non-functioning side. Cystoscopy should be carried out as soon as possible. Occasionally a stone is seen wedged in a ureteric orifice (fig. 656). If the necessary instruments are available,

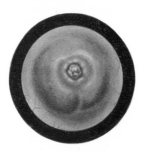

ureteral meatotomy or the passage of a stone dislodger may result in dis-impaction of the calculus. If the stone cannot be extricated or a catheter passed beyond it, nephrostomy should be performed. Usually the ureteric orifices are normal. In the not un-common anomaly of congenitally absent kidney, only one ureter is present. An attempt is made to pass an olivary-ended catheter into the renal pelvis on the side believed to be obstructed. If the catheter can be manipulated beyond the stone, dark urine drips from the catheter. Failing this, a large stiff ureteric catheter may cause a stone at the uretero-pelvic junction to be displaced into the renal pelvis. The contralateral side is also catheterised ; occasionally in cases belonging to groups 2 and 3 urine drips from both catheters. In the event of successful catheterisation, usually unilateral, the cystoscope having been removed, the ureteric catheter is strapped to the corresponding thigh. Every six hours the lumen of the catheter is irrigated with a weak antiseptic solution such as 1 per cent. mercurochrome, and as long as the catheter drains, it is left in position for several days. As soon as the blood urea approaches normal limits further X-ray examinations are carried out, and with the decrease of gaseous shadows the stone may be visualised. If it is still not seen, excretory pyelography will enable the stone to be delineated, after which the catheter is removed. If it is not expelled spontaneously within twenty-four hours after removal of the catheter, pyelolithotomy or ureterolithotomy, according to the position of the stone, is carried out.

Not infrequently during the first or second day of successful ureteral catheterisation the catheter becomes blocked, and must be removed. Removal of the catheter in these circum-stances may result in (a) renewal of the anuria ; (b) continuance of the passage of urine ; (c) occasionally by the spontaneous expulsion of the stone.

FIG. 656.—Stone im-pacted in the ureteric orifice as seen through the cysto-scope.

When a ureteral catheter fails to relieve the obstruction, or the catheter becomes blocked and after its removal excretion of urine again ceases, nephrostomy (fig. 657) or pyelostomy is undertaken. When the obstructing stone is readily accessible, it may be removed at the same time.

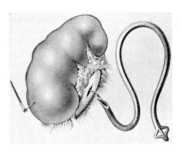

Fig. 657.—Cabot's method of performing nephrostomy.

If the kidney explored is found to be hopelessly diseased, nephrostomy must be performed upon the other side.

When the obstruction has been relieved, either by ureteric catheterisation or operation, the after-treatment includes giving a diuretic (p. 613). In cases where nephrostomy has been necessary, preparations should be made for blood transfusion, for sometimes the hæmorrhage from the incised œdematous kidney is excessive.

Anuria due to Sulphonamide Crystalluria.—Sulphapyridine and sulphathiazole in the presence of an acid medium are changed into acetyl salts which are insoluble. These crystals (fig. 658) are deposited in the kidney

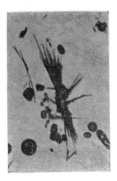

Fig. 658.—Acetylated sulphapyridine crystals resemble small wheat sheaves.

tubules and ureters. The condition is now infrequent, and occurs mainly in patients with partial obstruction to the kidneys, and in those who have become dehydrated from excessive sweating or vomiting.

Treatment.—When a patient undergoing sulphonamide therapy develops renal colic and oliguria, the drug should be withheld and the high fluid

Hugh Cabot, 1872-1945. Surgeon, the Mayo Clinic, Rochester, U.S.A.

intake further increased.   Should anuria supervene, firm deep massage is carried out on each ureter, from above downwards.   The lower ends of the ureters are then massaged per rectum.   If this is not followed by the passage of urine, there should be no delay in performing cystoscopy and attempting to catheterise the ureters.   Provided the catheters can be inserted, the kidney pelves are washed out with 2·5 per cent. sodium bicarbonate solution.   Ainsworth-Davis has had success with dislodging the crystalline mass with a spiral stone extractor (see p. 657).   As an alternative means to cystoscopic manœuvres, many favourable results have followed splanchnic block anæsthesia (see p. 613).   When none of the above measures are successful, unilateral or bilateral pyelostomy must be performed.

Anuria due to Accidental Ligation of the Ureters.—This is a hazard of hysterectomy.   Bilateral pyelostomy should be performed in the first instance.   Only when the patient is out of immediate danger should a plastic operation to reconstruct the ureters be performed.

Anuria due to Involvement of both Ureters in a Neoplastic Process, e.g. Carcinoma of the Cervix.—Nothing can be done in these cases, except bilateral nephrostomy.

John   Creyghton   Ainsworth-Davis,   Contemporary.   Urological   Surgeon,   Bolingbroke Hospital, London.

CHAPTER XXVII
THE KIDNEYS AND URETERS

EMBRYOLOGY

In human embryos the metanephros, or permanent kidney, appears as a bud from the lower end of the Wolffian duct. This bud grows backwards and upwards behind the peritoneum to the lumbar region (fig. 659). The stalk of the bud forms the ureter and its dilated extremity the kidney pelvis. Not infrequently the bud is duplicated or the stalk becomes bifurcated, giving rise to congenital anomalies which will be discussed. Commencing with an embryo of six weeks and continuing to a fœtus of five months, Kampmeier (1923) showed histologically that outgrowths of the primitive renal pelvis divide repeatedly to form collecting tubules. Each division is spoken of as a generation of collecting tubules, e.g. 1st generation, 2nd generation. Each collecting tubule is capped by mesoblast, which is the anlage of the glomerulus and the convoluted tubule. The first three or four generations are not permanent, but persist for a short period as cystic structures. Normally they degenerate and disappear. It is the persistence of these provisional structures which gives rise to the cysts of polycystic kidneys. If one cyst only fails to degenerate, it gives rise to a solitary cyst of the kidney.

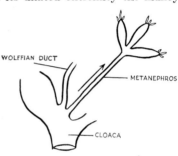

FIG. 659.—The metanephros.

The fœtal kidney is at first lobulated, but in the human organ the lobules become welded together by the growth of a new cortex beneath the capsule.

CONGENITAL ABNORMALITIES

(a) Of the Kidney

One Kidney may be Absent.—Sometimes pyelography reveals only one functioning kidney, and at cystoscopy only one ureteric orifice is present; at others a ureter and pelvis are present on the non-functioning side, but renal parenchyma is almost or entirely absent. In either of these circumstances the functioning kidney is hypertrophied. An absent or congenital atrophic kidney is present in at least 1 : 1,200 individuals; some authorities estimate the incidence as higher.

Ectopic Kidney.—A kidney is arrested in some part of its normal ascent, usually at the brim of the pelvis. The palpable lump that results may give rise to diagnostic perplexity. A subvariety of this anomaly is *con-*

Kaspar Wolff, 1733–1794. German anatomist.
Otto F. Kampmeier, Contemporary. Professor of Anatomy, University of Illinois, U.S.A.

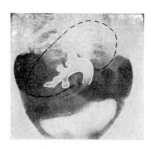

FIG. 660.—Excretory pyelogram showing a congenital solitary pelvic kidney.
(*M. O. Zucker.*)

genital solitary pelvic kidney. When such a kidney (fig. 660) becomes inflamed, it gives rise to supreme difficulties in diagnosis ; for instance, it may be mistaken for an appendix abscess.

Unilateral fusion (*syn.* **crossed dystrophia**) is rare. Both kidneys are situated in one loin. One kidney carrying its own blood-vessels, and with the ureter opening into the bladder in a normal position, crosses the middle line, and its upper pole fuses with the lower pole of the normally placed kidney. In this instance both kidney pelves are situated one above the other medial to the renal parenchyma (unilateral long kidney). In some cases the pelvis of the crossed kidney faces laterally (unilateral S-shaped kidney (fig. 661)).

Horse-shoe Kidney.—The most median subdivisions of the primary metanephric bud of each side fuse, and the kidneys fail to ascend completely. The suprarenals, being developed separately, are in their normal positions beneath the diaphragm.

The abnormality occurs once in every 1,000 necropsies (Zondek). It is more common in the male, the ratio being 8 to 3. In the majority of cases the bridge which joins the lower poles lies in front of the fifth lumbar vertebra. Exceptionally, it is the upper poles of a horse-shoe kidney that are fused.

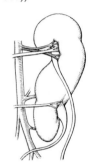

FIG. 661.—Unilateral S-shaped fusion of the kidneys.

Clinical Features.—Horse-shoe kidneys are notoriously prone to become diseased, largely because the ureters are angulated as they pass over the fused isthmus (fig. 662). This produces

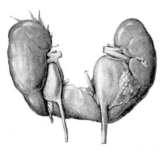

FIG. 662.—Horse-shoe kidney. Note the ureters passing in front of the fused lower poles.

urinary stasis ; consequently simple infection, tuberculosis, and calculus formation are common complications. On pyelography the most characteristic finding is that the calyces are reversed in position, i.e. directed inwards towards the vertebral column (fig. 663). Incidentally, the lower calyces are inclined to be more closely approximated to one another than is normal.

Theodor Zondek, Contemporary. Polish Physician.

Treatment.—In cases giving rise to pain, or when chronic simple infection is present, division of the isthmus followed by nephropexy of each half of the organ is usually curative. The operation is conducted extraperitoneally, for some leakage from the divided isthmus is to be expected. When one half of a horse-shoe kidney is irreparably diseased, e.g. the seat of tuberculosis or neoplasm, hemi-nephrectomy should be performed provided the remaining half has adequate function.

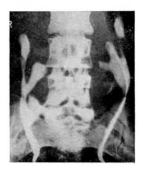

Fig. 663.—Pyelogram of a horse-shoe kidney. The calyces are directed towards the spinal column. (*A. Jacobs.*)

Congenital Cystic Kidneys (*syn.* **Polycystic Kidneys**).—In 18 per cent. the condition is associated with congenital cystic liver ; occasionally the pancreas is affected similarly. The disease is hereditary and can be transmitted by either parent.

Pathology.—The organs may become enlarged enormously. While the usual contour of a kidney is preserved, the surface presents an appearance which has been likened to a bunch of grapes. On section the renal parenchyma is riddled with cysts of varying sizes (fig. 664), some containing clear fluid, others thick brown material, and still others coagulated blood.

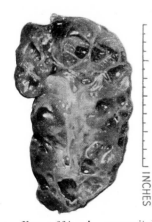

INCHES

Fig. 664.—A congenital cystic kidney removed for profuse hæmaturia.

Clinical Features.—In the Fœtus.— The kidneys may be so large as to obstruct labour. A quarter of the cases are stillborn or die shortly after birth.

In the Child.—The bilateral swellings of congenital cystic kidney must be distinguished from those of bilateral Wilms's tumour (p. 677). In cases of congenital cystic kidneys presenting during this period, renal rickets often develops a few years before the final uræmia.

In the Adult.—The condition is slightly more common in women than in men. There are five clinical types :

(a) *Insidious.*—The large knobby kidneys when discovered in the course of a routine examination can hardly be mistaken.

(b) *Renal Insufficiency.*—The patient presents himself on account of anorexia, headache, and indefinite gastric symptoms associated with a high blood-pressure. There is usually polyuria of low specific gravity.

Patients with congenital cystic kidneys pass abundant urine containing a slight trace of albumin but neither casts nor cells. The behaviour to renal function tests is curious. Usually there is considerable delay in the excretion of indigo-carmine, while the blood urea may be normal, or elevated but slightly.

Symptoms of uræmia often commence suddenly during middle life ; only a quarter of all cases survive the age of fifty.

(c) *Pain* is either due to the weight of the organ dragging upon its pedicle or to tension within the cysts. The pain is usually a dull ache in the loin, but may take the form of renal colic.

(d) *Renal Swelling.*—One kidney contains larger cysts than the other, and gives rise to physical signs similar to those of a renal new-growth.

(e) *Hæmaturia.*—In about 25 per cent. of cases, as a result of over-distension, one of the cysts ruptures into the renal pelvis and causes hæmaturia. Usually the hæmaturia lasts for a few days, and recurs at varying intervals. Sometimes it is profuse.

The most usual complication of congenital cystic kidneys in adult life is infection.

Pyelography.—Excretory pyelography is the best means of forming the diagnosis in the majority of instances, but if the concentration of dye is insufficient to cast a clear shadow retrograde pyelography may be necessary, in which case only one side should be injected, the other being deferred for a week lest uræmia be thereby induced. The shadows of the kidneys are enlarged in all directions. The renal pelvis is elongated and may be compressed. The calyces are also elongated and narrowed.

Treatment.—In the majority of cases the treatment is medical and is that of chronic insterstitial nephritis. By exposing the kidneys and puncturing the cysts (Rovsing's operation) the onset of renal failure can sometimes be postponed.

So improved by bilateral Rovsing's operation was one of our patients who was admitted in a state of uræmia, that two and a half years later he was serving in the Life Guards !

Thorkild Rovsing, 1862–1927. Professor of Surgery, University of Copenhagen.

Solitary Cyst of the Kidney.—Small cortical cysts, usually solitary, are often seen at necropsy. Small cysts cause no symptoms. Occasionally such cysts attain a large size. They can usually be excised without sacrificing the whole organ.

Aberrant renal vessels are found on the left side more frequently than on the right ; in females more often than males ; unilateral examples are three times more common than bilateral.

There are four anatomical varieties (fig. 665) :

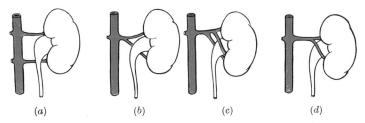

(a) (b) (c) (d)

Fig. 665.—Varieties of aberrant renal vessels (see text).
(*After F. L. Gill.*)

(a) is the true polar artery originating from the aorta and entering the lower pole of the kidney. This is a common type.

(b) is also a true polar artery, originating as an early division of the renal artery.

(c) There are two inferior branches of the main renal artery and sometimes the pelvi-ureteric junction is caught by them in a scissors grip.

(d) The renal artery divides close to, but outside, the hilum and the inferior branch may obstruct the renal pelvis.

A large aberrant renal artery may supply from one-quarter to one-third of the renal parenchyma, and division or ligation of such an artery amounts to a corresponding loss of active renal tissue. Obstructing aberrant renal *veins* may be divided because the venous collateral circulation is very generous.

While they sometimes give rise to symptoms early in life, in a number of instances the first symptoms appear during the third decade—the period of life in which nephroptosis often commences.

Aberrant renal vessels are a potent source of hydronephrosis (p. 636).

(b) Of the Renal Pelvis and Ureter

Duplication of a renal pelvis is the commonest anomaly of the upper renal track and is found in over 4 per cent. of patients examined by pyelography. It is usually unilateral, and is somewhat more common on the left side than on the right.

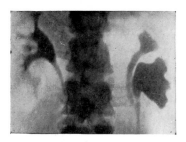

FIG. 666.—Pyelogram showing a kidney with a double pelvis.

The upper renal pelvis is comparatively small (fig. 666) and drains the upper group of calyces ; the larger lower renal pelvis drains the middle and lower groups of calyces.

Duplication of a Ureter.— Double ureters are present in addition to double renal pelves in about 3 per cent. of cases submitted to pyelography. The ureters may join, usually in the lower third of their course, and have a common orifice into the bladder (fig. 667). Less frequently the duplicated ureters open independently into the bladder (fig. 668), in which case

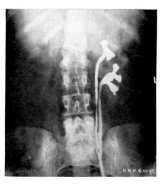

FIG. 667.—Double ureter. Instrumental pyelogram.

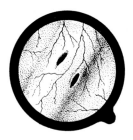

FIG. 668.—Duplication of a ureter as seen through the cystoscope.

the ureter draining the upper pelvis crosses its fellow, and opens below and medial to it. The explanation of this is embryological. The lower ureter in duplication is the first to have an independent orifice on the new-formed trigone. The upper ureter gains a lower and medial opening into the bladder later in development (the Weigert-Meyer law).

A kidney with a double pelvis, and especially one with a double ureter, often has a double blood-supply. Sometimes a groove at the junction of the upper third with the lower two-thirds on the convex border marks the division.

Clinical Features.—While in many instances the existence of a double renal pelvis or a double ureter is found accidentally

Carl Weigert, 1845–1904. German Pathologist and Histologist.
Georg Hermann Meyer, 1815–1892. German Anatomist.

in the course of an investigation of the urinary organs, the anomaly of double ureter, in particular, has a higher rate of associated pathology than normal, the commonest being hydronephrosis, calculus formation, and tuberculosis. The lower ureteric orifice is sometimes the seat of a congenital or acquired stricture, or a fold of mucous membrane at the site of bifurcation may obstruct one ureter. Hydronephrosis with hydro-ureter follows if the obstruction is allowed to persist. Chronic pyelonephritis is liable to supervene in the obstructed (usually the upper) renal duplication.

Treatment.—Except when ureteric meatotomy can be performed in early cases of a stricture of a ureteric meatus, cystoscopic means of relieving the obstruction are unsatisfactory, especially in cases of bifid ureter, because a ureteric catheter cannot be made to enter the smaller bifurcation. Heminephrectomy with ureterectomy is indicated in cases of hemihydronephrosis, and occasionally in pyelonephritis affecting one half of the double kidney. For persistent renal pain denervation of the renal pedicle (see p. 641) with separation of the ureters sometimes proves successful. In cases of tuberculosis and neoplasm commencing in one half of a double kidney, complete nephrectomy must be carried out.

Ectopic Ureteric Orifice.—Should a second ureteric bud arise from the Wolffian duct later than usual, the accessory ureter is prone to become implanted in an ectopic position. This is a rare anomaly. In the male the aberrant opening may be situated at the apex of the trigone, in the posterior urethra, in a seminal vesicle, or in an ejaculatory duct. As the ectopic opening is situated above the sphincter urethræ the male patient is continent of urine, but chronic pyelonephritis is prone to supervene in the renal tissues served by the ectopic ureter.

In the female an ectopic ureter opens into the urethra below the sphincter urethræ (fig. 669) or into the vagina, and causes intractable incontinence of urine.

The diagnosis can nearly always be made from the history alone. A girl or woman who has dribbled for as long as she can remember, despite the fact that she has a desire to void, and does urinate, has an ectopic ureteric orifice. The diagnosis is confirmed in the following manner :

The existence of a double ureter is determined by excretory pyelography. Posterior urethroscopy after the intravenous injection of indigo-carmine is the means of ascertaining that the patient has an ectopic ureter in the male. In the female the demonstration of the opening is often extremely difficult because it is guarded by a valve. Nevertheless, the incontinent

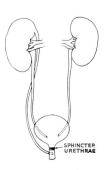

Fig. 669.—Ectopic ureter.

urine, coloured with the indigo-carmine, can be recognised easily on swabbing the vestibule.

Treatment.—Often, in the male, no treatment is necessary. In the female hemi-nephrectomy is usually advisable, because that portion of the kidney draining into the ectopic ureter is chronically infected. Such treatment is also indicated in the male when urinary infection persists in spite of conservative measures. In the female, if it can be shown that the urine draining from it is sterile, implantation of an ectopic ureter into the bladder has been carried out successfully.

Post-caval Ureter.—The right ureter passes behind the inferior vena cava (fig. 670) instead of lying to the right of it. This is liable to give rise to obstructive symptoms. If the symptoms warrant it, the ureter can be divided near the bladder, withdrawn from behind the vena cava, and reimplanted into the bladder.

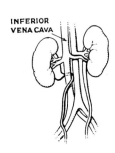

INFERIOR
VENA CAVA

FIG. 670.—Post-caval ureter.

Ureterocele is due to congenital atresia of a ureteric orifice which causes a cystic enlargement of the intramural portion of the ureter. Usually the walls of the cyst are composed of mucous membrane only, but occasionally the muscle coat is also included.

The condition is sometimes found on urinary investigation in children, particularly female children suffering from the symptoms of recurrent pyelonephritis. Often the condition is not recognised until adult life. Women are more often affected than men, and in 10 per cent. of cases the condition is bilateral. A prominent symptom is frequency of micturition, but there may be renal colic and occasionally hæmaturia. In many long-standing cases secondary infection is present. A ureterocele can sometimes be displayed on the film of an excretory pyelogram late in the series, after the bladder has been emptied. The cystoscopic findings are characteristic : when the wall consists of mucous membrane there is a translucent cyst over which blood-vessels radiate (fig. 671) ; in the rare variety containing muscle in the wall, the cyst is opaque. In either case the cyst is

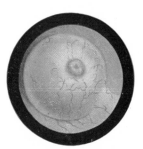

FIG. 671. — Right-sided ureterocele. (*Ainsworth-Davies.*)

seen to dilate quickly with each efflux of urine ; it then slowly collapses.

Treatment.—(*a*) Fulguration of the wall of the cyst with a diathermy electrode. Ten days later the coagulated area commences to slough, and eventually leaves a wide but normally functioning ureteric orifice ; (*b*) the alternative method is to excise the cyst wall with a McCarthy's prostatic resector (p. 733). In advanced unilateral cases associated with a hydro- or pyonephrosis and dilatation of the whole of the ureter, nephro-ureterectomy should be carried out.

Ureteric Prolapse.—The ureteric mucous membrane prolapses through the ureteric orifice into the bladder. Occasionally the muscle coat is included, in which event the condition is an intussusception of the lower end of the ureter. The stenosis produced is slight, and is mainly due to accompanying œdema. Repeated dilatations with ureteric bougies are curative.

Congenital atresia of the ureteric orifice (*syn.* **pin-hole ureteric meatus**) is a precursor of ureterocele, and is found in children undergoing cysto-scopic examination for renal colic or frequency of micturition. Usually the opening is so small that the finest ureteric catheter cannot be made to enter the ureter. Ureteric meatotomy (see p. 657) often remedies the condition.

Congenital megalo-ureter may be unilateral (fig. 672) or bilateral, and in late stages is accompanied by hydronephrosis. Often the condition is symptomless until infection has occurred. If, however, the patient experiences pain, a diagnosis can be made before the onset of infection. The ureteric orifice on the affected side is normal in size and shape, but it is immotile, the efflux being a continuous trickle instead of inter-mittent ejections. A ureteric catheter passes easily. Excretory pyelography shows the whole length of the ureter greatly dilated.

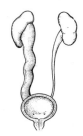

Fig. 672.—Uni-lateral congenital megalo-ureter.

Treatment.—In unilateral cases, if a subcutaneous injection of eserine causes contraction of the ureteric musculature, as shown by pyelography, division of the corresponding hypogastric nerve is sometimes followed by resumption of ureteric muscular activity. In infected cases, transurethral meatotomy and drainage of the dilated ureter with a ureteric catheter for about six weeks has been found to be effective (Lowsley). When the renal parenchyma is severely damaged nephro-ureterectomy is curative. In bilateral cases occasionally presacral neurectomy is successful. Bilateral meatotomy is likely to prolong life, but eventually increasing renal failure and pyelonephritis prove fatal.

INJURIES TO THE KIDNEY

Injuries to a kidney incurred in civil life are very seldom the result of an open wound. Blows or falls upon the loin are the most fruitful sources of renal injuries. Blows from in front, crushing accidents, and falls on the buttocks or feet all add their quota (fig. 673).

The degree of injury varies considerably from a small subcap-sular hæmatoma to a complete tear involving the whole thickness

Joseph F. McCarthy, Contemporary. Urologist, Post-Graduate Hospital, New York.
Oswald S. Lowsley, Contemporary. Formerly Director, Department of Urology, James Buchanan Brady Foundation, New York.

of the kidney (fig. 674) ; in addition, the kidney may be partially
or wholly avulsed from its pedicle.   Tears of the renal paren-

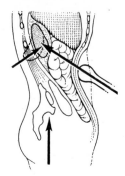

FIG. 673.—With a blow from behind, the
kidney is thrown against the liver.   With a blow
from in front, it is liable to be impinged against
the twelfth rib.   As a result of a fall on the
buttocks, the vascular pedicle may be damaged.
(*After Papin.*)

chyma follow the lines of the uriniferous tubules (fig. 675).
The whole of one pole may be detached. The injury is nearly

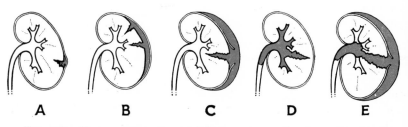

A   **B**   **C**   **D**   **E**

FIG. 674.—Various types of renal injuries : A, small subcapsular hæmorrhage ; B, large subcapsular hæmorrhage ; C, cortical laceration with perinephric
hæmatoma ; D, medullary laceration with bleeding into the renal pelvis ; E,
complete rupture.   (*After P. Adams.*)

always extraperitoneal, except in children below the age of
ten years in whom there is little, if any, perinephric fat ; consequently the peritoneum, being intimately related to the
kidney, is liable to be torn in addition to the renal capsule,
allowing blood and urine to pour into the peritoneal cavity.

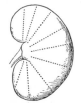

FIG.   675.—
Diagram to
show the usual
lines of rupture
of the kidney.

Clinical Features.—Rarely there is superficial
bruising, but there is likely to be considerable
local pain and tenderness.

Hæmaturia is a cardinal sign of a damaged
kidney, but it may not make its appearance until
some hours after the accident. If the hæmorrhage
is profuse, it is liable to be followed by clot colic.

Severe Delayed Hæmaturia.—Sudden profuse

hæmaturia may occur between the third and the fifth days in a patient who appeared, up to that time, to be progressing favourably. Delayed severe bleeding is due to a clot becoming dislodged.

Meteorism.—In many cases of renal injury, abdominal distension comes on about twenty-four to forty-eight hours after the accident. This is probably due to bruising of the overlying colon.

A perinephric hæmatoma should be suspected if there is even a slight flattening of the normal contour of the loin (fig. 676).

Fig. 676.

MANAGEMENT AND TREATMENT

The patient should be put to bed. It is imperative to keep a frequent pulse-chart, and to save all specimens of urine, duly labelled with the time of voiding. A cloth having been laid across the abdomen, sandbags are placed on either side of the patient in order to keep the trunk at rest. Morphia is administered, and if hæmaturia is severe or shock is considerable, a drip blood transfusion is commenced. If facilities exist, an excretory pyelogram should be arranged as soon as the patient has recovered sufficiently from the shock. On the injured side there may be an absence of excretion, extravasation of dye into the perirenal tissues, enlargement and irregularity of some of the calyces, or a normal outline. This form of examination is particularly valuable in demonstrating the presence or absence of a functioning kidney on the contralateral side.

Conservative treatment is continued if, after the patient recovers from shock, the pulse-rate remains steady and the hæmaturia lessens in amount. Penicillin and sulphatriad are given to prevent infection. A close watch must be kept on the patient for several days ; only when the hæmaturia ceases entirely, pyelography shows a normal outline on the injured as well as the uninjured side, and the local tenderness and rigidity abates, can the vigil be relaxed. The patient should be kept in bed for one week after the hæmaturia has ceased.

Operative Treatment.—If conservative measures are continued in patients in whom rigidity and tenderness persist for several days, after the expiration of about a week a certain number of them will develop a palpable swelling in the loin ; this is either a perinephric hæmatoma or a collection of blood and urine, some-times referred to as a pseudo-hydronephrosis. Drainage of this blood or blood and urine should be undertaken through a high McBurney incision. When the peritoneum is reached it is displaced medially with the finger. In this way the collection of fluid is entered and drained.

Exploration via the lumbar route is indicated when the hourly pulse-rate is rising, when the hæmaturia fails to abate after twenty-four hours and, in the opinion of many, when local tenderness and rigidity in the loin persist after twenty-four hours, and especially if there is an increasing area of dull-ness, or when a swelling is palpable. When an urgent operation has been decided upon and facilities for pyelography are not available, the presence of a functioning kidney on the contra-lateral side can often be confirmed by chromo-cystoscopy. When the kidney is found to be ruptured in several places or the kidney pedicle is damaged, nephrectomy must be undertaken. Small tears can be closed over a piece of oxycel, which promotes hæmostasis. Larger single rents in the middle of the kidney are best dealt with by performing nephrostomy through the rent and suturing the kidney on either side in the manner described. In laceration confined to one pole of the kidney, partial ne-phrectomy may be practicable.

When a sole existing kidney is sufficiently damaged to neces-sitate exploration, it must be repaired, if possible. Failing this, the wound is packed firmly with gauze in the hope that not only will the bleeding be controlled, but possibly the ruptured kidney may heal.

Laparotomy.—When, following an abdominal injury, there are signs of intraperitoneal hæmorrhage or peritonitis, lap-arotomy should be performed if the patient rallies from the initial shock. In the case of a child with intraperitoneal rupture of the kidney, abdominal nephrectomy is undertaken. In adults intraperitoneal rupture of the kidney is rare, and when it occurs it is associated with injury to other organs. Simultane-ous splenectomy and left transperitoneal nephrectomy has been carried out successfully on numbers of occasions when both the left kidney and the spleen have been found to be ruptured, but the mortality of cases of rupture of the kidney with damage to the liver or hollow organs, which are not infrequently

Charles McBurney, 1845–1913. Professor of Surgery, College of Physicians and Surgeons, New York.

further complicated by fractured ribs, pelvis, or vertebræ, is very high.

Complications after Renal Injuries

Urinary infection and infection of a perirenal hæmatoma are largely prevented by chemotherapy and antibiotics.

Clot retention is a troublesome complication in cases with severe hæmaturia. The clot in the bladder can sometimes be removed by means of a Bigelow's evacuator ; if this is not effective, suprapubic cystostomy and removal of the clots is sometimes necessary.

RARE INJURIES

Rupture of a hydronephrosis may occur after a trivial injury, or even spontaneously. It usually results in a perirenal extravasation of fluid, but rupture into the peritoneum has occurred.

Aneurism of a renal artery is usually a recent or remote rare complication of injury to a kidney. The most frequent symptom is pain in the renal region, and when the aneurism is large a non-tender swelling will be felt. Only occasionally is it pulsatile, in which event a bruit may be heard. In most cases the diagnosis is made on X-ray examination, which shows a shadow in relation to the pelvis of the kidney. Pyelography demonstrates that the swelling is extrarenal with the renal pelvis displaced laterally. Attacks of hæmaturia are not uncommon, and are probably due to congestion of the renal parenchyma. The aneurism may rupture into the peritoneal cavity or into the perirenal tissues, when the condition is rapidly fatal.

Treatment by nephrectomy and excision of the aneurism has been successfully undertaken on a number of occasions. In a few cases a saccular aneurism has been resected with preservation of the renal vessels and the kidney.

Rupture of a ureter can occur as the result of an accident causing hyperextension of the spine. The clinical diagnosis is impossible until a diminished quantity of urine is passed, followed by a swelling in the loin or iliac fossa. Excretory pyelography shows a diffuse shadow below the kidney on the injured side, and makes early diagnosis possible. In such circumstances a ureteric catheter is passed by a cystoscope, and through an appropriate incision the lower end of the ureter containing the catheter is readily recognised. The upper end of the ureter is found, and the end of the ureteric catheter is passed into it. End-to-end anastomosis is carried out over the catheter, which is left in place for six days. In late cases the extravasated urine is drained in the first instance, and provided the contralateral kidney is healthy, nephrectomy is undertaken a few days later.

Surgical injury of a ureter or both ureters is considerably more common than the foregoing and most often occurs during the course of a difficult hysterectomy. Preliminary catheterisation of the ureters prevents such accidents, for with catheters within them, the ureters can be felt and seen unmistakably. A ureter may be ligated, divided, or crushed in forceps. If division is recognised at the time of the operation, sometimes after trimming the cut edges obliquely, the ends can be united over a ureteric catheter. When the ends of the ureter cannot be brought together with-

Henry J. Bigelow, 1816–1890. Surgeon, Massachusetts General Hospital, U.S.A.

out tension, implantation of the proximal end of the ureter into the bladder should be carried out.

In many instances the accident is not recognised at the time of the operation, and because ligation of a ureter often leads to painless atrophy of the corresponding kidney, the accident may go unrecognised, or only become apparent if the patient subsequently undergoes a urological investigation. Sometimes, three or four days after the operation, the patient exhibits pain and tenderness in the loin with an elevation of temperature, when an excretory pyelogram shows an absence of excretion on the injured side. More commonly there are few, if any, symptoms until the tenth or fourteenth post-operative day, when a urinary fistula develops, usually into the vagina or occasionally (in cases of subtotal hysterectomy) through the abdominal incision. When a fistula is present, excretory pyelography will demonstrate the presence and the state of the kidney on the opposite side, and usually a slight hydronephrosis with dilatation of the ureter on the injured side. If the diagnosis is made before the development of a fistula cystoscopy is performed, and if a ureter has been ligated, a ureteric catheter passed into the ureter on the non-functioning side will become arrested about 1 inch (2·5 cm.) from the ureteric orifice. In these circumstances the best procedure is to expose the lower third of the obstructed ureter extraperitoneally, and divide it immediately above the occlusion. After freeing the ureter for 3 or 4 inches (7·5 or 10 cm.) its proximal end is implanted into the bladder, after which suprapubic cystostomy is performed. Ten days later the suprapubic tube can be removed, for by this time the bladder in the region of the implantation will have healed. In cases where the function of the contralateral kidney is defective, if implantation of the ureter into the bladder is impracticable, permanent nephrostomy on the injured side is likely to preserve the function of a kidney which otherwise is doomed to become a pyonephrosis. In cases of anuria following ligation of both ureters during hysterectomy an attempt is made to pass ureteric catheters, when both ureters will be found to be occluded. Bilateral nephrostomy is likely to save the patient's life if it is not deferred too long. Cases are on record where normal micturition has recommenced several weeks after bilateral nephrostomy, the explanation being that the ureters were ligated with catgut which in due course was absorbed and the continuity of the ureters became re-established. In the absence of this fortunate occurrence the ureters have been successfully implanted into the bladder. If one ureter has been ligated at too great a distance from the bladder to permit anastomosis, after the success of the unilateral anastomosis is assured, nephrectomy has been performed on the remaining nephrostomised kidney.

MOVABLE KIDNEY (*Syn.* NEPHROPTOSIS)

In many normal individuals the lower pole of the right kidney, and sometimes the left, can be felt. Three degrees of movable kidney are recognised :

First Degree.—The lower half of the kidney can be felt between the fingers during inspiration, and the kidney recedes during expiration.

Second Degree.—The fingers can be passed above the upper pole during inspiration and retained there during expiration.

Third Degree.—The kidney is freely movable within the abdomen.

The last is rare, and likely to be a floating kidney, which is a congenital abnormality in which the kidney and its pedicle have a complete peritoneal investment.

Ætiology. — Especially in second-degree movable kidney, repeated pregnancy and rapid loss of fat are predisposing factors. Movable kidney is often but a part of a general visceroptosis.

Clinical Features.—Women are ten times more often affected, and in 90 per cent. of cases the unduly mobile organ is on the right. In 25 per cent. of cases the condition is bilateral. Various clinical types are encountered.

Symptomless Type.—A mobile kidney may be found in the course of a routine examination. Such patients are usually those with a long, thin abdomen, and they have at least some degree of general visceroptosis. On no account must the patient be informed of the accidental finding, or she will probably become a member of the neurotic group.

Painful Type.—There is a dragging pain in the right side which is worse after standing for a long period and more pronounced when the patient is menstruating. The pain is relieved by lying down, and this is a notable and characteristic feature.

Crises.—Dietl was the first to draw attention to the serious attacks of acute abdominal pain which occasionally arise from a movable kidney. These crises are of two kinds :

(*a*) *Renal Crises.*—The commencement of the ureter becomes kinked or rotation of the renal pedicle occurs. A temporary hydronephrosis develops, with vomiting and renal colic. Suddenly the kink is rectified, and the pain passes off. Sometimes cessation of the pain is followed by polyuria. Repeated attacks may result in permanent hydronephrosis.

(*b*) *Pseudo-biliary Colic.*—The second part of the duodenum being an intimate extraperitoneal relation of the kidney, it will be appreciated that when the right kidney falls the duodenum can be dragged upon, and as a consequence the common bile duct becomes kinked. This will give rise to an attack of biliary colic with jaundice.

Neurotic Type.—Neurosis is often an accompaniment of a movable kidney. In such cases the symptoms are out of proportion to the clinical and pyelographic findings.

Joseph Dietl, 1804–1878. Professor of Pathology and Therapeutics, Cracow. In his later years achieved fame as a politician.

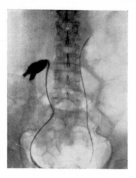

FIG. 677. — Profound nephroptosis with kinking of the ureter and distension of the renal pelvis. Nephropexy indicated.

Treatment.—*Palliative Treatment.*—In cases where there is no pyelographic evidence of hydronephrosis, and especially when general visceroptosis is present and in patients of the neurotic type, palliative measures are employed. Rest in bed with a fattening diet, together with massage and exercises, improves or effects a cure in many cases. When general visceroptosis is present, a well-fitting abdominal belt is of great service.

Indications for Operation.—(1) When renal or biliary crises have occurred. (2) When pyelography shows enlargement of the kidney pelvis and kinking of the ureter (fig. 677) and there is an alteration in the position of the kidney when films are taken in the upright and prone positions.

Nephropexy.—There are many varieties of technique. One in common use is as follows :

The kidney is exposed by the lumbar route and delivered into the wound. The pelvi-ureteric junction and the ureter are examined in order to verify that there are no adhesions or obstructions to the outflow of urine. The perinephric fat is removed, and also the fat and fascia from the quadratus lumborum and upper part of the psoas. The capsule is excised from the greater part of the posterior surface of the kidney (fig. 678). Three catgut sutures are inserted through the non-decapsulated convex border of the kidney and through the lateral part of the quadratus lumborum. Before tying any of the sutures they are pulled sufficiently taut to bring the bared area of the kidney against the muscle. If it is observed that there is neither kinking nor tension of the ureter, they are tied. If these requirements are not fulfilled, the sutures are removed from the muscle, and passed at a higher or lower level. It is not advisable to insert the uppermost suture above the twelfth rib, owing to the risk of penetrating the pleura. The wound is closed, with drainage if necessary, and the patient kept in bed for at least four weeks.

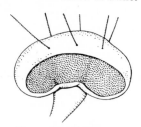

FIG. 678.—Kidney prepared for nephropexy. Showing the area of capsule removed from the posterior wall and the positions of the sutures.

HYDRONEPHROSIS

A hydronephrosis is an aseptic dilatation of the whole or part of the kidney due to a partial or intermittent obstruction to the outflow of urine.

Pathology.—The pathological changes that occur differ in some respects according to whether the kidney has an extrarenal or an intrarenal pelvis (fig. 679), the former being much

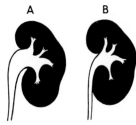

A   **B**

Fig. 679.—

(*a*) Extrarenal.

(*b*) Intrarenal.

more common.   In a kidney with an extrarenal pelvis, at first the pelvis alone becomes dilated (pelvic hydronephrosis (fig. 680)).   As time goes on, if the obstruction is not relieved the

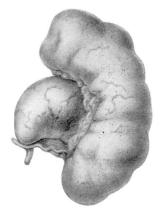

Fig. 680.—Pelvic type of hydronephrosis caused by aberrant renal vessels.

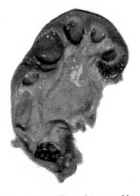

Fig. 681.—Renal type of hydronephrosis. The greater part of the renal parenchyma has been destroyed. Note the cluster of calculi in the lower pole.

calyces become increasingly dilated and the renal parenchyma is progressively destroyed by a process of pressure atrophy.   In a kidney with an intrarenal pelvis the destruction of the parenchyma (fig. 681) occurs more rapidly.   In either case, it is sometimes a matter of years before the diagnosis is made, by which time the kidney may be merely a lobulated sac containing pale uriniferous fluid of low specific gravity.   On bisecting the specimen longitudinally a series of compartments representing the dilated calyces will be found.   Only rarely is there no renal tissue remaining, although often the amount is small.

In the beginning a hydronephrosis is open, that is, urine can escape from the dilated pelvis down the ureter. Often it becomes intermittent ; finally it is closed.

Hydronephrosis may be unilateral or bilateral.

Unilateral hydronephrosis is either constant or intermittent, and always due to some form of *ureteral* obstruction. Usually the obstruction is at the pelvi-ureteric junction ; when it is situated in a lower part of the ureter, the ureter above the obstruction also becomes dilated.

Bilateral hydronephrosis is generally the result of some form of *urethral* obstruction, but it can also be caused by simultaneous partial occlusion of both ureters.

When, as is usually the case, the obstruction lies in the urethra, muscular hypertrophy of the bladder occurs, and the ureters, by reason of this hypertrophy, are partially obstructed in the intramural portion of their course, resulting in bilateral hydronephrosis.

ÆTIOLOGY

Unilateral :

1. There is a kink, valve, or stenosis of congenital origin at the pelvi-ureteric junction.

2. Congenital atresia of the ureteric meatus has been considered already (see p. 627).

3. A calculus in the ureter or a small calculus in the renal pelvis. The latter often gives rise to intermittent hydronephrosis.

4. Aberrant renal vessels were formerly considered to be a common cause of hydronephrosis. In a large number of cases of pelvic hydronephrosis an artery, or more usually a vein, is present over which the commencement of the ureter is kinked. In many instances this is not an aberrant vessel, but a normal inferior renal artery or vein which has been displaced downwards by the enlarged renal pelvis bulging between it and the middle renal vein or artery and vein. In these circumstances the displaced vessel, while adding considerably to the rapid increase in the size of the hydronephrosis is not the cause of the condition. Less frequently a true aberrant artery passing to the lower pole of the kidney is found obstructing the pelvi-ureteric junction, when it is extremely probable that the abnormal artery is responsible for the hydronephrosis.

5. Movable kidney is a rare cause of hydronephrosis.

6. Stricture of a ureter may be inflammatory following removal of a stone by any means if the stone was lodged for a considerable time in one portion of the ureter. It also sometimes follows anastomotic operations upon the ureter or trauma to the ureter during a pelvic operation.

7. Neoplasm of a ureter, or a neoplasm of the bladder which involves one ureteric orifice.

8. A diverticulum of the bladder sometimes presses on the lower end of the ureter in relation to it.

9. Chronic infection of the genital organs. Prostatitis and seminal vesiculitis in the male, and cervicitis in the female, can spread via the peri-ureteric lymphatics to the renal pelvis, and give rise to atonic dilatation of the renal pelvis in the upper part of the ureter (Winsbury-White). Untreated, the inflammation may give rise to cicatricial contracture at the pelvi-ureteric junction.

10. Achalasia. Apart from achalasia of the ureteric orifice, hydronephrosis in the absence of any cause has been attributed to neuromuscular inco-ordination at the pelviureteric junction.

Bilateral :

When due to lower urinary obstruction, the cause may be :

(*a*) **Congenital** : (1) Atresia of the urethral meatus or, very rarely, phimosis.

(2) Hypertrophy of the verumontanum, a valve, or a septum in this region, all of which are rare.

(*b*) **Acquired** : (1) A neoplasm of the bladder which involves both ureteric orifices. Occasionally a large diverticulum of the bladder compresses the lower ends of both ureters.

(2) Prostatic enlargement, fibrosis, or carcinoma.

(3) Inflammatory or traumatic urethral stricture.

(4) Carcinoma of the cervix and sometimes of the rectum involving both ureters.

Clinical Features

Unilateral hydronephrosis is twice as common in females as in males, and occurs slightly more often on the right side than on the left. Usually the condition remains latent until the patient is between twenty-five and thirty-five years of age,

Horace Powell Winsbury-White, Contemporary. Surgeon, St. Paul's Hospital, London.

although symptoms appearing earlier in life are not uncommon. Various types are encountered :

1. **Insidious.**—Pain is slight ; often there is only a dull ache or a sense of weight in the loin. On examination an enlarged, sometimes a greatly enlarged, kidney is found. In these cases the obstruction is usually at the pelvi-ureteric junction.

2. **Attacks of renal colic** occur. Often there is no palpable swelling.

3. **Intermittent Hydronephrosis.**—After an attack of renal colic with its accompanying abdominal rigidity passes off, a swelling in the loin is found. Some hours or days later, after the passage of a large quantity of urine, the pain is completely relieved and the swelling disappears.

Bilateral Hydronephrosis

1. **Due to lower urinary obstruction.**—There is little to call attention to the hydronephrosis except, perhaps, a dull ache in the loins. The symptoms are overshadowed by those of the causative lesion. There is often polyuria of low specific gravity containing a small quantity of albumen. The kidneys are unlikely to be palpable because before the hydronephroses become large enough to be felt, signs of uræmia set in.

2. **Due to Concomitant Ureteric Obstruction.**—This is rare compared with the foregoing varieties. Symptoms similar to those described under unilateral hydronephrosis are present, sometimes on one side and at others on the contralateral side or, what is more frequent, there are signs on one side only, and pyelography reveals some degree of hydronephrosis on the contralateral side as well as the affected side. Symptoms and signs may become manifest in the remaining kidney after its fellow has been removed for hydronephrosis.

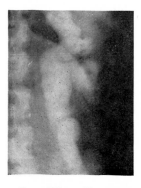

FIG. 682. — Excretory pyelogram in a case of pregnancy.
(*D. Baird.*)

3. **Due to Pregnancy.**—Dilatation of the ureters and renal pelves occurs in every case of pregnancy. Both renal pelves and ureters are affected, but the right side to a much greater extent than the left. The dilatation commences during the first few weeks of gestation, and reaches its zenith between the fifth and sixth months (fig. 682). It then remains stationary until after delivery, when involution occurs within two to twelve weeks. The condition is due to

atony of the ureteric musculature brought about by the hormone progesterone. Possibly pressure of the fœtal head on the ureters plays some part during the last months of pregnancy. The main importance of the condition is when infection supervenes (p. 661). Exceptionally the hydronephrosis persists.

Pyelography.—The diagnosis can often be made with certainty by *excretory pyelography.* When the hydronephrosis is advanced, films taken six to twenty-four hours after the injection may show a hydronephrotic kidney which was imperceptible on films taken at the routine times. As a rule, the earliest pyelographic manifestation of a hydronephrosis is dilatation of the renal pelvis, for in the majority of cases the pelvis is extrarenal. The next change is decreasing concavity and then flattening of the minor calyces and dilatation of the major calyces, which are the first changes when the pelvis is intrarenal. In moderate-

FIG. 683.—The progress from normal to clubbing of the minor calyces in hydronephrosis, as seen radiologically. (*After Macalpine.*)

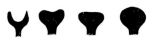

sized hydronephroses the minor calyces become convex and finally club-shaped (fig. 683) and the major calyces considerably broadened. In advanced cases there is extreme dilatation of the renal pelvis and the calyces, or no excretion of opaque media. *Retrograde pyelography* (fig. 684) is only required when the results of excretory pyelography are inconclusive or when a clearer definition of an extrarenal pelvis is required to determine if a conservative operation is feasible.

Treatment.—When possible, the cause is removed. *Nephropexy* is curative in a small number of cases of hydronephrosis due to a movable kidney. *Nephrectomy* is indicated in advanced unilateral hydronephrosis when the contralateral organ is unimpaired. *A plastic*

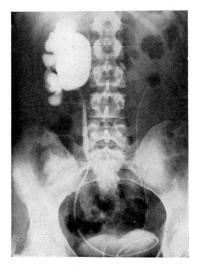

FIG. 684.—Retrograde pyelogram of a hydronephrosis showing a greatly enlarged pelvis and dilated calyces.

operation is indicated in early or moderate cases of hydrone-phrosis with an extrarenal pelvis.   Of many procedures, the following are most often employed.

Reconstruction of a Hydronephrosis (von Lichtenberg).—The affected kidney having been displayed, the upper third of the ureter and the renal pelvis is dissected.   A renal vein overlying the pelvi-ureteric junction can be divided, but an artery in this situation, whether aberrant or not, should be preserved, for if it is divided some degree of renal necrosis follows. The anastomosis about to be described is made in front of such an artery.   The upper end of the ureter is divided just below the pelvi-ureteric junction. The ureter is then dilated with bougies until it will accommodate a number 7 English catheter. The ureter is laid aside temporarily, and the redundant renal pelvis is excised (fig. 685 (*a*)).   A fine hæmostat is made to pierce the renal parenchyma from within, outwards through the lowest calyx, and

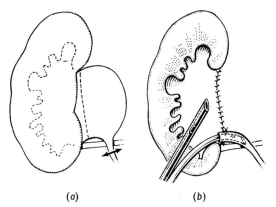

Fig.   685.—Recon-struction of a hydrone-phrosis. (*a*) Portion to be excised. (*b*) The edges of the renal pelvis sutured together and to the ureter containing a catheter at the extreme lower extremity of the suture line, combined with nephrostomy.

(*a*)   (*b*)

the jaws are opened to grasp the whistle-tipped ends of a number 7 and a number 10 English catheter.   The tip of the latter remains in the interior of the kidney to serve as a nephrostomy tube, while the former is drawn through sufficiently to permit it being passed into the upper ¾ inch (2 cm.) of the ureter, to which it is attached by a fine catgut stitch.   By pulling on the distal end of this catheter, the extremity of the divided ureter is made to lie just within the much-reduced renal pelvis.   Using 00 plain catgut sutures, the end of the ureter containing the catheter is stitched to the extreme lower end of the renal pelvis ; the remainder of the cut edges of the renal pelvis are approximated by interrupted sutures (fig. 685 (*b*)). Each catheter is stitched to the renal capsule at its point of exit from the lower pole of the kidney.   The lumbar wound is closed with drainage of the perinephric space, each of the emerging catheters being anchored to the skin by a stitch.

After-treatment.—Urinary infection is combated by sulphonamide and penicillin.   The catheter draining the interior of the kidney is irrigated at very frequent intervals (using not more than 4 ml. of normal saline) until bleeding has ceased.   The skin stitches are removed on the tenth day and those anchoring the catheters on the twelfth.   When it becomes loose, the catheter splinting the pelvi-ureteric junction is removed and two or three days later the nephrostomy tube is likewise removed.   Nephrostomy leakage should cease in a few days.

A   von Lichtenberg, Contemporary.   Late Professor of Urology, Berlin.

Nephro-plication (Stewart) has been followed by remarkably good results in cases of hydronephrosis due to aberrant or displaced renal vessels. The dilated renal pelvis and the commencement of the ureter are dissected from these vessels, and any adhesions between the terminal part of the ureter and the renal pelvis are divided. After squeezing the renal pelvis, pent-up urine passes down the ureter. The collapsed renal pelvis, with its attached ureter, can now be made to take up a position anterior to the obstructing vessels. In order to maintain this position and carry the aberrant vessels from contact with the renal pelvis, the two poles of the kidney are approximated. A kidney whose interior is dilated and whose parenchyma is consequently thinned is more amenable to folding than is a normal organ. Ribbon catgut or a strip of fascia lata is threaded through slots cut in the renal capsule. The encircling band is tightened sufficiently to approximate the medial aspects of the poles, when the ends of the ribbon catgut are tied together, or the ends of a fascial strip are sutured to one another (fig. 686). In this way the moulded kidney is returned to its bed with the aberrant or displaced vessels nearly approximating the renal vessels and removed from a position in which they can interfere with the pelvic outlet. The operation is applicable to early and moderate-sized hydronephroses in the circumstances mentioned, when, on unravelling the S-shaped bend in the extreme upper end of the ureter, no stricture is visible.

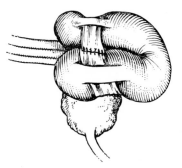

FIG. 686.—Nephro-plication completed using a band of fascia.
(*After Wilfred Adams.*)

Renal sympathectomy (*syn.* denervation of the kidney) is often successful in relieving pain associated with small hydronephroses when no cause for the condition can be discovered. An incision that gives ample access to the renal pedicle is necessary. After the kidney has been exposed and delivered into the wound the renal pedicle is freed from surrounding fat, so that the individual vessels are in full view. Commencing at least 1 inch (2·5 cm). from the hilum of the kidney, the delicate fibrils of the sympathetic plexus and connective tissue which lies between the vessels are dissected, picked up with fine dissecting forceps, and divided, and again divided near the hilum of the kidney. The process is repeated until all the vessels are cleared from these elements. During the dissection the left forefinger is placed behind the pedicle, and if hæmorrhage occurs from one of the renal veins, it can be controlled by forward pressure of this finger until the bleeding-point can be secured by a hæmostat. When the renal artery has been stripped as cleanly as possible, it is painted with 10 per cent. carbolic acid, which whitens sympathetic nerve fibres, thus enabling nerves that have been overlooked to be recognised and removed. The operation is concluded by clearing both aspects of the renal pelvis, the ureteric junction, and the upper inch (2·5 cm.) of the ureter of nerve fibres and strands of connective tissue. As a result of the operation, pain is relieved, and after the passage of many months the hydronephrosis often becomes less and less ; ultimately the pyelogram shows a normal outline.

Permanent nephrostomy must be performed when the oppo-

Henry Hamilton Stewart, Contemporary.   Surgeon, Royal Infirmary, Bradford, England.

site kidney is absent or diseased, although even in this instance, if feasible, it may be preferable to attempt a conservative operation.

Complications of a Hydronephrosis

1. *Infection* = Pyonephrosis.

2. *Hæmorrhage into the Sac.*—Severe hæmaturia sometimes accompanies this complication.

3. *Rupture* (see p. 631). These complications are tabulated in order of frequency.

RENAL CALCULUS

Ætiology.—Considerable light has been thrown upon the cause of renal and other urinary calculi. The subject is a large and complicated one, and the following is a résumé of recent work upon this problem.

1. *Geographical.*—In Britain, the Eastern Counties, Derbyshire, West-morland, and North Wales are districts where the incidence is high. Abroad, the condition is very common in Holland, eastern France, the Valley of the Volga, Palestine, and Egypt. Southern China and northern India have been known for centuries as regions where urinary calculus is prevalent. Evidence has been produced to show that urinary calculi become more frequent in areas affected by economic distress. Children were commonly affected with urinary calculus a century ago, but throughout Europe, probably due to an improved diet, the incidence of stone in children has decreased enormously.

2. *Dietetic.*—By a deficiency of vitamin A renal epithelium sustains serious injury, and it seems probable that desquamated epithelium forms a nidus around which the stone is deposited. From a study of economic conditions in the " stone areas," it is evident that the inhabitants suffer from dietetic imbalances. There is not only a deficiency in vitamin A, but sometimes a hypervitaminosis D, and often a grossly improperly constituted diet in general.

3. *Renal Infection.*—Infection favours the formation of urinary calculi. Both clinical and experimental stone formation is common when the urine is infected with a urea-splitting streptococcus, staphylococcus, or proteus organisms. The predominant bacteria found in the nuclei of urinary calculi are the staphylococcus and colon bacillus. A calculus which follows infection of the kidney is known as a secondary renal calculus ; a primary renal calculus is one unaccompanied by infection, although infection may supervene as a result of such a calculus.

4. *Faulty Renal Drainage.*—Stones are prone to occur in patients with a stricture of the uretero-pelvic junction or other obstruction to the free passage of urine.

5. *Hyperparathyroidism*, although very rare, occurring perhaps in 0·2 per cent. of cases, is a sufficiently frequent cause of renal calculus to warrant consideration. In cases of multiple or recurrent urinary calculi this cause should be eliminated by biochemical tests (p. 226). Hyperparathyroidism results in a great increase in the elimination of calcium in the urine. It has been aptly remarked that these patients pass their skeleton in their urine. In cases of hyperparathyroidism the parathyroid adenoma (p. 226) should be removed before urinary calculi are treated.

The first operation of nephrolithotomy was performed by Ambroïse Paré (1509–1590). His patient was a criminal condemned to death by hanging, instead of which Paré removed two stones from his kidney. Fifteen days later the patient was cured, secured his remission, and was given a grant of money.

6. *Prolonged immobilisation*, especially when occurring as the result of a fracture or disease of bone, is prone to result in skeletal decalcification and an increased output of calcium in the urine. This, combined with the baneful mechanical effects of recumbency on renal drainage (fig. 687), favours the deposition of calcium phosphate calculi. In uninfected cases spontaneous dissolution of the calculi sometimes occurs.

Irreversibility.—With the possible exception of the above, and small cystine calculi, a renal calculus is an irreversible colloidal adsorption product : irreversible because it cannot be dissolved in its original solution ; colloidal because it has entered into organic combination with some col-

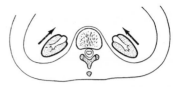

Fig. 687.—In prolonged recumbency the fact that the urine has to travel uphill from the kidneys to the bladder is a potent cause of urinary stasis and consequent stone formation. (*After McEarchen.*)

loidal substance such as fibrin ; adsorption because a colloidal solution will take up more crystals than an inorganic solution.

Randall's Hypothesis.—As a result of careful histological work, Randall seems to have proved that the initial lesion in many cases of renal calculus is an erosion at the apex of one of the renal papillæ. On this erosion are deposited urinary salts.

Varieties.—Stones found in the kidney belong to one of the following types, a mixture of the first two being especially common.

Oxalate Calculus (calcium oxalate).—Popularly known as the mulberry stone, it is covered with sharp projections. These cause the kidney to bleed, and altered blood is precipitated on the surface of the stone.

Fig. 688 shows two oxalate calculi. The larger one removed from the right kidney and the smaller from the left of the same individual. The

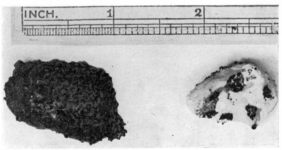

Fig. 688.—Oxalate calculi removed by operation.

larger is black, owing to altered blood. The smaller is beginning to be discoloured around its sharp projections. These specimens illustrate clearly the process by which the oxalate calculus changes its complexion.

An oxalate calculus, which is usually single, casts an exceptionally good shadow radiologically, and this is fortunate, for

Alexander Randall, Contemporary. Professor of Urology, University of Pennsylvania.

often, by virtue of its rough surface, it gives rise to symptoms when comparatively small. A calcium oxalate stone is very hard, and on section is laminated concentrically.

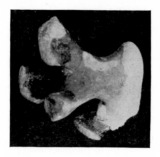

FIG. 689. — Phosphatic calculus. Note its branched nature (staghorn calculus).

Phosphatic calculi (usually calcium phosphate, though sometimes combined with ammonium magnesium phosphate and, rarely, the latter only) are smooth and dirty white. In an alkaline urine they enlarge rapidly, and often fill the renal calyces, taking on their shape (staghorn calculus, fig. 689). Because they are smooth, these calculi give rise to few symptoms until they have attained a large size. By reason of their size, rather than their density, they are demonstrated readily by X-rays.

Uric acid and urate calculi are hard and smooth, and since they are usually multiple, are typically faceted. Their colour varies from yellow to reddish brown. Pure uric acid calculi are not opaque to X-rays, but absolutely pure uric acid calculi are uncommon ; the majority contain enough oxalate crystals to render them opaque. Calculi of ammonium and sodium urate are sometimes found in children. They are yellow, soft, and friable, and unless they contain impurities, they do not cast an X-ray shadow.

Stones composed entirely of bacteria are very uncommon. They are soft and usually multiple.

Cystine calculi are usually round and multiple, but may assume a cast of the renal pelvis and calyces (fig. 690). These stones are soft like beeswax, but cast a good X-ray shadow, because of the sulphur they contain. Yellow when first removed, they change on exposure to a greenish hue. Cystine stones are rare, and only occur in subjects with that inborn error of metabolism, cystinuria.

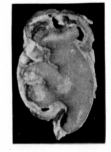

FIG. 690.—Cystine calculus of the staghorn variety which has destroyed the renal parenchyma.

Xanthine calculi are rarer still. They are smooth and round, brick red in colour, and show a lamellar structure.

Indigo calculi are exceedingly rare. Blue in colour, they are derived from indican.

Clinical Features.—Fifty per cent. of patients with renal calculus present between the ages of thirty and fifty, although symptoms may appear during childhood, or be postponed until late in life. Males are more frequently affected than females, the ratio being 4 : 3. The symptoms of renal calculus are very variable, and the nature of the condition is sometimes obscure until an X-ray examination has been made.

Quiescent Calculus.—Some stones, especially those composed mainly of phosphates, lie dormant for a long period, the patient being unaware of their presence. There is progressive destruction of the renal parenchyma, and secondary infection occurs eventually in most instances.

Pain is the leading symptom in 75 per cent. of cases.

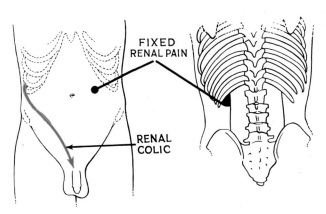

FIXED RENAL PAIN

RENAL COLIC

Fig. 691.—The usual distribution of renal pain.

Fixed renal pain is located in the renal angle posteriorly (fig. 691), in the hypochondrium anteriorly, or in both situations simultaneously. It is often worse on movement, particularly on walking upstairs. The patient may be unable to sleep on the affected side (Fenwick).

Renal colic is an agonising pain passing from the loin to the groin, coming on suddenly, causing the patient to draw up his knees and roll about. It is often accompanied by vomiting, profuse sweating, and pallor. During an attack the temperature is subnormal, the pulse quickened, and there is rigidity of the lateral abdominal muscles but not, as a rule, of the rectus abdominis. The colic usually lasts for several hours, but may continue for more than twenty-four hours. The condition is often due to a stone entering the ureter (p. 653), but also occurs

Hurry Fenwick, 1856–1944. Surgeon, London Hospital.

when a stone in the renal pelvis temporarily blocks the pelvi-ureteric junction.

Abdominal examination in an interval between attacks of renal colic is often completely negative. In patients with a dull, fixed pain there is often tenderness over the affected kidney, especially if it is infected. Only when a calculus-containing kidney becomes the seat of a hydronephrosis or pyonephrosis of considerable size does it give rise to a palpable swelling.

Hæmaturia.—Infrequently profuse hæmaturia is a leading, or the only, symptom. Hæmaturia usually occurs in small amounts (enough to render the urine "smoky") during or after an attack of pain. In about half the cases of calculus there is no blood in the urine, either to the naked eye or microscopically.

Pyuria.—In any case of renal calculus of considerable standing, infection of the kidney is liable to supervene, and pus will be found in the urine in varying amounts. When a large phosphate calculus is present, the passage of turbid urine, which on examination is found to be full of pus cells, is sometimes the chief symptom.

INVESTIGATION OF A SUSPECTED CASE OF RENAL CALCULUS

Radiography.—Before the examination the alimentary canal must be cleansed by the administration of a *vegetable* purgative, for minerals in the intestine cast a shadow (fig. 692). The whole urinary tract, both kidneys, their ureters, and the bladder must be examined in every case. When a renal calculus is branched there is no doubt concerning the shadow it casts. If a shadow is cast which *may* be a calculus in the kidney, and exposures made during full inspiration and expiration show that the opacity moves with the kidney downwards in inspiration and upwards in expiration, and measurements from the lower pole of the kidney to the opacity remain stationary, then there is no doubt that the shadow is intrarenal.

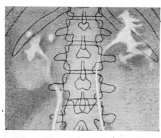

Fig. 692.—The two shadows in the region of the right kidney were mistaken for calculi. They were due to enteric-coated pills of ammonium chloride. (*After Kretschmer.*)

The most characteristic location for a renal calculus is opposite the spinous process of the first lumbar vertebra (pelvis of kidney, fig. 693).

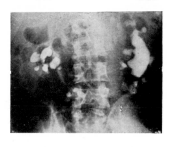

The following structures and substances from time to time cast a shadow which at first sight may appear to be a stone :

(i) A calcareous lumbar or mesenteric lymph node.

(ii) A concretion in the appendix or gall-stones in the gall-bladder.

(iii) Drugs in the alimentary canal, e.g. bismuth, Blaud's pills.

(iv) Phleboliths.

(v) The ossified tip of the twelfth rib.

(vi) A chip fracture of the transverse process of a lumbar vertebra.

(vii) Calcified tuberculous lesion of the kidney.

(viii) A calcified suprarenal gland.

Fig. 693.—Radiograph showing both kidneys full of stones. The patient, a man of forty-two, stated that he had enjoyed good health until one week before he came under observation.

A doubtful shadow in relation to the kidney often can be proved to be extrarenal by a lateral X-ray which shows it lying anterior to the bodies of the vertebræ, and therefore anterior to the kidney. Such is the finding in calcified mesenteric lymph nodes, a gall-stone, and opacities in the alimentary tract.

Excretory pyelography is of great assistance in confirming that the opacity is intrarenal, and also determining in which part of the kidney the stone is situated (fig. 694). It is also of great

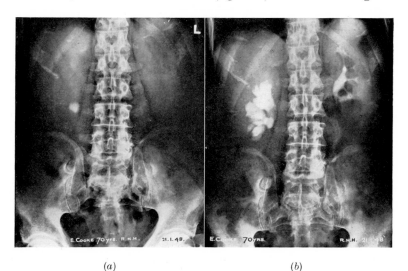

(a)   (b)

Fig. 694.—(a) Plain X-ray showing a renal calculus. In which part of the kidney is it situated? (b) Same case. Excretory pyelogram. The stone is located in the pelvis of the kidney. Pyelostomy indicated.

Pierre Blaud, 1774–1858. Physician of Beaucaire.

service in revealing the presence and normality or otherwise of the contralateral kidney.

The presence of a non-opaque calculus usually can be demonstrated by pyelography, for it causes a filling defect in the shadow cast by the medium. A similar defect is seen in papilloma of the renal pelvis (p. 681). Retrograde pyelography may be required to give a clearer delineation before these two conditions can be distinguished.

Cystoscopy.—If there is a urethral stricture or prostatic obstruction, it will be revealed by instrumental examination. Except in long-standing cases associated with infection, when evidence of cystitis is present, the appearance of the bladder wall is normal. The efflux from the affected side is increased if the stone lies irritating the renal pelvis, or decreased when a stone is blocking the pelvi-ureteric junction, or when the parenchyma has been largely destroyed. The ureters should be catheterised and a specimen of urine from each kidney sent for bacteriological examination. This will determine if infection is present, and if so whether it is confined to the affected kidney.

Treatment of Renal Colic.—Morphia $\frac{1}{4}$ to $\frac{1}{2}$ gr. (15–30 mg.), together with atropine $\frac{1}{100}$ gr. (0·6 mg.) are given to relieve pain. If it recurs, and the stone has proved by radiography to be in the ureter, antispasmodics (p. 656) are of more value.

OPERATIONS FOR THE REMOVAL OF RENAL CALCULI

Pre-operative Treatment.—If urinary infection is present, streptomycin is given during the twenty-four hours immediately preceding the operation. Should the urine contain staphylococci, penicillin is administered also.

All the operations about to be described have certain features in common. Via a lumbar incision (p. 682) the kidney is exposed and delivered on to the surface. In the small number of cases when delivery is impossible, the choice of procedure is more limited and the operation more difficult. An X-ray film that clearly shows the calculus or calculi should be displayed in an illuminated viewing-box in the operating theatre. The stone or stones removed should coincide in every respect with the X-ray findings. Failure to account for some part of the shadow calls for a further search in the interior of the kidney.

In specially equipped clinics it is possible to radiograph the exposed kidney. This ensures against any stone or portion of stone being left behind, and consequently reduces the number of so-called recurrences.

At the conclusion of all the operations to be described the kidney is replaced in its bed, and the lumbar wound closed with drainage of the perinephric space. If nephrostomy has been performed, the tube is either brought through the lumbar incision or through a stab incision ; in either event it is anchored to the skin with a stitch.

Pyelolithotomy is indicated when a stone (it is usually solitary) lies in the renal pelvis. This operation has a wide application, for in nearly 50 per cent. of cases a renal calculus is situated within the pelvis of the kidney. It is also sometimes possible to remove a stone or stones from a calyx by this route. The posterior wall of the renal pelvis is dissected free from its surrounding fat. The kidney is grasped in the left hand so that the tips of the index and middle fingers lie beneath the renal pelvis, making it more prominent while the thumb anteriorly prevents the stone slipping into one of the calyces. An incision is made on to the stone in the long axis of the renal pelvis (fig. 695). The stone is removed with gall-stone or special forceps, care being taken to avoid breaking it. If pyelography showed a stone in a calyx, it is located by a finger introduced into the renal pelvis. If the stone is accessible, it can be grasped in forceps and removed by this route. After a stone has been removed via the renal pelvis, a bougie is passed through the pelvi-ureteric junction in order to dilate a possible stricture, and at the same time any adhesions present in this neighbourhood are freed, or an obstructing vein is divided. When the kidney has been proved to be uninfected, the incision in the renal pelvis is closed completely by interrupted sutures of fine plain catgut, a flap of fatty tissue being brought over the suture line. If the kidney is infected, nephrostomy (p. 617) is performed before closing the incision in the renal pelvis.

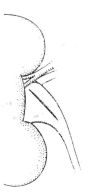

FIG. 695.—Showing the extent and direction of a pyelotomy incision.

Coagulum Pyelolithotomy is especially valuable in cases of multiple small calculi in the renal pelvis and calyces. The posterior aspect of the renal pelvis is exposed. A small incision, just large enough to admit a number 12 French rubber catheter, is made in the renal pelvis near the pelvi-ureteric junction. After the catheter has been introduced and the urine drained away, the interior of the kidney is irrigated with saline solution. A specially prepared solution of human fibrinogen is injected through the catheter while the assistant simultaneously injects one-tenth the amount of a freshly prepared solution of thrombin by a syringe, the needle of which is passed through the wall of the catheter. In this way the two substances are intimately admixed as they enter the renal pelvis. At this juncture the catheter is clamped. After an interval of six minutes, to allow the fibrinogen to coagulate, the catheter is removed and the incision in the renal pelvis enlarged. The coagulum partly extrudes itself, and can be lifted out with the stones and débris enmeshed within it.

Nephrolithotomy is indicated (1) when a calculus or calculi lies within an intrarenal pelvis, or the pelvis cannot be displayed because the pedicle is short, or because of adhesions due to a previous operation ; (2) when the calculus can be palpated through the cortex ; (3) a branched calculus, when the state of the opposite kidney precludes nephrectomy.

An incision into the renal parenchyma is accompanied by considerable hæmorrhage, which is lessened by digital compression of the renal vessels maintained by an assistant. Also with a view to reducing hæmorrhage, the renal parenchyma is incised with a diathermy knife just behind and parallel to the most prominent part of the convex border of the kidney (Brödel's line). As the terminal branches of the anterior and posterior renal arteries meet along this line, no large artery is divided, thereby minimising the amount of subsequent cortical necrosis. The incision, usually about 1 inch (2·5 cm.) long, is made over that calyx containing the stone or stones, which are removed with lithotomy forceps. When only a small incision has been necessary and the kidney is uninfected, the renal incision can be closed by interrupted catgut sutures passing through the kidney substance but not penetrating the calyx, and tied over a piece of oxycel or muscle to enhance hæmostasis. If the incision is large, and in all cases where infection is present, nephrostomy is carried out by placing a small de Pezzer catheter through the incision into the renal pelvis. The incision is then closed on either side of the tube in the manner just described.

Pyelonephrolithotomy is a valuable means of removing a calculus situated deeply in a calyx, especially if such a stone is present in addition to one in the renal pelvis, and in cases of stones situated in more than one calyx. Pyelotomy is performed, and a finger is introduced into the pelvis, and the calyx containing the stone is palpated. If pressure is exerted on the corresponding convex border of the kidney, even a small stone can be palpated. An incision is made through the parenchyma as described for nephrolithotomy, and with the finger pressing on the calculus from within, it is readily grasped by lithotomy forceps introduced through the cortical incision, and withdrawn. In cases where stones lie in other calyces the procedure may be repeated, making two, or even three, cortical incisions. The incisions are closed as described under nephrolithotomy and pyelolithotomy respectively. If drainage of the interior of the kidney is necessary, the catheter is introduced through the cortical incision, or if there are more than one, through the most dependent.

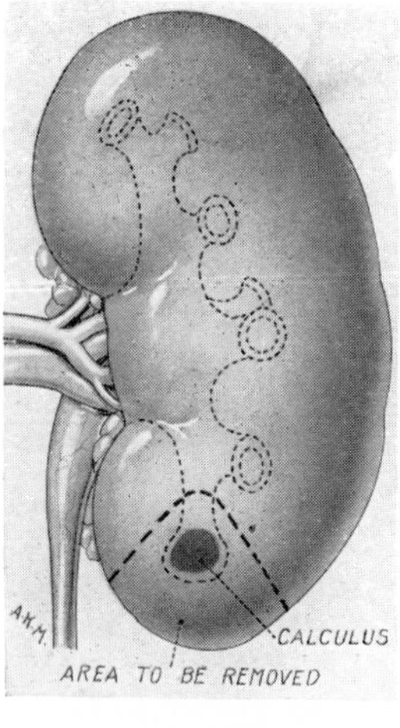

Fig. 696.—Resection of the lower pole calyx.
(*After O. S. Lowsley.*)

Partial Nephrectomy.—When the stone is in the lowermost calyx—a fairly common position—resection of the lower pole of the kidney (fig. 696) is often a wise step. If the dilated calyx is not removed, its dependent position encourages further stone formation.

Nephrectomy is indicated when the contralateral organ has been proved to be perfectly healthy and the stone or stones have destroyed much of the renal

Max Brödel, Contemporary. *Pathological artist, Johns Hopkins University, Baltimore.*
Joseph Hyrtl, 1811–1894. *Professor of Anatomy, Vienna, also described the line.*

parenchyma. Large branched calculi are notorious for recurring, and if the other kidney is healthy, nephrectomy is often the best course to adopt in such cases.

Post-operative Treatment.—In non-infected cases a prophylactic course of sulphatriad is given for a week, together with alkalis and a high fluid intake. If a nephrostomy tube has been inserted, it is managed in the same way as that described on p. 617. In infected cases the interior of the kidney is irrigated through the nephrostomy tube frequently, until the bleeding has ceased, and thereafter two or three times a day with solution G and streptomycin 1 : 1,000. The tube is retained for at least fourteen days. Streptomycin and, if necessary, penicillin, is administered systemically. These measures, by eradicating infection and dissolving phosphatic débris, greatly reduce the incidence of recurrence.

Excessive hæmorrhage sometimes occurs, usually about the fourth day after an operation which necessitated incising the renal parenchyma. Blood transfusion and the administration of morphia are sometimes sufficient to tide the patient over this complication. Should hæmorrhage continue in spite of these measures, the lumbar wound must be reopened. In cases where the contralateral organ is healthy, nephrectomy is the best method to adopt. In other circumstances, placing a strip of oxycel in contact with the cut renal parenchyma of the reopened kidney, and resuture, together with nephrostomy, if that procedure has not been performed already, may prove successful.

Treatment of Renal Calculi by Dissolution.—Most renal calculi, because they are irreversible colloidal compounds, cannot be dissolved. The exceptions are (a) occasionally non-infected calcium phosphate recumbency calculi undergo spontaneous dissolution with a high fluid intake ; (b) small cystine stones dissolve in an alkaline urine. A dose of sodium citrate solution (p. 663) three times a day is sufficient to clear the urinary tract of these calculi (Wesson) ; (c) small phosphate calculi can be dissolved by bringing them in direct contact with solution G :

Monohydrous citric acid .	32·3 gm.
Anhydrous magnesium oxide	3·8 gm.
Anhydrous sodium carbonate	4·4 gm.
Distilled water . .	ad 1,000 ml.

The main field of usefulness of this solution is after the removal of branched calculi when the fluid, injected repeatedly through a nephrostomy tube, can be relied upon to dissolve calculous débris. Although attempts have been made to dissolve phosphate calculi by injecting this fluid into the renal pelvis by way of a ureteric catheter or, more efficiently, by a double lumen ureteric catheter which permits a continuous flow, the measure has been found to be without value, except in isolated instances of phosphate gravel.

Treatment of Bilateral Renal Calculi.—Usually the kidney with the better function is operated upon first, the operation on the contralateral side being postponed for two or three months. Exceptions to this rule are (a) if there is pain on one side, that side is operated upon first, for pain usually signifies that the stone is obstructing the outflow of urine from the kidney, the function of which will become increasingly impaired ; (b) if

Miley B. Wesson, Contemporary. Urologist, San Francisco, U.S.A.

there is a pyonephrosis on one side this should be treated by nephrectomy, or, if the patient's condition is poor, by nephrostomy.

PREVENTION OF RECURRENCE

Frère Jacques, that famous lithotomist of the Middle Ages, used to say, " I have removed the stone, but God will cure the patient." With the advance of knowledge our responsibilities do not end with the mere removal of the stone ; provision must be made to prevent recurrence.

Recurrent calculi can be divided into two varieties :

(*a*) *False Recurrence.*—A fragment overlooked at the time of the operation is the parent of a new stone.

(*b*) *True Recurrence.*—The following constitute the more important precautions for the prevention of true recurrence.

The stone should be analysed so that by a proper diet and vitamin intake the patient may render his urine unfavourable to the formation of a similar stone. There should be a high fluid intake in all cases, regardless of the chemistry of the stone. In cases of multiple or recurrent calculi hyperparathyroidism must be excluded.

Uric-acid and Urate Calculi.—Those meats and fish rich in purin should be avoided. Sufficient sodium bicarbonate is given to keep the urine slightly alkaline.

Calcium Oxalate Calculi.—A diet adequate in calcium and magnesium is necessary. Hammersten has shown that the solubility of calcium oxalate is influenced by magnesium ions. Rhubarb, berries, plums, spinach, and tomatoes, which are rich in oxalate, can be taken if they are accompanied by a dose of calcium, or $\frac{1}{2}$ pint (300 ml.) of milk, because under these conditions oxalates are precipitated as an insoluble calcium salt in the intestine, and are not absorbed (Barrett).

Phosphate Calculi.—Excessive alkalinity of the urine should be treated by giving ammonium chloride or other urinary acidifier.

Cystine Calculi.—Sulphur-containing proteins such as meat or fish are prohibited, and proteins with a low sulphur content substituted. Carbohydrates and fats are unrestricted. The urine must be kept alkaline permanently, and to this end sodium citrate and sodium bicarbonate are given in sufficient quantities, the patient testing the reaction of his urine night and morning.

In all types of calculi accompanied by infection, no effort should be spared to render the urine sterile, and keep it sterile.

If there is any factor that predisposes to urinary stasis, be it a ureteral stricture, an enlarged prostate, or a urethral stricture, this should be remedied.

Complications of Renal Calculus

1. *Migration.*—The calculus may pass into the ureter, p. 653.

2. *Urinary Obstruction.*—Hydronephrosis (p. 634) or calculous anuria (p. 614) can arise.

3. *Infection* is a constant danger. All grades from a mild pyelonephritis to pyonephrosis are possible.

URETERIC CALCULUS

A stone in the ureter nearly always has its birth in the kidney, but authentic cases of primary ureteric calculus are on record.

Frère Jacques, 1651–1719. Itinerant Italian lithotomist, after serving as a trooper in the French army, adopted semi-religious habit and cut for stone in the bladder.

When it enters the ureter the calculus is rounded or oval in shape. Should it become arrested in its descent to the bladder, in time it becomes enlarged and elongated, resembling in shape a date stone (fig. 697). In 90 per cent. of cases the stone is single.

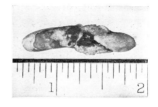

FIG. 697.—Ureteric calculus removed by operation.

Clinical Features.—When a stone descends into the ureter there is an attack of renal colic, which is repeated at longer or shorter intervals, until the stone is ejected into the bladder or becomes impacted in the ureter. There are five locations of anatomical narrowing of the ureter where a stone is liable to become arrested (fig. 698).

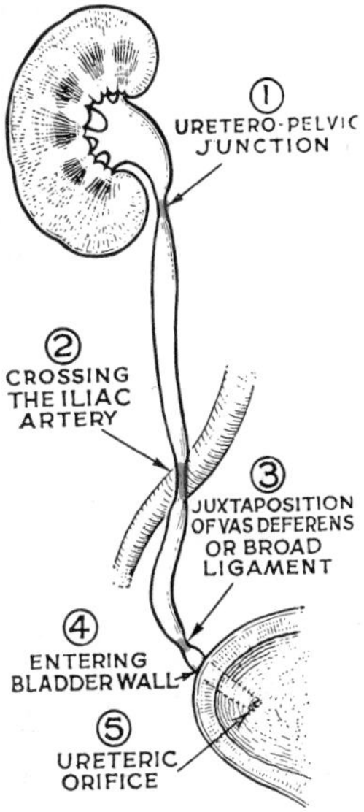

Renal Colic.—A stone in the upper third of the ureter produces symptoms identical with those of a stone blocking the pelvi-ureteric junction (p. 646). When a calculus enters the lower third of the ureter the colic it produces often commences anteriorly at a lower level than the kidney, and is frequently accompanied by pain referred along the two branches of the genito-femoral nerve, to the testis in the male (fig. 699), the labium majus in the female, and to the anterior surface of the thigh in both sexes. The testis usually becomes retracted by spasm of the cremaster, and tender, the tenderness persisting for half an hour or more after the colic has ceased. The stone having entered the intramural portion of the ureter, the pain is referred to the tip of the penis

FIG. 698.—Normal anatomical narrowings of the ureter. (*After C. C. Higgins.*)

① URETERO-PELVIC JUNCTION

② CROSSING THE ILIAC ARTERY

③ JUXTAPOSITION OF VAS DEFERENS OR BROAD LIGAMENT

④ ENTERING BLADDER WALL

⑤ URETERIC ORIFICE

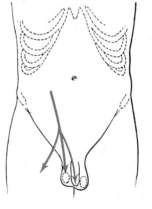

FIG. 699.—Radiations of ureteric colic produced by a stone in the lower third of the ureter.

in the male, and in both sexes there is strangury. In more than 50 per cent. of cases the stone is passed spontaneously.

Impaction.—When a ureteric calculus becomes impacted the attacks of colic pass off and give place to a dull pain, usually in the iliac fossa, for the calculus most often becomes impacted in the pelvic portion of the ureter. The pain is increased by exercise, and relieved by rest. Such pain varies in intensity and is often associated with back-ache due to distension of the renal pelvis. Complete cessation of pain sometimes occurs by the stone forming for itself a false diverticulum in the wall of the ureter by a process of pressure necrosis ; subsequent perforation of the ureter occurs but rarely. Early in the attack complete cessation of pain, without passage of the stone, usually signifies complete obstruction of the lumen of the ureter and temporary cessation of renal function. Occasionally, if the stone is not removed within a fortnight, this is permanent, and the kidney atrophies.

Hæmaturia.—Some degree of hæmaturia is usual after an attack of renal colic, and it lasts for a few hours or a day. It is sometimes so slight as to require microscopic identification.

Abdominal Examination.—There is tenderness and often rigidity in some part of the line of the ureter. On rare occasions a stone in the lower end of the ureter can be felt on rectal or vaginal examination. The principal difficulty on the right side is distinguishing the symptoms and signs produced by a ureteric calculus from those of acute appendicitis. The presence of blood in the urine does not necessarily rule out appendicitis, for an inflamed appendix lying in juxtaposition to the ureter can give rise to ureteritis which causes hæmaturia.

Radiography.—Occasionally a typical elongated shadow in the line of the ureter renders the diagnosis undoubted ; more often either no shadow is seen, owing to the small size of the stone and obscuration of it by intestinal gas shadows, or a shadow is seen which may or may not be a ureteric calculus.

Excretory Pyelography.—If the pyelograms show normal excretion on the affected side and the differential diagnosis between renal colic and acute appendicitis is at stake, immediate appendicectomy should be performed, for when a calculus is present in the ureter invariably the pyelograms display some aberration on the affected side. Soon after an attack of renal colic there is often either no excretion on the affected side or insufficient excretion to delineate the ureter. Forty-eight hours later, in most instances a good shadow of the pelvis and the ureter is obtained, and if an opacity seen on the plain X-ray film is a ureteric calculus, it will be shown to lie within the shadow of the ureter. A stone not visible in the plain X-ray may become outlined in the ureter by the contrast solution. A varying degree of hydronephrosis and dilatation of the ureter is often apparent after a stone has been impacted for a week or more.

Cystoscopy.—When a calculus is in the upper part of the ureter no abnormality is present in the bladder, although after an intravenous injection of indigo-carmine the efflux from the affected side is increased soon after impaction and later decreased, especially if the stone has given rise to some degree of hydronephrosis. When a calculus has reached the lower third of the ureter, or sometimes when it is at a higher level, the ureteric orifice becomes patulous and its immediate vicinity bespattered with minute petechial hæmorrhages. As the calculus descends to just above the bladder wall these hæmorrhagic spots coalesce to form larger, bright red extravasations in the mucous membrane, usually above the ureteric orifice. The stone having entered the intramural portion of the ureter, the ureteric orifice becomes grossly œdematous. Finally, the calculus may be seen pouting through (fig. 656). The passage of an opaque catheter provides much information, and in conjunction with radiography confirms the diagnosis with precision. Especially when the efflux is increased, a catheter sometimes passes into the renal pelvis without hindrance, or if arrested, after partial withdrawal and reinsertion (fig. 700). More often, especially when the efflux is diminished, a catheter fails to pass the obstruction and a radiograph shows the tip of the catheter abutting on the lower margin of the calculus.

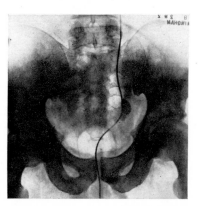

Fig. 700.—Stone in the ureter. Catheter passed alongside the stone.

Retrograde pyelography is seldom required. The only indications for its employment are when there is doubt concerning a shadow being a ureteric calculus and excretory pyelography shows absence or ineffective delineation of the corresponding renal pelvis and the ureter. It sometimes proves a means of displaying the presence of a ureteric calculus non-opaque to X-rays.

Treatment.—*Expectant.*—If the calculus as shown by radiography is small, and the patient is having attacks of renal colic, there is a good chance that it will pass naturally. The patient is encouraged to drink large quantities of bland fluid ; urinary antiseptics and anti-spasmodics are prescribed. The treatment is controlled by repeated radiographs and pyelography.

While the initial attack of renal colic is often severe enough to necessitate giving morphia and atropine, if the stone has been shown by radiography and pyelography to be situated in the ureter, and is of such a size that it may be expected to pass naturally, one of several anti-spasmodics which help to relieve the pain by relaxing the voluntary musculature of the ureter is substituted. Among the best in this respect are Trasentin (Ciba Laboratories) 2 ml. (100 mg.) twice daily, Pethidine (B.P.C.) 2 ml. (100 mg.) intravenously three times a day, or Tinct. ammi. visnaga[1] (British Drug Houses Ltd.), drachms 2 (8 ml.) in a tumblerful of water three times a day before meals. The patient should be encouraged to drink large quantities (at least 5 pints (3 litres) in twenty-four hours) of bland fluid. The urine should be rendered alkaline (p. 663). The continuation of the treatment is decided by repeated radiographs and a weekly pyelogram. Expectant treatment should not be attempted in the presence of infection and not continued when there is little change in the position of the stone after three or four weeks, or when pyelography shows an increase in the size of the renal pelvis and the ureter above the stone.

Immediate and complete relief of pain is afforded by paravertebral block anæsthesia of the twelfth dorsal to the second lumbar sympathetic ganglia of the affected side with 10 ml. of 1 per cent. procaine.

Instrumental Treatment:

Before and after treatment by instrumentation, sulphonamide should be given.

---

[1] Ammi Visnaga (Linn.) is a wild Eastern Mediterranean plant that has long been used by the local inhabitants as an antispasmodic for renal colic.

Ureteric Catheterisation.—A small stone half a centimetre or less in diameter arrested in any part of the ureter often passes after ureteric catheterisation. The catheter may be left in position for twenty-four to forty-eight hours, and 1 ml. of sterile liquid paraffin injected up the catheter before it is removed. This very frequently results in the stone being passed within a few hours or days. Five per cent. procaine injected into the ureter at the time of passing the catheter, and at intervals, often controls pain and overcomes spasm. In the presence of severe renal infection, if the catheter can be manipulated beyond the stone, the drainage afforded often prevents the development of a pyonephrosis. In this instance pelvic lavage with acriflavine 1 : 2,000 is employed in addition to systemic administration of antibiotics.

The following measures are specially suited to a calculus impacted in the intramural portion of the ureter or that part which is immediately adjacent to the bladder.

Ureteric Meatotomy.—The ureteric orifice is the narrowest part of the whole ureter. By enlarging the opening a stone is often permitted to pass. When the stone is not engaging the orifice but is situated in the commencement of the intramural portion of the ureter or within 1 inch (2·5 cm.) of the bladder, Ogier Ward's instrument is effective. Through an operating cystoscope the instrument is passed ½ inch (1·25 cm.) up the ureter and its concealed blade is made to transfix the ureteric cusp (fig. 701). With the cutting diathermy current the meatotome is withdrawn into the bladder, leaving the cusp divided and its edges coagulated.

The spiral stone dislodger (fig. 702) can be used alone or in conjunction with meatotomy performed in the above manner.

Releasing a Stone Imprisoned at the Meatus.—When a stone is just inside the meatus, or pouting through it, the anterior wall overlying the calculus can be divided by

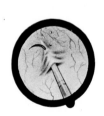

Fig. 701.—Ogier Ward's electro-surgical ureteric meatotome. Meatotomy in progress.

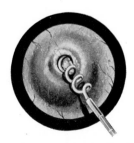

Fig. 702.—Welland Howard's spiral stone dislodger in action.

R. Ogier Ward, Contemporary. Surgeon, St. Peter's Hospital, London.
Henry Welland Howard, Contemporary. Associate Professor of Urology, Oregon University, U.S.A.

the more simple type of meatotome shown in fig. 703, thus releasing the stone, which sometimes falls into the bladder forthwith.

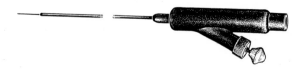

FIG. 703.—Diathermy meatotome, the platinum point of which can be protruded or withdrawn into its insulating sheath.

Operative treatment is indicated :

(*a*) When it is judged that the stone is too large to pass naturally.

(*b*) When expectant and instrumental treatments have failed.

(*c*) There is increasing dilatation of the renal pelvis and calyces.

(*d*) When infection is present.

Uretero-lithotomy.—The patient should be radiographed just prior to the operation, in order to detect any change in the position of the calculus. *When the stone is impacted in the lower two-thirds of the ureter but above the spine of the ischium.* This operation is described first because it is the commonest situation for a ureteric calculus requiring operative removal. With the patient in the dorsal position, an incision is made from a point 1½ inches (3·75 cm.) above the anterior superior iliac spine to the middle of Poupart's ligament. The external and internal oblique muscles are divided in the direction of their fibres, likewise the transversus. The peritoneum is then gently mobilised by gauze dissection until the dilated ureter is found adhering to its under-surface. The stone is sought by palpation, and, if possible, is milked upwards or downwards to a convenient point for extraction. When this is not possible the ureter is opened and the stone drawn out by a scoop or forceps. Occasionally the stone is so

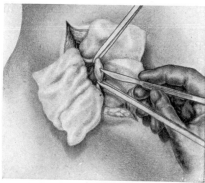

FIG. 704.—Uretero-lithotomy.

firmly impacted that the only course is to incise the ureter directly over it. This practice, however, should be avoided whenever possible, for the ureter's lining membrane is ulcerated at this spot, and is less likely to heal quickly than when the incision is made through healthy tissue. The opening into the ureter is always longitudinal (fig. 704), and after extraction of the stone the ureteric incision is closed by interrupted sutures of number 0 plain catgut. The lower end of the wound is drained down to the incision in the ureter, care being taken that the drainage tube does not impinge upon the iliac vessels. The drainage tube should be shortened on the third day and removed on the fourth, provided there is no leakage of urine. *When the stone is impacted in the upper third of the ureter*, an incision similar to that for exposing the kidney (p. 682) is made ; it can be prolonged downwards if necessary. The preliminary passage of a ureteric catheter helps in quick identification of the ureter during the operation. *When the stone is impacted in the juxtavesical or intramural portions of the ureter*, a mid-line, sub-umbilical extraperitoneal approach is often employed, the patient being in Trendelenburg's position. The peritoneum is stripped from the dome of the bladder and from the side wall of the pelvis. A dissection is then made between the posterior surface of the bladder and the wall of the pelvis. Often at this stage the stone will be felt. If this is not possible, the ureter must be located where it crosses the iliac vessels, and traced downwards.

INFECTIONS OF THE KIDNEY

Renal infections arise in one of the following ways :

1. **Hæmatogenous.**—From the colon, infected tonsils, carious teeth, or from cutaneous infections, particularly boils or a carbuncle.

2. **Ascending along the lumen of the ureter** from the bladder. This occurs only in cases of long-standing lower urinary obstruction with dilatation of the ureters when, as a result of vesico-ureteral reflux, infected urine may be carried from the bladder to the renal pelvis. Another possibility is that motile organisms, e.g. B. coli, ascend along the dilated ureters.

3. **Ascending along the peri-ureteral lymphatics** from the genital organs.

Bacteriology.—In order of frequency, the infecting organisms are B. coli, B. (lactis) ærogenes, staphylococcus, streptococcus, Proteus vulgaris, Ps. pyocyaneus, and (rarely) S. typhi or S. paratyphi. In 75 per cent. of cases coliform organisms (which include B. coli and B. (lactis) ærogenes) are present. Mixed infections are not infrequent.

For purposes of treatment it is important to distinguish Gram-positive from Gram-negative bacteria.

Gram-positive organisms include :	*Gram-negative organisms include :*
Staphylococcus (aureus and albus)	B. coli
Streptococcus (usually fæcalis ; occasionally hæmolyticus or viridans).	B. (lactis) ærogenes
	Proteus vulgaris
	Ps. pyocyaneus
	S. typhi
	S. paratyphi

In the presence of the common B. coli infection the urine is acid, as it is also in many types of streptococcal infection. Staphylococci or Proteus vulgaris split urea, releasing ammonia, which causes the urine to become alkaline.

Friedrich Trendelenburg, 1844–1925. Professor of Surgery, Leipzig.
Hans Christian Joachim Gram, 1853–1938. Professor of Medicine, Copenhagen.

PYELONEPHRITIS

It is now conceded generally that renal infection, by whatever route it originates, is never confined to the renal pelvis. In hæmatogenous infection the renal parenchyma is attacked first, and often the infection spreads to the renal pelvis. In ascending infection the bacterial inflammation is not limited to the renal pelvis ; it implicates the calyces, the pyramids, and at least some part of the adjacent parenchyma. It is, therefore, more correct to discard the term " pyelitis " in connection with the latter type of infection, in favour of the more accurate designation " pyelonephritis."

ACUTE PYELONEPHRITIS

Acute pyelonephritis without retention of bladder urine is seen more commonly in women and children than in men, and it occurs very much more often on the right side than on the left. Rarely it is bilateral.

Clinical Features.—Sometimes there are prodromal symptoms of headache, lassitude, and nausea. The onset is sudden, often commencing with a rigor. There is acute pain in the flank and the hypochondrium. In a minority of cases the pain radiates from the loin to the groin (renal colic). The temperature rises to 102 or 103° F. (38·8 or 39·5° C.), and is remitting. Soon after the onset, increased frequency of micturition sets in, and when, as is often the case, the urine is acid, micturition is accompanied by a scalding pain in the urethra. On examination there is tenderness in the hypogastrium and in the angle between the last rib and the erector spinæ, accompanied by a varying degree of muscular rigidity. In the early stages, when it is imperative to make a correct diagnosis, the urine is clear macroscopically.

Bacteriological Examination of the Urine.—A catheter specimen in the female or a mid-stream specimen in the male should be collected in a sterile bottle ; the urine is centrifuged and examined microscopically. In early acute pyelonephritis there are typically a few pus cells and many bacteria. It should be noted that the presence of coliform bacilli without pus cells is not confirmative evidence of pyelonephritis, for these organisms are often present in the urine, especially in women, without giving rise to symptoms. When pyelonephritis has been present for twenty-four hours or more, the urine is often cloudy and pus cells abound. In all cases the investigation includes culture of the specimen as well as an examination of the sediment stained by Gram's method.

Severe Cases.—There are repeated rigors and the temperature rises to 104 or 105° F. (40 or 40·5° C.), often without a corresponding rise in the pulse-rate. There is vomiting, sweating, and great thirst, and the patient looks and feels ill. The blood culture, if the specimen is taken soon after a rigor, often gives a positive result. After some hours the pain is localised in one, or rarely both, loins. Urine is scanty and highly concentrated, and may be teeming with coliform organisms and pus cells, in which case the diagnosis is simplified. In hæmatogenous coccal infections the organisms and pus cells do not appear in the urine until the infection has spread from the cortex to the medulla—a matter of many hours, and sometimes several days. As the abdominal rigidity abates, often the enlarged affected kidney can be felt.

Differential Diagnosis.—When the symptoms and signs are typical the diagnosis is straightforward. In other circumstances there may be difficulty in distinguishing the condition from pneumonia, acute appendicitis, and acute cholecystitis. The urgent need is to differentiate acute appendicitis from right-sided pyelonephritis. The fact that the pain commenced in, and did not pass to, the right side greatly favours the latter condition. Excretory pyelography may prove of assistance, for in early acute pyelonephritis limited to the right kidney the concentration of medium in the renal pelvis and calyces on the affected side is often so poor that no shadow, or a very indefinite shadow, is cast.

Pyelonephritis of Pregnancy.—In spite of the fact that the hydronephrosis and hydro-ureter of pregnancy are perfect prerequisites for the development of infection, pyelonephritis occurs in only 2 per cent. of pregnancies. The condition usually develops between the fourth and sixth months of gestation, and is slightly more common in primiparæ than multiparæ. After the second pregnancy it is unusual. In 90 per cent. of cases the right side alone is affected. The initiating causes are often chronic urethritis or a cervical erosion. The symptoms do not differ from those of pyelonephritis occurring in the non-parous. As a rule, with appropriate treatment symptoms abate, and within a week the patient looks and feels well, but the urine may or may not still be infected. In about 10 per cent. of cases the disease runs a more severe and protracted course, and occasionally it results in abortion or premature delivery. In all patients who have had pyelonephritis of pregnancy, periodic examinations of the urine are necessary during the puerperium, for if the infection has not been eradicated recrudescence of the symptoms is liable to occur during this period. In a few instances the infection lies dormant during pregnancy and manifests itself only during the puerperium, generally within the first week.

Pyelonephritis of infants and children is most common under the age of two years, when the sexes are equally affected. In older children it occurs much more frequently in females than in males. Often the infection commences acutely with rigors, the temperature rising to 103 or 104° F. (40 or 40·5° C.) remittently. In infants attacks of screaming due to colic occur. Slight terminal hæmaturia is sometimes present. In a number of instances a clue to the origin of the infection is apparent ; in females vulvitis extending around the external urinary meatus ; in circumcised males atresia with or without meatitis ; in the uncircumcised, balanitis. Older children may complain of lumbar pain. In chronic cases increased frequency of micturition and slight intermittent pyrexia are the usual symptoms, but an examination of the urine to account for otherwise unexplained pyrexia may be the means of directing attention to the urinary track.

Pyelonephritis with retention of bladder urine occurs most frequently in men suffering from prostatic obstruction or stricture of the urethra, and in cases of fracture of the spine with injury to the spinal cord (p. 879). To a lesser extent it may arise as a complication of retention of urine following operations. The retention is not necessarily complete and the patient may be able to urinate, but there is a varying amount of residual urine, from a few ounces to several pints. In the great majority of cases the infection is bilateral. Occasionally the condition arises spontaneously, but most often it is an ascending infection following the passage of a catheter, or other instrument, or operations on the lower urinary track. The old name for this condition was "surgical kidneys," and in the days of unsterile catheterisation it was frequent and dreaded.

Pathology.—At post-mortem examination the kidneys are enlarged and miliary abscesses can be seen beneath the capsules. On bisection there are numerous yellow streaks of pus in the parenchyma radiating from the medulla to the convex border. The renal calyces, pelvis, and ureters are dilated.

Clinical Features.—The symptoms are similar to those of severe acute pyelonephritis without retention, but in addition, depending upon the amount of renal damage by back pressure, there will be superadded varying degrees of uræmia. There is rigidity and tenderness in both loins, though often more in evidence on one side than the other.

TREATMENT OF ACUTE PYELONEPHRITIS

If the urine is acid, as it is in the common coliform infections, alkalinisation of the urine has a very beneficial effect in relieving the symptoms and in inhibiting the growth of these organisms. The following mixture, given four-hourly or more often, is efficacious :

R	Sodium Citrate .	.	.	.	.	gr. 20 (1·3 gm.)
	Sodium Bicarbonate .	.	.	.	gr. 20 (1·3 gm.)
	Syr. aurantii	.	.	.	.	q.s.
	Aq. ad	.	.	.	.	. to ½ ounce (15 ml.)

Tinct. Hyoscyamus, minims 20 (1·2 ml.), can be added to the mixture with advantage, to diminish pain.

We have found that to alkalinise the urine rapidly an intravenous injection of 10 ml. each of an isotonic solution of sodium lactate and a saturated solution of sodium bicarbonate (ampoules ready for use can be obtained from Crookes Laboratories) is very effective in ultra-acute cases.

If pain is severe, one of the anti-spasmodics (p. 656) is given and heat is applied to the affected loin by fomentations, an electric heating pad, or antiphlogistine.

The patient should be encouraged to imbibe large quantities of bland fluid, about 5 pints (3 litres) in the twenty-four hours. In severe cases with vomiting or dehydration, intravenous saline and glucose should be given until the dehydration has been rectified and the vomiting has ceased.

When the bacteriological report on the urine is to hand, treatment with a urinary antiseptic should be commenced. For mild and moderately severe cases the first of the under-mentioned is used. For severe cases the second is recommended. According to the bacteriology, one of the remainder is indicated, usually when the infection has resisted treatment by the first two agents.

Urinary Antiseptics.—The following are in common use :

Sulphonamides.—Sulphamezathine and sulphatriad (a combination of sulphathiazole, sulphadiazine, and sulphamerazine) have proved to be particularly satisfactory in urinary infections. The latter has the advantage of almost eliminating the risk of sulphonamide crystaluria. The dose is 1 gm. four-hourly by mouth for the first two days, both by night and by day.

During the third and the fourth days four doses are given in the twenty-four hours, and on the fifth and sixth days three doses. Most coliform infections are susceptible to these sulphonamides, the B. coli regularly so. Some strains of Proteus are also eradicated. Gram-positive organisms and Ps. pyocyaneus are nearly always resistant.

Streptomycin is exceedingly efficacious in all gram-negative infections, and at the same time it is inimical to most staphylococci and streptococci. Before commencing treatment with this antibiotic the urine should be rendered alkaline, as streptomycin is much more active in an alkaline than in an acid medium. Streptomycin is administered by intramuscular injection in doses of 0·5 gm. twice daily for three days. Streptomycin is the most powerful of the urinary antiseptics, and it often renders the urine sterile within three days. Should any strain of organism survive this onslaught it becomes extremely streptomycin-resistant, and a second course of this antibiotic is ineffective except in the rare event of the infection being a new one. It is profitable, therefore, to employ streptomycin as a first method of attack only in cases of great severity. In other circumstances it should be employed after failure of sulphonamides to eliminate the infection.

The main complication arising from the use of streptomycin is damage to the eighth cranial nerve resulting in vertigo and deafness, which persist for two to four months, after which time compensation usually occurs.

Penicillin is most effective in gram-positive infections. The usual dose is 200,000 units intramuscularly at intervals of eight hours for three to six days. Penicillin is more active in an acid urine, therefore alkalinisation should cease before it is administered, and if necessary ammonium chloride 1 gm. four-hourly substituted.

Aureomycin has a wide range of therapeutic activity. It is effective against gram-positive, and also most gram-negative, organisms, with the exception of Proteus and Ps. pyocyaneus. The administration is oral, 0·5 gm. four-hourly before meals. The course of treatment extends over a week. This antibiotic engenders nausea and sometimes vomiting, which is relieved somewhat by giving aluminium hydroxide, 10 gm., with each dose of aureomycin.

Chloromycetin is effective in most gram-negative urinary

infections, except Ps. pyocyaneus and some strains of Proteus. The drug is given by mouth. The usual initial dose is 1 to 2 gm., followed by a maintenance dose of 0·5 gm. six-hourly for seven to ten days. There are no toxic effects attributable to this drug.

Mandelic acid and its salts have been largely replaced by antibiotic treatment. Contraindications to this form of therapy are impairment of renal function, and infections producing ammoniacal decomposition of the urine. It is often curative in coliform infections and those caused by streptococcus fæcalis. Ammonium mandelate 2 gm., together with 1 gm. of ammonium chloride, is given six-hourly. Fluids are restricted to $2\frac{1}{2}$ pints (1·5 litres) in the twenty-four hours. The treatment is continued for a week.

CHRONIC PYELONEPHRITIS

Chronic pyelonephritis can occur insidiously or follow an attack of acute pyelonephritis. In the majority of instances the symptoms are those of cystitis, combined with intermittent lumbar pain. At others there are no localising symptoms, but rheumatic pains in various parts of the body, particularly over the lower part of the back. In such cases attention is directed to the urinary organs by finding pus in the urine. Chronic pyelonephritis can occur with or without retention of bladder urine.

Investigations.—The following investigations are carried out in chronic cases, and in acute cases after the acute phase has subsided with treatment by a sulphonamide or an antibiotic.

Such investigations are directed to unfolding a cause of obstruction to the upper or lower urinary track, and/or a source of infection, which is present most often in the genital organs or the urethra.

(*a*) *Clinical.*—The kidneys are palpated for tenderness and enlargement, and the bladder for chronic retention of urine. In middle-aged or elderly males the prostate is examined for enlargement or fibrosis. Especially in male children, atresia of the meatus or meatitis is sought.

(*b*) *A plain X-ray* of the urinary tract will reveal or eliminate the presence of a urinary calculus.

(*c*) *Excretory Pyelography.*—In chronic pyelonephritis and after an attack of severe acute, or recurring acute pyelonephritis, changes in the pyelographic shadow will be manifest. Some of these are similar to those of early hydronephrosis, but they are more unequally distributed. Although the calyces become flattened or clubbed, this is more in evidence in one part of the kidney than another. Persistent poor definition in one group of calyces is presumptive evidence of chronic infection. In cases of longer standing the renal pelvis becomes slightly dilated, but unlike hydronephrosis, the dilatation of the calyces predominates. Radiographs taken in the prone and the upright positions will determine or disprove the existence of nephroptosis, which is sometimes a cause of defective drainage of the renal pelvis. In a few cases of chronic pyelonephritis the upper part of the ureter is slightly dilated. As a result of a severe acute infection where the parenchyma has been the seat of widespread suppuration, there results chronic sclerosing pyelonephritis, which is recognised in the pyelogram by greatly dilated and deformed calyces with or without dilatation of the renal pelvis.

A film of the bladder filled with medium will occasionally reveal a diverticulum, while a film taken after micturition will demonstrate residual urine, if such is present.

(d) Examination of the cervix uteri with a speculum often displays cervicitis or cervical erosion. Examination of the secretion expressed by prostatic massage sometimes accounts for the presence of infection. If no infection is found in these situations, a possible focus in carious teeth or infected tonsils is excluded later.

(e) *Cysto-urethroscopy* should not be undertaken in cases of prostatic obstruction when there is sufficient residual urine to render the bladder palpable. After the instrument has been passed residual urine, if any, is measured. In both sexes examination of the urethra may show chronic urethritis or the presence of a stricture. In the female urethro-trigonitis is commonly found. Hitherto unconfirmed obstruction to the prostatic urethra by an enlarged middle lobe or median bar may be demonstrated. Evidence of cystitis is the most common cystoscopic finding. The ureteric orifice, or orifices in bilateral cases, is sometimes seen pouting, œdematous, or gaping. Some delay in efflux is usual on the affected side. Ureteric catheters are passed and specimens collected from each kidney. These specimens are examined for cells and bacteria. By these means it is ascertained whether the infection is bilateral or unilateral. In male children valves or stricture in the posterior urethra, or an enlarged verumontanum, are sometimes found.

Treatment.—When an obstructive lesion is found in any part of the urinary passages, after controlling infection as far as possible by a urinary antiseptic, the obstruction is removed. Local treatment of a focus of infection, when present, greatly helps in preventing recurrence of pyelonephritis.

PYONEPHROSIS

The kidney is converted into a multilocular sac containing pus or purulent urine, with a varying amount of renal parenchyma in its walls. A pyonephrosis can result from infection of a hydronephrosis, following pyelonephritis or, most commonly, as a complication of renal calculus (calculous pyonephrosis). As a rule the condition is unilateral. Like a hydronephrosis, it may be open or closed ; sometimes the occlusion is intermittent.

Clinical Features.—In the more usual open pyonephrosis there is pyuria, often obvious to the naked eye. There is constant pain in the affected loin, worse at night, and a renal swelling is palpable. When the condition arises as an infection of a hydronephrosis the swelling may be a large one. When the pyonephrosis is open an evening rise of temperature to 99 or 100° F. (37·2 or 37·7° C.) is usual ; if the pyonephrosis becomes closed, the temperature is considerably higher. Pyuria, when present, gives rise to cystitis, and the symptoms of that condition may be the chief complaint.

Investigation.—A plain X-ray may reveal the presence of a calculus. Excretory pyelography shows the same vagaries as advanced hydronephrosis, in that the shadow of the dilated renal pelvis and calyces is long delayed and may be absent. Cystoscopy often reveals chronic cystitis with a purulent efflux from the affected side. In closed cases the bladder is likely to be normal and the passage of a ureteric catheter may be arrested, most usually at the pelvi-ureteric junction, or may pass the obstruction and give exit to purulent urine.

Treatment.—In early cases of infection of a hydronephrosis, by the use of urinary antiseptics and the passage of a ureteric catheter to drain infected urine from the renal pelvis, it is occasionally possible to reconvert the pyonephrosis into a hydronephrosis. In most unilateral cases if, as is frequently the case, anæmia is present, as soon as the patient's general condition has been improved nephrectomy is undertaken. When the capsule is densely adherent to the surrounding structures subcapsular nephrectomy is performed. Rarely, when the patient's general condition cannot be improved, nephrostomy is carried out, a measure to be avoided if possible, because it renders subsequent nephrectomy more difficult. When the condition arises in a sole existing kidney, or in cases of bilateral pyonephrosis, permanent nephrostomy is the only measure which can be adopted.

CARBUNCLE OF THE KIDNEY

The source of origin of the organism is usually a cutaneous lesion, such as a boil, carbuncle, or whitlow, and the staphylococcus aureus is conveyed to the kidney via the blood-stream.

Morbid Anatomy.—On splitting open the kidney there is a necrotic mass of tissue involving the parenchyma (fig. 705).

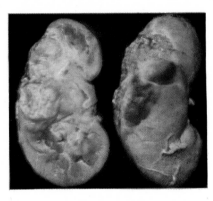

FIG. 705.—Carbuncle of the kidney.

Ætiology.—There is often a history of injury such as a blow upon the loin. If such a blow occurs while the patient is suffering from a cutaneous staphylococcal lesion, a carbuncle of the kidney is liable to develop.

Clinical Features. — Men are more frequently affected than women, and the right side more often than the left. There is an ill-defined, tender swelling in the loin, persistent pyrexia, and leucocytosis. In early cases the urine contains neither pus cells nor organisms, but after a few days, with much centrifuging staphylococci can sometimes be isolated. Pyelography often shows compression or obliteration of a group of calyces, an appearance which does not differ from adenocarcinoma of the kidney.

Treatment.—Penicillin has proved curative in a large proportion of cases. In a few resolution does not occur. An extensive carbuncle which resolves is sometimes followed by chronic sclerosing pyelonephritis. When resolution fails to occur the kidney must be exposed, the carbuncle incised with a diathermy knife, and the perinephric space drained. Although this conservative operation is often successful, a persistent discharging sinus sometimes follows which can only be remedied by secondary nephrectomy. Primary nephrectomy is indicated only when the major part of the kidney is involved by the carbuncle.

PERINEPHRIC ABSCESS

A perinephric abscess can arise in many ways. The most common are depicted in fig. 706. Other causes are infection of a perirenal hæmatoma and an extension from a pyonephrosis or a renal carbuncle. A tuberculous perinephritic abscess arises from advanced tuberculosis of the kidney or from tuberculosis of nearby vertebræ.

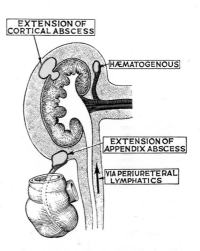

FIG. 706.—Sources of perinephric abscess.

Clinical Features.—The classical symptoms and signs of a perinephric abscess are a high, swinging temperature, rigidity, tenderness, and fullness in the loin. If the suppuration commences in the lower part of the perinephric fat, localising signs present early, but when perirenal suppuration is confined to the upper portion of the perinephric fat which lies beneath the lower ribs, it produces no visible swelling, and even rigidity and tenderness may be absent. The leucocyte count is always raised, often to 20,000 per cmm. As a rule no pus or organisms are present in the urine, even if a ureteric specimen is examined. X-ray examination often shows obscuration of the psoas shadow, with one or more of the following additional signs— scoliosis with concavity towards the abscess and elevation and immobility of the diaphragm on the affected side.

There are no characteristic early signs on excretory pyelography, except :

Mathé's sign. Absence of the downward displacement that occurs in the erect posture in every normal kidney. Two radiographs, one in the lying posture and one in the erect posture, during excretory pyelography are required.

Charles P. L. Mathé, Contemporary. Urologist-in-Chief, St. Mary's Hospital, San Francisco.

Later the kidney may be shown to be displaced, especially forwards, if a lateral view is obtained.

Treatment.—A lumbar incision large enough to enable the surgeon to open up pockets both above and below the kidney is made. At the same time the surface of the kidney is palpated for an unruptured cortical abscess, which, if present, should be incised. A specimen of pus having been obtained for bacteriological examination, the wound is closed with ample drainage. Appropriate antibiotic treatment follows.

RENAL TUBERCULOSIS

Ætiology.—There is abundant evidence that the original renal lesions are multiple and bilateral. They arise as juxtaglomerular microscopical cortical foci, which sometimes heal uneventfully. When symptomatic renal tuberculosis arises

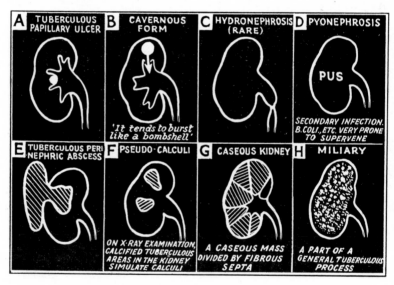

Fig. 707.—Blackboard sketches of types of tuberculous kidney (macroscopic pathology).[1]

it does so in one kidney only, in the great majority of cases. A group of foci coalesce and discharge pus and tubercle bacilli along one set of tubules, and the apex of the pyramid which gives exit to the discharge becomes ulcerated. Alternatively,

[1] G is called the "cement kidney" by the French. It is Nature's method of performing nephrectomy.

and somewhat less frequently, a larger abscess, having become walled off temporarily in the parenchyma, bursts into a calyx.

Course.—Once established as a visible lesion, renal tuberculosis disseminates to other parts of the kidney, and is sometimes confined to the organ for months or years. More often it spreads along the ureter to give rise to tuberculous cystitis, and eventually the second kidney becomes implicated by infection ascending along the peri-ureteral lymphatics, or by vesico-ureteral reflux. In the male, renal and genital tuberculosis are frequently associated, often before the bladder and posterior urethra are involved, in which event the genital infection probably occurs in the following way : an urgent desire to micturate causes the internal sphincter to open and the voluntary closure of the external sphincter prevents the escape of urine. At this moment infected urine is forced under pressure into the mucosal crypts of the prostate and into a common ejaculatory duct (Wells).

Clinical Features.—Rare during childhood, renal tuberculosis reaches its zenith between twenty and forty years of age. Men are affected twice as commonly as women, and the right kidney somewhat more commonly than the left.

Frequency.—The earliest symptom is frequency of micturition. Often this is the only symptom. It is progressive, the patient complaining that over a period of months frequency has increased both by day and by night.

The causes of the persistent, progressive, and unremitting frequency are, in order of sequence :

1. Polyuria. The output of the inflamed kidney is increased.
2. Irritation of the bladder by caseous débris passed down the ureter.
3. Tuberculous cystitis.
4. Increasing diminution of bladder capacity from fibrosis.
5. Secondary infection.

Pyuria.—In early cases the urine is pale and slightly opalescent. The presence of pus cells without organisms in an acid urine is extremely suggestive of tuberculous urinary infection. It is very unlikely that tubercle bacilli will be found in a single bladder specimen.

If renal tuberculosis is suspected but tubercle bacilli cannot be demonstrated, the patient should bring a twenty-four-hour specimen of urine. The sediment of this specimen is examined. Lowenstein's culture has made it relatively easy to cultivate tubercle bacilli. Whereas formerly, when animal inoculations were employed exclusively, it took six weeks

Charles Alexander Wells, Contemporary. Professor of Surgery, University of Liverpool.

before the diagnosis could be confirmed, by cultural methods the result is obtained in about three weeks.

In no field of medicine can the diagnosis be more exact. The microscope demonstrates tubercle bacilli in 72 per cent., the guinea-pig test in 94 per cent., and the culture medium in 98 per cent.

Chronic Epididymitis.—Aching in a testis may be an early symptom.

Painful Micturition.—Once tuberculous cystitis has set in, micturition becomes increasingly painful. First there is suprapubic pain if the bladder cannot be emptied immediately ; later a burning pain accompanies micturition, and when secondary infection has occurred there is superadded agonising pain after micturition referred to the tip of the penis or to the vulva, often associated with terminal hæmaturia (strangury).

Renal pain is often absent throughout the complete process of destruction of the kidney. Sometimes the patient complains of a dull ache in the loin.

Hæmaturia.—In 5 per cent. of cases the disease is ushered in with severe painless hæmaturia occurring from an ulcer situated on a renal papilla. During the hæmorrhage, and after it has ceased, investigations may or may not demonstrate the presence of a renal lesion and tubercle bacilli in the urine. In the latter event more typical symptoms usually commence some months later. Apart from the terminal hæmaturia or cystitis, macroscopical hæmaturia occurs only occasionally.

Constitutional Symptoms.—A continuous slight loss of weight is usual. Evening pyrexia to 99° F. (37·3° C.) occurs when the disease is fully established. A high temperature is indicative of a secondary infection by another organism, or disseminating tuberculosis.

On Examination.—It is unusual for a tuberculous kidney to be palpable.

When a patient with renal tuberculosis has an enlarged kidney which can be felt, it is by no means certain that this kidney is the one which is diseased, for compensatory hypertrophy sometimes renders the healthy kidney both large and tender.

The line of the ureter, and (in the male) the prostate, vesicles, vas, and epididymis should be examined for thickening, which bespeaks tuberculous invasion of these parts.

Investigation :

A plain X-ray sometimes shows areas of calcification in the kidney.

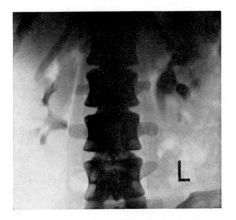

Fig. 708.—Excretory pyelogram in a case of tuberculous left kidney. Showing incomplete definition of the lower calyces and dilatation of the middle and upper calyces.

(*H. P. Winsbury-White.*)

Excretory pyelography reveals fairly well-established pathological changes. In these the evidence it produces concerning the diseased kidney and the opposite kidney is of supreme importance. The earliest change to be recognised is persistent irregularity and slight dilatation of a calyx. More gross lesions of the cavernous type are readily apparent. The affected ureter is often dilated, usually irregularly. In late cases the contralateral ureter often becomes dilated from obstruction to its intramural part by the cicatrised bladder. This is not necessarily an indication of disease in the opposite kidney. A series of excretory pyelograms that show an undoubted unilateral lesion, together with apparent normality of the kidney and ureter on the opposite side, is considered by some to suffice in making the diagnosis and determining operative treatment.

Cystoscopy.—When frequency is the only symptom, and that has not been present long, the bladder and the ureteric orifices are normal. The more frequent efflux and a delay in excretion of indigo-carmine may indicate which side is diseased. A unilateral cloudy efflux is sometimes observed before any vesical involvement. In 10 per cent. of cases there is an absence of efflux on the affected side, and no pathological changes in the bladder. These are examples of a closed ureter leading to so-called autonephrectomy, or a pyonephrosis. Hyperæmia around a ureteric orifice is the earliest cystoscopic sign of vesical involvement. Infiltration follows, and the affected ureteric orifice becomes raised in relation to the bladder wall. Tubercles appear, usually externally to the ureteric orifice, and over its intramural projection. Next they appear in the fundus of the same half of the bladder. By confluence of these tubercles, a tuberculous ulcer, which is irregular in outline, may form. Such an ulcer is seen near the affected ureteric orifice and often also in the fundus of the bladder. Later bulbous œdema frequently surrounds and hides the ureteric orifice, which can only be detected by the efflux of indigo-carmine. In long-standing cases, as a result of sclerosing peri-ureteritis, which causes shortening of the ureter, the ureteric orifice becomes displaced upwards and its mouth remains open (fig. 709). As the disease progresses the capacity of the bladder becomes increasingly diminished. At any stage, if a secondary infection supervenes, the intense generalised inflammation of the bladder wall obliterates many of the characteristic features described above.

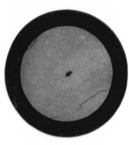

FIG. 709. — Golf-hole ureter. It fails to close between the effluxes.
(*Newman.*)
(*British Journal of Surgery.*)

Bilateral ureteric catheterisation should be carried out in early cases and the urine from each kidney examined for pus and tubercle bacilli. In later cases, when the appearance of the excretory pyelogram is characteristic, ureteric catheterisation can be limited to the supposed sound side, for confirmation or disproval that this side is free from infection. The catheter should be passed no farther than the middle third of the ureter, for fear of transmitting infection to the kidney.

Retrograde pyelography is necessary to establish the diagnosis in early cases. Appearances, such as shagginess of a calyx or an abscess of the parenchyma connected to a calyx by a narrow neck, are often displayed by this method when excretory pyelograms appear normal.

Examination of the Lungs.—An X-ray of the thorax and examination of the sputum, if present, should be undertaken to exclude active pulmonary tuberculosis.

Treatment:

Operative Treatment.—In cases when the infection has been proved to be unilateral, nephrectomy should be undertaken. Because in many cases the ureter is involved also (figs. **710** and

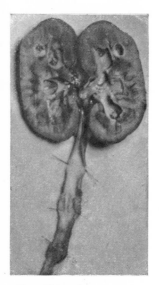

FIG. 710.—Cavernous type of renal tuberculosis. Note the abscess in the upper pole and the dilated ureter.

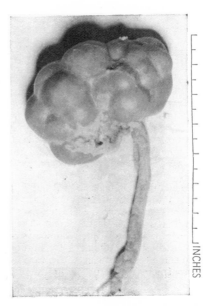

FIG. 711.—Tuberculous pyonephrosis. Nephro-ureterectomy.

711) the operation of nephro-ureterectomy, in which, through a separate incision, the ureter is divided and ligated at its entrance to the bladder before commencing lumbar nephrectomy, is the operation of choice. By total removal of the ureter a possible source of continued infection of the bladder is removed, and the incidence of post-operative wound infection and sinus formation is reduced. Nephrectomy is also indicated in cases of bilateral tuberculosis when one organ is much more diseased than the other, provided the renal function tests on the less involved side are satisfactory. Unless the lesion in the remaining kidney is a very small one, a cure cannot be expected in these circumstances, but often the symptoms are ameliorated.

Sanatorium Treatment.—Even when there are no pulmonary manifestations, six to twelve months' post-operative sanatorium treatment is beneficial.

Treatment by streptomycin is indicated in the following circumstances :

1. Tuberculous pyuria without a demonstrable renal lesion.
2. In bilateral cases unsuitable for operative treatment.
3. After nephrectomy when (*a*) tuberculous cystitis is present ;

(b) the remaining kidney is involved ; (c) a sinus develops in the scar.

A course of streptomycin (preferably dihydrostreptomycin) for tuberculosis is 0·5 gm. two or three times daily for sixty days.

ABACTERIAL PYURIA

That sterile pyuria indicates urinary tuberculosis is almost axiomatic. Nevertheless, there is a small group of cases of abacterial pyuria which is definitely non-tuberculous. The symptoms simulate renal tuberculosis very closely, and it is only when repeated examinations of the urine fail to reveal tubercle bacilli or other bacteria, and cultures and guinea-pig innoculations are negative, that the diagnosis can be made. Pyelography may be normal, or show one or both renal pelves and ureters dilated. Cystoscopy shows a severe cystitis and often diminished bladder capacity. The cause has been attributed to a virus, but in some cases spirilla have been found in the urine when examined by dark-ground illumination. Occasionally amœbiasis is responsible.

Treatment.—In many cases the condition is cured by neoarsphenamine 0·3 gm. injected intravenously weekly for four weeks. Great improvement is often noted after the first dose. Aureomycin has proved successful in some resistant cases. In rare instances, when amœbiasis is responsible, treatment with emetine hydrochloride is likely to eradicate the infection.

HYPERTENSION AND A RENAL LESION

Renal ischæmia regularly produces increased arterial tension. It has been established with reasonable certainty that ischæmia of the renal parenchyma leads to the formation of a vasopressor substance. Too often cases are labelled essential hypertension without a thorough urological examination. Sometimes in a case of hypertension a unilateral diseased kidney is demonstrated and nephrectomy is followed by permanent lowering of the blood-pressure. The most amenable lesion in this respect is sclerosing pyelonephritis. Occasionally patients with renal tuberculosis, a renal neoplasm, or renal calculi with infection, have been permanently benefited, in so far as hypertension is concerned, by removing the diseased kidney.

NEOPLASMS OF THE KIDNEY

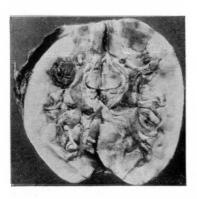

FIG. 712.—Angioma of the kidney. The kidney was excised for profuse painless hæmaturia.

Benign Neoplasms

Adenoma.—Pea-like cortical adenomata are sometimes found at necropsy. They give rise to no symptoms during life, and are of academic interest only.

Angioma is usually of the venous type, and may give rise to profuse hæmaturia. Fig. 712 shows a kidney containing a venous hæmangioma. The patient, who was a woman of thirty-five, had attacks of painless hæmaturia extending over five years.

Hans Wilbolz, 1873–1940. Professor of Urology, Berne. First described abacterial pyuria.

Truly benign tumours of the kidney are so rare that a good rule is " *all neoplasms of the kidney which can be recognised clinically should be considered malignant and treated as such.*"

MALIGNANT NEOPLASMS

Clinically neoplasms of the kidney are divided into two classes :

Those occurring in children between the ages of one and five.

Those occurring in adults after the age of forty.

Between the ages of five and forty malignant neoplasms of the kidney are rare.

THOSE OCCURRING IN CHILDREN

Wilms's tumour (*syn.* embryonal adenosarcoma ; nephroblastoma) is a mixed tumour arising from the connective tissue of the kidney. In early infancy such tumours are sometimes bilateral. More common is a unilateral neoplasm appearing between the ages of two and three. Exceptionally a tumour appearing in adult life is proved by histological examination to be a Wilms's tumour.

Clinical Features.—The symptomatology is always the same. An abdominal tumour appears and progresses rapidly, while the general health deteriorates. Hæmaturia does not occur until late in the disease. Examination of the abdomen reveals a mass which may be enormous (fig. 713) ; the bulk of the tumour is on one side of the abdomen. Wilms's tumour tends to grow within a capsule, pushing the rest of the kidney away ; thus the reniform shape of the kidney is lost early. As a rule the diagnosis presents but little difficulty. It is, however, necessary to differentiate the tumour from a congenital hydronephrosis, and on the left side an enlarged spleen has to be excluded. Pyelography will show gross deformity of the calyces and often of the renal pelvis also.

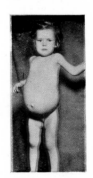

FIG. 713.—
Wilms's tumour.

Wilms's tumour metastasises early, usually to the lungs, but also to the regional lymph nodes and the liver.

Histologically these neoplasms are composed mainly of two types of cells—epithelial and connective-tissue. Cartilage, bone, and smooth or striped muscle fibres are occasional findings. The epithelial and connective-tissue cells exist side by side, but one is usually predominant. Thus the tumour is composed of mixed cellular elements, some of which are

Max Wilms, 1867-1918. Professor of Surgery, Heidelberg.

radio-sensitive and some radio-resistant. Consequently, the radio-resistant elements show an unabated continuance of activity in spite of radiotherapy.

Treatment.—A pre-operative course of deep X-ray therapy is given. In many cases this causes diminution in the size of the tumour, but it also causes leucopenia and anæmia. Therefore, in the interval of four weeks that elapses between irradiation and the operation, blood transfusion, as necessary, is carried out. Nephrectomy is then performed. If the tumour has not decreased greatly in size, the abdominal route is chosen ; otherwise lumbar nephrectomy is undertaken. As soon as the wound has healed post-operative irradiation is given. The operative mortality is about 20 per cent. In spite of irradiation, metastases prove fatal within two years in about 90 per cent. of cases.

THOSE OCCURRING IN ADULTS

1. **Adenocarcinoma** (*syn.* Grawitz tumour ; hypernephroma) is the commonest neoplasm of the kidney (78 per cent.). It arises in the cortex, possibly from a pre-existing adenoma, probably *per primam* in cells of the uriniferous tubules.

Pathology.—A tumour of moderate size is spherical in shape, and it often occupies one or other pole, the seat of election being the upper pole ; less often it is in the central portion of the kidney. On section it is characteristically yellow (due to lipoid) ; less often it is dull white, or semi-transparent. Hæmorrhagic areas are often seen. The tumour is divided into numerous lobules by fibrous septa (fig. 714). The larger the tumour the more extensive is central hæmorrhage and necrosis.

Microscopical Structure.—The most common appearance is solid alveoli of cubical or polyhedral clear cells, with deeply stained small rounded

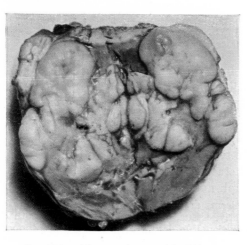

FIG. 714.—Adenocarcinoma of the kidney.

Paul Grawitz, 1850–1932. Professor of Pathology, Greifswald, Germany.

nuclei and abundant cytoplasm containing lipoids, cholesterol, and glycogen. The cells may also be arranged in the form of papillary cysts or tubules. In a much smaller percentage the cells are granular (dark). Clear and dark cells can co-exist in different parts of the same tumour. In all cases the stroma is scanty but rich in large blood-vessels, the walls of which often appear in places to consist of tumour cells.

Spread.—As the tumour enlarges it encroaches upon a group of calyces. It is prone to grow into the renal veins. Pieces of growth become detached, and are swept into the circulation when metastases become disseminated, particularly to the lungs and bones. Sometimes when a secondary growth appears in a long bone it is the only metastasis for a long time—sometimes a year or more.

While spread by the blood-stream predominates, spread by lymphatics also occurs, in some cases before the former. If the tumour bursts through the renal capsule into the perirenal tissues, it then metastasises to the lymph nodes in relation to the hilum of the kidney, and from there to the pre-aortic and other lymph nodes.

The following table shows the sites of these metastases, and is founded upon statistics compiled by A. P. Graham :

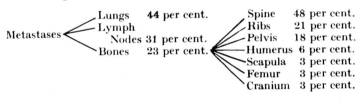

Metastases		
Lungs	44 per cent.	
Lymph Nodes	31 per cent.	
Bones	23 per cent.	

Spine	48 per cent.
Ribs	21 per cent.
Pelvis	18 per cent.
Humerus	6 per cent.
Scapula	3 per cent.
Femur	3 per cent.
Cranium	3 per cent.

Less commonly the liver, the brain, or the contralateral kidney is involved.

Clinical Features.—Men are more often attacked than women, the ratio being 2·5 : 1. Typically the first sign is painless, profuse, intermittent hæmaturia. Clot colic may follow. Pain in the loin may be the leading symptom. Occasionally the first manifestation is a palpable renal swelling. In the male over thirty-five years of age a rapidly oncoming varicocele is a suspicious sign of a malignant kidney tumour.

Atypical Cases.—(*a*) In no less than 33 per cent. of cases the primary growth remains " silent," the patient presenting because of some manifestation of secondary deposits such as a painful

Albert Parker Graham. Surgeon, Hines Memorial Hospital, Cook County, Illinois, U.S.A.

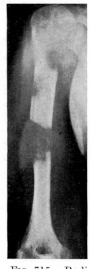

FIG. 715.—Radiograph showing metastases from a Grawitz tumour.

enlargement of a bone, a spontaneous fracture, persistent cough, or hæmoptysis. (*b*) There is a type in which persistent pyrexia is the only symptom, there being no infection to account for the temperature.

Differential Diagnosis.—(*a*) Hæmorrhage into a hydronephrosis, (*b*) congenital cystic kidney with hæmaturia, or (*c*) a solitary cyst of the kidney, can simulate a renal neoplasm to a point of nicety.

Early Diagnosis.—By the time a patient has the classical triad of symptoms, viz. hæmaturia, pain, and a palpable renal tumour, he nearly always has metastases. It is therefore of paramount importance to endeavour to make an early diagnosis and any one of these symptoms calls for a thorough renal investigation. Patients with painless hæmaturia, or hæmaturia which is not accompanied by symptoms of acute cystitis, should be examined cystoscopically while the bleeding is in progress. If blood is seen issuing from one ureteric orifice, and there is a clear efflux from the other, the information gained is of considerable value, but is by no means conclusive evidence of a renal neoplasm. Extremely suggestive is bleeding occurring from a palpable kidney. The early diagnosis rests almost entirely on pyelography. Excretory pyelography is seldom conclusive in early cases, because of lack of precise definition, and in late cases because there is poor or no concentration of the medium. At all times it is of great value in determining the function of the other kidney. Retrograde pyelography is often required owing to the better delineation it gives. The principal changes in the pyelogram of a kidney which is the seat of an adenocarcinoma are :

1. Filling defects due to invasion of one or more of the minor or major calyces. Very characteristic is failure of the medium to enter one major calyx.

2. Elongation and compression of one or more calyces and sometimes of the renal pelvis. This gives rise to what is known as the " spider leg " deformity (fig. 716). In congenital

cystic kidneys the "spider legs" are broader, more clearly cut, and involve the whole kidney ; moreover the condition is bilateral.

3. Displacement of the renal pelvis and the distorted calyces downwards in growths occupying the upper pole. Growths of the lower pole often displace the ureter inwards.

4. In advanced cases (which may give no shadow on excretory pyelography) the interior of the calyces and renal pelvis are so encroached upon that they are represented by a few, irregular, widely separated, medium-filled opacities.

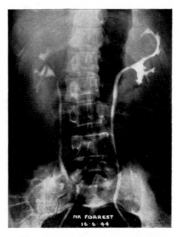

Fig. 716.—Retrograde pyelogram in a case of a Grawitz tumour of the left kidney. The only symptom was one attack of painless hæmaturia.

Treatment.—In cases without secondary deposits—and in this connection a radiograph of the thorax should always be performed—the treatment is nephrectomy with the removal of the perinephric fat. The abdominal or thoraco-abdominal routes (p. 684) offer certain advantages, notably that the pedicle can be ligated before the organ is handled, thereby minimising dissemination of the growth. Whichever route is chosen, the renal vein should be ligated as near as possible to the inferior vena cava, for in 10 per cent. of cases there is an extension of the growth into this vein.

Pre-operative irradiation often renders large tumours smaller. In inoperable cases, and in the presence of secondary deposits, this is the only form of treatment. Deep X-ray therapy often results in dramatic regression of a secondary growth, but improvement is usually only temporary and there follow other secondary growths less radio-sensitive.

Prognosis.—Statistical studies show that the size of the tumour is unimportant. Some of the largest growths have been followed by a permanent cure. In operable cases about 50 per cent. of the patients are alive and well after three years.

2. **Papilloma of the renal pelvis** (fig. 717) is similar in structure to papilloma of the bladder. It tends to invade the kidney

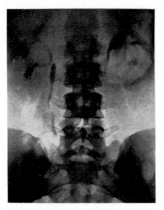

FIG. 717.—Pyelogram show-ing a papilloma of the renal pelvis.

(*Carl Krebs, Aarhus, Denmark.*)

proper, and to take on malignant characteristics. It also spreads down the ureter and may invade the bladder. Papillomatous growths of the renal pelvis constitute 9 per cent. of renal neoplasms.

Clinical Features.—Hæmaturia is often continued for months at a time. A renal swelling is absent, except in rare cases where the pelvi-ureteric junction becomes occluded and a hæmonephrosis results, in which event there is lumbar pain. Occasionally renal colic occurs from blood clot passing down the ureter.

Nephrectomy *with ureterectomy* is the correct treatment. The intramural portion of the ureter should be fulgurated thoroughly after the ureter has been divided as close as possible to the bladder wall.

3. **Squamous-celled carcinoma of the renal pelvis** is extremely rare, and appears to be preceded by leukoplakia. The condition is usually found associated with a renal calculus. Unless nephrectomy is performed early, the tumour spreads by direct infiltration of the perirenal tissues, and from thence to the pre-aortic lymph nodes.

Primary neoplasms of the ureter are also rare. Like those of the renal pelvis, they can be papillomata, papillary carcinoma, or squamous-celled carcinoma. The symptoms are identical with those of a neoplasm of the renal pelvis, although hydronephrosis, hæmonephrosis, and pyonephrosis are more frequent accompaniments. Occasionally a portion of a papillomatous growth can be seen protruding from a ureteric orifice. Usually the diagnosis is made by pyelography. The treatment is nephro-ureterectomy.

EXPOSURE OF THE KIDNEY

A lumbar approach is usually employed for all operations on the kidney, with the possible exception that some other route may be preferable for nephrectomy in the case of large neoplasms and, in the opinion of some, for all neoplasms.

The Oblique Lumbar Incision (Morris).—The patient is placed on the sound side, the lower limb of that side being flexed at the hip and the knee, while that of the opposite side is extended and supported by a pillow. The arm on the affected side is bandaged to an arm-rest, the other arm being flexed with the hand lying near the face. The bridge of the operating table is raised so as to throw the affected loin into prominence. Further exaggeration of this position can be obtained by lowering the head and the foot of the table. The incision commences at the angle

Sir Henry Morris, 1844–1926. Surgeon, Middlesex Hospital, London.

between the twelfth rib and the erector spinæ, and extends downwards and forwards to a point ½ inch (1·25 cm.) above the anterior superior iliac spine (fig. 718). The incision is deepened through the subcutaneous fat, and the first muscle layer is displayed. This is composed of the latissimus dorsi with some of the fibres of the underlying serratus posticus inferior in the upper part of the wound, and the external oblique in the lower part of the wound. This layer is incised in the length of the incision and the next layer, comprising the internal oblique, is likewise incised, care being taken to preserve the subcostal nerve, which may be en-

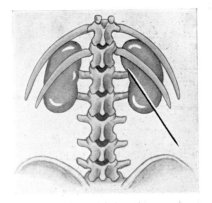

FIG. 718.—Morris's incision.

countered here or between this and the following layer. The third layer consists of the lumbar fascia (transversus aponeurosis) in the upper third of the incision and the transversus muscle in the lower part of the incision. The lumbar fascia is picked up in dissecting forceps and a small incision made into it. Extraperitoneal fat extrudes. Two fingers of the left hand are inserted beneath the fascia, which displaces the extraperitoneal fat and the peritoneum, while the fascia and the transversus muscle are divided in the length of the incision. In the upper third of the wound the extraperitoneal fat is displaced forwards, and the perirenal fascia (fascia of Zuckerkandl) comes into view. The fascia is picked up with dissecting forceps and incised well posteriorly, near the quadratus lumborum, the better to avoid opening the peritoneum in error. The incision in the renal fascia can be readily enlarged by traction with the fingers, and the lemon-yellow perirenal fat is displayed. As a rule the perirenal fascia and fat can be stripped easily from the renal capsule with the fingers, after which the kidney is delivered into the wound. If considerable adhesions are encountered, or if the kidney is too large to be withdrawn (or a combination of these circumstances) the first requirement is better access. This can be furnished by severing the lumbo-costal ligament, which extends from the neck of the last rib to the transverse processes of the first and second lumbar vertebræ. This permits the twelfth rib being dislocated upwards and nearly always entails ligation of the subcostal vessels, which were severed when the ligament was cut. Alternatively, the twelfth rib can be excised subperiosteally. A low reflexion of the pleura may be wounded during either of these procedures. It should be repaired immediately by sutures tied over a piece of fat, to prevent cutting through. Adhesions binding the kidney to the perirenal capsule, the peritoneum, or the diaphragm can now be rendered visible, clamped and cut proximal to the kidney, the distal ends being ligated. Such bands are encountered particularly at the poles of the kidney. Once freed from adhesions, the kidney is delivered. The peritoneum is occasionally wounded while mobilising the kidney ; the edges of the peritoneum are picked up and closed by a purse-string suture.

NEPHRECTOMY

Lumbar Nephrectomy.—The renal pedicle is cleared of fat so as to display its vascular components. The ureter is isolated and divided between

Emil Zuckerkandl 1849–1910. Professor of Anatomy, Vienna.

ligatures with a diathermy knife, as far from the kidney as possible. If there are aberrant vessels passing to the lower pole, these are divided between hæmostats and the distal end ligatured. Two, or if the pedicle is of such a length to permit it, three long curved hæmostats are applied to the pedicle, care being taken not to include the renal pelvis, which is retracted between the two most superficial hæmostats, if three have been applied, or between the hilum and the more superficial hæmostat if two were employed. A length of number 3 or 4 chromic catgut is tested for its tensile strength, and is passed beneath the deepest hæmostat. As the first knot approaches the pedicle the assistant loosens and then removes this hæmostat. The knot is tied. A second ligature is applied by transfixion beneath the remaining hæmostat, and as the second knot of this transfixion ligature is tied the assistant gradually loosens and removes this hæmostat. Only when it is certain that hæmostasis is complete are the ends of the ligatures cut.

Abdominal nephrectomy is employed in cases of rupture of the kidney complicated by an intraperitoneal lesion, and for large neoplasms. In the case of the latter, a sandbag placed under the affected loin helps to keep hollow viscera from the field of operation. A long upper paramedian incision is made, and at the level of the umbilicus a transverse extension is carried through the rectus muscle and the muscles of the lateral abdominal wall. When the peritoneum has been opened, the first step is to mobilise the colon medially by incising the peritoneum over its lateral aspect. By gauze dissection the colon and the attached peritoneum are pushed gently towards the middle line and the kidney is exposed. On the right side the duodenum is also mobilised. The renal vessels can be ligated close to the aorta and inferior vena cava before the kidney is handled ; this is advantageous in preventing detachment of an extension of the neoplasm into the renal vein.

CHAPTER XXVIII
THE URINARY BLADDER

ACUTE RETENTION OF URINE

ACUTE retention is usually, more correctly speaking, acute on chronic retention, for it seldom occurs unheralded.

Ætiology.—The condition is comparatively rare in women and children, and the most frequent causes are :

In the male :
> Prostatic enlargement.
> Urethral stricture.
> Acute urethritis.

In the female :
> Retroverted gravid uterus.
> Disseminated sclerosis.
> Hysteria.

In the male child :
> Atresia of the meatus and phimosis.
> Urethral or vesical calculus.

Other causes :
Post-operative retention.
Blood-clot in the bladder.
Foreign bodies in the bladder, urethra, or around the penis.
Rupture of the urethra.
Tumours of the bladder.
Spinal injuries and diseases, e.g. tabes dorsalis.
Ropy mucus from cystitis.
Muscular atony from advanced age, over-distension of the organ, or certain poisons, notably belladonna.

The patient has not passed urine for some hours, and is unable to do so. The full bladder can be recognised by palpation and percussion above the symphysis pubis. An attempt is made to elicit the cause of the retention. The floor of the urethra is palpated for induration of a stricture, the prostate is examined, and the reflexes are tested.

It is of paramount importance never to relieve, or attempt to relieve, acute retention and forthwith send the patient home. He must always be confined to bed immediately, and kept

S.P.—42

there for at least twenty-four hours after relief has been obtained. Once the patient is at home, or in hospital, if the general condition is good, the effect of administering a dose of morphia (to allay anxiety) and a hot bath (to promote cutaneous hyperæmia) is tried. In a proportion of cases the patient is able to pass urine into the bath. If this fails, catheterisation is attempted. This should always be performed with full aseptic ritual. A soft rubber catheter, e.g. a Foley's catheter (fig. 719), is used ; if this is unsuccessful, and the case is one of a suspected enlarged prostate, a large bi-coudé gum-elastic catheter (fig. 720) is tried. On the other hand, should the case be one of stricture, a gum-elastic olivary catheter (fig. 721) is selected.

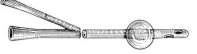
FIG. 719.—Foley's catheter.

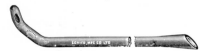
FIG. 720.—Bi-coudé catheter.
(*The bevel indicates the direction of the bend at the opposite end of the catheter.*)

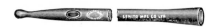
FIG. 721.—Olivary catheter.

Once a catheter has entered the distended bladder the urine must be let out slowly, a few ounces at a time. While decompression is in progress the catheter may be fixed temporarily in the urethra, and in order to control the flow of urine a stopper is inserted into its mouth. Four ounces of urine are permitted to escape each hour until the bladder is empty. The catheter is then removed.

Decompression of the bladder can be carried out more evenly and more slowly, which is most desirable, if the mouth of the catheter is connected with the dripper of an intravenous saline apparatus (fig. 722).

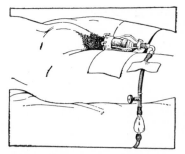
FIG. 722. — Decompression of the bladder using the dripper of an intravenous saline apparatus.

If, after a reasonable attempt with catheters, the bladder has not been entered, one of two courses may be adopted, according to circumstances.

Frederic Eugene Baisal Foley, Contemporary. Urologist, Miller and Ancker Hospitals, St. Paul, U.S.A.

1. **Suprapubic Catheterisation.**—Under local or general anæsthesia the front of the distended bladder is exposed by a short suprapubic incision. Into the distended bladder is thrust a Malécot's catheter (fig. 723) stretched upon an introducer, of which there are several patterns. Fig. 724 illustrates Bailey's bladder perforator which introduces the catheter without allowing the urine to gush forth (fig. 725). The cave of Retzius is

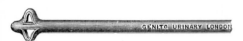

Fig. 723.—Malécot catheter.

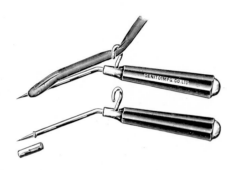

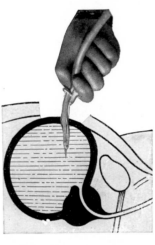

Fig. 724.—Apparatus for inserting a Malécot catheter into the exposed overfull bladder.

Fig. 725.—Introducing a suprapubic catheter into the exposed overfull bladder by means of the bladder perforator.

provided with a drain and the wound is then closed. The end of the catheter, which has been clipped, is connected to an intravenous saline dripper as shown in fig. 722. This allows the overfull bladder to be emptied slowly and steadily.

2. **Suprapubic Puncture with a Hollow Needle.**—Suprapubic puncture is a useful method of relieving acute retention when catheterisation has failed or the apparatus for introducing a suprapubic catheter cannot be obtained readily. The danger of this method is that if the bladder is allowed to refill after it has been punctured, leakage into the cave of Retzius may occur through the puncture hole. Used as a purely temporary expedient under extenuating circumstances, suprapubic puncture is a sound method of relieving urgent retention of urine.

RETENTION WITH OVERFLOW

Retention with overflow is referred to also under the headings of " false incontinence " (see below) and " prostatic enlargement " (see p. 722).

The general principles which govern the treatment of this condition are similar to the foregoing, but decompression of the bladder must be carried out exceedingly slowly.

Achille Malécot, M.D., Paris, invented his catheter in 1890.
Anders Retzius, 1796–1860. Professor of Anatomy, Stockholm,

POST-OPERATIVE RETENTION OF URINE

This is a frequent and troublesome condition, and while it can occur after any operation, it is more liable to do so after rectal and lower abdominal operations. Furthermore, proctoclysis definitely favours such retention.

Treatment.—The rectal tube, if present, should be removed. Potassium acetate, which is a parasympathetic stimulant and a diuretic, is prescribed : ½ oz. (15 ml.) of 1–15 solution of liquor potassii acetatis by mouth. The patient is reassured and placed on a *warm* bed-pan, if necessary, and the sound of a running tap is helpful. Failing this, an injection of Moryl (carbachol) can be prescribed, provided no operation, after which increased peristalsis is undesirable, has been performed. If these expedients fail, catheterisation must be resorted to.

INCONTINENCE OF URINE

Incontinence of urine is divided into two main varieties—*false* and *true*.

False Incontinence.—The bladder is full, the dribbling from the meatus being the overflow. False incontinence is observed chiefly in association with chronic retention from an enlarged prostate. It is met with also in some cases of injury or disease of the spinal cord interfering with the centre for micturition.

True Incontinence is subdivided into two clinical varieties :

(*a*) The urine dribbles away without further distending the bladder.

(*b*) The bladder becomes partially distended, but the patient exercises inadequate control over the organ.

Type (a) is the result of extensive damage to the compressor urethræ. Difficult labour, rupture of the urethra, and perineal prostatectomy account for a certain number of cases. The remainder are due to organic spinal or cerebral disease.

Treatment.—Various plastic operations, such as the formation of a new sphincter by using the gracilis muscle or a strip of fascia, are sometimes successful.

Type (b).—The chief sufferers are women and children.

In Women.—It is not uncommon for women who have borne children to lack complete bladder control, due to over-stretching of the internal sphincter or damage to the pubo-cervical fascia in labour. Expulsive acts, such as laughing or sneezing, may be sufficient to cause an escape of urine (stress incontinence).

Treatment.—Many operations have been devised for stress incontinence. Some cases are remedied by anterior colporrhaphy. Millin's retropubic fascial sling operation gives good results in appropriate cases.

Terence Millin, Contemporary. Surgeon, All Saints' Hospital, London.

In Children.—This embraces that well-known clinical entity, nocturnal enuresis. The patient wets his bed. Normal micturition by day and by night should be established by the age of three years. Nocturnal enuresis is usually a continuance of infantile bed-wetting. Occasionally it commences months or years after voluntary micturition has been established. In 4 per cent. of cases involuntary micturition is only diurnal ; in 12 per cent. of cases it is both nocturnal and diurnal. In all patients who have reached the age of four or over, some anatomical cause for the involuntary micturition should be sought :

1. The urine should be examined for pus and organisms.

2. Phimosis or atresia meati, if present, should be corrected ; likewise vulvitis or vaginitis.

3. Radiography and excretory pyelography may reveal a hydronephrosis, an ectopic ureteric orifice, or a urinary calculus.

4. Urethroscopy sometimes shows inflammation of the verumontanum, in which event periodic dilatation with a urethral bougie is beneficial.

5. Thread worms should be eliminated.

6. Enlarged tonsils and adenoids may cause partial asphyxia during sleep.

7. Epilepsy and other mental disorders can cause enuresis.

EXSTROPHY OF THE BLADDER (*Syn.* ECTOPIA VESICÆ)

There is an absence of the lower abdominal and the anterior vesical walls.

Ætiology.—The condition has been explained by a forward displacement of the cloacal membrane preventing the development from mesoblast of the anterior abdominal wall between the umbilicus and the genital tubercle. Another explanation is that the deformity is the result of intrauterine rupture of the fœtal bladder due to a congenital and complete urethral stricture.

Clinical Features.—It has been estimated that this congenital abnormality occurs once in 50,000 births. The condition may be complete or incomplete. In the more common complete ectopia the deep red posterior bladder wall protrudes through the defect (fig. 726) because of the pressure of the viscera behind it. On lifting up the exposed mucous membrane, which bleeds readily, the paler, wet trigone is

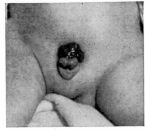

Fig. 726.—Ectopia vesicæ.

displayed, and effluxes of urine from the ureteric orifices can be seen. There is a well-defined line of demarcation between the protruding mucous membrane and the adjacent skin, and, especially after reducing the extruded bladder wall, the firm edge of the hernial ring can be felt beneath the muco-cutaneous junction. Usually the umbilicus is displaced downwards ; occasionally it is involved in scar tissue at the upper margin of the defect. The sex ratio is about 8 males to 1 female. In the male the completely epispadiac penis is broader and shorter than normal. There is often cryptorchidism, when the scrotum is rudimentary. In the female the clitoris is cleft and the labia minora are separated anteriorly, exposing the vaginal orifice. In both sexes there is separation of the pubic bones (fig. 727). The gait is similar to the waddle of a patient with bilateral congenital dislocation of the hips. In the rare incomplete form the pubes are united and the external genitalia are more normal.

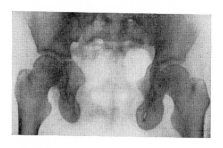

Fig. 727.—Showing the separation of the pubes in a case of ectopia vesicæ.
(*Professor Grey Turner.*)

If the condition remains untreated there are recurring attacks of pyelonephritis, and patients rarely survive the age of thirty years. Those who do so sometimes develop carcinoma in the ectopic bladder. Ectopia vesicæ is often associated with other congenital abnormalities.

Treatment.—The colon is sterilised with phthalylsulphathiazole. The left ureter is implanted into the pelvic colon and the right into the upper part of the rectum. Both ureters can be implanted at one stage, as described on p. 719, or the extraperitoneal route can be employed, when each ureter is implanted singly. The best time to perform the operation is between the second and fourth years.

Excision of the extroverted bladder is undertaken about a year after successful ureteric implantation. The mucocutaneous junction is incised and the mucous membrane excised. This can be followed by some form of plastic reconstruction of the mons veneris in the female or of the penis in the male. If the extroverted bladder is not excised, carcinoma is liable to develop in its mucous membrane.

ANOMALIES OF THE URACHUS

(See the Umbilicus, p. 602.)

DIVERTICULUM OF THE BLADDER

Ætiology.—It is disputed as to whether diverticula of the bladder are congenital or acquired. In most cases both factors probably play a part. A diverticulum rarely occurs unless there is prostatic or urethral obstruction. As only a small proportion (about 6 per cent.) of patients with obstruction to the lower urinary track develop a diverticulum, those that do so must possess a congenital weakness of the bladder wall at the point through which the diverticulum protrudes, or even a small vesical bud in this situation. The associated obstructive lesion is, in order of frequency, stenosis of the bladder neck (occasionally congenital hypertrophy, but usually inflammatory fibrosis of the internal sphincter), benign enlargement of the prostate, fibrous prostate, or urethral stricture.

Pathology.—The cavity of the diverticulum is lined by mucous membrane continuous with that of the bladder, unless severe infection has converted it into granulomatous tissue. The wall is composed of fibrous tissue, varying in thickness, with a few muscle fibres scattered through it, but insufficient to render it capable of contraction. Muscle fibres are sometimes more abundant around the orifice of the diverticulum, and may enable the ostium to open and contract, but this is unusual. There is often a considerable amount of fat around the sac. The majority of diverticula are single, but sometimes two or more are present. The mouth of the diverticulum is usually situated above and to the outer side of one ureteric orifice. Occasionally it is near the middle line behind the interureteric ridge, and rarely in the apex of the bladder. The size varies from that of a hazel nut to a sac larger than the bladder itself, the average (fig. 728)

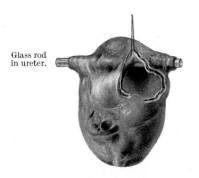

Glass rod in ureter.

Fig. 728. — Diverticulum of the bladder excised in the case of a man of twenty-nine. (⅓ scale.)

being the size of a tangerine orange. As a diverticulum at the seat of election enlarges, it does so in a downward direction and develops a short neck, which overlies the corresponding ureter and may drag upon or compress, and thus obstruct, that structure.

Complications

1. *Recurrent Cystitis.*—As the pouch cannot empty itself, there remains a stagnant pool of urine within it—concealed residual urine. Once this becomes infected, it continues to reinfect the main cavity of the bladder. In long-standing cases peridiverticulitis causes dense adhesions between the diverticulum and surrounding structures.

2. *Vesical calculi* due to stagnation and infection are present in 20 per cent. of cases, most often in the main bladder cavity, sometimes in the diverticulum as well, less often in the diverticulum only. On rare occasions a dumb-bell calculus fills the diverticulum and projects into the bladder.

3. *Hydronephrosis and hydroureter*, consequent upon implication of the lower end of the corresponding ureter, are liable to be followed by pyelonephritis and pyonephrosis.

4. *Neoplasm.*—A papilloma or a carcinoma may be situated wholly within the diverticulum or arise from the edge of the orifice. Only in the latter case is the neoplasm visible on ordinary cystoscopy.

Clinical Features.—The patient is nearly always a male (98·5 per cent. of cases). While most of the patients with this condition are between fifty and seventy years of age, it is not uncommon at an earlier age. Exceptionally the patient is a child. There are no pathognomonic symptoms of vesical diverticula ; they are those of lower urinary track obstruction, recurrent cystitis, or pyelonephritis. Hæmaturia (due to cystitis, vesical calculus, or, rarely, a neoplasm) is a leading symptom in one-third of cases. In a few instances of uncomplicated cases micturition occurs twice in rapid succession. Nevertheless this phenomenon is also sometimes encountered in prostatic obstruction and tabes dorsalis. Rarely a large diverticulum is felt per rectum, or, in cases of chronic retention of urine, two swellings are recognised rising out of the pelvis, one being the bladder and the other the diverticulum.

Cystoscopy is the usual means of discovering the diverticulum. Most often the orifice of the diverticulum is seen as a clear-cut hole about the diameter of a lead pencil, the depths of the diverticulum being black and unilluminated. Trabeculation is usually present only in the neighbourhood of the orifice (fig. 729). With inadequate distension of the bladder, the mouth of the diverticulum is sometimes seen closed, when the mucous membrane around the potential orifice is thrown into radiating pleats (fig. 730) or the track of the opening is visible; therefore it is important to have the bladder fully distended while searching for a diverticulum. In heavily infected cases much irriga-

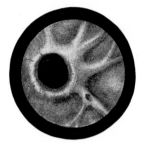

Fig. 729. — Cystoscopic appearance of the orifice of a diverticulum of the bladder.

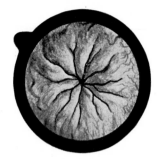

Fig. 730.

tion is necessary before a clear view of the bladder wall can be obtained. It is sometimes possible to pass an endoscope into the diverticulum and examine its interior.

Excretory pyelography will not only exclude or reveal implication of the upper urinary track, but in many instances the accompanying cystogram will give information regarding the size of the diverticulum.

Retrograde cystography is employed when the former fails to show the pouch clearly. The bladder is emptied of urine, and filled with about 15 oz. (500 ml.) of 5 per cent. sodium iodide solution. Radiographs taken before (fig. 731) and after micturition show the dimensions and position of the diverticulum clearly.

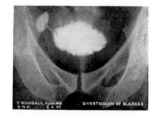

Fig. 731. — Diverticulum of the bladder shown by cystography.

Indications for Operation.—A vesical diverticulum gradually increases in size, and once infected the infection cannot be permanently eradicated. Therefore, unless the pouch is small, empties, and is uninfected, it should be removed, usually before the associated obstructive lesion is treated.

Pre-operative Treatment.—When, as is usually the case, the urine is infected, suitable preparative antibiotic treatment is given. In the presence of gross sepsis and retention of urine, it may be necessary to tie in a catheter for forty-eight hours at a time, and give bladder washes. Only in exceptional cases, when the infection cannot be controlled by these means, is suprapubic cystostomy indicated, and then a second tube should be passed into the diverticulum and stitched to the orifice so that both cavities can be irrigated frequently. Suprapubic cystostomy renders subsequent diverticulectomy more difficult.

Combined intravesical and extravesical diverticulectomy is the operation that is most frequently practised. Cystoscopy is performed, and a large ureteric catheter is passed up the ureter on the affected side, and left in place, 8 oz. (250 ml.) of lotion remaining in the bladder. With the patient in the Trendelenburg position, the anterior bladder wall is exposed through a 5-in. (13 cm.) suprapubic incision. The peritoneum is dissected upwards, and that side of the bladder bearing the diverticulum is cleared from surrounding structures with the fingers until some part of the pouch is brought into view. The bladder is then incised in the middle line near its dome, and emptied by suction. The interior of the diverticulum is packed with a strip of gauze, and with the fingers of one hand in the bladder and the recti muscles widely retracted, the diverticulum is freed from surrounding structures by gauze and sharp dissection. Usually the neck of the diverticulum can be separated from the ureter, and when the pouch is free it is severed from its attachment to the bladder with a diathermy knife. The resulting defect is closed in two layers. The cystostomy incision is sutured around a Malécot catheter, and the abdominal wall is closed, leaving a ½-in. (1·25 cm.) drainage tube in the extravesical space which housed the sac.

An alternative method, which is helpful when the sac is densely adherent, is to carry the incision in the bladder down to the rim of the diverticular orifice, then to detach the diverticulum, together with its fibrous rim. With hæmostats applied to the neck of the detached diverticulum, and a finger inside it, dissection of it with gauze and scissors, keeping close to the sac, is much facilitated. Occasionally the ureter is so incorporated in the wall of the neck that it must be severed and the proximal end reimplanted into another portion of the bladder.

HERNIA OF THE BLADDER

A portion of the bladder protruding through the inguinal or femoral hernial orifice occurs in 1·5 per cent. of such hernias treated by operation (Wakeley). The condition is relatively frequent in femoral and direct

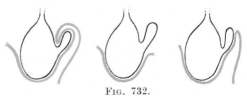

Fig. 732.

inguinal herniæ, but the total number of cases occurring in connection with indirect inguinal herniæ is greater because the latter type of hernia is so much more common. The disposition of the protrusion of the bladder in the hernia varies, and in order of frequency is :

Sir Cecil Pembrey Grey Wakeley, Contemporary. Senior Surgeon, King's College Hospital, London. President, Royal College of Surgeons of England.

(*a*) *Intraperitoneal.*—The protruded portion of bladder lies wholly within the hernial sac, usually along with other contents.

(*b*) *Extraperitoneal.*—There is no sac, the hernia being composed solely of a pouch of bladder.

(*c*) *Paraperitoneal.*—An extraperitoneal vesical protrusion lies on the medial side of the hernial sac.

The great majority of herniæ of the bladder are discovered during operations for hernia. In the paraperitoneal variety usually the peritoneal sac can be peeled off the bladder by gauze dissection ; if this can only be partially accomplished, the sac must be ligated below its neck. The intraperitoneal variety causes but little difficulty, for the bladder protrusion can be readily reduced into the peritoneal cavity. The extraperitoneal variety is liable to be mistaken for a thickened peritoneal sac, and opened, in which case escape of urine should be obvious.

Clinical Features.—Usually there are no symptoms referable to the bladder, unless there is prostatic or urethral obstruction, when, in a few cases, in order to empty the bladder completely the patient finds it necessary to exert pressure on the hernia. Suspicion of a bladder hernia can be confirmed by cystoscopy or cystography.

Accidental Wounding of the Bladder during an Operation for Hernia.— When recognised at the time, the wound in the bladder should be closed by a double layer of sutures, and either an indwelling catheter is retained for a week or temporary suprapubic cystostomy is substituted. If the accident is not recognised at the time, unless early operation is undertaken to repair the rent and drain the prevesical space or peritoneal cavity, as the case may be, combined with suprapubic cystostomy, the outlook, especially in the rare intraperitoneal variety, is grave.

BLADDER FISTULÆ

Vesico-vaginal Fistula.—Leakage of urine from the vagina is usually due to a vesico-vaginal fistula ; more rarely the fistula is uretero-vaginal (see below).

Ætiology

1. Injuries received during difficult labour are no longer the commonest cause, except in countries where native women do not receive proper obstetric care.

2. Injuries sustained during gynæcological operations, notably total abdominal hysterectomy ; more rarely during a vaginal hysterectomy.

3. Malignant disease or necrosis following radium treatment. Usually the growth is in the cervix, but occasionally it is in the urethra.

In both obstetric and gynæcological cases the leakage of urine can follow immediately after delivery or operation, but when it is due to necrosis of tissue, the leak may not make its appearance for five to twelve days.

Clinical Features.—There is incontinence of urine from the vagina, and, as a consequence, excoriation of the vulva. Digital examination of the vagina reveals a localised thickening on its anterior wall. On inserting a bivalved speculum, urine will be seen escaping from an opening in the anterior vaginal wall. It is usually possible to pass a bent probe from the vagina into the bladder. Cystoscopy is often difficult, owing to the contraction of the bladder from cystitis and the escape of urine from the fistula ; however, usually the tip of the probe that has been passed can be seen transitorily, emerging through an area of granulation tissue.

Closure of the Fistula by the Vaginal Route.—As a rule, the patient should be placed in the lithotomy position, but if the fistula is drawn behind the symphysis pubis, better access can be obtained by placing the patient's knees on a low stool with the abdomen and thorax resting on the operating table. While the postero-vaginal area is retracted with a Sims' speculum, the vaginal edges of the fistula, especially above and below, are excised widely. The scar tissue in the edges of the bladder wall is also excised, but a minimum of the latter structure is removed—just enough to reveal an oozing surface devoid of scar tissue. When feasible, the reparative stitching should be carried out in the long axis of the vagina. Mattress sutures of silkworm gut or tantalum wire are used. These traverse the bladder wall (but not its mucosa) and the whole thickness of the vagina. If necessary an incision is made on either side parallel to the original incision to relieve tension on the suture line. The operation is concluded by inserting a whistle-tipped catheter through the urethra into the bladder, and keeping it in position by stitching the catheter to the lowest vaginal stitch. All blood and clot is irrigated from the bladder. As soon as the patient has been returned to bed the catheter is connected to a suction drainage apparatus, and this form of drainage is continued for fourteen days. If the vaginal suture line encroaches upon the urethra, it is better to withhold a catheter in the urethra and to perform vaginal cystostomy through an incision at the extreme upper end of the vagina ; this drainage is maintained for a week. After this time the urethra will have healed sufficiently to permit drainage by an indwelling urethral catheter.

Uretero-vaginal Fistula.—Like a vesico-vaginal fistula, if an intravenous injection of indigo-carmine is given, a swab in the vagina will be stained blue, but unlike a vesico-vaginal fistula, if the dye is injected through the external urinary meatus into the bladder, the vaginal swab will not be coloured, and on cystoscopy the bladder is normal.

Treatment.—The treatment indicated will depend on the excretory pyelographic findings. If the kidney on the affected side is comparatively normal, if possible the freed proximal end of its ureter should be implanted into the bladder. When the corresponding kidney shows evidence of hydronephrosis or infection, and the other kidney is healthy, nephrectomy on the fistulous side is the best treatment.

Vesico-Intestinal Fistula

Congenital.—A fistula between the membranous urethra and the rectum complicates nearly half the cases of imperforate anus in the male. In the female, the bowel does not open into the urinary passages, but into the posterior wall of the vagina.

Traumatic.—Very occasionally a vesico-intestinal fistula follows a severe fracture of the pelvis.

Inflammatory.—Colonic diverticulitis is the commonest cause, others being Crohn's disease, pelvic appendix abscess, tuberculous peritonitis, and suppurative parametritis.

Neoplastic.—Carcinoma of the pelvic colon ulcerating into the bladder or, more rarely, carcinoma of the bladder ulcerating into the colon or rectum.

Clinical Features.—In addition to intractable cystitis, the patient passes gas per urethram (pneumaturia). Occasionally fæcal matter or particles of food are passed with the urine, and more rarely still urine is passed via the bowel. There is often an inflammatory or neoplastic mass to be felt in the recto-vesical or uretero-vesical pouch.

Cystoscopy.—That a vesico-intestinal fistula is present may be obvious (fig. 733). If the fistula is small and its edges smooth, it is likely to be inflammatory. An attempt should be made to pass a ureteric catheter through the communication, and if successful, to inject sodium iodide,

Marion Sims, 1813–1883, while a country practitioner at Montgomery, Alabama, was the first to succeed in closing a vesico-vaginal fistula.

which will render the segment of bowel involved radio-opaque. Other methods of investigation which may help in determining accurately the situation of the fistula are retrograde cystography and a barium enema.

Treatment.—The establishment of a defunctioning colostomy above the fistula brings about remarkable improvement in most cases, for no more gas and fæcal matter enters the bladder and the cystitis responds quickly to urinary antiseptics. After two or three weeks the fistula should be investigated by injecting lipiodol into the distal end of the colostomy loop and also by further cystoscopy. Inflammatory fistulæ rarely heal spontaneously. If the general condition improves, a further operation is undertaken to separate the fistulous communication between the bladder and the bowel, and if the lesion is inflammatory the opening in each viscus is closed and patched with omentum. In inflammatory cases temporary suprapubic cystostomy is performed after separating and closing the two viscera. After the cystostomy wound has healed, a third operation to close the colostomy can be undertaken. In neoplastic cases palliative colostomy is usually all that can be carried out.

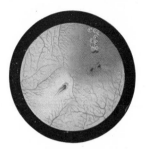

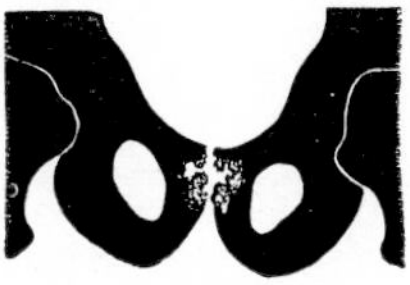

Fig. 733. — Cystoscopic view in the case of a vesico-intestinal fistula. Bubbles of gas can be seen issuing from the orifice of the fistula.

Osteo-vesical Fistula.—When necrosis of the pelvic bones, notably the pubis, causes a communication with the bladder there results what may be called an osteo-vesical fistula (fig. 734). Such a fistula follows rupture of the bladder associated with fractured pelvis, inadequately treated in the first instance, or as a result of a gun-shot wound. Excision of the fistula, which is often a very difficult procedure, is the only hope of a cure.

Fig. 734.—Typical X-ray appearances in osteo-vesical fistula.

RUPTURE OF THE BLADDER

Rupture of the bladder may be :

Extraperitoneal (20 per cent.).

Intraperitoneal (80 per cent.).

Ætiology

(a) *External Violence*

Blows or falls when the bladder is full, particularly when the patient is inebriated.

As a complication of fractured pelvis.

As an accident in herniotomy, usually the lower operation for femoral hernia, unrecognised at the time.

(b) *Internal Violence.*—Rupture of the bladder has occurred as a result of the use of the evacuator after litholapaxy ; during transurethral resection of the prostate and of growths of the bladder ; and as a complication of difficult labour.

(c) *Spontaneous rupture* has been recorded in cases of gangrenous cystitis, tuberculous cystitis, carcinoma of the bladder, and in chronic retention of urine.

In all injuries to the trunk the first point to ascertain is whether the patient has passed urine since the accident. The initial shock in cases of intraperitoneal rupture of the bladder may be slight. Except in utter smashes and perforation by fragments of bone, no rupture is possible unless the bladder is full.

Extraperitoneal Rupture (fig. 735).—Almost invariably, extraperitoneal rupture of the bladder is a complication of a fractured pelvis. Extravasation occurs into the prevesical space, causing

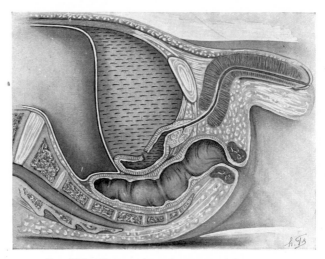

Fig. 735.—Extraperitoneal rupture of the bladder.

a tender swelling above the pubes ; later the extravasated urine passes up the anterior abdominal wall between the fascia transversalis and the peritoneum, causing necrosis of the connective tissue. It is impossible to distinguish this lesion from an intrapelvic rupture of the urethra (see p. 758) until the parts have been displayed by operation.

Intraperitoneal Rupture.—Shock is usually present, and some hours may elapse before symptoms develop. This is followed by an intense desire to micturate, but either no urine is passed, or only a few drops of blood-stained urine with great effort. The spasms come on at intervals. In spite of the fact that the patient has passed little or no urine since the accident, there is no dullness above the pubes corresponding to a distended bladder. If the amount of urine in the peritoneal cavity is considerable, shifting dullness may be elicited. Rectal examination often reveals a bulging of the recto-vesical pouch. Usually the symptoms and signs of peritonitis appear early, but when the urine is sterile they may not develop for many hours, or even a few days.

Confirming a Suspected Diagnosis.—The easy passage of a catheter with the withdrawal of a little blood-stained urine is a most characteristic finding. There are, however, two notable exceptions : (*a*) when the perforation is a small one, the bladder may contain a considerable amount of urine ; (*b*) the catheter may pass through the rupture and evacuate urine from the peritoneal cavity.

The most reliable confirmation of the integrity or otherwise of the bladder is obtained by examining the thirty-minute film after excretory pyelography.

Treatment.—It is abundantly clear that when there are reasonable grounds for suspecting rupture of the bladder, operation should be undertaken without delay.

Intraperitoneal Rupture.—Lower laparotomy is performed. Urine is removed by suction, after which the patient is placed in Trendelenburg's position. The edges of the rent, which is usually situated in the posterior part of the dome of the bladder, are trimmed and sutured by two layers of interrupted catgut stitches, and the operation completed by stitching a large drainage tube into an extraperitoneal suprapubic incision in the bladder. The latter ensures intravesical tension being kept minimal during the healing of the bladder wound. If the case is an early one, the peritoneum may be closed completely, otherwise suprapubic peritoneal drainage is necessary.

Extraperitoneal Rupture.—Suprapubic cystostomy is performed, and the prevesical space drained. It is unnecessary to attempt to suture the tear, which heals readily in these circumstances.

Prognosis.—When operation is performed within twelve hours the mortality is approximately 11 per cent. ; when operation is delayed to twenty-four hours the mortality rises to 55 per cent. As in the days of ancient Greece, when the condition was regarded as inevitably fatal, without operation the mortality is 100 per cent.

VESICAL CALCULUS

Ætiology of vesical calculus is, in most respects, similar to that of renal calculus. Prostatic obstruction is overwhelmingly the most common associated lesion. In Europe during the present century there has been a

---

In 1839 Dr. Walther, a general practitioner of Pittsburg, successfully sutured the ruptured bladder of a blacksmith.

remarkable diminution in the incidence of stone in the bladder in children, due to improvement in their diet.

Composition and Cystoscopic Appearance.—Most vesical calculi are composite, but have one component in excess, and assume the appearance of that variety. In two-thirds of cases the stone is solitary. A primary stone is one which develops in aseptic urine. It often, but not necessarily, originates in the kidney and passes down the ureter to the bladder, where it enlarges. Secondary stones occur in the presence of infection, and belong to the third of the following groups :

1. *Uric acid and urate calculi* are round or oval, fairly smooth or slightly bossed, and vary in colour from pale yellow to light brown. They may be single or multiple.

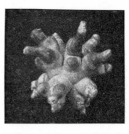

Fig. 736. — "Jack-stone"[1] calculus. This type of vesical calculus is typically found in a post-prostatic pouch.

2. *Oxalate calculus* grows slowly, is usually of moderate size, and is solitary. Its surface is uneven and often spicu-lated ; sometimes it bristles with spines (fig. 736). Although calcium oxalate is white, the stone is usually brown or black because of deposits of blood pigment upon it.

3. *Phosphatic calculus* is composed of triple phosphates and occurs in urine infected with urea-splitting organisms. It grows rapidly and often attains a large size. In some instances it occurs on a nucleus of one of the foregoing types of calculus ; much more rarely on a foreign body. Sometimes the nucleus is desquamated epithelium and bacteria. When single, the stone is round ; when multiple, it is faceted. It is dull white in colour, and comparatively soft.

4. *Cystine calculi* are rare, and are due to an error of metabolism. Although waxy in consistency, they are radio-opaque on account of their sulphur content. Hexagonal crystals are found in the urine.

A vesical calculus is usually free to move in the bladder. It gravitates to the lowest part of the organ, which is the bladder outlet, when the patient is erect or sitting. In the recumbent position (as also at cystoscopy) the stone occupies a position behind the interureteric ridge. Less commonly the stone is wholly or partially fixed in a diverticulum or a post-prostatic

[1] " Jack-stone." The kernel of the fruit of the jack tree. The stones are used in a game by boys in America.

pouch. In either of these situations the stone may be partially or completely hidden from view.

Clinical Features.—Males are eight times more often affected than females.

Latent.—When a stone is situated in a post-prostatic pouch or a diverticulum of the bladder, it is usually discovered unexpectedly at cystoscopy or on X-ray examination.

Typical.—Frequency is a common, and the earliest, symptom. Unlike other forms of frequent micturition, it is not much in evidence during the night. After micturition the patient does not feel fully satisfied that the bladder is empty. *Pain* is most in evidence in cases of spiculated oxalate calculus. It occurs at the end of micturition, and is usually referred to the tip of the penis or the labium majus ; more rarely to the perineum or suprapubic region. Pain and discomfort are much in evidence during exertion, and are aggravated by jolting movements, such as are occasioned when riding in a vehicle, or on going downstairs. If the patient lies down the symptoms tend to pass off, for the stone falls away from the sensitive portion of the bladder, the trigone. Thus he usually sleeps peacefully through the night. In young boys screaming and pulling at the penis with the hand at the end of micturition is suggestive of vesical calculus. *Hæmaturia* is characterised by the passage of a few drops of bright red blood at the end of micturition, and is due to the stone abrading the vascular trigone—a fact which also accounts for the pain. *Interruption of the urinary stream* during the act occurs in about 17 per cent. of cases. This symptom is not pathognomonic of vesical calculus, but when it occurs in addition to typical symptoms, it strengthens the clinical diagnosis. *Acute retention of urine* from a vesical calculus is extremely uncommon in adults, but not so in children.

As a stone increases in size it becomes less mobile, and in the rare event of the absence of considerable secondary infection, a large calculus may cause remarkably few symptoms.

Masked.—The symptoms of a concomitant persistent cystitis may overshadow those that might be occasioned by the stone.

Rectal or Vaginal Examination, when accompanied by abdominal palpation, occasionally enables a vesical calculus to be felt. Unless the stone is large, rectal examination is negative in the adult male, but in a female or child a calculus of moderate size can often be felt.

Examination of the urine will reveal blood, and possibly pus or crystals typical of the calculus, e.g. " envelope " in the case of oxalate stones, or hexagonal plates with cystine calculi.

Radiography.—In at least 92 per cent. of cases vesical calculus can be demonstrated on an X-ray film. Radiographs of the whole of the urinary track should be taken and excretory pyelography carried out. The former will reveal or disprove the presence of renal or ureteric calculi, while the latter will determine the functional capacity of the kidneys and the presence or absence of hydronephrosis or pyelonephritis.

Cystoscopy is essential for the final diagnosis. Frequently, on

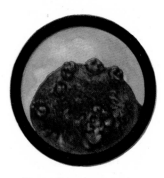

Fig. 737.—A stone in the bladder as viewed by a cystoscope.

introducing the sheath of the cystoscope, a significant " click " will be felt when a free-lying stone comes in contact with the instrument. As described already, cystoscopy usually determines the composition of the calculus (fig. 737). Stones non-opaque to X-rays can be seen. If the X-ray shows more stones than are counted on cystoscopy, a diverticulum must be carefully sought (Ogier Ward). The bladder wall is inspected. In primary calculus a septic cystitis is basal; in secondary calculus the cystitis is universal, but is still most severe at the seat of the stone. In appropriate cases the bladder neck is examined for prostatic enlargement, median bar, or fibrous prostate.

Litholapaxy.—For several days before the operation a sulphonamide is administered to reduce infection of the bladder as far as possible. While blind litholapaxy is preferred by those who have had much experience with the solid lithotrite, its only advantage is that, by reason of its solidity and greater strength, harder stones can be crushed than is the case with an instrument that contains a light and telescope incorporated in its shaft. Canny Ryall's cystoscopic lithotrite enables the stone, and such fragments as are necessary, to be seized under vision. The instrument, with its obturator in place, is introduced into the bladder, and rotated so that its closed jaws point downwards. The obturator is removed and the bladder is irrigated with boric lotion by means of two 6-oz. (200 ml.) syringes until the lotion is returned clear. The bladder is then filled with not more than 10 oz. (300 ml.) of the solution, and after inserting the telescope, the stone is

Ronald Ogier Ward, Contemporary. Senior Surgeon, St. Peter's Hospital, London.

seen. The screw on the handle of the instrument is turned, and the jaws thereby opened. The distal blade is hooked over the centre of the stone (fig. 738) and the proximal movable blade is advanced by rotating the screw handle so that the stone is grasped firmly. The ocular end of the lithotrite is depressed, and the calculus is lifted away from the bladder wall. After withdrawing the telescope slightly, to prevent damage to the light bulb, the screw is slowly turned, breaking the stone. Large fragments are crushed into small ones by repeating the manœuvre. With the jaws closed, the lithotrite is rotated so that the jaws point upwards, and after removing the telescope and allowing the lotion to escape, the instrument is withdrawn.

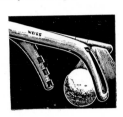

Fig. 738.—A cystoscopic lithotrite.

Evacuation of the Fragments.—When the crushing is finished, an evacuating cannula (fig. 739), the largest that the urethra will take, is passed, and 6 oz. (200 ml.) of lotion are introduced into the bladder. The evacuator (fig. 740), filled with lotion and with its tap closed, is fitted on to the cannula. The tap is opened and the bulb is elevated so as to depress the beak of the cannula towards the base of the bladder, after which the bulb is slowly compressed. As the bulb expands,

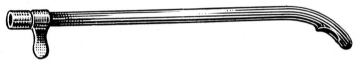

Fig. 739.—An evacuating cannula.

the returning lotion carries with it sand and fragments of the stone which, being heavier than the lotion, drop into the glass receptacle. Compression of the bulb and aspiration is continued until no further fragments fall. The beak of the cannula is turned to the left and to the right, and suction is applied in these situations. Two evacuators should be used to save time in emptying and recharging when the glass receptacle becomes full, or the lotion cloudy.

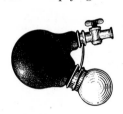

Fig. 740.—Freyer's evacuator.

If at any time the bulb fails to expand, this may be due to blocking of the eye by bladder mucosa, in which event release can be effected by further compression of the bulb and slight rotation of the instrument. Blockage of the cannula by fragments of the stone can sometimes be remedied in the same way, but more often they must be dislodged by detaching the evacuator and passing the obturator of the cannula. When no more fragments can be aspirated, the evacuator is detached and the bladder is irrigated with a syringe until the lotion is returned clear. The cystoscopic lithotrite is reintroduced, and if no fragments remain, a Foley's or Harris's catheter is passed and retained for forty-eight hours. The catheter is connected to a sterile bottle and bladder irrigations with a weak antiseptic solution are carried out twice daily during this period.

Contraindications to litholapaxy: (1) a large stone; (2) a moderately large oxalate stone which is too hard to crush; (3) vesical diverticulum; (4) prostatic obstruction; (5) a urethral stricture that cannot be dilated

Frère Jacques de Beaulieu, 1651–1714, was the most famous journeyman lithotomist. He mainly practiced the perineal operation using a bread-knife.

sufficiently ; (6) severe cystitis that fails to respond to urinary antiseptics ;
(7) contracted bladder ; (8) impaired renal function ; (9) foreign body
heavily encrusted ; (10) when the patient is below ten years of age ; (11)
a very small stone, which should pass naturally.

A stone associated with an enlarged prostate can be removed in the
course of a suprapubic or retropubic prostatec-
tomy. When the stone is associated with a median
bar or fibrous prostate, it is removed by preliminary suprapubic cystostomy, prior to transurethral resection.

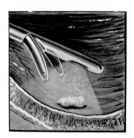

Suprapubic Lithotomy.—The alternative to
litholapaxy is removal of the stone through a
suprapubic incision, after which the bladder is
closed with drainage (suprapubic cystostomy).
Other necessary operations on the bladder can
be carried out at the same time, unless infection
has not responded sufficiently to urinary anti-

Fig. 741.—Young's cysto-
scopic rongeur.

septics. A very small stone sometimes can be
removed by means of an evacuator after passing
the largest-sized cannula commensurate with the
calibre of the urethra. For stones too large to pass through the cannula,
but small enough to pass through the urethra, Young's cystoscopic
rongeur is the ideal instrument (fig. 741).

FOREIGN BODIES IN THE BLADDER

A piece of catheter or bougie may become broken off and remain in the
bladder. The variety of foreign bodies which have been removed from the
bladder is astonishing. We have removed at various times a manicure
stick, a hair clasp (fig. 742), several hairpins, and a lump of candle grease.
The presence of such objects in the bladder is usually accounted for by
sexual perversion, or attempts to produce a miscarriage. Occasionally a
foreign body enters through the wall of the
bladder, e.g. a piece of rubber tubing after cystostomy ; unabsorbable sutures used in an extravesical pelvic operation. The diagnosis rests on
radiography and cystoscopy.

Complications of a Foreign Body in the Bladder
1. Cystitis, which is the most common complication.
2. Perforation of the bladder wall.
3. Vesical calculus.

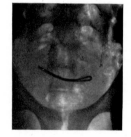

Treatment.—The foreign body may be removed
per urethram by means of an operating cystoscope, if this is feasible. Young's cystoscopic
rongeur is valuable for removing long, narrow
objects. When the foreign body is heavily encrusted, penetrating the bladder wall, or accom-

Fig. 742.—A hair clasp
in the bladder.

panied by severe cystitis, the suprapubic route should be chosen. A foreign
body composed of paraffin wax can be dissolved by the introduction of
equal parts of Xylol and water into the bladder for half an hour.

CYSTITIS

The transitional epithelium of the bladder is resistant to
infection, and may remain healthy for a considerable time, in
spite of a heavy infection of the urine. Some additional pre-

*Hugh Hampton Young, 1870–1945. Surgeon, The Buchanan Brady Urological Institute of
the Johns Hopkins Hospital, Baltimore.*

disposing factor must usually be present before the bladder becomes infected.

Predisposing Causes

1. By far the most important is incomplete emptying of the bladder, such as occurs in prostatic obstruction, urethral stricture, stenosis of the external urinary meatus, diverticulum of the bladder, pregnancy, cystocele, and diseases and injuries of the spinal cord.

2. The presence in the bladder of a calculus, foreign body, or neoplasm.

3. Lowered general resistance from intercurrent disease and avitaminosis.

Avenues of Infection

1. *Descending* from the kidney along the lumen of the ureter.

2. *Ascending* from the urethra probably occurs frequently. The shortness of the urethra is held responsible for the comparatively frequent occurrence of cystitis in females. Undoubtedly the passage of urethral instruments is a source of cystitis in both sexes. This does not necessarily imply that these instruments are unsterile at the time they are passed—for that must be exceptional—but rather that instrumentation starts up a latent infection in the posterior urethra.

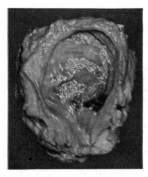

3. *Lymphogenous.*—The rich lymphatic network at the base of the bladder communicates with the prostate (fig. 743), the seminal vesicles or the cervix uteri, and the rectum, and provides a path by which organisms can reach the bladder from these commonly infected structures.

4. *From Adjacent Structures.*—Fistulous communications with the intestine, the vagina, and the Fallopian tube, or by suprapubic cystostomy.

5. *Hæmatogenous.*—Metastasis from a distant focus is exceptional. Interstitial cystitis is regarded as a probable example.

Fig. 743.—Acute cystitis. The patient, aged forty-four, died of ascending pyelonephritis. The primary focus was acute prostatitis, and pus around the prostate can be seen in the specimen.

Bacteriology.—The organisms responsible are conveniently divided into :

(a) *Those occurring in an Acid Urine.*

—B. coli ; Ps. pyocyaneus ; tubercle bacilli ; gonococcus ; B. typhosus.

(b) *Those occurring in Alkaline Urine.*—Staphylococci ; streptococcus ; Proteus vulgaris.

The presence of pus cells without organisms calls for repeated examination for the tubercle bacillus and the gonococcus.

Having eliminated these as the cause, the condition may be one of abacterial cystitis.

By far the most common infecting organism, especially in women, is the B. coli.

Clinical Features.—The severity of the symptoms varies greatly ; those of acute cystitis are usually the more distressing, but some chronic cases vie with them in intensity.

Frequency is the outstanding symptom.   It is in evidence both during the day and at night.   The desire to empty the bladder occurs from every hour to every few minutes, and often it is so urgent that if the bladder cannot be emptied forthwith, incontinence results.

Pain varies from mild to agonising.   When the inflammation is mainly confined to the dome of the bladder the pain is referred to the suprapubic region, while when, as is often the case, it is mainly situated in the trigone, it is referred to the tip of the penis, the labia majora, and the perineum.

Hæmaturia.—The passage of a few drops of blood-stained urine or blood-stained débris at the end of micturition is a frequent accompaniment.   Less often the whole specimen is blood-stained, but more so at the end (hæmorrhagic cystitis).

Pyuria is always present, except in some cases of trigonitis and interstitial cystitis (see later).   If urine is passed into two glasses, the second is the more cloudy.

Pyrexia.—In chronic cases the temperature is usually normal ; in acute cases, unless the cystitis is secondary to pyelonephritis, it seldom rises above 100° F. (37·7° C).

On examination there is tenderness over the bladder suprapubically, per rectum, or per vaginam.   In the acute stage it is necessary to differentiate between cystitis secondary to pyelonephritis and primary cystitis.   Excretory pyelography is the only method of investigation permissible at this stage, and a normal pyelogram eliminates a renal origin of the infection. Absence of tenderness over the renal angles and a normal or slightly elevated temperature also points to a non-renal origin. The absence of a urethral discharge or a tender swelling of the prostate eliminates a primary focus in the urethra or the prostate. A mid-stream specimen of urine in the male, or either a mid-stream specimen (after cleansing the vulva) or a catheter specimen in the female should be sent for bacteriological examination.

Treatment.—In the acute stage, if the urine is acid, it is rendered alkaline by giving four-hourly the same mixture as that advised on p. 663, to each dose of which is added minims 20 (1·2 ml.) of Tinct. hyoscyami and minims 10 of Tinct. belladonnæ, if pain is much in evidence. Once the urine has become alkaline a sulphonamide or, in more severe infections, streptomycin, is administered. When pyogenic cocci, are present, penicillin is administered. If the urine is alkaline,

> Ammonium Chloride, grains 20 (1·2 gm.)
> Extract. Glycyrrhizæ Liq. minims 25 (1·5 ml.)
> Water to ½ oz. (15 ml.)

is given four-hourly.

After seven to ten days resolution should occur. If terminal micturition continues to be painful after this time, daily instillations into the bladder with a catheter of one or two ounces of 1 : 5,000 solution of acriflavine, gradually increasing the strength to 1 : 1,000, are often soothing.

SPECIAL FORMS OF CYSTITIS

Chronic trigonal cystitis is a common form of chronic cystitis in women, and is usually associated with chronic urethritis. Cystoscopy shows increased vascularity of the trigone, œdema of its mucous membrane (most marked towards the apex) and, in severe cases, there is a pseudo-membrane limited to the trigone. In 90 per cent. of cases polypus formation is seen in the internal urinary meatus, or in the nearby posterior urethra. The urine is sterile in 10 per cent. of cases ; the remainder contain a few pus cells and B. coli, but even if the bladder urine is infected, ureteral specimens are sterile, showing that the infection is not a descending one. The urethra is commonly narrow—25 F. or less, instead of the normal 35 F. In such cases the cervix uteri should be examined for evidence of cervicitis, or a cervical erosion, which is often the primary source of infection.

Treatment.—Urethral polypi should be destroyed by light fulguration and the urethra dilated, if necessary. Cervicitis or a cervical erosion should be treated by excising the glandular tissue of the cervix with a diathermy loop.

Interstitial Cystitis (*syn.* **Hunner's Ulcer ; Elusive Ulcer**).— The lesion appears in the roof of the bladder as a star-shaped area of intense congestion, which rapidly fissures as the bladder is distended, and leads to bleeding. The ulcer, if ulcer it may

Guy L. Hunner, Contemporary. Adjunct Professor of Gynæcology, Johns Hopkins University, Baltimore, U.S.A.

be called, is situated mainly in the submucosa and muscle coats (fig. 744). In over half the cases the urine is sterile ; in the remainder it contains ordinary pyogenic bacteria. The bladder capacity becomes much reduced, and frequency about every

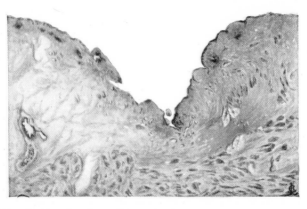

FIG. 744.—Section showing a Hunner's ulcer treated by partial cystectomy. The patient, a woman of forty-five, suffered from intractable cystitis for six years.

hour, both day and night, is the leading symptom. Pain, relieved by micturition and aggravated by jarring and over-distension of the bladder, is the second most characteristic symptom. In 60 per cent. of cases moderate hæmaturia is a leading symptom. Occasionally the hæmaturia is violent ; one of our patients was admitted with her bladder distended with blood-clot. In about 80 per cent. of cases the patient is a female and the average age is about fifty years.

Gangrenous cystitis is a rather rare and dangerous form of cystitis which usually commences acutely, but may occur in the course of chronic cystitis. It results as a combination of infection of the vesical mucous membrane and thrombophlebitis of the vesical venous plexus. The bladder mucosa sloughs in pieces, or as a whole cast, and in the latter event it is liable to give rise to retention of urine. In a female the slough may pass per urethram, but in the male particularly, this form of cystitis must be treated by suprapubic cystostomy.

Tuberculous Cystitis.—Primary tuberculous cystitis probably never occurs ; it is almost invariably secondary to a tuberculous focus elsewhere in the genito-urinary tract, notably in a kidney.

Pathology.—Cystoscopy shows that early tuberculosis of the bladder nearly always commences around one ureter or in the neighbourhood of the trigone, which suggests that it is spread from the kidney or the prostate, etc. In long-standing cases there is much fibrosis, and the capacity of the bladder is so much reduced that it has earned the name of " thimble " bladder.

Treatment.—After nephroureterectomy for renal tuberculosis, the symptoms of tuberculous cystitis usually abate. In about 10 per cent. of cases, when the bladder is much reduced in capacity and the seat of tuberculous ulceration, these symptoms continue. Streptomycin has proved a great advance in the treatment of tuberculous cystitis, and also if any irremovable complications such as tuberculosis of the remaining kidney, or tuberculosis of the prostate, exists. When tuberculous contracture of the bladder is present and threatens to implicate the sole-existing kidney by back pressure, provided excretory pyelography shows that its ureter is relatively slightly dilated and the renal function tests are satisfactory, implantation of the remaining ureter into the bowel often proves most beneficial, and relieves the constant pain of micturition. When the remaining ureter is enlarged, and is associated with a small ulcerated tuberculous bladder, cutaneous ureterostomy often increases the length of the patient's life, provided the ureterostomy tube is sterilised and supervised regularly. Instead of hourly, painful micturition, the patient can rest through the night.

Abacterial Cystitis.—Cystoscopy shows a generalised cystitis, least marked in the region of the trigone, and, in contradistinction to tuberculosis, no change is seen at either ureteric orifice, and there are no tubercles. The urine collected by ureteric catheterisation is usually normal, although in a few cases pus is found in the specimen of one side. Similarly, excretory pyelography occasionally shows slight dilatation of the pelvis and ureter on one side, but this examination is usually negative. The clinical features, probable ætiology, and treatment are discussed on p. 705.

Alkaline encrusting cystitis is a rare condition occurring particularly in elderly women, and due to urea-splitting organisms, staphylococcus and Proteus vulgaris. A deposition of phosphates occurs on the mucosa of the bladder, and the urine smells strongly of ammonia. The symptoms are those of chronic cystitis of many years' duration, and the passage of necrotic material, phosphatic crystals and sometimes, but seldom, pus and organisms. Radiography occasionally shows a partial or complete outline of the bladder. Cystoscopy performed under spinal or general anæsthesia shows encrustations, usually limited to the base and the sides of the bladder. Removal of the encrustations with forceps through an operating cystoscope, and afterwards light fulgurating of the resulting raw areas, is of value. Daily irrigations of the bladder with solution G (see p. 651) or half per cent. acetic acid, controls some cases. In a very heavily encrusted bladder, suprapubic cystostomy should be performed, together with curettage of the bladder mucosa. Connecting the suprapubic cystostomy tube with a tidal lavage apparatus containing dissolvent solution sometimes clears up recalcitrant cases.

Cystitis Cystica.—Glands are not found in the normal vesical mucosa. Under the influence of chronic inflammation, the surface epithelium sends down buds, resulting in minute cysts filled with clear fluid, most abundant on the trigone. Most of the cases are seen in women, and the urine usually contains pus, commonly the colon bacillus. An adenocarcinoma may originate in one of these cysts.

Leukoplakia is rare, and is due to cornification of the most superficial layers of the vesical epithelium. It is usually seen in the floor of the bladder, and is characterised by islands of greyish-white epithelium, the surroundings being intensely red. With this condition the bladder, which sometimes harbours a vesical calculus, becomes contracted.

Typhoid cystitis may complicate the convalescence of an attack of typhoid fever. The treatment is that usual for cystitis, and the symptoms may abate, yet typhoid bacilli may continue to be passed in the urine, e.g. the notorious case of " Typhoid Mary." It is a public duty to be certain that the patient is bacteriologically, as well as symptomatically, cured.

BILHARZIASIS OF THE BLADDER

Geographical Distribution.—The disease is endemic in the greater part of Africa, throughout Palestine, Syria, Arabia, Iran, and Iraq. It is met with frequently in Portugal and in Greece, and in the islands of Madagascar, Mauritius, and Cyprus. Dwellers along the valley of the Nile have suffered from time immemorial. The condition also occurs along the shores of some of China's great lakes. Marshes or slow-running fresh water provide a favourable habitat for the particular fresh-water snail (Bullinus contortus) which is the intermediate host.

Mode of Infestation.—The disease is acquired while bathing or standing in infected water. Agricultural workers in districts where bilharzia is rife become infected and reinfected time and again. The free-swimming bifid tailed embryos (cercariæ) of the trematode Schistosoma hæmatobium penetrate the skin by their motile and erosive secretory powers. Losing their tails, they enter the venous system to reach the liver and the portal radicles, where they sustain themselves by living on erythrocytes, and differentiate into males and females. Here the larger male trematode embraces the smaller female, and fertilises her. Unlike S. mansoni and S. japonicum, which migrate to the veins of the rectum, the paired S. hæmatobium have an affinity for the vesical venous plexus, which they reach through anastomotic channels between the mesenteric veins and those of the ureters. When approaching the smaller radicles of the plexus near the bladder, the male is discarded and perishes, while the slender female moves on until she enters a submucous venule so small that she completely blocks it. She now proceeds to lay about twenty ova in a chain, and after each is deposited, by slightly withdrawing herself, the venule contracts upon the ovum. Each ovum is provided with a terminal spine which penetrates the vessel wall. Aided by muscular contraction of the bladder, and perhaps by secreting lytic fluid, some of the ova reach the lumen of the bladder ; others die incarcerated in the mucous membrane. A heavily infected subject passes many hundreds of ova a day. In 10 per cent. of cases ova are excreted in the fæces also. If the ova reach fresh water, the low osmotic pressure of the new environment causes the shell to burst and there emerges the miracidium, which is ciliated. To survive, the miracidium must reach and penetrate the intermediate host within thirty-six hours. Within the snail's liver the miracidium enlarges and gives rise to myriads of daughter cysts, broods of which are set free on the death of the snail. A single miracidium thus begets thousands of cercariæ to complete the life-cycle.

Clinical Features.—After penetration of the skin there may arise urticaria, which lasts for about five days and sometimes recurs (swimmer's itch). After an incubation period ranging from four to twelve weeks, high evening temperature, sweating and asthma, together with leucocytosis and eosinophilia of over 10 per cent. sometimes lasts several weeks. Usually an asymptomatic period of several months supervenes before the ova laid in the bladder wall find egress and occasion the typical early sign and symptom of intermittent, painless, terminal hæmaturia.

Examination of the Urine.—The last few millilitres of an early-morning specimen of urine are collected and centrifuged. It is essential that all receptacles be absolutely dry. The ovum is recognised without staining (fig. 745) under the low-powered microscope. Examination on several consecutive days may be required. Even so, a negative result does not

---

Theodor Maximilian Bilharz, 1825–1862, working at the Kasr el Aimy Hospital, Cairo, discovered this parasite.
Sir Patrick Manson, 1844–1922. Physician, Dreadnought Hospital, Greenwich.

exclude bilharziasis, especially in patients no longer resident in bilharzial districts.

Cystoscopy.—Dependent on the length of time the disease has remained untreated, cystoscopy will reveal one or more of the following :

Bilharzial tubercles are the earliest specific appearance. The tubercles are somewhat larger (the size of a pin's head) and more yellow than those of tuberculosis.

Bilharzial nodules are due to the fusion of tubercles in the presence of secondary infection. They are larger and greyer than the foregoing.

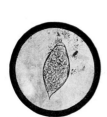

Fig. 745.—A bilharzia ovum.

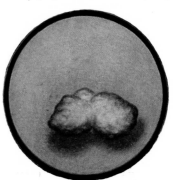

Fig. 746.—Bilharzial papilloma.
(*N. Makar.*)

" *Sandy patches* " are the result of calcified dead ova with degeneration of the overlying epithelium. They occur in the first instance around the ureteric orifices. Considerable calcification of this nature is visible on the radiograph.

Fibrosis is mainly the result of secondary infection. The capacity of the bladder becomes much reduced.

Ulceration is relatively uncommon ; when present, an ulcer is usually solitary. It is a result of sloughing of mucous membrane containing dead ova.

Granulomata.—Bilharzial masses due to an aggregation of nodules form. They are sessile and respond to medical treatment.

Papillomata are distinguished from the foregoing by being more pedunculated (fig. 746) and there is no response to medical treatment.

Carcinoma is a common end result in grossly infected Egyptian patients.

Treatment.—Sodium antimony tartrate (tartar emetic) given intravenously in saline solution on alternate days, commencing with $\frac{1}{2}$ grain (30 mg.) and, depending on the reaction, working up to $2\frac{1}{2}$ grains (150 mg.) until a total of 25 grains (1·6 gm.) has been given, kills the trematodes and the ova. The general toxic reactions following the administration of this drug are considerable, and if any of the solution is spilled in the tissues outside the vein, local necrosis follows. Fuadin ‚a trivalent antimony compound, is far less toxic, but is not as certainly curative. Ampoules of a 7 per cent. solution are available for injection intramuscularly, commencing with 1·5 ml. and working up to 5 ml., ten to fifteen injections constituting a course. These drugs are curative, although it takes months for dead ova to be expelled, but they do not confer any immunity to subsequent reinfestation.

John Christopherson, Contemporary. Physician, London and Egypt, revolutionised the treatment of bilharziasis by the intravenous injection of tartar emetic.
Napoleon's troops who served in his march to the Pyramids suffered from hæmaturia.

Complications requiring special treatment are secondary bacteria cystitis, urinary calculi (especially vesical and ureteral, which are very common), stricture of the ureters which affects the last inch (these often respond to cystoscopic dilatation, but may require open operation), papillomata and carcinomata, which are treated as such. Prostato-seminal vesiculitis, like tuberculosis of these structures, is made worse by prostatic massage, and general treatment alone must be employed. The fibrosis of the bladder neck that follows usually requires transurethral resection. Bilharzial urethral strictures are often accompanied by fistulæ, and can only be cured by excision of the fistulous tracks and that part of the urethra bearing the stricture after preliminary suprapubic cystostomy.

NEOPLASMS OF THE BLADDER

Over 95 per cent. of primary tumours of the bladder originate in its mucous membrane ; the remainder are connective-tissue growths—angioma (the least uncommon), myoma, fibroma, and sarcoma. These are too rare to merit description in this work. Secondary involvement of the bladder by extension of a malignant neoplasm of a neighbouring organ, viz. the prostate, the uterus, the pelvic colon, or the rectum, is not an uncommon late complication. Only on rare occasions are the first symptoms and signs referable to the bladder. In these the pelvic colon is the usual site of the primary growth and the symptoms are those of cystitis. Cystoscopy reveals a circumscribed area of intense cystitis, usually on the left side of the fundus. If the diagnosis is not made and treatment carried out at this stage, a vesico-intestinal fistula results (p. 696).

PRIMARY EPITHELIAL TUMOURS OF THE BLADDER

Ætiology.—Apart from the facts that epithelial tumours of the bladder occur in aniline dye workers thirty-three times more frequently than in other persons, that they are a common complication of vesical bilharziasis in Egypt, and that occasionally carcinoma of the bladder develops in a patch of leukoplakia, nothing is known as to the cause of tumours of the bladder. That bacterial cystitis is not usually a precursor is evident by the fact that the commonest vesical tumour—the papilloma—commences in an uninfected bladder.

Classification

Benign—Villous papilloma.
Malignant—Malignant papilloma.
　　　　　　Nodular carcinoma.
　　　　　　Carcinomatous ulcer.
　　　　　　Adenocarcinoma ⎱ Rare.
　　　　　　Endometrioma ⎰

Pathology

Benign Villous Papilloma.—The earliest stage of a primary growth is not seen cystoscopically, but it can be surmised from the appearance of minute secondary growths, each of which presents as a red projection of mucous membrane the size of a pin's head, which later becomes tufted. From these tufts spring villi—long, finger-like projections composed of transitional epithelium on a centre composed of a capillary vessel with a minimum amount of fibrous tissue supporting it. Thus the fully developed papilloma appears like a red sea anemone with delicate tentacles eddying to and fro with every movement of the bladder contents. Usually the tumour is pedunculated, the pedicle is slender and its central core of fibrous tissue and blood-vessels springs from the submucosa. Much more rarely it is sessile, the villi then taking origin from the mucous membrane. By far the most frequent location of a primary villous papilloma is above and to the outer side of one ureteric orifice, and as the growth increases in size, the latter may be obscured from view. The ureteric orifice is sometimes mechanically occluded by the neoplasm and some degree of hydronephrosis and hydroureter results. The growth may remain localised for a considerable time, for months or even years, gradually increasing in size ; on rare occasions it may fill the greater part of the bladder. We have removed a papilloma arising from a single stalk weighing nearly 3 lb. (1·5 Kg.). Size without any of the changes about to be described is not necessarily a sign of malignancy. At any time during its evolution other, less mature growths may appear. When the bladder is examined cystoscopically for the first time multiple growths are present in over one-third of cases. Daughter growths are often situated at points of contact of the

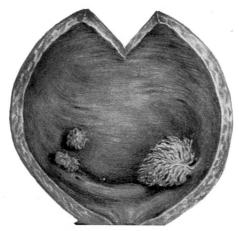

Fig. 747.—Multiple papillomata of the bladder.

bladder mucosa with the neoplasm when the bladder is empty (fig. 747). At other times they are situated near the parent growth, and probably arise from the detachment of small portions which become implanted on the bladder mucosa. Every villous papilloma is potentially malignant, and when open operation is undertaken precautions must be taken to prevent implantation of cells in the abdominal wall, for if they gain this situation they take on a malignant character.

Malignant Papilloma.—Malignant change in a papilloma is characterised by the appearance of more than one of the following alterations : (*a*) the villi become stunted, closely packed, and swollen ; (*b*) the growth becomes sessile (90 per cent. of villous papillomata are pedunculated); (*c*) the bladder wall immediately adjacent is more vascular and œdematous ; (*d*) the surface of the growth becomes ulcerated, shows areas of necrosis, or becomes encrusted with urinary salts.

Multiplicity of the growth is not necessarily a sign of malignancy, provided the daughter growths are limited to two or three. When general papillomatosis has occurred, they are certainly malignant, as also when a papilloma at the ureteric orifice is secondary to papilloma of the renal pelvis and ureter. The latter is rare, but it should be always excluded by excretory pyelography. A bladder tumour accompanied by cystitis that does not respond to urinary antiseptics is nearly always malignant. Malignant papillomata infiltrate the bladder wall, but they rarely spread beyond it. Lymphatic metastases occur late.

Nodular Carcinoma.—Instead of being tufted, the surface is bald from the outset. The tumour, which is sessile, becomes lobulated, is deep red, and bleeds on being touched. It is liable to become covered with a powder of phosphates. Later the surface becomes ulcerated in places. The typical situation of this growth is similar to that of the papilloma. Untreated, the growth infiltrates the bladder wall and surrounding structures. Lymphatic metastases occur earlier than is the case in malignant papilloma. Nodular carcinoma is the second most common form of carcinoma of the bladder.

Carcinomatous ulcer is similar in appearance to carcinomatous ulcer elsewhere, and occasionally it arises in a patch of leukoplakia. This type of growth occurs in the base of the bladder and on the trigone, and it infiltrates the muscle wall of the bladder, and spreads to the prevesical tissues. This is the most malignant carcinoma of the bladder. Lymphatic metastases occur early, at first to the nodes along the external and common iliac vessels, then to the paraortic lymph nodes, and from there to the mediastinal nodes ; sometimes the cervical nodes become implicated. Occasionally spread occurs by the blood-stream to the lungs, liver, and very rarely to bones.

Adenocarcinoma occurs in the fundus of the bladder of relatively young patients. It is believed to arise in the remnants of the urachus.

Endometrioma is characterised by a localised, smooth, vascular projection on the bladder wall, sometimes containing chocolate-coloured cysts ; and at other times translucent cysts of a bluish hue. The tumour enlarges and bleeds during menstruation.

Clinical Features

Benign Tumours.—Painless, bright red, intermittent hæmaturia is the only symptom for a long period. The hæmaturia may last for a few hours, or a few days, and then it ceases. After an interval of weeks or months, bleeding recurs ; as time progresses the intervals become shorter and the hæmaturia more severe and of longer duration. Eventually the resulting anæmia may be so severe as to necessitate blood transfusion. Clot retention sometimes occurs, as also dysuria from the growth being carried to the internal urinary meatus. A slight ache in one loin is not uncommon, and usually signifies a commencing hydronephrosis. Occasionally, when papillomata are multiple or large, there is frequency of micturition from a feeling of incomplete emptying of the bladder. Bimanual rectal or vaginal examination is entirely negative. In 80 per cent. of cases painless hæmaturia remains the only symptom and sign.

Malignant Tumours.—In the large majority of cases the initial symptom is intermittent hæmaturia, which eventually becomes continuous. Occasionally (in carcinomatous ulcer) the first symptoms are those of severe cystitis. Sooner or later in all cases cystitis supervenes, and painful, frequent, blood-stained micturitions are the dominating symptoms in established cases. As time goes on strangury occurs at the end of each act of micturition. A late manifestation due to nerve involvement is pain referred to the suprapubic region, the groins, perineum, the anus, or down the thighs.

Bimanual rectal or vaginal examination may enable the growth to be felt. It is a truism that if a growth of the bladder can be felt per rectum it is never innocent. It will be noticed in fig. 748 that the trigone and the lateral walls are most frequently attacked by malignant disease.

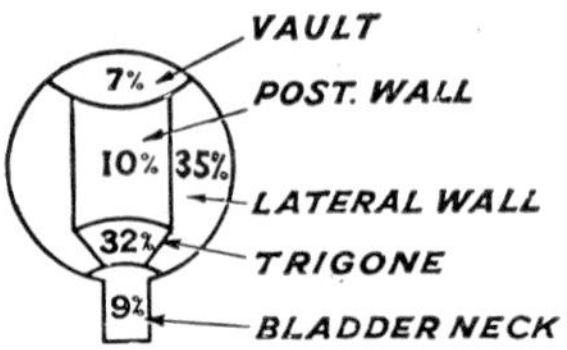

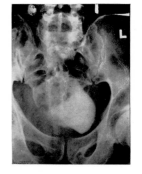

Fig. 748.—Sites of carcinoma of the bladder.
(*American Urological Association Statistics.*)

Radiography and Excretory Pyelography.—A plain X-ray occasionally shows a faint shadow of an encrusted neoplasm of the bladder. Excretory pyelography will reveal a hydronephrosis or pyelonephritis, if present. The accompanying cystogram displays gross deformity of the bladder caused by an advanced neoplasm (fig. 749). This information must be co-related with cystoscopic findings, for retained blood-clot can cause a filling defect.

Cystoscopy is the mainstay of diagnosis. It should be performed in every case of hæmaturia. The main cystoscopic appearances have been fully described under Pathology.

Transurethral biopsy is regarded by many as not always reliable, for it is the base, and not the superficial part of the tumour, that gives most information regarding malignancy. The specimen is obtained by a resectoscope, or by special cystoscopic forceps.

Treatment

Cystodiathermy.—The standard treatment of benign papillomata is coagulation diathermy applied by an electrode through an irrigating cystoscope. A small solitary papilloma can be treated satisfactorily,

Fig. 749.—Cystogram in a case of malignant papilloma of the right side of the bladder.

employing local anæsthesia of the urethra, the patient being ambulatory. For larger growths a general or spinal anæsthetic is given which permits more massive fulguration, but necessitates in-patient treatment. If daughter growths are present, they are fulgurated first.

The electrode is made to impinge upon the surface of the tumour, and the current is switched on. Blanching and coagulation occur in that part of the tumour in contact with the electrode, with the formation of bubbles of hydrogen. When a considerable number of villi have been destroyed the electrode is withdrawn, and applied to another area. Often the electrode adheres to the fulgurated tissues, and on withdrawing it pieces of coagulated tissue are adherent to it, and the electrode must be removed and scraped. The process is repeated (fig. 750) until all the growth has been destroyed or the medium becomes too cloudy for further progress. At the close of the operation the bladder is washed out with 1 : 4,000 silver nitrate, and 3 oz. (100 ml.) of the solution are left in.

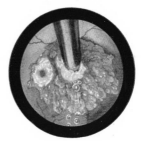

FIG. 750.—Cystodiathermy of a papilloma of the bladder.

The patient is given urinary antiseptics and re-cystoscoped in four weeks' time, when further treatment is carried out if necessary. Large papillomata can be destroyed more effectively by Kidd's diathermy cystoscope (fig. 751) than with relatively small electrodes. When the growth is situated in the region of the bladder neck a resectoscope can be used to excise the growth. After the papilloma has been destroyed, cystoscopically or by open operation, it is essential that the patient be examined cystoscopically at intervals commencing at three months and, if there is no recurrence, gradually lengthening

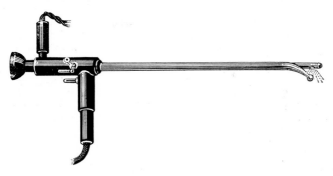

FIG. 751.—Kidd's diathermy cystoscope.

to one year. In 30 per cent. of cases there is no recurrence. In 50 per cent. of cases there is a recurrence, either at the site of the original lesion or in another part of the bladder, but the recurrences can be kept under control with regular cysto-diathermy. In 15 per cent. the rate of recurrence is high (more than ten new growths a year) and in 5 per cent. high and low rates of recurrence are exhibited at different times in the course of the disease (Deming).

Francis Seymour Kidd, 1878–1934. Surgeon, The London Hospital.
Clyde Leroy Deming, Contemporary. Professor of Urology, Yale University, U.S.A

Diathermy through the opened bladder is undertaken :

1. When a villous papilloma is very large.

2. When it is doubtfully malignant.

(*a*) *Excision of a Papilloma.*—The bladder is distended with 1 : 4,000 silver-nitrate solution and the viscus is exposed by a suprapubic incision. The contents of the bladder having been evacuated by a trocar and cannula, which permits suction of the fluid contents (fig. 752) so that

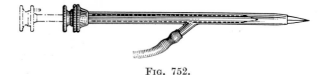

Fig. 752.

none is spilled, the edges of the abdominal wall are covered with packs soaked in silver-nitrate solution or 60 per cent. alcohol, as a precaution against contamination of the wound by detached tumour cells. The bladder is opened, and after placing the patient in Trendelenburg's position, a self-retaining retractor is inserted. The surface of the tumour is lightly coagulated (with the object of prevention of detachment of cells). It is then picked up with toothed dissecting forceps as near the bladder wall as possible. An innocent tumour can be elevated so that there is a substantial pedicle of normal mucous membrane. This is excised with the diathermy needle. After coagulating bleeding-points, the margin of the mucous membrane is approximated by sutures of plain catgut and the incision in the bladder is closed with drainage of the bladder and the prevesical space.

(*b*) *Fulguration* with a flat or ball electrode, without excision, is substituted for the above when the growth is sessile.

Partial cystectomy is indicated when the growth is definitely malignant, but is situated in such a position that it can be excised with 1 inch (2·5 cm.) of healthy bladder around it, and in endometriomata conforming with these conditions. After exposing the bladder, the first step is to mobilise the organ. The prevesical fat is dissected from either side of the urachus so as to enable this structure to be clamped, ligated, and divided. The lateral walls are dissected from the peritoneum, exposing the terminal ends of the ureters. That side of the bladder containing the growth is freed, so that the finger can reach well beyond infiltration of the growth. During this stage of the operation the peritoneum may be inadvertently opened, in which case the hole is closed by a purse-string suture. As a result of mobilisation a large part of the bladder can be drawn out of the wound. The bladder is emptied, opened, and the incision into it is extended to within 1 inch of the growth with the diathermy knife. The

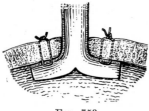

Fig. 753.

growth, with a surrounding inch of the whole thickness of healthy bladder wall, is excised. If the growth is situated near a ureteric orifice, the ureter should be divided before the excision is carried out, in which event, after the excision has been completed, the lower end of the ureter is bisected for ½ inch (1·25 cm.), and transplanted into the bladder, preferably through a stab incision (fig. 753).

Edwin Beer, 1876–1938. Surgeon, Mount Sinai Hospital, New York. Introduced fulguration of bladder tumours in 1910.

The defect in the bladder is closed by an inner continuous suture and an outer layer of interrupted sutures, provision being made for the introduction of a Malécot catheter. The abdominal wall is closed with drainage of the prevesical space by a piece of corrugated rubber.

Implantation of the ureters into the bowel is undertaken (*a*) as a palliative measure in inoperable cases and (*b*) as a preliminary to total cystectomy.

Uretero-intestinal Anastomosis (Grey Turner).—The preparation of the colon is the same as that described on p. 435. Both ureters are transplanted at the same operation, unless the general condition of the patient is poor, as is often the case when the deviation of the urinary stream is performed as a palliative measure. The abdomen is opened by a right lower paramedian incision. The patient is then placed in the Trendelenburg position and the small intestine is packed away from the pelvis. The right ureter is sought as it crosses the common iliac artery just above its bifurcation, when it may be discernible through the parietal peritoneum, or obscured by retroperitoneal fat. An incision is made through the overlying peritoneum in the line of the ureter, from the pelvic brim to near the bladder, and the ureter is identified and surrounded by a ring forceps. Suspended by the latter, the ureter is dissected from its bed for 2½ in. (6·25 cm.) towards the bladder, where a hæmostat is applied across it. The ureter is cut across proximal to the hæmostat, and its distal stump is ligated. The extremity of the mobilised portion of ureter is trimmed obliquely and one end of a double-needled chromic catgut suture is passed along its lumen for ⅓ in. (8 mm.), and out of the wall, the suture being tied so lightly that it cannot strangulate any of the ureteric tissues. The prepared, mobilised ureter is wrapped in a swab and the cut edges of the parietal peritoneum are approximated. The left ureter is next isolated and divided on the left side of the pelvic colon. It is passed beneath the mesocolon and made to emerge from the parietal peritoneum on the right side of the pelvic colon, and it is then prepared for transplantation as was its fellow. The edges of the peritoneum having been approximated on the left side of the colon, suitable areas on the right anterolateral surface of the colon are selected for the transplantation of each ureter. They should enter the colon obliquely without tension or looping, the left lying 1½ in. (3·75 cm.) higher than the right. The right ureter is transplanted first. A line 1½ in. long, extending downwards and to the right side of the anterior longitudinal band, is demarcated by stay sutures, and put on the stretch. The peritoneal and muscular coats are incised, but not the mucous membrane. In order to expose an elliptical area of mucous membrane, the beak of a blunt hæmostat may have to be introduced into the submucosa, and its blades opened. Bleeding-points

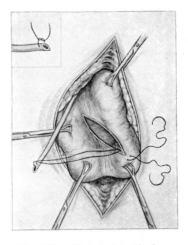

FIG. 754.—Uretero-intestinal anastomosis. The suture being passed through the wall of the pelvic colon. Inset shows the method of attaching the suture to the cut end of the ureter.

George Grey Turner, 1877–1951. Professor of Surgery, Postgraduate Hospital, London.

having been controlled, a tiny incision is made into the extreme lower end of the exposed mucous membrane. One needle of the ureteric suture, then the other, is passed into the lumen of the bowel and brought out by piercing its wall $\frac{1}{2}$ in. (0·6 cm.) lower down, the second needle emerging a $\frac{1}{4}$ in. lateral to the first (fig. 754), so that when the suture is tied the end of the ureter is pulled into the lumen of the bowel and fixed against its inner wall. The incision in the outer coats of the bowel is approximated over the ureter. A second layer of sutures, commencing beyond the fixation stitch, buries the first line of sutures. When it has been ascertained that the ureter is not compressed by the stitches (if obstructed, the ureter is likely to distend above the last stitch) the long ends of the last stitch are brought through the edges of the parietal peritoneum ; after this stitch has been tied the ureter has no intra-peritoneal course. The left ureter is implanted in the

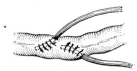

Fig. 755.—Disposition of the ureters in relation to the pelvic colon.

same way, $1\frac{1}{2}$ in. above the right (fig. 755). After the omentum has been laid over the field of operation, the patient is brought to the horizontal position and the wound is closed, usually without drainage. A rubber tube $\frac{1}{2}$ in. (1·25 cm.) in diameter is passed into the rectum and retained by a stitch at the anal margin. The tube is removed on the third day or, before, if it causes discomfort. There must be a large fluid intake ; if vomiting or nausea are present, intravenous saline and glucose is given. If anuria or oliguria supervene, treatment is as described on p. 612.

Total cystectomy is indicated in cases of diffuse papillomatosis and extensive papillary or nodular carcinomata involving the base of the bladder. A rubber catheter is tied in, and the bladder is filled with 1 : 1,000 silver-nitrate solution, the catheter being then spigoted. With the patient in Trendelenburg's position, the bladder is exposed through a median subumbilical incision. The pre-liminary stages of the operation are directed to freeing the bladder from its peritoneal attachments. The urachus is divided between hæmostats, and the upper end is ligated, but the lower end is left attached, to act as a retractor. If separation of the peritoneum from the bladder is impracticable, the peritoneum is opened along its anterior reflection, and incised again where it is attached pos-teriorly, these superior edges being united to reconstruct the peritoneal cavity (fig. 756). It is now possible to strip the ex-traperitonealised bladder from its postero-lateral fascial attachments, the lateral ligaments containing the superior vesical vessels being ligated and divided. At this stage the bladder is emptied through the catheter and the dissection of the posterior wall of the bladder from the rectum is carried as low as possible, the

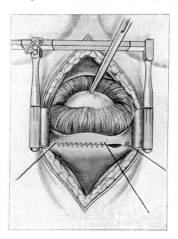

Fig. 756. — Total cystectomy. Exteriorising the peritoneum.

inferior vesical vessels being ligated on either side. Attention is then directed
to the prevesical space ; when veins are seen crossing the anterior aspect of
the prostate they are divided and coagulated. The pubo-prostatic ligaments are divided and their accompanying vessels ligated. With the
finger, the membranous urethra and the apex of the prostate are separated
from the fascia of Denonvillier, the catheter in the urethra acting as a guide.
The membranous urethra is then severed with a long scalpel or a diathermy
knife, the urethral catheter being divided with curved scissors. The
prostate is seized with a volsellum and dissected from the underlying
fascia, bleeding being controlled temporarily by packing. Upward dissection is continued and the seminal vesicles are freed from the rectum.
At the upper and outer extremity of each seminal vesicle lies the vas, with
its accompanying vessels. This pedicle is ligated on each side and the freed
bladder removed. Bleeding vessels are secured and ligated, but those
situated deeply near the cut urethra are best coagulated with diathermy.
The cut urethral catheter can be left in situ to act as a drain. Any enlarged lymph nodes along the iliac vessels are removed. The abdominal
wall is closed with drainage. The drains are removed after about forty-
eight hours.

Radiotherapy.—The radio-sensitivity of epithelial tumours of the
bladder is low.

Open Destruction of the Growth Combined with Insertion of Radon Seeds.—
In the opinion of some, for localised invasive tumours, open excision of the
growth with a cutting diathermy loop and coagulating diathermy to control
bleeding, followed by implantation of radon seeds in the base of the tumour
and in the margin 1 cm. around it (so as to achieve a dosage of 7,000 r)
is preferable to partial cystectomy. Closure of the bladder with urethral
catheter drainage can be substituted for suprapubic drainage.

Deep X-rays sometimes control the hæmaturia, and in a few cases retrogression of the tumour occurs. Severe increase in symptoms of cystitis
constitutes the chief disadvantage of this form of treatment.

Charles P. Denonvillier, 1808–1872. Professor of Anatomy, Paris.

CHAPTER XXIX
THE PROSTATE AND SEMINAL VESICLES

BENIGN ENLARGEMENT OF THE PROSTATE

BENIGN enlargement of the prostate occurs in men over fifty years of age ; most often between sixty and seventy. In isolated instances the patient is under the age of fifty. These facts refer to white races, in whom the condition is very common. In Indians prostatic enlargement is less frequent, and occurs more often in the younger age-groups. In Negroes prostatic enlargement is rare, while in Mongolians it is exceptional.

Ætiology.—For many years considered to be a hypertrophy, and later an innocent neoplasm (an adenoma, a fibro-adenoma or a fibro-myoadenoma), the enlargement is now regarded as an involutionary hyperplasia akin to chronic interstitial mastitis, and due to an imbalance of hormones secreted by the testes. Normally, the preponderant testicular hormone is androgen, but a small quantity of œstrogen is secreted. In cases of enlargement of the prostate the output of œstrogen (female) hormone exceeds that of the androgen (male) hormone. Prostatic enlargement can be produced in experimental animals by injection of œstrogen. Nevertheless, prostatic enlargement in man is unaffected by the administration of male hormones.

Surgical Anatomy.—A prostate the seat of adenomatous hyperplasia has three capsules. From within, outwards, there is a covering of compressed fibro-muscular tissue (the remnants of the normal gland) which can be termed the " surgical capsule." Next there is the anatomical capsule, external to which lies the prostatic sheath of pelvic fascia. Between the prostatic sheath and the anatomical capsule lies the prostatic venous plexus (plexus of Santorini).

Pathology.—There is hyperplasia of the connective tissue stroma and of the submucous glands of the base of the trigone (the subcervical glands) and those of the prostatic urethra. Often disease commences in the subcervical glands, in which event that portion of the prostate lying between the common ejaculatory ducts and the prostatic urethra—the middle lobe of the prostate—becomes enlarged. If the submucous glands of the prostatic urethra are involved, the lateral lobes enlarge also. It is common for the enlargement to remain confined to the middle lobe. It is also common for the lateral lobes and the middle lobe to become enlarged (fig. 757). More rarely the lateral lobes enlarge and the middle lobe is unaffected.

Giovanni Domenico Santorini, 1681–1737. Italian Anatomist.

Occasionally one lateral lobe is enlarged and the other macroscopically normal, but in this instance it is usual for the middle lobe to participate. The anterior lobe or isthmus of the prostate is involved in only one per cent. of cases. The so-called posterior lobe, which is a thin lamella of prostatic tissue covering the back and most of the lateral surfaces of the gland, does not take part in benign enlarge-

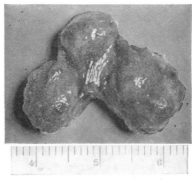

Fig. 757.—Trilobed enlargement of the prostate. Specimen enucleated by suprapubic prostatectomy.

ment. As the prostate enlarges extravesically it tends to displace the seminal vesicles, so that instead of lying on the base of the bladder, these structures become a direct posterior relation of the upper limit of the prostate. Intravesically an enlarged middle lobe insinuates itself within the cervical sphincter (fig. 758). Sometimes both lateral lobes also project into the bladder, so that when viewed from within, the sides and back of the internal urinary meatus are surrounded by an intravesical prostatic collar. The enlargement occurs mainly in that portion of the prostate situated above the level of the verumontanum and common ejaculatory ducts, the remainder of the gland becoming compressed so as to form a false (the so-called " surgical ") capsule from within which the pathological portion can be enucleated. The ratio of fibrous tissue overgrowth to glandular hyperplasia varies considerably. When the hyperplasia is mainly glandular (so-called adenoma) the prostate may become two or three times its normal size, sometimes larger. In prostates with considerable fibrous hyperplasia the enlargement is not so much in evidence, and the term fibro-adenoma is descriptive.

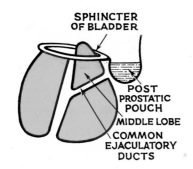

SPHINCTER OF BLADDER

POST PROSTATIC POUCH

MIDDLE LOBE

COMMON EJACULATORY DUCTS

Fig. 758.—The surgical subdivisions and relationships of the prostate.

SECONDARY EFFECTS OF PROSTATIC ENLARGEMENT

On the Urethra.—That portion of the urethra lying above the verumontanum becomes elongated, sometimes to as much as twice its normal length. The canal is compressed laterally, so that it tends to become an antero-posterior slit. The normal posterior curve often becomes so exaggerated that it requires a coudé, bicoudé, or even a fully curved metal catheter to negotiate it. When one lateral lobe becomes enlarged predominantly, lateral distortion of the prostatic urethra occurs.

On the Bladder.—The musculature of the bladder hypertrophies to overcome the obstruction. When viewed from within, bands of muscle fibres can be seen standing out— *trabeculation* (fig. 759). Between these hypertrophied bundles

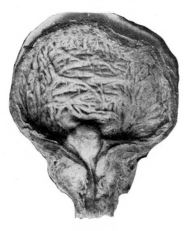

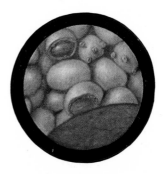

Fig. 759.—Trabeculation of the bladder from prostatic obstruction. (*Aschoff.*)

Fig. 760.—Calculi in a post-prostatic pouch behind the hypertrophied middle lobe of the prostate as viewed through the cystoscope. (*Young.*)

there are shallow depressions—potential diverticula, but because they are shallow the process is termed *sacculation*. One of the saccules (rarely two or more) may continue to enlarge, and form a true diverticulum.

When the middle lobe projects upwards into the bladder it acts as a dam to the last ounce or so of urine, which remains in what is termed the post-prostatic pouch. Stones are prone to develop in this stagnant pool of residual urine (fig. 760).

The enlarged prostate may compress the prostatic venous plexus, and the resulting congested veins (vesical " piles ") at the base of the bladder are apt to cause hæmaturia.

Unless the obstruction is relieved, a time comes when muscular tone gives out ; muscular hypertrophy dwindles, and eventually gives place to atony, the tired muscle making no attempt to overcome the obstruction.

On the Ureters and Kidneys.—Increasing intravesical pressure, or perhaps in some cases direct pressure of the intravesical portion of the prostate on the ureteric orifices, causes gradual dilatation of the ureters, and hydro-ureters are followed by some degree of bilateral hydronephrosis. When decompensation of the bladder hypertrophy occurs, the sphincter mechanism around the ureteric orifices ceases to function, permitting reflux of urine from the bladder into the dilated ureters. Chronic interstitial nephritis with increasing damage to the renal parenchyma is a frequent accompaniment of the back-pressure effects of prostatic obstruction. As a result of ascending infection from the bladder, or more rarely from the blood-stream, acute or chronic pyelonephritis supervenes.

On the Sexual Organs.—In the early stages of prostatic enlargement there is increased libido. Later impotence is the rule.

Clinical Features.—*Frequency* is the earliest symptom of an enlarged prostate. At first it is nocturnal, the patient being obliged to get up to micturate twice or more often during the night, usually commencing at 2 or 3 a.m. Frequency at this stage is probably due to eversion of the sensitive prostatic mucous membrane into the bladder by the intravesical enlargement of the prostate. The frequency becomes progressive, and is then present both by night and by day. When the vesical sphincter becomes stretched a little urine escapes into the normally empty prostatic urethra, causing an intense reflex desire to void, and urgency is added to the frequency. Later, as residual urine increases, frequency becomes more and more in evidence, and there is terminal dribbling.

Dysuria.—The patient finds it useless to strain (cf. urethral strictures and fibrous prostate (pp. 763 and 630)). Rather, he must first wait patiently, with a relaxed abdomen, for the stream to start. When it does start, the stream, instead of being projected, tends to fall vertically.

Pain is absent, unless cystitis or acute retention of urine supervenes. When hydronephrosis commences there may be a dull pain in the loins.　A feeling of weight in the perineum, or a fullness in the rectum, are occasional complaints.

Acute retention of urine may be the first symptom to impel the patient to seek relief because of the intense pain it produces. It often comes on after indulgence in alcoholic liquors, partic-

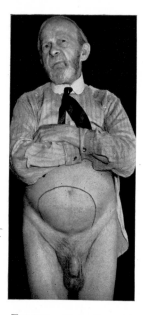

ularly when he goes out of doors on a cold night, or it may supervene after confinement to bed on account of some inter-current illness.

Retention with Overflow.—The patient comes complaining that urine is constantly dribbling away.　It is exceptional for him to have noticed the swelling caused by the distended bladder and he experiences no pain (fig. 761).

Hæmaturia.—The first symptom may be alarming hæmaturia, due to rupture of a varicose vein at the base of the bladder, or from an erosion on the engorged prostate.　More often the hæmaturia consists merely of a drop of blood at the beginning or at the end of micturition.

Renal Insufficiency.—The patient presents himself with one or more of the signs of renal failure (see p. 615).

Fig. 761.—Retention with overflow.　The patient's only complaint was that he " wet his trousers."　Note the overfull bladder.

Examination.—The act of micturition should be watched, if possible.　Loss of projectile power is significant.　The urine is collected into two glasses.　The mere inspection of it is of some service.　It is later examined chemically, and if not crystal clear, a mid-stream specimen is sent for bacteriological examination.

The patient then lies on a couch and the abdomen is examined. In patients with a long history, varying degrees of chronic retention of urine will be found on palpation, percussion, and sometimes on inspection.　The renal areas are palpated for tenderness and possible enlargement of the kidneys.　The state of the tongue is noted ; a dry brown tongue and a urine of low specific gravity is indicative of a considerable degree of renal failure.　The external urinary meatus is examined to exclude atresia meati, and the epididymides are palpated for signs of recent or remote inflammation.

Rectal examination is carried out in the knee-elbow position, and in the absence of a full bladder, bimanually in the dorsal position. In benign enlargement affecting the lateral lobes, increase in their size is evident. They are smooth, convex, and typically elastic, but because all grades of fibro-adenomatosis occur, the fibrous element may give the prostate a firm consistency. The rectal wall can be made to move over the prostate. On bimanual palpation an intravesical lobe can sometimes be felt. By exerting pressure on the apex of the prostate by the finger in the rectum, a gland which is the seat of benign enlargement can be made to move. Residual urine in a post-prostatic pouch can sometimes be felt as a fluctuating swelling above the prostate.

The nervous system is examined by testing the reflexes, and reactions of the pupils to eliminate a neurogenic lesion. Tabes and disseminated sclerosis give symptoms similar to those of prostatic obstruction.

The cardiovascular system should be investigated by a physician before operative treatment is undertaken. At the preliminary examination the blood-pressure is measured.

Examination of the Blood.—A blood urea estimation, a blood count, and a Wassermann reaction are all important, the first two being essential.

Excretory pyelography is only omitted if the patient shows clinical signs of renal failure, or if the blood urea estimation is high. It affords a great deal of information without resorting to instrumentation. It is an excellent test of renal function ; it will exclude or confirm the presence of hydro-ureters and hydro-nephroses ; a vesical diverticulum, if present, may be shown ; if a film is taken after micturition, residual urine will be revealed. Sometimes an intravesical enlargement of the prostate is outlined by the medium.

A preliminary radiograph may show a renal calculus, or a stone in the bladder, or in a diverticulum thereof. Stones in a post-prostatic pouch are sometimes not evident until cystoscopy has been performed.

Cysto-urethroscopy.—When the rectal findings are negative, when a differential diagnosis must be made between urethral stricture and a fibrous prostate, or when there is a history of hæmaturia, cysto-urethroscopy must be performed in order to

make the diagnosis. When the diagnosis of prostatic enlargement can be established on clinical and radiological grounds,
the investigation is unnecessary. Instrumentation should be
avoided when the bladder is palpable above the pubes, and
when there is considerable urinary infection which persists in
spite of urinary antiseptics. If cysto-urethroscopy is necessary
to make or confirm the diagnosis, and there is no contraindication to instrumentation, it is best performed as an immediate
preliminary to operation, if operation is found advisable.

The patient having been instructed to empty his bladder
immediately before the examination, the amount of residual
urine present in the bladder is
measured after the instrument has
been passed and its obturator withdrawn. After irrigation, if necessary, the bladder is distended. The
bladder is first examined. Trabeculation and sacculation is the
prominent finding. The presence
of cystitis will have been anticipated by the examination of the
urine. Normally it is impossible to
see the posterior edge of the internal urinary meatus and the left
and right ureteric orifices at four and eight o'clock, respectively,
in the same cystoscopic fields. In cases of moderate enlargement of the middle lobe this becomes possible (Marion's sign,
fig. 762). When the intravesical projection is great the ureteric
orifices and the inter-ureteric ridge are hidden completely
beneath the prostatic shelf. When it can be seen, the interureteric ridge is frequently hypertrophied and broadened.

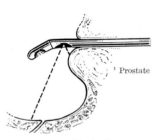

FIG. 762.—Marion's sign.

INDICATIONS AND PREPARATION FOR PROSTATECTOMY

When frequency seriously interferes with sleep, and when
there is residual urine apparent by excretory urography, if
there is no contraindication, prostatectomy is advised. Acute,
and acute-on-chronic retention of urine, or retention-with-
overflow, are all frequent reasons for surgical intervention. In
cases of acute retention of urine due to prostatic enlargement
prostatectomy can be carried out within a few hours if the
general condition is good, provided the blood urea does not
exceed 60 or at the most 70 mg. per cent., and there is no

*Jean-Baptiste Camille-Georges Marion, Contemporary. Professor of Urology, Faculty of
Medicine, Paris.*

obvious urinary infection. In order to relieve the pain and to obtain necessary information concerning the state of the urine, the retention must be relieved by a urethral catheter or, as some prefer, by suprapubic puncture with a hollow needle.

In cases of chronic retention of urine and retention-with-overflow the tendency is to avoid urethral catheterisation altogether, and thus prevent urethritis (and the danger of an ascending infection) which so commonly ensues if an indwelling urethral catheter is retained for more than forty-eight hours, or intermittent catheterisation is practised. Using a watertight stab puncture by one of the methods described on p. 687, a catheter is introduced into the bladder. Most advise that for the first twelve hours the bladder should be decompressed slowly. The catheter is then connected to a sterile bottle and bladder washes of acriflavine 1 : 8,000 are given twice daily until the general condition is improved and the renal function tests are satisfactory. Suprapubic cystostomy is also indicated in patients with acute retention of urine in the presence of serious urinary infection, affections of the myocardium, or considerable hyperpiesis. Severe hæmaturia or clot retention calls for suprapubic cystostomy rather than immediate prostatectomy, for in a very high percentage of cases bleeding ceases after the bladder has been drained, and this affords time for blood transfusion and more thorough investigation. It happens rarely that the bleeding continues at the time of the cystostomy, when immediate prostatectomy is the best means of controlling the hæmorrhage. In cases of prostatic obstruction complicated by an infected vesical diverticulum, prostatectomy should not be undertaken until the diverticulum has been excised, and the infection overcome (see p. 698). After the bladder has been drained for any of the above conditions, while waiting for the renal function to improve, the patient should be given a high fluid intake (6 pints (3·5 litres) per day), an alkaline mixture, and a short course of sulphonamide together, if necessary, with other urinary antiseptics. Many patients can be rendered fit for prostatectomy in fourteen days. Others require a longer period. When, after three weeks or a month the tests are still unsatisfactory, the patient can be fitted with a suprapubic belt, the catheter of which is changed at fortnightly intervals until he is fit to undergo prostatectomy.

TREATMENT

Open Operation

Freyer's operation is still employed, usually in cases where preliminary suprapubic drainage has been necessary and a patient with an enlarged prostate is unfit for a more prolonged operation. The operation is carried out blindly through a 2-inch (5 cm.) suprapubic incision. The adenomatous tissue is enucleated with the finger. As a rule hæmorrhage is not as copious as that encountered during a one-stage operation because, as a result of draining the bladder, periprostatic congestion is diminished, and warm irrigations are sufficient to arrest the bleeding. When considerable hæmorrhage persists the prostatic cavity is packed, preferably with oxycel.

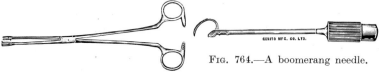

FIG. 764.—A boomerang needle.

FIG. 763.—Harris's ligature carrier.

The bladder and the abdominal wall are closed around a large rubber tube, and a drain is placed in the prevesical space. After five days the tube is removed and some form of suprapubic box is worn until the wound heals, which takes about sixteen days.

Harris's Operation.—The incision in the abdominal wall is similar to that described for the retropubic operation. The bladder is opened widely, and the prostate is enucleated. The prostatic cavity is packed and the patient is placed in the Trendelenburg position. A self-retaining bladder retractor is inserted, and the packing is removed. Arterial hæmorrhage is largely controlled by stitches passed through the posterolateral edges of the prostatic rim by means of a ligature carrier (fig. 763) and a boomerang needle (fig. 764). A large boomerang needle is inserted in the middle line behind the interureteric bar to emerge low in the floor of the prostatic cavity, and a No. 2 plain catgut suture is drawn through these structures. When this suture has been tied, not only does it still further decrease bleeding, but it lines the greater part of the floor of the prostatic cavity with mucous membrane. Two obliterative sutures are then passed through the anterior part of the prostatic rim, leaving an opening that

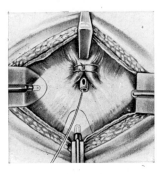

FIG. 765.—Harris's operation. Reconstruction of the prostatic bed has been completed.

will admit the index finger. A whistle-tipped catheter is passed from the external meatus by means of an introducer. The tip of the catheter is transfixed with a silkworm-gut stitch, the ends of which are brought out on to the surface (fig. 765) and temporarily secured by a hæmostat. At this stage the Trendelenburg position is exchanged for the horizontal. When hæmostasis is perfect, infection absent, and renal tests unimpaired, the bladder is closed completely, leaving a small rubber drain in the prevesical space. In other circumstances a small Malécot catheter is introduced through the upper part of the bladder incision. The edges of the abdominal wall and the skin are united. Finally, the ends of the

Sir Peter Freyer, 1852–1921. Indian Medical Service. Later Surgeon, St. Peter's Hospital, London.
S. Harry Harris, 1881–1937. Urologist, Lewisham Hospital, Sydney, Australia.
Achille Malécot, M.D., Paris, invented his catheter in 1890.

silkworm-gut suture are anchored at skin level by a button, or by transfixing and tying them over a piece of rubber tubing. The urethral catheter
is connected to a sterile bottle at the side of the bed and frequent small
irrigations are necessary to ensure that the catheter does not become
blocked by clot. When a suprapubic drain has been inserted, two-way
irrigation renders this complication improbable. If the urine is clear, the
suprapubic tube is removed on the fourth day,
and the catheter on the tenth.

Retropubic Prostatectomy (Millin).—A transverse incision 3 inches (7·5 cm.) long is made
1 inch above the pubis, or a vertical incision of
a similar length is employed. In either event
the aponeurosis is incised vertically and the
recti are separated. The retropubic space is
opened up with the forefinger, the extravesical
fat being drawn upwards. A self-retaining
retractor is inserted and its median blade adjusted so as to push the bladder upwards and
backwards (fig. 766). Veins superficial to the
prostatic sheath, if present, are divided between

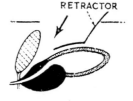

RETRACTOR

Fig. 766.—The approach
to the prostate in retropubic
prostatectomy.

hæmostats and their ends coagulated by touching each hæmostat with the
diathermy. The anterior aspect of the prostatic fascial sheath is cleared
of fat, using a small swab on a holder. A length of gauze 4 inches (10
cm.) in width is packed into each lateral recess with long dissecting
forceps. Having defined the junction of the bladder with the prostate
by palpation, using a long-handled scalpel, a transverse incision convex
downwards is made over the right lobe of
the prostate 1 cm. below the bladder neck.
The incision passes through the fascial sheath,
its contained prostatic venous plexus, and
the capsule of the prostate. There is much
venous hæmorrhage, and in order to visualise
the line of section, mechanical suction is
essential. The incision is deepened until
white adenomatous tissue is displayed. All
three capsules—the surgical, the anatomical,
and the pelvic fascial sheath—which are
closely applied to one another, have now
been traversed, and for simplification they
will be described collectively as "the
capsule." Using long, curved, blunt-pointed
scissors, the lower flap is undermined, and a
pair of T-shaped forceps is applied to the
lower edge of the capsule, and the bleeding is
largely controlled. The left half of the
capsule is dealt with similarly, and the left

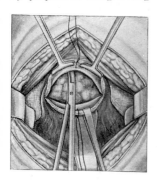

Fig. 767.—Retropubic pro-
statectomy. Dividing the
urethra within the prostatic
capsule. (*After Millin*.)

and right incisions are joined. If there is arterial bleeding from the upper cut
edge of the capsule, the vessel is picked up in a hæmostat, and coagulated. The
upper edge of the capsule of the prostate is grasped with volsellum forceps,
and a stay suture is inserted. A similar stay suture is passed through the
lower flap. Using the scissors referred to already, a plane of cleavage is
found between the adenomatous tissue and the prostatic capsule, and the
former is separated from the latter both distally and laterally. The
urethra is cut across within the capsule, keeping as near to the adenomatous mass as possible (fig. 767). The retractor, the T-forceps and

Terence Millin, Contemporary. Surgeon, All Saints' Hospital, London.

volsellum are removed. With the inferior flap elevated by traction on its stay suture, the forefinger is introduced into the prostatic cavity and hooked around the lower limits of the adenomatous tissue, which are enucleated from their posterior attachment to the capsule and the under-surface of the trigone, allowing the mass to be delivered into the prevesical space. Traction is then exerted on the upper stay sutures, and with closed scissors the adenomatous tissue is bluntly dissected from the vesical sphincter. It is often possible to recognise, clamp, divide, and coagulate the main prostatic blood-vessels entering the mass on either side. The cuff of vesical mucous membrane still attached to the mass is divided with scissors, enabling it to be removed. The prostatic bed is packed and the retractor is replaced without the median blade. By exerting traction on the stay sutures, the prostatic bed is inspected after withdrawing the packing, while the nozzle of the sucker is directed into the cavity. Loose tags are excised, and small nodules of prostatic tissue that remain are removed. Bleeding-vessels are picked up with a hæmostat, and coagulated. The prostatic bed is packed again, and the bladder neck is examined, using Millin's spreader. The posterior lip of the bladder neck is seized with forceps, and a generous wedge of the middle of the trigone is excised with scissors. The packing is again removed from the prostatic cavity, and after sealing any vessels that may require it, a whistle-ended catheter, usually 20 French, mounted on a stilette is introduced from the external meatus as far as the prostatic bed, from which it is advanced into the bladder. The lateral packs are removed and the edges of the capsule are united by a continuous strand of No. 1 chromic catgut, using a boomerang needle, the two stay sutures being tied together as a reinforce-ment. Having cleared the retropubic space of blood and clots, the retractor is removed, and the abdominal wall is closed, leaving a corrugated rubber drain in the prevesical space for forty-eight hours. The catheter is fixed to the skin of the penis by means of a silkworm-gut stitch, supplemented by two pieces of adhesive strapping applied longi-tudinally to the penis and wound around the shaft of the protruding catheter. The after-treatment is similar to that described in Wilson Hey's operation.

Wilson Hey's Operation.—The bladder is opened through a large suprapubic incision. A gum-elastic bougie with a long nylon thread attached is passed from the bladder to the external urinary meatus, where it is pulled through by an assistant, who places a hæmostat on the thread at the external urinary meatus. The thread should be long enough to leave at least 6 inches (15 cm.) lying on the towels at the lower end of the wound. The prostate is freed from its capsule as far as possible with the finger, after which the patient is placed in full Trendelenburg's position. Each ureteric orifice is identified with a probe. With a diathermy needle the trigone is excised to within $\frac{1}{2}$ inch (1·25 cm.) of the ureteric orifices, the interureteric bar being included, and the seminal vesicles being cut through during the process. The prostatic urethra is divided $\frac{1}{2}$ inch above its junction with the membranous urethra, care being taken not to cut the nylon thread. The freed prostate is removed and its bed is inspected through the large opening. Every bleeding-point is sealed in turn by picking it up in a fine-pointed diathermy hæmostat. All tags, remnants of the false capsule, and outlying pieces of prostatic tissue are excised with scissors. When the cavity is as dry as possible, clots are removed and 5 per cent. sodium-citrate solution is instilled into the cavity. A rubber tube 5 mm. in diameter with holes so cut in its proximal end that one will lie in the prostatic cavity and the

Wilson Harold Hey, Contemporary. Consulting Surgeon, Manchester Royal Infirmary.

other (in addition to the terminal opening) in the bladder, is passed retrogradely by means of the original nylon thread. The bladder is closed securely in three layers, after which the abdominal wall is closed with drainage of the cave of Retzius. The indwelling tube is retained in the same manner as that described for retropubic prostatectomy. After ensuring that the tube is free from clot, several ounces of 5 per cent. sodium citrate are left in the bladder, and a spigot is inserted into the end of the tube. The vasa are usually divided between ligatures through separate small incisions. The spigot is removed in two hours and the tube is connected to a bottle beside the bed, all the necessary apparatus being sterile. Should the tube become blocked with blood-clot, $\frac{1}{2}$ ounce (15 ml.) of

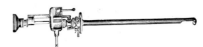

Fig. 768.—McCarthy's endoscopic prostatic resector.

sodium-citrate solution containing 1 : 500 formalin is injected. The tube is removed in two days, or before that time if it is not fulfilling its function.

Transurethral resection of the prostate is indicated particularly in obstruction due to an enlarged middle lobe, a fibrous prostate, or a median bar. Preliminary drainage by an indwelling catheter or a suprapubic tube may be required, and the adequacy of renal function and freedom from gross infection is just as necessary in this form of operation as in the open method. Transurethral resection is, however, better suited to frail patients.

McCarthy's resectoscope (fig. 768) is the instrument most often employed.

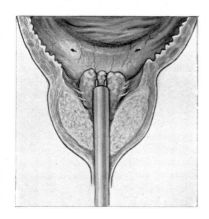

Fig. 769.—Transurethral resection showing the loop commencing to remove a strip from the middle lobe of the prostate. (*After R. M. Nesbit.*)

The operation is preceded by cystoscopy, unless this has been performed already, and it is often the cystoscopic findings that determine whether resection or open operation is the more desirable procedure. The instrument is passed with the patient in the lithotomy position. The larger of the two sheaths, with its obturator, is introduced into the urethra. If it fails to pass easily, the smaller is substituted. When the anterior urethra is narrow or strictured, perineal urethrostomy is sometimes required in order to admit the instrument. The obturator is removed and the bladder is irrigated with sterile water. The carrier, with its telescope lamp and electrode, is passed down the sheath, the cutting loop being in the retracted position. The irrigation inlet is connected to a reservoir of sterile water, and the outlet with a pail. The obstructing area of prostate having been located, the loop is advanced beyond it into the cavity of the distended bladder. With the cutting current switched on, the loop is slowly withdrawn through the obstructing tissue (fig. 769) by rotating the pinion handle. On completing the cut, the current is switched off and the inlet is closed. The carrier is removed and the contents of the bladder received

Joseph F. McCarthy, Contemporary. Urologist, Post-graduate Hospital, New York.

into a kidney dish. The strip of tissue excised will either be adherent to the end of the loop, or it will be swept out in the water. The process is repeated until sufficient prostatic tissue has been removed, or bleeding becomes troublesome. Each strip must be retrieved and accounted for. Hæmostasis is effected, after substituting a ball electrode for the cutting loop and a coagulating for a cutting current, by touching bleeding-points with the ball. When sufficient of the middle lobe has been removed the operator should be able to look down into the bladder when the telescope in the posterior urethra is at the level of the verumontanum. When necessary, strips are cut from the lateral lobes, but here the cutting loop should not transgress the margin of the bladder outlet. After sufficient tissue has been resected the bladder is inspected for fragments of prostatic tissue which, when present, can be removed by means of a Bigelow's evacuator or a special similar type of instrument that can be fitted to the sheath of the resectoscope. The operation is concluded by inserting a rubber whistle-tipped catheter or a Foley's catheter. The latter has the advantage that it is self-retaining and the balloon is of some hæmostatic value. The post-operative treatment resembles that of other operations upon the prostate which rely entirely upon a urethral catheter for drainage. The catheter is removed about the fourth day.

Punch Prostatectomy.—The Thompson punch is a direct-vision cysto-urethroscope containing a tubular knife which can be moved back and forth, the sheath having a fenestrum near the distal end of the opposite side of the beak. When the tubular knife is in the forward position it closes the fenestra. The instrument is passed and the bladder neck and the prostatic urethra are examined. When the tubular knife is drawn back, obstructing tissue at the bladder neck or in the prostatic urethra will project into the fenestrum (fig. 770). The knife is advanced and the

Fig. 770.—Punch prostatectomy. The fenestrum engaging the tissue of the middle lobe.

tissue engaged is cut from before, backwards. This cylinder of prostatic tissue is washed into the bladder, and from thence out of the wide irrigation outlet. Bleeding is controlled by introducing a diathermy electrode along the channel for it contained in the sheath of the instrument. An advantage of this method is that there is less necrotic tissue left behind than when the excavation is performed by a cutting current.

After-treatment in all operations of prostatectomy includes a high fluid intake and a course of alkalis, sulphonamide, and penicillin.

COMPLICATIONS OF PROSTATECTOMY

Hæmorrhage.—The loss of blood during and in the immediate post-operative period may be considerable ; consequently the blood of all patients about to undergo prostatectomy should be grouped and arrangements made whereby suitable donor blood is available. When there has been sufficient loss of blood to cause a considerable fall in blood-pressure, either during the operation or later, blood transfusion should be given. If secondary hæmorrhage due to infection of the prostatic bed occurs, it usually does so between the sixth and twelfth post-operative days, and may also call for blood transfusion. The local management of post-operative hæmorrhage differs in the various operations. In all, the foot

Frederic Eugene Baisal Foley, Contemporary. Urologist, Miller Hospital, St. Paul, U.S.A.
Gershom Joseph Thompson, Contemporary. Head of Urology Section, Mayo Clinic, Rochester, U.S.A.

of the bed is raised and an injection of morphia or omnopon is given. In operations which depend entirely on a urethral catheter for drainage, irrigations of 3·8 per cent. sodium citrate solution by means of a 2-oz. (60 ml.) rubber bulb syringe are undertaken should the catheter become blocked with clot. If this does not dislodge the clot, injection of the solution with, and suction by, a more powerful bladder syringe is employed. Should this prove ineffective, 1 oz. (30 ml.) of glycerin of pepsin injected into the bladder and allowed to remain there for half an hour, by its digestive action may enable disintegrated clots to be evacuated. If all these means fail, the patient must be taken to the operating theatre, where, under anæsthesia, after removing the urethral catheter, all clots can be cleared from the bladder by means of a Bigelow's evacuator after passing a large cannula. In a few cases where the patient's general condition is poor, it is more expeditious to perform suprapubic cystostomy. Clot retention does not necessarily follow excessive bleeding. In the more persistent, but less precipitant, forms of reactionary or secondary hæmorrhage, the passage of a Foley's catheter, which is strapped to the thigh after the balloon has been inflated, often effects hæmostasis by pressure on the prostatic bed. Irrigations of warm saline solution should be continued until they are returned almost clear.

When hæmorrhage is considerable after transurethral resection of the prostate and the bladder becomes full of clots that cannot be dislodged by a syringe, the patient is anæsthetised in the operating theatre, and after removing clots with an evacuator the resectoscope, furnished with its electrode, can be inserted and bleeding-points in the prostatic bed coagulated.

Hæmorrhage following operations in which suprapubic drainage has been employed can often be controlled by warm irrigations of normal saline, or other solutions. If the hæmorrhage is severe and occurs some days after the suprapubic tube has been removed and the wound has healed, or nearly healed, the opening into the bladder must be enlarged under anæsthesia. After clots have been evacuated, bleeding usually ceases with irrigation. If, however, the bladder washes remain highly blood-stained, the prostatic cavity must be packed, preferably with oxycel.

Infection.—The routine employment of sulphonamide and penicillin before operation and during the post-operative treatment has considerably reduced complications consequent upon infection of the prostatic bed, although they still occur, especially if blood-clot is permitted to collect there.

Epididymitis.—Many surgeons ligate and divide the vasa deferentia either at the commencement or the end of every operation of prostatectomy. This measure almost eliminates post-operative epididymitis, but a localised inflammation of the spermatic cord or a small abscess at the site of the division sometimes occurs.

Acute Pyelonephritis.—Ascending pyelonephritis can often be combated by streptomycin, but when serious infection occurs in the presence of kidneys already the seat of some degree of hydronephrosis, it may prove fatal.

Renal Failure.—Oliguria or anuria which does not respond to treatment by intravenous fluid therapy is often associated with the above, or is the result of operating upon a patient with impaired renal function. It is the most lethal complication of prostatectomy.

Extraperitoneal perforation of the bladder is an occasional accident during transurethral prostatectomy. The perforation occurs at the neck

Henry J. Bigelow, 1816–1890. Surgeon, Massachusetts General Hospital, U.S.A.

of the bladder, usually posteriorly on one or other side of the middle line, where the wall of the bladder is thin ; the prostatic capsule, being tough, resists too deep resection. When the patient is under low spinal anæsthesia, immediately the perforation occurs he complains of great suprapubic pain, often radiating towards the epigastrium. Such symptoms appearing after the patient has regained consciousness from a general anæsthetic are more difficult to interpret. When perforation of the bladder is suspected, immediate suprapubic cystostomy and drainage of the prevesical space should be carried out. If this operation is delayed more than twelve hours the prognosis becomes grave, except in a few instances when extravasation occurs slowly with the formation of an abscess in one inguinal region.

Thrombosis and embolism are not more frequent than in other operations, since early rising has been adopted in the modern operation.

Cardiac and respiratory complications are prevented by suitable pre- and post-operative treatment, but they occur more frequently than in most other operations owing to the advanced age of many of the patients.

LATER COMPLICATIONS

Osteitis pubis is a rare complication of suprapubic and retropubic prostatectomy. It is probably due to pricking of the periosteum during the operation, or to a spread of infection from the prevesical space. The symptoms do not appear until two or more weeks after the operation. There is great pain over the pubes, radiating to the buttocks and down the inner side of the thighs, with inability to walk more than a few steps owing to agonising spasmodic contractions of the adductor muscles. Tenderness is present over the pubic bones, and often over the tubera ischii. Radiography shows irregular rarefaction of the ischio-pubic rami, and widening of the symphysis ; these changes only appear after the symptoms have persisted for about three weeks. This exceedingly painful state continues for many weeks. Spontaneous cure with recalcification of the rarefied bone and bony ankylosis of the symphysis occurs after several months. Vitamin B in large doses hastens resolution. Short-wave diathermy is of doubtful value ; X-ray therapy is more efficacious.

Post-operative stricture is rare after those operations in which the posterior lip of the internal urinary meatus is either excised or sutured to the prostatic bed. More common now are strictures of the anterior urethra following the passage of a wide-bore resectoscope or punch.

FIBROUS PROSTATE AND MEDIAN BAR OBSTRUCTION

account for at least 25 per cent. of cases of benign prostatic obstruction. Many different names have been given to this condition—obstruction at the bladder neck, *prostatisme sans prostate*, and dysectasis, i.e. failure of the bladder neck to open —are all descriptive terms.

Ætiology.—In the majority of cases the condition is an aftermath of chronic prostatitis. There is a rare congenital form of median bar obstruction which gives rise to severe symptoms in youth, or earlier.

Pathology.—The glandular and muscular tissues of the prostate become infiltrated with fibrous tissue, which ultimately replaces them, the sphincter vesicæ being involved in the process. When the middle lobe is especially affected, stretching across the dorsal aspect of the internal urinary meatus and obstructing it, there is a bar or dam (fig. 771) composed of fibrous tissue covered by the epithelial lining of the bladder. The musculature of the trigone is much hypertrophied from endeavouring to open the vesical orifice, and there is often a deep pouch behind the interureteric ridge. Not all fibrous prostates giving rise to obstruction are associated with a median bar ; nearly as common a cause of obstruction is fibrous infiltration and contraction of the supramontine periurethral musculature, with similar involvement of the sphincter vesicæ.

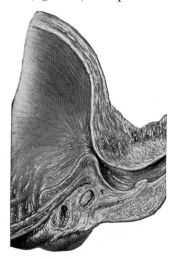

FIG. 771.—A median bar causing " prostatic " obstruction. (*Young.*)

Clinical Features.—The symptoms are similar to those of prostatic enlargement, and often by the time the patient presents there is a large amount of residual urine. Points of dissimilarity are (*a*) there is often a history of prostatitis for which the patient has received treatment ; (*b*) straining helps to expel the urine, and as a consequence an inguinal hernia into a preformed sac may be an additional or the main complaint ; (*c*) hæmaturia is rare. Patients with an acquired median bar obstruction are somewhat younger than those with benign prostatic enlargement, or the symptoms date back before the fiftieth year, but in cases of fibrous prostate *per se* this slight discrepancy in age does not appertain.

Rectal Examination.—The prostate is either normal in size or smaller than normal. In an average case it is distinctly harder than normal, and more fixed. When, as is sometimes the case, the prostate feels very hard, the differential diagnosis between a fibrous prostate and carcinoma is impossible without several of the aids described under carcinoma of the prostate.

Cysto-urethroscopy is essential in order to confirm the diagnosis and distinguish the condition from stricture of the urethra. It may be necessary to dilate the urethra with metal bougies before the cysto-urethroscope can be passed. The changes in the bladder wall are in all respects similar to those seen in prostatic enlargement. The walls of the prostatic urethra do not fall apart when the irrigation is turned on, and the internal urinary meatus does not expand. When a median bar is present it is seen as a narrow projection at the posterior margin of the internal urinary meatus, the floor of the bladder falling away steeply towards the hypertrophied and often shortened trigone. When the patient is asked to micturate, or the bladder is further distended, the trigone remains immotile and the steep angle between the floor of the bladder and that of the urethra persists. On the urethral side of the ridge the verumontanum is drawn up, so that it lies at the base of the shelf, thereby shortening the urethra.

Treatment.—Minor degrees of fibrous prostate unassociated with a median bar sometimes respond satisfactorily to intermittent dilatation by bougies and treatment of the chronic prostatitis, if such is still active. With this exception, operation is always needed. Transurethral resection of the obstructing tissue is usually followed by satisfactory results. Owing to the narrowing of the posterior urethra (and, in many cases, of the anterior urethra as well) the smaller sheath of the resectoscope must be employed. In a few cases when the urethra is too small to admit the resectoscope, an open retropubic operation is a good alternative. The obstructing prostatic tissue is approached by a vertical incision through the prostatic capsule, instead of the transverse incision which has been described.

PROSTATIC CALCULI

may be found within the prostate gland (endogenous) or a urinary calculus, commonly a ureteric calculus, is arrested in the prostatic urethra (exogenous). The latter is considered on p. 652. Endogenous prostatic calculi, which are usually composed of calcium phosphate but sometimes of oxalate or carbonate, together with about 20 per cent. of organic material, cast a well-defined radiological shadow. Various clinical types are encountered :

1. **Symptomless.**—Occur in an otherwise normal prostate, and are common in men over forty years of age. The stones, which are small and not, as a rule, very numerous, are dis-

covered on radiography, often for a non-urological condition. Such calculi are calcified corpora amylaceæ.

2. Incidental.—Small prostatic calculi are not uncommonly encountered during prostatectomy for an enlarged prostate. Usually, but not invariably, they are seen in a preliminary radiograph. Such calculi are situated between the surgical capsule and the pseudo-adenomatous portion that is enucleated.

3. Associated with Chronic Prostatitis (*syn.* Calculous Prostatitis).—The severity of the symptoms varies greatly. At first they are those of chronic prostatitis. The stones are small and impalpable. Rarely they are seen in one or more of the mouths of the prostatic ducts during urethroscopy, or grating is experienced during the passage of a metal bougie. When the stones are numerous and larger they often replace the major part of the prostatic gland, which is the seat of fibrosis. The symptoms are then those of prostatic obstruction, and the patient is usually over fifty years of age. On rectal examination the stones are often felt as irregular, intensely hard nodules which are difficult to distinguish from carcinoma of the prostate, although in the latter condition the organ is likely to feel more fixed. On rare occasions crepitus makes the diagnosis certain at the clinical examination.

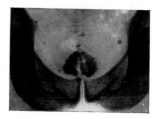

Fig. 772.—Radiograph showing prostatic calculi.

On radiography these stones often form a horseshoe (fig. 772) or a circle. Calcification in a healed tuberculous prostate can simulate prostatic calculi. The past history with signs of treated epididymitis will eliminate the former. Occasionally a large solitary stone occurs, often at a comparatively early age, when it is the sequel of a cavity in the prostate produced by a prostatic abscess.

Treatment.—When the calculi are small and the symptoms are mild, the treatment of chronic prostatitis by prostatic massage and a course of sulphonamide often keeps the patient free from symptoms for months at a time. Transurethral resection of the fibrous prostate will release multiple small calculi as the strips of prostatic tissue are excised, and many of them are removed by irrigation at the time of the operation. Others are passed per urethram at a later date. When

symptoms of prostatic obstruction are present, and a radiograph shows the prostate is riddled with stones, they can be
removed by the retropubic route.

After incising the capsule of the prostate longitudinally, the urethra is
incised and the catheter, previously inserted, is withdrawn until its tip
lies in the membranous urethra. Using a sharp curette, all the calculi
and as much as possible of the infected prostatic tissue is removed.
The bladder neck is then exposed, and a generous wedge of the posterior
lip is resected with curved scissors. The operation is concluded in a
manner similar to that of retropubic prostatectomy.

CARCINOMA OF THE PROSTATE

In the British Isles the annual death-rate from carcinoma of
the prostate has doubled in the past twenty years. About
16 per cent. of cases of prostatic obstruction prove to be due to
carcinoma, to which must be added a number in whom the first
and main symptoms are due to metastases. Carcinoma of the
prostate commences in one of the following ways :
  (a) In the posterior lamella of the normal gland ;
  (b) Diffusely in one or other normal lateral lobes ;
  (c) In association with benign enlargement.

Pathology.—The carcinoma is spheroidal celled, with a varying degree of tubule formation. As in other situations, the
more anaplastic it is, the greater the malignancy.

Local Spread.—Commonly a growth commencing in the
posterior part of the gland breaks through the prostatic capsule
and prevented (at least temporarily) from extending backwards
by the strong fascia of Denonvillier, grows upwards to involve
the seminal vesicles. Further upward extension causes compression on the lower ends of the ureters. Growths commencing in the lateral lobes involve the prostatic urethra early.
In advanced cases the base of the bladder is invaded. Occasionally a carcinoma of the prostate implicates the rectum. In
some cases distant metastases occur while the primary growth
is small and still confined to the posterior lamella of the prostate.

Involvement of Lymph Nodes.—(a) Via lymphatics passing
along the sides of the rectum to the nodes along the internal iliac
vein and in the hollow of the sacrum. These nodes lie in close
association with the sacral nerve plexuses. (b) Via lymphatics
which pass over the seminal vesicles and follow the vas deferens
for a short distance to drain into the nodes along the external
iliac vein.

From both these situations the retroperitoneal nodes, and later the mediastinal nodes, and occasionally the supra-clavicular nodes become implicated. Only rarely are the inguinal nodes involved.

Hæmatogenous metastases occur particularly in bones, and the bones affected in order of frequency are shown in fig. 773. The rami of the pubis, the ischium, the ilium, the sacrum, and the lower lumbar vertebræ are all common sites. The frequent proximity of skeletal metastases to the primary growth has

been attributed to reversed flow from the vesical venous plexus to the vertebral and osseous pubic veins during coughing, sneezing, etc. Bone metastases are typically sclerotic, resulting in increased density of bone, but osteolytic metastases causing bone destruction are not uncommon. Metastases occasionally occur in the skin. In late cases the lungs, the liver, the kidney, and the brain are involved in that order of frequency.

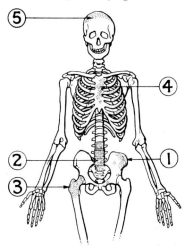

Fig. 773.—Sites of location, in order of frequency, of secondary carcinoma of the prostate in bones. (*After Swift Joly.*)

Clinical Features.—In the majority of cases the patient is over fifty-five years of age, but it is not very unusual for the disease to appear between forty-five and fifty-five years of age, in which event the growth is usually highly malignant.

Type 1. The Pathological.—The symptoms and signs are identical with those of benign enlargement. At histological examination 2 to 5 per cent. of prostates removed in the belief that they were benign prove to contain one or more areas of carcinoma.

Type 2. The Clinically Doubtful.—In a number of instances the symptoms and signs are similar to those of benign enlargement or fibrous prostate, but a hard nodule or increased fixation of the gland favours the diagnosis of carcinoma.

Type 3. The Clinically Certain.—The patient complains of pain in the perineum or suprapubic region, in addition to symptoms of prostatic obstruction. On rectal examination (see below) the findings may leave no doubt as to the diagnosis.

Type 4. The Occult.—Urinary symptoms are absent or slight. Pain in the back, or sciatica, is the main symptom. Bilateral sciatica in an elderly man is most often due to metastases from carcinoma of the prostate. Œdema of one or both legs, paraplegia, or a spontaneous fracture are occasionally due to metastases from a carcinoma of the prostate.

Rectal Examination.—Irregular induration in a part or the whole of the gland with decreased mobility is suspicious of carcinoma. Obliteration of the notch between the seminal vesicles, or of the groove between the lateral lobes, adds to the suspicion. If, in addition, the induration extends to one or more of the following situations (*a*) beyond the lateral limits of the gland, causing obliteration of the lateral sulci, (*b*) to the lymphatics above and lateral to the seminal vesicles, or (*c*) to the membranous urethra, the diagnosis is certain.

Radiological examination to exclude or confirm the presence of prostatic calculi or pelvic or lumbar skeletal metastasis is always necessary.

Serum Acid Phosphatase.—When the estimation is above 10 King-Armstrong units per 100 ml. of blood, it is strong confirmative evidence that the patient has carcinoma of the prostate with secondary deposits. Patients with carcinoma of the prostate and skeletal metastases often have a high serum alkaline phosphatase estimation as well. The same finding may be registered by patients suffering from Paget's disease of bone, but in the latter condition the alkaline usually greatly exceeds the acid phosphatase. A reading between 5 and 10 K-A units of serum acid phosphatase is suspicious of carcinoma of the prostate. There are, however, many exceptions to the test. In only about 40 per cent. of patients suffering from carcinoma of the prostate is the phosphatase estimation raised above normal (1 to 4 K-A units).

Additional Aids to Diagnosis in Doubtful Cases.—One or two of the following procedures are often required to confirm or disprove doubtful cases :

1. *Malignant Cells in the Prostatic Secretion.*—Some surgeons refrain from massaging the prostate, which may be the seat of malignant disease, and

Earl J. King and Arthur Riley Armstrong, Contemporaries. Co-workers at the Department of Medical Research, Banting Institute, University of Toronto.
Sir James Paget, 1814–1899. Surgeon, St. Bartholomew's Hospital, London.

prefer to rely on centrifuging an early morning specimen of urine which, however, only occasionally gives positive findings. In about 70 per cent. of cases of carcinoma of the prostate, malignant cells are found in a stained specimen of a prostatic secretion obtained by prostatic massage.

2. *Cysto-Urethroscopy.*—When there is a history of hæmaturia, this examination is essential. There is often a grating sensation as the prostatic urethra is traversed. With the instrument in place, deep induration in the prostate is more readily appreciated by a finger in the rectum, and fixation of the gland becomes more evident. Puckering of the apex of the trigone, submucous nodes in the base of the bladder, or ulceration of an intravesical projection are late manifestations. In earlier cases there are no pathognomonic visible signs.

3. *Needle Biopsy.*—Turkel's instrument is used as follows. Under pentothal anæsthesia the needle, with its cannula, is inserted in the middle line between the anus and the bulb of the urethra, and with the left index finger in the rectum its point is directed to the suspicious node. The cannula is removed, and the fine tubular trephine is passed through the needle. With the finger in the rectum hooked over the upper border of the prostate, the gland is pressed on to the trephine, which is rotated (fig. 774). Syringe suction is applied to the trephine, which is removed, as also is the needle. Bleeding from the puncture in the perineum soon ceases with pressure. The column of tissue 1 mm. in diameter is thrust from the trephine into the specimen bottle by a stilette. Histological examination of the fragment by a skilled pathologist gives accurate information.

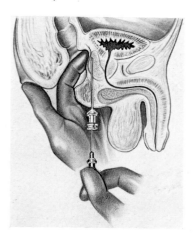

FIG. 774.—Obtaining a specimen of prostatic tissue by means of Turkel's needle.

4. *Transurethral Biopsy.* — Transurethral resection of the prostate has the advantage of removing the obstruction and providing large pieces of tissue, but it may not reach the posterior lamella of the prostate, which is commonly the seat of early carcinoma.

TREATMENT

Excluding those in whom prostatectomy is performed for supposedly benign enlargement, in under 5 per cent. of patients is the carcinoma confined to the prostate when the patient first presents.

Palliative treatment consists in (*a*) castration to remove the main supply of androgen, and (*b*) the administration of œstrogen.

Bilateral subcapsular orchiectomy is performed through a central scrotal incision. The tunica albuginea is incised and all the spermatogenic tissue is removed (fig. 775) by gauze dissection and, if necessary, a

Eric Francis Turkel, Contemporary. Urologist, Gamble Clinic, Greenville, Mississippi, U.S.A.

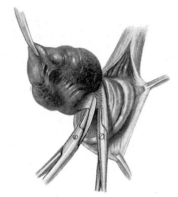

Fig. 775.—Subcapsular orchiectomy in progress.

sharp curette. After hæmostasis has been effected a prosthesis of acrilic resin is inserted, and the edges of the tunica albuginea approximated over it.

Stilbœstrol is given orally, 15 mg. per day for four or five days, and then 6 mg. daily for the next few months. In favourable cases this can be followed by a maintenance dose of 2 mg. for years. When the serum acid phosphatase is raised this form of treatment causes it to fall, which is an index of a favourable response. In some cases stilbœstrol causes painful enlargement of the breasts, with pigmentation of the areolæ, the median raphé of the scrotum, and any cutaneous scar. When the pain is severe, or when the hormone causes nausea and vomiting, the stilbœstrol must be discontinued, or some other œstrogen such as hexœstrol or dienœstrol is substituted; these, however, are not so potent.

According to their response to this treatment patients can be divided into three groups :

Group 1. No effect is registered ; the patient goes downhill rapidly.

Group 2 (the majority).—The pain is relieved promptly, the appetite improves, the primary tumour softens and becomes smaller. Metastases often disappear or become smaller (fig. 776). In over 70 per cent. of this group, after a varying period from several months to two years, the disease recommences. The unfavourable course of the recurrence is not significantly altered by increasing the dose of stilbœstrol.

Group 3.—The patient remains in good health for several years. In a few instances there has been no recurrence for five years or more.

Radical Treatment :

Retropubic Total Prostatectomy.—A No. 18 French rubber catheter is passed from the meatus into the bladder, and a spigot is inserted into the lumen. The prostate is displayed as described for retropubic prostatectomy. The apex of the prostate is freed laterally and posteriorly from the underlying fascia of Denonvillier, mainly with the finger and a swab on a holder, the indwelling catheter helping to define the membranous urethra. A long curved aneurism needle carrying a stout silk ligature is passed beneath the apex of the gland, enabling the ligature to be drawn through. The apex of the prostate is grasped on either side by long Allis forceps, the catheter is partially withdrawn, and the ligature is tied tightly proximal to the forceps. The urethra is divided between the ligature and the forceps. The posterior aspect of the prostate is separated from the fascia of Denonvillier from below upwards, and until the attach-

Charles P. Denonvillier, 1808–1872. Professor of Anatomy, Paris.
Oscar Huntington Allis, 1843–1921. Surgeon, Presbyterian Hospital, New York.

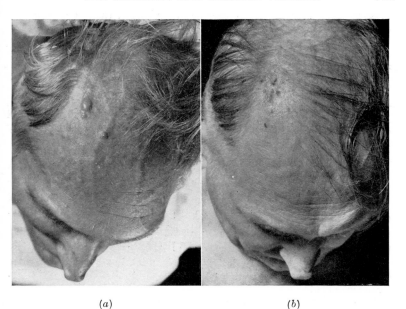

(a)   (b)

FIG. 776.—(a) Metastases of prostatic carcinoma of the scalp. (b) Thirteen
months after orchiectomy. (C. Huggins.)

ment of the fascia to the seminal
vesicles and the base of the bladder is
encountered. The fascia is incised transversely. Each seminal vesicle is freed
and the vas, with its vessels, is ligated
and divided. After still further separating the base of the bladder from the
fascia, the anterior wall of the bladder
is opened transversely to expose the
trigone. Thereafter the circumference
of the base of the bladder is transected
just below the trigone (fig. 777). The
mass, consisting of the whole prostate
(except its extreme apex), the seminal
vesicles, and a cuff of the base of the
bladder, is removed. Using a boomerang needle the depleted trigone is united
to the stump of the prostate and the
membranous urethra with fine catgut
sutures. The urethral catheter is advanced into the bladder. As the circumference of the cut edge of the
bladder is vastly greater than that of
the urethra, there remains a large
anterior defect which is closed vertically
from below, upwards (fig. 777 inset).
A Malécot catheter is introduced

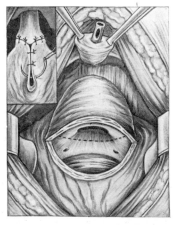

FIG. 777.—Retropubic prostatectomy. The prostate, with its
fascial sheath intact, has been
dissected from the fascia of Denonvillier and amputation at the bladder neck is in progress. Inset:
Closure of the large anterior defect,
after uniting the membranous
urethra to the cuff of the base of
the bladder. (After Millin.)

*Charles Huggins, Professor of Surgery, Chicago, and his co-workers introduced the treatment
of carcinoma of the prostate by orchiectomy and stilbœstrol in 1941.*

through a stab incision in the more proximal part of the anterior bladder wall before completing closure of the defect.

Wilson Hey's operation with a wider excision of the rim of the prostatic cavity than in his operation for benign enlargement is another method of removing a carcinoma of the prostate.

SARCOMA OF THE PROSTATE

Sarcoma of the prostate is so rare as to be of little practical importance. It usually occurs in boys, and must be distinguished from a large vesical calculus, with which it has been confused. The prognosis is practically hopeless.

PROSTATITIS

In both acute and chronic prostatitis the seminal vesicles are infected in a large percentage of cases, and when, as is usually the case, the prostatic urethra is involved also, there is a triad of pathological conditions, to wit: posterior urethritis, prostatitis, and seminal vesiculitis. Symptoms due to the infection of any one of these structures may predominate.

Acute prostatitis, always relatively uncommon, has become rare since gonorrhœa, its most frequent precursor, has been treated by penicillin. Even when acute prostatitis is preceded by gonorrhœal posterior urethritis, it is generally found to be associated with other organisms. Acute prostatitis may be due to a primary infection by staphylococci, streptococci, or B. coli, either singly or mixed, and while a urethral origin of the infection is far more frequent and may be activated by the passage of a urethral instrument, the infection is sometimes hæmatogenous.

Clinical Features.—As a rule there are symptoms of urethritis, and pus is present in both the initial and terminal specimens of urine. The characteristic early symptom is a feeling of heaviness in the perineum and the patient cannot sit comfortably for any length of time. Later there is pain in the perineum which passes to the tip of the penis during micturition. Pain on defæcation is also a symptom. When the seminal vesicles are involved, blood-stained nocturnal emissions are superadded. In severe cases the temperature rises to 102° F. (38·9° C.) or more, and there are rigors. In cases of hæmatogenous infection the pyrexia and general malaise often overshadow the local symptoms at the commencement of the attack, and as there is no urethral discharge and there may be a negative result to culture of the urine, the diagnosis is difficult. In established cases a rectal examination reveals a large, tender prostate, and often one seminal vesicle is more distended than the other.

Treatment.—Appropriate antibiotic treatment, together with sitz baths, often results in resolution of the inflammation.

Prostatic Abscess.—In addition to the foregoing symptoms and signs, there are one or more areas of softening to be felt in one or both lateral lobes. Painful micturition may give place to acute retention of urine. Sometimes the abscess bursts into the urethra when a catheter is passed, or while rectal examination is in progress. As this is not an invariable termination, and a prostatic abscess may track to the perineum or, very rarely, burst into the rectum, it is better to open the abscess. The older method, which gives satisfactory results, is by the perineal route. With a catheter in the urethra and the patient in the lithotomy position, a curved incision is made in front of the rectum. The dissection is carried below the bulb of the urethra. The swollen prostate is felt, and forceps are plunged into the abscess cavity. The retropubic approach may be substituted. A more chronic abscess can be opened per urethram with a resectoscope.

CHRONIC PROSTATITIS

Chronic prostatitis is a common condition occurring usually in late middle life, and there is often no history of previous gonococcal urethritis. The organisms most frequently encountered are the B. coli, staphylococcus, and streptococcus.

It is well established that chronic prostatitis may be a focus of infection that produces metastatic manifestations in other parts of the body; also that the prostate itself can become infected from distant foci such as carious teeth, infected tonsils, or furunculosis.

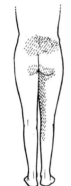

FIG. 778.— Sites of pain in chronic prostatitis.

Type 1.—The symptoms are predominantly urinary, frequency of micturition heading the list. Pain is usually mild, and referred to the perineum or the rectum. It may be aggravated by sitting on a hard chair. Occasionally relief is obtained by pressure on the perineum.

Type 2 is silent prostatitis. Arthritis, myositis, neuritis, and sometimes iritis and conjunctivitis, are only explained when pus from the prostate has been obtained. Particularly common is lower back pain, sometimes extending down the legs (fig. 778); such pain is usually attributed to lumbago or a strain at work, and many sufferers from prostatitis receive orthopædic treatment and physiotherapy without benefit.

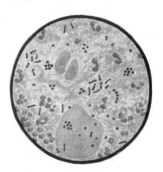

FIG. 779.—Film of prostatic fluid from a case of chronic prostatitis. Stained Gram plus basic fuchsin. Numerous pus cells, staphylococci, streptococci, and diphtheroid bacilli. (Oil immersion × 1,000.)

Type 3 comprises symptoms of sexual dysfunction, e.g. premature ejaculations, prostatorrhœa, and impotence. Hæmospermia (bloodstained emissions) should immediately suggest vesiculitis.

Diagnosis.—Digital examination of the prostate reveals a somewhat enlarged nodular boggy or indurated organ. The infected ducts may be temporarily occluded by débris, and two or three prostatic massages are often required before the presence of pus can be demonstrated (fig. 779).

Urethroscopy reveals inflammation of the prostatic urethra, and pus can often be seen exuding from the prostatic ducts. The verumontanum is likely to be enlarged and œdematous.

Local Treatment.—Massage of the prostate per rectum is the most important measure, the prostatic secretion and the contents of the seminal vesicles being emptied thereby. Usually eight strokes on each side are given, at first twice a week and then at lengthening intervals, as improvement sets in. In the later stage of treatment, which usually must be prolonged over months, urethral dilatation serves to open the prostatic ducts and permits better drainage. This can be followed with advantage by irrigation of the bladder with acriflavine 1 : 5,000.

In rebellious cases, canalisation of the vasa, which allows irrigation of the seminal vesicles, often clears up an infection which defied other methods.

General Treatment.—One or more courses of sulphonamide, penicillin, or streptomycin—according to the infecting organism —assists in eliminating the infection.

Long-standing chronic prostatitis terminates in fibrous prostate and median bar obstruction. Prostatic calculi are also the result of long-continued chronic prostatitis.

COWPERITIS

The diagnosis of Cowperitis is often wanting for lack of a simple examination. On passing the forefinger into the rectum and placing the thumb first

one on one side and then on the other of the median raphe of the perineum, Cowper's glands can be palpated (fig. 780). In acute cases the least pressure causes excruciating pain. In this way the condition is differentiated from an ischio-rectal or periurethral abscess.

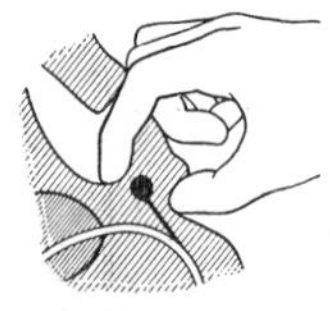

Treatment.—In acute cases penicillin, together with rest in bed, often culminate in resolution. When suppuration occurs, incision and drainage is the proper course. If a fistula develops, it is necessary to excise the remnants of the gland.

Fig. 780.— Palpating an enlarged gland of Cowper.

TUBERCULOSIS OF THE PROSTATE AND SEMINAL VESICLES

Tuberculosis of one or both seminal vesicles is more common than tuberculosis of the prostate, and is often discovered when examining a patient with chronic tuberculous epididymitis, there being no symptoms referable to the internal genitalia.

William Cowper, 1666–1709. London Surgeon.

On rectal examination the affected vesicle is found to be nodular and tender. When the prostate is involved there are one or more well-defined nodules, most often near the periphery of the upper or lower border of one or both lateral lobes. Less frequently a larger solitary mass is felt occupying a more central position. The patient, who is rarely over forty or under twenty years of age, may occasionally present with a urethral discharge as the first symptom. Then the diagnosis has to be made from gonorrhœa and abacterial urethritis entirely on bacteriological findings, for the prostate at this stage may feel normal. At other times the symptoms are a mild ache in the perineum, blood-stained ejaculations, or both. In later cases when the posterior urethra becomes involved from extension of tubercles from the prostate or by the discharge of a prostatic abscess, there is painful, frequent micturition and sometimes terminal hæmaturia. Even in cases without urinary symptoms a complete urological examination is necessary ; genital tuber-culosis is associated with renal tuberculosis in at least 30 per cent. of cases. In due course tuberculous seminal vesiculitis may lead to congestion and œdema of the base of the bladder, and later to a basal cystitis. If a cold abscess forms in the prostate it is felt as a slightly tender, soft swelling. Like other prostatic abscesses, it usually ruptures into the urethra, more rarely through the perineum, or into the rectum. Occasionally an abscess of the prostate or seminal vesicle bursts into the bladder ; later at cystoscopy a ragged, deep ulcer is seen alongside the trigone.

Treatment.—On no account must a tuberculous prostate or seminal vesicle be massaged. Urethral instrumentation should be avoided, or reduced to a minimum in order to confirm the diagnosis. Sanatorium treatment is essential. Streptomycin may be tried, but is usually ineffective. Tuberculin is more successful. If a prostatic abscess forms, it is better to evacuate it by the perineal route than to permit it to rupture spontane-ously.

Considerable involvement of the prostate, which goes on to suppuration, is a comparatively unfavourable form of genito-urinary tuberculosis. On the other hand, tuberculous seminal vesiculitis and non-suppurative tuberculosis of the prostate usually heal after other associated lesions in the kidney or epididymis (either or both of which are present in nearly 100 per cent. of cases of tuberculous involvement of the seminal vesicles and prostate) have been eradicated.

SEMINAL VESICULOGRAPHY

It is sometimes necessary to know if the common ejaculatory ducts are patent. This information can be obtained by catheterising the common ejaculatory ducts through a special posterior urethroscope. Sodium iodide is then injected up the catheter and a vesiculograph taken. The same information can be obtained more easily by vasotomy and injection of an opaque medium (fig. 781).

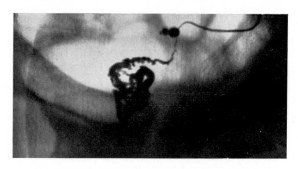

Fig. 781.—A seminal vesiculogram.

CHAPTER XXX
THE URETHRA AND PENIS

THE DEVELOPMENT OF THE URETHRA

From the internal urinary meatus to the sinus pocularis (uterus masculinus) the urethra is developed from the urogenital sinus. This portion of the male urethra corresponds to the entire female urethra. From the sinus pocularis to the fossa navicularis the male urethra is derived from the medial labial folds, which also form the corpus spongiosum (fig. 782). The urethra traversing the glans is the last to be developed, and is formed by the down-growth of a solid pencil of epiblast, which becomes canalised shortly before birth.

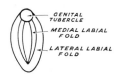

Fig. 782. — The male and female external genitals are undifferentiated until the end of the *third* month.

CONGENITAL ABNORMALITIES OF THE URETHRA

Meatal Stenosis.—The external urinary meatus, normally the narrowest part of the male urethra, is often the seat of congenital stenosis which is associated with phimosis. In the circumcised, meatal stenosis may also be acquired or increased by fibrosis following meatal ulceration. All degrees of narrowing are encountered. When the opening is reduced to a pin-hole, back-pressure effects on the whole urinary system result. Pin-hole meatus is occasionally a cause of enuresis, and at any time of life it may result in chronic retention of urine (fig. 783). In cases of chronic urethritis some degree of meatal stenosis hinders drainage of the urethra, and meatotomy is required. Frequently this operation is necessary before full-sized urethral instruments or a cystoscope can be passed.

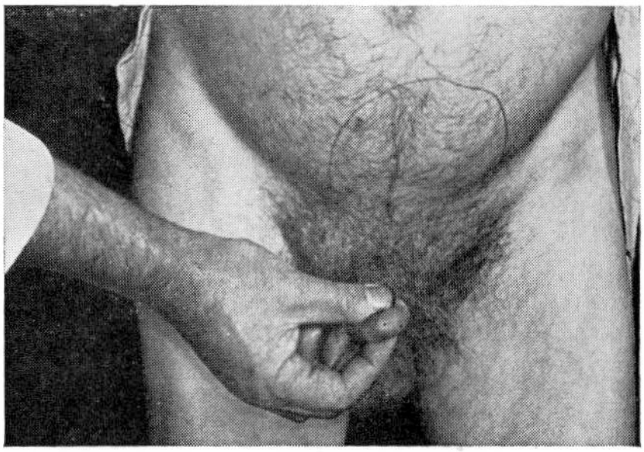

Meatotomy.—A fine-pointed scalpel is introduced into the urethra and a cut is made in a downward direction. In infants and children a metal bougie of suitable calibre is passed into the meatus each day for four or five days, and weekly dilatation for a month must be practised.

Fig. 783.—Pin-hole meatus causing chronic retention of urine in a man of fifty-one. Relieved by meatotomy.

In adults it is preferable to unite the cut edges of the urethra and the skin of the glans with two or three sutures, which control hæmorrhage and prevent the lips of the meatus from uniting. Dilatation on two occasions at weekly intervals is usually all that is necessary in this instance.

Congenital Strictures and Valves.—Congenital strictures occur particularly at the points where the developmental component parts of the urethra fuse. Thus they are found in the region of the sinus pocularis and the fossa navicularis. If the stricture is complete, or nearly so, the infant dies soon after birth, and necropsy shows bilateral hydronephrosis. Congenital strictures of moderate calibre are occasionally met with in infancy and childhood, and give rise to a train of ill-health, predisposition to attacks of recurrent pyelonephritis, and sometimes a fatal termination from uræmia. The most puzzling variety of congenital stricture takes the form of symmetrical valves, which allow the ingress of a bougie, but obstruct the outflow of urine. The treatment of a stricture is similar to that of an inflammatory stricture. Valves must be destroyed by diathermy excision through an operating urethroscope. In very young boys perineal urethrotomy is performed. Thus, by by-passing the narrow pendulous urethra a urethroscope of a calibre of 16 or 18 French can be introduced. After the valves have been destroyed by fulguration, a No. 10 Foley's catheter is left in place until the third post-operative day.

HYPOSPADIAS

Hypospadias is the commonest congenital malformation of the urethra, and it occurs once in every 350 males (Mayo). The external meatus is situated at some point upon the *under-*surface of the penis or in the perineum.

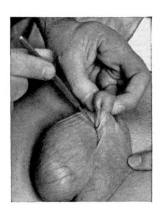

Fig. 784.—Penile hypospadias. The patient passes urine through the orifice demonstrated by the probe.

There are various degrees of the deformity which can be classified as follows :

Glandular Hypospadias. — There is an ectopic opening on the under-surface of the glans, separated from a blind depression at the normal site of the external urinary meatus, or from the ectopic meatus a channel runs forwards through the glans to the tip of the penis.

Coronal Hypospadias.—The meatus is situated at the junction of the under-surface of the glans with the body of the penis.

Penile Hypospadias.—The meatus opens at some part of the under-surface of the penis (fig. 784).

Peno-scrotal Hypospadias.—The urethra opens at the junction of the penis with the scrotum.

Perineal Hypospadias.—The scrotum is split and the urethra opens between its two halves. This variety is sometimes associated with bilateral maldescended testes, in which event the sex of the child may be difficult to determine.

Glandular hypospadias is its most frequent variety, and is due to a failure of canalisation of the glans (see embryology). The other varieties have been attributed to failure of the medial genital folds to fuse. They are now looked upon as an absence of the urethra and corpus spongiosum distal to the ectopic orifice, the absent structures being represented by a fibrous cord. In all except the first variety the penis is curved in a

Frederic Eugene Foley, Contemporary. Urologist, Miller Hospital, St. Paul, U.S.A.
W. J. (1861–1939) and C. H. (1865–1939) Mayo. Surgeons, Mayo Clinic, Rochester, U.S.A.

downward direction. The farther away the opening is from the normal position, the more pronounced is the bowing. In all cases the prepuce is deficient on its under-surface.

TREATMENT

In glandular hypospadias no treatment is necessary unless the opening is too small, in which case meatotomy is performed. In other forms plastic operations, of which there is a great variety, are carried out. Many of these operations are dependent upon utilising the prepuce. On this account circumcision should never be performed in these varieties of hypospadias.

Straightening the penis is undertaken, preferably between the ages of two and three years. In coronal hypospadias this can be accomplished by making a transverse incision above the ectopic meatus and excising the band of connective tissue that tethers the urethral opening to the base of the glans. The incision is then sewn up longitudinally. In more distal ectopic openings on the shaft of the penis an inverted Y- or Z-shaped incision provides enough local skin to cover the defect after the anchoring band has been excised. In cases of peno-scrotal and perineal hypospadias the curve is too pronounced to be remedied by the methods described, and additional skin must be provided on the ventral surface. This is usually accomplished by transferring the prepuce from the dorsum to the ventral aspect of the penis by one of a number of plastic procedures. Ombrédanne's flap is one such measure which, in other circumstances, is used as a covering for the reconstructed urethra.

All operations of straightening the penis cause the ectopic opening to become displaced farther back ; thus a coronal hypospadias becomes a penile, and a penile a peno-scrotal, and so on.

RECONSTRUCTION OF THE URETHRA

Ombrédanne's Method.—A catheter, lubricated with glycerin, is introduced into the urethra and anchored to the glans with a stitch. An oval purse-string suture of silk is inserted, the base of which extends as far from the ectopic opening as the apex, which lies on the under-surface of the glans. The breadth of the area enclosed should be one-third the circumference of the penis. An incision is made through the skin and subcutaneous tissue outside the lateral and inferior margins of the purse-string (fig. 785 (A)). The skin and the purse-string suture are dissected from the base towards the ectopic meatus, care being taken to avoid opening the urethra as the ectopic meatus is approached. Distal to the ectopic meatus the skin bearing the purse-string is undermined inwards for a short distance, and the purse-string is drawn moderately tight (fig. 785 (B)). The cutaneous bag so formed is the new urethra. The prepuce is now stretched by two stay sutures passed through the lateral parts of its free extremity. The lateral edges are incised, as also is the inner layer near the corona. The inner layer is dissected from the outer layer so as to form a single epithelial sheet, the raw surface of which faces the glans. A Y-shaped buttonhole incision is made at the base of this flap (fig. 785 (c)), avoiding visible blood-vessels. The ends of the purse-string suture and the glans

Louis Ombrédanne, Contemporary. Surgeon, Hôpital des Enfants Malades, Paris.

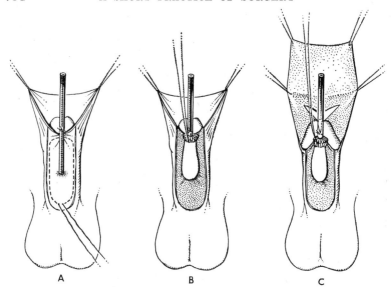

Fig. 785.—Ombrédanne's operation. (a) Purse-string suture inserted and flaps outlined. (b) Flaps dissected up and purse-string tightened. (c) The opposing layers of the prepuce have been separated to form a continuous sheet, and a Y-shaped incision made into the base of the flap.

are brought through the aperture. The flap is trimmed as necessary and is sutured so as to provide a covering for the whole of the defect on the ventral surface of the penis. The rim of the glans and the pouch are sutured to the edges of the Y. The purse-string suture can be used to suspend the penis to a light metal bridge strapped to the thighs for five days, or the purse-string can be withdrawn and the penis wrapped in a gauze bandage soaked in Masticol. Three months later another small plastic operation is carried out to advance the meatus to the tip of the penis.

When the ectopic meatus of a penis straightened by utilising the prepuce is situated at the peno-scrotal junction or behind that point, the construction of the new urethra is more complicated.

Blair's method consists in constructing a new urethra from broad-based flaps fashioned from the outer walls of the defect, sutured in the middle line over a catheter, and providing a covering from the skin of the scrotum. At a second stage the penis is freed from the scrotum and the open proximal end of the new urethra is anastomosed to the ectopic opening. Urine is diverted from the anastomotic line by performing perineal urethrostomy until healing is complete.

McIndoe's Method.—A special trocar (made in various sizes), the tip and handle of which unscrew, leaving a hollow interior, is used. A piece of

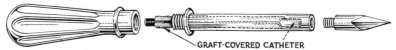

GRAFT-COVERED CATHETER

Fig. 786.—McIndoe's trocar. A piece of gum-elastic catheter surrounded by a skin graft, the raw surface of which lies outwards, is being inserted into the barrel of the instrument.

Vilray P. Blair, Contemporary. Emeritus Professor of Clinical Surgery and of Oral Surgery, Washington University, U.S.A.
Sir Archibald McIndoe, Contemporary. Plastic Surgeon, St. Bartholomew's Hospital, London

gum-elastic catheter that fits the interior of the trocar (which should be twice the size of the proposed urethra) is covered by a Thiersch graft cut from the inner surface of the upper arm. The graft-covered catheter is passed into the trocar (fig. 786), which is then assembled. A stab incision is made just distal to the ectopic meatus and another on the tip of the glans. The loaded trocar is thrust subcutaneously from the posterior incision until the point emerges at the tip of the penis. The point is then unscrewed, as also is the handle. The distal end of the catheter is grasped firmly with forceps and the barrel of the instrument is withdrawn from the posterior wound, leaving the catheter and skin graft in place. A rubber catheter is passed into the bladder through the ectopic meatus, and retained for forty-eight hours, to prevent escaping urine from contaminating the graft. On the tenth day the piece of gum-elastic catheter is removed and the grafted tunnel is syringed with a mild antiseptic. Thereafter a fresh piece of catheter is inserted. Special bougies with detachable ends, preventing slipping out, are an advantage. The process is repeated at weekly intervals for six months, and at no time should the bougie be left out of the new urethra for more than a few minutes. The second stage of the operation is similar to the second stage of Blair's operation.

EPISPADIAS

Unlike hypospadias, epispadias is exceedingly rare. There are epispadia glandis, epispadia penis, and epispadia totalis, which is usually associated with ectopia vesicæ. Epispadia glandis is the rarest type of this rare malformation. The urethral orifice is situated on the dorsum, and the penis is usually curved upwards. Plastic operations to rectify the twist and restore normality can be undertaken.

ULCERATION OF THE URETHRAL MEATUS

Ulceration of the meatus in young male children (fig. 787) is a common clinical entity. It is never found in the uncircumcised. It is common after circumcision, though an interval of three to eighteen months may elapse between the operation and the onset of symptoms. Lack of protection given by the prepuce is the initial cause. Friction of the clothing and ammoniacal urine are important secondary ætiological factors. The ulcer causes a *scab* to form which closes the meatus, and the child can only urinate by bursting this scab. This process is usually accompanied by pain and screaming, and a few drops of blood may be passed. Ulceration and scab

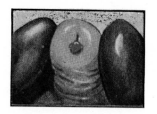

FIG. 787.—Ulceration of the urinary meatus in a child of one and a quarter years.
(*H. P. Winsbury-White.*)

formation alternate, and if neglected, cicatricial contracture of the meatus may result eventually in an acquired pin-hole meatus.

The meatal ulcer syndrome is considered by Campbell to be due to stenosis of the meatus. Many consider that the ulcer precedes the stenosis.

Treatment.—Meatotomy, followed by intermittent dilatation of the meatus, is curative so regularly as to support Campbell's hypothesis. If there is an associated ammoniacal dermatitis the diapers should be washed, not with soap, but with a saturated solution of boric acid. The baby itself is washed with the same solution, no soap being used. Ascorbic acid, 50 mg. (gr. 1) daily, is prescribed.

Karl Thiersch, 1822–1895. Professor of Surgery, Leipzig.
Meredith Fairfax Campbell, Contemporary. Professor and Head of Department of Urology, College of Medicine, New York.

RUPTURE OF THE URETHRA

Rupture of the urethra is divided into two distinct classes

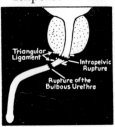

FIG. 788.—Showing the two distinct varieties of rupture of the urethra.

—rupture of the bulbous urethra, and rupture of the membranous urethra (*syn.* intrapelvic rupture) (fig. 788). Each is again redivided into complete and incomplete.

RUPTURE OF THE BULBOUS URETHRA

Rupture of the bulbous urethra is the more common accident. Almost without exception there is a history of a fall astride a projecting object. In days gone by, the common cause was falling astride a beam on board a sailing ship. To-day a loose manhole cover accounts for a number of cases (fig. 789).

Clinical Features. — The triad of signs of a ruptured bulbous urethra is urethral hæmorrhage, a perineal hæmatoma, and retention of urine, to which may be added a fourth—pain.

Preliminary Treatment and Investigation.—If the accident is suspected, in order to prevent the possibility of extra-

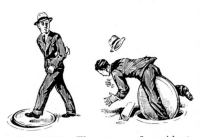

FIG. 789.—The type of accident which results in rupture of the bulb of the urethra. (*After O'Conor.*)

vasation, *the patient should be told not even to try to pass urine.* No attempt should be made to catheterise him until he is in the operating theatre, where asepsis can be assured, and operation can be undertaken in necessary cases. When circumstances are extenuating, and the bladder is full, it should be emptied by suprapubic puncture until the patient can be admitted to a surgical service, where the following investigation is undertaken. The urethra is washed out carefully, and a gum-elastic bi-coudé catheter of moderate size passed along the penile urethra, the beak of the catheter being directed strictly to the *roof* of the urethra. An attempt is made to pass the catheter gently through the damaged bulbous urethra.

If the rupture is incomplete, the catheter will pass onwards into the bladder.

If the rupture is complete, the catheter cannot be passed farther than the bulb, and its arrest synchronises with a flow of blood.

Treatment.—*Incomplete Rupture*

The bladder is distended with warm lotion and suprapubic cystostomy is performed by introducing a No. 28 Malècot catheter into the bladder through a short incision above the symphysis pubis. If there is considerable swelling of the perineum, as well as bruising, an incision is made in the middle line of the perineum and blood and blood-clots are evacuated. By avoiding the use of an indwelling urethral catheter subsequent stricture formation is considerably minimised. The after-treatment is similar to that of complete rupture.

Complete Rupture

Suprapubic cystostomy is performed and a metal bougie is passed through the internal urinary meatus and held in position by an assistant. The patient is then placed in the lithotomy position and a second bougie is passed from the external urinary meatus. An incision is made in the middle line of the perineum. Both ends of the ruptured urethra can readily be identified by the bougies they contain. Bleeding vessels having been ligated, the bougies are removed from the field of operation and the roof of the urethra is united with two or three fine catgut sutures. The perineal wound is packed lightly with ribbon gauze soaked in penicillin solution, and the skin is approximated by a stitch at each end, leaving the remainder open. The patient is taken down from the lithotomy position and the bladder is closed around a Malécot catheter. The suprapubic wound is closed in layers, leaving a corrugated rubber drain in the prevesical space.

After-treatment.—The patient is given a six-day course of sulpha-triad, and penicillin is administered systemically. The bladder is irrigated twice a day with 1 : 4,000 acriflavine solution. The perineal wound is syringed with the same solution and protected by a dry dressing until it heals by granulation. The prevesical drain is removed at the end of forty-eight hours. On the fourteenth day a well-lubricated metal bougie (12/14 for an adult) is passed from the meatus. If the bougie enters the bladder readily, the suprapubic drainage tube is removed. If any difficulty or bleeding ensues, the Malècot catheter is left in place for a further week. The urethra is dilated at weekly, then longer, intervals until it can be shown by urethroscopy and urethrography that no stricture is present.

COMPLICATIONS OF RUPTURE OF THE BULBOUS URETHRA

Subcutaneous extravasation of urine occurs in complete rupture if the patient attempts to pass urine (see p. 761).

Stricture.—This common complication is largely due to super-added sepsis, often introduced by attempts to pass a catheter or tying in a catheter in cases of incomplete rupture.

Both these complications are largely preventable, and in this connection it is well to bear in mind the words of Rutherford Morison : " Rupture of the urethra is one of the most serious of accidents, and unless your skill can prevent the development of a stricture, you are presiding at the opening of a lifelong tragedy."

Achille Malècot, M.D., Paris, invented the catheter in 1890.
Rutherford Morison, 1853–1939. Professor of Surgery, University of Durham, Newcastle upon Tyne.

RUPTURE OF THE MEMBRANOUS URETHRA (*Syn.* **INTRAPELVIC RUPTURE**)

Intrapelvic rupture of the urethra, which occurs in the membranous portion near the apex of the prostate (fig. 788), is almost invariably a complication of a fracture of the true pelvis or dislocation of the symphysis pubis. However, only about 6 per cent. of cases of fractured pelvis are thus complicated. Blood, and later urine, are extravasated into the prevesical space and, because the pubo-prostatic ligaments are torn, the prostate and the bladder become displaced backwards and upwards, thus producing wide separation of the ends of the severed urethra (fig. 790).

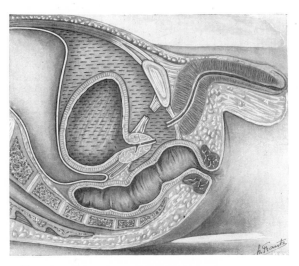

Fig. 790.—Intrapelvic rupture of the urethra. Note the displacement of the bladder backwards, due to the tearing of the pubo-prostatic ligaments.

Clinical Features.—Signs of shock and those of a fractured pelvis prevail for some hours. Urethral hæmorrhage is usually trivial in amount, or may be absent. Often it is only when the patient has not passed urine since the accident and hypogastric pain increases that signs of rupture of the urethra become manifest. On abdominal examination an ill-defined swelling is felt in the hypogastrium, usually more in evidence on one side than the other. In some cases the rounded dome of the distended bladder can be distinguished from the swelling caused by the prevesical extravasation. Per rectum the prostate cannot be felt ; the area normally occupied by it is tender and unsupported.

Investigation.—As in the preceding type, investigation should be undertaken in the operating theatre whenever possible. One should be mindful lest the passage of the catheter into the prevesical space and the withdrawal of a few drachms of blood-stained urine be mistaken for an entry into the bladder.

Treatment.—The first step is to make a suprapubic incision which opens the prevesical space. As a rule it is only after this has been done that it is possible to distinguish between an extraperitoneal tear of the bladder (see p. 698) and an intra-pelvic rupture of the urethra. The guiding rule is, if the bladder is even moderately distended, the lesion must be situated below the vesical sphincter. Thus the diagnosis of intrapelvic rupture of the urethra is confirmed. Direct suture of the urethra is difficult, yet it is imperative to bring into direct apposition the widely separated ends of the urethra. Usually this can be accomplished in the following way. The bladder is opened suprapubic-

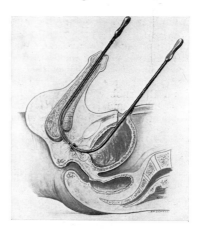

Fig. 791.—Intrapelvic rupture of the urethra. Showing the tips of the metal bougies in contact.

ally and a metal bougie is passed through the internal meatus to the seat of the rupture. Another metal bougie is passed from the external meatus until it comes in contact with the first. The two bougies are manipulated until their tips touch (fig. 791). By slowly withdrawing the first bougie and steadily advancing the second, while keeping their tips in contact, it is usually possible to guide the second bougie past the seat of the rupture into the bladder. The first bougie is withdrawn and a piece of plain rubber tubing of such a size as to fit tightly is threaded on to the beak of the second bougie, which is withdrawn, carrying with it the rubber tubing. Outside the external urinary meatus the bougie is separated from the rubber tubing, and to the latter is fastened, by means of a stitch, the tip of a Foley's catheter. By pulling on the vesical end of the rubber tubing the tip of the Foley's catheter is drawn into the bladder, where it is disconnected from the rubber tube. The bag of the Foley's catheter is inflated. The bladder is closed around a Malècot catheter and the suprapubic wound is closed, leaving two small rubber tubes—one passing to the right and one to the left of the prevesical space.

In rare instances when the above method of guiding the lower bougie into the bladder fails, the patient should be placed in the lithotomy position and a curved para-rectal incision, with its convexity forward, is made in the perineum. The beaks of the bougies passed from the bladder and from the external urinary meatus are readily accessible in the perineal wound, and by threading the ends of a piece of rubber tubing of suitable size (usually 22 French) on to the beaks of the bougies, the tube can be drawn upwards through the suprapubic incision and downwards through the external urinary meatus. By attaching the tip of a Foley's catheter to the lower extremity of the rubber tube with a stitch, the tip of the Foley's catheter can be drawn into the bladder, where it is disconnected from the rubber tube, which has served its purpose as a pilot. The perineal wound is packed lightly and partially closed. The remaining steps of the operation are the same as those described above.

During the operation the patient will receive either a blood transfusion or a plasma infusion, to combat shock. If, after completing the above measures to correct the urethral displacement the patient's condition remains good, a plaster cast can be applied to immobilise the pelvis (p. 1054). In other circumstances this is deferred for forty-eight hours, or longer.

After-treatment.—Traction is applied to the Foley's catheter, either by attaching one end of a length of silk to the margin of its butt end and to the other a 2-lb. (1 kilogram) weight, which hangs over the bed-rail (fig. 792), or by strapping the catheter to

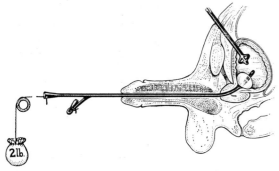

Fig. 792.—Method of correcting backward displacement of the prostate and approximating the ends of the ruptured urethra by traction on a Foley's catheter.

the thigh or the overlying plaster cast. The traction is maintained for twelve days, thereby closely approximating the torn ends of the urethra. After traction has been discontinued the catheter is left in the bladder for a further fourteen days. A course of penicillin and sulphatriad, as detailed for rupture of the bulbous urethra, is given; thereafter usually a small dose of sulphatriad (2 gm. daily) is sufficient to keep the urine sterile. Details of bladder washes and irrigation of the perineal wound (if any) are similar to those given for rupture of the bulbous urethra. About the twenty-sixth day the urethral and bladder catheters are removed. When the wound or wounds have healed (about a month to six weeks later) instrumentation by bougies is commenced. If correct urethral alignment has been attained, the membranous urethra shows but little tendency to stricture formation.

EXTRAVASATION OF URINE

The extravasation may be superficial or deep.

In order to understand the limitations of superficial extravasation, it is necessary to comprehend the limitations of Colles's fascia.

Colles's fascia is the deep layer of superficial perineal fascia. It is attached posteriorly to the base of the triangular ligament, by curving round the transversus perinei muscles. Laterally it is attached to the anterior lips of the rami of the pubes and ischia. Anteriorly it is continuous with the dartos of the scrotum and Scarpa's fascia.

Scarpa's fascia is the deep layer of the superficial abdominal fascia. It is continuous with the anterior border of Colles's fascia, and is fused inferiorly with the deep fascia of the thigh just below Poupart's ligament.

Superficial extravasation occurs in neglected cases of complete rupture of the bulbous urethra, i.e. when operation is not undertaken within twelve to twenty-four hours.

The extravasated urine cannot pass (1) behind the middle perineal point, because of the fusion of Colles's fascia with the anterior triangular ligament; (2) into the thighs, for Scarpa's fascia blends with the pubic portion of the fascia lata just distal to Poupart's ligament; (3) into the inguinal region, because of the intercolumnar fibres and fascia of the external oblique.

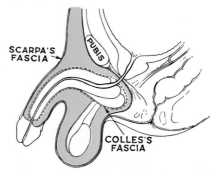

FIG. 793.—The fascial planes concerned in superficial urinary extravasation.

Abraham Colles, 1773–1843. Surgeon, St. Stephen's Hospital, Dublin. Professor of Surgery for thirty-two years.
In the United States of America Scarpa's fascia is known as Buck's fascia.
Gurdon Buck, 1807–1877. Surgeon to the New York Hospital.
Antonio Scarpa, 1747–1832. Anatomist and Surgeon, Venice.
François Poupart, 1661–1709. Anatomist of Paris.

It therefore must pass (1) into the scrotum ; (2) beneath the superficial fascia of the penis ; (3) up the abdominal wall beneath the deep layer of the superficial fascia (fig. 793).

Treatment.—Multiple incisions are made in the infiltrated tissues of sufficient depth to penetrate the limiting fascia. By the time extravasation has occurred it is unlikely that the urethra can be repaired in the way described already (see p. 757), for the sutures would cut out of the œdematous inflamed tissues. It is therefore often advisable to adopt the sutureless operation of Rutherfurd. Suprapubic cystostomy is performed and a metal bougie is passed through the internal urinary meatus. The patient having been placed in the lithotomy position, another metal bougie is passed from the external urinary meatus to the perineum, and perineal section is carried out. A Foley's catheter is introduced from the external urinary meatus into the bladder in the same way as that described for intrapelvic rupture of the urethra, and the bladder is closed around a Malécot catheter. The perineal wound is left widely open. The urethral catheter is removed after three or four days. In other respects the after-treatment is similar to that for complete rupture of the bulbous urethra.

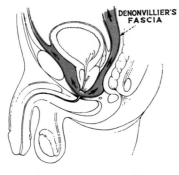

FIG. 794.—Area occupied by extravasated blood and urine in the case of rupture of the deep urethra.

Deep extravasation (fig. 794) occurs in the case of extraperitoneal rupture of the bladder, rupture of the ureter, intrapelvic rupture of the urethra, and after suprapubic puncture, when the bladder has been allowed to refill. The urine spreads in the layers of the pelvic fascia, or in the retroperitoneal tissues.

Treatment.—When extravasation is proceeding from the bladder, it is necessary to drain the cave of Retzius, and to perform suprapubic cystostomy. The treatment of the various conditions which are associated with deep extravasation are considered in their appropriate sections.

URETHRITIS

While gonorrhœa (see p. 41) is the most frequent cause of urethritis, it should be clearly understood that no case of

Henry Rutherfurd, 1861–1929. Surgeon, Glasgow Royal Infirmary.
Charles P. Denonvillier, 1808–1872. Professor of Anatomy, Paris.
Anders Retzius, 1796–1860. Professor of Anatomy, Karolinska Institutet, Stockholm.

urethritis should be regarded as due to a Neisserian infection until it has been proved bacteriologically. Non-specific urethritis is most commonly due to the staphylococcus albus, diphtheroids, and streptococci, in that order. Gram-negative organisms are occasionally found. Appropriate antibiotic treatment, together with (in chronic cases) urethral irrigations and dilatation by bougies, rids the patient of the infection.

Non-bacterial urethritis also occurs; the following are examples:

Trichomonas Vaginalis.—Approximately 16 per cent. of males suffering from non-gonococcal urethritis are suffering from trichomonas infection. As in the female, it is only by examining at once as a " hanging-drop " preparation a specimen of the discharge that this organism (fig. 795) will be found regularly. An important consideration in treatment is alkalinisation of the urine. Prostatic massage, preceded by an instillation into the bladder of 1 per cent. gentian violet, followed by irrigations of potassium permanganate solution 1 : 6,000, together with urethral dilatation, eventually cures this often resistant infection. Examination of the female partner is essential, as relapses due to reinfection are common.

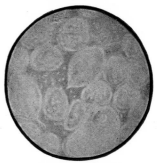

FIG. 795.—Trichomonas from a urethral discharge.

Reiter's syndrome is characterised by a triad of symptoms—urethritis, arthritis, and conjunctivitis. The urethral discharge is abundant and purulent, accompanied by but little frequency or pain. The arthritis is manifested by severe pain in the large joints of the limbs. It is usually polyarthritic and flitting. The conjunctivitis is profusely purulent, and it is sometimes associated with iritis. The condition is due to a filterable virus. It seems certain that Reiter's disease is not a venereal disease.

Treatment is often unsatisfactory. Penicillin is without value. Some cases have responded to arsphenamine; others to streptomycin or chloromycetin. Rest in bed for six weeks at least is necessary.

URETHRAL STRICTURE

Urethral strictures are conveniently divided into the following varieties :

Congenital.

Traumatic.

Inflammatory — Post-gonorrhoeal(90 per cent.).
— Post-urethral chancre.
— Tuberculous.

Post-operative — Prostatectomy.
Amputation of the penis.

Albert Ludwig Siegmund Neisser, 1855–1916. Professor of Skin and Venereal Diseases,
University of Breslau.
Hans Reiter, Contemporary. Professor of Hygiene, University of Berlin.

Post-gonorrhœal stricture may be situated in any part of the anterior urethra, but is most frequently situated (*a*) in the bulb (70 per cent.); (*b*) at the peno-scrotal junction; (*c*) in the distal part of the spongy urethra, in that order. The membranous and prostatic parts of the urethra are exempt.

Owing to the more effective treatment of gonorrhœa, stricture of the urethra is becoming less common.

Multiple strictures are very frequent, and in a urethroscopic study of eighty-seven consecutive cases we found that in over 30 per cent. the stricture was triple. Abraham believes that multiple strictures are a misnomer, and that every untreated urethral stricture is a spiral ; only after it has been traumatised by bougies is this difficult to make out. In his opinion nearly all strictures are right-handed spirals, each spiral decreasing in size towards the bladder, and it is the spirals which are described as multiple strictures. When there are two strictures the deeper is the narrower ; when there are three strictures the deepest is the narrowest. If a stricture in the penile urethra has a very narrow orifice, there is seldom another stricture behind it.

Pathology.—Following inadequately treated gonorrhœa, infection persists in the periurethral glands, and spreads to the periglandular tissues, which become infiltrated with round cells and fibroblasts. There is metaplasia of areas of the columnar cells of the mucous membrane into squamous cells, and from time to time the superficial layer of cells desquamates, giving rise to urethral flakes in the urine. Gradually the infiltrated periurethral tissues contract with the formation of scar tissue, localised thrombophlebitis of the corpus spongiosum playing a part in the more dense varieties. While in the bulb the fibrosis is most in evidence in the roof of the urethra, in the penile urethra it predominates in the floor. Most strictures develop during the first year after gonorrhœal infection, but they may not give rise to dysuria for ten to fifteen years.

Clinical Features.—In a stricture of large calibre there are few symptoms other than those of the occasional passage of urethral threads and a varying amount of urethral discharge (gleet), most in evidence in the early morning. Often these symptoms are neglected. The leading symptom is dysuria. In contradistinction to prostatic obstruction, the patient finds he must strain to empty the bladder. Another distinguishing feature is the patient's age. He is often considerably younger than the prostatic sufferer, or the symptoms of dysuria date back to some time prior to the fiftieth year. As the calibre of the stricture diminishes the urinary stream becomes increasingly narrow, and eventually is projected with so little force that it drops almost immediately. Micturition is prolonged, and after it has seemingly ended dribbling occurs. This is due to urine trickling from the dilated urethra above the stricture. Frequency of micturition, at first during the day and then both by day

J. Johnston Abraham, Contemporary. Consulting Surgeon to the Lock Hospital, London.

and by night, is another common complaint, due either to incomplete emptying of the bladder at each act of micturition, or to cystitis, or both. In long-standing cases it is often possible to palpate the stricture from without as an induration in the urethral floor. The evil effects of urethral obstruction upon the bladder, ureters, and kidneys are similar to those of prostatic obstruction, and consequently it is unnecessary to reiterate them. Untreated, sooner or later retention of urine supervenes. Sometimes acute retention sets in while the stricture is still of moderate calibre ; it is then due to super-added œdema of the urethral mucous membrane in the neighbourhood of the stricture, brought about by voluntary retention, alcoholic excess, or recrudescence of local infection. In other cases narrowness of the stricture results in increasing inability to expel residual urine, and acute-on-chronic retention, or retention-with-overflow supervenes.

Urethroscopy renders the diagnosis of urethral stricture very precise.

The stricture can be seen as a white scar of fibrous tissue, and its position in the urethra, the size of its contained lumen, and its dilatability can be judged (fig. 796). Often a stricture encircles the whole urethra, and the lumen is more or less centrally placed, but from time to time a variety of urethroscopic appearances is noted in individual cases ; for instance, the stricture may take the form of a crescent.

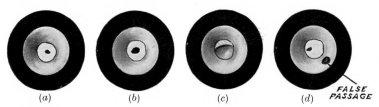

(a)   (b)   (c)   (d)   FALSE PASSAGE

Fig. 796.—Urethroscopic appearances. (a) Fine-bore stricture. (b) Moderate-bore stricture. (c) Crescentic stricture of the roof. (d) Stricture with false passage.

False passages may be seen. They are recent penetrations of the urethra in front of the stricture due to unskilful attempts to pass a sound. False passages are particularly liable to bleed, and it is of paramount importance to cease æro-urethroscopy if urethral hæmorrhage occurs, for fatal air embolism has resulted from air being pumped into the cavernous tissue through a urethral wound.

Urethrography is another valuable measure for investigating certain strictures of the urethra. By this means it is possible to gain information concerning the length of a stricture, of dilatation or diverticulum formation above the stricture, or

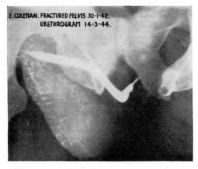

FIG. 797.—Urethrogram showing a stricture of the membranous urethra following fracture of the pelvis.

failure of the medium to pass a stricture (fig. 797). The patient lies on the X-ray couch half-way between the left lateral and the supine positions, with the lower leg flexed at the hip and the right leg extended. Ten to 15 ml. of warm iodised oil or uropac solution is instilled slowly into the urethra by means of a syringe, using but little pressure. The X-ray film is exposed while the last few millilitres of the solution are being injected.

TREATMENT BY DILATATION

Intermittent Dilatation.—Dilatation at regular intervals is a satisfactory form of treatment in the majority of instances, provided the patient attends regularly for treatment. Two doses of 1 gm. of sulphatriad taken with an alkali are given prior to the dilatation, preferably at four-hourly intervals. This dose is repeated eight-hourly for the next two days. Before each dilatation the glans penis and the meatus are cleansed, and the anterior urethra washed out with a mild antiseptic. Dilatation should be carried out under local anæsthesia. Few urethral strictures are impassable, but it often requires patience to insinuate even the finest urethral guide.

Gum-elastic bougies (*syn.* French bougies) (fig. 798) should be the

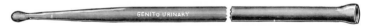

FIG. 798.—Gum-elastic bougie.

standard instruments in the early stages of treatment of all but the very finest strictures. It is usual to commence with a No. 10 French, and if this cannot be passed, progressively smaller bougies are employed. Eventually it may be necessary to resort to filiform bougies.

Filiform bougies are gum-elastic bougies varying in size from 1 to 3 French. If one fails to pass, it is often valuable to insert several as far as the stricture. By manipulating each back and forth, one may be made to pass the stricture (fig. 799). To distend the urethra with sterile olive-oil and apply a penile clamp to the glans penis adds to the chances of success of the foregoing method, because obstructing folds of mucous membrane are separated by the oil distension. If this method fails, it is sometimes possible to pass a filiform bougie through the stricture under the vision afforded by a urethroscope. If any bleeding has been occasioned by the attempt to pass bougies, urethroscopy should be postponed for several

FIG. 799.—"Faggot" method of introducing bougies through a stricture.

days. Only when even a filiform bougie cannot be passed on three successive occasions is a stricture held to be impassable.

Filiform Bougies with Followers.—Filiform bougies furnished with threaded hollow mounts at their proximal ends are to be preferred, because screw-ended gum-elastic bougies of a larger size can be attached and guided

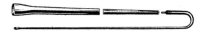

FIG. 800.—Filiform bougie with follower.

by the filiform through the stricture. In this way many strictures of very small calibre can be dilated sufficiently to render subsequent dilatations less arduous.

By means of gum-elastic bougies a stricture is dilated up to the size of 14 French. Thereafter metal bougies are to be preferred.

Lister's metal bougies (*syn.* English Bougies) (fig. 801) are indicated

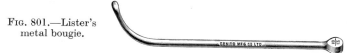

FIG. 801.—Lister's metal bougie.

after the second or third attendance of the patient, when it has been proved that the stricture is responding to dilatation by the French bougies. Metal bougies of a smaller size than 7/9 English should not be used, for fear of making a false passage.

Kollmann's dilator (fig. 802) is used in the last stages of treatment to

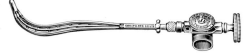

FIG. 802.—Kollmann's curved urethral dilator.

fully dilate the stricture. This instrument is also particularly useful in post-prostatectomy strictures. The illustration shows a curved Kollmann's dilator. The straight pattern is used for strictures placed more anteriorly.

In strictures of very small calibre dilatation should be carried out twice a week. In most instances it is sufficient for the patient to attend for treatment at weekly intervals until the calibre of the urethra is nearly normal, when the interval is lengthened. If the stricture shows but little tendency to contract, the intervals are lengthened. If full calibration has been obtained, the intervals between dilatations can be extended to

Lord Lister, 1827–1912. Professor of Surgery at Glasgow, Edinburgh, and London.
Arthur Kollmann, Contemporary. Urologist, Leipzig.

six months, and finally to one year. A few strictures are cured by full dilatation, but in the majority the patients must be kept under supervision for the remainder of their lives.

Continuous dilatation necessitates some days of in-patient treatment, but it is of immense benefit in cases where little or very slow progress is made by intermittent dilatation. It is also an excellent form of treatment in cases where there is considerable residual urine, or retention-with-overflow, and cases of acute retention unrelieved by a dose of morphia and a hot bath when a filiform bougie can be passed. Having inserted a filiform bougie, around its base is tied a silk ligature, the ends of which are fastened to the penis with adhesive plaster. The patient passes urine alongside the bougie for twenty-four hours. At the end of that time usually a very small gum-elastic coudé catheter can be passed. This is fixed in position, and each succeeding day a larger catheter is inserted. The bladder is irrigated twice daily with acriflavine solution, and sulphonamide and penicillin are given during this treatment, which usually lasts for a week. Such excellent progress accrues that subsequent intermittent dilatation progresses smoothly. In a number of instances continuous dilatation obviates the necessity for operative treatment.

OPERATIVE TREATMENT

Internal urethrotomy is indicated in cases of resilient stricture of the bulbous or penile urethra, particularly multiple strictures, which can be dilated with difficulty but contract within a few days. Before internal urethrotomy is undertaken renal function must be tested and proved satisfactory, and urinary infection controlled as far as possible by a sulphonamide and an antibiotic. The filiform guide of the instrument is passed through the stricture, and in cases where it is known that this part of the procedure is difficult, the guide is passed before a general anæsthetic is administered. On to the base of the guide is screwed the staff of the instrument, with its obturator in position. The well-lubricated staff is made to follow the guide, which curls up within the bladder. The wings of the staff are firmly held by an assistant in the middle line at an angle of 45° from the horizontal. The obturator is removed, and into the groove it occupied is passed a triangular knife (fig. 803). The penis is stretched

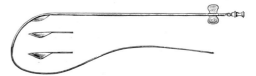

Fig. 803.—Thomson-Walker's urethrotome.

with the left hand behind the corona, and the knife, which has a bevelled apex so that it cannot cut the normal urethra, is advanced along the groove until it meets the stricture. By a sharp thrust of the knife the stricture is divided. As the knife is withdrawn its posterior edge cuts the stricture again. The staff, with its attached guide, is removed and large metal bougies up to 14/16 English are passed. A No. 14 gum-elastic catheter is tied into the urethra and retained for three days, during which time bladder washes are given twice daily. Internal urethrotomy is but a prelude to intermittent dilatation by bougies, which should be commenced fourteen days after the operation.

Suprapubic cystostomy with gradual decompression of the bladder is required when retention of urine cannot be relieved by urethral instrumentation. With the relief of retention reduction of congestion and

Sir John Thomson-Walker, 1870–1937. Surgeon, St. Peter's Hospital, London.

œdema of the strictured portion of the urethra ensues, and a week or ten days after the bladder has been decompressed it is often possible to insert a bougie via the external urinary meatus through a previously impassable stricture, in which event treatment is by continuous dilatation.

Retrograde Bouginage.—When the stricture remains impassable from below after three weeks of suprapubic drainage, retrograde bouginage can be tried. A special guide provided with a screw at its base, instead of the usual hollow thread, is required. By means of the screw the special guide is fitted to an ordinary guide. An operating irrigating cystoscope is passed through the suprapubic incision after placing a piece of thick rubber tubing around its shaft, so as to provide a more or less watertight junction at the suprapubic opening. The bladder is distended with saline solution and the tip of the special guide is passed via the cystoscope into the internal urinary meatus. Usually the guide can be made to traverse the prostatic and membranous urethræ with ease. After some manœuvring of insertion and withdrawal, the stricture of the bulbous urethra can sometimes be passed, and by further advancement the tip of the retrograde bougie appears at the external meatus. The cystoscope is removed and the retrograde bougie is drawn through the urethra until the base of the ordinary guide emerges from the external meatus. The retrograde bougie is unscrewed and an ordinary follower substituted. By passing followers of increasing size the stricture can sometimes be dilated sufficiently for a small gum-elastic catheter to be passed, and treatment by continuous dilatation is instituted.

External urethrotomy is indicated in cases of stricture of the bulbous urethra impassable both from below and above. A metal bougie is inserted through the internal urinary meatus as far as the stricture, and held in place by an assistant. The patient is transferred to the lithotomy position. A Wheelhouse's staff (fig. 804) is passed from the meatus

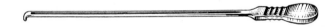

FIG. 804.—Wheelhouse's staff.

to the stricture, and an incision is made in the perineum in front of the stricture on to the groove of the instrument, which is then rotated through 180° so that its hook engages and retracts the anterior end of the open urethra. With the tip of the retrograde bougie acting as a guide, the face of the stricture is at once apparent and can be divided. One end of a piece of No. 22 French rubber tubing is threaded on to the beak of the bougie and withdrawn through the suprapubic incision, where it is detached from the bougie. The Wheelhouse's staff having been removed, the metal bougie is passed from the external meatus to the perineal wound, and the other end of the rubber tube is threaded on to the tip of the bougie. By withdrawing the bougie the distal end of the rubber tube is drawn along the urethra through the external urinary meatus. The perineal wound is packed lightly, and partially closed. The bladder is sutured around a Malècot catheter and the protruding portion of rubber tube, as also is the suprapubic incision. A safety-pin is placed through the rubber tube an inch from the external urinary meatus, and another safety-pin 2 inches (5 cm.) above the closed suprapubic wound. Redundant tubing beyond the safety-pins is cut away. The safety-pins ensure that the tube cannot be pulled out either from above or from below (fig. 805).

Claudius Galen Wheel'ouse, 1826–1909.   Surgeon, General Infirmary at Leeds, England.

After-treatment is similar to that described for complete rupture of the bulbous urethra, except the rubber tube is passed to and fro once a day, and changed each week by means of attaching a length of silk to it and drawing a larger tube along the urethra to protrude through the cystostomy wound. The process is repeated until the perineal wound has healed, when both the tube and Malècot catheter are removed. After the suprapubic wound has healed intermittent dilatation by bougies is commenced.

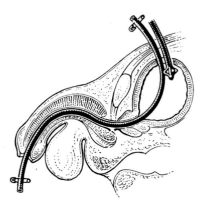

FIG. 805.—External urethrotomy with suprapubic cystostomy and an indwelling urethral rubber tube.

Excision.—Excision is indicated, particularly in long-standing, very indurated, solitary strictures of the bulbous urethra, especially those connected with a urethral fistula. Preliminary suprapubic cystostomy is carried out fourteen days before the perineal operation. An inverted Y-shaped incision is made in the perineum and after dividing the central tendon of the perineum, the bulbo-cavernosus muscle is incised. The urethra in front of the stricture is opened in the same manner as that described in external urethrotomy. With a bougie passed through the internal urinary meatus the limits of the stricture are defined. The urethra is divided at the face of the stricture and that portion of the urethra containing the stricture is excised. If necessary, the corpus spongiosum containing the urethra can be mobilised from the corpora cavernosa distally, to allow approximation of the cut ends of the urethra without tension. The roof of the urethra is united in a manner similar to that described in complete traumatic rupture of the bulbous urethra. The after-treatment is also similar.

OTHER CAUSES OF URETHRAL STRICTURE

Congenital stricture has been considered on p. 751.

Traumatic stricture follows unskilful or delayed treatment of rupture of the bulbous urethra. If dilatation is unsatisfactory, the question of excision of the stricture should be considered, especially in boys.

The so-called stricture following rupture of the membranous urethra is often not a stricture at all, but a complete loss of continuity of the urethra (see fig. 790). It can sometimes be remedied in much the same manner as that described for the excision of a urethral stricture. Urinary continence cannot be guaranteed after such an operation.

Post-operative Stricture.—A stricture develops in about 4 per cent. of cases after prostatectomy, irrespective of the method employed for the removal of the prostate. The stricture is usually situated in the proximal end of the prostatic urethra, but it can occur in other parts of the urethra from trauma due to the passage of the large calibrated panendoscope, or from urethritis due to an indwelling catheter.

In many cases the stricture can be dilated by regular intermittent dilatation. When the stricture takes the form of a shelf at the junction of the bladder with the prostatic bed, the bladder must be opened and the shelf excised.

Post-operative stricture can also follow partial or complete amputation of the penis. Methods of avoiding this complication are given in the section dealing with these operations. Regular dilatation is satisfactory.

COMPLICATIONS OF URETHRAL STRICTURE

1. Retention of urine (see p. 685).

2. Urethral diverticulum.

3. Periurethral abscess.

4. Urethral fistula.

5. All the attendant evils of " back pressure," culminating in bilateral hydronephrosis, combined with a susceptibility to urinary infection and an increased liability to urinary calculus.

6. Hernia, hæmorrhoids, or rectal prolapse may be induced by the straining.

URETHRAL DIVERTICULUM (*Syn.* URETHRAL POUCH)

Urethral diverticula are of three varieties :
1. Congenital.
2. Due to increased intraurethral pressure behind a stricture.
3. Due to the long-continued presence of a urethral calculus.

In many cases the pouch can be seen (fig. 806), and those which are not obvious at first become so when the patient interrupts the stream of urine.

Treatment is excision of the sac and removal of the cause if it is obvious.

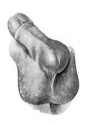

Fig. 806.—A urethral diverticulum.

PERIURETHRAL ABSCESS

Periurethral abscesses (fig. 807) are of two main varieties :

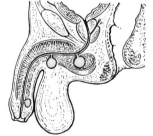

Fig. 807.—The commonest situations of a periurethral abscess. (*After Papin.*)

Penile periurethral abscess arises as an infection of one of the glands of Littré, and is usually a complication of acute gonococcal urethritis. A tender induration can be felt on the under-surface of the penis. Left to nature, the abscess frequently bursts externally, and a urinary fistula may result.

Treatment.—The passage of a bougie often causes the abscess to burst into the urethra. When this is unsuccessful, a ureteric meatotome is passed through a urethroscope and the abscess is opened by diathermy. When an abscess lies behind a stricture of the urethra it must be opened externally.

Bulbous periurethral abscess runs a variable course. Its most acute form, formerly termed periurethral abscess with

Alexis Littré, 1658–1726. Teacher of anatomy in Paris.

extravasation of urine, is better termed periurethral phlegmon, because in 50 per cent. of cases there is no stricture of the urethra present. Of the remainder, the majority have a passable stricture, while in the minority the stricture is impermeable (Rolnick). Consequently, in the majority of cases there is no reason why *urine* should extravasate. The condition is due to a spreading cellulitis by streptococci and anaerobic organisms invading the same cellular plane as that of superficial extravasation of urine (see p. 761).

Clinical Features.—There is pain in the perineum, considerable elevation of temperature, repeated rigors, and a rapid pulserate. In early cases the tenderness and swelling is limited to the perineum. Later, often in a matter of hours, the scrotum and then the penis become œdematous. From thence the infection spreads beneath the superficial fascia of the abdominal wall.

Treatment.—Pre-operative and post-operative penicillin and streptomycin greatly lower the mortality of the condition. The perineal abscess should be opened and incisions deep enough to traverse the superficial fascia are made into the scrotum, penis, and abdominal wall, if that is involved. When there is partial or complete retention of urine, if the infection is limited to the scrotum and the penis, after changing gloves and instruments, suprapubic cystostomy should be performed. If the superficial layer of the abdominal wall is implicated, it is best to drain the bladder by performing external urethrotomy. It should be noted that the abscess usually communicates with the urethra by a minute opening which cannot be found, and the urethra must be sought and its floor incised after passing an instrument from the external urinary meatus.

After-treatment.—In addition to antibiotics, intravenous saline and glucose may be beneficial if the patient is dehydrated, and should be continued for forty-eight hours if the output of urine is satisfactory. After instilling hydrogen peroxide into them, the various incisions are irrigated with weak potassium permanganate solution. Later Sitz baths of the same solution are given. When the infection has been overcome and the wounds commence to granulate, the stricture of the urethra, if present, is treated by one of the methods described already.

Chronic periurethral abscess is nearly always situated in the perineum, and is associated with much periurethritis. It is almost invariably the result of a long-standing stricture of the bulbous urethra. The abscess should be opened, together with various pockets which are often present. Later the associated stricture must receive thorough treatment. The condition is liable to be complicated by a urethral fistula which occurs either spontaneously or as a result of incision of the abscess.

Harry C. Rolnick, Contemporary. Professor of Urology, Medical School, Chicago.

URETHRAL FISTULA

The most frequent cause of an acquired external urethral fistula is bursting or incision of a periurethral abscess. When the opening is situated in the penile urethra or at the peno-scrotal junction, the amount of urine that escapes at each act of micturition is often small. A fistula following a periurethral abscess of the bulbous urethra can be either single or multiple. In the latter case the fistulæ originate behind a tight stricture and the patient passes most or all of his urine through the various fistulæ (watering-can perineum). A fistula can also follow external urethrotomy for stricture when there is another stricture situated distally.

Treatment.—A small fistula often closes spontaneously after repeated dilatation of the urethra. Searing the track with the diathermy needle often encourages closure. Occasionally a plastic operation is necessary. Temporary suprapubic cystostomy, by resting the urethra, aids in the success of such a procedure. When there is a fistula in the perineum, especially one with several openings associated with a solitary but unyielding stricture of the bulbous urethra, the following operative treatment is advised : suprapubic cystostomy is performed and the patient is given sulphonamide and penicillin. Three weeks later the fistula or fistulæ are dissected up until the floor of the urethra is reached. The stricture is then excised (see p. 770).

URETHRAL CALCULUS

Calculi occur less frequently in the urethra than in any other part of the urinary track. A urethral calculus can arise primarily in the urethra behind a stricture or in an infected urethral diverticulum. Such stones are composed of phosphates. Less rarely a calculus which has migrated from the ureter becomes arrested in the prostatic, bulbous, or penile portions of the urethra.

Clinical Features.—In the case of a migratory calculus arrested in the urethra there is a history of an attack of renal colic two or three days previously. During micturition the patient experiences sudden pain in the urethra and the stream of urine ceases abruptly. A few drops of blood-stained urine follow, and then there is retention of urine. In cases where the calculus becomes impacted in the penile urethra (often in the fossa navicularis) the stone can be palpated readily through the floor of the urethra. When the stone has been arrested in the prostatic urethra a rectal examination usually reveals a tender, hard nodule in the middle line of the prostate, generally near its apex. A calculus forming behind a urethral stricture often does so without causing much additional discomfort and it sometimes attains a considerable size before giving rise to retention of urine, or painful dysuria. In some cases such a stone can be felt easily ; in others, owing to periurethral thickening, its presence is not suspected until it is seen at urethroscopy, or a grating sensation is experienced on passing a gum-elastic bougie or a characteristic click is heard if a metal bougie has been employed. In all but superficially placed calculi giving rise to acute symptoms, radiography is necessary to confirm the presence, and particularly to reveal the size, of the calculus before commencing treatment.

TREATMENT

Migratory Calculus.—When the stone is impacted in the prostatic urethra a general anæsthetic is given and a metal bougie is passed. Nearly always the stone can be pushed back into the bladder, where it can be crushed by litholapaxy and the fragments evacuated. If much bleeding has been occasioned by the displacement of the stone into the bladder, drainage by an indwelling catheter and bladder washes for a few days will enable cystoscopic litholapaxy to be carried out. Alternatively, the stone can be removed at once by performing suprapubic cystotomy. Occasionally a small stone can be removed from the deeper parts of the urethra by means of special forceps through a posterior urethroscope. A stone impacted in the scrotal or pendulous penile urethra can sometimes be worked forward after the canal has been dilated under local anæsthesia. The urethra must be occluded behind the stone by digital pressure before the solution is injected, and kept occluded. A penile clamp prevents the solution escaping from the meatus. A stone impacted in the fossa navicularis, or worked forward to this position, can be removed by urethral forceps or by inserting a bent probe behind it. Meatotomy is often required to permit the stone being withdrawn. When a stone cannot be worked forward, external urethrotomy should be performed. In these circumstances the urethra can be closed in layers after the stone has been extracted.

Primary Calculus.—Provided a bougie can be passed beyond the stricture and the stone, a calculus behind a stricture is sometimes expelled after the stricture has been considerably dilated, or it can be removed by urethral forceps. When a bougie cannot be passed, external urethrotomy should be performed and the stricture dilated. The wound is left open and dilatation continued at regular intervals. In these circumstances there is a possibility of a urethral fistula continuing for months, but it generally closes if the stricture is kept fully dilated. A stone of considerable size in the prostatic urethra can be removed, either by the suprapubic or the retropubic route. A stone or stones occupying a diverticulum of the urethra should be removed, together with the diverticulum.

NEOPLASMS OF THE MALE URETHRA

BENIGN

Polypi are usually multiple and occur most frequently in the region of the verumontanum. As seen at urethroscopy, each polypus is a pale, finger-like projection with blood-vessels coursing over it. Polypi are never found without chronic infection. Sometimes, if the infection can be cured, the polypi disappear ; conversely, if polypi are destroyed, chronic urethritis, which previously resisted treatment, often responds to it. Possibly this condition should be classified as a granuloma.

Papillomata similar to those on the glans penis sometimes occur within the fossa navicularis occasionally associated with the external variety. Papillomata also occur in the prostatic urethra. When they are situated very near the internal urinary meatus they sometimes take on a malignant change. The symptom is hæmaturia immediately before micturition.

Angioma is rare. The hæmaturia to which it gives rise is often profuse, and may occur independent of micturition.

Treatment of all the foregoing is by diathermy coagulation through a urethroscope.

MALIGNANT

Carcinoma is rare. More than half the cases occur in the pendulous urethra ; the remainder are divided between the bulbous and the membrano-prostatic portions. In a number of instances a urethral stricture is antecedent to the carcinoma. Spread occurs to the inguinal lymph nodes if the penis becomes involved. Distant metastases are uncommon. The symptoms are those of stricture of the urethra, combined with muco-purulent, and later a sero-sanguinous, discharge. If the neoplasm arises in the pendulous portion of the urethra, induration and sometimes a lump can be felt. Early cases often simulate an inflammatory stricture, but the free hæmorrhage which occurs on instrumentation is a very suspicious sign. In the deeper parts of the urethra the first manifestation is sometimes an indolent periurethral abscess which both fails to heal and the periurethral thickening increases rather than decreases after draining the abscess. Biopsy then establishes the diagnosis.

Treatment.—When the growth is in the penile urethra, complete amputation of the penis can be carried out. This is followed by irradiation or dissection of regional lymph nodes. For growths of the deep urethra suprapubic cystostomy followed by interstitial radium causes temporary regression of the growth.

THE FEMALE URETHRA

Urethritis.—Acute urethritis is usually due to gonorrhœa. Chronic urethritis may be due to gonorrhœa or to other organisms, and in its severe forms is a urethro-trigonitis. The symptoms are frequency, pain on micturition, urgency, terminal hæmaturia, and low back pain. The diagnosis is made by urethroscopy. Urethral polypi are frequently present.

Treatment.—In addition to urinary antiseptics, local treatment is necessary. Intermittent dilatation of the urethra, by promoting drainage of infected foci within the urethra, often helps to eradicate the infection. If polypi are present, the condition is seldom remedied unless they are removed by fulguration. Swabbing the urethra with 10 per cent. solution of silver nitrate is also helpful.

Stricture.—An adult female urethra which fails to admit freely a 20 French bougie is the seat of a urethral stricture.

The causes are urethritis, not necessarily gonococcal, and trauma as the result of difficult labour. Inflammatory stricture is situated at the external meatus ; traumatic stricture usually affects the middle or posterior part of the urethra.

Sometimes the stricture will only admit a guide, and in these cases particularly, acute retention of urine is prone to occur. Dilatation of the stricture yields satisfactory results. In the more serious cases treatment by continuous dilatation is advisable. The recognition and treatment of a stricture often clears up an obscure case of dysuria.

Calculus impacted in the female urethra is exceptional. When it occurs it can be removed by grasping it with forceps while a finger on the anterior vaginal wall presses it forward.

Prolapse of the urethra is rare. Over 50 per cent. of cases occur in female children in whom the condition is congenital. The remainder are seen in women past the menopause suffering from chronic urethritis, when the cause is probably continual straining on micturition, combined with loss of tone of the urethral wall.

Clinical Features.—Frequency of micturition is usual. There is local discomfort in proportion to the degree of the prolapse, especially on walking. The prolapse becomes more evident when the patient strains. When the prolapse is complete the opening of the urethra is central; when it is partial, the opening is eccentric.

Treatment.—Mild cases can often be cured by making one or more linear grooves in the long axis of the mucous membrane of the urethra with a diathermy coagulating current. Subsequent contraction of the scar reduces or obliterates the prolapse. More advanced cases are treated by excision of the prolapse and uniting the cut edges of the urethra with fine catgut sutures. In complete prolapse excision and suture must be preceded by transfixing the whole thickness of the prolapse as far from its extremity as possible with four catgut sutures placed at equidistant intervals. The mucous membrane is then excised distal to the sutures, which prevent retraction of the mucous membrane into the canal. The cut edges of the skin and mucous membrane are then united.

Urethral Diverticulum (*syn*. **Urethrocele**).—Although rare, diverticulum of the urethra is more common in females than in males. The majority of cases occur in parous women, and in these the condition is due to injury to the floor of the urethra during difficult labour. A small, uninfected pouch may be symptomless. As the diverticulum increases in size, inability to pass all the urine at one time, or dribbling after micturition, occurs. Once infected—and infection is almost inevitable if the diverticulum is not completely evacuated at each micturition—recurrent attacks of cystitis perpetuated by reinfection from the diverticulum continue in spite of antibiotics and chemotherapy. On digital examination a swelling can be felt on the anterior vaginal wall in the line of the urethra, and when it is compressed, urine, usually obviously purulent, is expressed. If the beak of a curved metal bougie is passed along the floor of the urethra, it can often be made to enter the sac. In 10 per cent. of cases a stone forms in the diverticulum. Occasional hæmaturia is then sometimes a symptom.

Treatment.—When the diverticulum is grossly infected its fundus should be widely opened into the vagina. Excision of the opened sac, after urethral irrigations and urinary antiseptics have overcome the infection, is undertaken. With a bougie in the urethra the diverticulum is excised and the floor of the urethra in the vicinity of the defect is separated into its two layers, urethral mucous membrane and vaginal wall, which are united separately. An indwelling catheter is retained for a week.

BENIGN NEOPLASMS

Urethral caruncle is common in middle-aged and elderly women. The condition presents as a soft, raspberry-like, pedunculated, granulomatous mass about the size of a pea, attached to the posterior urethral wall near the external urinary meatus. Histologically it is composed of highly vascular connective tissue stroma infiltrated with polymorphonuclear leucocytes and covered by squamous epithelium.

Clinical Features.—There is frequency of micturition, and often great pain during and after micturition. Terminal hæmaturia often occurs, and there may be an independent blood-stained discharge. The condition can be diagnosed on inspection, although it must be differentiated from prolapse of the mucous membrane. With a probe it can be determined that the protrusion arises from a pedicle attached to the posterior urethral wall. The mass is exquisitely tender and bleeds readily.

Treatment. — The pedicle should be divided flush with the floor of the urethra with a diathermy needle, using a cutting current, after which that portion of the urethra from which it arose is coagulated with the diathermy current in order to prevent recurrence. The chronic urethritis with which the condition is always associated should be treated by intermittent urethral dilatation until the patient is symptom-free.

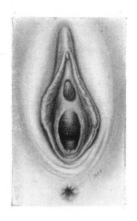

FIG. 808.—A urethral caruncle.

The benign neoplasms which occur in the male urethra are also found in the female urethra.

MALIGNANT NEOPLASM

Carcinoma, like that occurring in the male, is rare. The growth is either urethral or vulvo-urethral. The latter commences as a tumour which looks like a caruncle ; consequently after removal a caruncle should be subjected to microscopical examination. Vulvo-urethral carcinoma soon spreads to the vestibule, when there is no mistaking the indurated ulcer. Carcinoma commencing within the urethra originates in its distal third, and gives rise to dysuria, hæmaturia, and sometimes retention of urine. The induration accompanying a carcinoma of the urethra usually serves to distinguish it from an innocent tumour.

Treatment.—Suprapubic cystostomy, followed by radium, is generally employed. If subsequent fibrosis obliterates the urethra, the suprapubic cystostomy must be permanent, or the ureters can be transplanted into the colon.

PHIMOSIS

is usually due to congenital narrowing of the preputial orifice, often associated with an unduly long foreskin. The condition can be acquired as a result of chronic or acute inflammation of the under-surface of the prepuce (posthitis) which is invariably accompanied by some degree of inflammation of the glans (balanitis). At any time of life if the foreskin cannot be retracted smegma accumulates beneath it, and some degree of balano-posthitis results.   In extreme examples of congenital phimosis, when the patient micturates the prepuce balloons out first, and a thin, weak stream of urine follows.   Dysuria with residual urine, hydro-ureters, and hydronephroses are rarely due to phimosis, but more often occur as a result of atresia meati which may lie hidden by the phimosis.   Minor degrees of phimosis in early infancy can be treated by regular retraction of the prepuce.   In other circumstances circumcision is indicated.

CIRCUMCISION

In an Infant.—(*a*) The parts are washed with soap and water, and painted with a non-irritating antiseptic, e.g. metaphen.   If it is not possible to cleanse the post-coronal sulcus of contained smegma, the preputial orifice should be devulsed with a hæmostat.   A pair of sinus forceps is applied obliquely to the prepuce, parallel to the corona, just beyond the tip of the penis, and the skin distal to the forceps is excised with scissors close to the forceps, which are then removed.   The outer layer of the preputial skin retracts, leaving the glans covered by the inner layer, which is divided in the middle line anteriorly by introducing a blade of delicate scissors between it and the glans.   Each leaf of the deep layer of skin (formerly called the mucosa) is excised, leaving a narrow collar around the corona. The frænal artery usually requires ligation, as well as several small vessels on the dorsum.   The cut edges of the deep and superficial layers are approximated with fine catgut sutures.

(*b*) **Using Bone Forceps.**—The penis is cleansed with soap and water. The tip of the prepuce is grasped laterally by a small hæmostat, and sufficient traction is applied to it to permit thorough breaking-down of adhesions between the prepuce and the glans with a probe.   When all adhesions have been broken, after exerting suitable traction on the now freed prepuce, a pair of bone forceps are applied just distal to the glans, with their V-shaped surface towards the infant.   Momentary pain is experienced, but it lasts only a few seconds.   After three minutes the superfluous tissue is severed with a sharp scalpel, just distal to the instru-

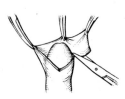

ment.   There is no hæmorrhage, and the superficial and deep surfaces of the preputial stump become sealed together throughout their circumference sufficiently to allow them to be placed behind the corona, where they are fixed with a dressing of a wisp of wool soaked in tinct. Benzoin co.

(*c*) **In adolescents and adults** the following method is preferable.   The prepuce is retracted until its tense orifice is apparent, or until the tip of the glans comes into view, and on to the edge of the prepuce are placed three hæmostats, one in the middle line ventrally and two on either side

FIG.   809.—Performing circumcision by the flap method.

of the middle line dorsally.   The prepuce is then slit up in the middle line dorsally to within ½ inch (1·25 cm.) of the corona.   The under-surface of the prepuce having been completely separated from the glans and the corona, the layers of each flap are excised (fig. 809), keeping ½ inch distal

---

Apparently circumcision did not originate among the Jews : they took the custom from either the Babylonians or the Negroes, probably the latter.   It has been practised in West Africa for over 5,000 years.

to the corona. The superficial layer is retracted and bleeding-points are secured and ligated. The inner layer of the prepuce having been trimmed to ⅛ inch (0·3 cm.) from the corona, the two cut edges are approximated accurately with fine interrupted catgut stitches.

In both operations the cut edges in the immediate vicinity of the frænum can be neatly drawn together by a mattress suture.

PARAPHIMOSIS

The tight prepuce has been retracted, but cannot be returned, and it is constricting the glans which is engorged and œdematous. The diagnosis is apparent at a glance.

Treatment.—A pad of cottonwool soaked in a mixture of 0·1 per cent. adrenalin and 10 per cent. cocaine can be applied for fifteen minutes, when, in a small proportion of early cases, reduction can be accomplished with ease (fig. 810). If this is unsuccessful, a general anæsthetic must be given, and the constricting band is incised, and the

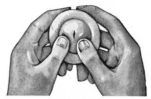

FIG. 810.—Reducing a paraphimosis.

narrow cuff of skin which formed the constricting band is excised. There is now no obstruction to reduction, and there remains only to remove a broad cuff of normal skin on the proximal side of the gap and unite the cut free edges, thus performing circumcision.

INFLAMMATIONS

BALANO-POSTHITIS

can occur at any age from an accumulation of smegma which sets up irritation and permits pathological organisms to flourish. It is greatly favoured by phimosis which, however, may be caused by the condition. The symptoms of balano-posthitis due to retention of smegma are mild itching and burning. Provided the prepuce can be retracted, the diagnosis and treatment are simple. By thoroughly cleansing the post-coronal sulcus of smegma and epithelial débris the condition subsides in a few days. When the prepuce cannot be retracted the bacteriological examination of any discharge is advisable. By syringing with a mild antiseptic beneath the prepuce it may be possible to overcome the inflammation, after which circumcision is carried out. It is unusual for non-venereal balano-posthitis not to respond to this measure, and it is also very exceptional for there to be any constitutional disturbance. In cases that do not respond quickly a V-shaped dorsal slit should be made.

HARD CHANCRE (*Syn.* HUNTERIAN CHANCRE)

The penis is the site of election of a primary chancre (see p. 34).

ACUTE EROSIVE BALANO-POSTHITIS

is sometimes called the fourth venereal disease. The surface of the glans and post-coronal sulcus, together with the under-surface of the prepuce (it usually occurs in the uncircumcised) become eroded in small areas, which appear white. In more severe cases the erosions are succeeded by ulcers with reddened borders and a yellowish-white slough, in which event constitutional symptoms will be in evidence. The condition is due to Vincent's organisms (coarse fusiform bacilli and spirilla, occurring together), which are found in smears taken from the purulent exudate and are probably transmitted by infected saliva. In exceptionally severe cases gangrenous patches appear and destroy large portions of the glans. Ultra-acute cases associated with gangrene, and known as phagadæna, are now rarely encountered. Local and general treatment with penicillin is curative.

LYMPHOGRANULOMA INGUINALE (*Syn.* LYMPHOGRANULOMA VENEREUM)

is caused by a filtrable virus, and although predominantly a tropical disease, it is commonly encountered in temperate climates, especially in countries where there is a mixed population of white and negro races. The disease has become increasingly widespread outside the tropics.

The primary lesion is a fleeting herpetic eruption occurring in some part of the genitalia, *in males* generally in the post-coronal sulcus, but sometimes on the inner surface of the prepuce ; *in females* the lesion is occasionally in the anterior part of the vulva, more commonly on the vaginal wall or cervix. The lesion occurs twenty-four to forty-eight hours after sexual intercourse. The vesicles are painless, and often escape notice.

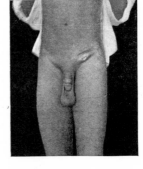

The Secondary Lesion.—In both sexes the secondary lesion is accompanied by considerable constitutional symptoms, especially in white people. Pyrexia persists for several weeks. By the time the chronic stage is reached there is a severe secondary anæmia.

In the Male.—About three weeks after infection a lymph node in one or both groins enlarges, usually in the medial part of the groin. The infection spreads to other nodes, and periadenitis occurs. A brawny mass presents, and increases in size. Untreated, it breaks down and discharges thick, yellowish-white pus free from organisms. The resulting sinus (fig. 811) or sinuses persist for months or years.

In the Female.—If the primary lesion lies

FIG. 811.—Lymphogranuloma inguinale. (*Professor F. A. R. Stammers.*)

Jean H. Vincent, 1862–1950. Professor of Epidemiology, Val-de-Grâce (Military) Hospital France.

Lymphogranuloma inguinale was first described in 1913 by Nicholas Durant and M. Faivre of Lyons.

in the anterior part of the vulva an inguinal bubo follows, as in the male. When, as is much more usual, the primary lesion is on the vaginal wall or cervix, œdematous thickening of the posterior vaginal wall occurs and at the same time the para-rectal lymph nodes enlarge and suppurate. As a result of this intense para-rectal inflammation, dense fibrosis of the rectal wall follows with the formation of a stricture of the rectum (p. 537). Elephantiasis of the vulva sometimes develops in chronic cases. Ischio-rectal abscess and rectovaginal fistula are not infrequent complications.

The diagnosis is proved by the Frei test, which consists in an intradermal injection of 1 or 2 minims (0·05 or 0·1 ml.) of an extract of macerated tissue taken from a lymphogranulomatous bubo or from the brain of a mouse inoculated with the virus. A positive reaction appears within forty-eight hours, and is a red papule of at least ¼ inch (0·6 cm.) in diameter.

Treatment.—In early cases sulphathiazole 1 gm. three times a day for fourteen days, followed by 1 gm. twice a day for six weeks, has proved effective in some instances, but in all cases, especially those seen late, aureomycin is more regularly curative.

CHORDEE

Chordee is due to an inflammatory effusion into the corpus spongiosum or corpora cavernosa. As a consequence the erect organ is bent down-wards or laterally. In the acute stage erections are very painful. Chordee is not a common condition, and is usually a complication of acute gonococcal urethritis.

Treatment.—An ethyl-chloride spray is useful in preventing erection, but painful. The best method is to prescribe stilbœstrol 6 mg. daily. After the acute attack has subsided the cavernous tissue is sometimes left permanently damaged by fibrosis, causing deformity of the organ.

PERSISTENT PRIAPISM

The penis remains erect, and is painful. Most often the erection is due to idiopathic thrombosis occurring in the prostatic venous plexus. Less frequently it is associated with leukæmia or sickle-celled anæmia. Second-ary malignant deposits in the corpora cavernosa, or in the pelvis, account for about 7 per cent. of cases. In another, completely different category are cases of priapism due to spinal injury or disease.

Diagnosis.—A low spinal anæsthetic will cause priapism of neurogenic origin to abate temporarily. A differential blood count is advisable.

Treatment.—Local applications are useless. Suitable sedatives must be prescribed, but they only dull the pain. Anticoagulants should be ad-ministered. Repeated aspiration of the corpora cavernosa is of value. When this fails, or is unsatisfactory, a small incision into a corpus cavernosum should be made, and blood and blood-clot evacuated. When gangrene threatens, early amputation is advised.

INDURATIO-PENIS-PLASTICA

Induratio-penis-plastica (*syn.* Peyronie's disease) appears as a slowly developing painless induration of the penis, and can be recognised readily by palpation. Usually the patient is over forty. Its ætiology is unknown, although some consider that the condition is a manifestation of granuloma

---

William Frei, Contemporary. Formerly Professor of Dermatology, Berlin.
François de la Peyronie, 1678–1747. Physician to Louis XIV.

inguinale (p. 780).   Treatment is far from satisfactory.   Cures have been reported following the use of radium in small doses.   Excision of the pathological fibrous tissue is sometimes successful.

PENILE HERPES

Herpes zoster, following the course of the ilio-inguinal nerve, may attack the penis, but it is very rare.   Catarrhal herpes is more common, and vesicles are present on the glans penis.   The chief importance of the condition is the liability to its being confused with venereal infection.

Treatment is an application of simple boric lotion.   The condition soon clears up, but catarrhal herpes is apt to recur

INJURIES

FRACTURE OF THE PENIS

Fracture of the penis is a very uncommon accident.   Following trauma the erect organ suddenly becomes flaccid.   The extravasation of blood, which is considerable, causes great pain and swelling.   In recent cases incision, clearing out blood-clot, and suture of the ruptured corpus cavernosum has yielded good results.

STRANGULATION OF THE PENIS BY RINGS

Removal is prevented by venous engorgement.   Consequently aspiration of the corpora cavernosa may assist in removal of the ring in early cases, otherwise a ring cutter or a hacksaw must be employed.

NEOPLASMS

Papillomata are the commonest benign growths of the penis. They usually occur on the surface of the glans, and particularly

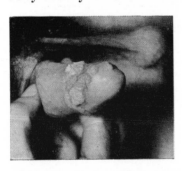

in the post-coronal sulcus.   When first seen they are usually multiple (fig. 812), implantation taking place, especially in the presence of phimosis or balanitis.   There is uncertainty as to their origin. Some consider that the condition is a venereal disease due to a virus infection.   Papillomata of the penis occur much more frequently in the uncircumcised than the circumcised.

FIG. 812.—Penile papillomata.

Treatment.—Circumcision should be undertaken in necessary cases.   When the growths are not extensive, painting them with 25 per cent. podophyllin resin in liquid paraffin is often effective, but such treatment is followed by a considerable local reaction, and is painful.   For this reason fulguration of the growths by diathermy at the time of circumcision is often preferable. For large papillomata, if there is even a suspicion of malignancy, radium treatment is advisable.

CARCINOMA OF THE PENIS

Ætiology.—Carcinoma of the penis is a condition in which the predisposing factors are fairly well defined. It is undoubtedly favoured by chronic balanitis secondary to phimosis. Furthermore, there are definite *pre*-carcinomatous states, viz. :

(*a*) **Leukoplakia of the glans** is exactly comparable to the well-known condition of the tongue.

(*b*) Long-standing penile papillomata.

(*c*) **Paget's Disease of the Penis** (fig. 813).—" I have seen a persistent rawness of the glans like a long-standing balanitis followed by cancer of the substance of the penis " (Sir James Paget). Because it is very rare, it is possible that penile Paget's disease escapes detection until an actual carcinoma has developed. Treatment is by radium.

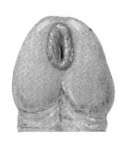

Fig. 813.—Paget's disease of the glans penis. (*Susman.*)

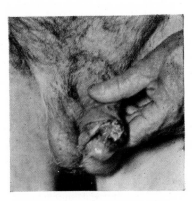

Fig. 814.—Carcinoma of the penis.

Pathology.—Two forms exist, the papilliferous (fig. 814) and the ulcerative. The papilliferous variety begins in a long-standing papilloma, while the ulcerative is often associated with leukoplakia of the glans. The growth is commonly situated on the dorsal surface of the glans or the nearby inner surface of the prepuce, less often in the neighbourhood of the frænum, and least often at the external urinary meatus. The growth remains purely local for a long time. The first spread is to the regional lymph nodes. Direct spread to the body of the penis is prevented for many months by the fascial sheath of the corpus cavernosum, but once this barrier becomes

Sir James Paget, 1814–1899. Surgeon, St Bartholomew's Hospital, London.

broken the growth extends more rapidly. Distant metastatic deposits are infrequent, even late in the course of the disease.

Clinical Features.—Penile cancer is extremely frequent among the Chinese and the inhabitants of Malaya. The condition is practically unknown amongst circumcised Jews. The patient is seldom under fifty years of age, and is nearly always uncircumcised. The progress of the disease is slow ; the first symptoms are a mild irritation and a purulent discharge from the prepuce. These symptoms are often neglected, and usually by the time the patient reports, sometimes more than a year after symptoms have appeared, there is a blood-stained, foul discharge. Pain is singularly absent. The inguinal lymph nodes are enlarged in over 60 per cent. of cases, but in only half of these is the enlargement due to secondary deposits, the remainder being due to sepsis. In a number of instances the prepuce cannot be retracted, and in order to view the lesion the prepuce must be slit up. In cases where the diagnosis is in doubt a biopsy should be performed.

Untreated, the whole glans becomes a fungating and particularly foul-smelling mass. Later, the inguinal lymph nodes fungate through the skin of the groin, and finally death relieves the victim, often suddenly, by torrential hæmorrhage following erosion of the external iliac artery.

Treatment.—**Radium** gives excellent results in cases of the papilliferous variety which have not extended around the majority of the circumference, and when there is no induration of the body of the penis. This form of treatment is also indicated in early ulcerative lesions.

Needles containing 1 mg. of radium are inserted at equidistant intervals into the base of the growth. Additional needles containing 0·5 mg. are inserted into a papilliferous growth. The needles are left in place for seven days, and a total dose of 7,000 r results. There is an extensive local reaction which subsides in two to three weeks, and healing occurs in about six weeks.

Partial Amputation.—A tourniquet is applied to the base of the penis. A ventral flap of skin and subcutaneous tissue is raised, the width of which is half the circumference of the penis, and the length equal to the diameter. A short dorsal flap is also fashioned. The flaps are dissected back to their fullest extent. The corpus spongiosum containing the urethra is divided ¾ inch (1·9 cm.) from the base of the flaps. The corpus spongiosum is dissected from the corpora cavernosa until the level of the base of the flaps is reached. The corpora cavernosa are divided at this level. The dorsal artery and vein are ligated, and mattress sutures are passed as shown in fig. 815 and tied. The tourniquet is then removed. If hæmostasis is not complete, additional sutures or ligatures are applied as necessary. Near the base of the ventral flap a small circular incision is made through which the urethra is passed. The flaps are united by interrupted sutures. The urethra is split longitudinally for ½ inch (1·25 cm.) and each half is united by a suture to the edge of the circular incision. A Foley's catheter is passed into the bladder and retained for five days, in order to keep urine away from the newly-constructed meatus.

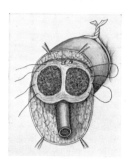

FIG. 815.—Partial amputation of the penis.

Complete amputation includes the separation and removal of the corpora cavernosa from the pubic bones and division of the corpus spongiosum as far back as to leave at least ½ inch protruding from the skin wound. This is the best treatment for advanced cases.

The Treatment of Associated Enlarged Inguinal Lymph Nodes.

—As these may be entirely inflammatory, it is permissible to wait for at least three weeks after the local lesion has been dealt with by one of the methods described. If the nodes are inflammatory, they will decrease in size or disappear with antibiotic treatment. If they remain unaltered at the end of this period, or do not undergo complete resolution within a further period of two or three weeks, they are best dealt with by dissection. If the enlarged nodes are massive and fixed (inoperable), irradiation causes some temporary regression.

CHAPTER XXXI

THE TESTES AND THE SCROTUM

CONGENITAL ABNORMALITIES

Supernumerary testis is exceedingly rare. The accessory testis is small, and in the majority of instances communicates with a common epididymis. Usually it occurs on the left side. The diagnosis can only be made with certainty at operation.

Anterior inversion is said to be present in one in every twenty males. The epididymis is in front, and the body of the testis and the tunica vaginalis behind. When the organ is diseased this anomaly causes much confusion in diagnosis, and is referred to on p. 811.

Imperfect Descent of the Testis.—This important subject must be discussed fully.

IMPERFECT DESCENT OF THE TESTIS

Under this heading are included two conditions :

Incomplete Descent.—The testis is arrested in some part of its path to the scrotum.

Maldescended (*syn.* **Ectopic Testis**).—The testis is abnormally placed outside this path.

Development of the Testes.—The testes develop below the kidneys in the upper part of the cœlomic cavity behind the peritoneum from the genital fold which lies medial to the mesonephros (Wolffian body). The primitive testis as it increases in size is attached to the posterior abdominal wall by a mesentery, the mesorchium, which contains the testicular blood-vessels, derived from the aorta at the level of the twelfth dorsal segment, and the testicular nerves which come from the tenth dorsal segment. A reflection of the mesorchium attaches the testis to the mesonephros. About the tenth week of intra-uterine life some of the transverse tubules of the mesonephros unite with the rete testis to form the vasa efferentia ; others remain rudimentary. The larger portion of the Wolffian body disappears, but the Wolffian duct becomes the epididymis and vas deferens. About this time the testis becomes attached to the lower part of the ventral abdominal wall by a

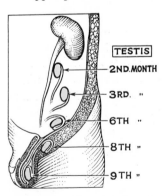

FIG. 816.—The migration of the testicle. It should reach the scrotum shortly before birth.

fold of peritoneum called the inguinal fold.   Within this fold lies mesoblast which, during the fourth month, becomes fibromuscular tissue.   This is the gubernaculum, which becomes attached above to the pole of the testis, while below its actively proliferating cells grow downwards through the abdominal wall to become attached to the subcutaneous tissue of the skin which later forms the scrotum.   The outwardly growing gubernaculum carries with it a funnel-shaped protrusion of peritoneum—the processus vaginalis—and a prolongation of every layer of the abdominal wall.   The testis passes through the internal and external abdominal rings during the seventh and eighth months of fœtal life, and it reaches the bottom of the scrotum just before birth.

The gubernaculum (= a rudder) was first described and so named by John Hunter, who evidently believed that its function was to guide the testis into the scrotum.   There is no evidence to support the view that the gubernaculum exercises traction upon the testis ; why and how the testes descend is still problematical.   Possibly intra-abdominal pressure due to accumulated meconium rises sufficiently by the eighth month to expel the testis down the inguinal canal.   The gonadotropic hormone of the pituitary gland has an influence on the development, and possibly on the migration, of the testis.   Normally the left testis descends a little earlier than the right.   Failure of a testis to develop fully unless it is housed in the scrotum or subcutaneously has been attributed to the slightly higher temperature to which a retained testis is subjected, or to compression of such a testis.

Obstacles to Descent :

1. Bands or adhesions attaching the spermatic vessels to the internal abdominal ring.   Remedied by division of these bands.

2. Shortness of the spermatic vessels.   Often remedied by mobilising the peritoneum by a finger passed into the retroperitoneal space, a manœuvre which abolishes the wide outward curve of these vessels. When the spermatic artery runs directly from the aorta to the internal abdominal ring, often as much as 1 inch (2·5 cm.) can be gained.

3. Shortness of the vas (very rare).   Sometimes remedied by division of the deep epigastric artery.

4. Adherence of the tunica vaginalis of an ectopic testis to tissues outside the line of normal descent.   Easily remedied by dividing the tunica from these structures.

INCOMPLETELY DESCENDED TESTIS

Pathology. — An incompletely descended testis fails to develop.   In adolescence it remains the same size as its scrotal counterpart in early childhood.   About the time of puberty another change is noticed in the incompletely descended organ ; the body of the testis and the epidydimis begin to separate.   By the time early manhood is reached this separation is unmistakable (fig. 817).   The external secretory mechanism of the imperfectly descended organ never functions normally.

Sir Astley Cooper rightly taught that patients with bilateral retained testes were usually sterile, whereupon

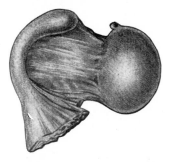

Fig. 817.—Characteristic separation of the epididymis from the body of a maldescended testis. Specimen from a man of twenty-three.

John Hunter, 1728–1793. Surgeon, St. George's Hospital, London. Founder of the Hunterian Museum.
Sir Astley Cooper, 1768–1841. Surgeon, Guy's Hospital, London.

one of his pupils, a cryptorchid, left the room and committed suicide. At the necropsy which followed, motile spermatozoa were demonstrated. It is therefore unsafe to deny the possibility of parentage to those with retained testes.

Nevertheless, the power of spermatogenesis of the imperfectly descended organ is usually negligible ; on the other hand, its internal secretory activity approaches normal. Even in cryptorchids, secondary sexual characters appear.

If an incompletely descended testis is brought down satisfactorily *before puberty*, it usually develops and functions fully.

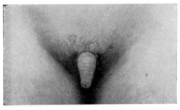

Fig. 818.—A cryptorchid at puberty.

Clinical Features.—The right side alone is affected in 50 per cent. of cases, the left alone in 30 per cent., while double arrested descent occurs in 20 per cent. The testis may be :

1. Retained within the abdomen extraperitoneally, usually just above the internal abdominal ring, but occasionally at a higher level. When both testes are within the abdomen the condition is known as cryptorchidism.

2. In the inguinal canal.

3. Just outside the external abdominal ring—a very common situation.

Only occasionally does a testis reach the scrotum by its own initiative if it has failed to do so by the end of the first year.

The condition is usually symptomless in infancy and childhood. Sometimes the absence of one or both testes is noticed by the child's parents. More often the condition remains unrecognised until a routine examination is made by the school medical officer. At or after puberty one complication or another often directs attention to the deformity, but it may only be discovered at a medical examination for entrance to one of the public services.

Retractile Testis.—Very frequently during infancy the testes are mobile, each being withdrawn by the contraction of the cremasters into the superficial subinguinal pouch (fig. 819), a

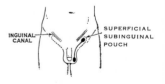

Fig. 819.—Mechanism of mobile testis.
(*After D. Browne.*)

Denis J. Browne, Contemporary. Surgeon, Hospital for Sick Children, Great Ormond Street, London.

space lined by loose areolar tissue lying beneath Scarpa's fascia and superficial to the external oblique aponeurosis (Browne), or into the inguinal canal. The retraction occurs from very slight stimuli such as touching the thigh or abdomen, or even by exposure of the parts. Not infrequently this mobility continues during childhood on both sides, or less frequently on one side. At all times it is liable to be mistaken for incomplete descent, for the testes (or testis) are impalpable unless a special method of examination is undertaken, if necessary on several occasions. The condition should be strongly suspected if the scrotum is normal ; in imperfect descent the corresponding side of the scrotum is undeveloped. The pulps of two fingers are placed over the inguinal canal, exerting moderate pressure. By sliding the fingers down the inguinal canal a testis of the retractile type can be pushed into the upper part of the scrotum, where it is grasped between the finger and thumb of the other hand. *Only if the testis cannot be made to touch the bottom of the scrotum is it imperfectly descended.* When the testis can be placed temporarily in a normal position neither hormone nor operative treatment is necessary. In a matter of time (it may be delayed until puberty) the testis will take up a normal position permanently.

The Hazards of Incomplete Descent

1. *Sterility* in bilateral cases.
2. *Pain.* An inguinal testis is liable to repeated injury.
3. *Associated Inguinal Hernia.*—In over 80 per cent. of cases subjected to operation the processus vaginalis is found to be patent. Frequently an inguinal hernia, usually a bubonocele, is present on clinical examination, and in adolescent and adult patients it is often the hernia that causes symptoms. Although rare, an interstitial hernia is nearly always a complication of an incompletely descended testis. The testis proves an obstacle to the descent of the contents of the sac, and owing to increased pressure, the sac is forced between the layers of the abdominal wall.
4. *Torsion* of the spermatic cord.
5. *Epididymo-orchitis.*—Because appendicitis and incomplete descent of the testis can co-exist, right-sided epididymo-orchitis occurring in an incompletely descended organ is extremely difficult, if not impossible, to differentiate from appendicitis.

Antonio Scarpa, 1748–1832. Anatomist and Surgeon, Venice.

Occasionally epididymo-orchitis occurring in a retained abdominal testis gives rise to peritonitis.

6. *Atrophy*, which sometimes is associated with a testis in the inguinal canal, is usually attributed to repeated slight trauma, such as is occasioned by full flexion of the hip. Even before puberty a testis in this situation sometimes shows signs of atrophy.

7. *Increased liability to malignant disease* (see p. 811).

Hormone Treatment.—There are three varieties of substances having a gonadotrophic action : (1) a gonadotrophic hormone obtained directly from the anterior lobe of the pituitary gland ; (2) one obtained from blood serum of pregnant mares ; (3) one produced from the urine of pregnant women, e.g. Pregnyl. The last is the most potent.

The course of treatment should be given preferably between the ages of seven and eight years. The usual dose recommended is 500 international units given intramuscularly once a week until descent occurs, or until a total dose of 4,000 units has been given.

In many centres routine hormone treatment for incomplete descent of the testis has been abandoned because (*a*) in the majority of cases there is a mechanical barrier to descent ; (*b*) a potential or actual hernia is present so often ; (*c*) the injections are painful ; (*d*) if retractile testes are eliminated, the chances of successful hormone treatment are small (under 20 per cent.) ; (*e*) the treatment precipitates puberty.

The main indications for hormone treatment are cases of bilateral incomplete descent associated with hypogenitalism and obesity.

Orchiopexy.[1]—Most surgeons favour performing the operation about the age of seven or eight years. If herniotomy must be carried out much before this time, it is better to postpone orchiopexy, for in very early life the friability of the peritoneum makes separation of the spermatic vessels from it more difficult. After the age of puberty the percentage of successful operations, which at the optimum age approaches 80 per cent., falls considerably. In cryptorchidism one side should be operated on at a time, with an interval of six months between the operations.

The initial stages of all operations for orchiopexy are similar to those of

[1] The term orchi*d*opexy is etymologically incorrect (Torek).

Franz Torek, Contemporary. Surgeon, Lenox Hill Hospital, New York.

inguinal herniorrhaphy. The cord and the testis are freed from surrounding structures, and the upper part of the processus vaginalis is dissected from the cord, ligated and divided at the level of the internal abdominal ring, leaving the distal part of the processus attached. This is the most usual type of hernial sac accompanying incomplete descent of the testis. Other varieties of hernial sac are excised completely. Any gubernacular bands attached to the lower pole of the testis are divided. Near the internal abdominal ring all the coverings of the cord are divided ; every muscle fibre and fibrous band is severed, leaving only the vas and its blood-vessels and the spermatic blood-vessels. More often than not this provides sufficient length for the testis to be placed in the scrotum. If not, other methods referred to in " Obstacles to Descent " are invoked. When some components of the pampiniform plexus hinder mobilisation they may be divided in addition. It is most exceptional for the above measures to fail to elongate the pedicle sufficiently for the testis to be placed in the scrotum, and beyond it, if the operation is performed during childhood. The empty half of the scrotum is stretched thoroughly with the index finger passed into it through the inguinal incision.

The testis is retained in the scrotum by one of a number of ingenious methods, of which the following are the ones usually practised :

(a) *Ombrédanne's Operation.*—This operation is suitable for patients under the age of ten years. A suture is attached to the lower end of the tunica vaginalis of the mobilised testis, and the two ends are left long. A vertical incision about 1 inch (2·5 cm.) in length is made in the opposite side of the scrotum, ½ inch from the median raphé, and deepened until the corresponding tunica vaginalis is seen. Between this and the septum dartos a bed is prepared by blunt dissection. The free ends of the suture are seized in a hæmostat, which is passed through the inguinal incision into the scrotum. The tip of the hæmostat is thrust against the septum dartos, permitting a small incision to be made through the septum exposing the tip of the hæmostat and the suture it grasps (fig. 820). The hæmostat is opened and the ends of the suture are drawn through the scrotal wound. Before removing the hæmostat its jaws are opened sufficiently to stretch the tiny opening in the septum to about half the size of the testis, which is pulled through the opening into the opposite side of the

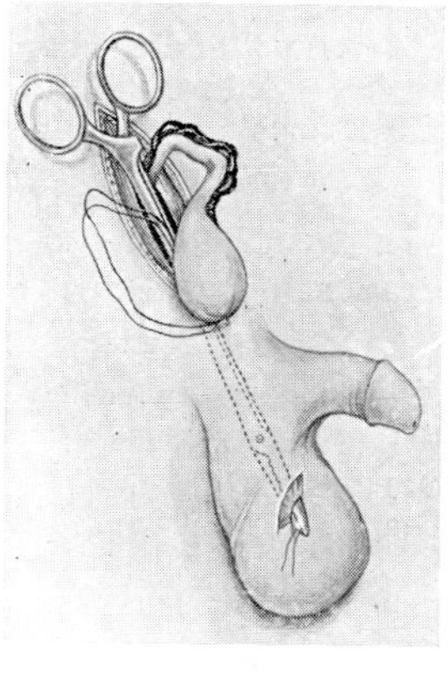

FIG. 820.—Method of passing the suture attached to the testis through the septum dartos and the skin of the opposite side of the scrotum.

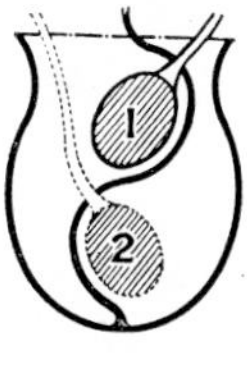

FIG. 821.—The disposition of the testes in relation to the septum dartos following bilateral Ombrédanne's operation.

scrotum by traction on the suture. The hole in the septum tends to contract, for its walls are elastic, and it requires only one or two sutures to close the septum around the cord sufficiently tightly to prevent the testis escaping from its new habitat, but not tightly enough to compress the cord (fig. 821). The scrotal and inguinal incisions are closed, the latter in layers.

Louis Ombrédanne, Contemporary. Surgeon, Hôpital des Enfants Malades, Paris.

(b) *The Keetley-Torek operation* is illustrated in fig. 822.   After six months or less the testis and the scrotum are freed from the thigh.

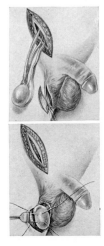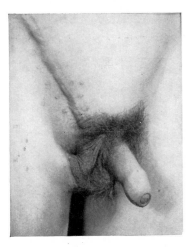

Fig. 822.—The Keetley-Torek operation.   Some months later, when the cord has become adequately lengthened, the scrotum and testis are detached from the thigh.

Orchiectomy is indicated when the other testis is normal, and the cord too short to allow replacement of the incompletely descended organ in the scrotum, or when the incompletely descended testis is hopelessly atrophic or diseased.

Orchio-cœlioplasty (abdominal replacement of the organ).   Only when the contralateral organ has been removed already and orchiopexy is found to be impossible is this measure justifiable.   Occasions arise when it is the only method of preserving a supply of internal testicular secretion and secluding an organ exposed constantly to injury.

MALDESCENDED TESTIS (*Syn.* ECTOPIC TESTIS)

An ectopic testis may be found :

1. Above and to the outer side of the external abdominal ring.
2. In the perineum.
3. At the root of the penis.
4. In Scarpa's triangle.

The first two positions are relatively common.

Unlike the imperfectly descended testis, an ectopic organ often develops fully.   Its main hazard is that, owing to its position, it is liable to injury.

Ætiology.—To explain the appearance of the testis in these anomalous positions, C. B. Lockwood advanced the ingenious theory of many gubernacular tails. His theory postulates that in ectopic testis the main scrotal tail becomes ruptured. As a consequence the testis, adrift from its usual mooring, follows one of the accessory rudders. Lockwood stated that the accessory gubernacula depicted in fig. 823 could be demonstrated in the fœtus, a claim which other workers have been unable to substantiate.

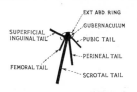

FIG. 823.—The " gubernacular tails " of Lockwood.

Treatment. — Of necessity, many ectopic testes have a comparatively long spermatic cord. On this account orchiopexy is performed easily.

TORSION OF THE SPERMATIC CORD (*Syn.* **TORSION OF THE TESTIS**) is not a common condition. It occurs with equal frequency in incompletely and fully descended testes, but seeing that incomplete descent is present in less than one per cent. of the male populace, the relative frequency in cases of incomplete descent is obviously higher.

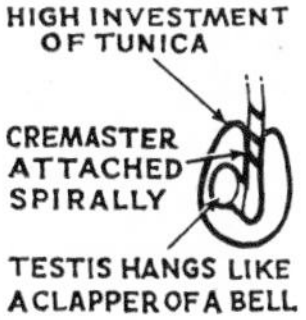

FIG. 824.—The predisposing factors of torsion.

Ætiology.—It is very doubtful if torsion can occur in a completely normal testis. In most instances the torsion takes place within a capacious tunica vaginalis, and the anatomical anomalies which predispose to rotation of the spermatic cord are shown in fig. 824. A testis which lies more horizontally in the scrotum than normal, and one whose spermatic cord is attached to the middle of the organ, is very prone to twist. Sometimes the testis is inverted, i.e. the hydatid of Morgagni is at the lower pole. Very occasionally torsion is extra-vaginal. Most often the symptoms arise while the patient is straining, but in a number of instances there is no exciting cause.

Clinical Features.—The highest incidence is between fifteen and twenty-five years of age, and the second most common age period is during infancy. The patient experiences sudden and agonising pain in the groin and lower abdomen, and vomits. Upon theoretical grounds one might think that the diagnosis is simple, but nothing could be farther from the truth, for it is practically impossible to distinguish *torsion of an imperfectly descended testis* from a strangulated inguinal hernia. The fact that the side of the scrotum is empty and œdematous is certainly in favour of the tender lump at the external abdominal ring being the testis with its cord twisted (fig. 825), but it is impossible to rule out a tense strangulated inguinal hernia until the parts have been displayed

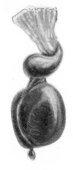

FIG. 825.— Torsion of the testis.

Alex. Roch?.)

by operation. *Torsion of a completely descended testis* is a less difficult problem. Sometimes the actual twists in the cord can be felt, thus establishing the diagnosis. At other times the condition can be mimicked exactly by a small, tense,

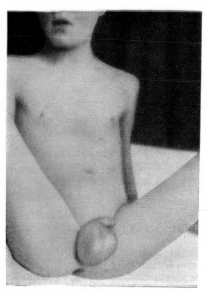

FIG. 826.—Torsion of a fully descended right testis in a boy aged fourteen. Mistaken for epididymo-orchitis.

strangulated hernia compressing the cord and causing congestion of the pampiniform plexus, the result of which is a tender, œdematous testis on that side. Torsion of the fully descended testis can also simulate closely acute epididymo-orchitis (fig. 826); even the temperature is raised slightly—99° F. (37·2° C.) after the lapse of a few hours. Elevation of the scrotum relieves the pain in epididymitis, but increases it in torsion of the spermatic cord (Prehn).

(See also Torsion of a Cyst of the Hydatid of Morgagni, p. 808.)

Recurrent torsion with spontaneous rectification occurs. We met with such a case in a young soldier. On the occasion upon which we saw him —the fourth attack within six months—spontaneous rectification took place in the jolting ambulance which conveyed him from his camp. As a result of the repeated interference with its blood-supply, the affected testis had become much smaller than its fellow. The excised testis was fibrotic.

Treatment.—Immediate operation is indicated. In early cases it may be possible to untwist the cord, and if the colour returns to normal to fix the organ in an anatomically correct position. As a rule, orchiectomy must be performed. It is well established that in cases where torsion occurs in a fully descended testis, the congenital abnormalities which permit twisting (see fig. 824) appertain to both sides. Particularly when a patient has lost a testis because of torsion, in due course the contralateral organ should be fixed in the scrotum (see fig. 827).

Douglas T. Prehn, Contemporary. Captain, U.S. Naval Medical Service.

EPIDIDYMITIS

Mode of Infection.—Most infections of the epididymis, particularly gonococcal, are secondary to infection of the corresponding seminal vesicle, which in turn is infected from the prostatic urethra. Usually it is considered the infection passes along the lumen of the vas. Some hold that the lymphatics which accompany the vas carry the infection from the prostate or the seminal vesicle to the epididymis. Many believe that tuberculosis and some non-specific infections of the epididymis are blood-borne, and that spread occurs from the epididymis along the vas to infect the vesicle and the prostate. In support of this theory is that in some early cases of tuberculous epididymitis there is no evidence of infection of the vesicle. Against it is the fact that infection commonly commences in the globus minor ; if it were blood-borne one would expect it to commence in the globus major, which is exceptional. In cases where the urine is infected, epididymitis may result from a reflux of urine down the vas, possibly as a result of a muscular strain with a full bladder.

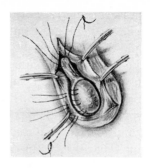

FIG. 827.—Method of anchoring the testis with non-absorbable sutures to prevent torsion.

In most cases of acute epididymitis infection does not spread to the body of the testis. This is also true of chronic infections, but if they remain untreated eventually the body becomes involved also (epididymo-orchitis).

ACUTE EPIDIDYMITIS

Acute Gonococcal Epididymitis.—Formerly very common, this has become comparatively rare since the introduction of sulphonamides and penicillin for the treatment of acute gonorrhœal urethritis. The epididymitis usually commences during the second or third week of posterior urethritis. In 90 per cent. of cases the infection is unilateral. The first symptom is pain in the groin and in the lower abdomen. The urethral discharge lessens ; pain then commences in the testis. The urethral discharge ceases, but the urine is hazy with pus cells. The temperature rises to 102° or 103° F. (38·9° or 39·5° C.) and the patient feels so ill that he goes to bed. On examination the scrotum is œdematous, some degree of secondary hydrocele is present, and the epididymis is exquisitely tender. In acute epididymitis a rectal examination is neither necessary nor desirable, as it may activate the primary focus in the vesicle or prostate. This part of the examination should be deferred until the acute stage is over, when it will be found that the prostate is enlarged and somewhat tender, as also is the seminal vesicle on the affected side. Later the skin of the scrotum may become reddened and adherent to the globus minor, but pure gonococcal epididymitis does not suppurate. After the fourth or fifth day the symptoms commence to abate, and by the eighth to tenth day the condition subsides. Induration of the globus minor may persist for months.

Treatment.—The patient must be kept in bed until the acute symptoms have abated. All local treatment of the urethritis must be discontinued. The scrotum is supported on a sling formed by broad adhesive plaster attached across the thighs

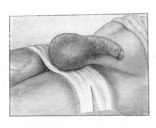

(fig. 828). Upon the sling is placed a nest of cottonwool, and in this the inflamed organ rests and an ice-bag or cooling lotions are applied. The urine is rendered alkaline, and a high fluid intake is necessary. An aperient is given, and sedation such as bromide or luminal is ordered. In severe cases morphia or omnopon is required to relieve the pain. If this is not effective, infiltration of the spermatic cord with 10 ml. of 1 per cent. solution

FIG. 828.—Treatment of acute epididymo-orchitis. A splint for the testicles. Broad adhesive is applied to the thighs as shown.

of procaine gives relief for twenty-four hours or more. Penicillin is administered—doses of 300,000 to 500,000 units per diem are required for five days or a week. When the inflammation commences to resolve, a well-fitting scrotal bandage is applied and the patient is allowed up. Usually the urethral discharge recommences, and after about a week local treatment of the posterior urethra, prostate, and seminal vesicles is continued until the infection has been eradicated.

Recurrent sub-acute gonococcal epididymitis does not often become chronic, but recurrent subacute attacks are not uncommon, due invariably to persistent infection in the corresponding vesicle. If the condition recurs in spite of penicillin therapy and prostatic massage during periods of quiescence, epididymotomy (exposing the epididymis) and incising pockets of pus with a tenotome and washing out cavities with proflavine solution, combined with vasotomy (tying a special small cannula into an incision in the vas) which enables the vesicle to be irrigated, clears up permanently infection which has resisted antibiotic treatment.

Acute non-specific epididymitis often arises as a complication of a urinary infection. The infecting organisms may be B. coli, streptococci, staphylococci, or pneumococci. Sometimes the condition is a complication of abacterial pyuria. Occasionally there is no urinary or urethral infection and the condition is blood-borne. The clinical features are similar to gonococcal epididymitis, but there is usually an absence of urethral discharge. Suppuration occurs frequently.

Treatment.—In addition to other measures detailed for acute gonococcal epididymitis, a sulphonamide is given by mouth. If the inflammation does not respond to these measures, streptomycin should be substituted. When suppuration occurs an incision to evacuate the pus must be made.

Acute Tuberculous Epididymitis.—There is sometimes an initial watery urethral discharge from tuberculous prostatitis. The epididymitis, although commencing acutely, is somewhat less painful than the foregoing varieties, but more or less acute inflammation is prolonged for weeks. The accompanying secondary hydrocele is of considerable size. Eventually the epididymitis culminates in abscess formation. If tubercle bacilli are absent from the pus on several examinations of the urine, and pyelography is negative, the diagnosis is extremely difficult, but the train of symptoms described suggests this condition. The effect of streptomycin should be tried. This variety of infection often invades the body of the testis, and more than one discharging sinus forms. Orchiectomy is then necessary. A few cases of chronic tuberculous epididymitis commence acutely.

CHRONIC EPIDIDYMITIS

Chronic tuberculous epididymitis is the most common form of chronic epididymitis ; indeed, nearly 90 per cent. of cases of chronic epididymitis are tuberculous. In the great majority of cases the disease commences insidiously. A slight ache in the testis or a trivial injury calls the patient's attention to the swelling in relation to the testis. An early manifestation is a discrete, hard, slightly tender nodule in the globus minor— rarely in the globus major. As the disease progresses other nodules appear, and eventually the entire epididymis becomes involved and is felt as a hard, craggy, often painless mass (fig. 829), situated behind the testis, which feels normal. In 30 per cent. of cases a secondary hydrocele is present. Rarely, when the testis is anteverted, these changes are found in front of the testis. Except in the very early stages of the disease

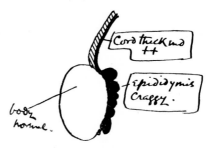

Fig. 829.—The physical signs recorded in a case of tuberculous epididymitis.

the corresponding vas can be felt distinctly thickened when compared with that of the opposite side. At a later stage it sometimes becomes beaded. Rectal examination reveals a thickened, and later an irregularly indurated, seminal vesicle of the corresponding side, and sometimes of the contralateral vesicle as well. The prostate is firm and in advanced cases contains one or more discrete nodules. In 20 per cent. of cases the patient first presents himself with a cold abscess in the lower and posterior aspect of the scrotum, or with a discharging sinus in this situation (fig. 830), which may have healed and reopened several times. Untreated, after a varying time—from a few months to several years—the contralateral epididymis becomes diseased and passes through the various phases from a solitary nodule to complete involvement of the epididymis, and finally pus formation, as did its fellow. Involvement of the opposite side is always preceded by tuberculous prostato-vesiculitis. In cases commencing acutely or subacutely, the body of the testis becomes implicated early.

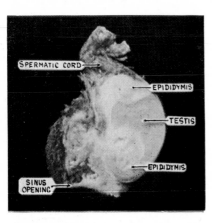

FIG. 830.—Advanced tuberculous epididymo-orchitis with scrotal sinus.

In the much more common chronic form the disease does not involve the body of the testis for a long period, often years. In under one-third of cases tuberculous epididymitis arises as a complication of urinary tuberculosis. The symptoms are then largely over-shadowed by those of frequent and often painful micturition. In these circumstances the tuberculous epididymis may be found on routine examination.

In all cases of chronic epididymitis the urine should be examined for tubercle bacilli, if necessary on several occasions, and pyelography should be undertaken. The lungs must be examined clinically and radiologically. In over 50 per cent. of cases there is no primary focus discovered. In some of these, when the disease is limited to a portion of the epididymis, it is extremely difficult to differentiate tuberculous from non-tuberculous epididymitis. If the condition fails to resolve after six or eight weeks, or if a second adjacent nodule appears, the condition should be treated as tuberculous.

Treatment.—In cases with active pulmonary involvement sanatorium treatment is necessary. The testes are supported. If an abscess forms it should be aspirated. Often gradual fibrosis occurs. If the pulmonary condition improves and the epididymitis remains stationary, epididymectomy may be considered advisable. In cases associated with a tuberculous kidney nephro-ureterectomy is performed, and sanatorium treatment, together with streptomycin, is necessary. Streptomycin is less effective in genital tuberculosis than in urinary tuberculosis. If the epididymis does not respond to these measures, epididymectomy should be performed. When tuberculosis is confined to the epididymis or, as is more common, to the epididymis and the corresponding vesicle, epididymectomy followed by six weeks' rest gives rapid and excellent results. After the epididymis has been removed, the infected vesicle undergoes fibrosis, or sometimes calcification. If there is any doubt about the excised epididymis being tuberculous, it should be submitted to histological examination. Caseous nodules are unmistakable macroscopically. Epididymectomy is also of value when both vesicles and the prostate are involved, but in this instance the vas on the opposite side should be divided between ligatures in order to minimise spread to the healthy epididymis. In such cases a period of sanatorium treatment is advisable.

Chronic non-specific epididymitis may be chronic from the commencement, or follow an acute attack. Chronic non-specific epididymitis can usually be distinguished from tuberculous epididymitis because in the former the involved portion of the vesicle is smoother. Thickening of the vas is not a prerogative of tuberculosis ; it occurs in any chronic epididymo-vesiculitis. In most cases associated posterior urethritis, vesiculitis, or prostatitis must receive treatment. In cases when tuberculosis cannot be ruled out prostatic massage must be eschewed. When support of the scrotum and antibiotic treatment bring no improvement after a month or six weeks, epididymectomy should be performed.

Epididymectomy.—When there is a sinus, or on palpation the epididymis is involved extensively, permission for orchiectomy should be obtained, as it is sometimes impossible to determine whether the body of the testis is implicated before the organ has been displayed. An incision is made from the external abdominal ring to below the testis. If a sinus is present, or the skin is adherent to the globus minor, the affected skin is included in an ellipse. The testis is withdrawn and the tunica vaginalis is opened. Commencing at the globus minor, the epididymis is separated from the body of the testis by blunt dissection, aided by the diathermy knife (fig. 831). The dissection of the epididymis from the testis proceeds upwards. The vascular pedicle entering the testis does so between the upper pole of the testis and the globus major, but it is possible to separate the globus major from the testis without injuring the spermatic vessels.

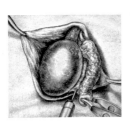

FIG. 831.—Epididymectomy. Commencing to detach the freed globus minor from the body of the testis.

The testis, with its vessels intact, is wrapped in a swab while the vas, still attached to the epididymis, is separated from the cord as far as the external abdominal ring. The vas is then divided between hæmostats near the epididymis, which is removed. The tip of the hæmostat containing the proximal end of the vas is thrust beneath the skin of the inguinal region and made to protrude about 1 inch (2·5 cm.) above the scrotal incision. A small nick is made in the skin over the tip of the hæmostat, and the latter, together with the vas, is pushed through. The end of the vas is grasped in a second hæmostat and the redundant vas is drawn on to the surface. This small incision is closed with two sutures, one of which passes through the outer coat of the vas. The protruding portion of the vas is allowed to separate at skin level, and it shrivels up and separates in about seven days. In this way infection of the scrotal wound from the lumen of the vas is prevented. The testis is removed from the swab and any bleeding vessels are ligated and oozing points controlled by diathermy coagulation. If hæmostasis is perfect, the scrotal wound is closed without drainage.

Orchiectomy is reserved for those cases where the body of the testis is involved. If such involvement is certain before the operation is commenced, retrograde orchiectomy similar to that for malignant disease of the testis is carried out. If the necessity for orchiectomy becomes apparent only after the testis has been displayed, after changing gloves and instruments, an incision is made over the inguinal canal, which is opened. The cord is ligated and divided near the internal abdominal ring. After the inguinal wound has been closed in layers the testis is removed through the scrotal incision, which can also be closed completely, if hæmostasis is assured. In either case it is advantageous to deal with the vas as has been described in epididymectomy.

ORCHITIS

occurs occasionally during many of the acute exanthemata.

Acute Orchitis of Mumps.—Although the epididymis is involved, it is customary to call the condition orchitis because the body of the testis is mainly affected.

Treatment.—If within forty-eight hours of the commencement

Robert Hamilton, Surgeon, King's Lynn, England, first described orchitis of mumps in 1761.

of the orchitis a small incision is made into the tunica albuginea, viscid fluid under considerable pressure gushes forth. A tube should be inserted for forty-eight hours. If this course is adopted, the temperature falls within a few hours, pain ceases immediately, and atrophy of the testis is prevented.

Syphilitic orchitis is now very rare. It occurs in congenital syphilis during infancy or childhood as bilateral orchitis (see p. 41).

Interstitial fibrosis is bilateral, symptomless, and leads to gradual destruction of the seminiferous tubules. The testes are not enlarged. They are harder than normal, and there is a gradual loss of testicular sensation.

Fibrosis of the testis is excelled only by meso-aortitis as the best macroscopical post-mortem evidence of syphilis. On bisecting the testis, scar tissue is seen within.

Gumma.—The condition is nearly always unilateral. The body of the testis enlarges slowly and painlessly. At this stage it feels extremely hard. Testicular sensation is lost, and there is nearly always an associated secondary hydrocele. Later there is softening anteriorly and the skin of the scrotum becomes

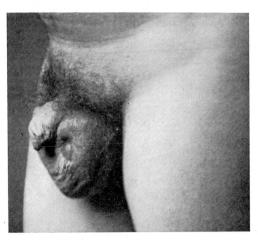

Fig. 832.—Gumma of the testis commencing to ulcerate.

inflamed, and a gummatous ulcer forms (fig. 832). The Wassermann reaction is strongly positive and the response to anti-syphilitic treatment is usually prompt, but so difficult is the diagnosis from malignant disease in the early stages that it is often better to perform orchiectomy than to risk the possibility of waiting to settle the issue by watching the effects of anti-syphilitic treatment in a case of possible malignant disease.

VARICOCELE

A varicocele is a varicose condition of the veins of the pampini-form plexus.   Between puberty and the age of thirty-five, from 5 to 10 per cent. of males have some degree of pampiniform varicosity on the left side (fig. 833).   In almost all cases it is the left side which is affected ; occasionally both sides are involved, but it is most exceptional for the right side to be affected alone.

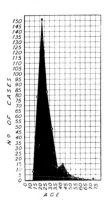

FIG. 833.—Age incidence of varicocele.
(*After Barney.*)

The cause of the predilection for the left side is obscure.   The following theories have been advanced :
1. The left spermatic vein enters the left renal vein at a right angle, while the right spermatic vein enters the vena cava obliquely.
2. The left testis is lower in the scrotum than the right.
3. A loaded sigmoid colon is liable to press upon and obstruct the left spermatic vein.
4. Most men " dress " on the left.

Clinical Features.—Usually symptoms are entirely absent.   In a proportion of cases the patient experiences a dragging pain on the left side.   When the varicocele is comparatively small and the symptoms are con-siderable, the probability of a neurosis being the real cause of the trouble should always engage the clinician's attention. The diagnosis of a varicocele is simple. The left side of the scrotum hangs lower than normal (fig. 834), and the impression gained on palpation of the varicose plexus has been aptly likened to a bag of worms. When the patient lies down and the scrotum is elevated, the veins will be emptied by gravity and the opportunity of comparing the size of the left testis with its fellow should be taken.   In long-standing cases of varicocele the left testis is somewhat smaller and softer than the right, due to a minor degree of atrophy.

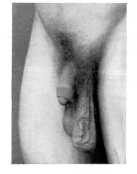

FIG. 834.—A large varicocele.

A comparatively rapid onset of a varicocele, due to pressure on the spermatic vein, is suggestive of a renal or suprarenal tumour, and in such cases the kidney region should be palpated (see p. 679).

Treatment.—A suspensory bandage, a cold bath in the morning, and reassurance that there is nothing to worry about is all that is necessary in most instances. Candidates for some public services must be operated upon to conform with the regulations. Cases in which the varicocele is large and the testis hangs low are often distinctly benefited by operation. Small varicoceles should be left alone or treated by injection.

Injection.—The injection treatment of varicocele is often successful. In most cases one treatment is all that is necessary.

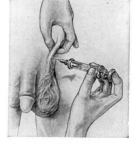

Fig. 835.—The treatment of varicocele by injection.

A small bunch of veins is taken up between the finger and thumb, and, using 2 ml. of a 5 per cent. solution of ethamolin, the injection is made from above downwards just below the external abdominal ring (fig. 835). The pampiniform plexus is entered at several points by a few short jabs of the needle. A suspensory bandage is worn for some weeks.

Operation.—An incision is made over the inguinal canal and the external oblique is divided in the line of its fibres. The spermatic cord is lifted from its bed and its coverings are divided. The venous trunks are isolated from other constituents of the cord, and ligated and divided near the internal abdominal ring. All the tributaries of the spermatic vein should be ligated. Anastomotic venules are sufficient to ensure adequate venous return. The wound is closed in layers. Post-operatively the patient wears a suspensory bandage for three weeks.

HYDROCELE

Congenital.

Acquired
{
  Primary, or idiopathic.

  Secondary, due to disease of testis
  {
    Acute.

    Chronic.
  }
}

A hydrocele is a collection of serous fluid in some part of the processus vaginalis, usually in the tunica.

Ætiology.—A hydrocele can appear in conjunction with some demonstrable pathological condition of the corresponding testis ; it is then termed a " secondary hydrocele." More often the condition arises spontaneously, and its pathogenesis is uncertain. The trend of current opinion attributes the effusion to trauma or to bygone low-grade bacterial epididymo-orchitis.

Hydrocele fluid is amber coloured, and registers a specific gravity of 1022 to 1024. It contains water, inorganic salts, 6 per cent. of albumin, and a quantity of fibrinogen. The last constituent confers upon the fluid a characteristic feature. If the contents of a hydrocele are allowed to run through a cannula into a receptacle, the fluid does *not* clot, but if a few drops of blood which have come into contact with cut tissues are stirred into even a large quantity of hydrocele fluid, the whole clots firmly. In old-standing cases the fluid is sometimes rich in cholesterol, and occasionally tyrosine crystals are found.

There are seven anatomical varieties of hydrocele.

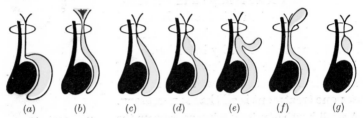

Fig. 836.—(*a*) Vaginal hydrocele. (*b*) Congenital hydrocele. (*c*) Infantile hydrocele. (*d*) Hour-glass hydrocele. (*e*) Bilocular hydrocele. (*f*) Abdomino-scrotal hydrocele. (*g*) Encysted hydrocele of the cord.

GOLDEN DIAGNOSTIC RULES FOR ALL HYDROCELES

99 *out of every* **100** *hydroceles are translucent. On examination it is possible " to get above the swelling."*

(*a*) *The vaginal hydrocele* is at least six times more common than all the other varieties put together. Vaginal hydrocele most often appears in middle-aged or elderly men, but it is not uncommon in early childhood, or indeed at any time of life. The condition is particularly common in tropical countries. The only complaint of the patient is the swelling, and occasionally he does not seek relief until the sac has attained enormous dimensions.

(*b*) *Congenital Hydrocele.*—The processus vaginalis communicates with the peritoneal cavity. Usually the communicating orifice is too small for the development of a hernia. When the scrotum is elevated the fluid disappears within the abdominal cavity, usually slowly, but it returns when the erect posture is resumed. Especially in bilateral cases, ascites or serous tuberculous peritonitis should be suspected.

(*c*) *Infantile hydrocele* does not necessarily appear in infants. The tunica vaginalis and the processus vaginalis are distended right up to the internal abdominal ring, but the sac has no connection with the general peritoneal cavity.

(*d*) *Hour-glass hydrocele* ⎫ are but variations of the foregoing,
(*e*) *Bilocular hydrocele* ⎬ and little more than pathological
(*f*) *Abdomino-scrotal hydrocele* ⎭ curiosities.

(*g*) *Encysted Hydrocele of the Cord.*—This fairly common condition causes some confusion in diagnosis. There is a smooth, oval swelling associated with the spermatic cord. When such a swelling is situated at the external abdominal ring, it is very liable to be mistaken for an irreducible inguinal hernia. If, with gentle traction upon the testis, the swelling moves downwards and becomes less mobile, the diagnosis of hydrocele of the cord is confirmed.

Hydrocele of the canal of Nück is a condition comparable to the foregoing. It occurs in females, the cyst being in relationship to the round ligament. Unlike a hydrocele of the cord, a hydrocele of the canal of Nück is always wholly, or partially, in the inguinal canal.

COMPLICATIONS OF A HYDROCELE

1. **Rupture** is usually traumatic, but may possibly be spontaneous. On rare occasions a cure results after absorption of the fluid.

2. **Hernia of the hydrocele sac** sometimes occurs in old-standing cases. Tension of fluid within the tunica causes herniation of a portion of the sac through some of the coverings of the testis (fig. 837).

3. **Transformation into a hæmatocele** may occur spontaneously, or as the result of trauma (see p. 808).

4. **Calcification** of the sac wall sometimes occurs in long-standing cases.

Treatment.—*Tapping.*—After transillumination, the swelling is made tense. A fine trocar and cannula, or what is often better, a lumbar puncture needle, is in-

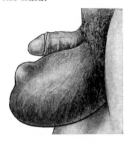

Fig. 837.—A hernia of a hydrocele through some of its coverings.

serted into an unquestionably translucent area. By this means the fluid is evacuated. After a varying interval the sac usually refills. Many patients seem content to be relieved at regular intervals in this way.

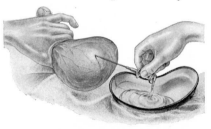

Fig. 838.—Tapping a hydrocele.

Tapping and injection is often effective in thin-walled hydroceles. The fluid is evacuated by tapping, and the interior of the sac washed out with normal saline. Two or three ml. of quinine-urethane are injected and the sclerosing fluid is massaged into every ramification of the sac. A suspensory bandage is worn. The fluid usually reaccumulates. One week later the process is repeated.

Anton Nück, 1650–1692. Anatomist, of Leiden, Holland.
Infection of a hydrocele caused the death of Gibbon, the historian.

If necessary, a third injection is given after an interval of three weeks.

Subtotal excision is the best means of insuring against recurrence, and it is the only method available for thick-walled hydroceles. An incision is made over the most prominent part of the swelling and the hydrocele and testis are separated from their coverings by gauze dissection. The sac is opened with a scalpel and its contents evacuated, after which the sac is split along its length. Each half of the tunica vaginalis is excised with a diathermy knife close to its reflection on to the epididymis. Usually a number of bleeding vessels must be secured by transfixion, or it may be necessary to insert a continuous running catgut suture along the cut edges to ensure hæmostasis. The testis is replaced and the wound is closed with drainage. The dressing is supported by a firm T-bandage. The drainage tube is removed after forty-eight hours.

Partial excision with eversion (Jaboulay's operation) is suitable for thin-walled hydroceles. Sufficient of the sac is excised to allow the cut edges to be united without tension behind the epididymis, so that the endothelial lining faces outwards. Occasionally recurrence follows this operation.

Complete excision of the whole sac is possible in the case of encysted hydrocele of the cord or a hydrocele of the canal of Nück.

RARER AFFECTIONS OF THE TUNICA VAGINALIS

Secondary Hydrocele.—Attention is again directed to the effusion into the tunica vaginalis which accompanies certain affections of the testis. It is a frequent associate of acute and chronic orchitis. It is nearly always present in the syphilitic affections of the testis, and occasionally complicates malignant disease of the organ. Often the question as to whether a hydrocele is or is not secondary to some underlying disease of the testis can only be settled after the hydrocele has been tapped. Secondary hydroceles rarely attain a large size, and in the case of acute orchitis they sometimes subside *pari passu* with the primary lesion.

Chylous hydrocele is seen in tropical countries, and is due to filarial parasites. Acute cases should be treated by rest, while chronic cases respond to the usual operations for hydrocele.

Hydrocele of a Hernial Sac.—The neck of a hernial sac may become plugged with omentum or by adhesions, and a hydrocele results.

CYSTS CONNECTED WITH THE EPIDIDYMIS

Spermatocele is a unilocular retention cyst derived from some portion of the sperm-conducting mechanism of the epididymis.

Ætiology.—It is not possible to dogmatise upon the exact origin of a spermatocele. A blocked vas efferens would account for the condition ; on the other hand, it is impossible to dispute a claim that a spermatocele

Mathieu Jaboulay, 1860–1913. Professor of Surgery, Lyons.

arises from one of those vestigial structures depicted in fig. 840, provided always that the remnant in question is connected with the sperm-conducting mechanism.

Clinical Features.—A spermatocele is nearly always situated in the head of the epididymis, and is therefore above and behind the body of the testis. Filled with fluid resembling barley water and containing spermatozoa, the swelling is typically softer than other cysts occurring within the scrotum but, like them, is translucent. Spermatoceles give rise to few symptoms, and are usually small and unobtrusive. Less frequently they are large enough to attract notice. Sometimes the patient presents himself because he believes he has a third testicle, but, as Sir Robert Liston remarked, "these patients flatter themselves in thinking they are unduly provided " (fig. 839).

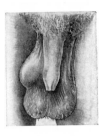

Fig. 839.—A large spermatocele.

Treatment.—Small spermatoceles should be left alone. Larger ones can be aspirated and injected, or excised.

Cysts of the Epididymis.—A cyst of the epididymis, filled with crystal-clear fluid (as opposed to the barley-water-like fluid of a spermatocele or the amber-coloured fluid of a vaginal hydrocele), is a common clinical entity.

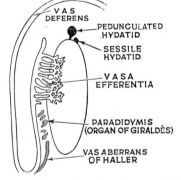

VAS DEFERENS
PEDUNCULATED HYDATID
SESSILE HYDATID
VASA EFFERENTIA
PARADIDYMIS (ORGAN OF GIRALDÈS)
VAS ABERRANS OF HALLER

Fig. 840.—Structures from which spermatoceles and other cysts of the epididymis arise.

Ætiology.—A cyst of the epididymis can arise as a retention cyst or a cystic degeneration of :

(*a*) The pedunculated hydatid of Morgagni.

(*b*) The sessile hydatid of Morgagni.

(*c*) The vas aberrans of Haller.

(*d*) The paradidymis, or organ of Giraldès.

(*e*) A blocked vas efferens.

Clinical Features.—Cysts of the epididymis (fig. 840) are usually found in middle life, and are often bilateral. They are translucent, tense, and often consist of an aggregation of a number of small cysts (fig. 841). Like spermatoceles, they are usually situated above and behind the body of the testis.

Fig. 841. —Cyst of the epididymis.

Sir Robert Liston, 1794–1847. Surgeon, Royal Infirmary, Edinburgh. Later Surgeon, University College Hospital, London.
Giovanni Morgagni, 1682–1771. Professor of Surgery, Padua. He held the chair for fifty-six years.
Albrecht von Haller, 1708–1777. Professor of Medicine, Surgery and Botany, University of Göttingen.
Joachim Giraldès, 1808–1875. Surgeon, Beaujou Hospital, Paris.

Treatment.—When large, or when symptoms are present, the cysts should be excised. Cautery excision minimises the occurrence of a post-operative scrotal hæmatoma. Owing to their multilocular nature, some cysts of the epididymis are unsuited to treatment by injection.

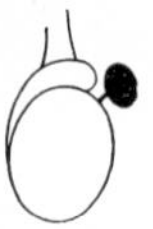

Cyst of one of the hydatids of Morgagni (fig. 842) is a separate clinical entity. It forms a small, globular swelling at the superior pole of the testis. It is usually unilateral, and in the case of the pedunculated hydatid it sometimes undergoes axial rotation and produces acute symptoms akin to those of mild torsion of the testis.

FIG. 842.—Cyst of the hydatid of Morgagni.

INJURIES TO THE TESTIS

1. Hæmatocele.—Hæmorrhage into the tunica vaginalis may result from a blow. It also sometimes occurs after tapping a hydrocele. Absorption of blood from the tunica vaginalis is slow and uncertain. It is far better to remove the blood and blood-clot promptly, and to perform at the same time an operation for the cure of the hydrocele. Hæmorrhage into a hydrocele may occur from a trivial injury, or even spontaneously. An old, clotted hæmatocele generally proves a diagnostic riddle. It is referred to on p. 811.

2. Laceration of the testis is a rare accident, and even when the damage is severe, repair is nearly always possible.

MALIGNANT DISEASE OF THE TESTIS

Pathology.—Tumours of the testis, which are invariably malignant, are relatively rare. They are classified most satisfactorily into two groups :

Seminoma, so named by Chevassu, is the commoner tumour of the testis. Macroscopically the cut surface is homogeneous, of a creamy consistency, usually pale yellow in colour (fig. 843), but sometimes pink. Occasionally fibrous septa give it a lobulated appearance. In rapidly growing tumours areas of necrosis may be present.

Microscopically the tumour is composed of either spheroidal or polyhedral cells, containing clear, pale cytoplasm with hyperchromatic nuclei, arranged in sheets separated by fibrous septa—an appearance resembling normal spermatocytes. In the more malignant varieties the cells are tightly packed, round and anaplastic. In both varieties lymphocytes are present in the septa.

The consensus of opinion is that this tumour is a carcinoma

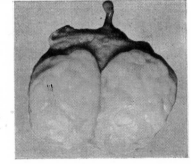

FIG. 843.—Seminoma of the testicle.

Maurice Chevassu, Contemporary. Chief of the Urological Department, Hôpital Cochin Paris.

derived from the seminiferous tubules.

Teratoma.—On section the tumour may be homogeneous ; more typically it shows cystic spaces (fig. 844) containing gelatinous fluid. Cartilaginous nodules are often present. The tumour is usually encapsulated and some of the compressed normal testis may remain, particularly at the upper pole.

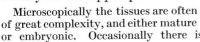

FIG. 844.—Teratoma of the testis containing solid and cystic areas.

Microscopically the tissues are often of great complexity, and either mature or embryonic. Occasionally there is remarkable differentiation, such as ciliated epithelium, non-striated muscle, intestinal epithelium, or thyroid tissue. A usual appearance is a mixture of lymphatic tissue, cartilage, and cysts, lined by squamous or cubical epithelium. Less commonly the cells are those of an undifferentiated carcinoma.

The tumour arises in the rete testis from toti-potent germ cells ; accordingly elements of hypoblast, mesoblast, or epiblast are often represented. Usually one of these predominates and attains malignancy. The most malignant teratoma is the chorion-epithelioma, which often gives rise to massive secondary deposits, while the primary tumour is so small that it is easily overlooked or impalpable. The least malignant is a dermoid containing sebaceous material and hair, but part of the tumour is usually solid and consists of cartilage, bone, and nerve tissue. Dermoid cysts are present at birth and grow slowly. Both chorion-epitheliomata and dermoid tumours are very rare.

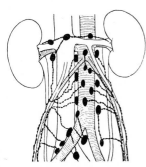

FIG. 845.—The lymphatic nodes into which the lymph from the testis drains.

(*After Jamieson and Dobson.*)

Spread.—Neoplasms of the testes metastasise in the following ways :

(*a*) Along the lymphatics of the spermatic cord. These lymphatic vessels drain into the lymph nodes situated along the aorta, from and including its bifurcation, to the level of the renal arteries (fig. 845). Secondary metastases in these retro-peritoneal lymph nodes often attain a considerable size. From the nodes around the renal pedicle lymphatic drainage is to the mediastinum, and from thence to the supraclavicular fossa.

(*b*) By way of the spermatic veins to the lungs.

(*c*) To the inguinal lymph nodes. This is rare, and only occurs when the scrotum has become infiltrated by the growth.

Clinical Features.—Clinically, there is no difference between the majority of seminomas and teratomas of the testis, although the age at which the growth appears is suggestive. Teratomas usually appear between twenty and thirty years of age, while seminomas are most often encountered between thirty and forty (fig. 846). Various clinical types are met with :

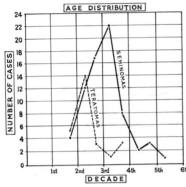

FIG. 846.—The age incidence of teratomas and seminomas of the testes.
(*T. M. Prossor's statistics.*)

1. **The Average.**—The patient states that he has noticed a swelling for several months, and it is increasing in size. In over 20 per cent. of cases there is a history of injury. It is generally conceded that injury merely calls attention to the testicular enlargement, and does not initiate the neoplasm. There is no pain in the early stages, but a sensation of weight is complained of when the testis has reached two or three times its normal size. Local pain is present in half the cases of some standing.

On Examination.—The body of the testis is found to be enlarged ; it tends to retain its normal shape and is hard, smooth, and heavy. Later one or more softer bosses may be palpable. Testicular sensation is lost early, but its presence depends upon the amount of normal testicular substance that remains. When a secondary hydrocele is present it is usually lax, and does not obscure the enlarged testis. Tapping the hydrocele should be avoided if enlargement of the testis can be determined without this measure. The epididymis is normal at first ; later it becomes so flattened or incorporated in the growth that it is imperceptible. The spermatic cord remains normal for a considerable time. It then becomes thickened, due to cremasteric hypertrophy and enlargement of its veins.

The vas is never thickened. Rectal examination reveals no abnormality in the prostate or seminal vesicles.

Next the sites of possible metastases (fig. 845) should be examined. The abdomen is palpated for secondary retro-peritoneal deposits, their most usual situation being just above the umbilicus on the same side, the opposite side, or both sides. The left supraclavicular region should be examined. A radio-graph of the thorax is essential.

2. **The predominant symptoms are due to metastases :** (*a*) the patient complains of abdominal or lumbar pain, and on examina-tion a mass is found in the region of the pancreas. (*b*) The patient, usually in the younger age group, complains of pain in the chest, dyspnœa, and perhaps hæmoptysis. Radiography shows multiple, rounded metastases of both lungs.

In either case the enlargement of the testis may not have been noticed by the patient, and is found at the clinical examination.

3. **More Exceptional Cases.**—The course of the disease varies very greatly. (*a*) In a few cases the neoplasm grows very slowly, the patient having noticed an increasing enlargement of the testis for years. (*b*) At the other end of the scale, in a matter of six or eight weeks the tumour rapidly increases in size, and radio-resistant metastases bring about a fatal termina-tion in a matter of weeks—the hurricane type (Gordon-Taylor). (*c*) A tumour in an imperfectly descended testis occurs in 14 per cent. of all cases of malignant disease of the testis. The testis is usually situated in the inguinal canal or in the superficial subinguinal pouch. More rarely it is within the lower abdomen. In a few instances the growth has appeared after the testis has been reposed in the scrotum by orchiopexy. (*d*) Gynæcomastia, either unilateral or bilateral, is a very rare accompaniment of testicular neoplasm. When it occurs the growth is usually a chorion-epithelioma, or other very highly malignant tumour.

Differential Diagnosis.—A gumma of the testis often presents symptoms and signs indistinguishable from those of a neoplasm, and a positive Wassermann reaction does not necessarily rule out the latter condition. An old clotted hæmatocele (fig. 847) also simulates a neoplasm in every respect clinically. Tuber-culosis in an anteverted testis may cause difficulty, but thicken-ing of the vas and involvement of the seminal vesicle is also often present, when chronic infection can be diagnosed with

Sir Gordon Gordon-Taylor, Contemporary. Consulting Surgeon, Middlesex Hospital, London.
August von Wassermann, 1866–1925. Director of the Institute for Experimental Therapy, Berlin.

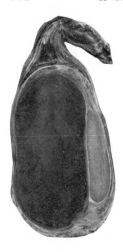

FIG. 847.—An old clotted hæmatocele. The long-standing pressure has flattened the testis.

certainty. Malignant disease of the epididymis occurs occasionally, and is usually diagnosed as tuberculosis in the first instance. Increase in size of the epididymis without involvement of the vas and the vesicle should favour early operation. As a rule the diagnosis can only be made on histological examination.

Hormone tests of the urine are very unreliable, and are often negative in early cases, and sometimes in late cases with metastases. In several reported cases the test has been positive in non-malignant intrascrotal swellings. A high positive reading (over 1,000 mouse units) when present is confirmatory evidence of malignant testis. In cases of chorion-epithelioma very high estimations (over 10,000 mouse units per litre of urine) are nearly always obtained.

Treatment :

Orchiectomy.—An incision is made over the inguinal canal and the upper part of the scrotum. The external oblique is incised, and the spermatic cord is doubly ligated and divided between the lower ligature and the hæmostat. The testis, with its coverings, is then excised. It is highly important to ligate the cord before manipulating the testis.

While the patient is under the anæsthetic the opportunity should be taken of palpating the relaxed abdomen for metastases.

Post-operative irradiation should be given in all cases. Not all seminomas are radio-sensitive and not all teratomas radio-resistant. It is not yet possible to determine beforehand, histologically or otherwise, which tumour will respond, except to state that chorionepithelioma and other tumours associated with a high output of gonadotropic hormone are unlikely to do so. Two courses of radiotherapy are given as a prophylactic measure ; more may be required in cases with established secondary deposits. The first course, delivered over thirty days, is to the lower para-aortic and iliac lymph nodes, both anteriorly and posteriorly, a total dose of 2,500 r being given. Six weeks later the upper para-aortic nodes also receive a similar dose.

Prognosis.—Patients in the fourth decade of life have the

best chance of prolonged survival. A history of pain is unfavourable. Seminomas, as a class, are accompanied by a better
prognosis than teratomas. When orchiectomy followed by
irradiation is carried out *before* metastases are demonstrable,
the five-year survivals are approximately 65 per cent. in cases
of seminoma, whereas in the case of teratoma they are between
45 and 55 per cent. Of all cases with metastases, about 15 per
cent. are alive after five years.

MALE STERILITY

The causes of male sterility are
as follows :

1. **Impotence.**—Inability to perform the sexual act may be due
to (*a*) Malformations or loss of
the penis. (*b*) Psychic causes, for
further information on which works
on sexual psychology should be
consulted.

2. **Absence of Spermatozoa in
the Semen.**—A cryptorchid is
usually potent, but sterile. Prolonged X-ray exposure is among
the causes of azoöspermia.

3. **Aspermia.**—Because of a
mechanical fault in the male
conducting apparatus, the semen
may not reach the vagina. Leading examples are a urethral fistula,
a tight stricture, and obliteration
by scar tissue of the lumina of both
vasa deferentia or both common

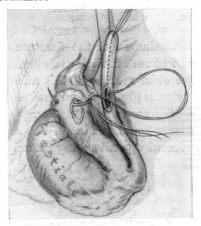

FIG. 848.—Vaso-epididymal anasto-
mosis with stainless-steel wire. (*Michelson.*)
(*Reproduced from " Surgery, Gynecology and
Obstetrics.*")

ejaculatory ducts. The commonest cause of male sterility is bygone
epididymitis, with its aftermath of cicatricial
obliteration of some part of the lumen of
the vas. When other means have failed,
operation (fig. 848) is occasionally successful.
By means of sutures of the finest wire the
epididymis is anastomosed to a healthy
portion of vas above the stricture.

THE SCROTUM

Sebaceous cysts are common in the skin of
the scrotum and are usually small and multiple
(fig. 849). Sometimes a large sebaceous
cyst suppurates, and when it does so the
odour emitted is particularly obnoxious. We
have seen a suppurating scrotal sebaceous
cyst mistaken for malignant disease, which
calls to mind Cock's peculiar tumour (see
p. 829).

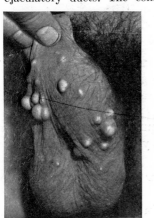

FIG. 849.—Sebaceous cysts of
the scrotum.

Edward Cock, 1805–1892. Surgeon, Guy's Hospital, London.

Idiopathic Gangrene of the Scrotum (*syn.* Fournier's gangrene).— Arises without apparent cause—first involving the scrotum, then extending along those planes so well known in urinary extravasation. The entire scrotal coverings slough, leaving the testes hanging exposed, bared to their tunica, though remarkably free from gangrene. The organisms responsible are varied, the most usual being a mixture of streptococcus, staphylococcus, and anærobic organisms.

Treatment.—Hot moist dressings of weak potassium permanganate solution are applied. Streptomycin preferably, or penicillin and sulphonamide, are administered. The gangrenous area is excised when demarcation occurs. If the infection spreads above the pubes, early incisions through the skin and superficial fascia are required. Even when the loss of scrotal skin is great enough to expose the testes, spontaneous healing usually occurs. Occasionally skin grafting is necessary. The mortality, formerly high, has been greatly reduced by antibiotic treatment.

Carcinoma of the Scrotum.—In days gone by this disease was almost confined to chimney-sweeps. At the present time the chief victims of this affection are mule spinners in cotton factories (fig. 850), and workers in tar, shale oil, and its products. Owing to improved factory conditions, there is a decreased occupational incidence, but occasionally the condition appears without a predisposing factor.

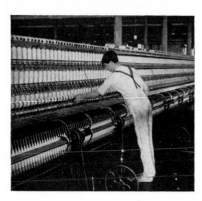

FIG. 850.—A mule spinner at work.
(*A. H. Southam.*)

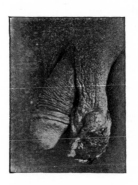

FIG. 851.—Carcinoma of the scrotum.
(*Macewen's "Textbook of Surgery."*)

Clinical Features.—The growth commences in a wart or an ulcer (fig. 851). As it advances it may involve the underlying testis.

Treatment.—The growth, together with a considerable margin of healthy tissue, is excised. The lymph nodes are treated in the same way as described in carcinoma of the penis.

Elephantiasis of the scrotum is confined to dwellers in tropical and subtropical countries, and is due to obstruction of the lymphatic vessels of

Jean Alfred Fournier, 1832–1914. Founder of the Venereal and Dermatological Clinic, St. Louis Hospital, Paris.
Chimney-sweep's cancer was first described by Percival Pott, 1714–1788. Surgeon, St. Bartholomew's Hospital, London.

the pelvis by filaria sanguinis hominis, with superadded infection and lymphangitis. The earliest manifestation is an attack of funiculitis with the development of a secondary hydrocele. Repeated attacks cause the scrotum to remain œdematous and the scrotal skin and subcutaneous tissue greatly thickens. In long-standing cases the scrotum becomes immense, and the penis is buried within it (fig. 852).

Treatment.—There is no medical treatment for the condition. Excision is carried out by making a circular incision around the neck of the scrotum through skin only. Two cutaneous short flaps are cut, one anteriorly extending from one external abdominal ring to the other, and one posteriorly. Very numerous blood-vessels are ligated. The base of each spermatic cord is exposed by making an incision over it, and isolated by a gauze loop passed beneath it. The root of the penis is likewise isolated. After applying powerful clamps to each half of the neck of the scrotum behind these structures, the testes are dissected from the mass and the hydroceles are incised and inverted. The penis is dissected from the tunnel it occupies, sparing, if present, the prepuce. The mass is cut away proximal to the clamps, securing bleeding vessels as they occur.

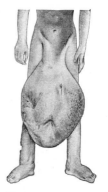

Fig. 852.—Filarial elephantiasis.
(*After Sir Frank Connor.*)

As a rule, sufficient normal skin is present in the flaps to fashion a new scrotum, which must be drained. If there is insufficient skin, the testes are implanted into the subcutaneous tissue of the thighs. In cases where the bared shaft of the penis cannot be covered by healthy prepuce, skin grafting is performed subsequently.

CHAPTER XXXII

THE SKIN

CALLOSITIES, CORNS, AND WARTS

A *callosity* is a localised hyperkeratosis due to prolonged pressure or friction. They are commonly occupational, e.g. a gardener's hands or the fingers of a violinist. In other cases they form over bony prominences, such as a hammer-toe. A callosity presents itself as a horny plaque which is yellowish-brown in colour. It is symptomless unless it occurs on the sole, in which case a callosity is often tender and causes discomfort on walking. If removal is desirable, the callosity can be shaved with a sharp scalpel or razor blade, or painted with collodion containing salicylic acid and ether (10 per cent. of each). Alternatively, a single dose of superficial X-rays (400 to 600 r.)[1] is often effective.

A *corn* (clavus) differs from a callosity in being more localised, and a horny plug of epithelial cells projects downwards into the corium. Pain is caused by the pressure of the horny plug on the sensory nerve endings. Hard corns occur over bony prominences, and are encouraged by ill-fitting boots. Soft corns result from maceration by sweat, and are found in the interdigital clefts. Plantar warts (verrucæ) are sometimes mistaken for corns, but warts are relatively soft and vascular.

Most corns yield to the chiropodist, provided that footwear is suitable. Skilled treatment is important in patients with diabetes or a poor peripheral circulation, as secondary infection may precipitate gangrene. Salicylic acid in collodion (20 per cent.) applied for a few nights, followed by soaking in hot water, is often effective in removing a corn. In obstinate cases the corn should be submitted to a single dose of superficial X-rays (1,000 r.).

A *wart* (verruca) is a localised overgrowth of the epidermis and papillæ, and is due to a virus infection. Verruca vulgaris,

---

[1] All radiations break up some of the molecules of the medium through which they pass into electrically charged particles. With a suitable circuit a measurable electric current is formed. The "r" unit is a physical one, and is that amount of radiation required to produce one unit of electricity as it passes through a unit volume of air.

the common wart, frequently occurs on the hands, particularly in children. They may grow as large as a pea, and are commonly multiple. The innumerable treatments recommended as " cures " indicate the uncertain effects of these remedies. As warts often disappear spontaneously, any treatment which is in use at the time will gain an undeserved reputation. The application of caustics, such as glacial acetic acid, phenol, or copper sulphate, all have their advocates. Curetting and cauterisation of the crater removes individual warts, but further crops may appear. X-ray treatment is often successful, and is usually administered in fractional doses of 100 to 200 r. at weekly intervals.

Verruca filiformis is a common disfigurement which appears on the eyelids, face, or neck in adults. It presents itself as a pointed excrescence, pinkish in colour, and some 3 to 4 mm. in length. If desired, they are snipped off with scissors and the base is touched with phenol applied on a sharpened matchstick.

Verruca plantaris occur on the sole and are usually multiple. They may be so tender as to render standing or walking exceedingly uncomfortable. They should be dealt with by curettage or superficial X-ray therapy. Radium should be avoided, as the resultant scar is sometimes tender, and necrosis of tissue may occur.

Venereal warts are discussed on p. 782.

ACUTE INFECTIONS

Boil (*syn.* furuncle).—A boil is due to infection of a hair follicle or sebaceous gland ; the offending organism is most commonly the staphylococcus aureus. A painful and indurated swelling appears which gradually extends. After two or three days the centre softens and a small slough is discharged with a bead of pus and in the large majority of cases the condition then subsides. A " blind boil " is one which subsides without suppuration.

A stye (*syn.* hordeolum) is due to infection of an eyelash follicle. Infection of a *perianal hair follicle* (perianal abscess) and consequent suppuration is likely to result in a blind external fistula. Furunculosis of the *external auditory meatus* is extremely painful, as the skin is attached to the underlying cartilage, and swelling is accompanied by considerable tension.

Complications of Boils :

(i) Cellulitis, which sometimes spreads extensively, especially in debilitated subjects.

(ii) Infection of the lymph nodes draining the affected part.

(iii) Secondary boils, due to infection of neighbouring hair follicles, or sebaceous glands.

Treatment consists in improving the general health of the patient, since boils are frequently associated with overwork, worry, debility, examinations, or other undermining influences. A small incision made into an indurated area is sometimes useful to relieve pain, but a firm elastoplast dressing is usually adequate and protects the inflamed area. Should softening occur around a hair follicle, particularly an eyelash (stye), removal of the appropriate hair allows the ready escape of pus. Penicillin, combined with chemotherapy if necessary, usually results in rapid improvement. Painting the surrounding skin with antiseptics, such as non-irritating dyes,[1] discourages the development of secondary boils. Local and general exposure to ultra-violet light is often advantageous, and fractional doses of superficial X-rays (50 to 100 r.) are valuable.

Carbuncle is an infective gangrene of the subcutaneous tissues, due to staphylococcal infection. It is uncommon before the age of forty, and men suffer more frequently than females.

Carbuncles often occur on the nape of the neck, as in this situation the skin is coarse and ill-nourished, and in some cases abrasions caused by a stiff collar encourage invasion by organisms (fig. 853). Carbuncles are especially liable to occur in diabetic

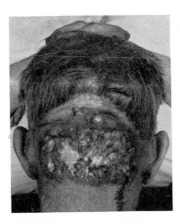

subjects, and the appearance of a carbuncle sometimes leads to the discovery of this disease. A blood-sugar curve will distinguish true diabetes from the transient glycosuria associated with the carbuncle.

The patient complains of tenderness and stiffness at the site of origin of the carbuncle. The subcutaneous tissues become painful and indurated, and the overlying skin is red. Unless the condition is aborted by

Fig. 853.—Carbuncle of the neck.

---

[1] A suitable paint is composed of mercuric chloride 1 per cent., malachite green 1 per cent., industrial methylated spirit 80 per cent., water q.s.

Carbunculus in Latin, Anthrax in Greek, is the word for charcoal. The Ancients saw in these conditions burning sores upon the skin—hence they likened them to charcoal.

prompt treatment, extension will occur, and after a few days areas of softening appear. The skin then gives way and thick pus and sloughs discharge. Infection sometimes extends widely, and fresh openings appear in the skin, and coalesce with those previously formed (fig. 854).

Carbuncles on the cheek or upper lip are particularly dangerous, owing to the risk of cavernous sinus thrombosis, via the facial and ophthalmic veins, or the deep facial vein and the pterygoid plexus (p. 130).

Treatment. — Penicillin is usually a specific remedy, and many carbuncles are aborted if penicillin is used in the early

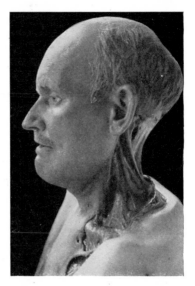

FIG. 854.—Extensive destruction of skin and subcutaneous tissue resulting from a carbuncle.

stages. Sulphatriad is also prescribed, bearing in mind that large doses are depressing in elderly patients. A paste composed of anhydrous magnesium sulphate (24 parts) and glycerine (11 parts) exercises a valuable osmotic effect if sinuses are present or sloughing has occurred. X-ray therapy yields good results ; it is applied either in one dose of 150 r., or in doses of 50 r. at intervals of two days up to 400 r.

These methods of treatment have rendered excision of a carbuncle, formerly much in vogue, rarely necessary, and surgical intervention is reserved for cases in which the carbuncle spreads rapidly in spite of treatment. Either the whole carbuncle, or else the portion which is spreading, is excised, preferably with a diathermy knife, and the wound is packed with gauze soaked in 1 : 1,000 flavine.

Attention is directed to improving the resistance of the patient by such means as fresh air, heliotherapy, vitamin B complex, and tonics including iron.

Small carbuncles are effectively treated by covering them firmly with elastoplast, which is untouched for some days.

For Carbuncles on the face, see p. 130.

CHRONIC INFECTIONS

Cutaneous tuberculosis is commonly seen in the form of lupus vulgaris. This disease usually occurs between the ages of ten and twenty-five, the face being the site of election for its commencement. One or more subcutaneous nodules appear, with congestion of the surrounding skin. On applying pressure with a glass tongue depressor the nodules are seen to be the colour of apple jelly. Induration spreads, and the skin is likely to ulcerate (fig. 855). The resulting ulcer tends to heal in one situation

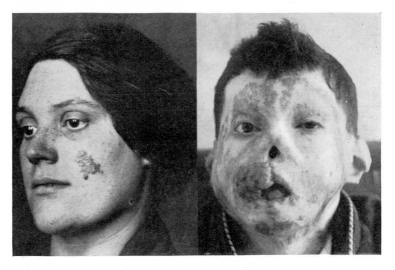

FIG. 855.—Early lupus vulgaris showing subcutaneous nodules.   Advanced lupus vulgaris. Carcinoma has developed on the upper lip.

as it extends to another. The healed portion is covered with a thin layer of epithelium, which is likely to re-ulcerate. The corresponding lymph nodes are liable to become affected by superimposed secondary infection, or less commonly by tubercle bacilli. The mouth and nose are sometimes attacked, either primarily or by extension from the face. Infection of the nose is followed by necrosis of underlying cartilage.

Treatment is directed towards improving the general health, and the administration of calciferol.

Local treatment, in the early stages, consists in exposure of the affected part to some variety of intensified light. A Finsen or mercury vapour lamp gives good results in the absence of ulceration, but prolonged treatment is necessary. When the

Robert Koch, 1843–1910. Professor of Bacteriology in Berlin; discovered the tubercle bacillus in 1882.
Niels Ryberg Finsen, 1860–1904. Danish physician ; founder of artificial heliotherapy ; received Nobel Prize for Medicine, 1903.

skin has ulcerated X-ray therapy is indicated, and cure is sometimes hastened by curetting the ulcer or scraping out persistent
nodules. Epithelioma is prone to occur in a lupus scar (p. 823).

Lupus verrucosis (*syn.* verruca necrogenica) is a tuberculous lesion of the skin, in which a circumscribed area becomes
irregularly nodular and indurated. The corresponding lymph
nodes are frequently affected, and present the usual features
of tuberculous nodes. When the condition is very localised it
resembles a wart, and the terms " anatomical tubercle " and
" butcher's wart " have been applied. The most expeditious
treatment is to excise the patch of affected skin and any
lymph nodes which are involved.

Tuberculin Tests.—As with suspected tuberculous disease in any part
of the body, skin tests are of some value (especially if negative) in establishing a diagnosis. Protein products derived from the tubercle bacillus
are either applied to the skin (Mantoux) or inoculated through a scratch
(von Pirquet). If positive, a reaction occurs in either test in forty-eight
hours, and lasts from one to four weeks.

Bazin's disease (*syn.* erythema induratum) is probably a tuberculous
condition which particularly affects adolescent girls. Symmetrical
purplish nodules appear, especially on the calves, and gradually break
down to form indolent ulcers, which leave in their wake pigmented scars.
The condition slowly responds to rest and general treatment.

NEW-GROWTHS

Papillomata are common tumours (p. 50).

Hereditary hæmorrhagic telangiectasis is a rare familial disease. It
is characterised by widespread development of telangiectases which tend
to bleed. Hæmorrhages from the gastro-intestinal tract may lead to
errors of diagnosis, but the cutaneous lesions and family history should
prevent mistakes. Bleeding from accessible tumours is controlled by
cautery or radium.

Basal-cell carcinoma (*syn.* rodent ulcer) commences in the
basal cells of the skin or in the cells of the sebaceous glands.
It rarely occurs before middle age, and is commoner in males.
Over 90 per cent. occur on the upper two-thirds of the face
(p. 143), and those which present themselves elsewhere are
often neglected by the patient in the early stages. At first the
growth appears as a pearly nodule, with one or two venules on
the surface. The epidermis is then eroded, and a small circular
or oval ulcer appears. As the ulcer extends, surrounding skin
is destroyed, and finally the deeper tissues and bone are invaded,
and air sinuses or even the dura mater are exposed (fig. 856).

A typical rodent ulcer presents the following features. The
edge is raised or beaded but not everted, as is the case with an

Charles Mantoux, Contemporary. Physician, Le Cannet, France.
Clemens Freiherr von Pirquet, 1874–1929. Professor of Children's Diseases, Vienna.
Pierre Antoine Ernest Bazin, 1807–1878. Dermatologist, Hôpital St. Louis, Paris.

epithelioma (fig. 857).   The floor is granular, and is occasionally covered by a thin layer of epithelium which extends over it from the adjacent margin.   This attempt at healing is merely temporary.   The base is less indurated than in the case of an

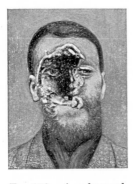

Fig. 856.—An advanced stage of rodent ulcer.

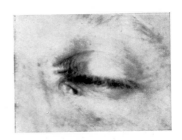

Fig. 857.—Early rodent ulcer, showing the typical rolled and beaded edge.

epithelioma, but secondary infection adds to the degree of induration.   Metastases do not occur, and lymph nodes are only enlarged as a result of secondary infection.

Microscopic section reveals masses or columns of epithelial cells which tend to spread in a lateral direction rather than downward, as in a carcinoma.   The cells vary in size and shape ; usually the peripheral cells are columnar, and arranged in a more or less definite layer.   The central cells are smaller and polyhedral, and although a few prickle cells are sometimes seen, cell nests are practically absent, owing to lack of keratinisation. Degeneration of central cells results in the formation of small cystic spaces.

Treatment.—Excision yields good results, but owing to the fact that most rodent ulcers occur on the face, this line of treatment is not often advisable, but should the lesion be situated on the trunk, limbs, or forehead, excision removes the ulcer in a satisfactory manner and the wound heals rapidly.

Formerly small ulcers or suspicious nodules were destroyed by carbonic acid snow, but this method has been replaced by radiotherapy.   For small lesions superficial X-rays (3,000 r. single dose), radium or radon (6,000 r. in three to four days) are equally good.   For large ulcers, daily fractional X-rays (5 × 1,000 r.)

may be used, but radium and radon, in the form of plaques or implants, give the best results except where bone or cartilage is invaded, in which case X-rays give a more uniform dose throughout the lesion.

If bone or cartilage is involved, surgical removal of the diseased tissue is usually advisable, as radiotherapy may cause necrosis.

Squamous-celled carcinoma (*syn.* epithelioma) presents itself either as a malignant papilloma, or a malignant ulcer, but there is no essential difference between the two types. They usually occur on exposed surfaces, especially in men whose occupation entails contact with irritating substances, such as dyes or tar (fig. 858) or whose skin is subjected to prolonged exposure to sun and wind, e.g. farmers and sailors. Occasionally it is seen in children who are so sensitive to light that they develop xerodermia pig-

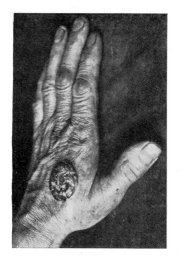

FIG. 858. — Squamous-celled carcinoma. The patient was a chemical worker.

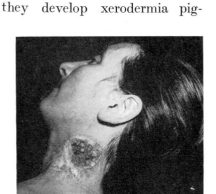

FIG. 859.—X-ray scar of the neck in which carcinoma has developed. (Marjolin's ulcer.) (*Professor Rendle Short.*)

mentosa, and in albino negroes in the tropics. Cancer of the scrotum is described on p. 814. Epithelioma occasionally develops on an old scar, especially if deficient in vitality or irritated by friction. Scars of old lupus are especially prone to malignant change, which is encouraged by the irritation of the otherwise remedial light or X-ray therapy (fig. 855).

An epithelioma which develops in a scar (*syn.* Marjolin's ulcer) (fig. 859) presents the following characteristics :
(i) It grows slowly, as the scar is relatively avascular.

René Marjolin, 1812–1895. Surgeon, Hôpital Sainte-Eugénie, Paris.

(ii) It is painless, as scar tissue contains no nerves.

(iii) Secondary deposits do not occur in the regional lymph nodes, as lymphatic vessels have been destroyed. When the ulcer eventually invades normal tissue surrounding the scar, it extends at a normal rate, and lymph nodes are then liable to be involved.

A typical epitheliomatous ulcer is irregular in outline, the edges are raised and everted. The base is indurated, and sooner or later becomes attached to the deeper structures. A sanious discharge occurs, which is increased in amount with the advent of secondary infection. The regional lymph nodes are involved, and are liable to undergo mucoid degeneration, to which secondary infection is often added.

Treatment.—If the situation of the ulcer allows such a procedure, wide excision is indicated ; the corresponding lymph nodes are removed either at the same time or at a subsequent operation.

In situations where excision is likely to lead to deformity, such as the orbital region, radiotherapy yields excellent results. The regional lymph nodes are removed if possible, but, if fixed, some degree of regression is obtained by radiotherapy. If radiotherapy is suitable, either radium or X-rays give good results, but short-distance low-voltage X-ray therapy (contact therapy) is preferable for small lesions, as its application is simple, and its effect localised. Also the time required for treatment is short, hospitalisation is avoided, and many patients can be treated with a minimum of expense.

Whether surgery or radiotherapy should be employed depends on the condition of the patient, and the size and attachments of the tumour. It is important that the treatment is adequate, otherwise the activity of the tumour may be stimulated, and metastases encouraged.

SEBACEOUS GLANDS

Sebaceous adenomata arise in connection with a sebaceous gland or cyst. These are usually seen on the face or scalp, and occur as slowly growing, well-defined tumours, which are firm in consistency. They were formerly believed to be a precursor of rodent ulcer, but malignant changes are uncommon.

Removal is indicated if the adenoma is unsightly, troublesome, or increasing in size.

A sebaceous cyst (*syn.* a wen) follows obstruction to the mouth of a sebaceous duct, and is therefore a retention cyst.

Sir Astley Cooper, 1768–1841. Surgeon to Guy's Hospital; was knighted for successfully removing a wen from the head of King George IV in 1821.

It commonly occurs on the face or scalp (p. 829), but can occur anywhere except the palms and soles, which are devoid of sebaceous glands.

A typical cyst appears as a hemispherical swelling, firm or elastic in consistency, and with no definite edge. It is more or less adherent to the skin, especially if it has been previously inflamed, or is subjected to pressure. The punctum of the obstructed duct can sometimes be seen on the summit of the cyst, and sebaceous material may be expressed from the duct (fig. 860). An uncomplicated cyst contains yellowish-white material composed of fat and epithelial cells, of a putty-like consistency.

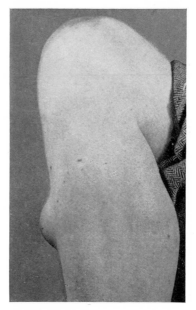

Fig. 860.—Sebaceous cyst of leg.

COMPLICATIONS

(i) *Infection.*—The cyst becomes enlarged and painful, and the overlying skin is red. After a few days the inflammation usually subsides, but recurrence is the rule. Recurrent attacks of infection cause the cyst wall to become adherent to surrounding subcutaneous tissue, and consequently more difficult to remove. The contents of an infected cyst become semi-liquid and often very foetid.

(ii) *Ulceration.*—An infected cyst occasionally breaks down and discharges its contents. A foul ulcerated surface remains, which superficially resembles a carcinoma, and to which the term Cock's " peculiar tumour " was formerly applied (fig. 861).

(iii) *Sebaceous Horn.*—The contents of a cyst sometimes slowly escape from the duct orifice and dry in successive layers on the skin. This " horn " is firmly attached at its base, and may grow several inches in length (fig. 862).

Removal of a sebaceous cyst is accomplished either by transfixion or dissection.

Edward Cock, 1805–1892. Surgeon to Guy's Hospital London.

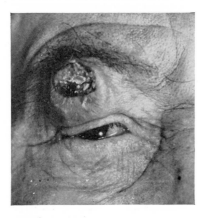

Fig. 861.—Cock's "peculiar tumour" on the upper eyelid.

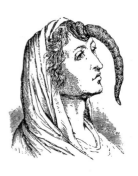

Fig. 862.—Sebaceous horn. (The owner, the widow Dimanche, sold watercress in Paris.)

Transfixion is useful if the cyst is not adherent. A bistoury is pushed beneath the cyst so as to emerge on the opposite side (fig. 863). The cyst and overlying skin are then divided.

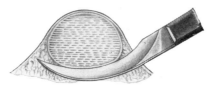

Fig. 863.—Transfixion of sebaceous cyst.

The contents are expressed and the cyst wall seized with artery forceps and avulsed, assisted by a few caresses with a scalpel.

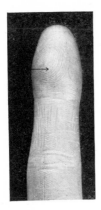

Fig. 864.—Implantation dermoid.

Dissection is necessary for cysts which have been previously inflamed or which are ulcerated. An incision is made over the cyst, the wall is defined, and if possible the cyst is dissected from adjacent tissue and removed intact. Unless the wall is completely removed recurrence is probable.

Implantation Dermoid (*syn.* implantation cyst).—These are due to the transplantation of squamous epithelial cells to the subcutaneous tissues by penetrating wounds, usually of a punctured nature. They are classically found in the fingers of women who sew assiduously (fig. 864). A painless, cystic swelling gradually develops, which is lined by squamous epithelium, and which contains débris that has undergone mucoid degeneration. They are readily excised.

AFFECTIONS OF THE NAILS

Paronychia is an infection of the cuticle, which is apt to extend beneath the nail-bed (see Chapter xxxix).

Ingrowing Toe-nail usually results from encasing sweaty feet in tight boots. The condition is encouraged by excessive trimming of the nail edges. As a result of pressure, the skin is displaced so that it overlaps the nail, and infection develops in

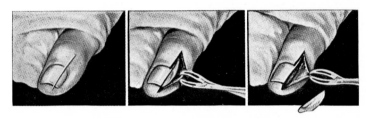

FIG. 865.—Wedge resection operation for ingrowing toe-nail.

the pocket thus formed. The established condition is surprisingly painful, and the patient can only limp. In the early stages relief of pressure, and meticulous daily packing of the pocket with a wisp of gauze soaked in a mild antiseptic, such as 1 : 1,000 flavine, usually prove successful. More advanced cases require wedge resection of the nail, overhanging skin, and

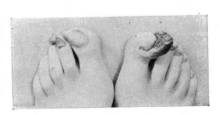

FIG. 866.—Onychogryphosis.

nail-bed (fig. 865). Even so, recurrence occasionally occurs, in which case the whole nail-bed is removed and the distal half of the phalanx is amputated. The toe pulp is turned upwards as a flap and stitched in position, and success is thus guaranteed.

Onychogryphosis is an overgrowth of a toe-nail, usually that of the big toe (fig. 866). It occurs in elderly people, especially if bed-ridden. Infection around the nail is an occasional complication. If necessary the nail and nail-bed are removed.

Subungual exostosis is considered in Chapter xli.

CHAPTER XXXIII

THE HEAD

THE SCALP

THE **scalp** consists of five layers—skin, subcutaneous tissue, epicranial aponeurosis (into which is inserted the occipito-frontalis muscle), a subaponeurotic areolar layer, and the pericranium. The scalp is well supplied with blood-vessels, and the walls of the arteries are adherent to the fibrous tissue in the subcutaneous layer. Therefore scalp wounds bleed freely, as the muscular coat of a divided artery cannot retract readily when the vessel is severed.

WOUNDS OF THE SCALP are treated by excision of the edges, the application of sulphonamide-penicillin powder, and suture with silkworm gut or braided nylon. In the case of tissue loss, a useful method of closing the gap consists in making a reversed " S " incision, by which means most defects in the scalp can be closed (fig. 867). Occasionally relaxation incisions are preferable (fig. 6).

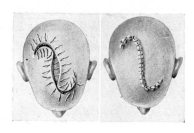

FIG. 867.

Owing to its rich blood-supply, wounds of the scalp heal readily, and portions of scalp which are avulsed retain their vitality in a surprising manner. Many cases are on record where the scalp has been avulsed almost completely, but after cleansing and suturing into position, union occurred in a satisfactory manner.

A HÆMATOMA OF THE SCALP situated under the epicranial aponeurosis spreads extensively, and is only limited by the attachment of the aponeurosis around the base of the calvarium. Should the hæmatoma occur under the pericranium, it is limited by the suture lines which border the underlying bone, and to which the pericranium is attached.

INFECTION OF THE SCALP is limited in a similar manner. If a wound involves the subaponeurotic areolar layer, infection is circumscribed only by the attachment of the epicranial aponeurosis, and may therefore extend from the superior curved line of the occipital bone behind to the supraorbital ridge in front, and laterally be bounded by the zygomatic arch, temporal ridge, and upper border of the mastoid process. Because extensive infection is possible, the subaponeurotic areolar tissue is sometimes termed the " dangerous area," and sinus thrombosis is liable to occur via the emissary veins. In the event of infection, chemotherapy is prescribed, and, if necessary, dependent incisions are made parallel to the main vessels and nerves, of sufficient depth to reach the areolar layer.

The following are the more important pathological conditions which affect the scalp :

Sebaceous cysts (*syn.* Wens), which are often multiple (fig. 868). If neglected, cysts may grow as large as hens' eggs, and when pressure interferes with the blood-supply to the overlying scalp the skin becomes bald.

Infection of these cysts is common, and when this occurs the contents are peculiarly putrid. Should the cyst break

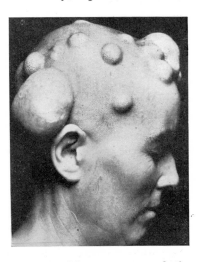

FIG. 868.—Sebaceous cysts of the scalp.

down, an ulcer results, formerly known as Cock's " peculiar tumour," which remotely resembles an epithelioma, but the edges are not everted, nor is the base indurated (p. 826).

Lipomata occasionally arise from the fatty tissue incorporated with the areolar layer, and therefore they lie under the epicranial aponeurosis. As they are only separated from the skull by the pericranium, pressure atrophy of the underlying bone follows in long-standing cases, and on pushing aside the lobulated edge of the tumour, the margin of a saucer-like depression in the bone is readily palpable (fig. 39).

Cirsoid aneurism is a rare condition, but of importance because of difficulty in treatment. It is due to dilatation of abnormal arteries, which open more or less directly into the veins. Capillary nævi are sometimes seen in the overlying skin. The

Edward Cock, 1805–1892. Surgeon to Guy's Hospital, London.

condition most commonly affects the superficial temporal artery and its branches, and as it increases in size the underlying bone becomes thinned, and the hair over the tumour falls out.   An X-ray may show perforations in the skull which indicate that part of the tumour is intracranial.   The tendency is for these tumours to enlarge slowly, so that eventually ulceration occurs and is likely to be followed by fatal hæmorrhage.

TREATMENT consists in extirpation of the tumour in the early stages.   If its size forbids such radical treatment, then the main vessels are ligated, often at successive operations.   Too long an interval must not elapse between operations, as collateral circulation is speedily established.   Ligation of one or both external carotid arteries is sometimes advisable as a preliminary step to local excision.

Dermoid cysts are most frequently seen over the external angular process (fig. 118).   They may not appear until the child is a few years old, and they occasionally communicate with the subdural space by a narrow neck, which passes through the underlying bone.   If such is the case, an impulse can sometimes be detected when the child coughs.   As this neck tends to constrict or close, it is wise to defer removal until after puberty, when there is less risk of opening the dura mater and the consequent possibility of meningitis.

Papillomata are common, and cause discomfort on combing the hair. Constant irritation of this nature, or the pressure of a hat, encourages the development of malignant changes.

Fibro-sarcoma has already been described (p. 60).

Epithelioma of the scalp is not common, and presents no special features.

Melanomata may be unrecognised, owing to the small growth being hidden by hair.   If malignant changes supervene, the appearance of secondary deposits should lead to the discovery of the tumour.

THE SKULL

Microcephaly is due to premature closure of the sutures ; the afflicted person is more or less an imbecile.   Removal of linear portions of the skull, or any other operation, is useless.

Macrocephaly is not necessarily associated with increased or diminished mental ability.

Oxycephaly (*syn.* Steeple head. Gk. oxus = sharp) is a condition in which the skull is egg-shaped following premature obliteration of sutures.   Most cases develop increased intracranial pressure, and blindness from secondary optic atrophy.   Tessellation of the skull, by making numerous trephine holes and connecting them with a Gigli's saw, is worth considering in cases of increasing intracranial pressure.

Scaphocephaly (Gk. skaphos = a ship) results from premature fusion of the sagittal suture. The forehead is tall, and the vault slopes downwards towards the occiput.

A meningocele is the protrusion of a pouch of dura mater through a congenital defect in the skull. The usual situations are the root of the nose, over the occipital bone, or in connection with the anterior fontanelle. Very occasionally they appear through the base of the skull, in which situation they have been mistaken for nasal polypi, and attempted removal has resulted in meningitis. A meningocele is present at birth, and forms a tense rounded swelling, which is translucent and sometimes pedunculated, and which occasionally yields an impulse when the child cries or coughs.

An *encephalocele* is a similar condition, but some portion of the brain is also extruded (fig. 869). Should this cerebral extrusion contain part of a ventricle, it is known as a *hydrencephalocele*. In this condition, and in an encephalocele, pulsation is usually present, but in many instances the child is still-born, or succumbs at an early age. Some degree of idiocy or deformity is likely to be associated with the misplacement of brain tissue.

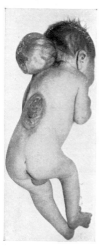

The **treatment** of a meningocele and of the conditions allied to it is primarily protection from injury and infection. Should the swelling increase in undue proportion to the child's natural growth, then an attempt should be made to remove it, and to close the cranial defect. Otherwise the enlargement will result in pressure atrophy of the skin and ulceration, followed by rupture and meningitis.

In the case of a small meningocele, growth of the skull may occlude the neck of the sac; in this case a cyst remains which is non-pulsatile and unaffected by coughing.

FIG. 869. — An encephalocele. A myelocele is also present.

INFLAMMATION OF CRANIAL BONES

Acute.—*Pericranitis* is likely to follow inflammation of the overlying areolar tissue. Necrosis of bone and thrombosis of emissary veins are troublesome and dangerous complications.

Osteomyelitis occurs as a result of :

(i) Direct infection, such as a compound fracture.

(ii) Local extension, as from the frontal sinus or mastoid antrum. Osteomyelitis occasionally results from an acute frontal sinusitis. The diploë is sometimes infected as a result of cellulitis of the scalp, and more rarely from an extradural abscess.

(iii) Blood-borne. As with acute osteomyelitis in any bone, an intraosseous extravasation of blood following trauma is liable to become infected by circulating organisms. Acute osteomyelitis of the skull is a serious condition. Infective thrombosis of emissary veins is likely to spread to the cranial sinuses, and meningitis and intracranial suppuration are other grave complications.

TREATMENT consists in the immediate administration of antibiotics. If infection occurs, or is already established, bone is excised, both tables being removed if intracranial infection is suspected. When acute infection abates, patience must be exercised to ensure that sequestra are separated before they are removed. When a probe indicates that a sequestrum is completely loose, the sinus is enlarged, and the dead bone lifted out.

Chronic.—*Tuberculous* disease of the skull is uncommon, but occasionally occurs in association with tuberculous lesions elsewhere. As with other bones, the infection commences either in the pericranium or in the medulla, i.e. the diploë. The diseased bone should be removed widely, otherwise abscesses are likely to form and erode the scalp. Secondary infection occurs at an early stage owing to the depth of the hair follicles.

Syphilitic pericranitis in civilised countries is now a rare affection. Localised swellings occasionally occur which are slightly tender and fixed to the bone. Under suitable treatment disappearance is usual, although a small bony swelling occasionally remains. Further stages are described in Chapter xliv.

NEW-GROWTH

Innocent tumours are rare. An ivory osteoma occasionally arises in the region of an air sinus or at the site of previous trauma (Chapter xliv).

Malignant new-growths resemble those of other bones. Pericranial sarcoma forms a bun-shaped tumour, the consistency of which depends upon its vascularity and rate of growth. Thus it may be pulsatile or of an almost bony hardness (fig. 870). Sarcoma or osteoclastoma very occasionally develops in the diploë.

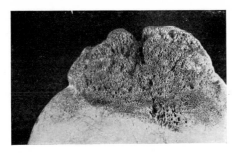

FIG. 870.—Osteosarcoma of the skull.

The commonest malignant tumour is secondary carcinoma. The breast, bronchus, and thyroid are most often the seat of the primary growth. Secondary growths of the skull are usually very vascular, and pulsate when the outer table is eroded. When examined casually they have been mistaken for sebaceous cysts, and attempts at removal cause considerable hæmorrhage !

FRACTURES

Vault.—These are caused by direct injury, indirect violence radiating from the base, or compression. This last cause operates when a degree of pressure is brought to bear on the skull which exceeds its limit of elasticity, and scalp is sometimes nipped by the fractured bone when the skull springs back to its former position.

Fractures of the vault are either fissured, depressed, or elevated.

(i) FISSURED.—A *simple* fissured fracture can only be definitely diagnosed by means of an X-ray. In every case of head injury which in the opinion of the surgeon may have been sufficiently severe to cause a fracture, a radiograph must be taken, partly as a guide to subsequent treatment, and also to show that " reasonable skill and care " has been observed, in the event of subsequent legal proceedings. The treatment of a fissured fracture is governed by the degree of associated injury to the brain. It usually suffices to confine the patient to bed for three weeks, and to add such length of convalescence as the mentality and occupation of the patient seem to require. This lengthy period is justified on the assumption that a force sufficient to fracture the skull must of necessity damage the brain. During this period of treatment, particularly in the early days, a careful watch is kept for the onset of such cerebral complications as compression or irritation.

Wilhelm Kónrad Roentgen, 1845–1923. Professor of Physics at Munich. Discovered X-rays in 1895.

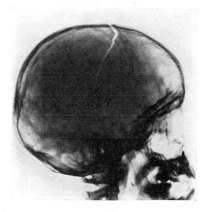

FIG. 871.—Fissured fracture of the vault. Complete recovery.

In the large majority of cases, in the absence of immediate complications, patients with simple fissured fractures make a complete and permanent recovery (fig. 871).

In about 5 per cent. of cases suffering from simple fissured fracture, subsequent complications develop. These include persistent headache, Jacksonian epilepsy, and mental deterioration. The complications are the result of injury to the brain at the time of the fracture, and are not likely to be prevented by operation. Surgical intervention is indicated only if clinical signs of increasing compression develop.

A *compound* fissured fracture has been mistaken for a normal suture line. A moment's reflection should be sufficient to decide whether the suspected lesion corresponds anatomically to a cranial suture, and furthermore, a suture line is irregular, and free from oozing blood. The majority of compound fissured fractures are visible at the bottom of the wound, but all scalp wounds should be explored adequately in order to exclude or discover a fracture.

As compound fissured fractures are potentially infected, emergency operation is necessary. The edges of the scalp wound are excised, and the wound rendered as aseptic as possible. The skull is opened with a small burr, which is placed in such a position that the bone to be removed incorporates the line of fracture. Any spicules of bone, loose fragments, or extradural clot are removed. If there is risk of subsequent infection owing to lapse of time since the injury, or to contamination of the wound, drainage should be provided. A prophylactic course of antibiotics is prescribed.

The prognosis of a compound fracture of the skull depends to some extent on associated injury to intracranial contents, and on the *integrity of the dura mater*. If this membrane is torn, a barrier to infection of the brain and meninges is removed, and inflammation of these structures is a grave possibility. Therefore, should a subdural hæmorrhage be revealed on opening the skull, the surgeon is called upon to decide whether the dura mater should be incised in order to evacuate the clot, or whether this procedure is unjustifiable on account of the risk of infection. No

John Hughlings Jackson, 1834–1911. Physician to the London Hospital.

definite rule can be laid down ; each case must be judged on its merits, and the graver risk, i.e. of compression or infection, avoided.

(ii) Depressed.—*Simple* depressed fractures are rare, as the scalp is relatively non-elastic, and an injury sufficiently severe to fracture and depress the bone is almost certain to lacerate the tough overlying scalp. A hæmatoma in the deeper

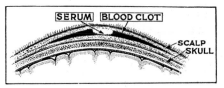

Fig. 872.—Hæmatoma simulating a depressed fracture.

layers of the scalp sometimes simulates closely a depressed fracture, as the blood clots round the periphery (fig. 872). On palpation, the margin of the clot resembles the edge of normal bone surrounding a depressed fracture, but the edge of the clot can sometimes be indented by the thumb nail. In the absence of intracranial complications no emergency treatment is required and an X-ray will distinguish the two conditions. The fracture, if present, is always much more extensive than is suggested by the radiograph.

The **treatment** of a closed depressed fracture depends on the extent of the depression and the site of the injury. Operation is not indicated if the fracture is small and no spicules which might pierce the dura mater are evident, provided that the affected site is not over an important cerebral area. Surgical interference is required if the fracture lies over the speech or motor areas, or if the X-ray suggests that spicules may have penetrated the dura mater, when a scar may form adhesions between the brain and membranes, with risk of subsequent epilepsy (p. 849).

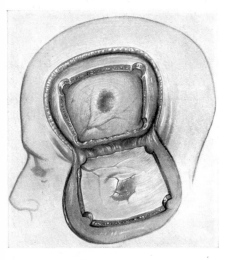

Fig. 873.—A depressed fracture exposed by an osteoplastic flap. Subdural bruising is revealed.

Operation.—Merely to trephine and elevate the depressed bone is quite inadequate, as a proper examination of the brain and membranes is not possible. An osteoplastic flap, which includes the fracture, is raised (fig. 873), and the depressed bone is either moulded into position or removed with suitable forceps. Attention is then directed to the dura, penetrating spicules are removed, and the membrane is then opened. The brain is inspected, and any exudate is removed or adhesions separated. If it appears that adhesions might re-form, it is wise to insert a sheet of cellophane between the brain and membranes. The flap is then replaced and the wound closed.

Pond-shaped depressions occur in infants, as a result of prolonged pressure of the head against the promontory during birth, or of direct injury during the first few months of life. If signs of compression are evident, or if no spontaneous elevation follows after a few months, the depression must be elevated.

The simplest method of performing this is by means of a guarded gimlet, i.e. silk is wound around the gimlet to within a quarter of an inch of its point. A small incision is made over the centre of the depression, and the skull is perforated by the gimlet. An aneurism needle is introduced through the aperture, and by this means traction is applied to the depressed bone. The elastic skull of the infant readily yields, and springs back to its normal position.

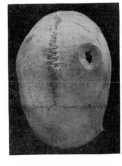

FIG. 874. — Skull found on the veldt in South Africa, showing depressed fracture, presumably compound. It was probably caused by a Zulu knobkerry.

Compound depressed fractures are the most common variety of injuries to the vault, but many are immediately or rapidly fatal, and so are of interest to the coroner rather than to the surgeon (fig. 874). Diagnosis is usually obvious, and if brain substance has escaped, it is unmistakable. Treatment is a matter of urgency, as infection rapidly becomes established. Operation is therefore undertaken as soon as possible, unless other injuries render the patient's condition so precarious that delay is advisable. The edges of the wound are excised and the deeper structures explored. If bone is completely detached, or grossly contaminated with dirt or foreign material, it is removed, otherwise the fragments are elevated, and the wound closed or drained according to circumstances. Antibiotics are prescribed.

HEAD WOUNDS DUE TO MISSILES

Improvised operations should not be performed, provided that the patient can be transported to a fully equipped hospital. Intracranial operations require preliminary X-rays and special apparatus, especially a continuous sucker. Local anæsthesia is not desirable, as patients are often restless or have other wounds which require attention. Pentothal is very suitable, and anæsthesia can be maintained by an intravenous drip of a 1 per cent. solution. Moist towels, wrung out in antiseptic solution, adapt themselves to the contour of the skull more readily than dry ones. Comatose patients require passive change of posture every few hours in order to prevent bed-sores, and incontinence necessitates frequent change of linen. Persistent post-operative restlessness is best combated by an intravenous injection of 3 ml. of undiluted paraldehyde, and tranquillity can be maintained by 1 ml. of this drug every 1 to 3 hours in an intravenous drip, according to requirements. Rehabilitation is essential, in order to minimise to the patient the importance of an injury to the brain, and he should be encouraged to undertake useful occupations as soon as his physical condition permits (Ascroft).

(iii) ELEVATED.—Elevation of a portion of the vault occasionally results from a blow with a heavy cutting instrument. Such fractures were not uncommon in former wars, when swords and cutlasses were used for other than ceremonial purposes. They are of necessity compound, and treatment is carried out on general principles.

Base.—Fractures of the base are caused by :

(i) *Direct Injury.*—The roof of the orbit is surprisingly thin, and has been perforated accidentally by umbrella ferrules, slate pencils, and other similar objects. A compound fracture of the base of the skull may result from discharge of a firearm through the mouth (as in cases of attempted suicide).

(ii) *Indirect Injury.*—A fall on the buttocks, or a blow on the jaw, sometimes transmits sufficient force to the base of the skull to cause fracture. Road accidents contribute a large number of cases. On rare occasions the condyle of the jaw is driven into the middle fossa.

(iii) *Irradiation.*—In some cases the fracture primarily affects the vault of the skull, and extends to the base.

(iv) *Compression.*—As in the case of the vault, a fracture of the base may be due to compression of the skull beyond its limit of elasticity.

Fractures of the base extend along the lines of least resistance, and therefore usually connect foramina. The line of fracture is deflected by buttresses of bone.

Clinical Features.—The essential features are :

(i) *Escape of cranial contents*, i.e. blood, brain, or cerebro-spinal fluid, which leaks along the torn dural sheaths of the nerves. Perilymph and endolymph escape if the fracture involves the internal ear, but are of no clinical importance.

(ii) *Injury to Cranial Nerves.*—All the cranial nerves are liable to be involved with the exception of the twelfth, as the anterior

P. B. Ascroft, Contemporary. Professor of Surgery, Middlesex Hospital, London.

condyloid foramen is protected by a stout ridge of bone, and the line of fracture is diverted into the foramen magnum.

Concussion, cerebral compression, and other injuries to the brain are not always associated with a fractured base, but are complications which commonly occur if the head injury is severe.

ANTERIOR FOSSA

(i) **Escape of Cranial Contents.**—Epistaxis occurs if the cribriform plate is involved. Should the fracture extend into the orbit, an effusion of blood follows.

This is distinguished from a " black eye " by the following features :
(*a*) The skin round the orbit is not damaged.

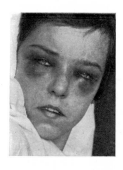

FIG. 875.—Fracture of the anterior fossa. Effusion of blood appeared twelve hours after injury. No bruising of skin.

(*b*) The orbital effusion occurs some hours after the injury (fig. 875).

(*c*) The eye is sometimes pushed forwards, as the extravasation occurs into the tissues at the back of the orbit.

(*d*) This extravasation impedes the action of ocular muscles, and movements of the eyeball are limited.

(*e*) Should subconjunctival hæmorrhage follow, the patch is wedge-shaped with the apex in front, and the posterior limit cannot be seen.

Cerebro-spinal fluid trickles through the cribriform plate, often in surprising quantities, a condition referred to as " traumatic rhinorrhœa."

Traumatic rhinorrhœa may persist for several weeks. Air may enter the cranial cavity when the patient blows his nose. In view of the ever-present risk of meningitis operative closure is indicated. By means of an intradural approach the rent in the dura is sealed with a patch of fascia lata, and the wound is closed.

Very occasionally, if the bone is extensively damaged, the brain extrudes into the orbit or nose.

(ii) **Injury to Nerves.**—The olfactory nerve is frequently torn, but unless its fellow is also damaged, the partial anosmia is likely to pass unrecognised. The optic nerve usually escapes injury even if the line of fracture passes through the optic foramen, on account of the relatively large size of this aperture. The third, fourth, first division of the fifth, and the sixth nerves may be involved as they pass through the sphenoidal fissure.

MIDDLE FOSSA

(i) **Escape of Cranial Contents.**—Epistaxis occurs if the fracture involves the basi-sphenoid. The muco-periosteum of the base of the skull, like that of the alveolar border of the jaws, is closely adherent to the bone, therefore a fracture is nearly always associated with laceration of the muco-periosteum, and is consequently compound.

Escape of cerebro-spinal fluid and blood from the ear is common. Slight bleeding originates from a torn tympanic membrane, or from separation of the bony and cartilaginous portions of the external auditory meatus. More serious hæmorrhage follows injury to the petrosal sinuses, the lateral sinus, or the middle meningeal vessels.

Brain substance very occasionally escapes through the ear or roof of the nose, and the prognosis is then gloomy.

(ii) **Injury to Nerves.**—The facial nerve is commonly injured at the time of the accident. In the majority of cases the involvement is only temporary, and is due to concussion, or extra- or intra-neural hæmorrhage. Occasionally the nerve is torn, and paralysis is permanent. In some cases paresis develops some weeks after the injury, owing to pressure on the nerve by fibrous tissue or callus. Spontaneous recovery in these cases is unlikely, but exploration may reveal a remediable condition. The eighth nerve is sometimes injured, in which case deafness follows. The sixth nerve, which passes across the middle fossa, is occasionally implicated, and internal strabismus results.

POSTERIOR FOSSA

(i) **Escape of Cranial Contents.**—Blood, cerebro-spinal fluid, or even brain may escape into the posterior part of the nasopharynx, through the basi-occiput. A common feature to be observed a few days after the accident is extravasation of blood in the suboccipital region. This appears either as a boggy swelling at the nape of the neck, or as a discoloration below the superior curved line, posterior to the mastoid process.

(ii) **Injury to Nerves.**—The ninth, tenth, and eleventh nerves are very occasionally damaged as they traverse the jugular foramen. As already stated, the hypoglossal nerve escapes injury, as it is protected by a bony buttress.

Treatment.—As in the case of all head injuries, the patient is confined to bed in subdued surroundings. Should epistaxis persist, dried blood is removed from the nose, penicillin and sulphonamide powder are insufflated, and the nares lightly packed with gauze moistened in a mild antiseptic. Escape of blood from the ear is treated on similar lines, except that a sterile pad is placed over the ear, as even light packing may obstruct the meatus and so predispose to cerebral compression. In very rare cases the flow of blood is so free and persistent as to indicate damage to a large vessel. The middle fossa is then explored through an opening in the skull above the ear, and efforts are made to deal directly with the bleeding sinus or artery, but the prognosis is almost hopeless.

HYDROCEPHALUS

Congenital hydrocephalus may be pre-natal, and so severe that labour is obstructed. It is due to obstruction of the cerebro-spinal fluid, and is usually associated with other abnor-malities. Other cases of so-called congenital hydrocephalus may be due to birth injury, and the arachnoid villi, through which cerebro-spinal fluid is absorbed, are obstructed by cor-puscles and extravasated blood (Cushing). Alternatively, organised blood may obstruct the circulation of fluid where it passes through narrow channels, such as the aqueduct of Sylvius or the foramen of Monro. The shape of the skull in the case of " congenital " hydrocephalus depends upon the stage of cranial development at the time of the onset of the condition. Should the exciting cause still be active after closure of the sagittal suture, the frontal and occipital regions are affected (fig. 876) ; if the lambdoid suture is closed when the disease commences, then bulging occurs chiefly in the frontal region. A ventriculo-gram shows the extent of ventricular dilatation (fig. 877).

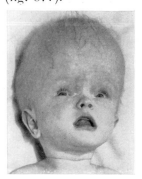

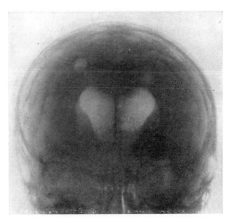

FIG. 876.—Congenital hydrocephalus.

FIG. 877.—A ventriculogram showing considerable dilatation of the ventricles. The " copper-beaten " skull is clearly shown.

François de la Boë (or Jacobus Sylvius, according to the Latinised form of his name), 1614–1672. Professor of Medicine, Leyden.

The **treatment** of this type of hydrocephalus is unsatisfactory, as is shown by the variety of operations which have been practised for its alleviation.

Such procedures as tapping a lateral ventricle, combined with elastic pressure or ligation of the common carotid artery, are useless. If ventriculography and the injection of 1 ml. of indigo-carmine into the ventricle indicate that the foramina in the roof of the fourth ventricle are obstructed, an attempt may be made to divide adhesions or to form an artificial foramen. Should the obstruction be at the level of the tentorial opening the fluid must either be short-circuited by opening the third ventricle so that it communicates with the subarachnoid space, or the choroid plexus is partially destroyed by transventricular fulguration, in order to diminish the amount of fluid secreted. Ventriculo-cisternostomy is sometimes indicated (p. 866). Operative measures are only justifiable in slowly progressive cases.

Acquired hydrocephalus may be due to over-secretion of fluid, inefficient absorption, or interference with the circulation. Two types result—obstructive or communicating.

Obstructive hydrocephalus follows interference with the circulation of the cerebro-spinal fluid. The commonest cause is a cerebral tumour, which, if situated in the mid-brain, is liable to compress the foramen of Monro or the aqueduct of Sylvius. Similarly a subtentorial tumour sometimes obstructs the foramina of Luschka or the fourth ventricle. Other causes are adhesions resulting from injury or inflammation. A rare congenital anomaly is the Arnold-Chiari malformation, in which a prolongation of the cerebellum extends into the spinal canal and so obstructs the return of fluid to the cerebral subarachnoid space.

Treatment depends on the cause. Tumours are dealt with according to circumstances. If adhesions are suspected, a subtentorial decompression is performed, and the cerebellum displaced upwards so as to expose the medulla. The cisterna magna is opened, and the bulging roof of the fourth ventricle incised. If no obstruction is demonstrated in the posterior fossa, the probable site is in the aqueduct of Sylvius. In such a case it may be advisable to remove the anterior wall of the third ventricle at a later operation, by the same route as for exposure of the pituitary gland.

Communicating hydrocephalus, in which there is no obstruction between the ventricles and the subarachnoid space, is due either to abnormality in the production or absorption of the fluid, or to obstruction to its circulation in the subarachnoid space. Otitis media or thrombosis of intracranial sinuses are predisposing causes. This condition is distinguished from obstructive hydrocephalus by manometry. Ventricular and lumbar punctures are performed, and different pressures are recorded in cases of obstruction, as distinct from communicating hydrocephalus, when manometric readings are approximately the same.

Treatment consists in dehydration by means of magnesium sulphate and restricted fluid intake, and lumbar puncture as required. Increasing pressure and threatened blindness necessitate a suboccipital decompression.

CEREBRAL INJURIES

The aphorism of Hippocrates that " no head injury is so trivial that it can be ignored, or so serious as to be despaired of " has been confirmed by succeeding generations.

Injuries to the brain include concussion, contusion, laceration, and compression. Frequently these co-exist.

Julius Arnold, 1835–1915. Professor of Pathological Anatomy, Heidelberg University.
Hans Chiari, 1851–1916. Professor of Pathological Anatomy, Strasburg University.
Hippocrates, 460–370 B.C. Established Greek medicine on a scientific and ethical basis.

CONCUSSION (*Syn.* STUNNING)

Theories.—(i) A blow on the head causes a momentary indentation of the elastic skull. This sudden reduction of the cranial capacity squeezes blood out of the skull, and a temporary cerebral anæmia results, with cessation of function.

(ii) Sudden reduction of the cranial capacity, and consequent pressure on the brain, compresses the cerebro-spinal fluid in the lateral ventricles. This is forced along the aqueduct of Sylvius, and a sudden wave of cerebro-spinal fluid impinges on the floor of the fourth ventricle, beneath which the vital centres are situated. This theory may be associated with the one above.

(iii) Punctate hæmorrhages are alleged to occur, but this theory introduces the possible features of compression also.

Clinical Features.—These vary with the intensity of the concussion, and include all grades of severity, from momentary dizziness to prolonged unconsciousness and death, although concussion alone is probably never fatal.

A summary of the features of a case of *moderate severity* is tabulated below, and for the purposes of comparison those of cerebral compression are included :

	Concussion.	*Compression.*
General condition	Unconscious, gradually regains consciousness, with, perhaps, cerebral irritation.	In a classical case concussion, then lucid interval, followed by increasing drowsiness and coma.
Appearance	Pale, with shallow respirations.	Flushed, respirations become stertorous and slow.
Pulse	Increased in rate and feeble.	Slow and " bounding." Rapid and feeble when cardio-vascular centre begins to fail.
Temperature	Subnormal.	At first raised on the side of compression.
Musculature	Relaxed, reflexes diminished or absent.	Varies on the two sides.
Sphincters	May be incontinent.	Become incontinent.
Pupils	Moderately dilated, equal, react sluggishly.	On side of injury, pupil contracts, and later dilates. The opposite side follows.

After a variable interval of unconsciousness, signs of reaction usually become evident, accompanied by photophobia. Respirations are deeper, the pulse increases in tension, and the face becomes flushed. The patient frequently turns on to his side, and the fact that he is in strange surroundings gradually dawns on his returning consciousness. Vomiting occurs as consciousness returns, and is due to cerebral hyperæmia, and consequent rise of intracranial pressure. Features of grave significance are the persistence of unconsciousness for more than twenty-four hours (this predisposes to pneumonia), a pulse which increases in rate and diminishes in tension, and pyrexia.

Treatment involves the seclusion of the patient in bed, with perhaps one low pillow. A cold compress is placed on the head and protected hot-water bottles round the body and limbs. Dentures are removed, and a catheter passed if necessary, as a full bladder promotes restlessness. The pulse is recorded at hourly intervals, and a careful watch kept for evidence of compression, which may develop with no intervening period of cerebral irritation. In cases of prolonged unconsciousness the patient should be nursed in the semi-prone position, the foot of the bed being raised, so that bronchial secretion and saliva can trickle out of the mouth. The feet are tied to the bed-rail by a bandage, to prevent the patient slipping up the bed (fig. 878). If coma persists for more than a few hours, associated compression is likely, and dehydration should be

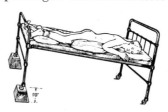

FIG. 878.—Coleman's postural drainage for the unconscious. The position is maintained by pillows, and bandages anchor the ankles to the foot of the bed.

practised (p. 858), so as to diminish cerebral œdema. Severe headache occasionally follows concussion, but it is usually relieved by the reduction of intracranial tension. In otherwise intractable cases a lumbar puncture is often effective.

A simple concussion recovers speedily, but in cases associated with cerebral contusion or other injury prolonged convalescence is needed, account being taken of the severity of the injury as measured by the duration of post-traumatic amnesia (P.T.A.). Also the mental make-up of the patient, the family history, and the amount of worry and concentration associated with his occupation deserve due consideration. The necessity for *supervised rehabilitation* is now widely and wisely recognised. This includes physical activity, occupational and mental exercises, and psychological encouragement.

CEREBRAL IRRITATION

is due to œdema, bruising or laceration of the cortex, and is particularly likely to follow falls on to the back of the head, in

Claude C. Coleman, Contemporary. Professor of Neurological Surgery, Richmond, Virginia.

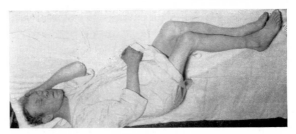

FIG. 879.—Cerebral irritation.   The patient has turned away from the light.

which the frontal lobes are damaged by *contrecoup.*

The patient is usually concussed for a variable period, and on his recovery he exhibits irritability of mind, and the body assumes a position of flexion (fig. 879).   Interference of any kind is resented verbally or even physically, and the patient remains curled up in bed, with the knees drawn up and the arms flexed. The temperature tends to be slightly but irregularly raised, and the pulse is normal in rate and low in tension, unless the condition is complicated by compression.   Improvement is indicated by a tendency for the patient to turn on the back, and to show an increasing tolerance to his surroundings.

Recovery may be apparently complete, but in these cases it is doubtful if the potential capabilities ever return to normal. More commonly some symptoms persist, such as irritability, depression, lack of concentration or judgment, and amnesia with reference to the accident or to events immediately before or afterwards.   In more severe cases dementia or other forms of insanity necessitate seclusion in a mental hospital.

Treatment demands a minimal amount of disturbance, but sufficient nourishment must be administered, and attention paid to the bladder and bowels, although excreta are often passed into the bed.   Sedatives are prescribed if necessary, and if tolerated, an ice-bag to the head is useful.   Dehydration by intravenous hypertonic solutions encourages absorption of cerebral œdema, and symptoms may thus be relieved.   The patient sometimes takes food if left by the bedside, and may use a urine bottle if one is left nearby within his field of vision.

CEREBRAL COMPRESSION

Compression immediately following trauma is due to depressed bone, extravasated blood, cerebral œdema, or a foreign body. If due to such conditions as depression of bone, evidence of compression is likely to follow the injury immediately. In other cases, such as compression following extradural hæmorrhage, concussion first occurs, followed by a period of improvement, after which the patient becomes drowsy, and lapses again into unconsciousness. Thus, an unconscious footballer was carried off the field of play, but recovered sufficiently to finish the match. Headache and drowsiness supervened, so that he retired to bed at an early hour, and later was found to be dead from middle meningeal hæmorrhage. Similar tragedies have occurred in police-stations, particularly as a head injury sometimes causes temporary excitement. Persons alleged to be drunk have been locked in cells, and the unconsciousness and stertorous breathing of compression mistaken for a drunken stupor. Therefore all cases of even minor concussion must be under observation for twenty-four hours.

If cerebral compression is due to middle meningeal hæmorrhage a boggy swelling is usually palpable in the temporal region, as the majority of cases are due to direct injury associated with fracture of the subjacent skull. Recognition of the resulting extracranial extravasation is valuable confirmatory evidence when middle meningeal hæmorrhage is suspected.

Middle meningeal hæmorrhage (fig. 880), although an uncommon condition, furnishes a typical example of compression ; the features of an established and classical case are as follows :

General Condition.—The concussed patient, after return of consciousness, becomes increasingly drowsy, and is more and more difficult to rouse. Coma follows, and unless the pressure is relieved, death is inevitable.

Appearance.—The face is flushed, and the facial muscles on the opposite side of the injury become paralysed, so that the cheek " flaps " as the patient

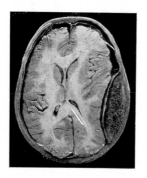

Fig. 880.—Extradural hæmorrhage, due to rupture of the middle meningeal artery.

breathes. Later both cheeks are paralysed. Respirations are deep, and when the palatal muscles are paralysed stertor follows. Breathing gradually becomes more difficult and laboured, and sometimes ends as Cheyne-Stokes's type.

John Cheyne, 1777–1836. A Dublin physician.
William Stokes, 1804–1878. Physician to the Meath Hospital, and Regius Professor of Medicine, Dublin.

Pulse.—The rate steadily falls, and the blood-pressure rises, so that the pulse is slow and bounding. This is due to efforts on the part of the cardio-vascular centre to maintain an adequate cerebral circulation. Eventually cerebral anæmia, due to the rising intracranial pressure, becomes so pronounced that the cardio-vascular centre fails. This is evinced by an abrupt rise of pulse-rate and lowering of blood-pressure, and death is then not long delayed.

Musculature.—Pressure on the cortex causes twitching and spasticity of the muscles of the face, arm, and leg on the opposite side of the body. As the pressure increases the motor cells are rendered anæmic and cease to function, so that the muscles innervated by them are flaccid and reflexes are lost. At the same time pressure is transmitted across the midline to the motor cells of the opposite side, and the consequent mild irritation causes spasticity of muscles on the side of the damaged vessel. As pressure of increasing intensity is transmitted across the brain, the cells on the opposite side of the injury cease to function, so that the muscles on the same side as the injury become flaccid (fig. 881).

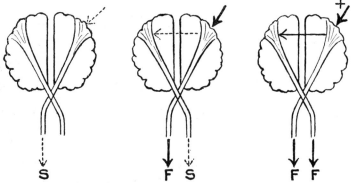

Fig. 881.—Diagram to illustrate effects of increasing unilateral pressure on the motor tracts. The dotted arrow indicates irritative pressure, and the dark arrow severe pressure. S = spastic, and F = flaccid paralysis.

Pupils.—Irritation of the third nerve causes the pupil on the side of the injury to contract. As pressure increases, paralysis supervenes, so that dilatation follows from unbalanced action of the sympathetic. Usually at this stage transmitted pressure to the other side causes irritation of the third nerve, so that the pupil becomes contracted. Eventually, increasing transmitted pressure causes paralysis of the opposite third nerve, and gradual dilatation supervenes, with finally dilatation and fixity of both pupils.

Temperature is sometimes unequal on the two sides of the body, being elevated on the opposite side to the injury. A sudden rise of temperature occasionally precedes death.

Sphincters.—As coma deepens, incontinence supervenes.

Treatment.—In any case of compression a careful examination must be conducted in order to determine the nature and site of the lesion. If possible a history is obtained of the details of any accident. The head is examined for evidence of injury or fracture, and the pupils and musculature may give some indication as to the site of the lesion. The localisation of the site of cerebral compression is often rendered difficult by *contre-coup,* i.e. bruising and laceration of the opposite side of the brain to the injury (p. 843). Damage to the brain as a result of *contre-coup* is frequently much more extensive than that which occurs at the site of injury. A lumbar puncture is sometimes of assistance in distinguishing extra- from intradural hæmorrhage ; in the latter case the cerebro-spinal fluid is likely to contain blood. A radiograph may localise the site of injury.

Surgical measures must be adopted without delay, appropriate to the type of injury. Depressed fractures are elevated, and efforts are made to discover and arrest intracranial hæmorrhage.

If it appears that the **middle meningeal vessels** are damaged, operation is undertaken as follows :

The head is shaved completely, and a point marked on the skull by means of a bradawl, either $1\frac{1}{2}$ or 2 inches (3·5–5 cm.) behind the external angular process, and above the zygoma. The actual measurement depends on the distance between the orbit and the ear, which varies considerably. This point lies over the anterior branch of the artery. It is wise at the same time to indicate the site of the posterior branch at the junction of two lines, one passing horizontally backwards from the upper margin of the orbit, and the other vertically upwards from the back of the mastoid process. A horse-shoe incision is made down to the bone, commencing $\frac{1}{2}$ inch (1·2 cm.) above the external angular process (to avoid the branch of the facial nerve which supplies the orbicularis palpebrarum and forehead muscles). The incision passes upwards for about 3 inches (7·5 cm.), and descends immediately in front of the ear. With a raspatory the scalp is separated from the skull, so that the teeth of the trephine will not be clogged with pericranium. The bradawl mark is identified, and the skull is opened with a $\frac{3}{4}$-inch (2 cm.) trephine or a burr. If the diagnosis is correct, blood-clot is encountered. This is disintegrated with a sharp spoon and washed away with saline, the opening being enlarged with nibbling forceps as necessary (fig. 882).

As the operation field is cleared the bleeding-point may be encountered, which is either the artery or vein. A fine, curved needle is passed under the vessel, carrying the thread with which both ends of the vessel are ligated.

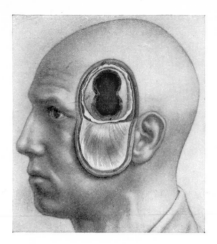

Fig. 882.—Middle meningeal hæmorrhage
(semi-diagrammatic).

Care must be taken not to pierce the dura mater, as cerebral veins are thin-walled and easily injured. Occasionally the vessel is found to be lying in a bony canal, which is then plugged with fibrin foam or a sharpened matchstick. Should no damaged vessel be found, the opening in the skull is enlarged downwards and forwards along the line of the artery, until the base of the skull is reached. If no bleeding-point is discovered and blood wells up from the middle fossa, it is probable that the base is fractured. Further attempts to find the bleeding-point should be abandoned in favour of ligation of the external carotid artery at the site of election, i.e. between the superior thyroid and lingual branches.

If no clot or hæmorrhage is displayed when the skull is opened, the opposite side should be explored. If no abnormality is revealed, the posterior branch on the original side is exposed by turning down a second flap behind the original one. The posterior branch is damaged in about 5 per cent. of cases.

The prognosis of middle meningeal hæmorrhage is poor, owing to the frequent association of other intracranial injuries. Failure of the dura mater to expand after removal of the clot is an unfavourable sign.

Intradural (*syn.* **subdural**) **hæmorrhage** sometimes results from laceration of cerebral veins or sinuses. The SUPERIOR CEREBRAL VEINS are those most frequently ruptured—a condition at least six times as common as middle meningeal hæmorrhage (G. C. Knight). The accident usually follows comparatively minor injuries in which the brain is jerked in an antero-posterior direction, e.g. a bump on the forehead. Symptoms may occur in a day or so, or be delayed for a few months, in which time a cyst develops. The cyst gradually increases in size as cerebro-spinal fluid is attracted to its interior by osmosis.

Persistent headache after a minor injury should always suggest the possibility of intradural hæmorrhage. If untreated, indefinite mental symptoms become increasingly evident, such as lack of concentration, inefficiency, and change of temperament. Increasing cerebral anæmia from pressure of the expanding cyst finally leads to torpor and coma. Localising signs are often absent, but the persistence of the headache after a slight injury demands exploration. Under local anæsthesia a small opening

G. C. Knight, Contemporary. Surgeon, West End Hospital for Nervous Diseases, London.

in the skull enables a diagnosis to be made, and permits of the evacuation of serum, or, in the later stages, of the contents of a cyst. If performed before the onset of stupor, the results are excellent.

Hæmorrhage from the *superior longitudinal sinus* is characterised by twitchings and spasms on both sides of the body, commencing in the lower limbs. This is due to pressure exerted by the extravasated blood interfering with the venous return from the upper part of the Rolandic areas, and as the congestion increases the spasms become progressively more widespread. If circumstances permit, the sinus is exposed and a piece of muscle is packed between it and the skull, so as to occlude the lumen of the sinus.

LATE EFFECTS OF BRAIN INJURY

After a severe head injury it is probable that the potential efficiency of the brain is always lessened. Such sequelæ as headache, neurasthenia, irritability, lack of concentration, impotence, epilepsy, etc., are common, and sometimes persist. In worse cases, such obvious mental deterioration follows that seclusion in a mental home is necessary. Impairment of sex function sometimes follows, varying from diminution of libido to complete impotence. One curious effect which occasionally follows a head injury is increased susceptibility to alcohol, and more than one unfortunate person has only discovered this when arrested for drunkenness after some very minor " celebration." Delayed apoplexy, described by Bollinger, may occur some weeks after injury. It is due to localised softening of the brain, and hæmorrhage occurs from a vessel in the degenerated area (fig. 883).

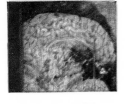

Fig. 883.—Cerebral hæmorrhage involving the occipital lobe. The patient was found dead in the street. Post-mortem showed that he died, not as a result of an accident, but from apoplexy.

Jacksonian epilepsy is due to local irritation of the brain, especially if a motor area is involved by a penetrating wound of the dura mater. Attacks of uncontrollable twitching occur, commonly in the hand or thumb. Twitching spreads to other groups of muscles, and eventually epileptic seizures develop, which are associated with unconsciousness. If medical measures fail, the affected area of the brain should be explored. Most commonly adhesions are found between the brain and dura. These are separated, any obvious scar is excised, and cellophane is inserted to prevent re-formation ; but only too often cortical fibrosis has already occurred, and the condition progresses. Idiopathic epilepsy is sometimes initiated by a head injury, but this condition can be distinguished from traumatic epilepsy by electro-encephalography.

THE BRAIN AND MEMBRANES

INFLAMMATORY CONDITIONS

Acute infective meningitis may result from compound fractures of the skull, osteomyelitis, or inflammation of an air sinus. In some instances the brain is inflamed in addition to the meninges. Blood-borne infections occasionally reach the meninges ; for instance, staphylococci in cases of acute osteomyelitis, or pneumococci following pneumonia.

The condition is ushered in with headache and vomiting. Severe consti-

Luigi Rolando, 1773–1831. Professor of Anatomy, Turin.
Otto Bollinger, 1843–1909. Professor of Pathology, Munich.

tutional symptoms follow, and if meninges over the convexity are affected, convulsions, delirium, and photophobia are in evidence. Should the base of the brain be chiefly involved, head retraction, papillœdema, and implication of cranial nerves are the main features. Lumbar puncture is performed in order to clinch the diagnosis and to identify the causative organism.

Treatment consists in dealing with any causative lesion, e.g. an infected middle ear. Lumbar puncture and intrathæcal penicillin administered daily (10,000 units) are valuable. Larger doses or more frequent injections irritate the cauda equina, and are apt to cause complications such as fits or retention of urine. Chemotherapy and antibiotics are administered according to the causative organism. If the patient survives the acute phase and a local abscess forms, this is drained provided that it is superficial, e.g. following a compound fracture. Deeper abscesses are aspirated as required and enucleated later (p. 852).

Extradural Abscess.—As in the case of abscesses elsewhere, an extradural abscess arises as a result of :

(i) DIRECT INFECTION, such as a compound fracture.

(ii) LOCAL EXTENSION from an accessory air sinus or the middle ear. In the case of the middle ear, infection most commonly reaches the extradural space by spreading through the tegmen tympani. Following a frontal sinusitis, a surprisingly large collection of pus may collect behind the frontal bone, infection having passed through the posterior wall of the sinus.

(iii) BLOOD-BORNE INFECTION accounts for a few cases. Thus the skull is occasionally affected by subacute osteomyelitis, and as a result an extradural abscess develops : the scalp in its turn becomes inflamed and œdematous. This condition was described by Percival Pott as a " puffy tumour," and a tender, œdematous, and adherent area of scalp, particularly if associated with cerebral symptoms, should raise the suspicion of an extradural abscess.

The SYMPTOMS of an extradural abscess depend upon its situation, size, and the rate at which it enlarges. Drowsiness, bradycardia, mental changes, and other evidence of cerebral compression are usual, and focal signs depend upon the site of the abscess.

Treatment consists in drainage, the method of approach depending on the cause of the abscess. If due to some pre-existing focus of infection, it is wise to deal with the cause, and follow the track along which infection has extended. Thus, if an abscess is apparently a complication of otitis media, the middle ear is explored, and the track of a sinus may thus be revealed.

Percival Pott, 1713–1788. Surgeon to St. Bartholomew's Hospital, London.

Similarly, local inflammation of the skull suggests a subjacent abscess if signs of intracranial infection supervene.

CEREBRAL ABSCESS

The usual cause of this condition is infection spreading from the middle ear or air sinuses. Less commonly such conditions as penetrating wounds, retained foreign bodies, or pyæmia cause a subacute abscess. On rare occasions the abscess is due to actinomycotic or amœbic infection.

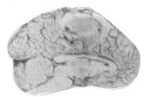

FIG. 884.—A cerebral abscess associated with bronchiectasis.

Abscess of the brain is an occasional complication of chronic pulmonary infection, such as bronchiectasis or empyema (fig. 884). In these cases the condition is usually of slow development, and the wall of the abscess may attain the thickness of up to ½ inch (1·25 cm.).

In the case of extension from the middle ear or frontal sinus, the inflammation usually spreads directly to the brain through the covering membranes, which become adherent to the bone. When the abscess is opened a layer of apparently healthy brain is frequently found between the cavity and the surface, in which case the infection has extended along the vessels entering the cortex. Occasionally an extradural abscess first forms, and if evacuation is delayed, infection is liable to extend through the membranes to the brain.

Clinical Features.—(i) *Signs of Infection.*—The temperature and pulse-rate are raised at the commencement, but as the abscess enlarges, so intracranial pressure rises also, with consequent lowering of temperature and slowing of the pulse. Therefore the chart frequently shows variations which depend upon whether infection or increased intracranial pressure is in the ascendancy. Leucocytosis is present, but its significance must be discounted if some other infective condition is also present.

(ii) *Increased Intracranial Pressure.*—Headache, irritability, drowsiness, and vomiting are commonly in evidence. Papilloedema, if it occurs at all, is a late sign, and is more marked on the side of the abscess. Bradycardia is variable, but is commoner than in the case of a tumour.

(iii) *Focal Signs.*—These depend on the site of the abscess. The more important signs are considered in connection with tumours (p. 854). In the case of abscesses due to otitis media, three out of five are in the temporo-sphenoidal lobe, and the remainder are in the cerebellum.

In every case of suspected cerebral abscess, it is obviously of great importance to examine all possible sources of infection. In many cases the probable cause of the mischief is evident, but it should be remembered that discharge from an ear may cease when intracranial complications develop. Also any hindrance to discharge, as by inspissated pus, predisposes to the extension of infection.

Treatment.—Drainage, formerly the recognised method of treatment of a cerebral abscess, has, in the majority of cases, been replaced by excision of the abscess after the acute stage of the infection has subsided (Northfield). For example, an abscess which complicates otitis media is no longer treated by opening the middle ear and enlarging the sinus until the brain is exposed, thus allowing evacuation of pus and drainage of the cavity. Neurosurgeons now regard the primary focus as of secondary importance, and means are taken to encourage the infection to localise. Localisation and subsequent enucleation diminish the risks of cerebral œdema and meningitis. Drainage is only indicated if the abscess is superficial, as in the case of one which follows a compound fracture.

In the early stages of cerebral inflammation antibiotics and chemotherapy are employed, and the infection may thus be overcome. If an abscess is suspected, a diagnostic burr-hole is made and aspiration may discover pus. In other cases ventriculography is useful, and if an abscess is disclosed by this method an osteoplastic flap should be reflected and the abscess aspirated. Progress is carefully observed, and if it is apparent that œdema is increasing, then further aspiration is necessary, with or without decompression. Aspiration is performed at intervals, and is combined with irrigation of the cavity. Electrolytic sodium hypochlorite (half-strength) is used, not only for its antiseptic properties, but also because it reduces the viscosity of pus and so permits more complete emptying of the cavity. When clear fluid is returned a small quantity of the antiseptic (5 per cent.) is injected into the cavity, so as to act as a bactericide and

D. W. C. Northfield, Contemporary. Neurological Surgeon, London Hospital.

also to stimulate fibrosis in the wall.   Thorotrast (1 to 2 ml.) is injected at one of the early aspirations, and a subsequent X-ray gives useful informa-tion concerning the size and precise posi-tion of the abscess (fig. 885).

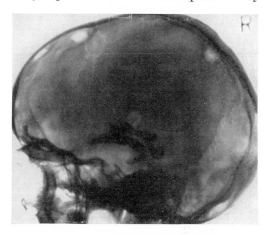

The abscess should be enucleated during the third month, as by then the wall is sufficiently tough to separate from sur-rounding brain tissue.   Too long a delay results in ex-cessive scarring around the cavity,

Fig. 885.—A temporo-sphenoidal abscess which was injected with thorotrast.   (*D. W. C. Northfield.*)

also the formation of loculi is encouraged.   Enucleation of a cerebellar abscess demands special care, as cranial nerves may be adherent to its wall.

INTRACRANIAL ANEURISMS

Two distinct types of aneurism occur:

(1) Congenital aneurism of an artery connected with the circle of Willis.   Leakage occurs, usually in early adult life, and causes a sub-arachnoid hæmorrhage.   A mild apoplectic fit, with ocular palsies, occipital headache and blood in the cerebro-spinal fluid, sug-gests the diagnosis.   An arteriogram is diagnostic (fig. 886).   If the patient survives, the hæmorrhage is likely to recur and may be fatal, so ligation and division of one common carotid artery should be considered after localisation of the aneurism by arterio-graphy (p. 101).   A more recent method of treat-ment is a direct attack on the aneurism, the neck of which is occluded with a silver clip.

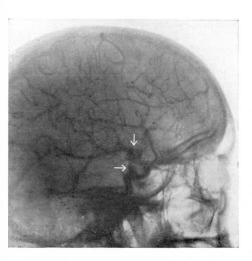

Fig. 886.—Arteriogram showing aneurisms of the circle of Willis.

Thomas Willis, 1621–1675. Professor of Natural Philosophy, Oxford. Afterwards practised as physician in St. Martin's Lane, London.

(2) Aneurism of the internal carotid artery, which usually follows fracture of the middle fossa. We have seen a case which followed severe vomiting in a girl fifteen years old. It may communicate with the cavernous sinus, and so be arteriovenous in nature (see p. 100).

CEREBRAL TUMOUR

Custom sanctions the inclusion of such conditions as cysts, gummata, tuberculomata, and chronic abscesses under the heading of cerebral " tumour."

Tumours arise in connection with the meninges, nerve sheaths, or in the cerebral substance. The commoner tumours are as follows :

Meninges.—Meningioma (*syn.* endothelioma, fibroblastoma, 12 per cent.), psammoma (calcified meningioma) (p. 64), tuberculoma, blood and arachnoid cysts.

Nerve Sheaths.—Neurinoma of the auditory nerve sheath (9 per cent.), fibro-sarcoma.

Brain.—Glioma (42 per cent.), gliomatous cyst, gumma, chronic abscess, secondary growths. Boeck's sarcoidosis occasionally involves the central nervous system.

Gliomata have been classified by Bailey and Cushing according to the stage of development of the cells from which the tumour arises. They arise from the cells which line the primitive neural groove. The malignancy of the tumour varies in proportion to the degree of reversion to the primitive type of cell. Gliomata occur most commonly in the frontal lobes and cerebellum, and three recognised types are :

Astrocytoma, which is the commonest, and as the name suggests is composed of star-shaped cells, which resemble adult neuroglial tissue. This type is comparatively benign, and after decompression the average period of survival is six years. Cystic degeneration commonly occurs owing to the relative avascularity of the tumour.

Spongioblastoma, which arises from a more primitive type of cell. They occur in middle life and usually arise in a cerebral hemisphere. These tumours are vascular, and are composed of round and spindle cells. The expectation of life after decompression is one year.

Medulloblastoma is uncommon, and usually occurs in children, most frequently in the region of the roof of the fourth ventricle. It grows rapidly and tends to spread along the meninges. Microscopically, it resembles a small round-celled sarcoma.

Clinical Features.—These depend on the actual site of the tumour and the disturbance produced by increased intracranial pressure.

(i) *Focal or Localising Features.*—A knowledge of the functions of different areas of the brain is essential for the accurate localisation of the site of a tumour. For example, a tumour which interferes with the cerebellum causes vertigo, nystagmus, inco-ordination, and a tendency to fall to the same side as the tumour, owing to ataxia and hypotonicity of muscles. Should

Percival Bailey, Contemporary. Professor of Neurosurgery, Chicago.
Harvey Williams Cushing, 1869–1939. Professor of Surgery, Harvard, and Stirling Professor of Neurology, Yale. The founder of modern cerebral surgery.

the Rolandic area be implicated, the corresponding muscles on the opposite side are rendered paretic, and if the cortex is irritated, spasms and twitchings precede the paresis. Involvement of Broca's area results in motor aphasia, and hemianopia suggests a lesion of the occipital lobe. The frontal area is relatively " silent," but not infrequently temperamental changes are noticed by relations, and the patient loses his natural buoyancy, frankness, and initiative (fig. 887). An acoustic neurinoma growing from the sheath of the eighth nerve is likely to cause tinnitus, followed by unilateral deafness and cerebellar disturbances. Recklinghausen's disease of nerves occasionally affects a cranial nerve.

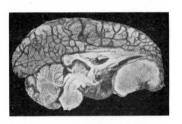

FIG. 887.—Meningioma arising in the frontal region.
(*W. R. Henderson. British Journal of Surgery.*)

(ii) *General Pressure Effects.*— These include headache, vomiting, papillœdema progressing to blindness, bradycardia, and retarded cerebration. The headache often wakes the patient in the early morning, and is aggravated by coughing and straining, which promote cerebral congestion. Vomiting occurs without warning, and is not preceded by nausea or related to food, but, like sea-sickness, sometimes follows change of posture. Papillœdema is especially prone to occur with subtentorial tumours, and is usually worse on the affected side. The symptoms of increased intracranial pressure are relieved by alimentary or intravenous dehydration.

Investigation.—The prognosis and treatment of a cerebral tumour depend upon its site and nature.

(i) **Site.**—The following methods of investigation assist in localising the tumour :

(*a*) *Palpation of the Head.*—In about 1 per cent. of cases some change in the skull is detected over the tumour. Hyperostosis occurs over a vascular tumour, while thinning or even erosion is sometimes evident if the tumour is avascular, as is a hydatid cyst.

(*b*) *Neurological examination,* which includes the cranial nerves and their nuclei, nerve tracts, reflexes, and cortical centres. In some cases this suffices accurately to localise the position of the tumour, as in the case of an auditory nerve tumour,

Paul Broca, 1824–1880. Anthropologist and Professor of Clinical Surgery, Paris.

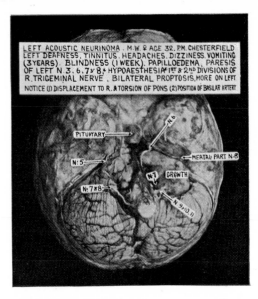

LEFT ACOUSTIC NEURINOMA . M.W. ♀ AGE 32. P.M. CHESTERFIELD
LEFT DEAFNESS, TINNITUS, HEADACHES, DIZZINESS, VOMITING
(3 YEARS). BLINDNESS (1 WEEK). PAPILLOEDEMA, PARESIS
OF LEFT N.3, 6, 7 & 8, & HYPOAESTHESIA 1ST & 2ND DIVISIONS OF
R. TRIGEMINAL NERVE , BILATERAL PROPTOSIS, MORE ON LEFT
NOTICE (1) DISPLACEMENT TO R. & TORSION OF PONS (2) POSITION OF BASILAR ARTERY

PITUITARY

N: 6

MEATAL PART N. 8

N: 5

N. 7

GROWTH

N: 7 & 8

N. 9, 10, 11

FIG. 888.—Neurological evidence of an auditory
nerve tumour.

which causes unilateral deafness and cerebellar symptoms (fig. 888).

(c) A *radiograph* occasionally demonstrates thickening or thinning which is not sufficiently advanced to be palpable. Some tumours are so calcified that they are opaque, as are a suprasellar cyst, or a psammoma. A calcified pineal gland or calcific plaques in the falx cerebri may be pushed across the midline by a tumour in the opposite side of the brain. Unilateral increase in the size, number, and tortuosity of meningeal vessels suggests an underlying tumour. An auditory nerve tumour, which grows slowly, characteristically expands the internal auditory meatus. A stereoscopic radiograph is a valuable help in visualising the site of an opaque tumour. A mottled appearance (" copper-beaten " skull) indicates prolonged increased

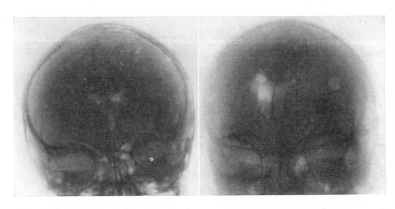

FIG. 889.—Normal ventriculogram. On the right a cerebral tumour has caused
displacement and dilatation of the right lateral ventricle.

intracranial tension, and is due to pressure by the convolutions (fig. 889). The outline of the lateral ventricle can sometimes be visualised in a ventriculogram following the injection of air through a small burr or trephine hole (fig. 890). The replacement of cerebro-spinal fluid by air must be accomplished very slowly, otherwise alteration of pressure may cause oozing from the choroid plexus.

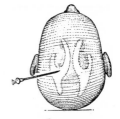

FIG. 890.—Ventriculography.

The danger of *ventriculography* increases with the degree of increased intracranial pressure. Sudden cerebral displacements following withdrawal of cerebro-spinal fluid are liable to cause impaction of the brain stem in the tentorial aperture, and arrangements should be made for operation to follow this investigation if necessary. However, the danger of opening the skull in the wrong place in the presence of increased pressure is greater than that of ventriculography (Norman Dott).

Encephalography is performed by replacing the cerebro-spinal fluid with air, which is introduced by lumbar puncture. By this means the subarachnoid space can be outlined, and abnormalities may thus be detected.

Electro-encephalography is sometimes of assistance in localising tumours. Electrical variations of the brain are recorded by cathode-ray apparatus. The periodicity of the waves is reduced and their amplitude increased when the electrode lies over a tumour.

Angiography is carried out by the injection of perabrodil into the internal carotid artery, during which procedure an X-ray of the brain is taken. The arteries are thus outlined, and vascular neoplasms or aneurisms may be detected and localised (fig. 886).

(ii) **Nature.**—(*a*) *The Age of the Patient.*—Tuberculomata occur in children, while meningiomata are usually found in young adults. Gummata and secondary deposits appear later in life. Cysts and chronic abscesses occur at any age.

(*b*) *History* is sometimes suggestive. Symptoms which slowly progress, perhaps for years, are probably caused by an innocent tumour, such as a meningioma. Intermittent symptoms, possibly varying with the general health of the patient, may be ascribed to a chronic infective condition or a tuberculoma. A malignant tumour, such as a medullo-blastoma or secondary carcinoma, causes symptoms which sometimes progress in an alarming manner. Chronic discharge from the ear is occasionally associated with a cerebral or cerebellar abscess.

(*c*) *General Examination of the Patient.*—In a child other signs of tuberculosis will suggest a tuberculoma. The presence of bronchiectasis should arouse suspicions of a chronic abscess. A

Walter E. Dandy, 1886–1946. Professor of Neurosurgery, Johns Hopkins University, U.S.A. Introduced ventriculography in 1918.
Norman Dott, Contemporary. Neurological Surgeon, Edinburgh Royal Infirmary.

gumma or secondary tumour would be suspected if other signs of syphilis or a primary growth are discovered.

(d) *Accessory Investigations.*—The W.R. must always be tested, and blood examination may also reveal eosinophilia or leucocytosis, which are suggestive of hydatid cyst or chronic abscess respectively. Examination of cerebro-spinal fluid is often of value, and evidence of syphilis or tuberculous disease is sometimes discovered. In the latter case an increase of small lymphocytes is found. In the presence of increased subtentorial pressure, only a few cubic centimetres of fluid should be withdrawn, otherwise the medulla is liable to be forced into the spinal canal, with risk of death from pressure on the cardio-respiratory centres. A pressure of over 200 mm. of fluid indicates pathologically increased pressure. Increase of the protein content is often associated with a spinal block.

TEMPORARY DEHYDRATION

The intravenous injection of hypertonic solutions, and, to a lesser degree, alimentary administration of magnesium sulphate, causes a dehydration of the tissues of both brain and tumour, with temporary amelioration of symptoms.

Intravenous injection of 50 to 100 ml. ($1\frac{1}{2}$–3 oz.) of 15 per cent. to 30 per cent. sodium chloride acts almost immediately, but the effect is limited to a few hours. As this evanescent effect is frequently followed by a period of increased intracranial pressure the patient should be under observation so that operation can be performed forthwith if necessary, since a second injection is often less effective. This temporary improvement is particularly valuable during the course of a prolonged operation. Intravenous administration of 50 to 100 ml. ($1\frac{1}{2}$–3 oz.) of sucrose (50 per cent.) exerts a less rapid effect than that obtained by sodium chloride, but the result is more lasting, and the risk of pulmonary œdema is negligible. Intravenous injection of hypertonic solution predisposes to local thrombosis, so a few ml. of normal saline should be injected prior to withdrawing the needle.

More gradual and prolonged decompression is obtained by the rectal administration of 6 ounces (200 ml.) of magnesium sulphate in 3 ounces (100 ml.) of water. The patient is recumbent and the pelvis is raised, and he is instructed to retain the increasing volume of fluid as long as possible. This procedure is carried out twice daily, and the maximum effect is evident after three or four days. Large doses of magnesium sulphate administered orally exert a similar, but less potent, effect. Needless to say, the fluid intake is restricted. The relief obtained by alimentary decompression is useful as a preliminary to clinical investigation, also distressing symptoms are relieved in inoperable cases and the final stages thereby rendered less burdensome.

Treatment

Palliative decompression for a supratentorial tumour has to a great extent been supplanted by more determined efforts to remove the tumour. The technique of neurosurgery and anæsthesia has so improved of recent years that more radical operations are now possible. Infiltrating malignant tumours are hopeless, but a large proportion of the more circumscribed growths, such as astrocytomata, can be excised or removed with a portion of adjacent brain. If the tumour cannot be removed, a decompression should be performed when the tumour is of slow growth. A decompression for a rapidly growing neoplasm results in a hernia cerebri, hemiplegia, etc., and merely prolongs the misery of the patient.

Subtentorial decompression is of value for tumours in the posterior fossa, and yields relatively better results than supratentorial decompression.

Craniotomy.—Local anæsthesia, with 2 per cent. novocaine, or intratracheal anæsthesia, are used. A flap incision is made over the suspected site of the tumour. This is best accomplished in stages. The assistant exerts digital pressure, with the fingers of each hand on either side of the proposed incision, and the surgeon incises the scalp between the fingers. Before the assistant relaxes pressure, the surgeon picks up the epicranial aponeurosis on either side with artery forceps at quarter-inch intervals. These are folded back so that the vessels in the scalp are bent on themselves, and each bunch of four or five forceps is secured by means of a rubber ring. By degrees the requisite incision is made, and an extensive exposure can be obtained almost bloodlessly with patience, and a large number of forceps. The scalp is separated from the skull just sufficiently to allow the application of a burr (fig. 891) to each corner of the proposed osteoplastic flap.

Brisk venous oozing occurs when the diploic area is entered, and a seeker or blunt end of a needle is useful in determining when the dura mater is reached.

When the four openings are completed the intervening bone between them is divided by means of a Gigli's saw. The dura mater is first separated from the skull, and a grooved introducer insinuated through adjacent holes.

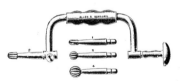

Fig. 891.—Hudson's burr.

The saw is passed along the groove, and the bone divided. The cut should be made so as to bevel the bone, so that in the event of replacement of the entire flap, there will be no tendency for the bone to sink beneath its normal level. The bone forming the base of the flap is only partially divided, as complete division will inevitably score the soft parts in the flap. When damage to the scalp appears to be imminent, the remainder of the bone is fractured by inserting a raspatory under the upper border of the bone flap, and applying leverage. The osteoplastic flap is now turned down, and,

Leonardo Gigli, 1863–1908. An obstetrician of Florence. Invented his saw for pubiotomy.

after examination for any abnormality of the bone, it is wrapped in gauze moistened with warm saline.

The exposed dura mater is inspected, and the absence or degree of pulsation is noted, also any local discoloration or congestion which sometimes accompanies a meningeal tumour. If the dura mater is tense and pulseless, intravenous hypertonic saline may be given, or a few ml. of cerebro-spinal fluid withdrawn from a lateral ventricle with a fine needle. The dura mater is then nicked with a tenotomy knife, and opened by a crucial incision. Any meningeal vessels which cross the path of the proposed incision are previously clipped or underrun and ligated with thread (fig. 892). If a

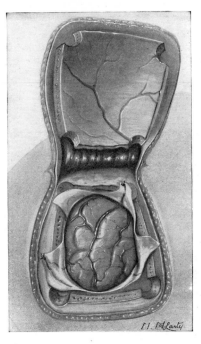

tumour is now exposed, its relations are ascertained, and if possible it is removed. A meningioma which lies in a depression in the cortex is readily excised with the portion of dura mater from which it grows. If no tumour is visible, the exposed convolutions are gently palpated, and any suspicious area is explored with a needle. If fluid is withdrawn, its character is noted. Probably it is either cerebro-spinal fluid from a distended lateral ventricle, which suggests a deep-seated tumour causing internal hydrocephalus, or else fluid from a gliomatous cyst. In the latter case the fluid is yellowish from altered blood, and slightly viscid in consistency. In either case discretion must be exercised in the withdrawal of fluid, and only sufficient removed to relieve excessive tension, otherwise oozing is likely to follow from the choroid plexus in the case of a ventricle, or from the wall of a gliomatous cyst. Radon seeds have been implanted in the wall of a cyst and in malignant tumours, with variable results.

Fig. 892.—The osteoplastic flap has been raised, and the dura mater incised after ligation of meningeal vessels.

In the few cases where a tumour is satisfactorily removed, the dura mater is sutured with fine silk, although many surgeons now consider this to be unnecessary. Even if part of the membrane has been excised, re-formation occurs within a few weeks, so that fascial grafts, which were formerly used to remedy the defect, are unnecessary. The complete osteoplastic flap is replaced and stitched securely in position, the silkworm or braided nylon sutures serving to control hæmorrhage.

In many cases the tumour is only partially removable (or possibly not discovered), or a cyst is merely aspirated. If considered advisable, the bone on the osteoplastic flap is then stripped from its pericranial attachment, and the soft parts stitched back into position. The craniotomy thus becomes a decompression.

Should a tuberculoma be suspected, general treatment, including streptomycin, is instigated, as these tumours are sometimes multiple, and also an attempt to remove them is liable to result in dissemination and tuberculous meningitis.

DECOMPRESSION OF THE POSTERIOR FOSSA

Intratracheal anæsthesia is advisable, and the head is completely flexed and suitably supported.

The incision most commonly employed is the " crossbow," the horizontal portion of which passes from the base of one mastoid process to the other at a level just below the superior curved lines. The vertical part of the incision passes downward in the midline from the external occipital protuberance to the level of the fourth or fifth cervical spinous process. Owing to division of the occipital nerves, this incision is followed by prolonged anæsthesia of the back of the scalp, and therefore some surgeons prefer a midline incision which commences at about the centre of the vertex and passes downwards to the fifth cervical spine. The soft tissues can be stripped sufficiently from the bone to allow adequate exposure.

In either case, muscles are separated from the bone with a raspatory until the mastoid processes are exposed laterally, and the posterior rim of the foramen magnum and the arch of the atlas are seen at the bottom of the wound. Free bleeding occurs from emissary veins, but is conveniently arrested with Horsley's wax or absorbable gauze.

A burr is applied to the skull in the angle between the superior curved line and the occipital ridge, and the skull is opened. This procedure is repeated on the opposite side, and by means of a Gigli's saw the intervening bridge of bone is removed. Entrance to the posterior fossa now having been gained, the occipital bone is nibbled away as far as the mastoid processes laterally, and downwards so as to include the rim of the foramen magnum. It is advisable also to remove the arch of the atlas so that subsequent backward bulging of the cerebellum will not compress the medulla against this bony ring, with consequent risk of respiratory failure owing to pressure on the medullary centre.

Should considerable intradural tension be present, as indicated by absence of pulsation, intravenous hypertonic saline should be given. The temporary decompression which results diminishes the risk of sudden backward displacement of the brain and pressure on the medulla.

The dura mater is now opened as follows. The occipital sinus is underrun with two sutures at the level of the foramen magnum, and divided between these ligatures, although in many cases pressure has collapsed and emptied the sinus. Incisions are now made in the dura mater in an upward and outward direction on either side, so that a triangular flap is turned upwards. The cerebellum is thus exposed, and the posterior fossa is open to exploration. The operation is completed by apposing and suturing the original scalp incision.

In the case of a tumour the site of which is known, such as an auditory nerve fibroma, the corresponding half of the posterior fossa is first removed. Should the tumour be irremovable, the bone on the opposite side is then nibbled away, and the arch of the atlas excised, so that a complete decompression is obtained.

X-ray therapy should be employed if growths known to be radio-sensitive are incompletely removed, or if exploration has only permitted a portion to be removed for section. Cranio-pharyngeal carcinoma, which invades the base of the skull, is highly radio-sensitive, and can be controlled for years. Similarly, eosinophil tumours of the pituitary regress with X-ray therapy, and acromegaly and associated visual defects often show striking improvement. On the other hand, chromophobe adenomata of the pituitary gland are radio-resistant. Increasing experience and refinements of

Sir Victor Horsley, 1857–1916. Surgeon to the University College Hospital, London. Died from heatstroke while on Active Service in Mesopotamia. One of the authors paid his last respects at the burial service.

technique offer increasing hope for those unfortunate patients who are condemned to suffer from a cerebral tumour.

PREFRONTAL LEUCOTOMY

Prefrontal leucotomy is performed through a burr hole in both temporal regions. After the introduction of a special knife the association fibres are divided as they pass backwards. The mortality is 2 per cent. and is mainly due to hæmorrhage, but in half the cases an unstable or even a maniacal patient is transformed into an unimaginative but useful person.

APOPLEXY

A " stroke " is due to one of three causes—cerebral embolism, thrombosis, or hæmorrhage. The differential diagnosis is important, as some measure of relief may be possible in suitable cases.

Cerebral embolism is usually associated with heart lesions. It can occur at any age from youth upwards, and emboli may have previously occurred in the brain or other situations. Treatment consists in dealing with associated auricular fibrillation if present, and an oxygen tent to prevent anoxæmia. As soon as possible, stellate block is performed on the appropriate side, and heparin is administered. Anticoagulants are subsequently prescribed.

Cerebral thrombosis usually occurs in patients past their prime of life, and, more often than not, is gradual in onset. " Softening " of the brain is commonly associated with renal deficiency, and some cases are hypertensive.

As is to be expected, pulmonary complications are apt to follow prolonged unconsciousness. Treatment therefore consists in provision of an oxygen tent, combined with stellate block and venesection in cases associated with unduly raised blood-pressure.

Cerebral hæmorrhage also occurs in those of riper years, and most cases have hypertension. The onset is sudden, and lumbar puncture usually reveals blood-stained fluid and increased tension, especially in severe cases.

The patient should be nursed in an oxygen tent, and measures such as intravenous hypertonic fluids are useful to reduce cerebral œdema and intracranial pressure. Stellate block is contraindicated.

THE PITUITARY BODY

Development and Structure.—This small body, which plays a part in metabolism out of all proportion to its size (5 to 10 grains), has been described as the leader of the endocrine orchestra (Pennybacker). It is composed of four portions :

Pars anterior, or anterior lobe, is developed from ectoderm in the roof of the stomadeum. It is composed of two varieties of cells, chromophobe and chromophil. The latter are either eosinophil or basophil, according to their staining reaction. The anterior lobe is well supplied with blood, and its secretion passes directly into the blood-stream.

Pars intermedia.—This portion, with the pars nervosa, comprises the posterior lobe. The pars intermedia is derived from cells of Rathke's pouch, and is represented by a narrow layer of tissue containing clear cells ; in the spaces between the cells colloid material is found, which contains granules. These granules pass through the pars nervosa into the third ventricle. Their function is unknown.

Pars nervosa, which arises as an outgrowth from the embryonic brain, and during fœtal life contains a cavity which communicates through the infundibulum with the third ventricle. It is only in mammalia that this portion becomes associated with the remainder of the pituitary body. The pars nervosa contains neuroglial and ependymal cells, and is less vascular than the remainder of the pituitary body.

Pars tuberalis.—This also is formed from an off-shoot of the embryonic pharynx. It comprises a mass of cells which encircle the pituitary stalk, and spread thence over the adjacent tuber cinereum, which is an eminence of grey matter forming part of the floor of the third ventricle, and from the centre of which the pituitary stalk, or infundibulum, is attached. The pars tuberalis is composed of vesicles which contain colloid material.

Function.—Many points regarding the functions of these various portions still require elucidation, but the main surgical importance of the gland is concerned with tumours.

CHROMOPHIL ADENOMA

In children these tumours cause gigantism, while patients whose epiphyses have united develop acromegaly (a term which implies enlargement of the extremities). Acromegaly (fig. 893) is characterised by thickening of the subcutaneous tissues, particularly of the face, hands, and feet, and overgrowth of certain bones (Chapter xli). Although acromegaly commences with hyperpituitarism it ends with hypopituitarism, as indicated by loss of sexual activity, deposition of subcutaneous

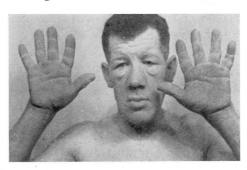

Fig. 893.—Acromegaly.

J. B. Pennybacker, Contemporary. Neurosurgeon, Radcliffe Infirmary, Oxford.
Martin Heinrich Rathke, 1793–1860. Professor of Zoology and Anatomy, Königsberg.

fat, and increasing asthenia, i.e. a frail giant. The patient usually presents himself complaining of impaired vision, due to pressure on the optic chiasma, which results in varying degrees of bilateral hemianopia. X-ray shows expansion of the sella turcica (fig. 894), which may eventually be so severe as

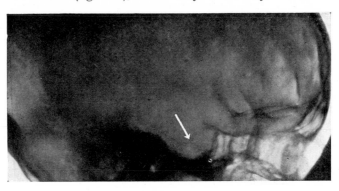

FIG. 894.—Enlargement of the sella turcica caused by a pituitary adenoma.

to compress the cavernous sinus and the third, fourth, and sixth cranial nerves. Headache, sexual impairment, asthenia, and diabetes mellitus are often associated conditions. The disease progresses slowly, and surgical intervention is rarely required except to preserve vision.

BASOPHIL ADENOMA

Basophil adenomata are more common than chromophil tumours. Loss of sexual function is an early symptom, accompanied with an increase of subcutaneous fat, which in the male often assumes a female distribution. The skin is smooth and supple, and the hair fine and silky. Visual disturbances occur sooner or later. Lowered metabolism results in loss of energy and a lowered blood-pressure. Expansion of the sella occurs eventually.

CUSHING'S SYNDROME

Cushing described a syndrome which is associated with a basophil adenoma of the anterior lobe, although a similar condition is sometimes due to adrenal dysfunction (adreno-genital syndrome (p. 230)). Females are more commonly affected. The first symptom is impotence in a male and amenorrhœa in a female. Fat accumulates on the trunk and head and neck, but the limbs remain normal. The hair is redistributed, and baldness of the scalp occurs while the face becomes hirsute. Pigmentation of the skin and kyphosis develop, and in the later stages there is rise of blood-pressure and glycosuria. Many cases improve with deep X-ray therapy.

Harvey Cushing, 1869–1939. Professor of Surgery at Johns Hopkins and Harvard Universities.

PITUITARY DECOMPRESSION

Surgical intervention is considered in the event of intolerable headache, or symptoms due to local pressure effects, especially progressive visual impairment or possibly neuralgia following involvement of the trigeminal nerve.

An *intrasellar* tumour can be approached by the trans-sphenoidal route, either under general or local anæsthesia. The inferior turbinate bones are removed, and submucous resection of the nasal septum allows approach to the sphenoidal air sinus. A special speculum is utilised in order to separate the muco-periosteal flaps, and the sphenoidal air cells are removed piece-meal, so as to open the sella turcica. This procedure gives access for drainage of a cyst, or allows subsequent expansion of a tumour in a downward direction, and so relieves pressure on the structures in the sella turcica and on the base of the brain. Owing to improvements in neuro-surgery this method is now rarely employed, as the transfrontal, intradural approach is a more radical procedure.

In most cases the tumour is approached through an osteoplastic flap, which is turned outwards in the frontal region. The operation should be performed on the side of the better eye. The head is extended over a sand-bag, and an osteoplastic flap is then turned outwards, hinged by the temporal muscle. Care must be taken not to open the frontal sinus while making the lower and inner burr-hole. Usually the intact muco-periosteum can be separated from the bone and pushed downwards. If the sinus is inadvertently opened, the osteoplastic flap can be completed, but the remainder of the operation must be postponed for ten days in order to avoid the risk of meningitis.

The exposed dura mater is then opened, and the frontal lobe is elevated from the floor of the anterior fossa. At this stage of the operation the patient's head should be hyperextended (Rose's position), so that the weight of the brain causes it to fall away from the anterior fossa. A retractor carrying an electric light is inserted, and the optic nerve is identified and followed backwards to the chiasma and sella turcica. The cyst or tumour is then removed, usually piecemeal, and perhaps with the aid of suction.

This method of approach has also been utilised to allow implantation of radon seeds into intrasellar tumours, with some measure of success. X-ray therapy is used after removal of a tumour. It is dangerous as a pre-operative measure, as resultant œdema of the brain in the presence of increased intracranial pressure may be fatal, and in any case increased pressure by the tumour on the optic chiasma is unwelcome.

CRANIO-PHARYNGEAL TUMOUR (*Syn.* RATHKE POUCH TUMOUR)

These tumours are derived from remains of the cranio-buccal pouch. The original cells are squamous in origin, and cystic degeneration commonly occurs, in which case the tumour becomes a cyst, and may contain adamantinomatous elements. These suprasellar tumours usually occur during the second decade. Symptoms are caused by local pressure effects, particularly upon the optic chiasma, or occasionally they extend directly upwards into the third ventricle. Hypopituitarism is usual, and if the tumour occurs early in childhood the Lorain

Frank Atcherley Rose, 1873–1935. Surgeon to the Throat and Nose Department, St. Bartholomew's Hospital, London.

type of dwarf is typical. Sexual development is retarded, and impotence or amenorrhœa is to be expected.

A radiograph is often conclusive in confirming the presence of a suprasellar tumour. The majority contain sufficient calcium to render themselves opaque to X-rays, and a stereoscopic radiograph indicates their exact position. At a later stage the dorsum sellæ and the clinoid processes are eroded, but there is no expansion of the sella turcica.

Treatment is difficult, although removal of some of the tumour or evacuation of fluid can be accomplished via the frontal approach as for a pituitary tumour. As the tumour is usually adherent, complete extirpation is impossible, and aspiration of a cyst gives relief only for a few months. A recent method of overcoming obstruction caused by a tumour which projects into the third ventricle is ventriculo-cisternostomy (Torkildsen). This procedure entails the passage of a polythene tube from the lateral ventricle to the cisterna magna, so as to by-pass the third ventricle, the aqueduct, and the fourth ventricle. Internal hydrocephalus is thus relieved, but any local pressure effects are unaffected.

Adeno-carcinoma very occasionally occurs in middle life, and consists of a vascular tumour composed of chromophobe cells. Adjacent bone is destroyed, and nerves are involved. If the patient survives for a sufficient period, metastases disseminate by the blood-stream.

It is probable that Milton suffered from a cranio-pharyngeal tumour, which caused blindness, mental depression, and altered personality. The tumour presumably calcified, and, although the blindness persisted, his mental state improved, and he then produced *Paradise Regained.*" (Lambert Rogers, Professor of Surgery, Cardiff.)

FRÖHLICH'S SYNDROME (*Syn.* DYSTROPHIA ADIPOSO-GENITALIS)

This disease was formerly considered to be due to deficiency of the pars nervosa in childhood, but neurophysicians are inclined

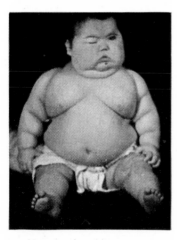

to exonerate the pituitary gland and to consider the syndrome to be hypothalamic in origin. The sexual organs are well-developed, and fat is deposited more or less generally, but particularly around the bust and hips (fig. 895). There is an increased sugar tolerance, and the basal metabolism is lowered. A gonadotropic hormone should be prescribed if puberty is delayed.

DERCUM'S DISEASE

This condition is alleged to be due to deficiency of the pars nervosa in adults. It usually

FIG. 895.—Fröhlich's syndrome.

Arne Torkildsen, Contemporary. Neurosurgeon, Rikshospital, Oslo, Norway.
Alfred Fröhlich, Contemporary. Formerly Professor of Pharmacology, University of Vienna. Described his syndrome in 1901.
Francis X. Dercum, 1856–1931. Professor of Neurology, Jefferson Medical College, Philadelphia.

affects females, and in addition to a general deposition of fat, local deposits also occur (fig. 896). These fatty tumours are sometimes painful, and in these cases the term "adiposis dolorosa" has been applied.

Asthenia is a troublesome symptom, and the presence of creatinuria suggests that this is due to abnormal muscle metabolism. Prostigmin affords great relief.

Diabetes insipidus follows derangement of the posterior lobe, and is characterised by the output of up to several gallons of urine daily, of extremely low specific gravity, combined with intense thirst. The condition may be familial, or occasionally follows

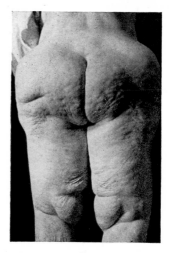

FIG. 896.—Dercum's disease (adiposis dolorosa).

head injuries or pressure by an adjacent tumour. Subcutaneous injections of pituitrin give relief for a few hours, during which remission the patient can sleep, but they often cause unpleasant symptoms of vasodilatation and hyperperistalsis. Oral administration is useless, but dried posterior lobe powder administered in the form of snuff is sometimes effective.

LORAIN'S SYNDROME

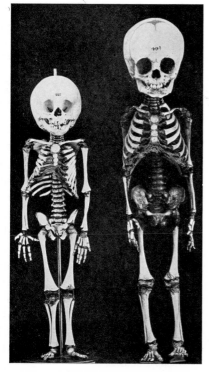

FIG. 897.—*Left.*—Skeleton of "Madame Crachami," who was exhibited as "The Sicilian Dwarf." Aged nine years, height 19·8 inches. An example of Lorain's syndrome. *Right.*—Normal infant, aged sixteen months. (*R.C.S. Museum.*)

Deficiency of the anterior lobe in childhood results in dwarfism (Lorain's syndrome) (fig. 897). Pituitary dwarfs are proportionate and graceful (which distinguishes them from cretins, rickety patients, and achondroplasics), therefore the skeleton is a miniature of the normal. Epiphyses unite at a later period than usual. Secondary sexual characteristics are absent,

Paul Lorain, 1827–1875. Physician, Hôpital de la Pitie, Paris.

and in the male the voice remains high-pitched, as the vocal cords do not lengthen. This condition is uncommon, but examples are sometimes exhibited at a circus.

TUMOURS OF THE PINEAL GLAND

These tumours are rare, and the diagnosis is often speculative. Sexua precocity is sometimes noted. In addition to the usual features of increased intracranial pressure, some degree of hypopituitarism follows pressure of the dilated third ventricle on the pituitary gland, a condition which is apt to occur in any case of obstructive hydrocephalus.

Attempts to remove such an inaccessible tumour are dangerous, and likely to cause structural damage, therefore ventriculo-cisternostomy or anterior ventriculostomy (incision through the anterior wall of the third ventricle) is performed, followed by deep X-ray therapy, as pineal tumours are radio-sensitive (Pennybacker).

J. B. Pennybacker, Contemporary. Neurosurgeon, Radcliffe Infirmary, Oxford.

CHAPTER XXXIV
THE SPINE

Sprains in connection with the spinal column are of common occurrence. Spinal ligaments are sometimes injured as a result of a sudden jolt, as in car or railway accidents. Fibres of spinal muscles are occasionally torn by excessive muscular contraction, as attempting to lift heavy weights, or damage may result from a direct injury. In either case severe localised pain follows, accentuated by any movement which stretches the damaged structure. Palpation reveals a tender spot, and if muscular fibres are torn, some bogginess, due to extravasation of blood, is often detected. An exact diagnosis is usually difficult, but an X-ray excludes or reveals injury to bone. Treatment consists in rest and cold applications, followed a few days later by massage and graduated movements. If the site of pain can be localised with accuracy, an injection of 5 ml. of procaine (2 per cent.) may cause immediate improvement (N.B., as with lumbago). The time required for complete recovery is often surprisingly long, particularly if litigation is pending ! In more severe injuries the ligamentum subflavum is occasionally torn, and hæmatorachis is then likely to follow. Laminectomy is sometimes indicated in these cases (p. 878).

DISLOCATION

A *true* dislocation can occur only in the cervical region, because the oblique and vertical directions of the articular processes in the dorsal and lumbar regions respectively do not permit of dislocation without fracture.

Dislocation following hanging occurs between the atlas and the axis. Forward displacement of the atlas follows rupture of the transverse ligament, or less commonly fracture of the odontoid process. Death occurs immediately owing to compression of the cord, and is due to shock and paralysis of all the muscles of respiration. Dislocation at this level has also occurred as a result of lifting a child by means of the hands encircling the neck from behind.

Dislocations at a lower level usually occur between the fourth and fifth (fig. 898) or the fifth and sixth vertebræ. The classical cause of this accident is diving

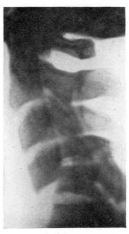

Fig. 898.—Posterior dislocation at the level of C4–C5.

into shallow water, which causes excessive flexion of the upper part of the spinal column. The inferior articular process of the fifth vertebra is forced over the front margin of the superior articular process of the sixth. The condition can occur on one or both sides.

If the dislocation is *unilateral*, the head is turned towards the opposite side, and all movements are restricted. Severe pain may be referred along the corresponding nerve root, which is nipped in the intervertebral foramen. The dislocation is usually readily reduced under general anæsthesia, by further flexion of the head, followed by lateral flexion towards the opposite side. If reduction fails, the joint should be exposed, and a minimum of bone removed in order to allow unlocking. If the dislocation is unreduced, pain and deformity will persist. Involvement of the spinal cord is uncommon in one-sided dislocations.

In *bilateral* cases associated damage to the cord often occurs, usually of a complete nature. In more fortunate cases, owing to the large size of the spinal canal, the cord escapes serious injury. The head is displaced forwards, and obvious deformity is present. Pain is referred to the neck, or arms, according to the site of injury, which is usually lower cervical.

Emergency reduction should be attempted, under anæsthesia, by means of a chin strap or halter. This is connected to a band which passes around the waist of the manipulator so that traction is applied when he leans backwards, and the hands are free for manipulation. If reduction is accomplished, traction is maintained for a week or so, and a plaster cast is then applied. Should manipulation fail, continuous skeletal traction is applied by means of a skull calliper.

As a last resort open operation is performed and a minimal amount of bone is removed from the articular processes until unlocking is possible. To prevent recurrence the spinous processes should be wired together. The head and neck are immobilised in plaster for six weeks.

Pathological dislocation of the atlanto-axial joint occasionally complicates a retropharyngeal abscess, or even tonsillitis. Flexion of the head and torticollis are obvious signs. The condition is confirmed by X-rays. Traction is required for a few weeks, followed by plaster fixation, and the pharyngeal abscess receives appropriate treatment (p. 238).

FRACTURES

Incomplete fractures are those which do not interfere with the continuity of the spinal column. They include fractures of the spinous and transverse processes, laminæ, and fissured or compression fractures of a vertebral body. Fractures of the processes or laminæ are usually due to direct violence. The most common situation for fracture of a spinous process is the dorsal region, where these processes are relatively long, and exposed to injury. Shovellers' fracture is a "stress" fracture of spinous processes which occurs in men who use a shovel excessively, especially if they are undernourished. Localised pain and perhaps crepitus suggest the nature of the injury, which is verified by a radiograph. Fracture of the transverse processes occurs most usually in the lumbar region, where these processes are long and comparatively unprotected. Injury to the corresponding kidney is a frequent accompaniment. Fracture of a lamina may be associated with depression of bone and consequent involvement of the underlying cord, when laminectomy is indicated.

Compression fractures of a vertebral body may cause immediate damage to the cord. In less severe cases persistence of pain demands an X-ray examination which reveals the nature of the injury. (N.B.—In many cases the compression is visible only in the *lateral* X-ray.) It is probable that most cases of Kümmell's disease are due to compression of the vertebral body at the time of injury, rather than to subsequent osteitis, as was formerly believed. Pain, deformity, or cord involvement leads to an X-ray examination, which reveals rarefaction and collapse of the body of a vertebra, usually in the lumbar region (fig. 899). Support to the spine

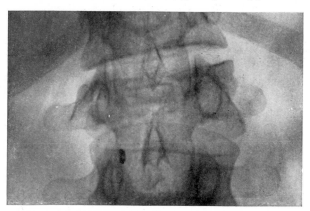

FIG. 899.—Kümmell's disease affecting the first lumbar vertebra.

is necessary for one year, although Albee's bone-graft operation finds favour with some surgeons.

Complete fractures arise as a result of direct or indirect violence. In the former case the injury occurs at any level, but fractures due to indirect violence are usually in the cervico-dorsal or dorso-lumbar regions. Separation commonly occurs through an intervertebral disc, which carries with it a portion

Hermann Kümmell, 1852–1937. Professor of Surgery, Hamburg.
Fred. H. Albee, 1876–1945. Professor of Orthopædic Surgery, Post-graduate Medical School, New York.

of the anterior superior lip of the vertebral body below; thus the injury is in reality a fracture-dislocation.

Damage to the spinal cord is due to the displacement forwards of the upper part of the spine, so that the cord is pressed against the body of the vertebra below the lesion. In the adult the spinal cord ends at the level of the lower border of the body of the first lumbar vertebra, hence lesions below this level can only be associated with injury to the cauda equina or some of its component parts.

The prognosis of fracture of the spine depends on the level and extent of injury to the spinal cord. If the cord is completely crushed the following changes occur:

(a) *Sensory.*—Complete anæsthesia at and below the level of the lesion, with hyperæsthesia of the segment above, due to irritation by effused blood and later by the disintegrating cord.

At a higher level dissociation of sensation occasionally occurs, due to blood passing upwards within the central canal of the cord and interfering with the adjacent fibres which conduct temperature and pain. This phenomenon therefore resembles the sensory changes associated with syringomyelia, and is of academic interest only.

(b) *Motor.*—Complete paralysis of all muscles below the site of the lesion. After spinal concussion (p. 879) has abated, spasticity and contractures supervene, as the lesion is of the upper motor neurone type. At the actual site of the lesion the anterior horn cells are crushed, and therefore flaccid paralysis occurs and continues in connection with the muscles supplied by that segment. This is followed by rapid wasting and the reaction of degeneration. The segment above the lesion is irritated by disintegration of the crushed cord, and therefore the muscles innervated by this segment are spastic.

(c) *Reflexes.*—All superficial and deep reflexes disappear below the level of the lesion, but after about three weeks, extensor responses reappear in an exaggerated form, and a " mass reflex " appears; in which case an effort to obtain a plantar reflex causes excessive contraction of the muscles of the leg and thigh, and possibly automatic emptying of the bladder and rectum. This " mass reflex " is an unequivocal sign that the cord is seriously damaged.

(d) *Visceral.*—During the period of spinal shock incontinence of urine is present. Subsequently, one of three types of bladder paralysis ensues, depending on the site of the lesion (fig. 900):

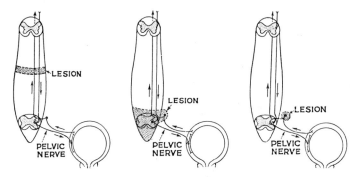

1. Reflex bladder.   2. Automatic bladder.   3. Atonic bladder.

FIG. 900.   (*After Nesbit and Gordon.*

(i) If above the conus, a reflex bladder results, and urine is voided periodically.

(ii) If the conus or cauda equina is injured, an automatic bladder follows, i.e. the bladder can be emptied by suprapubic pressure combined with straining, or by reflex stimuli such as scratching the inner side of a thigh.

(iii) If the sensory nerves to the bladder are involved, the organ becomes atonic. The internal sphincter is relaxed, and dribbling ensues. Permanent suprapubic drainage is usually desirable.

(*e*) *Trophic.*—Severe trophic changes are liable to occur in parts which suffer from deranged innervation. Bedsores may occur in spite of every care, and are often a contributory cause of death (p. 75). Similarly, cystitis in the case of a paralysed bladder may be followed by extensive sloughing of the mucosa, or ascending infection to the kidneys, which become riddled with abscesses (" surgical kidneys ").

The phenomena which follow cord injuries at different levels are summarised as follows :

Cervical.—If above the fifth segment all the respiratory muscles are paralysed, including the diaphragm, which receives its motor supply from the phrenic nerve, mainly the C4 segment.

If the fifth segment is injured, the arms, trunk, and legs are all paralysed, and the patient only breathes with his diaphragm. A lesion of the sixth segment results in the arms being abducted and externally rotated, with the forearms flexed and supinated (fig. 901). This position is due to irritation of the fifth segment, and consequent spasticity of the muscles innervated by it, the most important being the biceps, brachialis anterior, supinators, spinati, and deltoid. Similarly, a lesion through the seventh segment causes irritation of the sixth, with spasticity of the serratus

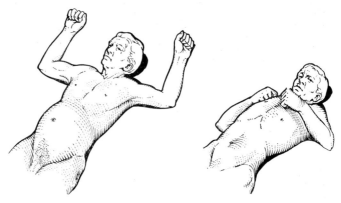

FIG. 901.—Irritation of fifth cervical segment. Abdominal distension is developing.

FIG. 902.—Attitude following irritation of the sixth cervical segment.

anterior, part of the pectorals, and the pronators ; consequently, the arms are drawn forwards and adducted, the forearms being flexed by the pronator teres and pronated by both this muscle and the pronator quadratus (fig. 902).

Dorsal.—Injury at the level of the second dorsal segment is liable to cause contraction of the pupils owing to irritation of the oculo-pupillary fibres, which leave the spinal cord at the segment above. Hyperæsthesia may extend along the inner side of the arms. At lower levels a band of hyperæsthesia is usually detected encircling the trunk, and is present one segment above the site of the injury. Destruction of the cord at any level above the mid-dorsal region results in paralysis of the abdominal muscles, but below this level the paralysis is partial, depending on the site of injury.

Lumbar.—The lumbar enlargement corresponds to the twelfth dorsal and first lumbar vertebræ, and it contains the centre for nervous control of the urinary bladder. An injury above this level prevents inhibitory impulses from the cortex reaching the centre, and after a period of retention, due to spinal shock, reflex micturition occurs. If the lumbar enlargement, or the nerves passing from it to the bladder (principally the third and fourth sacral), are damaged, then absolute incontinence follows from paralysis of the sphincter.

The centre for defæcation is also situated in the lumbar enlargement, and damage to this is followed by a patulous anus and incontinence.

Cauda Equina.—Injuries to the nerves in the spinal canal below the level of the lumbar enlargement give rise to a degree of disability which corresponds with the actual nerves involved. If the lesion occurs just below the formation of the cauda equina, the legs and perineal muscles are completely paralysed, and anæsthesia of the legs and a saddle-shaped area in the perineum is present. As mentioned above, the patient will suffer from true incontinence of fæces and urine. Injury at a lower level will not affect the nerves which arise from the upper lumbar segments, e.g. the femoral, obturator, genito-femoral, so that corresponding groups of muscles are spared, and anæsthesia of the legs is incomplete. If the femoral nerve is intact, sensation remains on the front of the thigh, and along the distribution of the internal saphenous nerve, i.e. the inner side of the leg and foot as far as the head of the first metatarsal.

Partial lesion of the cord occasionally occurs, in which case the motor elements are more liable to remain affected than the sensory. This is explained by the fact that the anterior portion of the cord suffers most, as it is pressed against the body of the vertebra below the injury, and this part of the cord is composed chiefly of motor fibres and anterior horn cells.

Clinical Features.—Evidence or history of an accident is usually obtainable. Neurogenic shock frequently accompanies the injury, but the patient may be able to state that he has severe pain in the back, girdle pains encircling the body, or that he " feels dead " below a certain level.

On examination, the utmost gentleness must be exercised in order to prevent further injury to a cord which is only partially damaged or to avoid injury to an undamaged cord. Deformity of the vertebral column may be noticed, but if the patient has been turned on to his back, " recoil " usually follows, and the spinal column regains its alignment. If the fracture is due to direct injury, bruising or local trauma is evident.

Paraplegia and anæsthesia extending from the level of the lesion are usually present, and are due either to spinal concussion, pressure on, or actual crushing of the cord. A more detailed examination is postponed until the patient is safely installed in a suitable bed and a programme has been outlined for his subsequent treatment. A radiograph should be taken, with due precautions regarding movement of the patient.

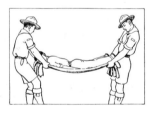

Fracture of the manubrium sterni may be associated with fractures in the dorsal region.

Fig. 903. — Transporting a patient with a fractured spine.

Treatment. — First-aid treatment necessitates transport of the patient, face downwards, care being taken that he is lifted without bending or torsion of the unstable spine (fig. 903). Intravenous morphia or other available sedative should be given to alleviate pain and anxiety. On arrival at his destination the patient should be placed in a bed provided with a "three-piece" mattress, which facilitates nursing, as the central portion can be withdrawn with a minimum of disturbance to the patient.

Symptomatic treatment is now instituted, while recovery from general or spinal shock is awaited.

Spinal shock should show some evidence of abatement at the

end of forty-eight hours. If no sign of recovery is evident after the expiration of this period, the prognosis is gloomy, and anxiety is confirmed by the subsequent development of the " mass reflex " (p. 879).

The treatment of the case now mainly resolves itself into nursing problems, care of the bladder, reduction of the fracture, and rehabilitation.

(i) **Nursing.**—The prevention of bedsores should be a constant preoccupation of the nursing staff ; and although these some-times develop in spite of every precaution, prophylactic meas-ures should never be relaxed (p. 75).

Attention to the bowels is necessary, and aperients or enemata are administered as required. If meteorism is allowed to occur, upward displacement of the diaphragm causes pulmonary embarrassment. Hypostatic pneumonia is a grave danger, particularly if important accessory muscles of respiration, e.g. abdominal muscles, are paralysed,when coughing and expectora-tion are hampered. Contracture of muscles is prevented by frequent passive movements of the limbs.

(ii) **Bladder.**—Overdistension of the bladder must be avoided, otherwise, if the spinal cord recovers, permanent paralysis of the bladder will remain, or if the cord be irremediably damaged, micturition will never become automatic.

Catheterisation is performed as a temporary measure. Utmost aseptic precautions must be taken, and irrigation of the anterior urethra with a weak antiseptic (e.g. oxycyanide of mercury 1 : 4,000) prior to catherisation is some safeguard.

Cystostomy is necessary as soon as it is obvious that retention is inevitable, i.e. if there is no sign of recovery in twenty-four hours. The opening in the bladder should be about 3 inches above the pubic symphysis. This " high " cystostomy facil-itates control of escaping urine, and obviates adherence of the bladder to the pubic bones, which delays subsequent spon-taneous healing or renders operative closure more difficult. Sul-phonamides or antibiotics will assist in preventing or controlling infection.

(iii) **Reduction.**—The fracture usually follows excessive flexion of the spine, and hyperextension corrects this deformity, and relieves any existing pressure on the cord or nerves. In most cases morphia and scopolamine are adequate, but if advisable pentothal or general anæsthesia is administered. Hyperextension is effected by laying the patient prone between two tables, the one which supports the head and arms being 12–18 inches higher than the table on which the legs and pelvis rest ; a sling, if available, gives comfortable support (fig. 904).

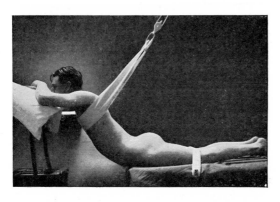

Fig. 904.—The spine is hyperextended by a band with block and tackle. The patient supports himself on a padded chair. The legs are strapped. The stockinette vest in this case has been omitted.

In special clinics an Abbott's frame and a canvas sling are used ; straps are applied to the patient's ankles, which can then be raised to the desired height. The trunk is covered with a stockinette vest, and the plaster is applied from the pelvis below to the axillæ above. A completely crushed vertebra consolidates slowly, so the jacket must be worn for from four to six months.

Acute dilatation of the stomach is a rare but important complication of hyperextension of the spine, as in that position the small intestine gravitates into the pelvis, and consequently the superior mesenteric vessels are rendered taut. In addition, the third part of the duodenum is thrust forward by the lumbar convexity ; this further encourages compression. Removal of the plaster may be necessary. Less severe cases of abdominal distension are usually relieved by cutting a window in the plaster.

Contraindications to Hyperextension.—In the following conditions (about 10 per cent. of cases), hyperextension may cause damage to the cord, therefore it is essential that adequate X-rays are taken to detect the precise nature of the fracture.

(i) Fracture-dislocation with locking of articular processes. The superior processes of the lower vertebra must be excised, as until this is done hyperextension merely stretches the cord.

(ii) Comminuted fractures which involve the neural canal. The spine is immobilised in the normal position with head traction if necessary.

(iii) Fractures due to hyperextension associated with rupture of the anterior common ligament, in which case the spine must be immobilised in slight flexion. An avulsed flake of bone suggests that the ligament is ruptured.

(iv) **Rehabilitation.**—The day after the plaster has been applied the patient should be trained to exercise the abdominal, spinal, and upper limb muscles, and, in the absence of paraplegia, the leg muscles as well.

A paraplegic patient is fitted with a spinal support and callipers about six weeks after the injury, and is best treated in a specialised rehabilitation centre.

Laminectomy as a rule yields disappointing results, but might be considered in the following instances :

(i) Paraplegia partially recovers and then " marks time." This suggests that complete recovery of function is prevented by some mechanical cause, such as depressed bone or blood-clot. This type of case yields the best results from operative treatment, especially if lumbar puncture indicates the presence of cerebro-spinal block (Queckenstedt's test). To perform the test the patient lies on one side, and following lumbar puncture the needle is connected to a manometer. The jugular veins are compressed above the clavicles, and no increase in the pressure (normally 110 to 150 mm. of water) indicates a subarachnoid block between the needle and the cisterna magna.

(ii) Damage to the cord is incomplete at the time of the accident, and remains stationary.

(iii) The cord lesion is incomplete or non-existent at the time of the accident, but progresses or develops later. An example of this type is the " gravitation paraplegia," described by Thorburn, due to hæmorrhage within the spinal canal filling the canal from below upwards. Laminectomy permits blood to be evacuated, and active bleeding will probably have ceased.

Laminectomy performed as a speculative measure in cases where paraplegia is complete from the time of the injury is to be condemned.

Complications.—Death may result from the following causes :

(i) Shock, which may be immediately fatal.

(ii) Cessation of respiration if the lesion is above the fifth cervical segment.

(iii) Hypostatic pneumonia may develop after a few days, especially if the lesion is sufficiently high to cause paralysis of abdominal and intercostal muscles.

(iv) Cystitis is prone to infect the kidneys, causing death from pyelonephritis (*syn.* surgical kidneys). Necropsy reveals the renal cortex and pelvis studded with abscesses and areas of acute inflammation.

(v) Allusion has been made to bedsores, which hasten death owing to toxic absorption.

Sequelæ.—Traumatic neurasthenia may persist, and the patient complains of lassitude and indefinite pains in the back. Cure sometimes follows satisfactory litigation.

In the case of men who follow laborious occupations, pain at

Hans Queckenstedt, Contemporary. Physician at Rostock, Germany. Described the test in 1917.
Sir William Thorburn, 1861–1923. Professor of Surgery, University of Manchester.

the site of the fracture, due to osteoarthritis, may delay them from returning to their former employment. Spinal fusion is sometimes curative.

Meningitis serosa circumscripta more commonly follows an injury of less severity than a fracture (p. 880).

INJURIES TO THE SPINAL CORD

The spinal cord is frequently implicated in association with injury to the vertebral column.

Spinal Concussion (*syn.* Spinal Shock).—In severe cases complete paraplegia and anæsthesia follow, and it is then impossible to distinguish concussion from a gross cord injury, e.g. a crush. In milder cases temporary paresis results, with weakness of sphincteric control.

Treatment is symptomatic, and consists in careful nursing, including attention to the skin, bladder, and bowels. If the case is merely one of concussion, some return of voluntary power or sensation is usually evident within forty-eight hours.

As time passes without improvement recovery is increasingly improbable, and the development of the " mass reflex " indicates destruction of the cord.

Hæmorrhage occurs either in the cord itself (hæmatomyelia), or as an extramedullary condition (hæmatorachis) ; in the latter case the blood escapes either into the cerebro-spinal fluid, or outside the dura mater, as in the case of a torn ligamentum subflavum. Extradural hæmorrhage may fill the spinal canal gradually from below upwards, causing progressive irritation of the cord, followed by paraplegia (Thorburn's gravitation para-plegia). Intradural hæmorrhage is shown by blood in the cerebro-spinal fluid following a lumbar puncture.

Hæmatomyelia causes symptoms which usually follow the injury immediately. Destruction of the anterior horn cells causes a flaccid paralysis of the muscles concerned, while irritation of the pyramidal tracts results in some spasticity of the spinal muscles or legs. Pain and irritation are much less in evidence than in cases of extramedullary hæmorrhage.

Hæmatomyelia in the cervical region sometimes results from com-paratively minor injuries. In the early stages symptoms and signs are often vague, and the patient may be suspected of malingering. Sub-sequently, obvious neurological signs, e.g. muscular wasting, present themselves, and are usually permanent.

Treatment in the first instance is symptomatic, and lumbar

puncture is useful in order to detect intradural hæmorrhage. Laminectomy may be considered (p. 895).

Meningitis.—Acute infective meningitis is likely to follow a penetrating wound, or may be a complication of septicæmia. Severe constitutional disturbances follow, with local and referred pain, hyperæsthesia, muscular spasms, and increased reflexes. Extension to the basal meninges is usual, and the only hope lies in an adequate course of penicillin and chemotherapy.

Chronic meningitis sometimes follows a local injury, and occasionally leads to the condition dignified by the title of " Meningitis serosa circumscripta." This is characterised by the formation of a subdural cyst or cysts, which, some months after the receipt of injury, give rise to features somewhat resembling a tumour. Laminectomy and evacuation of the cyst is followed by relief or cure.

Neurasthenia is a frequent sequela of spinal injury, and is either of the generalised type or referred particularly to the spine. In the latter case vague pains in the back, localised areas of hyperæsthesia, and girdle pains are the main features. The erstwhile term " railway spine " is now obsolescent, as motorbuses and cars contribute the majority of cases.

Treatment is often disappointing. Following adequate rest supervised rehabilitation is indicated, as in the case of head injuries (p. 843). Satisfactory litigation sometimes results in a cure, even in stubborn cases !

SPINA BIFIDA

Embryology.—During the second week of intra-uterine life a longitudinal furrow appears on the dorsum of the embryo, this groove being formed by infolding of the epiblast. The margins of the neural groove unite, so that it becomes converted into a tube, from which the nervous system is developed. This epiblastic tube becomes separated from the surface by mesoblast, which grows over it from either side, and from which are developed the vertebræ, spinal muscles, membranes, etc. (fig. 905). In each segment bars of cartilage appear on either side of the neural tube, which during the fourth month fuse with each other to form the vertebral arches. Failure of fusion of these arches gives rise to spina bifida, with which is frequently associated maldevelopment of the spinal cord and membranes. The incidence of spina bifida, excluding spina bifida occulta, is 0·1 per cent.

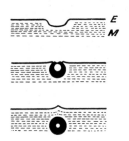

Fig. 905.—Development of the spinal cord. E = epiblast, M = mesoblast.

The types of spina bifida are as follows :

(i) *Spina bifida occulta* is due to failure of the neural arches to unite, but there is no protrusion of cord or membranes.

Frequently only one vertebra is affected, most commonly in the lumbo-sacral region. A local patch of hair, a nævo-lipoma, or a depression in the skin are suggestive of underlying bony deficiency. Occasionally the patient presents himself with nocturnal enuresis or low backache, the latter symptom being

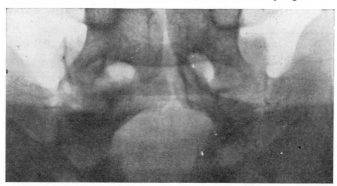

Fig. 906.—Spina bifida, showing cleft in the spino-laminar segment of the fifth lumbar vertebra, and absence of upper part of the sacrum. The patient complained of persistent low backache, especially after exercise.

due to lack of bone for adequate attachment of ligaments and muscles in a region subjected to heavy strain (fig. 906). Many cases are unsuspected until an X-ray is taken for some other reason.

(ii) *Meningocele.*—This is a protrusion of meninges through a

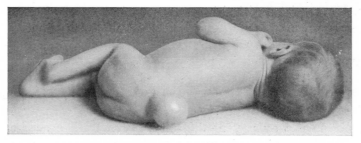

Fig. 907.—A typical meningocele, which was excised successfully.

defect in the spino-laminar segment (fig. 907). It contains only cerebro-spinal fluid.

(iii) *Meningo-myelocele.*—The normally developed spinal cord or cauda equina lies in the sac, and may be adherent to the posterior aspect. The cord or nerves can be seen as dark shadows on transillumination.

(iv) *Syringo-myelocele.*—The rarest type of spina bifida, in which the central canal of the cord is dilated, and the cord lies within the sac together with the nerves arising from it.

(v) *Myelocele* results from arrest of development at the time of closure of the neural furrow. An elliptical raw surface is seen, which represents the ununited groove, and at the upper end the central canal opens on the surface and discharges cerebro-spinal fluid (fig. 908).

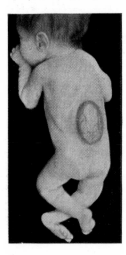

With the exception of spina bifida occulta, myelocele is the most common type of spina bifida, but many cases are stillborn, and therefore of no clinical interest. If the child is born alive, death ensues within a few days from infection of the cord and meninges. Gross talipes is obvious.

For practical purposes interest centres round meningocele and meningo-myelocele. The two conditions are distinguishable on transillumination, and a depression in the

FIG. 908. — Myelocele, with associated talipes.

skin due to adherent cord or nerves is sometimes seen in a meningo-myelocele. Interference with the spinal cord or nerves is often associated with either condition. This interference will be more severe in cases of meningo-myelocele, in which condition bilateral talipes with trophic changes is common, and in more advanced cases extensive paralysis of the legs and incontinence are present. In these cases no surgical intervention is indicated.

If associated nervous phenomena are present, the diagnosis of spina bifida is obvious. Cases of meningocele without nerve involvement may present difficulty, especially if occurring in the cervical region. Moreover, a fatty pad occasionally lies over the sac, and thereby masks its physical features.

Treatment.—Operation for meningocele or meningo-myelocele is advisable as soon as the surgeon is of the opinion that the child's strength and condition warrant the procedure (often within a few days of birth), otherwise the sac is liable to grow out of proportion to the growth of the child, and the overlying skin will become atrophic and ulcerate. If operation is considered inadvisable, the sac should be protected with a celluloid cup.

Some otherwise successful cases have subsequently developed hydrocephalus. However, most neurologists now consider that hydrocephalus is never caused by repair of a spina bifida, but that it is associated with the Arnold Chiari phenomenon (p. 841).

Operation entails exposure of the sac by means of an incision to one side of the midline. The sac is opened and redundant membrane excised. If the cord or nerves are adherent, they are either freed by dissection, or separated with a strip of attached membrane or skin and replaced in the vertebral canal. Membranes are sutured over the cord, the sutures being placed on the opposite side to that of the skin incision. Spinal muscles are approximated, and the wound is reinforced with flaps of sheath from the erector spinæ muscles.

A *complication* of spina bifida occulta consists of nervous phenomena arising during growth, usually between the ninth and twenty-fourth years (fig. 9). The explanation of this late development of symptoms is that a fibrous band, the membrana reuniens, connects the skin with either the spinal cord, nerves, or membranes. In the early months of fœtal life the spinal cord ends opposite the coccyx, at birth the cord extends to the third lumbar vertebra, and in adult life to the lower border of the first lumbar vertebra. Thus as the spinal canal grows away from the spinal cord traction is liable to be exerted by the fibrous band upon the membrane, nerves, or cord itself. The symptoms which follow include weakness or sensory disturbances in the legs, incomplete control of the sphincters, or perforating ulcers of the feet. An X-ray reveals bony deficiency.

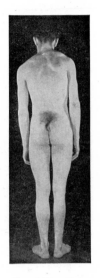

Fig. 909.—Spina bifida occulta with a tuft of hair, and wasting of the right leg due to traction on nerves in the spinal canal. Also right-sided Sprengel's shoulder.

(*R. L. Benison, F.R.C.S.*)

The onset of nerve symptoms is a definite indication for operation. On the under-surface of the skin or deep fascia a tough fibrous band is encountered, which is traced down to the point where it passes through the bony cleft and is attached to the dura mater. The dural sheath is opened and the band excised together with any fibro-lipomatous tissue which may be compressing the cord. Excision is followed by improvement in the nervous symptoms, especially if these symptoms have not appeared until adolescence.

INFLAMMATORY DISEASES

Acute osteomyelitis occasionally occurs, either in connection with the epiphysis of the body of the vertebra, or more rarely, with one of the epiphyses from which the neural arch develops. The main features are severe constitutional disturbances, associated with local pain and tenderness. Pain may also be referred along an adjacent spinal nerve. If the disease commences in a neural arch, some local evidence of inflammation is often detected, and invites exploration. Acute osteomyelitis of a vertebral body has been mistaken for spinal meningitis, acute appendicitis, acute pancreatitis, and other abdominal conditions.

As soon as the disease is suspected penicillin is administered, supplemented by chemotherapy if necessary. X-rays assist in determining the progress of the disease, and evacuation of pus or sequestrectomy is performed if necessary.

TUBERCULOUS DISEASE (Syn. POTT'S DISEASE)

More than half the cases are children in the first decade. Fortunately an increasing number of farmers are restricting their herds to tuberculin-tested cattle, which is the first step

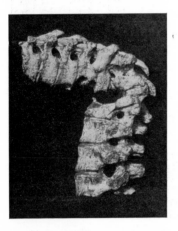

in the reduction of surgical tuberculosis. The most common region to be involved is from the tenth dorsal to the third lumbar vertebra, as stress strains are apt to affect the junction of two comparatively fixed parts of the spine. The disease commences either in the body of the vertebra (endosteal), or in the periosteum under the anterior common ligament.

The endosteal type nearly always affects children, and commences in the anterior part of a vertebra. This is due to the fact that the infection is blood-borne and the nutrient artery enters the vertebral body on the posterior aspect, so that organisms are arrested in the

Fig. 910.—Pott's disease, with gross angular curvature.

capillary loops by which the anterior part of the bone is nourished. As the epiphyseal plates are incomplete, infection readily spreads to adjacent vertebræ.

Owing to rarefaction and destruction the front of the affected vertebra collapses, but the posterior part is held rigid by interlocking of the articular processes, and an angular deformity results (fig. 910).

The periosteal type affects adults, and causes erosion of the anterior aspect of several vertebral bodies, so that a gradual curvature results.

Clinical Features.—These vary to some extent according to the site of the disease, but in any situation the following features are likely to be in evidence.

Symptoms.—These include lassitude, asthenia, and if the patient is a child, fretfulness, peevishness and loss of appetite.

Pain and deformity comprise the local symptoms, either of which may first be noticed. Pain occurs as a local ache, or is referred along the spinal nerves which correspond to the affected segments. Deformity occurs in the early stages if the bodies are affected, and is sometimes the first indication of the disease. Kyphosis is the most common type (fig. 911), but scoliosis occasionally occurs.

Signs.—A systematic examination of the whole of the spinal column must be made. Rigidity is a constant sign, and inability or unwillingness to bend the back is well demonstrated by requesting a patient to pick up an article from the floor, in which case the knees are bent and the patient assumes a squatting position. Active flexion, extension, and lateral rotation are attempted, and if no

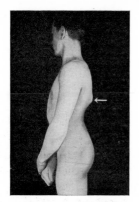

Fig. 911.—Kyphosis due to Pott's disease.

restriction of movement is discovered, the possibility of Pott's disease is remote.

Deformity is either a symptom or a sign, and if more than slight it has probably already been noticed by the patient or, if a child, by the mother or nurse.

Abscess formation is a common feature with Pott's disease (fig. 912) ; the site and extension depend upon the portion of the spine affected (*vide infra*).

Paraplegia is seen less frequently than formerly, owing to

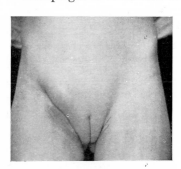

Fig. 912.—A psoas abscess pointing in the right groin.
(*Pybus.*)

earlier diagnosis and more efficient treatment. It is rarely if ever due to deformity, as the cord adapts itself to this slow process. It arises as a result of pachymeningitis, or pressure by granulation tissue, abscess, or possibly a sequestrum. Spasticity of the legs, with dragging of the feet on walking, is the first symptom of threatening paraplegia, and may even be the first evidence of spinal caries. Sensory disturbance and loss of sphincteric control follow.

Ninety per cent. of cases of paraplegia respond to extension of the spine, which can be obtained by recumbency on a Bradford frame or a plaster bed. Strapping extension to the legs may be necessary. If conservative methods are unsuccessful, *costo-transversectomy* should be considered. This operation involves excision of the vertebral end of the rib opposite the apex of the kyphosis, and the corresponding transverse process at its base. An abscess can thus be evacuated and pressure relieved. *Laminectomy* must be considered only as a last resort, as removal of the spinous processes and laminæ seriously weakens the spine if the bodies of the vertebræ are diseased, and the vertebral column is virtually transected. Collapse of the vertebral column and compression of the cord have followed this operation, which, if performed, must be combined with bone grafting, or else followed by prolonged support to the spine.

FEATURES OF THE DISEASE AT DIFFERENT LEVELS

Cervical Region.—The body of the second cervical vertebra is occasionally affected, or even the odontoid process, which represents the body of the atlas. Pain occurs in the distribution of the second cervical nerve, and the head is fixed owing to spasm of the suboccipital muscles. The transverse ligament or the odontoid process is liable to become eroded, and in either case the head may suddenly slip forwards with immediate fatal results.

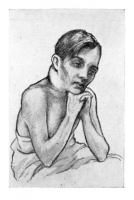

If vertebræ at a lower level are affected, pain is experienced over the distribution of the corresponding spinal nerves. A retropharyngeal abscess sometimes occurs, and may be seen or palpated (fig. 913). The pus erodes the longus colli muscle, and lies beneath the prevertebral fascia, and thus differs from an acute abscess (see p. 238), which is submucous.

The abscess either tracks laterally and appears in the posterior triangle, or in the case of the lower cervical vertebræ, it passes downwards beneath the fascia into the thorax. If allowed to extend, the prevertebral fascia is destroyed, and cases have occurred where the abscess has burst into the pharynx. Even if the patient is not suffocated secondary infection follows, with its attendant evils. Therefore a retropharyngeal abscess must be evacuated as soon as it is recognised, by an incision behind the sternomastoid muscle, which is displaced forwards with the carotid sheath. After evacuation the muscles, fascia, platysma, and skin are carefully and completely closed in separate layers. A radiograph of the upper four cervical vertebræ should be taken through the open mouth, so that the vertebral bodies are not obscured by the lower jaw.

FIG. 913.—Attitude assumed in Pott's disease of the cervical spine. The swelling is due to a retropharyngeal abscess.

Thoracic Region.—If the first dorsal vertebra is affected pain is referred along the inner side of the arm ; at a lower level intercostal neuralgia is likely, and abdominal pain and rigidity sometimes follow involvement of the eighth to the twelfth dorsal vertebræ (the appendix has been removed in such cases !).

Abscesses sometimes remain in the mediastinum, where they are visible in a radiograph. In other cases they track along an intercostal nerve, and either follow the posterior branch and so appear in the back, or pass forwards to come to the surface with the lateral cutaneous branch. The psoas muscle is attached to the twelfth dorsal body, and a psoas abscess may follow disease of that bone.

Lumbar Region.—Pain is referred to the lower part of the abdominal wall or down the lower limb. Abscesses are likely to appear in one of three situations—the lumbar region, the psoas sheath, or in the pelvis. A lumbar abscess is due to pus tracking along the posterior branch of one of the spinal nerves. It appears at the outer border of the erector spinæ muscle, or in the triangle of Petit.

The psoas muscle is attached to all the lumbar vertebræ, and an abscess within its sheath is common (fig. 914). The swelling is first palpable in the iliac fossa,

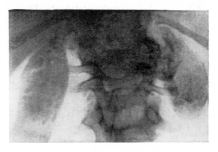

FIG. 914.—Old-standing tuberculous disease of the second lumbar vertebra, with calcified psoas abscesses.

whence the pus burrows beneath Poupart's ligament, on the outer side of the external iliac artery. Fluctuation can usually be transmitted from that portion of the abscess above the ligament to the collection of pus below, and vice versa. The abscess then may extend beneath the femoral vessels to appear at the saphenous opening, where it simulates a femoral hernia, especially as an impulse occurs on coughing owing to the contraction of the abdominal muscles compressing pus in the iliac fossa, and forcing an additional quantity downwards beneath Poupart's ligament. In later cases the abscess follows the external circumflex vessels, and appears in the region of the great trochanter.

A pelvic abscess occasionally follows disease of the lower lumbar vertebræ, and pus then either passes along the inferior hæmorrhoidal vessels into the ischio-rectal fossa, or escapes into the buttock through the sacro-sciatic notch.

Complications.—(a) *General.*—Miliary tuberculosis occasionally occurs, as it may with any active tuberculous affection. Should abscesses discharge on the surface secondary infection causes a varying degree of toxæmia, which, if prolonged, culminates in amyloid disease.

Prolonged recumbency and consequent decalcification of bone encourages the formation of renal calculi, which should be suspected if hæmaturia occurs. Adequate fluid intake and tilting the bed are prophylactic measures. Small calculi may disappear on resumption of the erect posture.

(b) *Local.*—Paraplegia has already been mentioned.

Abscess formation is not necessarily of serious import, and, with the exception of retropharyngeal abscess, no active measures are required, because the pus absorbs if the causative lesion responds to treatment. However, if the abscess is enlarging in size or threatening to involve the skin, steps must be taken to prevent rupture, which is inevitably followed by secondary infection. Aspiration is performed, usually with a

Jean Louis Petit, 1674–1750. Director of the Academy of Surgery, Paris.
François Poupart, 1661–1708. A Parisian anatomist.

wide-bore needle, which is thrust obliquely through adjacent healthy skin. In the case of a psoas abscess the puncture is made 1 inch (2·5 cm.) above and medial to the anterior superior iliac spine. In order to obtain a valvular puncture, the skin should be made to "slide" on the deep fascia before insertion of the needle. When evacuation is nearly complete the yellowish pus becomes pink in colour, owing to oozing from the unsupported capillaries in the granulation tissue of the abscess wall.

Pulmonary complications are encouraged by spinal deformity, as normal respiratory excursions are hampered by crowding of the ribs. Also kinking of the great vessels imposes an extra strain on the cardiac muscle. For these reasons few hunchbacks survive early middle age.

General Treatment.—This is conducted as for any tuberculous affection, and is best carried out at a recognised institution or sanatorium. Streptomycin appears to be of value.

Local Treatment.—Immobilisation of the spine is essential in order to encourage ankylosis. In some cases weight-extension is also applied in order to correct or minimise deformity.

Fixation of the spine is obtainable by two methods, conservative or operative.

CONSERVATIVE methods of obtaining immobilisation are numerous, and depend upon the age of the patient, the stage of the disease, and the preferences of the individual surgeon. If considerable deformity exists, treatment should commence with weight-extension, e.g. strapping is applied to each leg, and connected with a suitable weight by means of a cord passing over pulleys, which are fixed to the bottom of the bed. Counter-extension is obtained either by tilting up the foot of the bed, or by means of an axillary band which is fixed to the top of the bed.

Plaster of Paris jackets are applied when the deformity is overcome sufficiently, or if deformity is negligible treatment is commenced by the application of a jacket. If the disease affects the cervical spine, the jacket is continued well up under the chin in front and as high as the occipital tuberosity behind (fig. 915), while if the dorsal or lumbar regions are

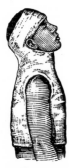

FIG. 915.—Plaster jacket for tuberculosis of cervical vertebræ.

affected the plaster extends from the axillæ to below the iliac crests. In all cases bony prominences are carefully padded, and a window is cut over the epigastrium to allow movement of abdominal muscles, and also to lighten the plaster. As the disease becomes quiescent less stringent methods of immobilisation are substituted. Thus a plaster bed is suitable for adults, and is moulded to the back while the patient lies upon his

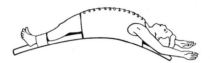

FIG. 916.—Whitman's frame, consisting of a double-inclined plane with corset and leg-pieces.

face. Further correction of any existing deformity can be obtained by means of pads suitably arranged. Children are conveniently treated by means of a Jones's or Whitman's frame, in which they can be transported as necessary, e.g. for sun or ultra-violet-ray treatment. As improvement progresses a modified apparatus is provided, so that the spine is supported while the patient can enjoy some liberty. A specially fitted celluloid jacket or a Taylor's brace is suitable, and if necessary an extension is fitted so as to steady the cervical vertebræ and support the head. These spinal supports are gradually discarded when pain and spasm have disappeared, and the patient's general health is satisfactory. Increasing sclerosis as seen by X-rays and a normal sedimentation rate are favourable features.

OPERATIVE TREATMENT.—This aims at supporting the spine by means of a bone graft from the tibia (Albee's operation), by which means practically complete immobilisation is secured.

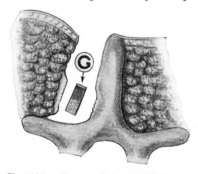

FIG. 917.—G = graft, inserted between spinous process and muscles.

The diseased portion of the spine, together with two vertebræ above and below, is exposed. The muscles, periosteum, and a flake of bone at the base of the spinous process are separated from the neural arch and spinous process of these exposed vertebræ (fig. 917). The bed so prepared is rendered hæmostatic by means of a hot saline pack. A graft of sufficient length is then cut from the subcutaneous surface of a tibia, by means of a double-bladed, electro-motor saw. Iced saline should be dripped on the saw during use to prevent the heat arising

Royal Whitman, Contemporary. Professor of Orthopœdics, New York Polyclinic.
Charles Fayette Taylor, 1827–1899. Surgeon, The Orthopœdic Hospital, New York.
Fred H. Albee, 1876–1945. American Orthopœdic Surgeon.

from friction exerting a deleterious effect upon bone cells. The graft is lifted from the tibia and fixed in the prepared bed by pressure of the separated muscles, which are firmly sutured back into position with stout catgut.

Until the wound has healed the patient is nursed in a box splint, which allows him to be turned on his face at intervals. In about fourteen days a plaster of Paris jacket is applied, and three months later this is removed and a celluloid jacket or other suitable support is fitted. After another six months this is gradually discarded, and cure should be effected about one year after the operation.

The value of Albee's operation has provided a fruitful subject for discussion. It certainly provides more efficient fixation of the diseased spine than conservative measures, and in satisfactory cases it is a time-saving procedure. The main objection is that if the disease progresses after operation a cavity results which is prevented by the graft from closing. Perhaps the general consensus of opinion may be summarised as follows :

Bone grafting should be considered, provided—

(i) The affected region is other than cervical. Fixation of the cervical region results in a permanently stiff neck.

(ii) The patient is sufficiently robust, and the skin of the operation field is healthy. (A tuberculous abscess can be incised, mopped out, and otherwise ignored.)

(iii) The patient has reached the age of at least ten years. In younger children time is of relative unimportance, and conservative measures are usually satisfactory. Also growth is impaired if spinal fixation is performed in growing children, and the graft may prevent collapse of vertebral bodies and so delay healing.

(iv) The disease is quiescent so that further bony destruction is improbable.

SPONDYLITIS

Widespread inflammation of the spinal muscles, ligaments, or bones occasionally occurs, due to various and sometimes obscure causes. Those which appear to be separate clinical entities are as follows :

GONOCOCCAL, resembles the periarticular type of arthritis which sometimes occurs in the feet. The spinal ligaments are chiefly affected, giving rise to pain and stiffness. Treatment is symptomatic, combined with eradication of the primary disease.

RHEUMATIC, which may be associated with myalgia, fibrositis, etc., elsewhere. Ligaments and muscles become stiff and contracted, but no marked bony changes are obvious in a radiograph.

OSTEOARTHRITIC, a painful and intractable condition which is predisposed to by injury, laborious occupations, exposure, and possibly by toxæmia from some focus of infection. It is commonly met with in elderly people, especially males. The pathological changes occurring in the spinal joints resemble those of osteoarthritis elsewhere, and in addition fibrosis of muscles and ossification of spinal ligaments occur. Manipulation is often beneficial in early cases, otherwise treatment is symptomatic.

Spondylitis deformans (*syn*. ankylosing spondylitis) is a crippling disease of unknown ætiology, which, clinically, occurs as two distinct types :

(i) Von Bechterew, which affects males, and often during adolescence. The cervical region is first affected, and the disease spreads to the remainder of the spine and the costo-transverse joints (fig. 918).

(ii) Marie-Strümpell, which affects both sexes and begins in middle life. It usually first involves the lumbar region, then spreads upwards along the spine, and eventually the hip and shoulder joints are affected.

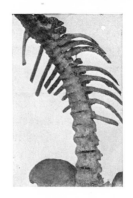

FIG. 918.—Advanced spondylitis, showing kyphosis and ossification of the anterior common ligament.

In both types the first symptom is pain, which is followed by stiffness and increasing deformity. Pain diminishes as ankylosis increases. Eventually the spine becomes completely rigid (" poker back," fig. 919) and deformity may be so extreme that the patient, while standing, cannot raise his eyes from the ground (fig. 1202).

In the early stages the discovery and eradication of a focus of infection may arrest the disease. Deep X-ray therapy is often of value, and in suitable cases spinal osteotomy should be considered (p. 1191).

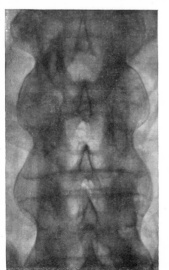

Sacralisation of the lowest lumbar vertebra is a condition which is now recognised as pathological. The transverse process of the vertebra is elongated, so that it is in contact with the lateral mass of the sacrum. Lateral flexion of the spine causes nipping of the soft tissues between the bones, or pressure on the fifth lumbar nerve which passes below the enlarged transverse process. The resulting pain is relieved by extension of the spine or by recumbency. A pelvic support sometimes relieves symptoms. Manipulation is occasionally useful, and osteopaths are well aware of the condition. Operative intervention and removal of part of the transverse process is sometimes advisable.

FIG. 919.—Ossification of the lumbar spine (*bamboo spine*).

Vladimir von Bechterew, 1857–1927. A Russian neurologist.
Pierre Marie, 1853–1929. Professor of Medicine in Paris.
Adolf von Strümpell, 1853–1925. A German physician.

TUMOURS OF THE VERTEBRAL COLUMN

INNOCENT TUMOURS are extremely rare, although chondromata, osteomata, and fibromata have all been reported. The symptoms which arise simulate those of extradural tumours, and a radiograph may demonstrate them.

MALIGNANT TUMOURS of the spine are primary or secondary.

Primary sarcoma is uncommon, and is most frequent in children and young adults. The neural arches are usually affected, and therefore a palpable swelling is often detectable. Complete removal of the tumour is rarely possible, and usually only palliative treatment, i.e. a spinal support, deep X-ray therapy, and analgesics, is possible.

Secondary deposits in the spine are unfortunately of common occurrence, and more than half the cases follow carcinoma of the breast. The other organs which, on becoming carcinomatous, often disseminate to bone, contribute their quota. These include the prostate, kidney, bronchus, and thyroid. Periosteal sarcoma of any bone may also give rise to a secondary deposit in the spine. Metastases nearly always affect the body of the vertebra.

In the large majority of cases pain is the first, and for a variable period, the only symptom. The pain occurs at the site of the disease, and later becomes girdle in type, or radiates along one or more limbs. Probably at this stage the patient is treated for lumbago, sciatica, abdominal disorders, and may even be subjected to operation. The pain increases in intensity and is aggravated by movement, so that the patient may remain crouched on a chair or huddled up in bed for hours at a time. Cord symptoms appear at any time. One of our patients, with no sign of vertebral involvement, developed complete paraplegia on the first occasion she left her bed after removal of a breast for carcinoma. More commonly the onset of paraplegia is ushered in with increased reflexes and spasticity, but cord involvement is usually complete in a few weeks, and is followed by cystitis, pyelonephritis, bedsores, and death.

TREATMENT of secondary deposits necessitates a support to the spine, analgesics, and possibly deep X-ray therapy. The antero-lateral tracts have been divided in order to relieve agonising pain. Welcome relief is sometimes obtained by intrathæcal alcohol (p. 898).

TUMOURS IN THE SPINAL CANAL

These are extradural or intradural, the latter being either extra- or intramedullary.

Extradural tumours are very rare, but neuromata, lipomata, and fibromata all occur. As these tumours are innocent and slowly growing, symptoms are present for a long period before pressure on the cord is sufficient to interfere with its function. Vague motor or sensory disturbances, which often remit and are variable, are suggestive of this condition.

Dumb-bell tumours are neuro-fibromata. Part of the tumour is extradural, and is connected with a larger paravertebral portion by a narrow isthmus which passes through an intervertebral foramen. Spinal compression eventually develops, necessitating laminectomy and excision. Erosion of an intervertebral foramen is a useful radiological aid to diagnosis.

Extramedullary growths, the most common spinal tumours, are meningiomata or neuro-fibromata, the latter arising from a nerve sheath. Paræsthesia followed by pain, due to irritation of a posterior root, is the first symptom. As a rule, a definite interval of some months elapses before cord symptoms appear, which may resemble those which arise from hemisection (Brown-Séquard syndrome), i.e. pressure of the tumour on one side of the cord causes motor paresis and loss of sensation on the same side of the body, while on the opposite side sensibility to pain and temperature is diminished, and possibly tactile sensation also.

As mentioned in connection with secondary deposits in the vertebræ, root pains often cause errors of diagnosis in the early stages.

Intramedullary Tumours.—The commonest is an ependymoma (which is a growth of the ependymal cells which line the central canal), but other varieties of gliomata and cysts also occur. More than half the intramedullary tumours occur in the cervical portion of the cord.

The symptoms which arise from an intramedullary tumour depend upon the site of its origin. Usually motor and sensory symptoms synchronise, e.g. paresis of one limb accompanied by sensations of heat or cold. Root pains are not likely to appear until later, so that intramedullary tumours are not usually painful in the early stages.

RECOGNITION OF THE LEVEL OF THE TUMOUR

A careful clinical examination is of paramount importance, and in some sites it is possible to locate accurately the affected segment. Accessory means of investigation include the electrical reactions of muscles, radiography, and lumbar puncture.

Charles-Edouard Brown-Séquard, 1818–1894. Successively Professor of Medicine in the Harvard and Paris medical faculties.

Clinical Examination.—May show sensory disturbances, paresis, and wasting of muscles, exaggeration or diminution of reflexes, and disturbed function of sphincters. Root pains and hyperæsthesia are among the most reliable signs of the upper level of the neoplasm, and of the side on which it lies. In addition to symptoms arising from interference with the ascending and descending tracts, disease of different segments of the cord gives rise to disturbances depending on the function of that particular portion.

The more important localising features are as follows :

Upper Cervical.—Tumours in this region are occasionally fatal from involvement of the phrenic nerve centres, and interference with the medulla oblongata sometimes causes cardiac irregularity and hyperpyrexia. Involvement of the oculo-pupillary fibres which pass down to their nucleus in the first dorsal segment results in myosis, narrowing of the palpebral fissure, and enophthalmos (Horner's syndrome). Neuralgic pains are likely to occur over the mastoid and occipital regions, the neck, supraclavicular or acromial areas, or down the arms.

Lower Cervical and Upper Dorsal.—Irritation or compression of the oculo-pupillary fibres is liable to occur if the tumour is situated at or above the first dorsal segment. Interference with the anterior horn cells from the fifth cervical to the first dorsal segments causes paralysis and wasting of characteristic groups of muscles (p. 920).

Examination of reflexes may yield valuable information. If the supinator reflex is absent the tumour is situated at the level of the fifth or sixth cervical segment, while absence of the triceps jerk indicates interference with the seventh segment. A tumour in the lower cervical or first dorsal area is likely to cause pain radiating down the arms. Below this level, intercostal neuralgia or girdle pains will probably be a prominent symptom.

Lower Dorsal.—Interference with the cord between the eighth and twelfth dorsal segments is likely to cause loss of upper or lower abdominal reflexes. Paresis of muscles is sometimes present, and if unilateral, a striking bulge of one-half of the abdominal wall is noticeable when the patient coughs.

Irritation of the seventh to the twelfth posterior roots causes a variety of abdominal symptoms, usually indefinite but persistent, and is a fruitful source of diagnostic errors.

Lumbar Cord.—Disturbances of the rectal and bladder sphincters are common. If the tumour is situated at or below the level of the second lumbar segment, one or both knee-jerks are diminished or absent. The cremasteric reflex is abolished if the tumour involves the upper part of the lumbar cord. Involvement of centres from which the lumbar plexus is derived causes paralysis and wasting of corresponding muscles. Owing to the comparatively small size of the lumbar and sacral segments of the cord, sacral nerves are commonly affected in addition to the lower lumbar.

Cauda Equina.—Pain occurs in the back, and extends to the perineum, genitals, and backs of the thighs. Sensory loss usually occurs over the distribution of the sacral nerves (saddle-shaped anæsthesia), and the lower the tumour is situated the smaller is the area of anæsthesia. Bladder and rectal disturbances are usual, and paresis of muscles depends upon the actual nerves involved.

Electrical Reactions.—Should pressure or infiltration by the tumour interfere with the anterior horn cells, then the muscles innervated by these cells undergo a lower motor neurone paralysis. Hence the absence of reaction of a muscle or group of muscles to faradic current may be an important clue to the situation of the tumour.

Radiography.—The introduction of 1 ml. of lipiodol into the cisterna magna was formerly used to demonstrate spinal block. It is now realised that lipiodol is an irritant to nerve roots, so pantopaque or myodil has superseded its use.

Cisternal Puncture.—A graduated lumbar puncture needle is inserted at the centre of a line joining the tips of the mastoid processes, and the cistern is reached at a distance of 4·5 to 6 cms. (1·8 to 2·5 inches). The needle should not be introduced to a greater depth for fear of injuring the medulla.

Pantopaque is injected and gravitates downwards until it is arrested by the tumour, and the site of the block can then be seen in a radiograph. This method is secondary in importance to clinical examination, and we have seen cases where a complete block was apparently present, but at operation no abnormality was discovered. Air or oxygen myelography is sometimes performed.

Lumbar Puncture.—If the tumour interferes with the cerebro-spinal circulation, the fluid below is frequently yellow in colour (xanthochromia), and contains an increased amount of protein, which is normally 20 to 30 mg. ($\frac{1}{3}$ to $\frac{1}{2}$ gr.) per cent. Examination of the intradural pressure by means of a manometer attached to the needle sometimes shows difference of pressure in the cisterna magna and the lumbar region. Although this is of little value in locating the site of a tumour, it is important in confirming its presence.

As spinal tumours increase in size, the natural result is that destruction of the cord occurs sooner or later. Laminectomy is performed as soon as a tumour is diagnosed and its situation located. The prognosis is much more favourable than in the case of cerebral tumours, as about 50 per cent. of spinal tumours are removable.

As in the case of cerebral tumours, the possibility of the lesion being syphilitic in nature must be borne in mind.

LAMINECTOMY

The indications for laminectomy are as follows :

1. **Traumatic.**—These are considered on p. 878.

2. **Inflammatory.**—Paraplegia complicating Pott's disease (p. 885).

3. Neoplasm.—Provided that the condition of the patient is satisfactory, laminectomy is performed for all tumours within the spinal canal. " Tumour " includes such conditions as tuberculoma and cysts. Occasionally new-growth of the spinal column justifies exploration.

4. Division of suitable posterior roots in order to overcome spasticity in Little's disease (fig. 920) is now practised by but few surgeons, as division of muscles and peripheral nerves, combined with physiotherapy, usually give better results.

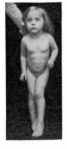

FIG. 920.—Spastic paraplegia, showing typical attitude and adduction of the legs.

5. **Cordotomy.**—Division of the spinothalamic tracts was devised for the relief of pain due to such conditions as an irremovable new-growth or spondylitis, provided that the cause of the pain is not at a higher level than the fifth dorsal segment. The cord is exposed above the site of the lesion, and the spinothalamic tracts are divided to a depth of 3–4 mm. as they lie between the denticulate ligament and the anterior root. A deeper incision will involve the pyramidal tract. If the pain is unilateral and not of visceral origin, the tract on the opposite side only need be divided. The patient must be warned against unconscious injury or burns of anæsthetised areas.

The tremor of Parkinson's disease is relieved by division of the whole of the lateral tract at the second cervical segment on the side affected (L. C. Oliver). The operation is only suitable for patient's under fifty with unilateral tremor, and who are mentally stable.

The immediate effects of the operation are total absence of tremor, hemiplegia on the same side, and loss of sensation to pain and temperature on the opposite side. Later a little tremor is to be found at times of mental stress, and the hemiplegia usually recovers almost completely, but the hemianalgesia and hemithermanæsthesia are permanent.

Operation.—If laminectomy is to be performed for the attempted removal of a tumour, the discrepancy between the level of the affected segment of the cord and that of the corresponding vertebra must be considered. It must be remembered that owing to the disparity in the length of the spinal cord and vertebral column, a segment in the cervical region lies one vertebra above its corresponding vertebral body. In the upper dorsal region the tumour will be two vertebræ, and in the lower dorsal three vertebræ, above the corresponding vertebral body.

In estimating these levels by palpation of the spinous processes, it must not be forgotten that in the dorsal region the processes overlap the vertebra below. Thus, presuming a tumour is localised to the ninth dorsal segment, it should be opposite the tip of the fifth spinous process, i.e. three vertebræ higher on account of the shortness of the cord as compared with the spinal column, and one vertebra higher because of the obliquity of the spinous process.

The patient is usually placed in the prone position, with a sandbag under the sternum and pelvis. If the laminectomy is exploratory, a midline incision is advisable, as it can be prolonged in either direction if necessary. Otherwise a flap is preferable. Muscles are separated from the spinous processes and neural arches with a raspatory and an occasional touch with a scalpel, and venous hæmorrhage controlled by means of hot

William John Little, 1810–1894. *Physician to the London Hospital.*
L. C. Oliver, Contemporary. *Neurosurgeon, Royal Northern Hospital, London.*

saline packs. When sufficient vertebræ are exposed the interspinous ligaments are divided, and spinous processes removed by means of angled bone forceps. The neural arches are then divided on either side with a Doyen's saw, which is guarded so as to avoid possible injury to the cord (fig. 921). Owing to the obliquity of the pedicles the direction of the saw-cut must be forwards and *inwards*. A small trephine and laminectomy forceps are favoured by some surgeons as a means of removing the laminæ. When the arches are

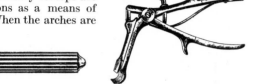

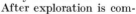

FIG. 921.—Doyen's saw.

FIG. 922.—Hudson's guillotine forceps for laminectomy.

divided the ligamentum subflavum is cut across above and below, and the laminæ removed. Projecting portions of neural arches are conveniently removed with a Hudson's guillotine, the blade of which cuts upwards, so as to avoid risk of injury to the cord (fig. 922).

The dura mater is now exposed, and the presence of a tumour, and the degree of pulsation or discoloration, are noticed. Unless some pathological condition is found the dura is opened. This is done by steadying the membrane with tenaculum forceps or a stitch, nicking it with a tenotome, and then slitting it up with guarded scissors, or by means of a grooved director and a scalpel. The divided dura is held aside by means of a stitch or mosquito forceps, and the exposed structures are inspected. A meningioma is excised together with the portion of dura from which it arises. If a neurofibroma is discovered, it is removed with a portion of the nerve sheath to which it is attached. Should it be deemed necessary to inspect the anterior part of the cord, one of the prolongations of the ligamentum denticulatum is grasped with forceps, and traction then permits of rotation of the cord. The cord is then incised vertically on the side of the tumour (fig. 923). An infiltrating tumour, such as an ependymoma, cannot be removed, but a vertical incision over it allows it to extrude, and symptoms may thereby be relieved.

After exploration is com-

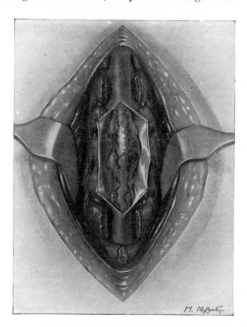

FIG. 923.—An intramedullary tumour exposed
by laminectomy.

Eugène Doyen, 1859–1916. Surgeon, Doyen Clinic, Paris.
William Henry Hudson, Contemporary. Surgeon, Atlanta, Georgia.

pleted the dura mater is closed with a continuous silk or linen suture, the spinal muscles are firmly sutured together, and the skin closed with interrupted stitches.

LUMBAR PUNCTURE

This procedure is adopted for the following reasons :

1. **Diagnostic,** e.g. meningitis, Wassermann reaction or gold test for syphilis, to disclose intradural hæmorrhage.   Also for the injection of pantopaque, or to assess the protein content, if a tumour is suspected.   Manometric readings are sometimes useful to assess the intradural pressure.

2. **Therapeutic,** in order to introduce some drug, e.g. penicillin for meningitis (p. 880), or for reduction of intrathecal pressure.

Relief of Pain.—Differential anæsthesia is produced by the injection of 0·75 ml. of absolute alcohol.   The pain-conducting fibres passing from the posterior root ganglia to enter the spinal cord possess a much thinner myelin sheath than fibres conducting other forms of sensation.   Consequently the pain fibres are more readily affected by alcohol.   The patient lies with the affected side uppermost, and a pillow is inserted so that the nerves to be destroyed are at the summit of the curve.   Lumbar puncture is performed, usually between L iv and L v, and the alcohol injected drop by drop during an interval of about two minutes.   The patient should lie on the side for about two hours, and then walk.   It is lighter than cerebrospinal fluid, and is rapidly fixed by the nerve fibres and therefore does not injure the cord.   Parasympathetic fibres are liable to be involved, so retention of urine occasionally occurs.   Some numbness of the leg is experienced, but is transitory.   This method is valuable for relieving intense pain due to malignant neoplasms, e.g. carcinoma of the cervix. If pain is bilateral, the procedure is repeated on the opposite side one week later.

3. **Anæsthesia:** stovaine, novocaine, spinocaine, and percaine ; each has its individual supporters.

Spinocaine is composed of novocaine (100 mg. in each ml.) and strychnine.   The dose varies from 1 ml. for children under six years of age to 3 ml. for adults.   A pressor substance, such as ephedrine gr. $\frac{1}{2}$—$\frac{3}{4}$ (30–45 mg.), is usually given intramuscularly in order to maintain the blood-pressure.

Percaine is used in a 1 : 1,500 solution in 0·5 per cent. saline.   The specific gravity of this solution is 1003, which is lighter than cerebrospinal fluid (sp. gr. 1006).   The average dose is 14 ml., which gives complete abdominal anæsthesia, but 10 ml. is usually sufficient for operations below the umbilicus.   After injection the patient lies on his face for five minutes so that the posterior roots are chiefly affected.   He is then turned on his back, and slight tilting downwards of the head of the table will help to fix the percaine caudalwards and counteract any fall of blood-pressure.

Catastrophes, such as incontinence of urine or damage to spinal nerves, occasionally occur.   These calamities are possibly due to an invisible crack in a phial, which, if submerged in spirit or other antiseptic, may allow some of the fluid to percolate into the interior. *Phials should always be submerged in coloured fluid,* and any phial which contains coloured contents is rejected.

Some premedication, such as omnopon and scopolamine, is safe and humane, but if the intercostal muscles are paralysed, depression of the respiratory centre is dangerous.

It will be remembered that at birth the cord extends to the third lumbar vertebra. In the adult it terminates opposite the lower border of the body of the first lumbar vertebra, and therefore the dural sac can be safely punctured at any site between the second lumbar interspace and the fifth lumbar vertebra. The nerves of the cauda equina are so arranged that a space of 2 mm. to 5 mm. in width exists between the roots on either side, and the needle usually passes between the nerves. Sudden pain in the leg indicates that the needle is in contact with a nerve, but this symptom is of no moment.

A line connecting the highest parts of the iliac crests passes over the fourth lumbar spine, so that a needle entered just above or below should pass through the third or fourth lumbar interspaces respectively (fig. 924). The depth to which the needle passes varies from 1 cm. in a small child to 10 cm. in a fat adult. If the patient is self-controlled, a small amount of local anæsthetic is desirable, although not imperative, but in the case of

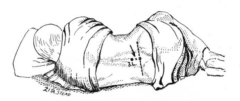

Fig. 924.—Lumbar puncture. (The site of puncture is usually between the third and fourth lumbar spines.)

children or patients afflicted with tetanus a general anæsthetic is necessary. Flexion of the spine widens the spaces between the neural arches. The needle used should be of medium bore (about 18 to 20 gauge), as the aperture resulting from puncture with a wide needle will allow subsequent escape of cerebrospinal fluid, with consequent persistent headaches, which, however, are usually relieved by the local application of diathermy. Also the bevel of the needle must be short, so that there is no danger of part of the opening remaining outside the dura mater, and resistance to penetration is more readily perceived with an abruptly bevelled needle. As the needle and stylet are entered the resistance of the tough ligamentum subflavum is encountered. A little extra pressure perforates this structure, and on withdrawal of the stylet the cerebro-spinal fluid should flow from the needle. If only a few drops of blood escape, in all probability the point of the needle is lying in the spinal canal outside the dural sheath, and the blood is escaping from the spinal veins. The needle should then be withdrawn, washed out in saline solution, and reinserted. A manometer, attached to the needle, is useful in estimating the cerebro-spinal pressure, the normal being from 60 to 120 mm. of water in the recumbent position, and about 20 mm. higher if the patient sits. The pressure is increased in such conditions as meningitis, cerebral or spinal tumour, and intracranial hæmorrhages. Care must be taken that not more than 15 ml. of fluid are removed in cases of increased pressure, otherwise the medulla is liable to become wedged in the foramen magnum with fatal consequences, owing to interference with the vital centres.

PROLAPSED INTERVERTEBRAL DISC

Herniation of the nucleus pulposus through the tough annulus fibrosus follows trauma, and usually affects men between the ages of twenty and forty. The central portion of the inter-vertebral disc, which is developed from the notochord, is of jelly-like consistency, and herniation of this substance may be associated with strain or injury.

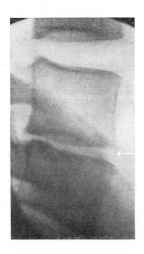

Fig. 925.—Narrowing of the intervertebral space between the fourth and fifth lumbar vertebræ.

The condition usually occurs in the lower cervical or lower lumbar regions. In either case symptoms are increased by coughing or sneezing, and the protein content of the cerebro-spinal fluid is raised. X-ray usually reveals narrowing of the intervertebral space (fig. 925). Owing to a clearer appreciation of the neurological signs, intradural injection of pantopaque, followed by an X-ray, is now but rarely necessary.

Cervical.—Prolapse of the disc at C.5–6 compresses the sixth root, and results in paresis and wasting of the biceps muscle, and paræsthesia or pain, which radiates down to the dorsum of the thumb and index finger. The disc at C.6–7 affects the seventh root, and gives rise to wasting of the triceps muscle and sensory disturbances, which spread down the arm to the middle finger. In either case other muscles are often affected. The majority of patients are relieved of symptoms by rest in bed for a month with the head flexed by pillows, and relaxation of paretic muscles. If symptoms persist, they usually respond to manipulation by rotation and hyperextension and fixation in a plaster of Paris cast. Operation is very rarely indicated.

Lumbar.—Prolapse occurs most commonly between L.5 and S.1, and gives rise to paræsthesia or pain, which radiates down the back of the thigh and leg to the outer side of the foot, with diminution or loss of the ankle jerk. The clinical features are more limited in distribution than in a case of sciatic neuritis, which is a comparatively rare condition, and pressure over the nerve is painless. Involvement of a disc at higher levels produces symptoms referred to the appropriate nerve, accompanied by low backache and spasm of the lumbar muscles.

In most cases attempts at toe-touching with legs rigid cause an exacerbation of pain. Patients occasionally adopt a postural scoliosis, as in this position pressure on the spinal nerve is relieved. In some cases compression of the internal jugular veins causes an exacerbation of symptoms. Herniation of the nucleus must be distinguished from such conditions as tuberculous abscess, secondary carcinoma, and a neuroma of the cauda equina.

Treatment consists in confinement to bed until symptoms abate, which is usually a matter of two to four weeks. A plaster jacket is applied for about two months, after which a spinal brace is worn for a further few months. The majority of cases are cured by this routine. Operation is indicated if symptoms persist or if severe pain recurs, as the prolapse may be irreducible. The disc is exposed by excision of the interspinous and interneural ligaments, with a minimum of bone. A standard laminectomy is contraindicated, as it encourages further collapse of the spine. Even after satisfactory removal of the prolapsed disc, symptoms are not always alleviated, as two conditions may persist. In long-standing cases prolonged compression of the nerve may have resulted in interstitial neuritis, or possibly osteoarthritis has affected the intervertebral joints. If these conditions are suspected, spinal fusion should be performed when the disc is removed, so as to afford complete rest to the affected segment of the spine.

SACRAL PUNCTURE

The sacral epidural space may be entered through the large triangular opening on the dorsum of the bone, and sacral anæsthesia obtained by the injection into the space of 20 ml. of 1 per cent. novocaine. Operations on the lower bowel and anal margin can then be performed painlessly, and some obstetricians practise this method in order to relieve the pains of child-birth, an additional advantage being that the infant is unaffected.

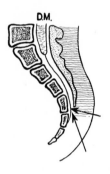

FIG. 926.—Indicating direction of needle.

To perform sacral puncture the median crest of the sacrum is palpated until the depression caused by the sacral opening is recognised. A lumbar puncture needle is introduced directly forwards until the ligaments covering the opening are pierced, after which the direction of the needle is changed so that it passes vertically upwards within the sacral canal (fig. 926). In order to ensure that the point of the needle is within the epidural space, it is wise to inject a few ml. of normal saline ; if the needle has not penetrated the canal, infiltration of the subcutaneous tissues will be evident, in which case it is withdrawn and a fresh attempt is made.

CHAPTER XXXV
NERVES
INJURIES

INJURIES of nerves are classified according to the extent of the damage to the sheath and nerve fibres. *Neurapraxia* is due to such injuries as concussion or contusion, and rapid recovery is the rule. *Axonotmesis* follows compression or crushing, when the sheath survives, but nerve fibres are damaged to a variable extent. Regeneration and functional recovery are usually more or less complete, but several months may elapse before the final result can be assessed. *Neurotmesis* occurs as a result of anatomical division by wounds or subcutaneous rupture, and the peripheral part of the nerve undergoes Wallerian degeneration.

NEURAPRAXIA

Contusion of a nerve is associated with an extravasation of blood within its sheath. Temporary paræsthesia and paresis follow, and recovery is usually complete.

Concussion follows vibratory effects, such as the passage of a missile of high velocity through tissues adjacent to the nerve. No apparent lesion of the nerve can be detected, and recovery is the rule.

AXONOTMESIS

Compression is caused by the pressure of crutches, tourniquets, fractures, bony abnormalities such as cervical ribs, splints, or incorrect posture on an operating table. The first symptoms are usually due to paræsthesia, and consist of numbness and tingling along the distribution of the nerve, followed by neuralgic pain. Paresis occurs later, but complete paralysis and wasting of muscles are uncommon unless the compression is prolonged. The pressure must be removed, and operative measures may be necessary, e.g. excision of a cervical rib, or freeing a nerve from callus. Sensory symptoms are thereby relieved, but if interstitial fibrosis has occurred as a result of prolonged pressure, motor disability is likely to persist.

Friction may interfere with function, owing to the development of a patch of fibrosis within the nerve. It is an uncommon cause of nerve injury, but sometimes follows cubitus valgus, in which case transposition of the ulnar nerve is required (p. 926).

NEUROTMESIS

Rupture of a nerve occurs as a complication of a dislocation, fracture, or of excessive stretching, as in the case of the brachial plexus. The sheath of the nerve sometimes remains intact (axonotmesis) when natural repair is to be expected.

Treatment consists in relaxing paralysed muscles, and in exploring the nerve if recovery does not commence within a reasonable time (p. 907).

Division of a nerve is either *complete* or *incomplete*. If division is complete, the results are immediate or remote.

Immediate.—After division of a mixed nerve there follows paralysis of muscles supplied by the nerve, a varying area of anæsthesia depending on the amount of overlap of neighbouring nerves, and vasomotor changes, the part supplied by the nerve becoming temporarily hyperæmic, but later colder and anæmic.

Remote.—(*a*) *Nerve.*—Retraction of the divided ends occurs, the intervening gap being filled with blood. This eventually organises, and during this process nerve fibres grow distally, and if unable to unite with divided peripheral fibres they become coiled up, the resulting mass of fibrous and nervous tissue forming a false neuroma. Distally, Wallerian degeneration occurs, the medullary sheath degenerates, and the myelin is removed by leucocytes within a month. Axis cylinders disappear, and neurilemma cells proliferate, so that the nerve is eventually represented by a fibrous strand containing neurilemma tubules.

(*b*) *Muscles.*—Paralysis, followed by wasting, occurs. Paralysed tendons will become stretched unless relaxation is rigorously maintained. Complete immobilisation is, however, harmful, as it results in stiffness from contracture of ligaments. All joints are therefore put through a full range of passive movement at least once a day.

Response to faradic stimulation is lost within three weeks, while galvanic response may remain for years, the contraction being sluggish, and the anodal closure is greater than the cathodal. This *reaction of degeneration* is of practical importance, as it indicates that suture is necessary for recovery.

Augustus Volney Waller, 1816–1870. English physiologist.

(c) *Sensation.*—Various objective sensory tests are applied in order to discover the extent to which sensation is impaired ; the more important are :

Touch.—The appreciation of light touch is tested by stroking the skin with a wisp of cottonwool. Pressure touch is investigated by pressure with a blunt object, and localisation of touch by asking the patient to indicate the point of contact.

Tactile Discrimination.—Blunt-pointed compasses, with a scale indicating the distance between the points, are used. The skin is sometimes touched with one point, and at other times by both. Records are noted concerning recognition of one or of two points, and in the latter case the distance separating the points.

Pain.—Superficial pain is tested by pricking the skin with a pin. Areas of anæsthesia or hyperæsthesia are discovered by drawing a pin or pencil along the skin, and requesting the patient to comment on altered sensation. Deep pain is elicited by squeezing a muscle or tendon.

Temperature.—Metal tubes are used, one of which is filled with ice, and the other with water at about 45° C. (113° F.). A higher temperature than this will be interpreted as pain.

Passive Movement.—The limb, or segment of a limb, is moved in a certain direction, and the patient is then asked to describe the position, or imitate it by moving the opposite limb.

Stereognosis.—An object in common use, such as a cork, is placed in the patient's hand, and he is asked to identify it.

Division of a mixed nerve causes a loss of all forms of sensation, which may be much less than the anatomical distribution of the nerve, owing to overlap of adjacent nerves.

(d) *Trophic and Vasomotor.*—Transient vaso-dilatation is followed by diminution of the circulation, so that the affected parts become cold and ulcers are prone to occur. The skin becomes dry and nails wrinkled, and absorption of small bones and ankylosis of joints eventually occur. In children, lack of growth of the affected limb is to be expected.

Closed injuries, i.e. those due to compression or traction, are treated by supporting the affected muscles in moderate relaxation, combined with routine movements of the appropriate joints. Massage is beneficial, but it must not be vigorous as the muscle fibres have lost their resiliency and are easily damaged.

Also, as they are insensitive, the patient cannot register a degree of pressure which would otherwise be painful. Galvanism is helpful in limiting the amount of wasting and in discouraging fibrosis.

Injuries due to traction are seldom suitable for exploration. If spontaneous recovery does not occur, then operation is unlikely to improve matters (e.g. brachial plexus, p. 919). Compression injuries should be explored if there is no evidence of recovery after a reasonable time.

Movements produced by unaffected muscles must not mislead the observer. Thus, in a case of radial paralysis, the fingers can be extended by the interosseous and lumbrical muscles, provided that the hand is supported. Also vicarious movements may be performed by adjacent muscles, e.g. in the case of division of the median nerve, the adductors of the thumb, acting in conjunction with the extensor ossis metacarpi pollicis, can produce opposition of the thumb.

H. J. Seddon *et al.* have endeavoured to calculate the rates of nerve regeneration, basing their results on the following clinical data :
(i) Tinel's sign—the course of the nerve is lightly percussed with a patella hammer, from below upwards. A tingling sensation is experienced when the level of regeneration is reached.
(ii) Measurement of the rate at which pain and touch sensibility return.
(iii) Observation of the times at which the function of muscles returns at different levels from the injury.
It appears that regeneration occurs initially at about 2 mm. a day, but the rate diminishes as time passes, so that after about three months it has slowed down to about 1 mm. a day. Other factors which influence the results of suture are discussed on p. 908.

Open Wounds.—Until recently it was considered that unless infection was inevitable immediate primary suture was the ideal treatment for a divided nerve. Surgeons with special experience of these injuries now recommend that the wound should be treated on accepted lines, i.e. excision and closure if possible, but that the nerve suture should be postponed until three or four weeks after the injury. If a divided nerve is encountered during excision of the wound, the ends are approximated by one stitch of fine silk, which prevents retraction during the period of delay. On no account should an attempt be made to identify or scrutinise a nerve in the vicinity. If only one end of a nerve is seen, then a suture should be inserted so as to fix it to adjacent muscle or fascia.

Luigi Galvani, 1737–1798. Italian physicist.
H. J. Seddon, P. B. Medawar, H. Smith. Peripheral Nerve Injury Centre, Oxford.
Jules Tinel, Contemporary. Physician, Hôpital Beaujon, Paris.

The advantages of early secondary suture over immediate primary suture are as follows :

(i) Primary suture usually requires enlargement of the wound by further incisions, so as to mobilise the nerve in order to allow approximation of the ends without tension. As the wound is potentially infected, exposure of previously uncontaminated tissues should be avoided.

(ii) The normal nerve sheath is a delicate structure, which is easily torn by the slightest tension, and accurate suturing is essential for the success of the operation. In addition, the sheath is often further weakened by longitudinal slits or tears. After about three weeks of the injury epineural fibrosis occurs and the sheath becomes thicker and tougher, consequently the insertion of sutures and accurate coaption of the nerve ends are greatly facilitated.

NERVE SUTURE

The two ends of the nerve are identified, the incision being prolonged sufficiently to expose the nerve well above and below the seat of injury, in such a position that its normal anatomical relations are not obscured by scar tissue. The two ends of the nerve are freed and " freshened " by means of a scalpel or a Bard-Parker knife. Scissors should not be used, as the nerve is crushed thereby. Slices are removed from the ends of the nerve until the projecting fibres are seen, and blood freely oozes from the cut surface. Apposition of the two ends is accomplished by the following manœuvres :

(a) *Mobilisation.*—The two ends are dissected from surrounding structures, care being taken to preserve important motor branches. Branches can often be stripped from the parent nerve in order to facilitate mobilisation.

(b) *Posture.*—The limb being held in a suitable position.

(c) *Transposition.*—The radial nerve is brought in front of the humerus, or the ulnar nerve in front of the internal condyle (p. 926).

(d) *Nerve Anchoring.*—If it is obvious that the two ends of a divided nerve cannot be brought together, on account of excessive loss of tissue or retraction, then the two untrimmed ends are approximated as closely as possible by tension stitches, the position of the limb being such that approximation is facilitated. Subsequently the nerve is stretched by gradually straightening the limb, and at a second operation the two ends are brought together. In some cases adequate suture can be performed while the limb is flexed, and extension is gradually regained.

(e) *Resection of Bone.*—This extensive procedure may be justifiable if nerve injury is associated with an ununited fracture, which also needs operative measures, e.g. in the case of the radial nerve and a fractured humerus.

Approximation having been obtained by one of the above procedures, sutures are introduced through the nerve sheath (fig. 927). Non-irritating material is used, such as fine black silk or tantalum wire. Catgut encourages fibrosis of the nerve. The suture line can be further supported

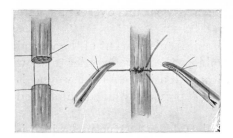

FIG. 927.—Primary nerve suture. Two sutures are passed through the sheath of the nerve in order to approximate the cut ends. The sheath is then sutured.

by painting with fibrin glue. Torsion of the nerve ends must be avoided, so that, as far as possible, proximal nerve fibres will join with their corresponding distal fibres. " Shunting " is thus avoided, and delay due to re-education of groups of muscles is obviated. If adjacent tissues are fibrosed, a new path can be constructed for the sutured nerve by opening a muscle sheath, and embedding the nerve among the muscle fibres, or a strip of fascia lata may be wrapped around the nerve and stitched in position. The limb is placed in a suitable position to prevent any strain on the sutured nerve, and a plaster cast may be advisable for a few weeks to immobilise the limb.

RESULTS OF NERVE SUTURE

This depends on many factors :

1. **Pre-operative.**—(a) *The Nerve Affected.*—Suture of nerves which supply muscles whose actions are intricate usually give disappointing results ; thus, recovery of palmar muscles, after suture of an ulnar nerve, may be negligible. On the other hand, muscles which perform coarse movements, e.g. those supplied by the radial nerve, often, to all appearances, recover completely. In addition, the radial nerve is mainly composed of motor fibres, hence there is little likelihood of motor fibres being " shunted " into sensory ones, with consequent wastage.

(b) *Infection.*—Not only causes delay before subsiding, but some degree of interstitial neuritis will result, and further damage to the nerve may be caused by contraction of surrounding scar tissue.

(c) *Time.*—Early secondary suture (p. 906) yields the best results, and further delay is detrimental.

(d) *Pre-operative Treatment.*—If muscles and tendons have been allowed to stretch, or if the tone of the muscles has been neglected, then the chances of recovery are correspondingly diminished.

2. **Operative.**—This consists of attention to the details already mentioned, e.g. hæmostasis, prevention of torsion and tension, preparation of suitable bed, and the use of non-irritating suture material.

3. **Post-operative.**—(a) *Absence of Infection.*—If the wound is already infected, or if infection supervenes, or being already present lights up again, then little improvement is likely.

(b) *After-treatment* consists in continuance of the relaxation of paralysed muscles, massage, electrical treatment, and muscular effort gradually increased as muscles recover their power.

(c) *Co-operation of the Patient.*—This important factor must receive due consideration, and the patient given every encouragement during his long and tedious rehabilitation.

(d) *Vicarious Movements.*—Although the physiological results of nerve suture may be poor, yet adjacent muscles often take upon themselves some of the functions of those which are paralysed, e.g. if the hamstrings are paralysed, and flexion of the knee thereby affected, the sartorius and gracilis muscles hypertrophy, and partially compensate for this deficiency.

Thus the functional result of a nerve injury is often more satisfactory than the physiological recovery would suggest.

In the case of successful suture of a nerve, apparent return of sensation is usually experienced within a few days, much to the surprise and gratification of the patient. He must be warned against optimism, as this phantom return disappears in two or three weeks. A pause of weeks or months occurs while the highly specialised sensory terminals and motor end-plates recover. Thus the time necessary for recovery depends to some extent on the site of injury and the length of nerve along which regeneration must occur. The first evidence of regeneration is a return of sensation. Motor recovery is slower than sensory. Even although motor recovery is disappointing, and restoration of sensation incomplete, yet trophic changes often improve to a marked extent, and healed sores and ulcers compensate to some extent for deficient motor and sensory recovery. As an example regarding the rate of recovery, an average length of time which lapses following primary suture of an ulnar nerve at the wrist would be six months for epicritic sensation, and up to two years for the paralysed muscles, the recovery of which will always be incomplete.

Irremediable Injury.—If suture is impossible on account of loss of tissue or wide separation of the ends of a divided nerve, the following procedures may be considered :

(*a*) *Nerve anastomosis*, e.g. part of the hypoglossal nerve is united to the distal end of the facial nerve. This method often results in improvement, but " successful " cases are sometimes associated with uncontrolled grimaces on movement of the tongue.

(*b*) *Nerve grafting* has produced encouraging results in selected cases, e.g. a gap in the facial nerve within its bony channel may be bridged by insertion of an autograft from the external cutaneous nerve of the thigh. Grafting of peripheral nerves is disappointing.

(*c*) *Tendon transplantation*, e.g. in the case of radial paralysis, tendons and muscles of the forearm may be transplanted into the extensor group. However, if proper relaxation of the extensor muscles has been consistently maintained, drop wrist should not occur, as the extensor tendons will not be over-stretched.

(*d*) *Arthrodesis*, e.g. in the case of injury to the sciatic nerve, arthrodesis of the flail ankle joint will render it stable and rigid.

(*e*) *Amputation*, for persistent sores and ulcers on the foot, particularly if growth is impaired. Sympathetic ganglionectomy might first be tried (p. 933).

Incomplete division of a nerve gives rise to a central or lateral neuroma. Effects vary according to the extent of the injury. Fibres supplying certain muscles are often constant in position, and hence are more liable to injury if their position exposes them to trauma. Thus partial division of the great sciatic nerve affects the external popliteal portion nine times more commonly than the internal popliteal, which passes down on the inner and deeper aspect of the great sciatic nerve.

Partial lesion of the median or internal popliteal nerves, or injury to their branches, may give rise to the distressing condition of *causalgia* (p. 935).

Injection lesions are due to accidental injection of therapeutic agents. They are more common in tropical countries where amœbiasis, schistosomiasis, and malaria are treated by intramuscular injections. The sciatic and radial nerves are usually

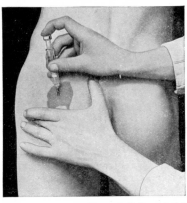

Fig. 928.—Intramuscular injection. The needle is inserted deeply into the upper and outer quadrant of the buttock.

(Burroughs Wellcome & Co.)

involved. Injections in the buttock should always be given into the upper and outer quadrant (fig. 928), and in the case of the arm into the upper half of the deltoid muscle.

CHAPTER XXXVI

SPECIAL NERVES

CRANIAL NERVES

THE **Olfactory Nerve** is liable to be injured by fractures passing through the cribriform plate, resulting in partial loss of smell (hyposmia), or anosmia of the corresponding side. Olfactory filaments are apt to be damaged as a result of occipital injuries (contre coup, p. 847).

The **Optic Nerve** may be damaged by fractures involving the optic foramen, or by compression by blood or inflammatory exudates in the orbit. Involvement by tumours or aneurisms is not uncommon. Blindness of the corresponding eye results, but contraction of the pupil occurs if the opposite retina is stimulated. The optic nerve is an outgrowth of the brain, and consequently gliomatous tumours occasionally arise in its substance.

The **Third Nerve** is sometimes involved by tumours, trauma, or aneurism, either in the skull, sphenoidal fissure, or the orbit. The following features are noticed :

(*a*) Ptosis of the upper eyelid, owing to paralysis of the levator palpebræ superioris.

(*b*) Proptosis, owing to paralysis of the majority of the ocular muscles, which normally exercise traction on the eyeball.

(*c*) Mydriasis, as the sympathetic fibres are unopposed, and cause unhampered dilatation of the pupil.

(*d*) Loss of accommodation, owing to paralysis of the ciliary muscle.

(*e*) Diplopia and external strabismus, with a slight downward inclination of the eyeball due to unopposed action of the external rectus and superior oblique muscles. Owing to their proximity, other nerves passing to the orbit are often affected. Involvement of the nerve sometimes occurs in cases of subdural hæmorrhage (p. 848).

The **Fourth Nerve** supplies the superior oblique muscle, and is rarely involved alone. Diplopia and deficient movement of the eye in a downward and outward direction may be noticed.

The **Fifth Nerve** or its branches are sometimes injured, and sensory disturbances follow (p. 1023).   The main surgical import-ance of this nerve lies in its susceptibility to neuralgia, or *tic douloureux*.   Trigeminal neuralgia occurs more commonly in females, and appears to be increasing in frequency.   Pain usually commences in the infra-orbital or inferior dental nerve, and extends to the remaining branches of the superior and inferior maxillary nerves, the ophthalmic division usually escaping.   Spasms of pain are precipitated by any external stimulus, such as a draught, brushing the teeth, or washing, and eventually the patient hardly dares to eat or speak.   The patient sometimes indicates " trigger zones," stimulation of which precipitates an attack.   The condition varies with the general health of the patient, and remissions occur, but the general tendency, at any rate for two or three years, is one of progress, so that the patient may become a morphomaniac or even suicidal.   Treatment consists in a thorough search for any source of reflex irritation, either dental, nasal, or ocular, and in the exhibition of analgesics, e.g. physeptone.   The patient must guard against exposure to cold or damp, and the general health must be maintained.   If the condition persists, injection or operation is indicated.

Injection is made into the Gasserian ganglion.   The needle is inserted immediately below the centre of the zygoma, and is passed backwards with a slight inclination upwards and inwards, for about $2\frac{1}{2}$ inches (6·25 cm.).   Local infiltration is used rather than general anæsthesia, as the patient's sensations are a guide to the position of the needle.   However, when the needle is in contact with the ganglion pentothal anæsthesia is a humane procedure, as the injection causes severe pain.   One ml. of 90 per cent. alcohol is injected just within the foramen ovale.   If the needle is inserted too far within the skull, or if an excess of alcohol is used, some of the fluid may trickle over the superior border of the petrous bone and damage the facial and auditory nerves.   Anæsthesia of the face, nose, and cheek indicates successful injection.   Relief follows immediately, and may last from six months to two years.   Repeated injections are often necessary, and are made with increasing difficulty on account of fibrosis around the foramen ovale, but each injection further destroys the nerve, and in any case the disease, having reached a climax, tends to decrease in severity. If injection fails to give relief, the sensory root of the Gasserian ganglion should be divided.

Division of the sensory root has superseded ganglionectomy, as it is a simpler procedure, and the motor root is spared.   The temporal fossa is exposed by a suitable incision and the skull is opened.   The dura mater is separated from the floor of the middle fossa until the middle meningeal artery is seen emerging from the foramen spinosum.   The foramen is plugged with wax or a matchstick, and the artery is divided.   The mandi-bular nerve is then identified as it passes backwards from the foramen ovale to the cave of Meckel. A special retractor (fig. 929) is inserted, and an incision is made in the dural sheath of the ganglion. The cerebro-spinal fluid which escapes is patiently mopped away with small swabs. The sensory root is then traced backwards to the apex of the petrous bone, and

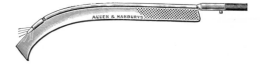

FIG. 929.—Retractor for exposure of Gasserian ganglion, with electric light.

is distinguished from the ganglion itself by its loose texture and parallel fibres. The root is supported on a blunt hook and divided with a suitable knife (fig. 930). Some surgeons prefer to avulse the sensory roots from the pons. The motor root lies deep to the sensory fibres, and if necessary for

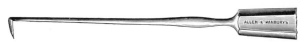

FIG. 930.—Angled knife for dividing the sensory root of the fifth nerve.

the purposes of identification it may be stimulated, so that the fibres of the temporal muscle exposed in the wound will contract. Complete and permanent relief follows an efficient operation. Temporary facial paralysis occasionally follows the operation, and is due to traction on the facial nerve via the great superficial petrosal nerve, which is displaced during approach to the ganglion.

The **Sixth Nerve** is slender, and has a long intracranial course. It is sometimes involved in cases of fractured base of the skull or prolonged intracranial pressure, and it may be interfered with in association with other ocular nerves, either in the cavernous sinus, sphenoidal fissure, or orbit. The external rectus muscle is paralysed, and internal strabismus results.

The **Seventh Nerve** is involved by a variety of causes :

1. *Intracranial.*—Lesions within the skull are supranuclear, nuclear, or infranuclear. Supranuclear lesions are due to injury, gumma, or new-growth. They are characterised by involvement of only the lower half of the face, as the occipito-frontalis and orbicularis palpebrarum muscles enjoy bilateral innervation. Nuclear lesions are due to hæmorrhage or thrombosis, the face on the same side being affected, and also the opposite arm and leg, as the motor decussation takes place at a lower level. An infranuclear lesion occasionally results from pressure of a tumour, e.g. of the cerebello-pontine angle, in which case involvement of the auditory nerve and cerebellum is usually evident.

Johann Friedrich Meckel, 178 1–1873. Professor of Anatomy, Obstetrics, and Botany, Berlin.

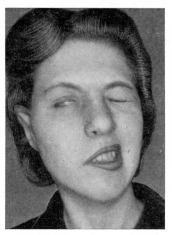

Fig. 931.—Right-sided facial paralysis following fracture through the middle fossa.

2. *Cranial.* — The commonest causes of involvement of the interosseous portion of the facial nerve are fractures of the base (fig. 931), and middle ear disease. In cases of fracture involvement may be immediate, usually due to hæmorrhage within the sheath of the nerve, in which case recovery is probable. Involvement after a few weeks is due to pressure by callus, and the prognosis is problematical. Facial paralysis as a complication of middle ear disease sometimes follows injury if an operation on the mastoid antrum is performed. Compression within the aqueduct of Fallopius occasionally follows chronic inflammation.

In cases of involvement of the cranial portion of the facial nerve, some paralysis of the palatal muscles may occur, due to interference with the petrosal nerves. Hyperacusis results from paralysis of the stapedius muscle, and if injury occurs between the geniculate ganglion and the canaliculus chordæ tympani, interference with the chorda tympani nerve will result in loss of taste in the corresponding half of the tongue.

3. *Extracranial.*—The facial nerve or its branches are sometimes injured outside the skull. The nerve itself is commonly involved by Bell's palsy. This condition is probably due to neuritis of the nerve, and may follow exposure to cold or a draught. Swelling within the sheath of the nerve extends into the stylomastoid foramen, and consequently the nerve is compressed within the bony canal. Absorption of exudate usually occurs before the pressure has damaged the nerve permanently, but in about 3 per cent. of cases complete paralysis remains, and in 5 to 10 per cent. some degree of paralysis persists. Tetanus arising from a wound in the distribution of the facial nerve sometimes causes paralysis, the cause being similar to that described above. Another possible explanation of Bell's palsy is virus infection. Malignant tumours of the parotid gland are likely to involve the facial nerve, and this is an important diagnostic sign in distinguishing simple from malignant tumours.

Gabriel Fallopio, 1523–1563.   Professor of Anatomy and Surgery, University of Pisa.
Sir Charles Bell, 1774–1842.   A Scots physiologist who became Surgeon to the Middlesex
*   Hospital.*

Branches of the facial nerve are injured either accidentally, e.g. by broken windscreens, or by ill-placed operation incisions. Needless to say, operations on the parotid gland for the removal of tumours or drainage of abscesses must be performed through incisions parallel to the main divisions of the nerve.

As a result of facial paralysis the face is flat and expressionless. The eye cannot be closed, and attempts to do so result in the eyeball being turned upwards and outwards (fig. 931). Corneal ulceration may follow from exposure. Epiphora occurs owing to drooping of the lower eyelid. Whistling is impossible, as the cheek merely flaps, and food collects between the gums and cheek. Treatment is directed to any cause, and the angle of the mouth should be supported by means of a malleable rod covered with rubber tubing. This is bent like an " S "; the upper curve hooks around the ear, and the lower passes into the mouth. Small strips of elastoplast applied under tension also form a very convenient method of preventing overstretching of the facial muscles (fig. 932). If considered advisable, and the services of a skilled dental surgeon are available, an intraoral splint can be fashioned from plastic material. Electrical treatment and massage are prescribed, and during recovery the patient should practise facial movements with the aid of a mirror. Hypoglossal anastomosis may be considered in otherwise hopeless cases.

In cases of Bell's palsy early decompression of the nerve by removal of part of the mastoid process reduces the risk of paralysis (Duel).

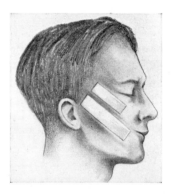

Fig. 932.—The application of strapping to prevent stretching of the facial muscles.

The **Eighth Nerve** may be involved in fractures of the middle fossa, or compressed by a tumour, e.g. of the auditory nerve sheath, in which case unilateral deafness, such as inability to hear the telephone, is sometimes the first symptom. Vestibular functions are sometimes impaired.

Ménière's disease is a paroxysmal disturbance associated with giddiness, nausea, and vomiting. If medical measures fail, the vestibular portion of the nerve is exposed through the posterior fossa and divided as it enters the internal auditory meatus.

A. B. Duel, Contemporary. Aural Surgeon, New York City.
Prosper Ménière, 1799–1862. Physician to the Institute for Deaf and Dumb, Paris.

The **Ninth Nerve** is occasionally injured by a fracture involving the jugular fossa. Some dysphagia may occur from paresis of the constrictor muscles, and trophic ulceration of the corresponding side of the tongue has been ascribed to injury of the glosso-pharyngeal nerve.

Glosso-pharyngeal neuralgia is characterised by severe explosions of pain either in the region of the tonsil, or deeply in the ear. The " trigger " zone is in the tonsillar area, and the diagnosis is clinched by the fact that cocainisation of the zone temporarily relieves the condition. In genuine cases the nerve must be divided. It is approached through the posterior fossa, and severed as it enters the jugular foramen.

The **Tenth Nerve** may be damaged in association with a fractured base, or crushed by a ligature which includes it as well as the internal jugular vein or common carotid artery. Œdema of the lung has followed in some cases, but injury to one vagus nerve is unlikely to cause more than a temporary tachycardia. In doubtful cases examination of the laryngeal muscles will reveal vagal injury. Irritation of the nerve by a ligature which is not sufficiently tight to interrupt impulses causes an intractable and distressing cough from laryngeal spasm.

The *recurrent laryngeal nerve* is extremely susceptible, and is often temporarily involved in operations on the thyroid gland or ductus arteriosus, either by traction, or pressure by traumatic œdema. Complete involvement sometimes follows division or inclusion by a ligature at operation, infiltration by neoplasm of the thyroid gland, and on the left side by pressure of an aneurism of the aortic arch. Partial involvement affects the abduction fibres, which are more susceptible than those which supply the adductor muscles, and thus if partial involvement is bilateral, stridor results, and tracheotomy may be required. Complete involvement results in paralysis of both abductors and adductors, and consequent paralysis of the corresponding vocal cord in the halfway or " cadaveric " position. The opposite vocal cord increases its range of mobility, so that it reaches across the midline and closes the glottis. The voice is adequate but somewhat monotonous.

Hysterical aphonia sometimes follows a sudden shock or violent emotion. It is readily distinguished from true paralysis by the fact that, although the patient can only whisper, yet coughing is readily performed on request.

The **Eleventh Nerve** is rarely damaged by fractures involving the jugular fossa. More commonly it is injured during operations on the neck, particularly in the removal of tuberculous nodes which often entirely surround the nerve. The nerve passes downwards and backwards at right angles to the centre of a line connecting the angle of the jaw and the mastoid process, and emerges from the posterior border of the sternomastoid muscle at the junction of the upper third and lower two-thirds ; it then passes across the posterior triangle, and disappears under cover of the trapezius muscle. Division of the nerve in the anterior triangle results in only partial paralysis of the trapezius and sternomastoid muscles, as the trapezius receives an additional supply from the third and fourth cervical nerves, and the sternomastoid from the second and third. If injury occurs in

the posterior triangle the trapezius alone is affected. On inspection, drooping of the shoulder is seen, and wasting of the trapezius is obvious (fig. 933). The integrity of the sternomastoid muscle is tested by placing a hand under the patient's chin and requesting him to flex his head. Palpation will then detect the rigid band of muscle if contraction is normal. Injury of the nerves to the trapezius results in inability to continue elevation of the arm after it is abducted to a right angle by the deltoid muscle. If the branches to the muscle from the third and fourth cervical nerves are intact, about 20 degrees elevation from the right-angled position is possible.

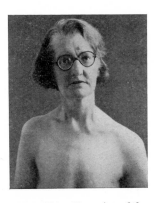

FIG. 933.—Drooping of the left shoulder and wasting of the trapezius muscle following division of the spinal accessory nerve. The swellings on forehead and face are soft fibromata—a common condition after middle age.

If division of the spinal accessory nerve is recognised at operation, primary suture should be performed. Secondary suture is unlikely to be successful on account of retraction of the ends and difficulty in identifying them in scar tissue.

The **Twelfth Nerve** escapes in fractures of the base of the skull, as the anterior condyloid foramen is protected by a bony ridge which diverts a fissure towards the foramen magnum. Nevertheless, it is commonly endangered in submental operations, especially those for removal of tuberculous nodes.

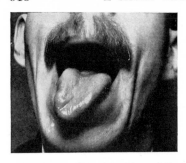

FIG. 934.—Hemiatrophy of the right side of the tongue following involvement of the hypoglossal nerve by syphilitic basal meningitis.

Hemiatrophy of the tongue occurs, the corresponding side of the tongue being shrivelled and wrinkled. On protrusion the tongue is pushed *towards* the paralysed side (fig. 934).

SPINAL NERVES

Injuries of the **Cervical Plexus** are uncommon, although muscular branches, e.g. to the trapezius and sternomastoid muscles, are occasionally damaged (p. 917).

The **Phrenic Nerve**, which arises from the third, fourth, and fifth cervical nerves, is commonly crushed or avulsed in order to reduce the size of the pleural cavity in such conditions as bronchiectasis, tuberculosis, or after repair of the diaphragm for a hernia.

Division of the nerve, as first practised, frequently gave disappointing results, for an accessory phrenic nerve arising either from the fifth cervical nerve, or the nerve to the subclavius, is present in 20 to 30 per cent. of cases and joins the main nerve between the first rib and the root of the lung. Thus *avulsion* replaced division, the nerve being exposed and divided. The distal end is seized with Spencer Wells's or similar forceps, which are rotated so as to withdraw the nerve from the thorax (p. 977). If only temporary paresis of the diaphragm is required, *crushing* is adequate (p. 977).

The phrenic nerve on the right side passes between a group of nodes below the inferior branch of the pulmonary vein, while the left phrenic has no such nodal relations. Involvement of the nodes secondary to malignant disease of the

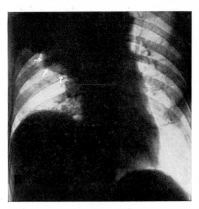

FIG. 935.—Elevation of the diaphragm following involvement of the right phrenic nerve by malignant lymph nodes. The primary bronchial growth is indicated by arrows.

Sir T. Spencer Wells, 1818–1897. London gynæcologist, popularised ovariotomy. His favourite motto was " Do to-day's work to-day."

lungs is an occasional cause of compression of the right nerve and consequent paralysis of the right half of the diaphragm (fig. 935).

Brachial plexus lesions are either complete or partial (fig. 936).

Complete lesions are rare, as an injury of sufficient severity to damage all the roots of the plexus will probably inflict fatal injuries on adjacent important structures.

In the event of a complete lesion, anæsthesia of the upper limb occurs except over areas supplied by the supra-acromial branches of the cervical plexus and the intercosto-humeral nerve. Complete paralysis of arm and scapular muscles occurs, except that in the case of tears of the plexus the lesion is usually distal to the site at which the nerve of Bell and the nerve to the rhomboids arise, and consequently the serratus magnus and rhomboid muscles escape.

Incomplete lesions, if due to stabs or cuts, are liable to affect any of the roots, the clinical features depending on the nerves divided. The commonest type of injury is due to traction or pressure, and affects either the upper or lower portions of the plexus.

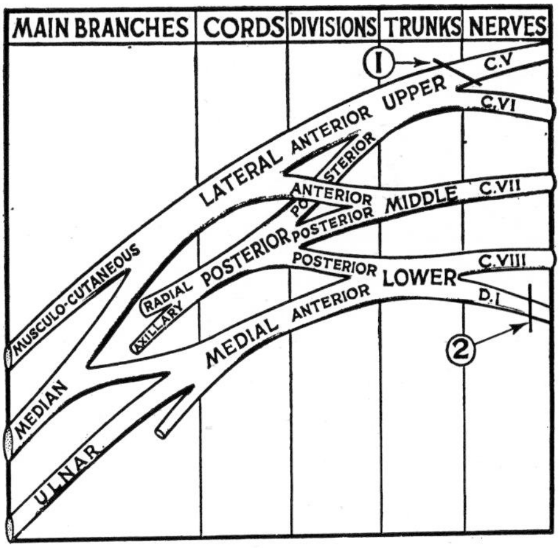

FIG. 936.—The brachial plexus, showing two classical sites for injury—see text.

Although the segmental innervation of the arm muscles is somewhat inconsistent, the following table summarises a distribution which is commonly accepted :

Nerve	Muscles
C. v	Rhomboids, spinati, deltoid, teres minor, biceps, brachialis, brachio-radialis, supinator brevis.
C. vi	Pectoralis major (clavicular head) and minor, subscapularis, coraco-brachialis, latissimus dorsi, teres major, serratus anterior, triceps, pronator teres, pronator quadratus.
C. vii	The extensors of the fingers, extensor carpi ulnaris and sternal part of the pectoralis major.
C. viii	The flexors of the wrist and fingers.
D. i	The small muscles of the hand.

Upper Lesion (Erb-Duchenne, fig. 936 (1)).—This injury is due to excessive displacement of the head, depression of the shoulder, or a combination of these two conditions. Thus, it not uncom-

William Erb, 1840–1921.   Professor of Medicine at Heidelberg.
Guillaume Duchenne, 1806–1875.   Practised medicine in Boulogne and Paris.

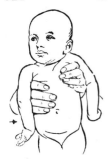

FIG. 937.—Erb's paralysis.

monly occurs during a difficult confinement, and in adults may be due to weights falling on the shoulder, or more commonly to a motor-bicycle accident. The fifth and sometimes the sixth cervical roots are involved. In the former case the muscles affected are the biceps, brachialis, brachio-radialis, supinator brevis, spinati and deltoid, and thus the limb, internally rotated by the unopposed subscapularis, hangs by the side with the forearm pronated, in the well-known " tip " position (fig. 937.) Sensory changes are absent if the fifth nerve only is involved, but if the sixth nerve also suffers, an area of anæsthesia is present over the outer side of the arm.

Lower Lesion (Klumpké, fig. 936 (2)).—The lower nerve trunk or the inner cord are injured either above the clavicle, e.g. by pressure of a cervical rib, or classically by inclusion with the sub-clavian artery in a ligature, or in the axilla, as by an unreduced dislocation of the humerus. In either case, the inner portion of the plexus is involved, and wasting of all the small muscles of the hand occurs, together with sensory changes along the inner side of the forearm and the inner three and a half fingers, owing to involvement of the ulnar and inner head of the median nerves.

Nerve roots may be avulsed from the spinal cord, as in the case of a falling person clutching at an object and hyper-abducting his arm, e.g. failing to obtain a foothold on a passing bus. The first dorsal root is usually affected. Paralysis of the intrinsic muscles of the hand results, with anæsthesia of the inner three and a half fingers in front, and inner one and a half behind. In addition, the oculo-pupillary fibres, which pass along the dorsal nerves to the rami communicantes, and so to the cervical sympathetic, are also affected, and Horner's syndrome follows (p. 938). Hæmorrhage sometimes occurs in the spinal cord following avulsion of the nerve root, and results in irrita-tion of the pyramidal tract and consequent spasticity of the leg on the same side.

Treatment.—Subcutaneous injuries are at first treated on expectant lines, paralysed muscles being relaxed. Thus, in the case of an Erb's paralysis, the arm should be fixed in a position of

Madame A. Klumpké, a neurologist of Paris.
Friedrich Horner, 1831–1886. Professor of Ophthalmology, Zurich; described his syndrome in 1864.

right-angled abduction and eversion, to relax the deltoid and spinati, the forearm being flexed and supinated in order to relax the biceps, brachialis, and supinators. Commonly, for convenience, the arm is merely bandaged across the chest, and ultimately recovery is the rule, but the price paid for convenience is prolonged paresis of the deltoid and spinati muscles, which are not relaxed in this position.

The commonest subcutaneous lesion of the plexus is intra-neural hæmorrhage (neurapraxia), in which case more or less complete recovery ensues. More serious lesions in which nerves themselves are torn may be explored, but the results are indifferent.

The brachial plexus is exposed by an incision along the posterior border of the sternomastoid. If necessary the incision may be carried backwards along the middle third of the clavicle or, if complete exposure of the plexus is desirable, the original incision is prolonged over the clavicle, which is drilled for subsequent wiring, and divided. The weight of the arm separates the ends of the divided clavicle, and the plexus is freely exposed. Three difficulties now confront the surgeon—identification, approximation, and accurate suturing. Identification is hampered by fibrosis and matting together of structures by organisation of extravasated blood. When torn nerves are recognised and dissected from their fibrous bed, approximation is difficult on account of retraction, and posture can give but limited assistance. Finally, rupture commonly occurs where nerves fuse or divide, so that accurate suture is a difficult problem in that it may be necessary to suture two roots to one trunk.

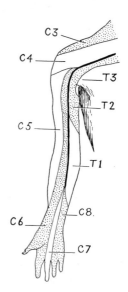

BRACHIAL NEURALGIA

This condition (*syn.* brachial neuritis) is comparable to sciatica in the leg. The cutaneous distribution of the cervical nerves is illustrated in fig. 938, and the muscular innervation is summarised on p. 919. Some of the more important causes of brachial neuralgia are as follows :

Spinal tumour (p. 892). Evidence of pressure on the cord is usually present, and Queckenstedt's test is commonly positive.

Prolapsed intervertebral disc (p. 900) is often difficult to distinguish from osteo-arthritis, but localised pain in the

FIG. 938.—The dermatomes of the upper limb.

Hans Queckenstedt, 1849–1918. A German physician.

neck, which often appears suddenly, and which is aggravated by coughing, suggests a disc lesion.

Osteoarthritis of the cervical spine causes neuralgia either as a result of pressure on a spinal nerve by an osteophyte, or from absorption of the disc and consequent compression of the spinal roots. The onset is gradual and symptoms intermittent, and radiography usually establishes the diagnosis.

Costo-clavicular syndromes are due to many conditions (p. 191). Sagging of the shoulder girdle, especially in middle-aged females who must of necessity carry heavy shopping baskets, is a common present-day cause. Exercises and physiotherapy directed to improving the tone of muscles which elevate the shoulder relieve the symptoms, and, if the husband is not available, a wheeled basket should be used for shopping.

PERIPHERAL NERVES

The **Circumflex Nerve** passes through the quadrilateral space, and winds around the shaft of the humerus about one finger's

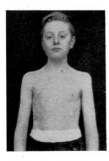

FIG. 939.—Wasting of the left deltoid muscle, due to bruising of the circumflex nerve.

breadth below the centre of the deltoid muscle. It is sometimes injured by a direct blow, or involved by a fracture or dislocation of the humerus.

The deltoid muscle is paralysed and wastes rapidly (fig. 939), and a patch of anæsthesia over the outer side of the arm distinguishes this condition from a partial lesion of the fifth cervical nerve. Paralysis of the teres minor is unrecognisable clinically.

Recovery commences in a few weeks if the cause of the compression is removed, provided that the arm has been supported in right-angled abduction.

The **Nerve of Bell,** or external respiratory nerve, arises from the fifth, sixth, and seventh cervical nerve roots. It may be injured by blows or carrying a heavy object on the shoulder, or during operations on the breast or chest wall, as it lies on the inner wall of the axilla. Paralysis of the serratus anterior allows " winging " of the scapula, i.e. the vertebral border and inferior angle are unduly prominent (fig. 940). The " lunge " stroke of fencing is dependent on the serratus anterior, and this and similar movements, such as pushing forward with the arm, are deficient. Owing to inability to rotate the scapula on the chest wall, difficulty is experienced in raising the arm above a right angle from a position in front of the body.

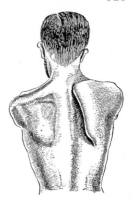

Suture of the nerve is sometimes possible. Otherwise, if disability warrants such a procedure, the scapula is steadied by a slip of pectoralis major muscle, which is detached from the humerus and fixed to the inferior angle of the scapula.

Fig. 940.—Winging of the scapula ; the patient is pushing against a wall.

The **Radial** or musculo-spiral nerve is commonly injured. The classical sites are the axilla and the radial groove.

1. Injury in the **axilla** follows :

(i) Crutch palsy : all crutches should have hand-grips, and their length should be carefully adjusted, especially if use is likely to be prolonged. Paresis has occurred after only four hours' use with crutches unsupplied with hand-grips.

(ii) Fractures and dislocations of the upper end of the humerus, or by attempts at their reduction.

(iii) Rarely by pressure of an aneurism, or new-growth.

Clinical Features.—(*a*) *Motor.*—The triceps and extensors of the wrist and fingers are paralysed, and consequently inability to extend the elbow, wrist, and fingers results, and drop wrist is present. If the hand is supported, as by resting it upon the table, extension of the fingers can be produced by the action of the lumbricals and interossei, which are inserted into the extensor expansions. The supinator and brachio-radialis are also paralysed, but supination is ably performed by the biceps. The supinator longus muscle is tested readily by endeavouring to flex the semi-prone forearm against resistance. If the muscle is active the contraction is visible, and the rigid muscle is easily palpable.

(*b*) *Sensory.*—Anæsthesia is commonly present over the back of the hand, thumb, and outer two and a half fingers, with the exception of the nail beds, which are supplied by the median nerve, but this area of anæsthesia is sometimes reduced to a patch over the ball of the thumb, owing to overlap by the musculo-cutaneous nerve.

(c) *Trophic.*—These are usually trivial.

2. Injury in the **radial** groove is due to :

(i) Pressure, e.g. of the arm on the edge of the operating table, especially in Trendelenburg's position, or as in " Saturday night " paralysis, due to the enjoyment of a heavy sleep with the arm over the sharp back of a kitchen chair. Prolonged application of a tourniquet is especially liable to compress the radial nerve, as it lies close to the bone, and possibly the median and ulnar nerves as well. For this reason a sphygmomanometer should always be used on the arm.

(ii) Fracture of the shaft of the humerus, immediate involvement of the nerve occurring in about 8 per cent. of cases. It is often overlooked owing to the more obvious fracture overshadowing the nerve injury, in which case involvement in callus is usually blamed, rather than oversight on the part of the surgeon.

(iii) The nerve is liable to be overstretched during operations on the humerus, e.g. in dealing with an ununited fracture.

(iv) " Intramuscular " injections of drugs have been given into the radial nerve.

Clinical Features.—(a) *Motor.*—These are similar to those following injury in the axilla, except that the triceps and anconeus muscles escape.

(b) *Sensory.*—If the external cutaneous branch escapes, anæsthesia will be limited to a patch over the ball of the thumb. Division of the radial nerve in the upper third of the forearm is symptomless. Below this position the musculo-cutaneous nerve joins the radial, and division then causes anæsthesia over the ball of the thumb.

(c) *Trophic.*—These are slight.

The *posterior interosseous nerve* may be injured as a result of fracture or dislocation of the upper end of the radius, or in operations performed to deal with these conditions. Paralysis of the extensors of the wrist and fingers results. The upper end of the nerve has been sutured with excellent results (fig. 941). If nerve repair is impracticable, good results are obtained by tendon and muscle transplant, e.g. the radial carpal flexor is transplanted to the extensor tendons of the thumb and fingers, and the pronator teres into the extensors carpi radialis longus and brevis.

The **Median Nerve** is classically injured at the wrist or elbow.

1. Injuries at the **elbow** are due to fractures of the lower end of the humerus or dislocations of the elbow joint. A tourniquet endangers the nerve at any level in the arm, in which case other nerves, particularly the radial, will also be involved.

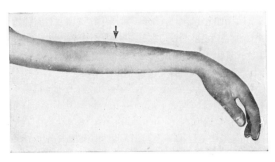

Fig.941.—Wrist-drop following an incised wound which divided the posterior interosseous nerve. The wound is indicated by the arrow.

Clinical Features.—(*a*) *Motor.*—The pronators of the forearm and flexors of the wrist and fingers, with the exception of the flexor carpi ulnaris and the inner part of the flexor profundus digitorum, will be paralysed. As a result of paralysis of the flexor carpi radialis the hand deviates to the ulnar side when flexed against resistance. The index finger cannot be flexed at the phalangeal joints—the " pointing index "—but flexion of the other fingers is performed by that portion of the flexor pro-fundus digitorum which is supplied by the ulnar nerve. Flexion of the terminal phalanx of the thumb is impossible, owing to paralysis of the flexor longus pollicis. The muscles of the thenar eminence are wasted and paralysed, and on inspection the eminence is flattened, so that the metacarpal bone of the thumb is apparently on the same plane as the other metacarpal bones—the so-called " simian " or " ape-like " hand. Paralysis of the two outer lumbricals is unrecognisable.

(*b*) *Sensory.*—Appreciation of touch is lost over the thumb and outer two and a half fingers in front, and posteriorly as far proximally as the middle of the proximal phalanges. Loss of response to pin-prick affects the terminal phalanges of the index and middle fingers, but sometimes a larger area is involved. Deep sensibility is lost over the terminal phalanges of the index and middle fingers.

(*c*) *Trophic.*—Obvious trophic changes are usually seen in the hand and affected fingers.

2. Injuries at the **wrist** are comparatively common, and are due to cuts from a variety of causes. Fractures of the lower end of the radius or dislocation of the semilunar bone sometimes cause injury to the median nerve.

Clinical Features.—(*a*) *Motor.*—The muscles of the thenar eminence are paralysed and wasted. The hand is " simian," and abduction and opposition of the thumb are lost. Attempts to oppose the tip of the thumb to the tip of the little finger result in flexion and adduction of the thumb, as the patient is unable to swing it across the palm.

(*b*) *Sensory.*—Sensory losses resemble those following an injury at the elbow. Muscular sense is not impaired if tendons are not severed. Thus, as no striking muscular deficiency occurs, and as no part of the hand is completely anæsthetic, a divided median nerve at the wrist is readily overlooked, particularly in those who use refinements of sensation but little, e.g. a horny-handed labourer.

(*c*) *Trophic.*—These occur, as with an injury at the elbow.

The poor prognosis of a divided median nerve is rendered even more gloomy if tendons are also severed.

Median Compression occasionally occurs as the nerve passes through the carpal tunnel. Paræsthesia, followed by wasting of the thenar muscles, suggests the diagnosis. Relief is obtained by division of the anterior annular ligament.

The **Ulnar Nerve** is also classically injured at the elbow and wrist.

1. Injuries at the **elbow** are due to the following causes :

(i) Fractures in the region of the internal condyle.

(ii) Excision of the elbow joint.

(iii) Cubitus valgus, due to old injury of the humerus and increase of the " carrying angle." Hence the nerve is unduly exposed, and friction occurs as the groove on the internal condyle becomes a pulley, and this continuous friction results in interstitial neuritis. This condition may occur many years after the original injury, and transposition of the nerve is required.

Anterior transposition of the ulnar nerve is sometimes required for friction (axonotmesis), following fracture of the internal condyle, pressure by an osteophyte, or recurrent dislocation of the nerve, and injury which results in loss of substance, so that approximation is thus rendered possible. The nerve is exposed by a curved incision with the concavity forwards, and the humeral head of the flexor carpi ulnaris is divided. Careful dissection is necessary so as to avoid injury to motor branches, and the internal intermuscular septum should be divided or excised, otherwise the nerve may be kinked by this structure when it is displaced forwards. A bed is then prepared in the flexor group of muscles and the nerve buried therein (fig. 942).

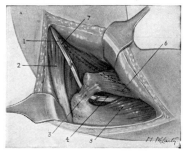

FIG. 942.—Anterior transposition of the left ulnar nerve.

1. Ulnar nerve.
2. Triceps.
3. Olecranon head of flexor carpi ulnaris.
4. Posterior ulnar recurrent artery.
5. Flexor profundus digitorum.
6. Superficial flexor muscles.
7. Inferior profunda artery.

(The dotted line represents the new course of the nerve.)

Clinical Features.—(*a*) *Motor.*—The flexor carpi ulnaris and inner portion of the flexor profundus digitorum are paralysed. Normally, on flexion of the wrist, the tendon of the flexor carpi ulnaris is readily palpable just above its insertion into the pisiform bone, but when the muscle is paralysed the tendon is impalpable, and wasting causes flattening of the inner border of the forearm. Weakness of the flexor profundus digitorum results in hyperextension of the little, ring, and slightly of the middle fingers at the metacarpophalangeal joints.

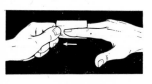

FIG. 943.—Test for weakness of the interosseous muscles.

Paralysis of the small muscles of the hand also results, with the exception of the thenar muscles and outer two lumbricals. Inability to abduct and adduct the fingers results, and the patient cannot grip a piece of paper placed between the fingers (fig. 943). If the patient pinches a piece of paper between his thumb and fingers the terminal phalanx of the thumb assumes a flexed position, as weakness of the flexor brevis pollicis permits over-action of the long flexor of the thumb (Froment's sign). Considerable wasting occurs, which is obvious in the interosseous spaces and along the inner border of the hand, the normal curve being lost (fig. 945).

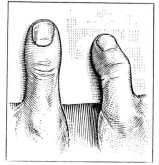

FIG. 944.—Froment's sign for right ulnar paresis.

Jules Froment, 1878–1946. Professor of Clinical Medicine, Lyons.

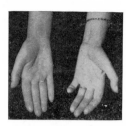

FIG. 945.—Wasting of the hypothenar eminence following injury to the left ulnar nerve.

(b) *Sensory.*—The appreciation of light touch is lost over the inner one and a half fingers in front and behind. Response to pin-prick is lost over the little finger and ulnar border of the palm.

(c) *Trophic.*—These changes are usually well marked.

2. Injury at the **wrist** is due to the same causes as those enumerated in connection with the median nerve. The ulnar nerve passes in front of the anterior annular ligament, and is damaged by more superficial injuries.

Clinical Features.—(a) *Motor.*—Paralysis and wasting of small muscles of the hand, as described above.

(b) *Sensory.*—The dorsal cutaneous branch of the ulnar nerve leaves the main trunk about 2½ inches (6·25 cm.) above the styloid process of the ulna. Sensation is therefore lost only on the anterior aspect of the inner one and a half fingers.

(c) *Trophic.*—Correspond to the area of sensory loss.

The **Twelfth Dorsal Nerve,** as in the case of the intercostal nerves, is sometimes implicated by severe neuralgia, which may be associated with herpes zoster. Neuralgia of the twelfth nerve is occasionally due to pressure by an elongated twelfth rib, and has been cured by removal of the costal tip. More commonly the nerve is implicated by a suture during a kidney operation, or by subsequent scar tissue. Resulting pain is occasionally sufficiently severe to necessitate exposure and excision of part of the nerve.

The **Ilio-inguinal Nerve** may be damaged on the right side in a gridiron incision for appendicectomy, although with care the nerve should be avoided. If drainage tubes are inserted through this incision, the resulting scar tissue may implicate the nerve. On the left side, injury to the nerve may follow iliac colostomy. Weakness of the conjoined tendon results, with consequent predisposition to the formation of an inguinal hernia (fig. 946).

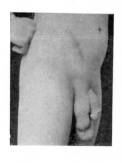

FIG. 946.—An inguinal hernia which followed appendicectomy with drainage through a gridiron incision, one year previously.

The **External Cutaneous Nerve** is occasionally compressed as it passes through the deep fascia of the thigh, especially in muscular subjects, e.g. rowers. The condition is termed meralgia paræsthetica, and resection of part of the nerve is sometimes necessary to rid the patient of pain or paræsthesia (fig. 947).

The **Sciatic Nerve** is occasionally injured by wounds, fractures, or "intramuscular" injection of drugs. The component nerves in the pelvis may be involved by fracture, tumour, or aneurism. Injury in the upper part of the thigh sometimes complicates deep wounds, or posterior dislocation of the hip joint. If the lesion is above the origin of branches to the hamstrings, the following features will be present :

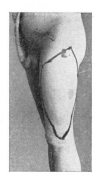

Fig. 947.—Area of anæsthesia following resection of the external cutaneous nerve. The scar of the operation is visible.

(*a*) *Motor.*—The flexors of the knee are paralysed, but some degree of flexion is possible owing to the action of the sartorius and gracilis muscles. Complete paralysis exists below the knee, and drop foot results from gravity.

(*b*) *Sensory.*—Complete loss below the knee, with the exception of the skin supplied by the long saphenous nerve, i.e. a strip along the inner side of the leg extending along the inner border of the foot to the ball of the big toe.

(*c*) *Trophic.*—Especially on the sole of the foot and toes.

Partial involvement of the sciatic nerve affects the external popliteal portion nine times as commonly as the internal popliteal (p. 909).

A fibrous band, which arises from the sacro-sciatic notch and reinforces the origin of the gluteus minimus muscle, occasionally causes pressure on the sciatic nerve, and consequent sciatica. The condition is analogous to a cervical rib exerting pressure on the brachial plexus, and when other causes of sciatica, notably a prolapsed disc, have been excluded, a search for the band beneath the pyriformis is justifiable.

The **External Popliteal Nerve** is injured as follows :

(i) Subcutaneous tenotomy of the biceps tendon.

(ii) Fracture or excision of the upper end of the fibula.

(iii) Pressure from plasters or splints.

Clinical Features.—(*a*) *Motor.*—Complete paralysis of the extensor and peroneal groups of muscles, with resulting talipes equino-varus.

(*b*) *Sensory.*—Anæsthesia on the outer side of the leg in its lower two-thirds, and of the dorsal aspects of all the toes, with

the exception of the outer side of the little toe, which is supplied
by the external saphenous (sural) nerve, as one contributory
branch—the sural communicating from the internal popliteal
nerve—escapes.

(c) *Trophic.*—Corresponding to the sensory loss.

The **Internal Popliteal Nerve** is but rarely injured on account
of its protected position. The calf muscles and muscles of the
sole are paralysed, and talipes calcaneo-valgus may result. The
sole is anæsthetic, and trophic changes usually severe. Causalgia occasionally follows a partial injury of the nerve, or injury
to one of its branches.

THE SYMPATHETIC NERVOUS SYSTEM

Anatomy.—The sympathetic nervous system is composed of preganglionic fibres, ganglionated trunks, and postganglionic fibres.

Preganglionic fibres are axons of the " connector " cells situated in the
lateral horns, which are present in the grey matter of the dorsal and upper
two or three lumbar segments of the spinal cord. These fibres are medullated
and pass from the anterior roots of the dorsal and upper lumbar spinal
nerves (white rami communicantes) and join the ganglionated trunk.
Here some form synapses, while others pass through the ganglia to reach
visceral ganglia and plexuses. Finally, preganglionic fibres pass to the
medulla of the suprarenal gland (which is developed from nerve tissue, the
medulla itself representing the synapse and postganglionic fibres).

The **ganglionated trunks** of the sympathetic lie upon the sides of the
bodies of the vertebræ, and extend from the skull to the coccyx. In the
cervical region the ganglia are condensed to three in number. The dorsal
ganglia number eleven or twelve, the upper one of which is closely connected
with the inferior cervical ganglion, and forms the stellate ganglion. The
lumbar and sacral ganglia usually number four in each region.

In addition to the ganglionated trunk, visceral ganglia also exist, e.g. the
cœliac, superior and inferior mesenteric. To these ganglia the splanchnic
nerves pass from the lower six dorsal ganglia of the sympathetic trunk.
These splanchnic nerves contain preganglionic fibres which have traversed
the ganglia of the sympathetic cord.

The **postganglionic** or second relay of fibres are non-medullated, and
originate in the trunk and visceral ganglia from cells (termed excitor cells)
fibres from which form synapses with the preganglionic fibres. These
postganglionic fibres innervate the sweat glands, pilomotor muscles, vessels, viscera, and other structures influenced by the sympathetic system.
In addition, from all the ganglia of the sympathetic trunk, two or more
grey rami communicantes pass to each spinal nerve.

A central sympathetic nucleus exists in the region of the hypothalamus,
and is influenced by stimuli from the higher centres. Clinical evidence
shows that a tumour which interferes with the anterior and superior portions of the thalami causes sympathetic derangement (Penfield).

The function of the sympathetic nervous system is to deal with emotional
and psychological emergencies. It is designed to prepare the animal for
defence. Thus the blood-pressure is raised and pulse-rate increased so as
to maintain the circulation at a high pitch of efficiency, and contraction

*Wilder G. Penfield, Contemporary. Professor of Neurosurgery, McGill University,
Montreal.*

of the spleen forces additional red cells into the circulation so as to assist in oxygenation, which is supplemented by dilatation of the bronchioles. The pilomotor muscles contract and cause the " hair to stand on end," which is a useful phenomenon in the case of an animal, as its apparent size and ferocity are increased. In order to maintain muscular efficiency glucose is set free from the liver, and exophthalmos and dilatation of the pupil widen the visual fields. The unstriped muscle of the intestine is inhibited in order to prevent waste of energy by peristalsis, and sphincters are contracted. Sweating assists in preventing a wasteful rise of temperature. The supply of adrenalin is increased so that the reaction already commenced by stimulation of the sympathetic is augmented and maintained.

The **parasympathetic** system has its origin in the brain and sacral region. Cranial parasympathetic fibres pass to the pupil, salivary glands, the heart, and alimentary canal, including its developmental outgrowths, i.e. lungs, liver, and pancreas. Parasympathetic impulses stimulate the secretion of saliva and cause contraction of the pupil. It is secretory and motor to the alimentary canal, and inhibitory to the heart.

The sacral portion of the parasympathetic system is concerned with the " emptying processes." Thus it supplies motor impulses to the rectum and bladder, and is concerned with penile erection.

The above summary explains two important clinical observations. Firstly, in cases of ileus a spinal anæsthetic frequently results in a copious motion, and in doubtful cases the effect of a spinal anæsthetic is a useful method of discriminating between mechanical and paralytic obstruction. The beneficial effects of spinal anæsthesia are due to paralysis of the inhibitory sympathetic fibres, with the result that the motor parasympathetic impulses are unopposed.

Secondly, the fall of blood-pressure which occurs during spinal anæsthesia is due to paralysis of the vaso-constrictor nerves. This can be to some extent counteracted by an intramuscular injection of ephedrine (gr. $\frac{1}{2}-\frac{3}{4}$).

INDICATIONS FOR OPERATION

I. To Improve Circulation

Sympathectomy, by removing the influence of vaso-constrictor fibres, allows dilatation of the corresponding blood-vessels. This chiefly concerns the smaller arteries, which contain a large proportion of unstriped muscle in their walls, and the large vessels are but little affected. Also pathological changes in the coats of the vessels are liable to impair very seriously their power of dilating, and therefore pre-operative tests are necessary in order to estimate their capacity for dilatation.

TESTS FOR VASODILATATION

(i) **Anæsthesia of the Sympathetic.**—In the case of the lower limbs a spinal anæsthetic which reaches to the level of the umbilicus inhibits vasoconstrictor impulses to the legs. An ordinary bath thermometer bandaged between the first and second toes will give a rough indication of alteration of temperature, but a precise method is by means of thermo-couples or special skin thermometers, which can be attached at different places and so indicate the condition of vessels at various levels.

Sympathetic fibres to the upper limb can be anæsthetised by injection from behind of 5 ml. of 1 per cent. novocaine below the necks of the first and second ribs. The stellate and upper dorsal ganglia are thus reached and vasoconstrictor impulses to the arm are interrupted. Intraneural injection of a peripheral nerve has the same effect over the area of distribution of the nerve. Thus the brachial plexus, or ulnar nerve at the elbow, can be injected with 2 per cent. novocaine and the effect upon the vessels noted.

(ii) **Heating the Body.**—The patient sits in a chamber constructed of non-conducting material so that his head and wrists or ankles protrude, the basis of the investigation being the estimation of the reflex dilatation produced by heating the body. The hands are cooled by immersion in water at 15° C (59° F.), the temperature of the room being maintained at that level, and the patient is sealed in the chamber. The temperature of the chamber is raised to 50° C. (122° F), and by means of an electric thermometer the effect upon the peripheral circulation is accurately estimated.

Thrombo-angiitis obliterans (*syn.* Buerger's disease) is a progressive condition, erroneously stated to be commoner in Russian Jews. It affects mainly the lower limbs, usually terminates in gangrene, and is associated with severe pain and sometimes with intermittent claudication. Two factors are present—vasospasm, and thickening of the arterial wall which may progress to obliteration. It is possible that the primary condition is one of spasm, which interferes with the circulation through the vasa vasorum, and consequently the nutrition of the arterial wall is impaired and degeneration follows.

In early cases measures are taken to preserve the nutrition of the limb and to keep the patient ambulatory. Warm stockings, avoidance of trauma to the feet, and gentle exercise within the limit of tolerance, are important. If the patient is handicapped by pain in the calf muscles division of the motor nerves to the gastrocnemius and soleus is helpful. As an alternative the tendo Achillis is divided, and so grateful is the patient for relief from pain that the disability seems slight. Intravenous injections of hypertonic saline (50–100 ml.) of 5 per cent. twice or thrice weekly are sometimes beneficial, as the resulting osmosis increases the blood-volume (Sibert).

If vasodilatation tests are satisfactory, lumbar ganglionectomy may eventually be required in order to relieve pain and promote the healing of ulcers; but prognosis must be guarded, as many cases after remarkable initial improvement are apt to relapse, although pain is usually greatly relieved. Finally, persistent ulceration or gangrene may necessitate amputation. Not infrequently the prognosis in a young patient is less rosy

Leo Buerger, 1879–1943. American urologist of Austrian birth. Mount Sinai Hospital, New York. Described his eponymous disease in 1908.
Samuel Sibert, Contemporary. Academy of Medicine, New York.

than in the elderly. Total abstinence from smoking is imperative.

Early cases of arterial spasm are sometimes improved by Padutin (Bayer Products, Ltd.). This is an active dilator substance, and is administered orally or intravenously. Another popular preparation is Priscol. Arteriosclerotic claudication in elderly patients is often ameliorated by lumbar ganglionectomy if the skin temperature rises with reflex heating.

Raynaud's disease is practically confined to females, and usually commences in early adult life. Paroxysmal attacks of vasospasm occur in the hands, and are precipitated by cold and occasionally by emotion. As a result the hands become cold and cyanosed, and are incapable of finer movements, the attacks being accompanied by aching pain of considerable severity. As the attack passes off the hands become red, and a burning sensation replaces the previous numbness. Eventually superficial necrosis occurs, the tips of the fingers undergo dry gangrene, and the distal parts of the terminal phalanges are absorbed (fig. 948). In some cases scleroderma affects the hands and face.

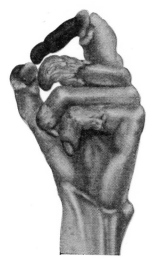

FIG. 948.—Gangrene in an advanced case of Raynaud's disease.

Early cases of Raynaud's disease must be distinguished from chilblains and vascular disturbances which are sometimes associated with the costo-clavicular syndrome.

The immediate results of ganglionectomy in Raynaud's disease are good, but after a few months the susceptibility to cold

A. G. Maurice Raynaud, 1834–1881. Physician, Hôpital Lariboisière, Paris.

returns, although cyanosis is not so severe as before the operation, and subjective symptoms are less marked. This partial relapse is an indication that the underlying cause of Raynaud's disease is not in the sympathetic system, but is due to some abnormality in the smaller arteries and arterioles ; sympathectomy apparently raises the threshold at which spasm occurs. From the practical point of view, ganglionectomy can be recommended as a palliative procedure in Raynaud's disease, especially if performed before the onset of scleroderma, ulceration, and absorption of the terminal phalanges.

Some surgeons endeavour to divide only the constrictor nerve fibres, in the hope that the unbalanced action of the dilators will encourage the arterial circulation. The sympathetic trunk is divided below the third thoracic ganglion, and the rami communicantes connecting the second and third thoracic nerves with the cord are severed. It is claimed (but not yet proved) that the results of this operation are more permanent.

Infantile Paralysis.—The improvement in the circulation which follows ganglionectomy encourages growth in the limb of a growing child. Trophic sores and ulcers are encouraged to heal, but in some cases the improvement has only been of a temporary nature.

Other Conditions.—Selected cases of scleroderma, in which the hands or face are principally affected, are improved by cervico-thoracic ganglionectomy. The pain and stiffness of polyarticular osteoarthritis are alleviated by a suitable ganglionectomy, and some cases of retinitis pigmentosa with narrowing of the visual field have improved after removal of the first and second cervical ganglia. Callous ulcers, such as those associated with trophic lesions or leprosy, sometimes respond to periarterial neurectomy, and indolent ulcers of the face often improve after excision of the superior cervical ganglion.

Perniosis may cause such disablement that sympathectomy is indicated, especially when the chilblains affect the toes.

II. Painful Conditions

In the case of hollow viscera, pain is probably caused by stretching of the muscular coat resulting from intravisceral tension, and similarly, increased tension in solid viscera stretches the fibrous capsule. The relief of pain which follows ganglionectomy in the case of the limbs is probably due to an increased blood-supply.

Visceral Pain.—*Bladder.*—The constant wearying pain of chronic cystitis is relieved by resection of the presacral nerve, which may be combined with division of the sympathetic cords. Carcinoma of the bladder (or uterus) is apt, sooner or later, to escape from the confines of the viscus and cause pain from invasion of the lumbo-sacral plexus and other structures, which is beyond the aid of sympathectomy.

Uterus.—Most cases of spasmodic dysmenorrhœa which resist less drastic measures are cured or relieved by presacral neurectomy. No untoward effects on uterine (including parturition) or bladder function have been recorded.

Renal Pain.—The diagnosis of sympathetico-tonus is confirmed if the pain is relieved by eserine. In these cases pyelography shows clubbing of the calyces. Stripping of the renal pedicle results in sympathetic denervation and restoration of neuromuscular balance.

Angina pectoris is relieved by removal of the upper five thoracic ganglia. In cases of difficulty the lower two, if out of reach, can be injected with alcohol. It was formerly alleged that to abolish pain was to remove a danger signal, but further experience disproves this. Equally good results appear to follow thyroidectomy, the possible explanation being that alteration in the circulation of thyroxine renders the nerve-supply to viscera, including the heart, less sensitive.

Causalgia is a condition in which paroxysmal attacks of pain follow an incomplete nerve injury, especially of the brachial plexus, sciatic or median nerves. In more than half the cases symptoms supervene immediately after the injury, in the remainder symptoms are deferred for any length of time up to two or three months. The immediate onset of symptoms suggests some reflex cause, and rules out infection as a necessary factor. The pain of causalgia is typically sympathetic in character, in that it is " burning," not easily localised, and varies with the patient's emotional state. Hyperæsthesia, wasting, and trophic changes are associated conditions. Either vasodilatation or vasoconstriction occurs, and pain is alleviated by cold (e.g. a wet sock or glove) or warm applications respectively. Sooner or later the patient loses his morale, and becomes introspective and unco-operative. Some cases of causalgia tend to recover gradually, but the condition is so distressing that surgical alleviation is highly desirable as soon as the condition is confirmed. Paravertebral block (either D2 and 3, or L1, 2, and 3) relieves the pain for a short time, and confirms the necessity for operation. Also during the interval of freedom it is possible to assess the extent of nerve involvement.

Treatment necessitates excision of the approximate ganglia. Periarterial sympathectomy gives variable relief, but is worthy of trial in a patient who is unfit for more drastic procedures.

III. Secretory Disturbances

Excessive sweating (hyperidrosis) is sometimes so distressing to the patient that he is willing to undergo surgical measures in order to obtain relief. Excessive sweating of the face, which is sometimes associated with emotional stress, is abolished by removal of the superior cervical ganglion. Sodden, offensive feet, the skin of which is cracked and painful, may be a genuine disability for which lumbar ganglionectomy is justified.

A parotid fistula, which fails to respond to cautery or radium, is encouraged to heal by avulsion of the auriculo-temporal nerve, which is exposed in front of the ear in relation to the superficial temporal artery. The parasympathetic secretory fibres are ablated, and the fistula closes.

IV. To Relieve Spasm

Retention of Urine.—The presacral nerve contains sympathetic fibres which act as motor nerves to the internal sphincter, but the act of micturition is not interfered with to any great extent by presacral neurectomy, although some temporary frequency sometimes results. Apparently the nerve restricts the action of the detrusor urinæ muscle. In certain cases of " cord bladder," where unbalanced action follows such injuries as partial lesions of the cauda equina, resection of the presacral nerve has been of value in restoring muscular balance. Proctologists often remove the presacral plexus when they perform perineal resection or radical removal of the rectum, which operations necessitate division of the nervi erigentes from the sacral plexus, which inhibit the internal sphincter. Presacral neurectomy thus obviates unbalanced action of the bladder sphincter, and consequent post-operative retention of urine.

Essential hypertension in patients who are below the age of fifty, and who have no impairment of the renal or cardiovascular systems, is often improved by bilateral resection of the splanchnic nerves together with the sympathetic trunks from the ninth thoracic to the first lumbar ganglia. Benefit results either from depression of the activity of the adrenal glands, or by dilatation of the splanchnic vessels and those of the lower limb, which thus provides a reservoir for blood. In our experience the fall of blood-pressure may be slight, but headache, palpitations, and dizziness are often relieved for many months to a few years.

OPERATIONS

Periarterial Neurectomy.—Leriche, who popularised this operation, performed it in the belief that all the sympathetic fibres pass to a limb in the adventitia of the main artery. It is now known that the arteries to a limb receive sympathetic fibres not only from the aortic plexus, which accompanies the main vessel, but also from mixed nerves which join the vessels at varying levels. Thus periarterial neurectomy does not remove all the vasomotor fibres passing to the limb.

Nevertheless, periarterial neurectomy occasionally yields satisfactory results, though these are less consistent than with ganglionectomy. Therefore the operation is more or less palliative, but it is sometimes of value in patients whose general condition is unsuited for the more extensive operation of ganglionectomy.

René Leriche, Contemporary. Professor of Clinical Surgery, Strasburg.

The operation is readily performed under local anæsthesia. The vessel is exposed for a distance of 2 or 3 inches (5 or 7·5 cm.), and the sheath and adventitious coats are divided and stripped off the vessel, which is conveniently rotated with an aneurism needle. Flooding the wound with saline reveals the sympathetic threads which are adherent to the muscular coat, and the last remnants of nerve fibres are destroyed by mopping the artery with 90 per cent. alcohol. Temporary contraction of the vessel follows an adequate neurectomy.

Presacral Neurectomy.—The patient is placed in the Trendelenburg position and the abdomen is opened by a subumbilical paramedian incision. The bifurcation of the aorta is exposed by a vertical incision through the overlying peritoneum, which is easily lifted from the vessel. The presacral nerves are usually represented by a plexus, and in order to ensure complete removal, all the nervous, fatty, and areolar tissues lying over the lower inch of the aorta and the sacral promontory are excised (fig. 949).

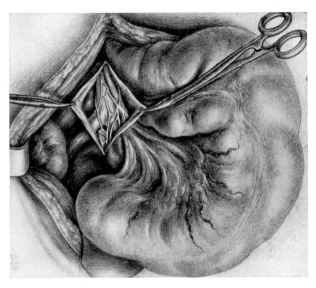

Fig. 949.—Displaying the presacral nerve. The presacral and inferior mesenteric sympathetic nerves (following the inferior mesenteric artery) are divided. (*After Learmonth.*)

Pre-ganglionic Cervico-dorsal Sympathectomy.—The operation is performed under either general or local anæsthesia, and a good forehead lamp is advisable. An incision is made ½ inch (1·25 cm.) above the inner half of the clavicle, and the clavicular part of the sternomastoid, the posterior belly of the omo-hyoid, and the scalenus anterior muscles are divided, the phrenic nerve being displaced inwards. The subclavian artery is thus exposed, and the thyro-cervical trunk is divided between ligatures. Occasionally the posterior scapular artery arises directly from the subclavian, in which case it also is ligated. The subclavian artery is depressed and Sibson's fascia is divided, so that the dome of the pleura can be displaced downwards and outwards. The stellate ganglion is then identified as it lies on the neck of the first rib (fig.

Francis Sibson, 1814–1876. Physician, St. Mary's Hospital, London.

950), the superior intercostal artery being on the outer side. The sympathetic trunk is traced downwards and divided below the third thoracic ganglion. All rami communicantes associated with the second and third ganglia and the nerve of Kuntz are meticulously divided. Deep bleeding-

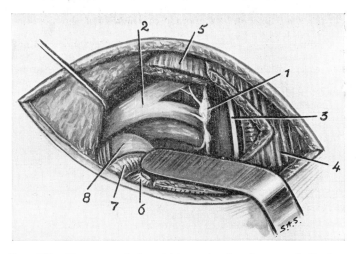

Fig. 950.—Exposure of the right cervico-dorsal sympathetic from the front.

1. Stellate ganglion.
2. Lower trunk of brachial plexus.
3. Phrenic nerve displaced inwards.
4. Partially divided sterno-mastoid muscle.
5. Divided scalenus anticus muscle.
6. Divided posterior belly of the omo-hyoid.
7. Subclavian artery displaced downwards.
8. Dome of the pleura.

points are best controlled by silver clips. A small drain is inserted for twenty-four hours. Not infrequently the ganglion on the opposite side is also removed at the same operation.

Cervico-dorsal ganglionectomy was formerly practised, and although somewhat easier to perform, a successful ablation was followed by Horner's syndrome, i.e. myosis, enophthalmos, ptosis, and hypoidrosis (diminished sweating) of the face and neck.

Lumbar Ganglionectomy.— *Unilateral ganglionectomy* is sometimes performe in cases where one limb has already been amputated for gangrene. The approach is extraperitoneal, and is similar to the exposure required for nephro-ureterectomy. The muscles are divided and the colon and peritoneum, to which the ureter clings, are stripped inwards so as to expose the inner border of the psoas muscle (fig. 951).

The sympathetic trunk lies on the side of the bodies of the lumbar vertebræ, and on the right side is overlapped by the vena cava. Lumbar veins are apt to cross the trunk superficially, and must be meticulously ligated as they pass directly into the adjacent inferior vena cava. (We have seen a case of fatal hæmorrhage from a lumbar vein.) The sympathetic trunk is divided on the side of the body of the fourth lumbar vertebra, and the trunk is traced upwards to below the duodenum on either side, where it is divided and resected.

Bilateral ganglionectomy is commonly performed transperitoneally. A left paramedian incision is made from above the umbilicus to an inch or two

Albert Kuntz, Contemporary. Professor of Histology, St. Louis University, U.S.A.

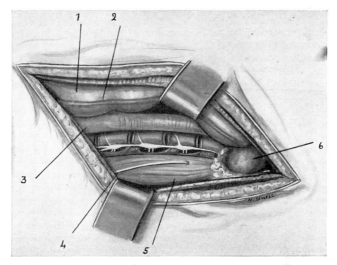

FIG. 951.—Left lumbar ganglionectomy.

1. Peritoneum stripped forwards, with ureter
   (2) adherent to it.
3. Aorta.

4. Genito-crural nerve.
5. Psoas.
6. Lower pole of kidney.

above the pubis. Intestines are packed off, and on the right side the posterior layer of peritoneum is incised vertically over the outer side of the vena cava. The mesenteric attachment is displaced upwards, together with the ileo-colic and right colic arteries. The sympathetic trunk lies under the outer border of the vena cava, and is divided above after displacement upwards of the duodenum. It is traced downwards until it disappears behind the right common iliac vein, when it is divided and resected.

On the left side exposure is gained by incising the peritoneum on the outer side of the pelvic colon. The bowel is stripped inwards together with the left colic vessels and ureter. The genito-crural nerve is seen emerging from the psoas, and eventually the inner border of the muscle is exposed. The sympathetic trunk is then identified as it lies on the vertebral bodies. It is divided above after displacement upwards of the duodenum, and is dissected downwards until it disappears underneath the left common iliac artery, where it is divided and removed.

Many surgeons now perform bilateral ganglionectomy through two separate incisions in the loins (as described for the unilateral operation), as the incidence of post-operative complications is diminished, and the duodenum can be more easily displaced forwards from the loin. Also, although two incisions are required, shock is diminished if the peritoneal cavity is unopened.

Thoraco-lumbar splanchnicectomy (Smithwick) has been considerably modified since its introduction for hypertension. The essential feature is removal of the sympathetic chain from about the eighth thoracic to below the third lumbar ganglion, with division of the splanchnic nerves.

The modified technique is briefly as follows. The patient is placed in the kidney position, and an incision is made from the lateral border of the erector spinæ muscle along the eleventh rib, and continued to the linea

Reginald H. Smithwick, Contemporary. Professor of Surgery, Boston.

semilunaris. The eleventh rib is excised, the flank muscles are divided, and the sympathetic chain is exposed by stripping up the peritoneum. It is divided below the third ganglion and freed in an upward direction to the internal arcuate ligament. This ligament and the crus of the diaphragm are incised upwards, and the greater splanchnic nerve is observed piercing the crus. The sympathetic chain is cleared to as high a level as possible above the diaphragm. The thoracic attack begins by opening the pleura at the posterior end of the wound. The lung is retracted upwards and the sympathetic chain is readily seen lying on the necks of the ribs, with the greater splanchnic nerve on the inner side. The pleura covering the chain is divided in the neighbourhood of the eighth ganglion, and the chain is dissected downwards with the greater splanchnic nerve until the upper part of the abdominal dissection is reached, and the lumbar and thoracic parts of the chain appear in continuity, and it is then resected with the splanchnic nerves.

Transpleural approach is preferable to stripping the pleura from the thoracic wall as less shock follows, and if hæmostasis is not absolute, a collection of blood in the pleural cavity is preferable to an extrapleural effusion, as it can easily be aspirated (A. M. Boyd).

Bilateral lumbar ganglionectomy may result in temporary postural hypotension, and bilateral removal of the first and second lumbar ganglia leads to sterility, but not to impotence (Learmonth). Sweating of the feet and legs is abolished after lumbar ganglionectomy.

A. M. Boyd, Contemporary. Professor of Surgery, University of Manchester.
Sir James Learmonth, Contemporary. Professor of Surgery, Edinburgh.

CHAPTER XXXVII

THE BREAST

THE NIPPLE

CONGENITAL ABNORMALITIES

Absence of the nipple is very rare, and usually it is associated with amazia.

Supernumerary nipples are fairly common, particularly in the male. Usually they occur along a line extending from the anterior fold of the axilla to the fold of the groin. This constitutes the milk line of lower mammalia. Unless the clinician is familiar with the anomaly, supernumerary nipples are frequently mistaken for moles or warts.

Retraction of the nipple is either recent or of long standing.

Long-standing retraction is due to :

1. Failure of evolution from childhood to womanhood.
2. Fibrosis following a mammary abscess or mastitis of infancy.

Non-protuberance of the nipple hinders an infant suckling at the breast. Clinical experience shows that a breast with long-standing retraction of its nipple is prone to abscess forma-

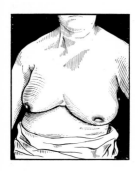

tion during lactation and to fibro-adenosis[1] at all times. The importance of long-standing retraction is dwarfed by the ominous diagnostic significance of recent retraction (fig. 952).

Recent retraction is a frequent accompaniment of scirrhus carcinoma.

Therefore the all-important question to put to the patient is : " How long has this nipple been retracted ? "

Cracked Nipple.—Want of care in the preparation for lactation and neglect of the hygiene of the nipple during lactation are the chief causes of this frequent condition. Its main importance lies in the fact that the crack may be the forerunner of acute suppurative mastitis.

FIG. 952.—Recent retraction of the nipple.

[1] The term fibro-adenosis has replaced the obsolescent " chronic interstitial mastitis," as it more accurately depicts the pathology of this disease.

Prophylaxis.—During the last two months of pregnancy the nipples should be hardened by gently rubbing them with a soft nail-brush every day (Sir Truby King), afterwards dabbing the nipple and areola with surgical spirit, which is allowed to evaporate. After suckling, the nipples should be washed and dried.

Treatment.—The mother should discontinue suckling at that breast until the fissure has healed, antiseptic dressings being applied. The breast must be emptied artificially at regular intervals.

Papilloma of the nipple presents the features of a cutaneous papilloma. It sometimes grows to a large size, but the pedicle is always narrow. The treatment is excision.

Retention Cyst of a Gland of Montgomery.—These glands, situated in the areola, secrete sebaceous material and, like sebaceous glands elsewhere, are liable to distension resulting from their orifices becoming blocked.

Chancre of the Nipple.—Wet nurses are not now employed, but in former days infection from the mouth of a syphilitic child sometimes occurred. It was noted that the mother of such an infant is immune to reinfection from her child. The majority of chancres of the nipple occur by infection from a buccal mucous patch in the mouth of a member of the opposite sex.

Eczema of the nipple is often bilateral, and presents features common to eczema elsewhere.

Paget's disease of the nipple must be distinguished from the foregoing. Paget's disease will be considered under the heading of " Carcinoma of the Breast " (see p. 955).

ABNORMAL DISCHARGES FROM THE NIPPLE

A milky discharge can sometimes be expressed long after lactation has ceased. It can be associated with a galactocele, but this condition is rare.

A clear serous discharge is associated usually with a retention cyst, consequent upon fibro-adenosis.

A blood-stained discharge is pathognomonic of duct papilloma or duct carcinoma. The former condition is more common than the latter.

A black or green discharge may be due to altered blood from the foregoing, but is much more frequently an accompaniment of retention cysts of fibro-adenosis. We have found that a dirty green discharge is usually due to polycystoma, and when the breast is removed it is found to be riddled with cysts containing the same material.

Sir Truby King, 1858–1938. Infant Welfare Authority, New Zealand.
William Montgomery, 1797–1859. Professor of Midwifery, Dublin.

A purulent discharge sometimes occurs in connection with a breast abscess.

THE BREAST

CONGENITAL ABNORMALITIES

Amazia.—Congenital absence of the breast may occur on one or both sides. It is sometimes associated with an absence of the sternal portion of the pectoralis major. Amazia is more common in males.

Polymazia.—Accessory breasts have been recorded in the axilla, groin, buttock, and thigh (fig. 953). They have been known to function during lactation.

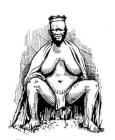

Gynæcomazia.—Hypertrophy of the male breast may be unilateral or bilateral. The breasts enlarge at puberty, and sometimes present the characteristics of a well-developed female organ. The subjects of this deformity are often virile. Chengwayo, chief of the Zulus (fig. 954), a gynæcomast, at the age of fifty-five, had forty wives and over a hundred children. Tribal tales of a father nurturing his motherless infant with milk from his own breast belong to the realms of mythology, but pseudo-lactation has been observed in rare instances, and a fluid akin to colostrum has been expressed.

FIG. 953. — An accessory and functioning breast on the left thigh. (*After Witkowski.*)

FIG. 954.—Chengwayo, from a photograph by Schujelot.

The treatment of gynæcomazia should be excision of the breasts, for their possessor is subject to ridicule. Enlargement of the breast often accompanies œstrogen therapy of carcinoma of the prostate.

DIFFUSE HYPERTROPHY

Diffuse hypertrophy of the breasts appears sporadically in otherwise healthy girls at puberty, and, less often, during the first pregnancy. The breasts attain enormous dimensions, and may reach below the knees when the patient is sitting. Except in those cases occurring during pregnancy, where it is possible that the enlargement will subside at the conclusion of lactation, surgical treatment should be undertaken,

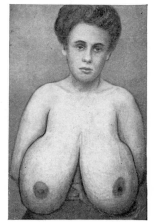

FIG. 955. — Congenital hypertrophy.

for the deformity and weight of the breasts are a real handicap to the patient (fig. 955). In many cases plastic reconstruction of the breasts can be performed. Occasionally the enormity is so great that the breasts are better excised, usually one at a time, but in young patients a plastic operation might be considered.

INJURIES OF THE BREAST

Injuries of the breast are rare and comparatively unimportant.

Hæmatoma, particularly a resolving hæmatoma, gives rise to a lump which, in the absence of overlying bruising, is difficult, if not impossible, to diagnose correctly until an exploratory incision has been made.

Milk fistula can follow an incised wound of a lactating breast or an operative incision. It usually heals spontaneously.

Traumatic fat necrosis may be acute or chronic. Following a blow or even indirect violence (e.g. contraction of the pectoralis major) or the administration of subcutaneous saline into the breast, a lump appears. In the absence of such a lead, the swelling is usually diagnosed as a carcinoma. A definite history of injury, especially that inflicted by subcutaneous saline solution, should bring the condition to the clinician's mind. On incising the mass the macroscopic picture is fairly characteristic. The chalky white area of necrotic fat is akin to the areas of fat necrosis seen in subsiding cases of acute pancreatitis.

ACUTE AND SUBACUTE INFLAMMATIONS OF THE BREAST

Mastitis of infants is at least as common in the male as in the female. Its ætiology is closely related to the lactation of infants. On the third or fourth day of life, if a mamma of an infant is pressed lightly, a drop of colourless fluid can be expressed ; a few days later there is often a slight milky secretion, which finally disappears in the third week. This is popularly known as " witch's milk."

The cause of mastitis of infants is not the ignorant maternity nurse " breaking the nipple strings," for it occurs in babies born in hospital. Furthermore, the misguided midwife presumably limits her activities to the female infant's breast ; and all who deal with the new-born appear to be agreed that mastitis of infants is, if anything, commoner in the male. Thus the midwife is exonerated. An ingenious explanation of this phenomenon is that the hormone which stimulates the mother's breast reacts also upon the newly formed mammary tissue of the fœtus. The infant with secreting breasts is liable to the same danger of a retrograde bacterial infection as its mother.

Mastitis of infants is essentially a physiological activity. It may lead to a true mastitis by retrograde infection. This true mastitis usually resolves ; occasionally it suppurates.

Mastitis of puberty is encountered frequently, usually in males. The boy, aged about fourteen, complains of pain and swelling in the breast. In 80 per cent. the condition is mainly or entirely unilateral. On examination the breast is enlarged, tender, and slightly indurated. The treatment is expectant. Suppuration never occurs. The symptoms usually disappear in fourteen days or so, but induration often persists for several weeks.

Mastitis from local irritation is now less common in women since high corsets strengthened with whalebone have been out of fashion, but it may be produced from a too tight elastic brassière. Mastitis from local irritation is by no means rare in men, and in this instance can usually be traced to pressure of a fountain-pen in the waistcoat pocket, or to the loss of a trouser button, which is compensated by hitching the braces buckle to a higher level (fig. 956). The treatment is to remove the cause. The substitution of a belt for braces is sound advice.

Mastitis from milk engorgement is liable to occur about weaning time, and it is sometimes confined to one portion of a breast. Unless the engorgement is relieved with a breast pump, an ascending bacterial infection may take place, the stagnant milk being a good medium for bacterial growth.

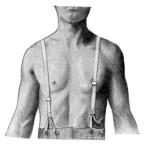

FIG. 956.—A frequent cause of mastitis in the male.

Mastitis of lactation is the commonest of all the acute inflammations of the breast, and in contradistinction to the others, it usually goes on to suppuration. The sufferer is often in the *first* month of her *first* lactation. Infection occurs in one of two ways:

(*a*) Staphylococci enter the lactiferous ducts and cause clotting of the milk. Within the clot the organisms multiply.

(*b*) Streptococci enter through a crack of the nipple. Inflammation proceeds apace in the interglandular tissues, and unless it is arrested, the infection spreads to the glandular mechanism.

Even upon the closest examination it is rare to find a cracked nipple. Clinical and bacteriological investigations leave little doubt that (*a*) is the commonest cause of an abscess of the breast.

" Cleaning the baby's mouth " with a swab is also an ætiological factor. The delicate buccal mucosa is excoriated by the process ; it becomes infected, and organisms in the infant's saliva are inoculated on to the mother's nipple.

The affected breast presents the classical signs of acute inflammation.

Treatment.—The patient should be confined to bed. If she is feeding her child, it must be weaned and the breasts emptied by a breast pump. The secretion of milk is minimised by giving saline aperients. A single intramuscular injection of 12·5 mg. of hexœstrol dipropionate inhibits lactation in a large percentage of cases. A second dose may be required (Prescott).

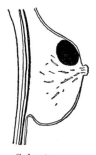

Fig. 957. — A simple form of breast pump.

Alternatively stilbœstrol 5 mg. t.d.s. can be prescribed. Large magnesium sulphate fomentations are applied locally. During this treatment the infected breast is examined daily. Occasionally resolution occurs, but in spite of chemotherapy and antibiotics in a large number of cases tenderness and induration become confined to one-quarter or, at the most, half of the breast, and an acute mammary abscess forms.

ACUTE MAMMARY ABSCESS

Most abscesses of the breast are of the intramammary variety (fig. 958), and it is lactating women who are the usual sufferers.

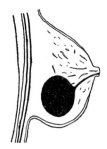
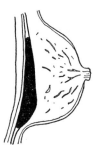

Subcutaneous.   Intramammary.   Retromammary.

Fig. 958.—Varieties of breast abscess.

Treatment.—It is seldom wise to consider incision until some localisation of the inflammation has occurred. The " closed " **method** of treatment offers many advantages.

Technique.—Under gas or pentothal anæsthesia an incision is made at the most dependent portion of the indurated area. The finger is inserted and loculi of the abscess cavity are broken down. Drainage tubes and dressings are then arranged as shown in fig. 959.

After-treatment.—Every four hours azochloramide or Dakin's solution is injected down the tube (fig. 960). The dressing is not disturbed for

Frederick Prescott, Contemporary. Research Director, Wellcome Research Institution.
Henry Drysdale Dakin, Contemporary. Director of the Herter Laboratory, New York.

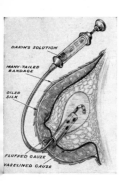

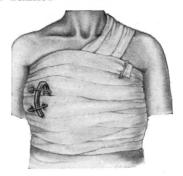

FIG. 960.—Method of applying the overall many-tailed bandage, and of fixing the end of the irrigating tube when not in use.

FIG. 959.—Azochloramide or Dakin's solution is injected down the small tube. The overflow runs out of the large tube and is absorbed by the gauze. The layer of vaseline gauze protects the skin from the irritating effect of the fluid.

twenty-four hours. The overflow is absorbed into the fluffed gauze. At the end of that time the many-tailed bandage is undone and the fluffed gauze changed. Provided the temperature chart is satisfactory, and the patient does not complain of discomfort, the inner dressing of vaseline gauze and the tubes are not disturbed. This labour-saving, pain-sparing régime is followed until the fourth or fifth day, when the dressings and tubes are removed.

Thenceforward the abscess cavity is washed out by means of a rubber catheter once or twice a day, gradually diluting the solution with saline day by day, until the wound granulates.

Penicillin treatment of breast abscess has proved useful, but has not replaced the necessity for drainage except in some early cases.

Chronic Abscess of the Breast.—Chronic abscess of the breast is often a very difficult condition to diagnose. *It simulates in many respects a carcinoma of the organ.* Removal and examination of the swelling is often the only means of determining this all-important differential diagnosis.

Retromammary Abscess.—Here the pus is situated in the cellular tissues behind the breast, and in practically all cases it has nothing to do with the breast proper. It arises from a tuberculous rib, infected hæmatoma, or possibly from a chronic empyema necessitatis, and treatment must be directed to the relief of these conditions, the breast being retracted as necessary from the field of operation.

Submammary Intertrigo.—On lifting up large, pendulous breasts in fat women it is not uncommon to find patches of intertrigo on the abutting skin surfaces of the breast and the chest wall.

Tuberculosis of the Breast.—Tuberculosis of the breast is comparatively rare. It may be associated with other tuberculous lesions. It usually takes the form of multiple chronic abscesses. The diagnosis rests on bacteriological and microscopical examinations. The usual treatment is amputation of the breast, but a trial may be given to streptomycin.

Actinomycosis of the breast is rarer still, and presents the characteristics of actinomycosis in other regions.

Syphilis of the Breast.—A primary chancre of the nipple has been referred to on p. 942. Secondary lesions of syphilis in the form of mucous patches are sometimes found in the submammary folds. In the second stage also both breasts may become swollen and painful, the condition being known as diffuse syphilitic mastitis. Gumma of the breast is very rare, and almost impossible to diagnose unless there are other evidences of syphilis.

CYSTS OF THE BREAST

Cysts of the breast are usually due to blockage of the secreting mechanism, either by fibrosis from without or obstruction from within the lumen. Occasionally cysts occur in the stroma.

Classification of Cystic Swellings of the Breast

1. **Polycystoma.**—The breast is riddled with cysts (fig. 961); one cyst may be large and the others insignificant. The condi-

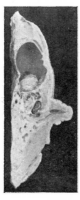

tion is frequently an accompaniment of fibro-adenosis. Less often, one sector of the breast is affected alone, when obstruction to a main duct near the nipple by a duct papilloma should be suspected.

2. **Cystadenoma** (serocystic disease of Brodie) (p. 954).

3. **Intracystic Papilliferous Carcinoma** (p. 958).

4. **Colloid Carcinoma** (p. 955).

5. **Chronic Abscess** (p. 947).

6. **Lymph Cyst.**
7. **Hydatid Cyst.**
8. **Hæmatoma** (p. 944).
9. **Galactocele.**—Galactoceles are usually single, and always date from lactation. They contain milk which may be inspissated, and in long-standing cases the walls tend to calcify.

FIG. 961.—Fibro-adenosis with cysts. The largest cyst contains an intra-cystic papilliferous growth.

Probably 75 per cent. of mammary cysts belong to group 1. Transillumination and aspiration are helpful aids in differential diagnosis.

MASTODYNIA

Slight discomfort in the breasts is not unusual in the premenstrual phase. When breast discomfort amounts to pain it is termed mastodynia. On palpation the breasts appear normal, but they are tender. Mastodynia is sometimes associated with a neuropathic temperament.

Treatment.—Hormone therapy is effective in genuine cases. Testosterone propionate in doses of 10 to 30 mg. daily has been followed by an amelioration of symptoms. In the case of young girls a much smaller dose is advised. Testosterone therapy is contraindicated during pregnancy.

FIBRO-ADENOSIS (Syn. CHRONIC INTERSTITIAL MASTITIS)

The term " chronic interstitial mastitis " is deep-rooted in British medical nomenclature, but the term is essentially erroneous. The condition is not a chronic inflammation. The modern conception is that it is due to an aberration of those physiological changes which occur in the mammary tissue at puberty and the menopause, and the condition is more accurately termed " fibro-adenosis " (Hedley Atkins).

Clinical Features.—Fibro-adenosis may occur at any age after puberty ; it is particularly common about the time of the menopause. Spinsters, childless married women, and multiparous women who have not suckled their children are the usual sufferers. This suggests that the condition is prone to appear in breasts which have been denied their intended function. The patient usually complains of pain in *one* breast, worse about the time of menstruation, or after using the arm. On examination both breasts are inclined to be what may be described as " lumpy." The breast complained of, when examined between finger and thumb, may contain a definite lump, but this is felt only vaguely with the flat of the hand. The lump is not adherent to the pectoral fascia nor to the skin. There is no recent retraction of the nipple, but sometimes there is a serous or dark-green discharge therefrom. A cyst, or cysts, may complicate or obscure the clinical picture. The axillary lymph nodes are frequently enlarged, and they are soft and often tender.

Pathology.—When sectioned with a knife the affected areas in the breast are white or yellow, but they never present the grey tones of carcinoma. Cysts of varying sizes filled with dark mucoid material are often seen in long-standing cases. Microscopically, it will be found that the interstitial tissues are swollen, and there is a round-celled infiltration. Fat and elastic tissue have largely disappeared. Later the interstitium is replaced by dense white fibrous trabeculæ. It is this fibrous tissue which compresses the ducts, thus favouring cyst formation. Often the epithelial lining is so compressed that it atrophies ; occasionally it hypertrophies and distends the acini.

After many decades of discussion the majority of surgeons and pathologists are now convinced that fibro-adenosis is *not* a precarcinomatous condition (Hedley Atkins). As the two

Hedley J. B. Atkins, Contemporary. Director, Surgical Department, Guy's Hospital.

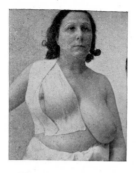

FIG. 962.—A method of supporting the breast by adhesive strapping.

conditions are common they occasionally co-exist as a coincidence.

Treatment.—In early cases without cyst formation and where the possibility of carcinoma does not arise, reassurance of the patient, strapping the breast (fig. 962), and hormone therapy often relieves symptoms, and in a certain number of cases the nodules disappear. In the present state of our knowledge it appears that testosterone is the most useful hormone, and about 5 mgms. in ointment are massaged into the affected breast nightly until symptoms are relieved. Improvement often follows pregnancy. Removal of a local cyst is sometimes advisable. If symptoms persist, or if the breast is riddled with cysts, local mastectomy is justifiable. A satisfactory method of removing the mammary gland in these cases is through a submammary incision. The breast, including its axillary tail, is dissected out, leaving the skin and nipple intact. After the mammary gland has been excised, a purse-string suture on the under-surface of the areola ensures eversion of the nipple. This operation, which is known as Gaillard-Thomas's, gives a very good cosmetic result, especially in thin women (fig. 963).

When the Diagnosis of Carcinoma is in Doubt.—There will always be cases where the clinician cannot be sure whether a

FIG. 963.—Result of submammary excision of both breasts for fibro-adenosis.

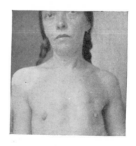

particular lump in the breast is a patch of fibro-adenosis or an early carcinoma. In doubtful cases it is wise to advocate operation without delay. The first step is to excise that part of the breast containing the lump, and to look at its cut surface

T. Gaillard-Thomas, 1831–1903. Surgeon, The Women's Hospital, New York.

(fig. 964). In many cases, a glance will suffice to indicate the nature of the tumour. *If it is fibro-adenosis,* local removal of the affected area is indicated. *If it is carcinoma,* the incision is closed, gloves and instruments are changed, and the operator proceeds to perform a radical excision of the breast.

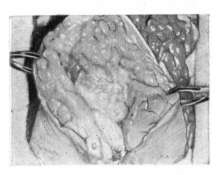

FIG. 964.—Macroscopic examination of a doubtful lump in the breast. In the lower part of the specimen the dead white appearance of fibro-adenosis is evident. In the centre there is a small carcinoma which is greyish-white and cuts like an unripe pear.

There remain a small number of instances in which by looking at the cut surface we are still in doubt. If facilities for immediate histological diagnosis by frozen section are not available, the surgeon should proceed to treat the case as one of carcinoma.

BENIGN NEOPLASMS OF THE BREAST

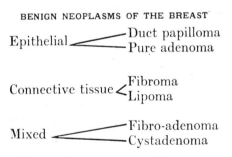

Epithelial —— Duct papilloma
—— Pure adenoma

Connective tissue < Fibroma
Lipoma

Mixed —— Fibro-adenoma
—— Cystadenoma

Duct Papilloma.—The majority of these tumours are single, but in some cases multiple papillary growths are found in the ducts. The usual single papilloma often has a stalk, and is situated in one of the larger lactiferous ducts.

Clinical Features.—The condition is rare before the age of twenty-five, and usually occurs in women between thirty-five and fifty. In the majority of cases a hæmorrhagic discharge from the nipple is the only symptom. Occasionally the discharge is serous and not bloodstained. On examination, a distended

NORMAL STRUCTURE, ADENOSIS, EPITHELIOSIS, CYSTIC HYPERPLASIA, AND NEOPLASIA OF THE BREAST

10–20 main ducts dilated just deep to the nipple forming milk reservoir; each drains a lobe which (embedded in fat) is made up of several lobules (encapsuled in fibrous tissue), each consisting of several gland fields (separated from one another by fibrous septa running in from the lobular capsule) which consist of terminal ductules (embedded in special loose connective tissue, different from and more lightly staining than that surrounding the gland fields and lobules). These ductules are absent before puberty, formed after puberty, expand during the premenstrual period, bud out into acini during pregnancy, actively secrete milk during lactation, and undergo involutionary collapse after lactation and during the menstrual period; they atrophy after the menopause.

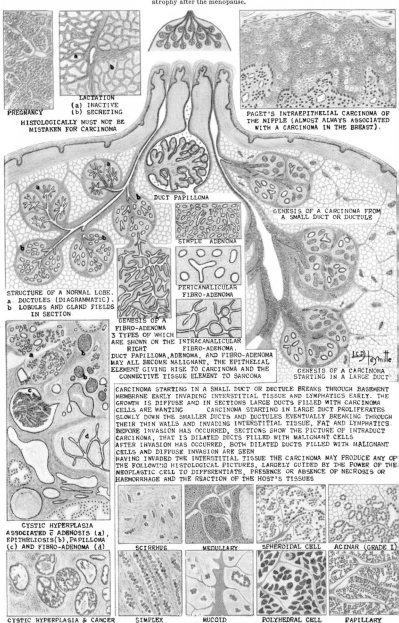

PREGNANCY

LACTATION
(a) INACTIVE
(b) SECRETING
HISTOLOGICALLY MUST NOT BE MISTAKEN FOR CARCINOMA

PAGET'S INTRAEPITHELIAL CARCINOMA OF THE NIPPLE (ALMOST ALWAYS ASSOCIATED WITH A CARCINOMA IN THE BREAST).

DUCT PAPILLOMA

GENESIS OF A CARCINOMA FROM A SMALL DUCT OR DUCTULE

SIMPLE ADENOMA

STRUCTURE OF A NORMAL LOBE.
a. DUCTULES (DIAGRAMMATIC).
b LOBULES AND GLAND FIELDS IN SECTION

PERICANALICULAR FIBRO-ADENOMA

GENESIS OF A FIBRO-ADENOMA 3 TYPES OF WHICH ARE SHOWN ON THE RIGHT

INTRACANALICULAR FIBRO-ADENOMA.

DUCT PAPILLOMA, ADENOMA, AND FIBRO-ADENOMA MAY ALL BECOME MALIGNANT, THE EPITHELIAL ELEMENT GIVING RISE TO CARCINOMA AND THE CONNECTIVE TISSUE ELEMENT TO SARCOMA

GENESIS OF A CARCINOMA STARTING IN A LARGE DUCT

CARCINOMA STARTING IN A SMALL DUCT OR DUCTULE BREAKS THROUGH BASEMENT MEMBRANE EARLY INVADING INTERSTITIAL TISSUE AND LYMPHATICS EARLY. THE GROWTH IS DIFFUSE AND IN SECTIONS LARGE DUCTS FILLED WITH CARCINOMA CELLS ARE WANTING   CARCINOMA STARTING IN LARGE DUCT PROLIFERATES SLOWLY DOWN THE SMALLER DUCTS AND DUCTULES EVENTUALLY BREAKING THROUGH THEIR THIN WALLS AND INVADING INTERSTITIAL TISSUE, FAT AND LYMPHATICS. BEFORE INVASION HAS OCCURRED, SECTIONS SHOW THE PICTURE OF INTRADUCT CARCINOMA, THAT IS DILATED DUCTS FILLED WITH MALIGNANT CELLS AFTER INVASION HAS OCCURRED, BOTH DILATED DUCTS FILLED WITH MALIGNANT CELLS AND DIFFUSE INVASION ARE SEEN HAVING INVADED THE INTERSTITIAL TISSUE THE CARCINOMA MAY PRODUCE ANY OF THE FOLLOWING HISTOLOGICAL PICTURES, LARGELY GUIDED BY THE POWER OF THE NEOPLASTIC CELL TO DIFFERENTIATE, PRESENCE OR ABSENCE OF NECROSIS OR HAEMORRHAGE AND THE REACTION OF THE HOST'S TISSUES

CYSTIC HYPERPLASIA ASSOCIATED c̄ ADENOSIS (a), EPITHELIOSIS(b), PAPILLOMA (c) AND FIBRO-ADENOMA (a)

SCIRRHUS   MEDULLARY   SPHEROIDAL CELL   ACINAR (GRADE I)

CYSTIC HYPERPLASIA & CANCER   SIMPLEX   MUCOID   POLYHEDRAL CELL   PAPILLARY

FIG. 965

(Designed and drawn by Dr. L. C. D. Hermitte.)

duct can sometimes be felt beneath the areola ; pressure upon it will cause a discharge from the nipple.

Treatment.—Amputation of the breast is usually unnecessary. After constriction of the nipple with a rubber band or ligature, in order to keep the affected duct distended, an incision which follows the junction of the skin with the areola through half its circumference (fig. 966) enables the distended duct to be dissected out. Often a stalked papilloma can be demonstrated to the naked eye.

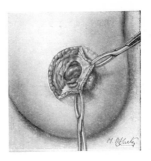

FIG. 966.—Method of displaying a distended lactiferous duct.

(*After Davidoff and Friedman.*)

In any case, the specimen should be submitted to microscopical scrutiny. Should the condition prove to be anything but a duct carcinoma, the patient will have been cured by the above, comparatively minor, operative procedure without any mutilation.

Fibro-adenoma of the breast is divided clinically into two varieties, the hard and the soft.

Hard fibro-adenoma is again redivided from the histological standpoint into *pericanalicular* fibro-adenoma, which is rare, and *intracanalicular* fibro-adenoma, which is common.

Clinical Features.—The patient is usually between the ages of fourteen and thirty, and she complains of a lump in the breast. Occasionally, there is more than one of these neoplasms present. On examination the lump is smooth, hard, and so freely movable that they have been termed " breast mice."

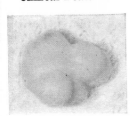

FIG. 967.—Fibro-adenoma of the breast enucleated.

Treatment is enucleation of the tumour (fig. 967); this is readily accomplished, because a fibro-adenoma is encapsulated and can be shelled out easily.

Soft fibro-adenoma again is a definitely localised tumour. Much rarer than the hard variety, soft fibro-adenomata occur in women about the age of thirty-five or forty. They are inclined to be bilateral and usually lie deeply in the breast. To the examining fingers they have the consistency of a lipoma. Occasionally cystic or sarcomatous changes occur.

Treatment.—As these neoplasms usually lie some depth from

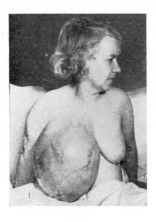

Fig. 968.—Serocystic disease of Brodie.
(*Professor A. Rendle Short's case.*)

the surface, they are best removed through a submammary incision.

Cystadenoma (*syn.* serocystic disease of Brodie) (fig. 968) is a rare affection which constitutes one of the massive tumours of the breast. The cysts are filled with fibro-papillomatous proliferations. The tumour tends to become sarcomatous. Excision of the breast is usually followed by an excellent result.

MASSIVE TUMOURS OF THE BREAST

This will be a convenient point at which to tabulate the massive tumours of the breast. They are :

1. Diffuse hypertrophy, which is usually bilateral.
2. Serocystic disease of Brodie.
3. Sarcoma.
4. Colloid carcinoma.

Each of these is considered in its appropriate section.

CARCINOMA OF THE BREAST[1]

There is no known cause of mammary cancer, and it can be stated with assurance that fibro-adenosis is not a predisposing cause. It is most improbable that injury plays any part in the production of the condition. Cancer very rarely attacks both breasts simultaneously. Only 1·5 per cent. of all cases of carcinoma of the breast occur in males. Women between forty and fifty years of age who have suckled children are its most frequent victims, but the disease is not rare in spinsters. It is estimated that about 2 per cent. of all women of the cancer age will develop malignant disease of the breast. While any portion of the breast may be attacked, the disease commences most frequently in the upper and outer quadrant (fig. 969). Unfortunately, so often the patient states that whilst washing she noticed a lump in her breast, but "took no notice of it because it was painless." It is computed that

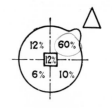

Fig. 969.—The relationship of carcinoma of the breast to the quadrants of the breast. (*Marshall and Higginbotham's statistics.*)

the average time between the patient noticing the lump and reporting it is eight months. Women should be urged to report to their doctors as soon as a lump in the breast is discovered.

[1] The importance of this subject becomes more evident when it is realised that 7,500 women die annually from this condition in England.

Sir Benjamin Brodie, 1783–1861. Surgeon, St. George's Hospital, London.

CLINICAL CLASSIFICATION OF THE VARIETIES OF CARCINOMA OF THE BREAST

(*a*) *From the alveoli*, and histologically a <u>spheroidal-cell</u>ed carcinoma :

Malignancy	Colloid carcinoma .	.	approx. 1 per cent. of all cases
	Atrophic scirrhus .	.	approx. 5 per cent. ,, ,, ,,
	Scirrhus .	.	<u>approx. 60 per cent.</u> ,, ,, ,,
	<u>Encephaloid</u> .	.	<u>approx. 16 per cent.</u> ,, ,, ,,
	Mastitis carcinomatosis .		approx. 2 per cent. ,, ,, ,,

(*b*) *From the ducts*, and histologically a <u>columnar-cell</u>ed carcinoma :

Duct carcinoma . . . . approx. 8 per cent. of all cases
Intracystic papilliferous carcinoma . approx. 2 per cent. ,, ,, ,,

(*c*) *Commencing in the skin of the nipple* and <u>histologically</u> disputed :

Paget's disease of the nipple . . approx. 1 per cent. of all cases

The percentages in the above tables are culled from the Ministry of Health reports on Carcinoma of the Breast, Nos. 28, 32, and 34.

Colloid carcinoma is the rarest form of carcinoma in group (*a*). It occurs in patients at about the same age as in the scirrhus variety. Tumours undergoing this gelatinous degeneration sometimes reach an enormous size, and translucent areas can be seen by transillumination. Contrary to what one might expect, the prognosis after operation is exceptionally favourable.

Atrophic scirrhus carcinoma is distinctly uncommon. It is seen principally in aged, thin women with small breasts. The cellular element of the growth is comparatively small, its main constituent being the fibrous stroma. Although steadily progressive, the disease runs a very chronic course, perhaps taking ten years to ulcerate through the skin, when it is inclined to grow somewhat more rapidly.

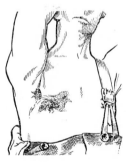

FIG. 970.—Atrophic carcinoma of the male breast of eight and a half years' standing.

This type of carcinoma is sometimes found in the male breast (fig. 970).

Scirrhus carcinoma is the leading <u>type of mammary cancer.</u> While it may commence in any portion of the breast, <u>the upper and outer quadrant (fig. 971) is the site of election.</u> Owing to an abundance of fibrous tissue the <u>lump</u> feels <u>very hard,</u> while its contour tends to be <u>irregular.</u> In its early stages it

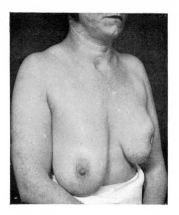

can be moved freely upon under-lying structures, and the skin can be made to move over it. Later it becomes tethered to the skin or to the underlying muscle, or to both. The im-portance of re-cent retraction of the nipple has been alluded to already (p. 941). *Peau d'orange* of the skin overly-ing the tumour (fig. 972) is another impor-

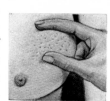

Fig. 972.—Early peau d'orange is made more obvious by pinching up the skin as shown.

Fig. 971.—Carcinoma of the breast. Note the elevation of the affected breast and the retraction of the nipple.

tant sign. Both these manifestations are comparatively late. The axillary lymph nodes are not palpable in the early stages, but they are microscopically invaded long before they can be felt.

Untreated, the growth eventually invades (fig. 973), and ulcerates through the skin and it may invade the thorax, while dissemination via the lymphatic and blood-streams finally determines the fatal issue. Two to two and a half years from the time the lump was first noticed is the average duration of life.

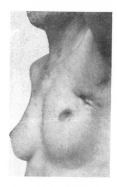

Fig. 973.—Scirrhus carcinoma of the breast invading skin.

If a breast containing a scirrhus carcinoma is cut with a knife so as to section the tumour, the following features will be noticed :

MACROSCOPICAL CHARACTERS

1. The growth cuts like an unripe pear, and may grate whilst being cut.

2. Usually *both* cut surfaces are found to be concave.

3. The colour of the cut surface is definitely grey (see fig. 964), and its appearance has been aptly likened to the interior of an unripe pear. Here and there will be seen a yellow spot, which is an island of fat undergoing degeneration.

4. On viewing the periphery of the sectioned tumour it will be found that there is not the slightest indication of a capsule. True to its name-sake, the crab, its claws have penetrated hither and thither into the breast tissue, and it is impossible to separate the tumour from the breast.

5. Expression of opaque cancer juice from the cut surface, dear to the old-time demonstrators of morbid anatomy, is no longer regarded as a characteristic feature of carcinoma.

Encephaloid carcinoma is usually found in women between twenty-five and thirty-five years of age with well-developed breasts. While presenting many characteristics of the foregoing variety, the epithelial element of the growth is in excess of its fibrous stroma. As a consequence the tumour does not feel so hard, and in advanced cases it may present semi-solid areas due to degeneration of masses of ill-nourished cells. This variety of carcinoma is not so intensely malignant as one is often led to believe. Statistics from all clinics show that the survival rate after operation is very little worse, or even a little better, than that of scirrhus carcinoma. Perhaps the relatively large size and rapid growth of the tumour impel the patient to seek relief earlier than in the case of scirrhus carcinoma.

Mastitis carcinomatosis occurs in the lactating breast and, according to the astute clinicians of former days, always in women of a florid aspect. Possibly a carcinoma has been present during the latter part of pregnancy, but it is fired into

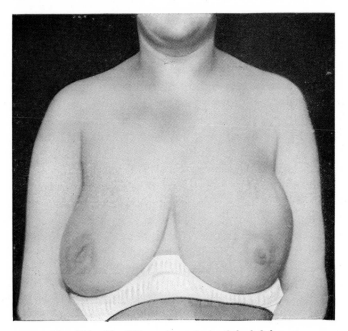

Fig. 974.—Mastitis carcinomatosis of the left breast.

extreme activity by the increased metabolism of its immediate host—the breast. It will be appreciated that the parasitic cells will take full advantage of the plentiful blood-supply destined for the milk-forming mechanism, and the result is an unbridled proliferation of cancer cells with very little fibrous reaction. This galloping form of mammary cancer often presents many of the signs of acute inflammation (fig. 974) and is sometimes mistaken for, and incised as, an abscess. The main distinguishing feature between the two conditions is the massive œdema which accompanies mastitis carcinomatosis. In spite of every effort to stay the course of the disease, mastitis carcinomatosis usually ends fatally within a few weeks or months.

Duct Carcinoma.—It is difficult, if not impossible, to tell from a clinical examination where a duct papilloma ends and a duct carcinoma begins. The leading symptom in both conditions is a blood-stained discharge from the nipple. A lump may be palpable behind the nipple or areola, and emerging from this there is usually a sector-shaped area of induration, viz. ◖. Obviously, the cause of the latter is distension of those alveoli drained by that duct which is blocked by the growth. On bisecting a breast containing a duct carcinoma, we have several times been able to trace the original stalk of the growth arising in one of the larger ducts behind the nipple. From this stalk delicate tendrils, like fine seaweed, could be traced along smaller ducts, the latter and their corresponding alveoli being dilated into a fine spongework by the growth and a blood-stained serous exudate. Histologically, the carcinoma is columnar-celled. According to Lockwood, this variety is " not less malignant than the other varieties of carcinoma," but as the lymph nodes are involved somewhat late in the course of the disease, and as it gives rise to alarming symptoms (bloody discharge from the nipple), which impel the patient to seek advice early, the prognosis after complete removal of the breast is usually good.

Intracystic Papilliferous Carcinoma (*syn.* disease of Réclus).—It is usually impossible to differentiate this condition from a simple cyst until its interior has been displayed. Within the cyst there is a cauliflower growth ———→ The prognosis after early operation is distinctly good.

Charles B. Lockwood, 1858–1914. Surgeon, St. Bartholomew's Hospital, London.
Paul Réclus, 1847–1914. Surgeon to the hospitals of Paris.

Paget's disease of the nipple is a persistent eczematous condition which does not respond to treatment and usually commences about the menopause. The nipple is slowly eroded

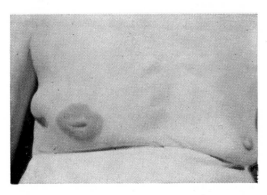

FIG. 975.—Paget's disease of the nipple, and an obvious carcinoma of the breast co-existent.

and eventually disappears. As the disease progresses the areola is involved (fig. 975), and the erosion continues to spread superficially for about two years, when definite signs of a malignant tumour within the breast become manifest.

Differential Diagnosis

Eczema	Paget's Disease
Bilateral.	Always unilateral.
Lactation.	Menopause.
Vesicles.	None.
Always itches.	Sometimes itches.

Theories of Causation.—Ever since Sir James Paget first described the condition, its exact nature has been the subject of dispute. Many of the older theories have been discarded.

Microscopically the eczematous area is characterised by the presence of large vacuolated cells with small deeply staining nuclei in the epidermis. At the present time two main theories exist :

1. That this change is due to a slowly growing intraduct carcinoma which infiltrates the skin by intra-epithelial spread along the ducts.

2. That the condition is a primary carcinoma of the skin.

The first theory is supported by the fact that in the majority of cases an exhaustive microscopic search reveals the presence of

Sir James Paget, 1814–1897. Surgeon, St. Bartholomew's Hospital, London.

malignant changes in the ducts (Donald Teare). Sooner or later a scirrhus carcinoma develops in the breast itself.

Treatment should be radical removal, which, if performed before there is a palpable lump in the breast, is accompanied by an excellent prognosis.

PHENOMENA RESULTING FROM LYMPHATIC OBSTRUCTION IN CASES OF MAMMARY CARCINOMA

Peau d'orange (see fig. 972, p. 956) is due to cutaneous lymphatic œdema. Where the infiltrated skin is transfixed by the sweat ducts it cannot swell. The characteristic pitted appearance, so well likened to orange peel by French observers, has become a classical physical sign of carcinoma of the breast. But it should be noted carefully that the same picture is occasionally seen over an abscess, particularly a chronic abscess, of the breast.

Early œdema of the arm which occurs within a few days of the operation is of little moment. It is a " traumatic " lymphatic obstruction following removal of lymph nodes and division of lymphatic vessels. Elevation and rest relieve the swelling, which is not usually so severe as to cause the patient much discomfort. It tends to improve as a collateral lymphatic circulation develops.

Brawny Arm (*syn. elephantiasis chirurgica*).—Swelling of the arm a few months after radical mastectomy indicates a neoplastic recurrence. The œdema is persistent and brawny (fig. 976), and is occasionally associated with inflammatory reactions. Most cases of brawny arm are due to lymphatic œdema, but in some cases venous obstruction is a contributory cause. The recurrences may be in the axilla, the supraclavicular region, or the mediastinum. Fore-quarter amputation is merciful in selected cases, especially in order to relieve the intense pain caused by involvement of the nerves in the axilla.

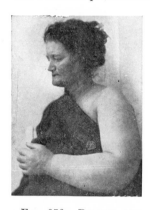

FIG. 976.—Brawny arm following radical mastectomy.

Serous effusion into the peritoneal or pleural cavities may be classed as one of the terminal events in hopeless cases.

While not entirely a phenomenon of lymphatic obstruction, this is a convenient place to mention a rare complication of carcinoma of the breast which is constantly in the mouth of the student, for no better reason than its fascinating name. We refer to " cancer en cuirasse." Here one side of the thoracic wall is studded with carcinomatous nodules, and the skin is so infiltrated that it has been likened to a coat of armour. The condition appears usually, but not necessarily, in cases with local recurrence after amputation of the breast. It is fortunately rare, and when seen the end is not far distant. It in no way merits that prominent position in the professional mind which it has so long enjoyed.

THE SPREAD OF MAMMARY CARCINOMA

(*a*) **Local Spread.**—The tumour increases in size, and invades other portions of the breast. It tends to involve the skin, and

Donald Teare, Contemporary. Pathologist, St. George's Hospital, London.

to penetrate the pectoral muscle (fig. 977), and even the chest wall.

(*b*) **Lymphatic spread** occurs in two ways: *by emboli*, composed of carcinoma cells, being swept along the lymphatic vessels by the lymphatic stream ; and *by permeation*, that is, actual growth

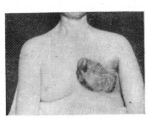

FIG. 977.—After eighteen months' treatment by a herbalist, carcinoma of the breast fungating through the skin.

of columns of cancer cells along the lumen of the lymphatic channels. By these means the axillary lymph nodes are involved. This occurs early. Later, the supraclavicular nodes, the mediastinum, and the sheath of the rectus abdominis are all possible stations for carcinoma cells journeying by this means. Finally, they may be found in lymph nodes even farther afield.

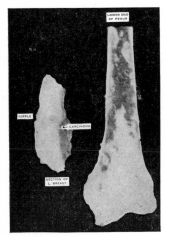

FIG. 978.—Secondary carcinoma in the lower end of the femur. The primary growth in the breast is shown also.

(*c*) **Spread by the Blood-stream.**—It is by this route that bones become invaded (fig. 978). In most instances it is also by way of the blood-stream that metastases arrive in the liver from the breast. It cannot be denied, however, that secondary deposits may also be carried to the liver via the lymphatics within the rectus sheath and the falciform ligament.

RADICAL MASTECTOMY

So far the best results in carcinoma of the breast have followed wide removal of the mammary gland, together with the structures which are likely to be infiltrated by carcinoma cells. The breast and associated structures are dissected *en bloc*, and the mass excised is composed of :

1. <u>The whole breast.</u>

Sir William Mitchell Banks, 1842–1904. Surgeon, Liverpool Royal Infirmary in Britain, and William S. Halsted, Professor of Surgery, Johns Hopkins University, Baltimore, were responsible for evolving the radical amputation of the breast as performed to-day. The operation is often known as " a complete Halsted."

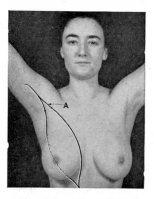

FIG. 979.—The incision for radical mastectomy. The part marked A is incised in the first instance, in order that the contents of the axilla may be dissected before the breast is removed.

2. A large portion of skin, the centre of which overlies the tumour, but always includes the nipple (fig. 979).

3. The fat and fascia from the lower border of the clavicle to, and including, the upper quarter of the sheath of the rectus abdominis, and from the manubrium to the anterior border of the latissimus dorsi.

4. The pectoralis major and its fascial sheath (its clavicular head is usually left).

5. The pectoralis minor and its fascial sheath.

6. The costocoracoid membrane.

7. All the fat, fascia, and lymph nodes of the axilla.

8. The fascia over, and a few of the more superficial muscle fibres of the anterior part of the external oblique, serratus anterior, the subscapularis, the latissimus dorsi (except its posterior surface), and the upper quarter of the rectus abdominis.

9. Sometimes the supraclavicular fat and fascia have to be removed in addition.

During the operation no effort should be spared to preserve :

1. The axillary vein.

2. The cephalic vein.

3. The nerve of Bell.

(4. The middle or long subscapular nerve should be retained if possible.)

During the operation the exposed chest wall must be protected by towels wrung out in hot saline. At the com-

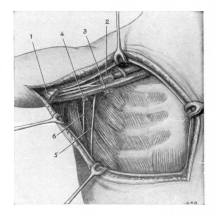

FIG. 980.—The field of operation after radical removal of the breast.

1. Divided sternal portion of pectoralis major muscle.
2. Divided pectoralis minor muscle at its insertion into the coracoid process.
3. Thoracic axis vessels.
4. Subscapular vessels.
5. Nerve of Bell lying on the serratus muscle.
6. Middle or long subscapular nerve passing latissimus dorsi.

Sir Charles Bell, 1774–1842. Surgeon, Middlesex Hospital, London, and founder of its Medical School

pletion of the operation the wound is drained in order to prevent blood accumulating.

If a wide area of skin has been sacrificed, it may not be possible to approximate the skin edges completely. A deficiency is left, which is later treated by skin grafting.

After operation the arm is supported upon a pillow until the wound has healed, and later carried in a sling until convalescence is complete. The movements of the arm after so extensive a loss of muscle are surprisingly good (fig. 981). If the axillary lymph nodes are involved, a course of prophylactic deep X-ray therapy should be given after the patient has convalesced from the operation.

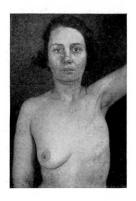

Fig. 981.—Patient two years after radical amputation of the breast for carcinoma.

Results.—Unlike some forms of malignant disease, where if the patient survives five years a permanent cure can be assumed, there is no such criterion in cases of carcinoma of the breast. Patients die of secondary mammary carcinoma as long as fifteen or twenty years after operation. It is, however, abundantly clear that when the axillary lymph nodes are not involved, the prospect of five years' survival is greater.

Survival Rate after Operation

	Three years	*Five years*
No axillary lymph node involvement	79 per cent.	69 per cent.
Axillary lymph node involved .	52 per cent.	30 per cent.

(*Jessop's compilation from University College Hospital cases.*)

On the whole, the prognosis is somewhat better than it was even ten years ago. This is due to earlier operation and improvements in deep X-ray therapy.

THE RÔLE OF RADIOTHERAPY IN THE TREATMENT OF MAMMARY CARCINOMA

While there are some differences in opinion as to details, a combined surgical and radiological attack is, at the present time, in vogue throughout the world for the treatment of comparatively early mammary cancer.

The following scheme is representative :

Stage 1.—The <u>tumour is localised</u> ; it is <u>mobile,</u> and <u>neither the skin nor the axillary lymph nodes are involved.</u> Here radical mastectomy, followed—as soon as the wound has healed—by a course of high-voltage X-ray therapy, is advised by some surgeons. 3,500–4,000r. is delivered to the whole of the operation area, including the axilla, the supraclavicular and anterior mediastinal regions. A <u>high survival rate</u> (<u>up to 84 per cent. of ten-year cures</u>) <u>can be expected</u>.

Stage 2.—The <u>tumour is attached</u> to underlying structures <u>and/or to the skin</u>. There are also <u>palpable axillary lymph nodes</u>. In these circumstances <u>preoperative irradiation,</u> delivering 2,500–3,500r. over three weeks to the involved area and the potential metastatic sites, not only cause a diminution in the size of the primary growth and the axillary lymph nodes, but it is believed to minimise dissemination of the neoplasm during the operation. Two or three weeks after the operation a post-operative course of irradiation is given similar to that described for stage 1.

Stage 3.—<u>When the tumour is fixed to the pectoral fascia and/or the supraclavicular lymph nodes or the contralateral axillary lymph nodes are involved</u>, <u>irradiation only is recommended.</u>

OTHER VIEWS ON THE TREATMENT OF CARCINOMA OF THE BREAST

(*a*) **Radium.**—A few surgeons (now very few) prefer radium to operation or combine operation with radium. When the former mode of treatment is favoured, the tumour, the surrounding breast and lymphatic drainage areas from the supraclavicular fossa above to the rectus sheath below, and from the axilla laterally to the anterior mediastinal lymph nodes medially, must be irradiated uniformly. Up to 100 mgms. of radium may be required in needles containing 1, 2, or 3 mgms. each and screened with 0·5 mm. of platinum. They are inserted parallel to each other ½ inch (1·25 cm.) apart, and by tying together the threads that are attached to the needles, they are held in position. The needles are left in place for several days, and then removed, hot fomentations being applied for twenty-four hours.

(*b*) **Local Mastectomy and Radiotherapy.**—Simple excision of the breast followed by deep X-ray therapy—a form of treatment which was given a trial some years ago—is again being used in some clinics. With the advance in knowledge of radiotherapy and the improved apparatus, it is believed that the results will be encouraging.

TREATMENT OF RECURRENCES AND SECONDARY DEPOSITS

Deep X-ray therapy causes to disappear, or retards the progress of, recurrences and secondary deposits in about one-third of cases. Examples are encountered—and not rarely—where extensive metastatic deposits are so radiosensitive that they melt away with this form of therapy. Another promising weapon is diethylstilbœstrol which, in a few cases, appears to be giving the same encouraging results as is the case in some instances of carcinoma of the prostate (see p. 633).

PROGNOSIS OF MAMMARY CARCINOMA

The following points are taken into consideration :

(i) **Age.**—As with most malignant neoplasms the younger the patient the worse the prognosis. This is especially so with regard to carcinoma of the breast, as the hyperæmia associated with the monthly periods (and even more so with lactation), encourages rapidity of growth.

(ii) **Sex.**—The prognosis in a male is practically hopeless, and recurrence is usual within a year whatever treatment is adopted. This gloomy outlook is due to lack of a buffer of fat, and in this connection it may be mentioned that the prognosis in a female is improved by plumpness, in fact, mastectomy is the only operation where the surgeon welcomes obesity.

(iii) **Type of Growth.**—As already mentioned, atrophic cancer may persist for years, whereas mastitis carcinomatosis is rapidly fatal. Columnar-celled carcinoma disseminates more slowly than the spheroidal-celled variety.

(iv) **Site of Growth.**—If the tumour is situated in the inner half of the breast, early involvement of the lymph nodes on the internal mammary vessels is probable. Growths in the lower and inner quadrant are apt to spread to the liver via the rectus sheath and falciform ligament.

(v) **Extent of Growth.**—On general principles involvement of the skin or fixity to the chest wall impairs the prognosis.

(vi) **Presence of Metastases.**—The significance of involvement of the axillary lymph nodes has already been referred to (p. 961). Although these nodes may be removed, their existence indicates that spread has probably occurred in other directions, e.g. to the supraclavicular or mediastinal nodes. Osseous, mediastinal, or other metastases are naturally of grave import.

SARCOMA

Sarcoma of the breast is usually of the spindle-celled variety, and it accounts for 1 per cent. of malignant tumours of the breast. Some of these growths arise in soft fibro-adenomata. It is difficult to differentiate from encephaloid carcinoma, but its growth is more rapid, and it is even softer than the latter. On incising the growth, its friable, pale consistency suggests the diagnosis. The condition is most often met with in women between the ages of thirty and forty. Metastases occur early, and usually determine a fatal issue in a comparatively short time. Even when the breast has been completely removed at an early stage in the disease, the prognosis is almost hopeless.

THE " FOLLOW-UP " OF CASES OF CARCINOMA OF THE BREAST

It is the duty of the surgeon to examine all his cases periodically so that the patient may be reassured if all goes well, or, in the event of recurrence, to enable the surgeon to prescribe such treatment as is applicable.

The following indicates a routine suitable for this periodic examination :

History.—This includes physical energy, general health, and any unexplainable cough. Also symptoms which the patient may ascribe to rheumatism, lumbago, or sciatica, which might indicate a secondary deposit in the humerus, spine, or femur. Gain in weight is not necessarily of good omen, as it may be due to such pathological conditions as brawny arm, serous effusions into the peritoneal or pleural cavities, or metastases in the liver.

Examination.—The operation field is examined for nodules. The axillæ, supraclavicular lymph nodes, and opposite breast are palpated. The hand and arm are examined for œdema. The chest is percussed and auscultated and the abdomen examined for evidence of enlarged liver or ascites. If considered necessary, a rectal or vaginal examination is made in order to detect pelvic or ovarian metastases.

Radiograph.—In doubtful cases a radiographic examination is made of the chest, or of any bones suspected of harbouring metastases.

CHAPTER XXXVIII

THE THORAX

INJURY TO THE LUNGS AND PLEURA

NON-PENETRATING

Compression of the chest (*syn.* traumatic asphyxia) occasionally follows such accidents as mining disasters, panics, or overcrowding, as at football matches. The flow of blood in the intrathoracic veins is obstructed, or the direction of the blood-stream may even be reversed. The veins of the head, neck, and arms become acutely engorged and capillaries rupture, so that the parts are dusky or purple in colour, owing to extravasated blood. Subconjunctival and submucous hæmorrhages also occur. Treatment is symptomatic, and the blood is absorbed in two or three weeks.

Contusion of the pleura results in dry pleurisy, and consequent pain on deep inspiration. If the lung also is contused, local extravasation occurs, causing a patch of consolidation (traumatic pneumonia). Hæmoptysis varies with the severity of the injury. Uneventful recovery is the rule, but the possibility of infection must be borne in mind.

Laceration of the lung is usually associated with fracture of one or more ribs ; but in some cases, especially in children, serious pulmonary injury is possible without fracture of the bony framework.

The immediate dangers are shock, severe hæmoptysis, or asphyxia following obstruction of main bronchi with blood. Subsequently the following conditions may develop :

Hæmothorax—which is accompanied by dyspnœa. The physical signs resemble those of a pleural effusion, and a rise of temperature is usual, as in any condition in which blood is extravasated. Bleeding diminishes as the lung collapses.

Pneumothorax—which yields a high-pitched note on percussion, with absent breath-sounds. Pneumothorax is usually associated with hæmothorax, and therefore adds to the dyspnœa, but at the same time assists in arresting hæmorrhage by exerting pressure on the bleeding lung.

Surgical emphysema is likely to occur if both the parietal and visceral layers of pleura are torn. The condition sometimes spreads widely. Affected tissues yield a soft crepitus on palpation, akin to that experienced when handling tissue-paper. The air is absorbed uneventfully in a few days.

Empyema—infection of a hæmothorax is always a possible danger, especially if the patient is bronchitic, or if the injury is associated with an external wound.

Treatment.—Morphia, preferably intravenously so that its action is immediate and controlled, is given to relieve pain, allay restlessness, and thereby discourage bleeding. The patient is kept at rest, and an ice-bag may be applied over the presumed site of injury. Inhalation of oxygen in high concentration relieves the dyspnœa and anoxia of the tissues. Needling should be performed if hæmothorax is suspected. The question then arises : Is hæmorrhage from the lacerated lung continuing ? Frequent pulse readings and blood-pressures must be taken. If these suggest that bleeding continues, a thoracotomy is indicated, so that the patient's life may be saved by direct arrest of the hæmorrhage. In most patients who survive the initial dangers, the bleeding ceases spontaneously, but the hæmothorax remains. In order to obviate the risk of infection, and discourage the subsequent formation of adhesions and thickening of the pleura, aspiration of the hæmothorax should be performed about the second or third day. (Blood in the pleural cavity does not clot unless the cavity is infected.) Aspirations sometimes require to be repeated, or a thoracoscope may be introduced through the chest wall and suction applied. Any subsequent collection of serous fluid responds to aspiration.

Careful attention to oral and dental hygiene will reduce the likelihood of empyema, and prophylactic penicillin should be administered.

PENETRATING

Puncture of the lung is likely to follow any penetrating wound of the chest, such as stab or gunshot wounds. A considerable degree of shock follows, and hæmoptysis indicates pulmonary injury. If a large opening is made through the chest wall the negative pressure in the pleural cavity disappears, and the lung collapses. Inspiratory efforts draw the mediastinum towards the uninjured side, which further embarrasses respiration by compressing the active lung. During expiration the contents of the mediastinum are pushed across to the injured side, and so to-and-fro movements or " flapping " results.

Dyspnœa, engorgement of veins of the neck, and increasing embarrassment of the heart are the obvious features of an open pneumothorax. Shock, cardiac failure, and hæmorrhage are the early dangers, and, if the patient survives, infection is likely to supervene (fig. 982). The treatment of a penetrating wound depends upon the urgency of the symptoms. In the case of an extensive wound the immediate necessity is to arrest any obvious hæmorrhage, and to pack the aperture with a suitable dressing. This is retained in position by means of adhesive strapping so

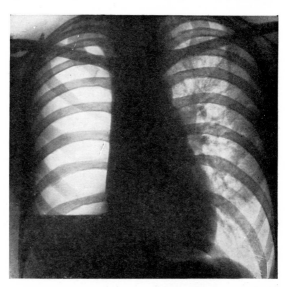

FIG. 982. — A pyopneumothorax, with a well-defined fluid level.

as to render the wound airtight. Intravenous morphia is given as soon as possible. If time and circumstances permit, the parietes should be approximated with a few stitches. Mediastinal " flap " is thus controlled, and a short interval is allowed for resuscitative measures. Under intratracheal anæsthesia the superficial wound is excised, and clots and any foreign bodies are removed from the pleural cavity. Lacerated portions of tissue are excised, and adjacent structures, such as the pericardium and diaphragm, are examined, bearing in mind that penetrating wounds of the thorax may also involve upper abdominal viscera. Sulphonamide and penicillin powder is insufflated, the wound is closed without drainage, and treatment is conducted as for a subcutaneous injury.

HERNIA OF THE LUNG (syn. PNEUMOCELE)

This condition occurs either spontaneously, or as a result of severe damage to the chest wall. In the former case Sibson's fascia yields, and a

Francis Sibson, 1814–1876. Physician to St. Mary's Hospital, London.

soft swelling appears behind the clavicle, which is readily compressible, but enlarges on coughing.   A pad with suitable straps should be applied if the swelling causes discomfort or increases in size.

CHYLO-THORAX

From time to time cases have been recorded where a wound has resulted in the outpouring of chyle into the pleural cavity ; enormous quantities have been aspirated.   Fortunately, the thoracic duct is usually lacerated in its upper portion, and there is a probability that small collateral vessels also empty into the subclavian vein.   For this reason some patients have recovered.

In cases of rapid deterioration, the chyle aspirated from the thorax should be injected into a vein.

INFECTIONS OF THE LUNG AND PLEURA

ACUTE EMPYEMA

Causes.—As with pus in any situation, empyema arises as a result of :

(*a*) Direct infection, as by penetrating wounds.

(*b*) Extension from neighbouring foci of infection, particularly pneumonic and subphrenic.

(*c*) Hæmatogenous infection (uncommon).

Clinical features are those of a pleural effusion combined with toxæmia.   The three cardinal signs of fluid in the chest are

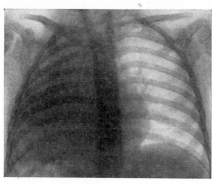

FIG. 983.—Posterior view of a generalised left-sided empyema.   The heart is displaced to the right.   (*Dr. J. E. A. Lynham.*)

diminished movement, a dull percussion note, and displacement of viscera, especially the heart (fig. 983).   Breath-sounds are usually inaudible, but are sometimes bronchial, especially in children. Leucocytosis is the rule.

Occasionally empyemata are localised or situated between the lobes, in which case X-ray is a valuable help in diagnosis.   If un-treated, and the patient survives for a sufficient length of time, the pus may erode a bronchus and be expectorated, or point through the chest wall, usually along one of the perforating branches of the internal mammary artery (empyema necessitatis).

Needling the chest is always necessary, both to confirm the

diagnosis and to allow bacteriological examination of the fluid, including the effect of penicillin on causative organisms. The skin and deep structures are infiltrated with 1 per cent. novocaine, which not only anæsthetises but also prevents pleural reflex shock. A fine needle is used, which is pushed into the pleural cavity. If no fluid is withdrawn, a large needle should be substituted, which is less likely to become obstructed by fibrin.

Treatment.—In bygone days practically all empyemata were treated by rib resection and drainage. During the influenzal epidemic of 1918, it was noted with regret that immediate drainage of empyemata associated with pneumonia (synpneumonic) carried a mortality of about 60 per cent. This was partly due to the fact that the effusion occurred, and was diagnosed, while the lung was still consolidated, and therefore unable to expand, also adhesions were weak or absent. Therefore rib resection caused an open pneumothorax, with consequent embarrassment of a heart on which great demands were already made, and the musculature of which was enfeebled by toxæmia. On the other hand, a pneumococcal empyema occurs at a later stage when consolidation has nearly or has already abated (post-pneumonic), and therefore the lung is expansile. Adhesions also have formed, and so walled off the pus to form a localised pleural abscess, and the general condition of the patient is improving.

The treatment of a streptococcal empyema consists in aspiration and partial replacement with penicillin solution. Sulphonamides are prescribed, and penicillin is administered parenterally. Cardiac embarrassment is relieved by aspiration, which is repeated as often as necessary, with penicillin replacement. If numerous aspirations cause infection of the chest wall, a catheter should be inserted under local anæsthesia and connected with a water-locked bottle. Breathing exercises are valuable. In most cases aspiration combined with penicillin and sulphonamide therapy is successful, but if the empyema persists, rib resection and drainage can now be performed with comparative safety.

Operation.—In the case of a generalised empyema, the most suitable ribs for excision are the ninth in the scapular line, or the eighth in the mid-axillary line. Drainage at a lower level is likely to be impeded by the diaphragm, and above this the scapula covers a portion of the ribs, and the opening is too high to be dependent. Care must be observed regarding posture. Either the prone position is adopted, or the patient is placed with the affected side projecting beyond the edge of the table, with a sandbag beneath the loin so as to turn him slightly towards the sound side. He should not be rolled over on the unaffected side in such a manner that the healthy lung is unable to expand.

Careful consideration must be given to the choice of anæsthetic. Gas and oxygen, cyclopropane, pentothal, or local infiltration are the methods of choice. If local anæsthesia is used, it is advisable to infiltrate and divide the skin and tissues so as to expose the required rib. The region of the intercostal nerve, which runs along the lower costal border, is then infiltrated with novocaine as far back as possible, and the process repeated to anæsthetise the nerves above and below.   An angled needle facilitates this step.

The incision is made either transversely along the axis of the rib, or vertically.   In the latter case the fibres of the latissimus dorsi are split, and the drainage tube can be inserted precisely opposite the opening in the pleura.   The periosteum is incised along the rib and separated from the superficial surface with a periosteal elevator.   By means of a Doyen's

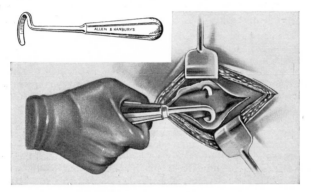

FIG. 984.—The periosteum of the rib is being stripped from the bone with a Doyen's raspatory (inset).

raspatory the periosteum and intercostal vessels and nerve are pushed off the deeper surface (fig. 984).   From 2 to 4 inches of rib are excised with rib shears the actual length depending on the size of the patient.   If an intercostal vessel is injured a further amount of bone is excised so that it can be securely ligated.   Sinus forceps are then thrust through the deep layer of periosteum and parietal pleura, and as pus escapes a finger is inserted into the opening, so as to control the gush of pus and prevent sudden movements of the mediastinum.

As the flow of pus diminishes, the finger is introduced into the lower part of the cavity so as to open any loculi, and flakes of fibrin, particularly noticeable in pneumococcal infection, are removed with sponge forceps. The *closed* method of drainage should always be employed. As compared with open drainage it presents the advantage that during inspiration air is not drawn into the pleural cavity, and consequently the negative pressure which encourages lung expansion is maintained.   Also frequent dressings, which are exhausting in a debilitated patient, are unnecessary.   The muscles and

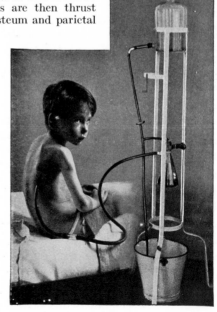

FIG. 985.—Closed method of drainage.

Eugene Doyen, 1859–1916.   Surgeon, Doyen Clinic, Paris.

skin are firmly sutured round the drainage tube, which is allowed to project some 3 or 4 inches. Collodion painted around the junction of the skin and tube assists in preventing air-entry. A glass connection is fitted into the drainage tube, and to the other end a rubber tube is attached sufficiently long to allow the free end to be submerged in a jar containing antiseptic solution, which is placed by the bedside. During inspiration the antiseptic rises in the tube, and on expiration pus is ejected into the antiseptic (fig. 985). After five or six days the drainage tube loosens, but by this time adhesions have formed round the sinus.

In the case of bilateral empyemata the side containing the larger collection of pus is drained, and the opposite side aspirated for a few days until the original wound is securely closed by adhesions.

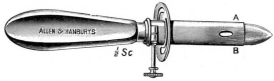

FIG. 986.—An empyema trocar for intercostal drainage.

In cases where the minimal amount of disturbance is desirable, as in the case of young children or debilitated patients, intercostal drainage can be obtained by means of a special trocar and cannula (fig. 986). If necessary, rib resection is performed after the immediate crisis has passed—that is, about ten days later.

MacMahon has devised a series of specialised exercises in which inspiration is emphasised rather than expiratory effort, and in the case of empyema breathing exercises are adopted with the spine curved laterally so that the sound lung is compressed and expansion of the collapsed lung correspondingly encouraged.

Interlobar empyemata, and those in apposition with the mediastinum or diaphragm, are unlikely to be diagnosed with certainty without the assistance of X-rays (fig. 987). They are the occasional cause of a symptomless temperature. The radiological appearance resembles that of a pulmonary abscess, but usually the definition is clearer in the case of an empyema. Although spontaneous cure sometimes follows rupture into a bronchus, delay is not advisable owing to the risk of subsequent bronchiectasis. As in the case of

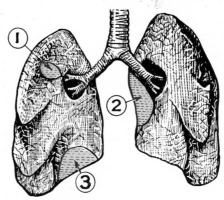

FIG. 987.
1. Interlobar empyema.
2. Mediastinal empyema.
3. Diaphragmatic empyema.

Cortlandt MacMahon, M.A. (Oxon), Contemporary. Instructor for Speech Defects and Breathing Exercises, St. Bartholomew's Hospital, London.

pulmonary abscess, exploratory needling as an aid to diagnosis is not advisable, owing to the risk of infecting the general pleural cavity. In suspicious cases penicillin and chemotherapy should be prescribed, bearing in mind that an empyema may thereby be rendered symptomless. Clinical examination and X-ray will disclose the abscess, which must be drained if persistent.

The affected portion of lung should be exposed by resection of a suitable rib. In the absence of adhesions, stitching the parietal and visceral pleuræ, and immediate drainage, usually results in extension of infection. It is wiser to pack gauze moistened with tincture of iodine into the wound, and allow adhesions to form between the two layers of pleura before drainage. A few days later the empyema is opened with a cautery or diathermy knife.

CHRONIC EMPYEMA

The term " chronic " is an arbitrary one regarding duration of time, but clinically it is applied to those cases which require subsequent surgical treatment in order to obtain healing.

Causes.—The majority of empyemata become chronic as a result of delay in the treatment of acute cases, or due to faulty or inadequate drainage.

The actual causes can be summarised as occurring in connection with the chest wall, the pleural cavity, or the lung, although in many cases more than one factor is responsible for chronicity.

(i) *Chest Wall.*—Drainage is inadequate. Either it is not dependent, or the opening is too small to allow free escape of pus. In other cases loculi are present, and continually reinfect the main cavity.

Fibrosis of intercostal muscles and thickening of the parietal pleura result in inelasticity of the parietes, and consequent delay in healing.

(ii) *Pleural Cavity.*—Foreign bodies are occasionally responsible for non-closure, and include drainage tubes and swabs. Should tuberculosis or actinomycosis be present, prolonged chronicity is inevitable.

(iii) *Lung.*—Expansion of the lung is hindered or rendered impossible by interstitial fibrosis or thickening of the visceral pleura. The thickened pleura also harbours organisms, and so is a source of reinfection. Bronchiectasis and lung abscess are not uncommon causes, and occasionally a chronic empyema is associated with a neoplasm.

Treatment.—Obviously it is essential to endeavour to discover the cause of delayed healing. A routine clinical examination of the chest may suggest the presence of fluid or of a neoplasm. A probe in some cases shows that the drainage is obviously inadequate, or detects the presence of a sequestrum or a foreign body.

A radiograph will demonstrate loculi containing fluid. Information regarding the extent and direction of the cavity or sinuses can be obtained by means of an X-ray after injection of lipiodol. The suspected presence of most foreign bodies, including tubes of red rubber (which contain sulphur, and are therefore opaque) is confirmed.

Bacteriological examination of the discharge is likely to show a variety of organisms, owing to mixed infection. The presence of tubercle bacilli or actinomycosis is of gloomy significance, and amyloid disease may eventually supervene.

Treatment in the first instance consists in the removal of a foreign body if such is present, and in securing adequate drainage. In some cases dilatation of a small sinus by laminaria "tents" will allow the introduction of a tube of adequate size. If necessary, portions of one or two ribs are removed, and loculi are opened so that they drain freely into the main cavity.

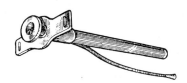

FIG. 988.—Two-way tube to permit of irrigation. (*Tudor Edwards.*)

Irrigation with penicillin may promote healing, and also, by softening the fibrous coating over the lung, encourages expansion (fig. 988). Irrigation cannot be used if bronchial fistulæ are present, as fluid trickles into the lung and causes violent coughing. When healing is proceeding in a satisfactory manner, the use of an appliance which exercises pressure on the chest wall will expedite closure of the cavity. Breathing exercises are important. Compensatory scoliosis, flattening of the chest, emphysema of the lung, and displacement of the mediastinum all contribute towards obliteration of the cavity.

If, after a reasonable trial of the above measures, progress is disappointing, more extensive measures must be adopted, so that the chest wall and lung are approximated. Either the chest wall is mobilised, or the visceral pleura dealt with so that the lung can re-expand.

OPERATIONS ON THE CHEST WALL

Estlander's operation, which consisted of subperiosteal removal of portions of overlying ribs, yields poor results, as the chest wall is also rendered immobile by indurated and fibrotic muscles and thickened parietal pleura. Schede therefore elaborated Estlander's operation and removed these structures, as well as the ribs and periosteum, with gratifying results. Avertin or pentothal is advisable, reinforced with gas and oxygen or local anæsthesia. Cyclopropane is excellent in skilled hands. A flap of skin and subcutaneous muscles is turned up, and shock and post-operative pain are diminished if the intercostal nerves corresponding to the ribs to be resected, together with the nerve above and below, are injected posteriorly with 90 per cent. alcohol. Schede's operation is now reserved for small empyemata situated laterally. Sauerbruch's method consists of an extensive thoracoplasty from above downwards, in two or three stages if necessary. Regeneration of periosteum is discouraged by mopping the beds of the ribs with 10 per cent. formalin or Zenker's solution.

PULMONARY TUBERCULOSIS

In a volume of this nature a summary of the surgical procedures for the treatment of pulmonary tuberculosis is all that can be attempted. However, it must be emphatically stated that surgery is only incidental in the general treatment and control of the patient.

Artificial Pneumothorax.—This is a simple procedure in the absence of adhesions and is performed when the disease is quiescent. Pneumothorax is indicated in cases in which one lung is comparatively healthy, provided that no advanced cardiovascular disease is present. The procedure is sometimes useful in controlling hæmoptysis. Air is injected into the pleural cavity through a needle, a manometer being used so that pressure can be regulated. When the puncture is made, a negative pressure and respiratory variations indicate that the needlepoint is in the pleural cavity. An initial dose of 250 ml. is injected and increased at subsequent sittings until the lung is adequately collapsed, as shown by radiography (fig. 989).

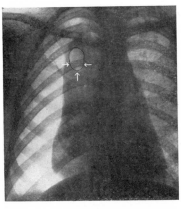

FIG. 989.—Posterior view of collapsed left lung, after artificial pneumothorax. The arrows indicate a cavity. (*Dr. J. E. A. Lynham.*)

Thoracoscopy with division of adhesions is a valuable adjunct to artificial pneumothorax, as adhesions prevent collapse of

Jacob August Estlander, 1831–1881. A Finnish surgeon.
Max Schede, 1844–1902. Professor of Surgery, Bonn.
Ernst Ferdinand Sauerbruch, 1877–1951. Professor of Surgery, Berlin.
Friedrich Albert von Zenker, 1825–1898. Professor of Pathology, Erlangen.

the lung. Two cannulæ are introduced between suitable ribs. A thoracoscope is inserted through one cannula, and a cautery through the other, so that the adhesion is divided under direct vision.

Extrapleural pneumothorax is useful if adhesions prevent an adequate artificial pneumothorax. One or more ribs are resected and the parietal pleura is stripped from the chest wall, so that permanent collapse results.

Phrenic Crush or Avulsion.—Local anæsthesia is desirable, provided the patient is old enough to be self-controlled. The nerve arises from the third, fourth, and fifth cervical nerves.

The nerve is exposed through a horizontal incision situated 1 inch (2·5 cm.) above the clavicle. The omohyoid muscle is drawn upwards, and the outer border of the scalenus anticus identified. On retraction inwards of the sternomastoid, the phrenic nerve is exposed by blunt dissection, and is seen passing downwards and inwards on the scalenus anticus. If crushing is performed the minimum of local disturbance is desirable, as it may be necessary to repeat the operation. If avulsion is indicated the nerve is divided, the lower end is seized with artery forceps, and by traction and twisting the nerve is avulsed. Usually about 4 inches of nerve are removed. An accessory phrenic nerve may arise from the nerve to the subclavius or directly from the fifth cervical nerve, and pass into the thorax in front of the subclavian vein. It joins the main nerve in the thorax, and is therefore removed by a successful avulsion. Some venous hæmorrhage may occur from rupture of tributaries of the internal mammary vein.

The maximum result of phrenic operations is to diminish the capacity of the corresponding pleural sac by about one-third. As the diaphragm loses its tone this amount increases. The diaphragm is sometimes partially supplied by the lower inter-costal nerves, in which case paralysis is incomplete. Dia-phragmatic adhesions and thickening of the pleura will also hamper elevation of the diaphragm.

Phrenic crush is particularly indicated as an accessory to artificial pneumothorax, especially if the lung is adherent to the diaphragm, or if pneumothorax has failed to collapse a thin-walled cavity. Also, when the lung is allowed to re-expand, the required degree of expansion is limited. After a crush temporary paralysis of the diaphragm lasts for about six to twelve months. Phrenic avulsion is sometimes performed as a preliminary to total thoracoplasty, as a less extensive operation is then adequate.

Pneumoperitoneum, which is especially useful when basal cavities are present, consists in injecting from 1,000 to 2,000 ml. of air into the abdominal cavity. The diaphragm is thus elevated and the lungs relaxed.

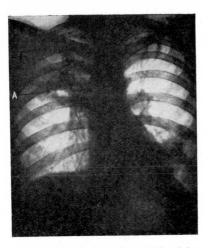 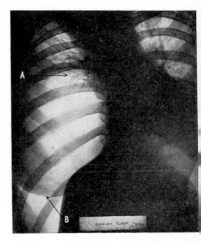

Fig. 990.—Tuberculosis of the right lung. Infiltration of apex, and cavity indicated by arrow (A).

Fig. 991.—Same patient after phrenic crush and pneumoperitoneum. The heart and liver are displaced, and the diaphragm (A) has risen to the third rib. B indicates the breast shadow.

(Drs. E. Clifford Jones and N. Macdonald, Clare Hall Sanatorium, Middlesex.)

The effects are augmented if combined with a phrenic crush. Refills are given as necessary, and patients suffer little inconvenience from their distension (fig. 991).

Thoracoplasty may be considered in cases of unilateral long-standing tuberculosis, especially if cavities are present, and provided that the patient is not suitable for more radical procedures. In such cases, if artificial pneumothorax has failed, thoracoplasty usually results in permanent collapse, and further local treatment is then unnecessary.

In bilateral cases thoracoplasty is contraindicated unless severe hæmorrhage occurs from one lung, in which case rib resection on that side is sometimes performed in order to arrest the periodic bleeding.

As a preliminary to the operation efforts must be made to improve the patient's general health. The operation should be performed only when the disease shows some response to treatment and after a careful survey of the general condition of the patient. A premature operation may result in dissemination of the disease.

Operation.—Sauerbruch's method is usually adopted. The complete operation consists in excision of the posterior ends of the upper eleven ribs as close to the costo-transverse joint as possible. The amount of each rib to be removed is approximately as follows : first rib, 3 cm. ; second rib,

6 cm. ; and from 10 cm. to 16 cm. for subsequent ribs up to the eighth, below which the length decreases. To avoid excessive shock the operation is usually done in stages, but owing to scar tissue fixing the ends of the ribs already divided, the amount of collapse is lessened. The interval between stages should not exceed three weeks, otherwise this fixation very seriously interferes with falling in of the chest wall.

The most desirable anæsthetic is cyclopropane, combined with oxygen. Induction is smooth, and the depth of anæsthesia can be quickly varied. Cyclopropane is non-toxic, non-irritating, and is rapidly excreted. A periscapular incision is made for the upper ribs, and the superficial muscles are divided. The arm is drawn forwards so as to displace the scapula and expose the subjacent ribs. The upper five or six ribs are excised, and special care is exercised in resecting the first rib, as the first dorsal nerve and superior intercostal artery pass across its neck. If the condition of the patient is satisfactory and a one-stage operation is intended, an oblique or J-shaped incision is made so as to expose the lower ribs. A firm bandage is applied in order to steady the mediastinum, and the patient is encouraged to cough freely so as to expel secretion.

Supplementary rib-resection operations are occasionally necessary if the original operation has been inadequate. If the disease is localised, the excision of a limited number of ribs may suffice.

Lobectomy and Pneumonectomy.—These measures are growing in popularity. Eradication of the disease is obviously the ideal treatment, and the patient is spared tedious years while the results of lesser measures are awaited. Also the risks associated with cavitation are abolished—it is estimated that 85 per cent. of patients with a persistent cavity succumb within five years.

The indications for these operations are briefly as follows (Price Thomas):
(i) Persistence of a cavity in spite of collapse treatment.
(ii) A tuberculoma, i.e. a caseous mass with no cavitation.
(iii) A primary lesion which is progressive.
(iv) Tuberculous bronchiectasis.
(v) Bronchial stenosis affecting the lower lobe (the upper lobe may drain efficiently after thoracoplasty).

ABSCESS OF THE LUNG

Causes.—The commonest cause (60 per cent.) of lung abscess is aspiration, during an operation, of foreign material, such as blood-clot, a tooth, part of a tonsil, or regurgitated food. The majority of abscesses follow operations under general anæsthesia. Other causes include unresolved pneumonia, pulmonary infarcts, massive collapse, aspirated foreign bodies (fig. 992), and penetrating wounds. An empyema is occasionally the result of a lung abscess, but rarely, if ever, the cause. A pulmonary growth occasionally presents itself clinically as a lung

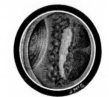

Fig. 992.—A mutton bone which had lodged in the trachea for two years.

(*J. E. G. McGibbon and E. T. Baker-Bates. British Journal of Surgery.*)

Sir Clement Price Thomas, Contemporary. Surgeon, Brompton Chest Hospital, London.

abscess, owing to infection of secretion which is pent up in an obstructed bronchus.

Clinical Features.—General signs and symptoms are evident, and in acute cases include a swinging temperature, cough, sweating, anorexia, and wasting. The breath is fœtid, and pain indicates involvement of the pleura. Physical examination of the chest usually reveals a local area of dullness, with diminished breath-sounds, and possibly signs of a cavity. In stout patients a small abscess is naturally difficult to locate with assurance. The commonest site is the lower lobe of the right lung.

An abscess is likely to rupture into a bronchus, in which case a copious amount of offensive, purulent sputum is expectorated. Shreds of lung tissue or elastic fibres can frequently be recognised. If the sputum is allowed to stand, three layers become evident; the upper of frothy mucus, the central turbid, and the lowest containing debris and pus cells. The sputum is frequently blood-stained, but obvious hæmoptysis is less common than with bronchiectasis. Clubbing of the fingers occurs in long-standing cases.

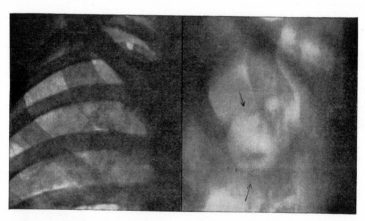

Fig. 993.—A case of pulmonary abscess, invisible in a straight X-ray.

Fig. 994.—The same case. By means of tomography the abscess is clearly demonstrated. The arrows indicate fibrous septa.

Radiography is of the utmost value, and films should be taken from the front, side, and back. The tomograph is especially useful in thoracic conditions (figs. 993 and 994). Appearances vary according to the acuteness or chronicity of the abscess, and whether an existing cavity contains pus or is partly air-filled. In acute cases respiratory movements are limited, and the portion involved appears as an area of irregular density, surrounded by a zone of slightly increased opacity, due to consolidation. In some cases a fluid level is discernible. In chronic cases the area of density is more circumscribed, and should air be present the upper portion of the cavity is translucent. Tomography will sometimes reveal an abscess which is unrecognisable in a straight X-ray.

The *tomograph* operates on the principle that the tube and the film-holder move in opposite directions during exposure. The movement is electrically controlled, and the tube is focused on the particular section of the organ regarding which information is required. The movement blurs structures which are superficial or deep to the plane of focus, and thus tissues in this plane are recorded with comparative clearness on the film. The tomograph is especially useful for thoracic conditions, in which the chest wall, breasts, and scapulæ are apt to overshadow the deeper structures in a straight X-ray.

Lipiodol is of little use, as even if the cavity is partially empty granulation tissue prevents entry of the oil. It is even stated that lipiodol may disseminate infection to other parts of the lung. Exploratory needling is never justified, owing to the risk of infecting the pleural cavity and consequent formation of an empyema.

The *complications* of a lung abscess include gangrene, empyema, either spontaneous or as a result of treatment, bronchopneumonia of the opposite lung following aspiration of pus, suppurative pericarditis, and cerebral abscess. (Camptoid)

Treatment.—Symptomatic treatment is necessary in acute cases. Antibiotic therapy, expectorants, sedatives, and posture, so that free expectoration is encouraged, all receive consideration. This treatment is continued so long as the abscess drains freely, and shows signs of resolution, but it is inadvisable to delay operation for longer than six weeks, as otherwise fibrosis and bronchiectasis may develop.

Operations.—*Bronchoscopy* with aspiration is the simplest form of treatment, but is unlikely to be curative as the opening into the abscess is usually small and difficult of access ; also it is apt to be obscured by granulation tissue. Aspiration is continued as long as improvement is maintained, and granulations can be discouraged by painting with 15 per cent. silver nitrate solution.

Phrenic avulsion or *artificial pneumothorax* are only indicated if the abscess is basal in position, recent in origin, and draining freely into a bronchus. Otherwise measures to induce collapse are risky, as the abscess may rupture through the friable lung and infect the pleura.

Pneumonotomy, in the absence of widespread fibrosis or bronchiectasis, is comparatively safe, and gives good result in selected cases. Unless urgent, or if obvious adhesions are present, the operation is performed in two stages.

Careful localisation is essential, and exposure is obtained by resection of portions of two suitable ribs and intercostal structures. The parietal and visceral pleuræ are encouraged to adhere by the insertion of gauze moistened with iodine. The wound is closed. Ten days later the wound is reopened, the gauze is removed, and the lung is explored with a needle. On discovery of the abscess, the needle is left in the cavity, and the intervening lung incised with a scalpel or diathermy knife. Pus is evacuated and loculi opened freely. The cavity is packed with gauze moistened with mild antiseptic, and the wound is partially closed. The gauze is removed on the third day, and the wound repacked daily until healed. Drainage tubes should not be used, as they are apt to erode the lung and cause secondary hæmorrhage.

Lobectomy, when the abscess is confined to one lobe, holds out the best prospect of cure, especially when the abscess is complicated by surrounding fibrosis or bronchiectasis, but the presence of other abscesses may forbid this procedure.

BRONCHIECTASIS

Causes.—Dilatation of the bronchial tubes may be congenital, but the commonest cause is unresolved broncho- or lobar-pneumonia. Aspiration of foreign bodies or mucus plugs and pressure on a bronchus by enlarged lymph nodes, tumours, or aneurisms occasionally result in bronchiectasis. A chronic lung abscess or long-standing tuberculosis is usually associated with some degree of bronchiectasis.

Clinical Features.—The usual symptoms are persistent cough and free expectoration, which varies in quantity according to the position of the patient. The sputum is usually frothy and fœtid, and on standing separates into three layers—froth, mucus, and debris. Loss of weight, or, in the case of a child, diminution in stature, is sometimes observed. Children often vomit swallowed secretion. Not infrequently intermissions occur, the patient being alternatively " dry " and well, or " wet " and ill. Hæmoptysis occurs in about 25 per cent. of cases, and clubbing of the fingers in approximately 50 per cent.

On examination of the chest the percussion note is dull over the affected area. Amphoric breathing and moist sounds may be heard, but vary according to the emptiness of the dilated tubes. Surrounding fibrosis may displace the heart, and in long-standing cases scoliosis develops.

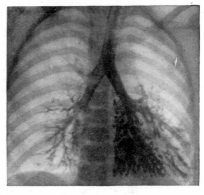

Lipiodol injection after postural emptying, with the patient in such a position that the oil gravitates to the affected area, is essential for detailed diagnosis. The bronchial tree is outlined, and the site and extent of the disease can be estimated (fig. 995).

FIG. 995.—Bronchogram in a case of bronchiectasis, following lipiodol injection.

Lipiodol is either introduced into the trachea, after cocainisation of the pharynx, or injected through the cricothyroid membrane with a special trocar and cannula.

Treatment.—Cure is impossible apart from lobectomy. Inhalations of creosote, expectorants, and postural coughing are palliative measures, and may render a patient comparatively comfortable, while the diminution of halitosis will be appreciated by his associates. If a foreign body is present it should be removed by bronchoscopy (but cure is not to be expected), and aspiration of secretion via a bronchoscope at intervals will relieve the symptoms. Cerebral abscess is a dreaded complication, as with other chronic pulmonary diseases.

Phrenic avulsion interferes with expectorative efforts, but if hæmoptysis is more than trifling, the loss of blood is often greatly reduced in patients unsuitable for lobectomy.

Lobectomy is the only procedure which can guarantee a cure, and the mortality in skilled hands is under 10 per cent. (fig. 996).

Operation.—The patient should be in bed for two or three weeks before the operation, so that by means of postural drainage the dilated bronchi can be emptied.

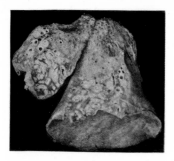

Fig. 996.—Lower lobe of left lung. Bronchiectasis. Lobectomy. (*Pathological Department, Sheffield Royal Infirmary.*)

The usual anæsthetics are gas or cyclopropane, combined with oxygen. Atropine is not injected, as it encourages obstruction in the healthy bronchi by plugs of mucus. Heavy premedication is valuable.

The incision follows the fourth or seventh intercostal space according to whether the upper or lower lobe is to be removed. The pleura is incised, and the posterior part of the rib above is excised so as to expose the underlying intercostal bundle, containing the nerve and vessels, which is then ligated and divided. A mechanical rib-spreader is introduced (fig. 1001), and the exposed lobe is freed from adhesions to the diaphragm, pericardium, and other lobe. Mass transfixation and division of tissues after the application of a tourniquet (fig. 997) is now rarely performed. If circumstances permit, the tourniquet is dispensed with, and individual vessels are ligated and divided. The bronchus is then cut across and sutured. This procedure obviates leaving a large and infected stump, which encourages an

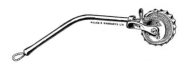

Fig. 997.—A lobectomy tourniquet.

empyema or fistula. Also, in suitable cases, it permits of separation of the blood-vessels to a portion of the lobe, so that a limited excision (segmental resection) can be performed. Packing and retractors are removed, and through-and-through stitches are inserted which encircle the rib above and the rib below. If necessary the ribs are apposed by means of rib

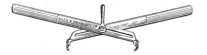

Fig. 998.—A rib approximator.

approximators (fig. 998). The intercostal muscles are then sutured, and the thorax is thus closed. The skin is retracted downwards so as to expose the second rib below the incision, and about 1 inch of the rib is removed. The skin and superficial muscles are then sutured, and the chest wall is pierced with a trocar and cannula through the gap in the rib. The trocar is removed and a self-retaining catheter is inserted along the cannula, which is then withdrawn. The catheter is connected with a closed-drainage system which removes serum or pus until the upper lobe undergoes compensatory expansion.

Small doses of omnopon or morphia are subsequently administered so that the patient can cough without excessive discomfort. An empyema occasionally complicates convalescence and may require drainage. A small bronchial fistula is a frequent but relatively unimportant complication.

INTRATHORACIC NEOPLASM

Benign

Mediastinum :
Subserous lipoma. Fibroma. Teratoma.
Dermoid, usually in the anterior mediastinum.
Retrosternal adenoma of the thyroid gland, often calcified.
Ganglio-neuroma.

Lung and Pleura :
Endothelioma, adenoma of bronchus.

Malignant

Primary

Mediastinum :
Lympho-sarcoma. Fibro-sarcoma.

Lung :
Hilum, i.e. bronchial carcinoma (common).
Parenchymatous, i.e. squamous-celled carcinoma arising in a terminal
bronchus, and not attached to the hilum (rare).

Secondary

Mediastinum :
Direct invasion, as from the breast.
Involvement of lymph nodes, e.g. thyroid or breast.

Lung :
Blood-borne metastases, usually sarcoma.

Benign mediastinal neoplasms give rise to signs and symptoms according to their size, position, and rate of growth. A benign tumour which grows slowly may attain insidiously the size of a fœtal head, as structures are gradually displaced and accommodate themselves in a surprising manner. Gradually increasing pressure, especially in children, is likely to cause deformity of the chest wall, owing to bulging of the ribs or even sternum.

A tumour in the upper narrow portion of the thorax is more likely to cause trouble from pressure on the œsophagus or trachea while it is still of comparatively small size. A typical example is the plunging retrosternal goitre with associated dyspnœa.

The symptoms and signs of a benign thoracic tumour naturally vary widely. In the case of a large growth, inspection reveals diminished movement and possibly deformity. Percussion over the tumour yields a dull note, and on auscultation breath-sounds are absent.

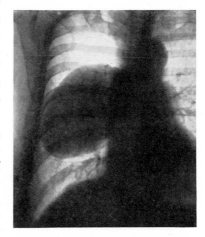

Fig. 999.—An intrathoracic fibro-lipoma, successfully removed.
(*Dr. L. Rau.*)

Radiography is of the utmost value. A straight X-ray reveals the tumour (fig. 999). Alteration in position of the tumour following an artificial pneumothorax, suggests that the tumour is attached to the lung or pleura. Lipiodol injection may reveal pressure collapse of part of the lung adjacent to the tumour.

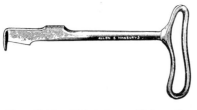

Fig. 1000.—Chisel for splitting the sternum.

Removal of a benign new-growth should always be contemplated, otherwise vital structures will eventually become compressed, with fatal results.

Approach to the *anterior mediastinum* can be obtained by partially splitting the sternum, a special chisel being used for the purpose (fig. 1000). Traction on either side gives a wide exposure. If a less extensive operation is adequate, the sternum is split to the third space, and then laterally, either on one or both sides as may be necessary. Incisions are carried through the intercostal spaces, the internal mammary vessels are ligated, and the two halves of the sternum are pulled apart.

A tumour situated in the *region of the hilum* is exposed by lateral thoracotomy. An incision is made along the fourth intercostal space from the angles of the ribs behind, to the costal cartilages in front. If the maximum amount of room is desirable, the fourth rib is excised subperiosteally. Mechanical rib spreaders are introduced (fig. 1001), and an excellent view of the corresponding side of the thoracic cavity is thus obtained. Intratracheal anæsthesia is necessary for these operations, in order to prevent pulmonary collapse.

A *benign adenoma of the bronchus* causes prolonged bronchial irritation followed by obstruction. Bronchoscopic examination reveals the tumour, which can usually be extirpated without difficulty.

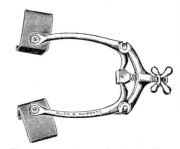

Fig. 1001.—A mechanical rib retractor.

Malignant.—Primary malignant tumours of the lung arise either in a main bronchus, or more rarely in the lung tissue itself, in which case they originate in a terminal bronchus (parenchymatous). The disease is apparently increasing in frequency, and in 1947 (the last figures available) it accounted for 19·7 per cent. of male deaths from carcinoma. Inhalation of petrol fumes and cigarette smoking are possible contributory causes.

Bronchial carcinoma must be recognised in the early stages if radical cure is to be given its rightful opportunity. Suspicions should be aroused when any change from normal habits occurs, especially an unexplained cough which is " brassy " and unproductive. Only too often this is dismissed as due to excessive smoking or " bronchial catarrh," until hæmoptysis or pleuritic pain compels adequate investigation rather than repetition of a sedative linctus. An attack of " asthma " arising in a patient of riper years, especially on change of posture, is very suspicious. Hæmoptysis is welcome in the early stages, as it drives the patient to the physician. Some cases originate as a pneumonia, which fails to resolve, or as " influenza."

In *early cases* clinical examination of the chest is often negative, but sometimes evidence of bronchial obstruction is detected. Examination of sputum, or preferably mucus aspirated during bronchoscopy, is frequently rewarded by the discovery of carcinoma cells. A radiograph, both lateral as well as postero-anterior (fig. 1002), is essential in all suspicious cases, as physical signs may be absent or equivocal. Unless the radiograph is entirely negative, bronchoscopy should be performed, and most growths can be visualised and a fragment removed for section. If these investigations are negative, and suspicions still unallayed, a bronchogram is indicated. Finally, aspiration biopsy through the chest wall occasionally establishes a diagnosis, and in skilled hands this procedure appears to be devoid of risk.

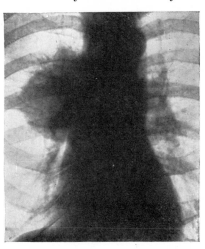

FIG. 1002.—Carcinoma of the right bronchus extending into the lung.

In the *later and hopeless stages* brisk hæmoptysis is likely to occur, and a purulent sputum indicates secondary infection. Loss of weight and deterioration in health soon follow. Secondary changes in the lung include bronchiectasis, and resorption collapse of a lobe owing to bronchial obstruction. A pleural effusion, usually blood-stained, is sometimes present, and is liable to infection.

Nerves are often involved, including the phrenic, left recurrent laryngeal, or sympathetic, in which case Horner's syndrome is manifest (myosis, ptosis, anidrosis, and enophthalmos). Pressure on veins is a late manifestation. Axillary and cervical lymph nodes are sometimes invaded, and secondary deposits in bones and brain are relatively common, and may lead to the discovery of the primary growth. Clubbing of the fingers and osteo arthropathy sometimes occur, especially if the growth projects into the mediastinum.

In established cases examination of the chest reveals diminished movement, dullness on percussion, altered or absent breath-sounds, and possibly evidence of effusion. Dilated veins are commonly seen, and evidence of nerve involvement is sometimes present.

Parenchymatous carcinoma is much less common than the bronchial type The tumour consists of a squamous-celled carcinoma, and is usually situated in the upper lobe. Symptoms are slow in appearance, and may be delayed until involvement of the pleura causes pain. Cough and expectoration are not in evidence until a bronchus is eroded, or compression results in bronchiectasis. A radiograph shows a shadow of somewhat unequal density, which closely resembles a lung abscess.

The **treatment** of bronchial carcinoma depends on early diagnosis, and results are becoming increasingly encouraging Unless obviously contraindicated, thoracotomy should be under taken with the object of performing pneumonectomy. Some temporary improvement may follow deep X-ray therapy Aspiration of fluid with or without air replacement sometimes diminishes discomfort. The insertion of radon seeds through a bronchoscope is liable to cause mediastinitis, but intubation with a radon tube or local removal helps to maintain an airway and so prevent atelectasis, with consequent relief of symptoms. Hypodermic injections of cocaine produce a humane euphoria

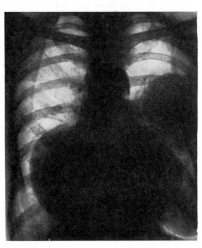

Fig. 1003. — Typical " cannon-ball " metastases in the mediastinum.

Johann F. Horner, 1831–1886. Ophthalmic surgeon, Zürich.

or cannabis indica extract (gr. i-iii t.d.s.) can be given orally.

Provided that the patient's condition is satisfactory, pneumonectomy should be considered.

OPERATION.—The chest is opened through a wide thoracotomy, and the lung is freed from adhesions. The pulmonary vessels and the bronchus are isolated, and ligated separately. The lung is removed, and the chest drained, as infection from the bronchial stump is probable. Recent figures show that in about a quarter of diagnosed cases thoracotomy is advised. Of these about half are found to be inoperable at exploration. The mortality of pneumonectomy is under 10 per cent. A successful pneumonectomy causes surprisingly little disability.

Secondary deposits in the thorax or lung are important from the standpoint of prognosis. They are usually readily demonstrable by X-rays (fig. 1003). Radiotherapy may cause some recession or arrest of growth.

HYDATID CYST

The lung occasionally harbours a hydatid cyst (fig. 1004), and this condition must be considered in the differential diagnosis of a doubtful intrathoracic neoplasm. The usual tests (p. 339) will, if positive, establish the diagnosis.

Thoracotomy is performed and the lung is carefully divided so as to expose the surface of the cyst. The cyst is then extruded from the lung by means of positive pressure anæsthesia, the patient being placed in such a position that gravity also assists in the extrusion of the unopened cyst (Price Thomas).

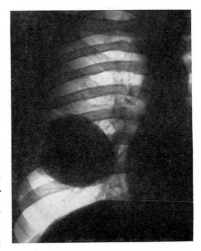

FIG. 1004.—Hydatid cyst of lung.
(*Professor Harold R. Dew, Sydney.*)

PULMONARY EMBOLISM

This dreaded complication is the cause of death in 0·1 per cent. of all major operations. In addition to these fatal cases, thrombosis of veins and emboli not infrequently delay convalescence and cause alarm and anxiety to both surgeon and patient.

The following predisposing causes favour embolus production:

Pre-operative.—*Age of Patient.*—Embolism is rare under the age of twenty. The common decades are the fifth and sixth.

Site of Operation.—Cholecystectomy and pelvic operations, particularly hysterectomy and prostatectomy, are most commonly associated with embolism. Operations on the upper

Sir Clement Price Thomas, Contemporary. Surgeon, Westminster and Brompton Hospitals, London.

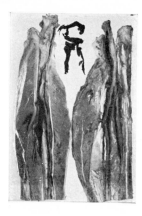

FIG. 1005.—Post-mortem specimen showing thrombosis of veins in the calf, and the lethal clot which was found in the pulmonary artery. (*R.C.S. Museum.*)

limbs and the head and neck are rarely complicated by embolism.

Posture.—It is now recognised that thrombosis originates in the veins of the calf or soles of the feet (fig. 1005). Therefore, in order that venous return is unhampered during the operation, the heels should be supported on a sandbag or a wedge of sorbo-rubber (fig. 1006). *This is essential when the type of patient or the nature of the operation predisposes to thrombosis* (fig. 1007).

Operative.—*Operative Trauma.*— Tearing or bruising of tissues, as by prolonged pressure of mechanical retractors, encourages the formation of thrombokinase.

Post-operative.—*Stasis.*—Post-operative shock and prolonged immobility of the patient favour venous stasis, and so encourage

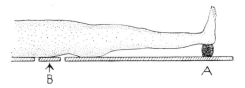

FIG. 1006.—A suitable heel support can easily be made from sorbo-rubber, mackintosh, and strapping. Routine use will save lives.

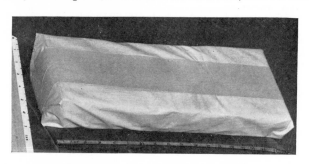

FIG. 1007. — Heel support in position.

intravenous clotting. After operations on the upper abdomen, diminution of the diaphragmatic excursion favours stasis in the abdominal veins. In this connection tight abdominal binders should be replaced by strips of adhesive strapping. Elevation of the foot of the bed encourages the return of blood from the lower limbs.

Infection.—It was formerly considered that infection of the operation field was almost a *sine qua non* in the production of pulmonary embolism. There is little evidence to support this, and Spilsbury in 120 necropsies, in which death was caused by pulmonary embolism, found infection present in only 25 per cent.

Dehydration.—Pre-operative limitation of fluids, hæmorrhage during the operation, and post-operative vomiting all lead to diminution of body fluids, and consequently predispose to thrombosis.

Detection of Thrombosis.—An otherwise unexplained elevation of temperature or pulse-rate is suspicious of deep thrombosis. Occasionally the patient complains of tenderness or aching in the calves, and slight swelling of the ankles may be observed. Homan's sign (tenderness of the calf on dorsiflexion of the foot) is less reliable than tenderness on deep pressure over the course of the posterior tibial and peroneal veins. In all cases in which thrombosis may develop the calves should be palpated daily, followed, if suspicions are aroused, by palpation of the soles, popliteal fossæ, and adductor regions. In doubtful cases a phlebogram taken after an injection of 20 ml. of diodone into a vein on the dorsum of the foot will reveal segmental or " mantle " shadows in the deep veins (R. S. Murley).

Clinical Features.—Pulmonary emboli occur in three more or less distinct degrees of severity.

(i) The patient experiences a sudden sharp pain which is aggravated by respiratory movements. Hæmoptysis follows, and on examination a small patch of dullness and crepitations are usually discoverable. Recurrences are not infrequent, but the prognosis is favourable. Doubtless many patients with less typical symptoms are diagnosed as basal atelectasis or other post-operative pulmonary conditions.

(ii) Sudden acute precordial pain occurs, with dyspnœa and cyanosis. After a period of acute distress, usually lasting for a few minutes, the patient succumbs.

(iii) The patient gasps, perhaps urgently requests a bed-pan, and dies almost immediately. The sudden desire to defæ-

Sir Bernard Spilsbury, 1885–1948. *Pathologist to the Home Office.*
John Homans, Contemporary. *Emeritus Professor of Clinical Surgery, Harvard University, Baltimore.*
R. S. Murley, Contemporary. *St. Bartholomew's Hospital, London.*

cate is possibly due to temporary obstruction of the common iliac vein by the clot, and consequent rectal congestion.

Thrombosis is most likely to be detected between the third and eighth days, and most cases of emboli occur towards the end of the second week.

Treatment.—*Pre-operative.*—The avoidance of purgation and of deprivation of fluids.

Operative.—Trauma must be reduced to a minimum. Self-retaining retractors should not overstretch the muscles for long periods. Unnecessary loss of blood must be prevented. Posture receives due consideration.

Post-operative.—The patient should be encouraged to drink freely. If vomiting is troublesome, rectal tap water or saline infusions are administered. Post-operative exercises discourage venous stagnation, and, in our opinion, exercises should be carried out much more frequently than is customary.

Within a few hours of the operation active flexion of the hip and knee joints should be performed every two hours. In addition, on the day following the operation the patient is encouraged to raise the buttocks by pressing the hands into the bed. A few slow and deliberate deep breaths should be taken at stated intervals so that the piston-like action of the diaphragm squeezes blood out of the abdominal veins. These exercises, with elaborations, if necessary, are continued until the patient leaves his bed, and, in addition to lessening the risk of embolism, they interest the patient, improve muscular tone, and shorten the period necessary for convalescence.

If thrombosis is suspected, anti-coagulant therapy should be instituted without delay (p. 92).

Treatment of an Embolus.—Mild cases are treated symptomatically, and anti-coagulant measures are instituted. Severe cases receive an immediate injection of atropine (gr. $\frac{1}{100}$) and papaverine (gr. 1), which relaxes arterial spasm, and these preparations should be at hand in every surgical ward (and, indeed, in every maternity bag), for emergency use. Heparinisation is begun without delay, and intravenous morphia and inhalation of oxygen are administered if necessary. Recurrent cases may require ligation of suitable veins.

Ligation of Veins.—If anti-coagulants are not available or efficient, or if laboratory control is inadequate or non-existent, ligation of veins should be contemplated. Thus the internal saphenous vein is ligated for superficial thrombosis which extends in spite of treatment. If considered necessary the common femoral vein is ligated, and the ligature should be below the junction of the internal saphenous vein so as to reduce the risk of subsequent venous œdema of the leg. If bilateral thrombosis occurs ligation of the inferior vena cava may prove a life-saving measure, and surprisingly little disability results. The vein is best exposed extraperitoneally through a transverse incision at the level of the umbilicus, on the right side.

Trendelenburg's operation for removal of the clot from the pulmonary artery is only contemplated if the measures outlined above are not available.

MASSIVE COLLAPSE OF THE LUNG

A day or two after general anæsthesia it occasionally happens that a large bronchus is blocked by a plug of sticky secretion. Hence a resorption collapse occurs in the regional part of the lung, with associated fever and unproductive cough. On physical examination the clinician finds impaired percussion note, absence of breath-sounds, and displacement of the heart *towards* the affected side. Many cases subside if the patient, while lying flat on the bed, is firmly rolled from side to side half a dozen times, but this may be impracticable after a serious operation. Failing this, bronchoscopy should be performed and the plug removed with forceps or by suction, otherwise a pulmonary abscess may result. The administration of carbon dioxide after an anæsthetic causes deep breathing and diminishes the likelihood of this complication ; but once the condition is established, deep breathing will suck the plug farther along the bronchus.

THE HEART AND PERICARDIUM

SUPPURATIVE PERICARDITIS

The causes of pyopericardium are as follows :

Direct infection, as by penetrating wounds.

Local extension, as from an adjacent empyema.

Blood-borne infection, which is the commonest cause, and classically occurs as a complication of acute osteomyelitis.

Pus in the pericardium, as is the case with any fluid, produces cardiac distress owing to heart tamponade (see p. 994). If a pyopericardium is suspected, the sac must be aspirated. The needle is inserted obliquely upwards through the fifth space, a full inch from the left border of the sternum, so as to avoid injury to the internal mammary vessels. If pus is withdrawn, pericardostomy should be performed, and a suitable course of chemotherapy and antibiotic therapy is prescribed.

PERICARDOSTOMY

Drainage is obtained either by the anterior or the inferior route. The former is the simpler method, but drainage is less dependent.

(*a*) *Anterior.*—The fifth costal cartilage is excised through a transverse incision. The internal mammary vessels are divided between ligatures, and fibres of the triangularis sterni muscle brushed aside. The pleura is displaced by distended pericardium and is not encountered. The pericardium is aspirated, opened, and drained.

An alternative method of exposing the anterior surface of the pericardium consists in trephining the sternum just above the xiphoid cartilage. The trephine hole is enlarged towards the left with nibbling forceps. The internal mammary vessels are not encountered, and the operation can be

Friedrich Trendelenburg, 1844–1925. Professor of Surgery, Leipzig.

performed under local anæsthesia. We have found this method to be very satisfactory.

(b) *Inferior.*—A vertical incision is made over the left costo-xiphoid angle. The rectus muscle is split and the peritoneal reflection pushed downwards. If the costo-xiphoid angle is narrow, part of the seventh costal cartilage should be excised. The superior epigastric artery is identified as it passes downwards between the costal and xiphoid origins of the diaphragm, and is divided between ligatures. The pericardium is then recognised as it bulges downwards, and is aspirated and drained. By this method dependent drainage is obtained with diminished risk of mediastinitis, although whichever method of drainage is adopted, pus is apt to become walled-off by adhesions in the transverse pericardial sinus.

WOUNDS OF THE HEART

The immediate causes of death are shock, hæmorrhage, and heart tamponade. This latter condition is due to compression of the heart by blood which has escaped into the inelastic pericardium, which prevents efficient diastolic filling. It is characterised by muffled heart-sounds, falling arterial blood-pressure, and rising venous pressure. Should the patient survive these risks operation is performed without delay so as to effect hæmostasis, repair injury, and obviate infection. The probable depth and direction of the wound are clues to the probability of cardiac injury. In the rare event of a weapon still being *in situ*, it should be withdrawn only at operation, as it is possibly acting as a temporary plug and so checking hæmorrhage.

An osteoplastic flap is rapidly turned outwards, containing portions of the fourth, fifth, and sixth ribs and costal cartilages, which are divided close to the sternum. If necessary part of the sternum is nibbled away. The internal mammary vessels are divided between ligatures, and fibres of the triangularis sterni separated. The exposed pericardium is slit from apex to base, and relief of pressure is likely to be followed by brisk hæmorrhage from the cardiac wound, which can be temporarily plugged with a finger. Interrupted catgut sutures are inserted, care being taken not to penetrate the underlying chamber. If possible sutures are tied in diastole, so as to reduce the likelihood of cutting out. In some cases a temporary stitch inserted through the apex is useful in steadying the heart. The pericardium is emptied of blood and clots, and the incision sutured. The track of the weapon or missile is excised, and adjacent structures are examined for any associated injury. The flap is stitched back into position, and drainage provided if infection is expected.

Prophylactic penicillin is prescribed and sulphonamides if necessary. The development of a cardiac aneurism is a rare sequel.

OTHER OPERATIONS ON THE HEART AND GREAT VESSELS

Cardiac massage may be a life-saving measure in cases of reflex cessation of the heart-beat which occasionally abruptly interrupts an operation. Unless beats are resumed as a result of a hot pack, or an intracardiac injection of 1 ml. of 1:1,000 adrenalin, massage must be performed immediately. If contractions are restarted within one minute recovery will ensue. After the lapse of two minutes vital centres in the medulla are likely to be irreparably damaged, and although the heart-beat may be restored death will probably occur in a few hours. Unless the abdomen is already open a rapid incision is made through the left rectus muscle, and the heart is manually compressed against the sternum every two or three seconds. Rigid asepsis is of less importance than rapid action.

Cardio-omentopexy.—Attempts have been made to improve inefficient cardiac circulation due to coronary thrombosis by fixing part of the great omentum to the anterior surface of the heart (O'Shaughnessy). Some patients were temporarily improved, but the end results do not appear to justify the operation.

Chronic Constrictive Pericarditis (Pick's disease).—This is an uncommon condition, probably tuberculous, in which the pericardium becomes fibrous or even calcified. It follows that the heart cannot adequately dilate during diastole, and chronic congestive heart failure is inevitable. Removal of the affected pericardium usually restores the patient to an active life.

Patent Ductus Arteriosus.—This abnormal connection between the aorta and the pulmonary artery sooner or later causes heart failure, and in 24 per cent. of cases becomes the site of an infective endocarditis. Ligation of the vessel (silk being used) yields excellent results, and is performed as soon as the diagnosis is made. Even when infective endocarditis is established, ligation and a prolonged course of penicillin usually results in cure, although some deficiency may result from destruction of the valves.

Coarctation of the aorta is amenable to surgical relief provided that the stricture is immediately distal to the origin of the left subclavian artery. Excision of the stricture and end-to-end anastomosis can then be performed without interfering with the cerebral circulation.

Congenital pulmonary stenosis produces cyanosis, dyspnœa, clubbing of the fingers, and typical murmurs. Patients rarely survive childhood. Division of the left subclavian artery and anastomosis of the proximal end with the left pulmonary artery shunts systemic blood to the lungs, and oxygenation of the blood is thus improved (Blalock). The optimum age for the operation is between three and ten years, and the mortality is less than 10 per cent.

Valvular Stenosis.—Valvulotomy in cases of pulmonary stenosis is performed with a special knife which is introduced through the wall of the right ventricle. Mitral stenosis is dealt with either by division of the valve via the right auricle or by the formation of an artificial opening in the interauricular septum. These operations are not performed until early middle age owing to the risk of further attacks of acute rheumatism, and the myocardium must be reasonably efficient.

Laurence O'Shaughnessy, 1900–1940. Surgeon, L.C.C. Cardio-vascular Clinic. Killed during the evacuation from Dunkirk.
Friedle Pick, 1867–1926. Professor of Laryngology, Prague.
Alfred Blalock, Contemporary. Professor of Surgery, Johns Hopkins University, Baltimore, U.S.A.

CHAPTER XXXIX

INFECTIONS OF THE HAND

INFECTIONS of the hand are still but imperfectly understood and, as a result, are sometimes treated badly. If the pages which follow are studied, digested, and remembered, it is unlikely that suppurative teno-synovitis will be left until the fascial spaces and even the arm are exten-sively infected ; that incisions will be made into the œdematous dorsum when the pus lies in the palm ; or that pulp infections by improper incision will be turned into suppurative tenosynovitis—all of which only too often have occurred in the past.

GENERAL PRINCIPLES OF TREATMENT

The four principles in the treatment of infections of the hand can be summarised as follows :

(i) Immediate administration of penicillin.

(ii) Early recognition of the presence of pus and its accurate localisation.

(iii) Suitable incision to evacuate pus.

(iv) Adequate after-treatment.

To consider these principles in some detail :

(i) *Penicillin* is administered without delay except in trivial or superficial infection. It must be remembered that penicillin can, by subduing local reaction, mask the presence of pus. This is of special importance in the case of tendon sheath infection, as the usual price to be paid for sloughing of a tendon is amputation of the finger.

(ii) Infections of most soft tissues begin as cellulitis and, unless the infection is controlled, suppuration will follow. The early detection of the presence of pus and its accurate localisation are of vital importance. Pus should always be suspected if the patient complains of throbbing pain which is worse when the limb is dependent, or if *the pain interferes with sleep*. Palpation of an inflamed area is best carried out with a blunt-pointed probe or a lead pencil rather than with the finger, as by this means the site of maximum tenderness can be detected more accurately.

(iii) Suitable incisions are described in the text, but there are three incisions which should never be employed :

(*a*) The skin of the pulp is attached to the base of the terminal phalanx by a fibrous sheet. If an incision for pulp infection is carried too far proximally (fig. 1008 (*a*)), this barrier will be divided and infection will

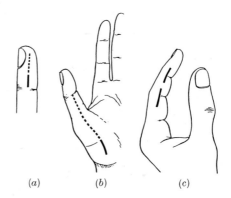

(*a*)   (*b*)   (*c*)

spread into the finger, with possible involvement of the flexor tendon sheath.

(*b*) If the radial bursa requires to be opened, it must be remembered that the branch from the median nerve to the thenar muscles passes outwards about 1 inch (2·5 cm.) below the distal crease of the wrist, therefore an incision must not be prolonged proximally into the palm so as to endanger the nerve (fig. 1008 (*b*)). Paralysis of the thenar muscles is a lifelong disability, or even a tragedy for those whose livelihood depends upon the intricate movements of the fingers and thumb.

(*c*) It is a surgical axiom that incisions should be avoided over areas of pressure, and nowhere is this more important than on the fingers. A scar over the radial side of the index finger (and to a lesser extent over the ulnar side of the little finger) may result in a painful disability for a prolonged period and, in addition, is often unsightly (fig. 1008 (*c*)).

(iv) After-treatment is discussed on p. 1005.

PARONYCHIA (*Syn.* WHITLOW)[1]

Organisms gain entrance through a " hang-nail," so that the tissues about the base of the cuticle become inflamed, usually on one side. Untreated, the inflammation tends to spread around the horse-shoe-shaped cutaneous margin. Suppuration follows frequently, and in many cases pus accumulates under the nail as well as beneath the cuticle.

Prophylaxis.—The loose tag of skin is cut off with scissors and the associated fissure is treated with a mild antiseptic and protected with a suitable dressing.

[1] The term " whitlow " means literally inflammation of the quick of the nail, but is loosely applied to any infection of the finger. Now that the types and sites of infection are clarified, the term " whitlow " should be abolished.

Treatment is early operation. Lateral incisions are made (fig. 1009 *a* and *b*) and a flap is turned back. In order to keep the flap elevated a wisp of vaseline gauze is inserted. Hot hypertonic saline dressings are applied to the whole finger three or four times a day for forty-eight hours, after which vaselined

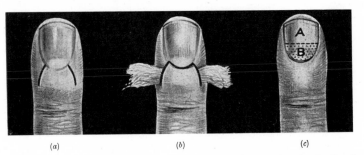

(a) (b) (c)

FIG. 1009.—Kanavel's operation. (*a*) Incisions for turning back the flap. (*b*) A wisp of vaseline gauze or glove drainage is used to maintain elevation of the flap. (*c*) When there is pus under the nail a portion (B) is removed and the part (A) is retained.

dressings are used until the wound granulates. In cases where there is pus under the nail the proximal (shaded) portion is removed (fig. 1009 (*c*)). The distal part which remains acts as a protection to the sensitive quick until the new nail grows, a process which takes at least two months.

Paronychia is a common and painful condition, but it seldom gives rise to complications.

INFECTION OF THE TERMINAL PULP COMPARTMENT

The pulps of the fingers and thumbs are subjected to more pricks, and therefore infections, than any other part of the body.

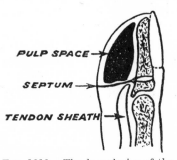

PULP SPACE →

SEPTUM →

TENDON SHEATH →

FIG. 1010.—The boundaries of the pulp space.

Nature has provided in this situation a closed fascial compartment which extends from the tip of the digit to the level of the epiphyseal line of the terminal phalanx (fig. 1010).

Clinical Features. — There is tenderness over the pulp. If suppuration occurs, the pulp becomes tense and swollen.

Treatment. — Early efficient

Allan B. Kanavel, 1874–1938. Professor of Surgery, North-Western University, and Surgeon, Cook County Hospital, Chicago. Was largely responsible for the proper understanding of infections of the hand.

drainage is imperative. *Incisions must on no account extend in a proximal direction farther than ½ inch (1·25 cm.) distal to the terminal flexor crease.* The "transfixion" operation fulfils these essential requirements. A tourniquet in the shape of a rubber catheter is placed around the base of the digit. Keeping ½ inch (1·25 cm.) distal to the terminal flexor crease (fig. 1010), two lateral incisions are made. A narrow-bladed scalpel is then inserted as shown in fig. 1011 B. A through-and-through rubber drain is left in position (fig. 1011 c) and the tourniquet removed. There is no need to disturb the dressing until the third day. Unless early and adequate drainage is instituted, necrosis of the diaphysis of the terminal phalanx occurs regularly. Armed with this knowledge, radiography during convalescence is essential. When the bone is involved the diaphysis of the terminal phalanx separates as a seques-

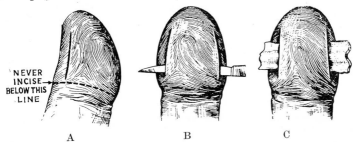

NEVER
INCISE
BELOW THIS
LINE

A B C

FIG. 1011.—The "transfixion" operation for terminal space infection.

trum two or three weeks later and the dead bone is easily withdrawn, after which the wound soon heals. This leaves a shortened phalanx with an ugly curved nail, but with full function of the digit.

Paronychia and infections of the terminal pulp compartment, together with boils on the dorsum of the hand and strictly limited superficial cellulitis, are the only types of infected hand which should be treated in the outpatient department or in the consulting-room. In the case of boils, removal of overlying dead skin will expedite healing. The more serious infections which we are about to consider must be admitted urgently and treated as major lesions.

SERIOUS INFECTIONS OF THE HAND

Grave infections of the hand fall into three categories :

1. Lymphangitis.
2. Suppurative tenosynovitis.
3. Fascial space infections.

LYMPHANGITIS

Organisms, almost always streptococci, gain entrance through an abrasion, which may be minute. The adjacent portion of the hand becomes swollen and painful within a few hours, and there is often considerable elevation of the temperature. Later, red streaks, so characteristic of lymphangitis, can be seen coursing up the arm. It is of cardinal importance to distinguish lymphangitis from suppurative tenosynovitis and fascial space infections. The latter require urgent operation, while in lymphangitis in its early stages incision is highly mischievous. Lymphangitis is discussed on p. 115.

SUPPURATIVE TENOSYNOVITIS

The essential signs of an infected tendon sheath are :
1. Swelling of the finger.
2. Flexion of the finger, with exquisite pain on extension.
3. Tenderness, maximally over the infected sheath (fig. 1012).

When the ulnar and/or the radial bursæ are involved, in addition to tenderness over the individual sheaths there is œdema of the whole hand, especially of the dorsum, and a fullness immediately above the anterior annular ligament. It should be noted that these two sheaths intercommunicate in a large percentage of cases, and often after an infection of one has been present for more than forty-eight hours the other becomes infected.

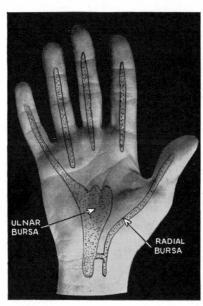

Treatment.—Early operation is imperative. An anæsthetic is administered ; the arm is held up for three minutes. After a tourniquet has been applied suitable incisions are made to drain the infected sheath.

In the case of a digit an incision somewhat to one side of the middle line (fig. 1014) is made ; the slightly lateral incision tends to obviate prolapse of the tendon.

FIG. 1012.—The surface markings of the flexor tendon sheaths.

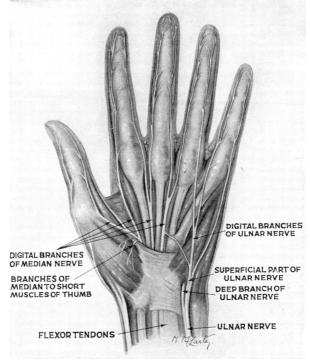

Fig. 1013.—
Showing the flexor tendons, their sheaths, and the nerves in relation, after removal of the palmar fascia.

(*After Spalteholz*.)

DIGITAL BRANCHES OF ULNAR NERVE

DIGITAL BRANCHES OF MEDIAN NERVE

BRANCHES OF MEDIAN TO SHORT MUSCLES OF THUMB

SUPERFICIAL PART OF ULNAR NERVE

DEEP BRANCH OF ULNAR NERVE

ULNAR NERVE

FLEXOR TENDONS

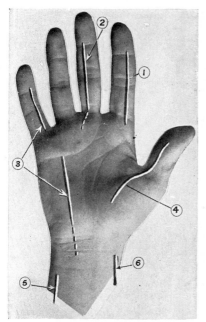

Fig. 1014

1. Incision for opening an infected tendon sheath. In most cases an incision on the ulnar side of the index finger is preferable.

2. When a lumbrical canal is infected in addition, the incision is prolonged into the appropriate web space.

3. Incisions for opening an infected ulnar bursa.

4. Incision for opening an infected radial bursa.

5. Incision for opening all infections of the forearm from the hand.

6. Counter-incision used in the case of infection of the forearm from the radial bursa.

In the case of the radial bursa the opening in the sheath can be followed downwards through the thenar eminence to within 1 inch (2·5 cm.) of the anterior annular ligament, but no farther, for the median branch to the thenar muscles crosses the sheath a little proximal to this point (fig. 1013).

For drainage of the ulnar bursa the incision passes along the radial side of the hypothenar eminence and can, if necessary, be prolonged through the anterior annular ligament (fig. 1014).

INVOLVEMENT OF THE FOREARM FROM THE HAND

Before proceeding further it is essential to understand that when a radial or ulnar bursa distended with pus bursts, pus travels up the forearm between the flexor profundus superficially and the pronator quadratus and interosseous membrane on the deeper aspect. It is here, in the space of Parona, that a quantity of pus can collect without giving rise to much swelling (fig. 1015). Therefore, in cases of infection of the radial and ulnar bursæ, if pus can be expressed by pressure over the wrist after the main sheath has been opened, it is essential that

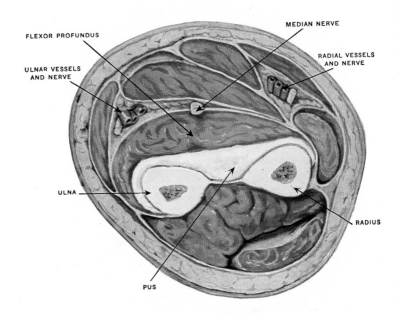

Fig. 1015.—Pus in the space of Parona.

Francesco Parona, 1861–1910. Surgeon, Hospitale Maggiore, Milan. Wrote of this space towards the close of the last century.

the forearm be drained in the following manner. The styloid process of the ulna is palpated and an incision is commenced $1\frac{1}{2}$ inches (3·75 cm.) above this point over the flexor surface of the ulna, and passes down to the periosteum. The incision is at least 2 inches (5 cm.) long. A hæmostat is thrust beneath the flexor tendons, and the jaws of the forceps are opened, as a result of which the proximal extremity of the infected bursa is ruptured thoroughly into the space beneath the flexor tendons. In the case of a radial bursa infection a counter-incision is made at the radial side (fig. 1014).

FASCIAL SPACE INFECTIONS

The Thenar Space

Boundaries (fig. 1016).

Palmar Aspect.— The palmar fascia.

Dorsal Aspect.— The adductor pollicis (transverse head).

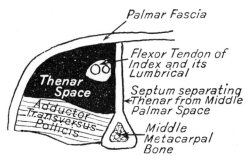

FIG. 1016.—The boundaries of the thenar space.

Ulnar Aspect.— A septum of strong fascia attached to the middle metacarpal bone. This septum separates the thenar from the middle palmar space.

Source of Infection.—The thenar space can be infected directly

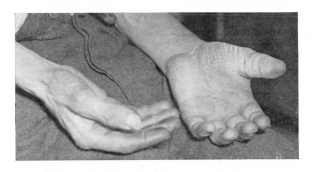

FIG. 1017.—Infection of the thenar space.

from a wound. Much more frequently it is involved by the bursting of an infected and untreated tenosynovitis of the index finger (fig. 1017).

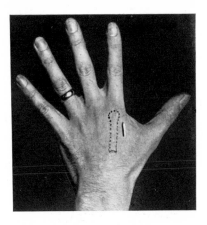

FIG. 1018.—Incision for draining the thenar space.

Clinical Features.—There is ballooning of the thenar eminence. Flexion of the terminal interphalangeal joint is considerable, but it lacks the resistance to extension so characteristic of infection of the radial bursa.

Treatment.—An incision is made on the dorsum (fig. 1018) and a hæmostat is passed into the space. This gives perfect drainage. It is essential to drain the infected flexor sheath of the index finger, if infection is present.

Middle Palmar Space (fig. 1019).

BOUNDARIES

Palmar Aspect.—Fascia separating it from the flexor tendons of the fingers and their lumbricals.

Dorsal Aspect.—Fibrous tissue separating it from the inter-osseous muscles.

Radial Aspect. — The fascial septum alluded to above separating it from the thenar space.

The middle palmar space has three diverticula which are the lumbrical canals. *It is overlapped on the ulnar side by the ulnar bursa, and therefore must never be incised directly,* otherwise the ulnar bursa will become infected.

Source of Infection.—Sometimes the space is infected directly by penetrating wounds or from osteomyelitis of the ring

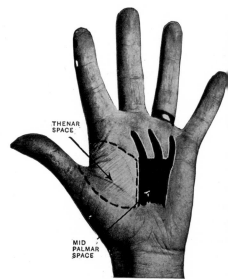

FIG. 1019.—The thenar space and the middle palmar space with its three diverticula, the lumbrical canals.

or middle metacarpal bones. Usually the space becomes involved from rupture of an infected tendon sheath of the middle, ring, or little finger.

Clinical Features.—Infection of the middle palmar space gives rise to those enormous hands which have been likened to a whale's flipper. The concavity of the palm is obliterated. Obliteration of the concavity of the palm with slight bulging thereof is almost pathognomonic of a middle palmar space infection.

Treatment.—The space is drained through a web space, usually between the middle and ring fingers (fig. 1020). A closed hæmo-

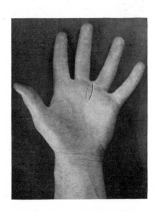

FIG. 1020.—The middle palmar space is drained by splitting a web space and inserting a hæmostat downwards under the flexor tendon. The middle palmar space must never be drained by a direct incision.

stat is inserted under the flexor tendon, and its blades opened widely. The necessity for treating the primary cause, if it is suppurative tenosynovitis, is again stressed.

AFTER-TREATMENT OF SERIOUS INFECTIONS OF THE HAND

Adequate after-treatment comprises measures to encourage or provide the maximum function should adhesions or loss of tissue diminish the usefulness of the thumb or fingers. Hypertonic saline baths are useful in order to promote hyperæmia and to relieve pain, provided they do not cause the skin and subcutaneous tissues to become swollen and sodden. Ten minutes' immersion three times a day is the maximum which should be permitted. If available, radiant heat should be substituted for baths or moist applications. Tendon-sheath infections may be followed by permanent stiffness, and in these cases the affected finger should be kept at rest in a semiflexed

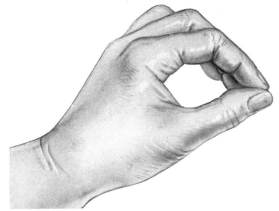

Fig. 1021.—The position of function which is also the position of rest for an inflamed hand. By the position of function is meant that, should the hand or any part of it become stiff, it is in this position that the hand will be most useful.

position, which will provide the best functional result should stiffness ultimately ensue (fig. 1021).

In addition, immobilisation of the hand is often advisable, especially in a case of suppurative tenosynovitis.

The wound itself is packed lightly with vaseline gauze. A piece of gamgee having been wrapped around the forearm, a length of Cramer wire is bandaged firmly to the dorsal aspect of the forearm. A suitable piece of sorbo sponge is placed between the Cramer wire and the dorsum of the hand. The incised finger is encased in a Viscopaste bandage without fixing it to the splint, but as the bandage reaches the base of the finger it is carried around the splint and the palm. The sound fingers are lightly bandaged to the splint in order to extend them.

The arm is elevated by suspending the end of the Cramer wire from an irrigator stand (fig. 1022). After the third day the hand is dressed, and with a little ingenuity the unaffected digits can be released from the bandage in order that the patient may exercise them.

If suppuration continues for more than fourteen days, the hand should be X-rayed for evidence of bone necrosis.

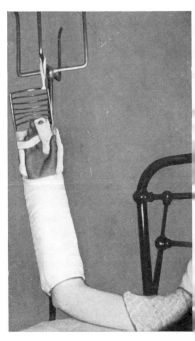

Fig. 1022.—A case of suppurative tenosynovitis being treated by immobilisation and elevation.

Sloughing tendon is a potent source of prolonged suppuration and much time will be saved by excising the diseased portion, care being taken to anchor its proximal end by sutures to prevent the cut end being carried into the forearm by muscular contraction and thereby spreading infection. Massage and exercises form an important part of the late after-treatment. In the case of fingers it should be remembered that total amputation of a digit is better from every point of view than a stiff finger, but amputation should seldom be undertaken until the infection has abated. The surgeon's watchword for the thumb in all lacerations and infections is always " Save all possible."

CHAPTER XL
INJURIES TO BONES

Contusion of a bone results in traumatic periostitis and an extravasation of blood under the periosteum. Resolution and absorption of exudates usually follow, but in more severe cases a permanent periosteal node may persist. As in the case of extravasated blood in any situation, if the resistance of the patient is low and infective foci exist, suppuration may ensue. A sub-periosteal abscess results, and unless opened without delay, the underlying bone may necrose.

Treatment consists in rest and cold applications, which exert a vaso-constricting effect and thus limit oozing. If infection threatens, systemic penicillin is prescribed. Fluctuation necessitates an incision down to the bone in order to evacuate pus.

FRACTURES

The treatment of fractures is now a highly specialised branch of surgery. In a book of this nature we can only outline the general principles. We are indebted to Sir Reginald Watson-Jones for a considerable amount of material in this chapter, and would refer readers who require more detailed information to his classical volumes on " Fractures and Joint Injuries."

A fracture is caused by direct violence, indirect violence, or muscular action. Predisposing causes are either general or constitutional disturbances, or local pathological conditions. Some of these conditions encourage a pathological fracture, which results from a degree of violence which would be insufficient to fracture a normal bone.

1. **General.**—(a) *Age.*—Fractures, especially greenstick, are common during the " toddling " period, when co-ordination and balance are being acquired. During the subsequent growing years separated epiphyses are common, and the prime of life predisposes to dislocations, sometimes associated with a fracture. Towards the end of life senile atrophy predisposes to fracture, e.g. intracapsular fracture of the neck of the femur.

(b) *Occupation.*—Chauffeur's fracture may occur as a result of a back-fire (fig. 1051). Stress fractures follow excessive strain on a bone, e.g. shoveller's fracture of the spinous process of a lower cervical vertebra, or march fracture (p. 1074).

(c) *General disease of bone,* such as osteitis deformans, generalised fibrocystic disease, and osteogenesis imperfecta.

Generalised fibrocystic disease is associated with parathyroid tumour and an increase of blood calcium. Removal of the tumour causes an immediate fall in the calcium content of the blood, and re-formation of bone (p. 227).

Sir Reginald Watson-Jones, Contemporary. Orthopædic Surgeon, London Hospital.

Osteogenesis imperfecta (*syn.* fragilitas ossium) is characterised by marked predisposition to fractures, which may be evident at birth, or manifests itself during childhood (p. 1098).

(*d*) *Neuropathic conditions*, such as tabes and general paralysis of the insane. Attendants in asylums are sometimes unfairly accused of being over-zealous when fractures occur in patients under their care.

2. **Local.**—(*a*) *Inflammatory conditions*, such as acute osteomyelitis (fig. 1090).

(*b*) *New-growth*, including local cysts and malignant growths, either primary or secondary.

(*c*) *Local atrophy*, e.g. tuberculous arthritis, infantile paralysis.

(*d*) *Erosion of bone*, as by an aneurism.

Fractures which are predisposed to by local causes are particularly likely to occur in bones which are unsupported, notably the femur, humerus, and clavicle.

VARIETIES OF FRACTURE

1. *Simple.*—The bone is broken in one place only, and no other important structures are injured. Sometimes the fracture is represented by a mere crack or fissure.

2. *Compound.*—The fragment communicates with the external air, either through the skin, lung, or mucous membrane.

3. *Complicated.*—Other important structures are injured, such as vessels, nerves, joints, or viscera.

4. *Comminuted.*—The bone is broken into more than two pieces.

5. *Impacted.*—One fragment is driven into the other, so that abnormal mobility will not be evident.

6. *Greenstick.*—The fracture is incomplete, the bone bending, so that it is partially fractured transversely and is further damaged by a longitudinal split. This type occurs in children.

7. *Spontaneous.*—The bone fractures as a result of violence insufficient to fracture a normal bone. This type is associated with local pathological conditions. " Fatigue " fractures are included in this group.

Clinical Features.—A history of injury is usually obtainable from the patient, or from a witness, and in some cases a distinct " crack " is audible. In serious injuries, which may occur following a traffic accident, the possibility of multiple fractures must not be overlooked. On examination some or all of the following clinical features can be recognised :

(i) *Pain.*—If the patient is conscious, and not under great emotional stress, pain is referred to the site of the fracture.

(ii) *Loss of function,* which varies with the individual bone, and may not be obvious if the fracture is impacted. Thus a patient with an impacted fracture of the neck of the femur may walk about for weeks, until the persistent ache or pain suggests the desirability of an X-ray examination. The result may prove an unpleasant surprise for all concerned !

(iii) *Deformity,* which is either longitudinal, lateral, or rotatory. The initial deformity is due to the direction of violence, contraction of muscles, and the influence of gravity, and the deformity is maintained by spasm of muscles, gravity, and extravasation of exudates.

(iv) *Abnormal Mobility.*—Is usually present, unless the fracture is of the greenstick or impacted variety.

(v) *Signs of Local Trauma.*—These may be absent or extensive. In the case of a simple fracture, extravasated blood usually reaches the surface in two or three days, possibly at some distance from the site of injury.

(vi) *Crepitus.*—This sign can be detected if the fragments are adjacent and not impacted. Obviously it must be sought for with gentleness and discretion, owing to consequent pain, and the possibility of causing further injury.

(vii) *X-ray Evidence.*—It cannot be too strongly emphasised that even in cases in which there is but the merest possibility that a bone is fractured, an X-ray of the whole bone should be taken in at least two planes. Otherwise the " reasonable skill and care " of the practitioner may be questioned, and no other branch of surgery is more damaging to a practitioner's reputation. A wise and experienced Irish surgeon taught his pupils that " bones are not filled with red marrow, but with black ingratitude."

UNION OF FRACTURES

The changes which occur around the ends of a fractured bone resemble those which result from any wound, but the ultimate result is the formation of bone.

As a consequence of the injury to blood-vessels at the time of the fracture, an extravasation of blood occurs around the fragments. After a few days absorption commences, and pigment from the disintegrated corpuscles stains the surrounding tissues. Connective-tissue cells proliferate, new blood-vessels are formed, and granulation tissue is found around the fragments. Osteoblasts, derived from the deep layer of the periosteum and from the bone itself, invade the granulation tissue, and callus, which gradually increases in density, is formed. If the fragments are adjacent, or a bridge of periosteum unites them, " ensheathing " callus is formed around the bone, and if the medullary cavities are adjacent, they are gradually connected by a bar of " internal callus." If the medullary cavities are separated from each other, they become sealed off by a layer of compact bone.

Owing to its comparative avascularity, the compact bone is the last to unite. If the bone unites in an anatomically correct position, the ensheathing and internal callus may practically disappear, so that, even when a dry bone is examined, it may be difficult to decide whether a fracture has occurred. Although callus formation is proceeding normally, some weeks elapse before sufficient calcium is deposited for the callus to be clearly seen in an X-ray. A high protein diet and an adequate intake of Vitamin C and D is advisable.

TREATMENT OF FRACTURES

The best results are only obtainable in a special fracture centre, where all but the simplest cases are under the care of fracture specialists.

First-aid treatment of fractured limbs necessitates fixation of the bone by improvised splints and transportation to a suitable place for subsequent treatment. The cardinal principle is to immobilise the joint above and below the fracture. Fractures of the spine, pelvis, and lower extremity should receive necessary attention at the site of the accident, prior to transport to hospital or elsewhere for treatment, to prevent further injury to adjacent soft parts ; and in the case of the lower limb, to avoid converting a simple fracture into a compound fracture.

Treatment of a simple fracture falls under three headings, i.e. reduction, fixation, and rehabilitation.

(a) **Reduction.**—This is necessary in all cases in which the displacement would impair the utility of the limb if uncorrected. If reduction is necessary it is effected with or without an anæsthetic, depending on the power of adjacent muscles and the associated degree of pain. It is important to place a limb in such a position that muscular relaxation is obtained ; thus, in the case of fractures below the knee, flexion relaxes the calf muscles, and facilitates manipulation of the foot. Clinical examination and probably X-rays have previously indicated the direction of the deformity, and traction and rotation are used in directions necessary to restore alignment. Reduction should be attempted as soon as possible because infiltration by exudates and their subsequent organisation render successful manipulation increasingly difficult. Unless reduction is obviously satisfactory, confirmation must be obtained by radiology, but a tape measure will always exclude longitudinal deformity.

Local anæsthesia is often adequate for the reduction of fractures, provided that rigid asepsis is maintained.

Method of Injection.—A 2 per cent. solution of novocaine in saline is commonly used, and is injected into the hæmatoma which surrounds the fragments, but if more than 25 ml. of solution is necessary a 1 per cent. solution is preferable in order to avoid toxic symptoms. A previous X-ray is advisable so as to locate the exact site of the fracture. The skin is sterilised, and a small subcuticular wheal is raised by injecting novocaine with a hypodermic needle (fig. 1023). A 0·8-mm. needle is inserted so that the point is adjacent to the fracture, and a 20-ml. syringe is attached to the needle. The piston is withdrawn, and the appearance of blood-stained fluid in the barrel indicates that the hæmatoma is reached. If no fluid is withdrawn the needle must be reinserted. When the hæmatoma is tapped an adequate amount of novocaine is injected. If necessary injections are made from different angles. Thus in the case of a Colles's fracture novocaine is injected from the flexor and extensor aspects of the wrist, and in the region of the avulsed styloid process of the ulna. The amount of novocaine required naturally varies with the site and extent of the fracture, but average quantities are from 10 ml. to 20 ml. After injection gentle pressure is maintained for five to ten minutes, by which time muscular spasm disappears and the parts can be manipulated painlessly. If necessary, a Steinmann's pin can be inserted after suitable injections of novocaine.

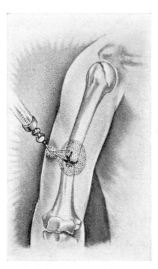

Fig. 1023.—Reduction under local anæsthesia. The dotted area represents the hæmatoma.

The use of local anæsthesia in simple fractures, as compared with a general anæsthetic, has the following advantages :

(i) The fracture can be reduced single-handed.

(ii) Local anæsthesia can be used in patients unsuited for a general anæsthetic, which is often of necessity deep and prolonged.

(iii) In cases associated with shock, pain is relieved and the fracture can be reduced without undue delay.

(iv) The patient can co-operate with the surgeon. Thus in the case of fracture of the humerus the patient can sit up, and even assist in the application of the splint or plaster.

(v) Reduction can be confirmed immediately by X-rays, and if necessary further manipulation can be performed during the period of anæsthesia, which lasts for about three hours.

(vi) Unless confinement to bed is necessary, the patient can depart as soon as satisfactory reduction is confirmed.

Local anæsthesia, as in any other circumstance, is unsuitable for young children and nervous patients. Also, unless an X-ray is obtainable before reduction is attempted, a general anæsthetic is advisable, unless the exact site of the fracture can be determined with reasonable exactitude.

Spinal, regional, or local anæsthesia yields excellent results in reduction of fractures. Spinal anæsthesia, especially in the case of compound or complicated fractures, is useful in selected cases for fractures of the lower extremity, although local anæsthesia is adequate in simple cases. Simi-

Fritz Steinmann, Contemporary. Professor of Surgery, Berlin.

larly, compound fractures of the upper extremity can be dealt with after injection of novocaine into the brachial plexus.

In the case of fractures of the shaft of long bones, manipulation sometimes fails, and traction is then necessary. Reduction can be obtained by heavy traction applied for a few minutes, or by skeletal transfixion and mechanical reduction. Heavy traction must not be used for the gradual reduction of a fracture, as weeks may elapse before it is recognised that the result will be unsatisfactory. It is a useful procedure for immediate reduction, after which traction or counter-traction should be just sufficient to prevent displacement. Skeletal transfixion with steel pins and machine reduction is apt to result in distraction and delayed union ; moreover, unless two pins are used in each fragment, rotatory deformity can occur, and there is a constant risk of infection along the tracks of the pins.

(*b*) **Fixation.**—If reduction is satisfactory, the fragments are maintained in their correct position until union has occurred, the length of time required depending on the individual bone and age of the patient. Thus the thick weight-bearing bones of the leg require a longer period of fixation than the arm or forearm bones, also fractures unite more quickly in children than in adults. The patient's weight and occupation also influence the time during which fixation is necessary.

Adequate fixation is now almost universally obtained by means of plaster slabs or casts, and splints are rarely employed. The fragments must be controlled without excessive compression of the limb, otherwise pressure sores, or interference with the circulation, are liable to occur.

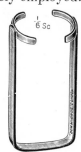

The limb must be inspected frequently after the application of splints or bandages, as further extravasation may occur, with consequent tightening of the bandages.

In many cases, provided that fixation can be maintained, the patient is encouraged to use a fractured limb. This " functional activity during treatment," strongly recommended by Böhler,[*] and use of a limb during union of a fracture stimulates the circulation and prevents atrophy of bone and muscles, and discourages stiffness

Fig. 1024.— Böhler's malleable walking iron, for incorporation in a plaster cast. A rubber heel is sometimes attached.

Lorenz Böhler, Contemporary. Director, Hospital for Accidents, Vienna.

and adhesions. Furthermore, the patient is often enabled to continue his occupation, and the convalescence is shortened (fig. 1024). Joints which need not be immobilised must be actively exercised but never passively stretched.

(c) REHABILITATION

Rehabilitation is the restoration of function of the injured structures, and the instillation of confidence in the mind of the patient. Rehabilitation clinics are now part of the normal hospital service in hospitals which deal with fractures. Under a trained supervisor a patient recovering from a fracture is encouraged gradually to regain the use of a limb by means of graded exercises and occupations, and to become less " fracture-minded." At the same time it is desirable that his anxieties be set at rest regarding his financial and domestic obligations, and, if possible, his future capacity for wage-earning. An understanding almoner is a great asset.

When patients are ambulatory, rehabilitation should occupy most of the day, in order to combat brooding and a spirit of despondency. Lectures and debates are useful for occupying the mind during periods of rest.

Active remedial exercises often require continued individual supervision, which may be impossible with a limited staff. In a fracture ward many patients can be trained as a " class," and carry out to music the movements most suitable for their respective conditions (fig. 1025). Those

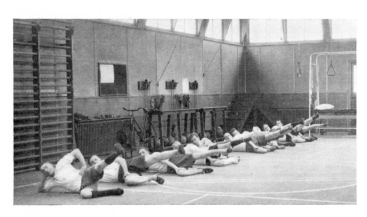

Fig. 1025.—A rehabilitation class.
(*Pilkington Bros., Ltd., St. Helens*).

who are debarred from limb movements can take part by participating in deep breathing exercises.

Bedridden cases are encouraged to occupy themselves with such handicrafts as basketwork, knitting, belt making, etc. For manual workers these occupations are mainly of a diversionary nature, but handicrafts are extremely useful for patients recovering from tendon or peripheral nerve injury, and in post-concussion cases.

More strenuous occupational therapy comprises such activities as boot-repairing, carpentry, gardening, etc., all of which require tools, suitable facilities, and a more or less skilled instructor.

Organised games play a very useful part in rehabilitation. Billiards, darts, quoits, skittles, etc., interest most patients. Competitions can be arranged, during the excitement of which a patient will often involuntarily exercise a limb far more efficiently than if he were conscious of his effort.

Vocational training is provided by the Ministry of Labour for patients who have suffered from permanent disability, as a result of which they cannot follow their original employment.

COMPLICATIONS OF A FRACTURE

The complications of a fracture are general and local.

1. General

(i) **Shock.**—The degree of shock following a fracture depends on the size of the bone or bones affected, the temperament of the patient, and the associated circumstances. As with any injury, a severe lesion may be almost unnoticed during a period of great excitement or mental stress. Simultaneous fracture of both femora is often fatal.

(ii) **Fat Embolism.**—A rare complication, which sometimes follows the shattering of a large bone, e.g. by a bullet or fragment of shell (p. 101).

(iii) **Hypostatic Pneumonia.**—This condition is particularly liable to occur in elderly patients who are confined to bed for more than a few days, particularly if they are " fat and wheezy."

(iv) **Aseptic Traumatic Fever.**—This is due to absorption of fibrin ferment from extravasated blood, as in the case of any injury where blood escapes into the soft tissues.

(v) **Delirium Tremens.**—This condition, fortunately much rarer than formerly, occurs in three stages :

(a) *Prodromal Stage.*—The signs of onset become evident on or about the third day. They are sleeplessness, semi-conscious muttering, anorexia, marked constipation, and tremors of the hands and tongue, which is heavily coated. The patient is restless, and the pulse usually shows considerable variations.

(b) *Stage of Violence.*—This follows the prodromal stage either gradually or abruptly. In the latter case, calamities are likely unless the condition has been anticipated. The patient suffers from delusions, sometimes of persecution, or perhaps with a reptilian background, and may inflict serious injuries on himself or others. Insensitiveness to pain is a marked feature, and we recall an incident in which a patient, scantily clothed in a nightshirt, escaped from hospital at night and dragged himself along for half a mile with a recently fractured femur.

(c) *Stage of Exhaustion.*—This is characterised by extreme feebleness, and is liable to terminate in coma and death. The pulse is raised, while the temperature varies, periodically becoming sub-normal. The prognosis is improved if sleep can be induced.

Treatment.—Delirium tremens sometimes occurs in the most unlikely

patients, but in cases where an alcoholic tendency is suspected, carefu
watch should be observed for the prodromal symptoms, as early recog
nition and appropriate treatment may prevent the onset of actual deliriun
and exhausting struggles. Sedatives and aperients are indicated, and a
moderate amount of alcohol is given, in the hope that it will prevent the
onset of delirium. Precautions are taken to obviate further damage to
the fracture, and if circumstances permit, a plaster of Paris casing shoul
be applied. The patient must be under continuous supervision, with
adequate assistance immediately at hand, and if delirium supervenes
continuous narcosis with paraldehyde, which is preferable to a strait-jacket
may be necessary.

(vi) **Crutch Palsy.**—All crutches should be supplied with a
suitable hand-grip, so that weight can be transmitted along the
arms, thus avoiding pressure on the axillæ. A drop-wrist, due
to pressure on the radial nerve, has followed only four hours' use
of crutches unsupplied with hand-grips.

2. Local

(i) **Bone.**—(a) *Slow Union.*—No arbitrary time can be fixed
as the period required for any individual fracture to unite
In the case of slow union there is no excessive separation of
the fragments, and sclerosis and decalcification do not occur
Slow union is encouraged by the same factors which predispose
to non-union, especially if excessive traction is applied during
reduction of the fracture, or if subsequent immobilisation is
incomplete. All cases of slow union will
eventually unite if the fragments are
completely immobilised for a sufficien
length of time.

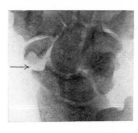

(b) *Delayed Union.*—Decalcification
occurs and in the scaphoid " cavita
tion " may develop (fig. 1026). Sclerosi
has not yet developed, and the fragment:
are separated by granulation tissue rathe
than by fibrous tissue. Complete and
prolonged immobilisation will usually be
rewarded by union. Delayed union is often associated with
inadequate reduction.

Fig. 1026.—Ununited
fracture of the scaphoid,
with cavitation.

(c) *Non-union.*—This term is applied to those fracture
which, in the opinion of the surgeon, will not unite by th
natural processes of repair and in which the X-ray reveal
sclerosis of the fractured ends (fig. 1027). The condition include
fibrous union, absolute non-union, and pseudoarthrosis, in

*David Livingstone, 1813–1874, suffered for thirty years from non-union of a compoun
fracture of the humerus, due to the bite of a lion.*

which a false joint is formed, the synovial membrane being represented by an adventitious bursa, which forms between the fragments (fig. 1028).

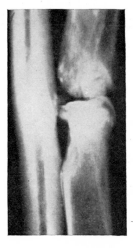

Fig. 1027.—Ununited fracture of the tibia, showing marked sclerosis.

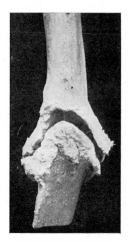

Fig. 1028.—A false joint following an ununited fracture of the shaft of the humerus.

Non-union is predisposed to by local and general conditions. GENERAL causes include old age, debility, conditions which exercise a devitalising effect on the bone marrow, e.g. malaria, syphilis, and some disorders of the central nervous system, such as tabes dorsalis.

LOCAL causes are numerous, and may be summarised as follows :

(i) Infection, which is primarily a cause only of delayed union, but if treatment of the infection prevents immobilisation non-union may result.

If the compound fracture can be adequately treated, the infection merely prolongs the time required for union.

(ii) Inadequate immobilisation is a common cause of non-union. Immobility must not only prevent the movement of fragments, but must also protect the cellular proliferation around the fractured ends from strain. Shearing or rotational movements are particularly harmful, as a plane of cleavage is thus created between the fragments, which become separated by fibrous tissue. As there is no continuity of callus between the fragments union is impossible, and eventually the ends of the bone become sclerotic. Since the importance of adequate and prolonged immobilisation has been recognised cases o non-union are now uncommon.

(iii) Impairment of the blood-supply only delays union, bu undue delay may result in impatience so that absolute immobi lisation is abandoned too early and consequently non-unior occurs. The union of fractures through the neck of the femur, the waist of the scaphoid, or the lower third of the tibia is often delayed on account of interference with vascular channels.

(iv) Excessive traction is apt to result from modern methods of mechanical reduction, or from the suspension of heavy weights from the limb for days and possibly weeks. This over-correction or distraction reduces the tone of muscles so that recoil does not occur and the persistent gap between the bones requires many months to bridge. " Late " reduction of fractures, or " moulding " the soft callus, by manipulation some weeks after injury, is to be condemned, as the granulation tissue forming around the fragments is thus lacerated, and the blood-supply so vital for callus formation is seriously impaired.

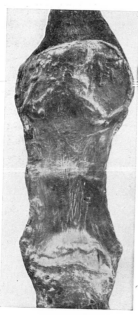

Fig. 1029.—Old fracture of the patella. The fragments are united by a band of fibrous tissue.

Traction, as distinct from distraction, is often necessary as a preliminary procedure, but the object in mind is to correct deformity within a day or so of injury, and then to immobilise the limb with the minimum of necessary traction. In the case of an unstable fracture of the tibia, transfixion of the fragments with a vitallium screw is often preferable to a traction pin and weight suspension.

(v) Interposition of soft parts prevents union because there is no continuous hæmatoma between the fragments. Thus in a transverse fracture of the patella, the raw surface of the proximal fragment is covered with the torn expansion of the quadriceps tendon (fig. 1029), and in some fractures of the femur due to direct violence one fragment may be driven into the belly of an adjacent muscle.

Interposition of soft parts which

cannot be remedied by manipulation requires an open operation so that the bony fragments can be brought into apposition.

(vi) Tumours of bone predispose to fracture ; in the case of secondary carcinoma, union may occur, but a fracture caused by sarcoma will not unite.

Treatment.—This is first directed to any cause which is amenable to treatment, and if necessary the general health of the patient should receive attention. Vitamin C is administered if necessary. Locally, as already stated, slow and delayed union are combated by efficient reduction and immobilisation for a further period. Bier's passive congestion (fig. 1030), by increasing the blood-supply to the affected part, is sometimes a stimulus to union.

If union does not occur, operative measures are indicated, the simplest being drilling of the bone ends, which opens up a new source of blood-supply. If this fails, the fracture is exposed and the ends are " freshened " and fixed, vitallium plates and screws being used if necessary. Bone screws or pegs are useful for bony processes. In the case of long bones bone graft is commonly used, either autogenous or cut from bone obtained from a " bank."[1] This not only acts as an internal splint which immobilises the fracture, but also supplies healthy bone cells, which reinforce those in the devitalised bone. An inlay graft from another bone is the most suitable line of treatment. A sliding graft from the same bone avoids an operation on a normal bone, but the graft should be wedge-shaped so that it is tightly impacted in the decalcified bed which bridges the fracture.

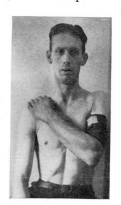

Fig. 1030. — Bier's passive congestion.

Gaps between bone fragments can be filled with bone chips derived from the iliac crest. These cancellous fragments rapidly acquire an adequate blood-supply, and good results have been obtained by this method, which is also useful in bridging gaps following fractures with loss of bone. Absolute immobilisation for an adequate period is imperative after such operations.

---

[1] Human bone can be stored, and retains its vitality for about a year.

Gustav Bier, 1861–1949. Professor of Surgery, Berlin.

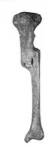

FIG. 1031.—
Mal-union of a
tibia. (*The patient
fell ninety feet from
the mast of a schooner,
and this was his only
serious injury.*)

(*d*) *Mal-union* (fig. 1031).—Although union in correct alignment is always desirable, particularly in the case of weight-bearing bones, yet in some cases malunion does not appreciably affect the function of a limb, e.g. most fractures of the clavicle unite in a faulty position, but the usefulness of the arm is unimpaired. If mal-union is likely to interfere with the function of a limb, reconstruction of the fracture is sometimes necessary, or osteotomy may be performed. Operations on bones should always be performed by the " no touch " technique.

(*e*) *Dis-union.*—This is a rare condition in which union is occurring in a satisfactory manner, but some grave constitutional disturbance, such as enteric fever, undermines the reparative powers of the patient, so that callus is absorbed.

(*f*) *New growth.*—Some surgeons consider that sarcoma occasionally results from a fracture, but the possibility of co-incidence is always a difficult factor to eliminate.

(ii) **Muscle.**—If fracture occurs in a bone clothed with muscle, some matting of the muscular fibres is liable to occur as a result of organisation of extravasated blood and exudates. Stiffness is prevented by actively exercising adjacent joints which do not require immobilisation. The two principles of complete immobilisation of the fracture and active use of the limb must be constantly borne in mind. Movements prevent atrophy of muscle, decalcification of bone, and a subconscious attitude of mind that the function of the limb may be seriously impaired.

Two complications in connection with muscles demand special mention.

(*a*) *Myositis Fibrosa* (*syn.* Volkmann's ischæmic contracture). —Sometimes occurs in the calf muscles, following injury to the main artery of the limb or an unduly tight plaster, but it is most commonly seen in connection with the flexor muscles of the forearm. In most cases the condition is due to contusion and spasm of an artery. Occasionally the artery is compressed by a fractured bone. Excessive flexion or too tight a plaster are contributory factors. Pain, blueness, and swelling of and inability passively to extend the fingers, and diminished or absent radial pulse are all danger signals. Diagnosis must be made at the earliest possible moment, and the first step in

Richard von Volkmann, 1830–1889. Professor of Surgery, Halle.

treatment is to block the brachial plexus with 2 per cent. novocaine. This will relieve arterial spasm, and any necessary manipulations of the limb can be conducted painlessly. If the fracture has not previously been reduced, reduction is performed forthwith ; otherwise the plaster is removed and the angle of flexion is diminished. A posterior plaster slab is then applied in order to immobilise the fracture. Unless the circulation obviously improves within two hours the artery is exposed at the site of injury and freed from any structure which is causing compression. An injection of papaverine gr. ii (100 mgm.) is given in order to overcome arterial spasm. If pulsation does not return, the damaged portion of the artery is excised between ligatures in the hope that reflex vasospasm will thus be abolished.

Threatened contracture should be prevented by suitable splinting, and early deformity can usually be corrected by this means. If contractures are established, sliding the muscles from the internal condyle improves the condition, but owing to replacement of muscle fibres by fibrous tissue stiffness and weakness inevitably persist.

A muscle-slide operation can only gain from ½ to ¾ inch (1·25 to 2 cm.), as further stretching will cause undue tension on the motor nerves. Tendon lengthening or resection of parts of the radius and ulna are unsatisfactory procedures. If further operation is necessary, excision of the proximal row of carpal bones is preferable.

(b) *Myositis Ossificans.*—Deposition of bone in a muscle consequent on a fracture most commonly occurs in the brachialis anticus (fig. 1032), but other muscles occasionally affected are the quadriceps and adductors of the thigh (fig. 1033). The condition is due to extensive laceration of periosteum and

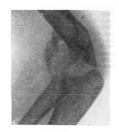

Fig. 1032.—Myositis ossificans.

muscle. Displaced bone cells find an agreeable nidus in the extravasated blood, and proceed to carry on their normal function of laying down new bone in the hæmatoma. After a period of four to six weeks an indurated mass is palpable in the muscle, and sufficient calcification will have occurred to be visible in an X-ray. Many cases are due to ossification of the anterior ligament of the elbow rather than to deposition of bone in brachialis anticus muscle.

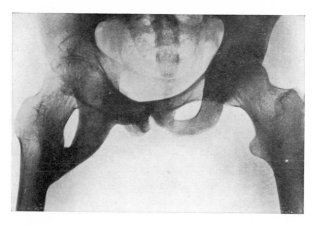

FIG. 1033.—Myositis ossificans. The bony bridge resembles an extra-articular arthrodesis, and most of the weight is conducted by this adventitious bone. Consequently atrophic changes have occurred in the head and neck of the femur. (*A good example of the law of Julius Wolff.*)   (*Colonel E. W. Hayward, Lahore.*)

Massage and passive movements merely stimulate the osteoblasts to increased efforts. The only treatment necessary is to prohibit passive stretching, and movement can be allowed to recover at its own rate by the patient's guarded activity (Watson-Jones). Complete immobilisation permits organisation of adhesions, and permanent stiffness is then probable. Operation is never indicated until at least a year has elapsed, and then only if the bony deposit limits movement of the joint.

(iii) **Joint.**—Either true or false ankylosis is liable to occur as a result of a fracture of the neighbouring bones.

TRUE ankylosis is usually of the *fibrous* variety, and is particularly liable to occur if the joint is implicated by a fracture, owing to organisation of blood. Limitation of movement may follow an excess of callus formation, as in fracture involving the elbow joint. *Bony* ankylosis can only occur when both or all the bones forming the joint are severely damaged.

FALSE ankylosis sometimes follows adhesions between muscle fibres, or fascial planes between the muscles. Myositis fibrosa has already been discussed. Limitation of movement as a result of adhesions of tendons in their sheaths is a complication particularly to be dreaded in the case of fractures in the region of the wrist or ankle, in which situations the tendons lie in close

Julius Wolff, 1836–1902, a German anatomist, pointed out that structures adapt themselves to the function which they are called upon to perform.
Sir Reginald Watson-Jones, Contemporary. Orthopædic Surgeon, London Hospital.

apposition with the bones. Thus, particularly in the case of a Colles's or Pott's fracture, early active movements of the toes and fingers are imperative, provided that the adjacent joints are immobilised.

Osteoarthritis must be mentioned as a sequela of mal-union of a fracture, particularly in the case of weight-bearing bones. Owing to alteration in the direction of the lines of stress, an unwonted strain is thrown on the joint, and the penalty exacted for this abuse is early degeneration of the joint above the fracture. Thus mal-union of a fractured femur in youth or early manhood is liable to be followed by osteoarthritis of the hip joint in middle age.

(iv) **Nerves.**—Nerves, particularly those which lie adjacent to bones, are liable to be involved as a result of contusion, traction, or laceration by the jagged fragments. Appropriate tests should always be carried out when the patient is first seen in order to test the function of any nerve which may have been injured.

Contusion, which gives rise to transient block (neuropraxia) is the commonest lesion, and recovery usually occurs within two or three weeks.

Axonotmesis, or lesion in continuity, occurs if a nerve is crushed so that the axis cylinders only are damaged. The sheath of the nerve is intact, so a good functional result is to be expected after a few months as axons reunite with a minimum of " shunting."

Neurotmesis, or complete division of the nerve, only occurs when there is considerable displacement of fragments. In the case of closed fractures neurotmesis is probable if no improvement occurs within three months, after which time exploration is desirable.

Nerves which are frequently injured at the time of the fracture are the ulnar, in the case of supracondylar fracture or separation of the lower epiphysis of the humerus, and the radial (8 per cent. of cases), as it lies in its groove on the humerus. The median nerve is occasionally injured, as it lies in front of the elbow and wrist, in connection with fractures of the lower end of the humerus and radius. The commonest nerve to be " involved in callus " is the radial, owing to its close relationship to the humerus (p. 924).

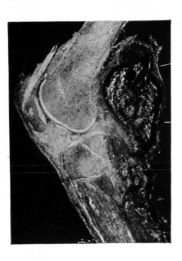

Fig. 1034.—False aneurism of the popliteal artery following fracture of the upper end of the tibia.

(v) **Blood-vessels.**—Arteries or veins are sometimes ruptured immediately at the time of the fracture. Extravasation of blood occurs, which, in the case of an artery, is liable to result in the formation of a false aneurism (fig. 1034). If the arterial wall is partially damaged, the weakened wall may subsequently yield and so form a true saccular aneurism.

Vessels are occasionally occluded by spasm due to bruising, or by the pressure of displaced fragments, e.g. pressure on the popliteal artery by the diaphysis of the femur in the case of separation of the lower epiphysis, which is displaced forwards. If the circulation of the limb is unsatisfactory after reduction of a fracture, exploration of the adjacent artery is often advisable (p. 1020).

(vi) **Skin.**—Pressure sores, as a result of the application of splints and plasters, should be avoided by reasonable care and foresight.

Pressure sores are encouraged by ridges or local pressure. Ridges are due to the uneven application of the bandage, or to the alteration of the position of a joint after the plaster has been applied. Local pressure occurs if bony prominences are unprotected, or if pressure is allowed to indent the casing before the plaster has set. Persistent localised discomfort or pain must not be ignored, and the gradual diminution of the pain should not lull the surgeon into a sense of false security, as it possibly indicates the onset of gangrene (as with gangrenous appendicitis). Recurrence of œdema of the digits after initial swelling has subsided usually indicates a pressure sore. If infection occurs it can be recognised by a local patch of warmth or discoloration of the plaster, and later by the odour which emanates from beneath it. When a sore is suspected an inspection window is cut in the plaster, and if no sore is discovered the gap is packed with cottonwool and firmly bandaged in order to prevent œdema. If a sore has occurred the window must be enlarged beyond the area affected, and suitable antiseptic dressings are applied.

(vii) **Infection.**—If the fracture is compound, and efforts to prevent infection are unsuccessful, then the general and local complications of infection supervene. Infection may also follow operative reduction and fixation. Locally, necrosis of bone and delayed union are probable, and the surrounding soft tissues may be involved by cellulitis, secondary hæmorrhage, or gas gangrene.

As a rule the general clinical manifestations of infection are not severe, as the open wound associated with a compound fracture provides an exit for inflammatory exudates.

More detailed accounts of the effects of local and general infection are to be found in the chapters dealing with the structures involved.

INDICATIONS FOR OPERATION

The indications for operative intervention in connection with a fracture can be classified as immediate, intermediate, or remote. The first group includes those cases in which an emergency operation is necessary, the second comprises fractures which require operative treatment after the lapse of a few days, while remote indications include surgical measures devised to combat late complications. These indications only refer to fractures of bones of the limbs ; such conditions as fractures of the skull, spine, or pelvis are considered in their appropriate sections.

(i) **Immediate.**—(a) *Complicated fractures,* as in the case of rupture of, or pressure on, the main vessels of a limb, may require operative interference in order to control hæmorrhage, or to diminish or obviate the risk of myositis fibrosa or gangrene.

(b) *Compound fractures* must be operated upon immediately in order to diminish the risk of infection. Each hour's delay allows infection to become more firmly established, and if much blood has been lost or a tourniquet has been applied, or if inadequate splinting has encouraged laceration of the soft tissues by jagged fragments, then the devitalised tissues are particularly susceptible to bacterial invasion. In severe cases a delay of six hours usually means some degree of infection.

The operation demands stringent aseptic technique, and should be conducted by the " no touch " method. The wound is excised (p. 10), and if an injury to an important nerve is suspected it should be identified, provided that little or no dissection is required. If ruptured, the ends are approximated by one non-absorbable stitch, so as to facilitate suture at a later date. Reduction is effected by the means most suitable for the individual fracture. Sulphonamide and penicillin powder is applied, and the wound is closed. If a denuded area remains as a result of skin loss, it is covered with tulle gras or vaselined gauze. The method of immobilisation to be adopted depends on the nature of the injury and the individual fracture.

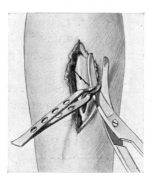

Fig. 1035.—Excising the wound edges in a compound fracture.

Winnett Orr's method of treating compound fractures is now established. The principles of treatment are drainage without dressing, and immobilisation until the fracture is united. After cleansing and shaving of the skin, the edges of the wound and damaged soft tissues are excised (fig. 1035). Reduction is obtained, e.g. in the case of the tibia, by transfixion of the lower end of the tibia and screw traction on a Hawley's table. The wound is insufflated with sulphanilamide powder, and packed with gauze impregnated with sterile vaseline. The limb is covered with gauze and wool, and encased in plaster of Paris, transfixion pins being included if necessary. A moderate rise of temperature for a few days is of no moment, and the plaster is left untouched for about a month. On removal it is found that the extruded gauze covers a granulating wound. The wound is redressed, and any sequestra which have separated are removed and further plasters are applied as necessary. The fœtid smell which emanates from the plaster can be diminished by spraying with Sanitas or nursing in the open air. The advantage of this method is that wide excision prevents pocketing, and repeated painful dressings, with the attendant risk of secondary infection, are abolished. The method is not infallible, and occasionally persistent pain or raised temperature necessi-

Hiram Winnett Orr, Contemporary. Surgeon, General Hospital, Lincoln, Nebraska, U.S.A.
George Waller Hawley, Contemporary. Consulting Surgeon, Norwalk General Hospital, Norwalk, Connecticut.

tates removal of the plaster, but the net results are encouraging.

If a compound fracture is associated with extensive damage to the soft parts, particularly the main vessels or nerves, then immediate amputation may be the most desirable line of treatment. This is especially the case in the lower limb, which possesses less vitality than the arm.

(ii) **Intermediate.**—(a) *Complicated simple fractures*—as when a large joint or an important nerve is involved. In the case of joint involvement, the advantages of operation are twofold. Firstly, blood-clot is evacuated, so that its organisation into troublesome fibrous adhesions is prevented, and secondly, mechanical fixation of the fragments is usually possible, so that early movements can be safely instituted without the risk of displacement recurring. For example, a fracture of the outer tuberosity of the tibia is exposed by a lateral incision, the blood in the knee joint evacuated, and lavage performed with saline solution if necessary. Either a bone peg or screw is inserted, or the fragments are approximated by a circumferential wire passed around the tibia (Capener), so that the tuberosity is held firmly in its normal position, and the tibial plateau thus restored. Active movements of the knee joint are commenced a few days later, and a full range of movement can confidently be expected. Injury to a nerve at the time of fracture may require subsequent operation (p. 1023). It is, of course, of paramount importance to test the functions of all nerves which might be implicated *before* immobilising the limb so that involvement is not overlooked. Paralysed or paretic muscles must be supported during the period which elapses while evidence of recovery is awaited.

(b) *Manipulation is not successful*—as in the case of wide separation of fragments, interposition of soft parts, or small bony processes which are not amenable to manipulation.

In some situations manipulation may fail to overcome existing deformity, e.g. fracture of the shafts of the radius and ulna at the same level. Unless adequate reduction is obtained, cross-union is likely to occur with consequent limitation of pronation and supination (fig. 1060).

(c) *Reduction is not maintained*, e.g. spiral fractures of the tibia are easily reduced, but displacement occurs immediately traction is relaxed. Continuous traction may result in

Norman Capener, Contemporary. Orthopædic Surgeon, Exeter, England.

slow union, hence internal fixation secures a satisfactory result in the shortest time. In other situations the nature of the displacement or an associated dislocation may require open reduction and perhaps internal fixation.

Operations designed to secure adequate reduction should be performed within a few days after the accident. If operation is delayed much beyond this period, organisation of extravasated blood and exudate, and, at a later date, the formation of callus, add considerably to the difficulty of apposing the fragments. Moreover, bony spicules are absorbed, and the ends of the fragments become rounded, which prevents interlocking of the fragments. When operation is performed at the end of a few days, the fragments usually dovetail in a sufficiently firm manner to render accessory fixation unnecessary. If, however, the fracture is unstable, mechanical methods, such as bone plates, are used to fix the fragments, especially in such situations where early movements are desirable.

(*d*) *Union is slow*—as in the case of subcapital fracture of the femoral neck. Although immobilisation by plaster spicas may result eventually in union, internal fixation is more certain and may save many months. Also in fractures of long bones where union is delayed, a bone graft may be a time-saving measure.

(iii) **Remote.**—(*a*) *Severe multiple injuries*—in some cases a fracture must, of necessity, be merely supported until the condition of the patient permits of attention being directed towards its treatment. Also fractures which occur in remote districts, or where transport is difficult, may be inadequately treated for a considerable time before expert attention is available. If extravasated blood and inflammatory exudates have begun to organise, attempts at manipulation are unlikely to be successful, and exposure and fixation of the fragments will be necessary.

(*b*) *Late complications affecting soft structures* sometimes occur, e.g. in connection with muscles, concerning which myositis fibrosa and myositis ossificans have already been mentioned. Nerves are occasionally involved (p. 1023). Rarely an aneurism, arterial or arterio-venous, demands surgical interference.

(*c*) *Non-union or mal-union* may require surgical intervention (p. 1016).

SPECIAL FRACTURES

FACIO-MAXILLARY

The **Superior Maxilla** is fractured as a result of a direct localised blow, or a portion of the alveolar border is broken off in efforts to extract a tooth. In the former case comminution is probable, and the fracture is frequently compound, on account of involvement of the maxillary antrum. If the fracture extends to the alveolar border, crepitus can usually be elicited and dental occlusion is impaired. Treatment consists in the application of lead lotion in order to discourage hæmorrhage, mouth-washes, and nasal irrigation. If the alveolar border is involved, a dental splint is advisable. Complications which sometimes follow are extensive extravasation of blood, surgical emphysema, infection, necrosis of bone, and aspiration pneumonia.

The **Zygomatic Arch** may be fractured and depressed by a direct blow. Unsightly deformity results, and anæsthesia of the cheek may occur owing to pressure on the infraorbital nerve. Pain on mastication is commonly noticed. If the arch cannot be elevated by digital pressure from within the mouth, a small incision is made at the hairy margin above the bone (fig. 1036), through which a blunt instrument is inserted. This is manipulated beneath the arch so that the fragments can be elevated. Reposition of the depressed arch should always be performed, otherwise the cheek is permanently flattened.

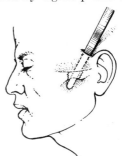

Fig. 1036.—Elevation of a fractured zygoma.

The **Nasal** bones are commonly fractured as a result of direct violence. The fracture usually occurs near their lower margin, but in more severe injuries the root of the nose may be driven in towards the base of the skull. In these cases the septum is commonly fractured and displaced. Epistaxis, considerable swelling, and surgical emphysema may result. Consolidation speedily occurs, hence replacement should be undertaken without undue delay, although reduction may be successful within two weeks of the injury. Under anæsthesia (e.g. pentothal) one blade of a pair of long forceps, protected with rubber tubing, is introduced into each nostril alternately, and the fragments levered into position. It may be necessary to exert external digital pressure on the fragment in the direction of the deformity, so as to disimpact it, before reduction is possible.

The **Inferior Maxilla** is usually fractured in one of four situations (fig. 1037).

(i) The *coronoid process* is sometimes fractured, diagnosis only being possible by means of a radiograph. Only slight displacement occurs, as the temporal muscle is inserted over the inner surface of the process and

so retains the fractured portion in position. Treatment consists in sup
porting the jaw for three weeks.

(ii) The *neck of the condyle* is occasionally fractured, in which case it is
displaced forwards and inwards by the pull of the attached external
pterygoid muscle. Localised pain occurs on movements of the jaw, and

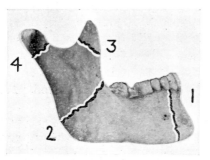

Fig. 1037.—Lower Jaw.

1. Commonest site, anterior to
the mental foramen, through the
canine fossa.

2. Through the angle or ascend
ing ramus.

3. Coronoid process.

4. Neck of condyle.

crepitus is detected by the patient or surgeon. Removal of the condyle
shortens the period of disability, and obviates the likelihood of adhesions
and consequent limitation of movement.

(iii) The *ascending ramus* may be fractured, usually in the region of the
angle of the jaw. Little displacement occurs, as the masseter on the
outside and internal pterygoid muscle on the inner aspect sandwich the
fragments between them. The injury is suspected on account of persistent
localised pain, and is confirmed by an X-ray. Mastication is limited to
soft food for three weeks.

(iv) The *body of the jaw* is the part most commonly fractured,
usually as the result of a blow with a fist. The fracture frequently occurs at the site of the socket of the canine tooth,
the cavity of which weakens the bone, and also this region is the
junction of two curves. As the mental foramen is situated
posteriorly, the inferior dental nerve and vessels are not implicated. Occasionally the fracture is bilateral, in which case the
central portion of the jaw is displaced downwards by the anterior
belly of the digastric muscle and the muscles attached to the
genial tubercles. Owing to the firm attachment of the muco-
periosteum to the bone, the fracture is nearly always compound.

Diagnosis is usually obvious as speech and swallowing are
impaired. Blood-stained saliva trickles from the mouth, and
irregularity of the line of the teeth is apparent. Crepitus can
be elicited with ease.

Treatment.—As a first-aid measure the fracture is supported
by a barrel bandage,[1] which is a great improvement on the

[1] So-called, as it is the method by which draymen secure barrels when lowering
them into vaults.

" four-tail " method, in that it supports the jaw without any backward pull, which pull maintains the deformity instead of overcoming it. A 2-inch (5 cm.) bandage is used. It is passed under the jaw so as to support it firmly, and tied in a simple knot over the vertex. The knot is then opened, and one loop is manipulated over the forehead, and the other over the occiput. The twist in the bandage on one side thus comes to lie above one ear, and on the opposite side the long end of the bandage is passed beneath the part encircling the head so as to form a corresponding twist. The two long ends are then tied over the vertex (fig. 1038).

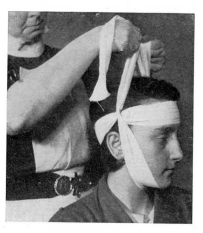

As soon as possible the patient is referred to the dental surgeon for fixation, the most satisfactory appliance being an interdental splint which fits over the teeth adjacent to the fracture. A corresponding splint is fitted to the upper jaw, so that fixation of the two splints secures immobilisa-

Fig. 1038.—The barrel bandage.

tion. Any obviously infected teeth, or an interposed tooth, are removed when the splint is being fitted.

As the fracture is compound, infection from the mouth is likely, particularly if pyorrhœa or infected teeth are present. Warm antiseptic mouth-washes are therefore used almost continuously. The diet is confined to fluids, which are taken temporarily through a rubber tube.

Complications are mainly due to infection. Thus necrosis of bone and delayed union are not uncommon, while submaxillary cellulitis may require operative interference. Aspiration pneumonia is a grave danger, particularly in old or alcoholic patients with pyorrhœa.

UPPER EXTREMITY

The **Clavicle** is the commonest long bone to fracture, indirect violence being the usual cause. Fractures occur in one of the following four situations (fig. 1039) :

(i) *Acromial Tip.*—This fracture is due to direct violence, such as a sharp blow on the shoulder. Separation occurs owing to contraction of

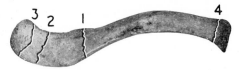

FIG. 1039.—Clavicle.

1. Commonest site, at junction of outer flattened and inner pyramidal portions.
2. Between the conoid and trapezoid ligaments.
3. Acromial tip.
4. Inner extremity, between the rhomboid ligament and sternoclavicular joint.

those fibres of the deltoid muscle which are attached to the fragment. If strapping is unsuccessful in retaining the fragment in position and relieving pain, then an operation should be undertaken, and the tip screwed or pegged in position.

(ii) *Acromial End.*—This fracture is also due to direct violence, but displacement is slight, as the fracture occurs between the trapezoid and conoid ligaments, and thus the two fragments are held in position. Localised pain and tenderness suggest the presence of the fracture, which often requires a radiograph for confirmation. The application of strapping and a sling for three weeks is adequate.

(iii) *Sternal End.*—This is the least common situation for fracture, and as a rule little deformity occurs, since the small inner fragment is steadied by the sternoclavicular ligament, and the outer fragment is anchored to the junction of the first rib and costal cartilage by the rhomboid ligament. The application of a sling for two or three weeks is usually all the treatment that is necessary.

(iv) *Greater Convexity.*—This is an exceedingly common fracture, and is usually due to indirect violence, such as falls on the hand or shoulder. It is frequently met with in the hunting-field and on the football ground.

A greenstick variety occasionally occurs in children, and is liable to be overlooked, but the definite localised tenderness and reluctance to move the arm should suggest the necessity for an X-ray. The frequency of fracture at this site is accounted for by the fact that it is the junction of two curves, also the bone on the outer side is flat and the inner side pyramidal, hence the internal architecture undergoes adjustment at this site. Subsidiary reasons are that the bone is weakened in this situation by the groove for the subclavius muscle, and also by the foramen for the nutrient artery.

Diagnosis is usually obvious, even at a distance, as the patient is seen supporting the elbow on the injured side with the opposite hand, and flexing his head to the affected side in order to relax the sternomastoid muscle (fig. 1040). The outer fragment is displaced in three directions—downwards by gravity, forwards by the pull of the pectoral muscles, and inwards by contraction of the muscles inserted into the bicipital groove, notably the latissimus dorsi. The inner fragment is tilted slightly upwards by the sternomastoid muscle, but the obvious projection of its outer end is due to displacement downwards of the lateral fragment.

If displacement is slight, all that is necessary is to place a pad in the axilla, steady the fragments by passing strapping over the site of fracture, and apply a sling for three weeks. If deformity is pronounced, the " three slings " method is adopted, which allows the arm to be free, the sleeve of the coat to be worn, and the joints of the arm, except the shoulder, to be freely mobile. Movements of the shoulder joint are encouraged ten days after the injury.

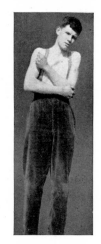

Fig. 1040.—Fractured clavicle.

" *Three Slings* " *with Collar and Cuff.*—Cottonwool is sewn into a 4-inch bandage so as to form a quoit-like ring. Two rings are necessary, and two holes are bored through each ring posteriorly, and rubber tubing is passed through the holes (fig. 1041). The patient is seated, and the rings are applied over the shoulders. The surgeon places his knee between the shoulders and braces the joints backwards. The rubber tubes are then tightly tied over a wool pad (fig. 1041). A collar-and-cuff sling is then applied. The tubing maintains the tension necessary to hold the fragments in position, while the sling supports the outer fragment. The patient must

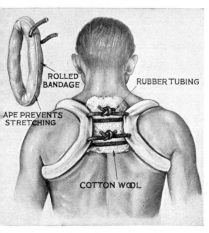

Fig. 1041.—Modified three-slings method.
(*Royal Northern Hospital.*)

ROLLED BANDAGE

RUBBER TUBING

TAPE PREVENTS STRETCHING

COTTON WOOL

attend twice weekly for adjustment, otherwise chafing of the
skin in the axilla, or œdema of the arm, may develop.

Average period of disability—heavy work eight weeks, light work five
weeks.

Some degree of mal-union is common, but no disability results.   In the
case of gross mal-union, excessive drooping of the shoulder girdle may
cause traction on the inner cord of the brachial plexus, which thus becomes
stretched over the normal first rib.   Similar symptoms to those caused by
a cervical rib are thereby produced.   Reconstruction of the fracture or
excision of part of the first rib may be necessary in order to relieve traction
on the plexus.   If fracture of the clavicle is caused by direct violence, the
subjacent structures are sometimes injured, e.g. the subclavian vessels
brachial plexus, or pleura.   In cases where fracture is due to indirec
violence, these structures are protected by the subclavius muscle and
prolongation of deep cervical fascia, which in this situation consists of a
dense, felted membrane.

Fractures of the **Scapula** occur in connection with the coracoid
process, acromion process, neck, or body
(fig. 1042).

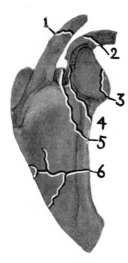

FIG. 1042.—Scapula.

1. Acromion process.
2. Coracoid process.
3. Portion of glenoid fossa.
4. Anatomical neck.
5. Surgical neck.
6. Stellate fracture of the
body.

(i) The *coracoid process*, on account of its
protected situation and sturdy structure, is
rarely fractured. The kick from a loosely held
gun, or other severe localised blow, occasionally results in a fracture, which may also
result from muscular contraction.   Owing
to extensive ligamentous attachments, only
slight displacement of the fragment is possible
and elevation and fixation of the arm for two
or three weeks is sufficient.

(ii) The *acromion process* may be detached
by localised direct violence.   Crepitus is
obtainable if a sufficiently large fragment is
detached.   Owing to the attachment of the
trapezius and deltoid muscles, separation is
usually slight, but if troublesome the
detached fragment should be fixed in position by a bone peg.

(iii) The *neck* of the scapula may be fractured through the articular surface, a small
fragment, usually including the origin of the
long head of the triceps, being separated
downwards.   Fracture also occurs through
the anatomical neck, i.e. running downward
from between the base of the coracoid process
and the glenoid fossa, or through the surgical
neck, in which case the fracture commences
above the suprascapular notch.   In either
case the articular surface is displaced downwards by the weight of the
arm.   On inspection some flattening of the shoulder is apparent, which
superficially simulates dislocation of the joint ; however, repositio
is easy, but the deformity recurs when support is withdrawn.   Some cases
are complicated by dislocation of the shoulder.

Treatment consists in elevating the shoulder by means of a large axillar pad or other suitable support. Movements of the shoulder joint are begun after about ten days, as stiffness is more to be feared than inaccurate apposition of the fragments.

(iv) Fractures of the *body* of the scapula are caused by severe and direct injury. Any degree of damage is liable to result, from a simple crack to a star-shaped comminution. In any case, little separation occurs owing to widespread muscular attachments, although extensive bruising commonly co-exists. Treatment consists in the application of cooling lotion and support by strapping and a sling. After a few days, active movements of the shoulder joint are essential.

Fractures of the **Humerus** (fig. 1043).

(i) *Upper End.*—Until recently fractures of the upper end of the humerus were classified as occurring either through the anatomical or else through the surgical neck. A more satisfactory classification is that of abduction or adduction fractures, which indicates the nature of the injury, and on this depends the treatment of the fracture.

Abduction fractures are the commonest type, and are always associated with fracture of the greater tuberosity. The fracture is impacted on the outer side. No manipulation is required, and the only treatment necessary is a sling. Active movements of the elbow, wrist, and fingers are begun forthwith, and movements of the shoulder after some ten days.

Adduction fractures are associated with outer angulation of the fragments, and impaction commonly occurs on the inner side. Reduction is usually advisable (except in the elderly or if displacement is slight), otherwise movement may be limited by the diminished range of abduction. Under anæsthesia the fracture is disimpacted and reduced by traction on the abducted arm ; the arm is then fixed in right-angled abduction either by means of a frame or plaster for about one month.

Fracture-dislocation.—This is a severe injury, and the shoulder joint is usually more or less disorganised. In elderly patients the shoulder should be abducted to about

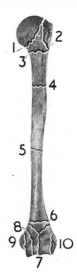

Fig. 1043.—Humerus.

1. Anatomical neck.
2. Greater tuberosity.
3. Surgical neck.
4. Shaft above the deltoid insertion.
5. Shaft below the deltoid.
6. Supracondylar.
7. Y-shaped into the elbow joint.
8. Internal condyle.
9. Internal epicondyle.
10. External condyle.

30 degrees for three weeks. In the case of young and active patients, if traction and manipulation fail, exploration is indicated, so that the dislocation can be reduced and bony fragments approximated.

Either *tuberosity* may be avulsed, the greater particularly in association with dislocation of the shoulder joint (fig. 1144). A

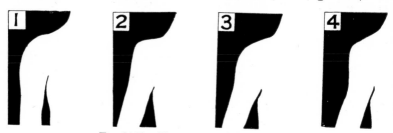

FIG. 1044.—The contour of the shoulder :
1. Normal—rounded and mobile. 2. Dislocation—angular and fixed. 3. Fracture—rounded and fixed. 4. Wasting of deltoid muscle (e.g. circumflex nerve palsy)—angular and mobile.

crack in the greater tuberosity merely requires a temporary sling. If the tuberosity is avulsed, the supraspinatus muscle is functionally inactive and approximation is important. As manipulation of the tuberosity is impossible, the head of the humerus must be in such a position that union will occur. This is obtained by fixing the arm in a position of right-angled abduction and external rotation for two months.

Separation of the epiphysis occurs between the ages of six and twenty. It is uncommon, owing to the conical shape of the diaphysis, which fits into the correspondingly cup-shaped epiphysis. Displacement is sometimes partial, and can occur in any direction. The signs resemble those of fracture, but the age of the patient and soft character of the crepitus are of assistance in distinguishing the conditions. Accurate reposition is advisable, otherwise limitation of movement is probable, and also interference with growth, particularly in young children. Manipulation often fails if separation is complete, as sometimes the cup-shaped epiphysis lies in such a position that it is impossible to appose the conical diaphysis ; while in some incomplete cases the diaphysis protrudes through the periosteum and so becomes buttonholed. In either case, the bone should be exposed by operation and manipulated under direct vision, or, in incomplete separation, division of periosteum will permit of easy reduction.

(ii) *Shaft.*—Fractures of the shaft of the humerus are usually easily recognisable, and deformity varies with the site of the fracture. Thus, if the fracture is just below the neck, the upper fragment is abducted by the supraspinatus muscle. If above the deltoid muscle, the upper fragment is drawn inwards by the muscles inserted into the bicipital groove, while the lower fragment is drawn outwards by the deltoid and upwards by the biceps and triceps. If fracture occurs below the deltoid, then the upper fragment is displaced outwards by the deltoid, and the lower inwards and upwards.

Immediate injury to the radial nerve occurs in about 8 per cent. of cases. Myositis ossificans developing in the brachialis anticus, and delayed union, are other not uncommon complications.

Treatment consists in the application of a U-shaped plaster slab from the axilla to below the elbow joint (fig. 1045), after which the arm is supported in a sling. Reduction under anæsthesia is rarely required, as the weight of the limb and plaster maintains the fragments in position. In the case of horizontal fractures deformity may persist, correction is then obtained by fixation of the arm in right-angled abduction by means of a plaster spica.

(iii) *Lower End.*—Fractures at this site are either supracondylar, transcondylar, fissured into the elbow joint, involve either condyle, or result in separation of the epiphysis.

Supracondylar fractures are usually due to falls on the hand, in which case the lower fragment is displaced backwards, and is pulled upwards by the triceps. If lateral displacement occurs as well, it is usually in an outward direction. The condition somewhat resembles a posterior dislocation of the elbow joint, but the following observations should prevent error :

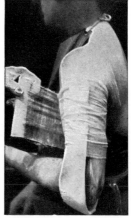

Fig. 1045.—A 3-inch (7 cm.) U-shaped slab extends from the axilla round the elbow to the acromion. It is fixed by one gauze and two plaster bandages.

(*a*) In the case of fracture the normal relationship of bony points around the elbow is unaltered (fig. 1146).

(*b*) Measurement from the acromion process to the external condyle is shortened in a fracture, as compared with the opposite arm.

(*c*) The anterior projection of the lower end of the upper fragment forms an obvious swelling or is palpable in the case of a fracture, while if a dislocation has occurred, the olecranon process is unduly prominent.

(*d*) A fracture can usually be readily reduced, provided the patient tolerates this procedure, but the deformity recurs.

(*e*) Crepitus is obtainable if a fracture is present.

Less commonly a fall on the back of the elbow causes a supracondylar fracture, with anterior displacement of the lower fragment.

In cases seen after a few hours' delay, extensive extravasation masks many of the above signs, and a radiograph is necessary for accurate diagnosis without discomfort to the patient.

Treatment consists in reduction under anæsthesia. Accurate reduction is essential, otherwise limitation of movement and cubitus valgus or varus are likely. Traction is applied to the forearm with one hand, and firmly maintained while the fragments are manipulated with the other. Lateral displacement must be corrected in full extension, and if the lower fragment is displaced backwards the elbow is flexed to about 45 degrees after reduction. Reposition is then confirmed by X-rays, preferably stereoscopic, as the lower end of the humerus is obscured by the radius and ulna. Re-manipulation is sometimes necessary. The condition of the circulation is then noted, and if the limb is congested, or the radial pulse weak, the forearm is extended towards a right angle. A posterior plaster slab is applied from the upper third of the arm to the knuckles, and is covered with a gauze bandage. The limb is then encircled with a light plaster bandage. The plaster slab and gauze bandage protect part of the front of the forearm from direct pressure by the plaster bandage, so that subsequent swelling can be accommodated without interference to the circulation. Finger and shoulder movements are begun at once, and the plaster is retained for four to five weeks.

Should the lower fragment be displaced forwards, reduction is effected as described above, and the elbow is immobilised in extension.

Transcondylar fractures, owing to the small size of the lower fragment, are difficult to maintain in position. Reduction should be performed under X-ray control, and a plaster is applied as for a supracondylar fracture. Maintenance of reduction is confirmed by subsequent X-rays.

T- *or* Y-*shaped fractures* are the result of a fall on to the point of the elbow. If complete separation has occurred, crepitus is usually obtained and X-rays give detailed information.

Traction and manipulation enable reduction to be obtained, and the elbow joint is immobilised in the optimum position (a little less than a right angle) consistent with maintenance of reduction. Open operation, formerly much in vogue for these fractures, is rarely necessary.

Separation of the lower epiphysis frequently occurs, and it is the commonest epiphysis in the body to separate. The line of separation, however, more commonly occurs on the diaphyseal side rather than actually through the epiphyseal cartilage. This accident can occur at any age up to sixteen or eighteen. At the age of five or six years the centre for the internal epicondyle appears, this centre remaining separate from the main epiphyseal mass, until about two years before union with the shaft. Hence from about six years until sixteen separation does not include the epiphysis for the internal epicondyle.

The signs and symptoms closely resemble those of a supracondylar fracture with forward displacement, with the exception that crepitus is softer. Treatment requires traction and immobilisation of the elbow, accurate reposition being essential, as any initial deformity may be magnified as growth continues. Particular care should be taken to maintain the " carrying-angle." Should cubitus valgus develop, involvement of the ulnar nerve may result (p. 926).

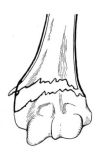

Fig. 1046.— Buttonholing of the periosteum by the jagged diaphysis.

Reduction by manipulation occasionally fails, owing to the jagged diaphysis buttonholing the periosteum (fig. 1046). Operation is then required, and a posterior incision exposes the site of injury, and after enlarging the buttonhole reduction is simple.

Fractures of the *condyles* are due to direct injury, and the elbow joint is implicated in both cases. Fracture of the internal *epicondyle* or separation of the epiphysis occasionally occurs, and does not involve the joint. If wide separation persists, and is not improved by manipulation, fixation by open operation

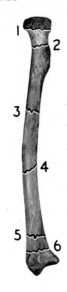

FIG. 1047.—Radius.

1. Transverse fracture of head.
2. Transverse fracture of neck.
3. Shaft, above pronator radii teres.
4. Shaft, below pronator radii teres.
5. Chauffeur's fracture.
6. Colles's fracture.

may be desirable. Fractures of the internal condyle are sometimes associated with injury to the ulnar nerve.

Average period of disability after fracture of the neck or shaft of the humerus—heavy work twenty-four weeks, light work fifteen weeks.

Fractures of the **Radius** are common (fig. 1047).

(i) Fractures of the *head or neck* occasionally occur, the former frequently being associated with injury to other bones forming the elbow joint.

There are three types of displacement :

I. The head may be impacted into the neck, so that the outer aspect is on a lower level than the inner, but the upper table is unbroken.

II. A vertical fracture through the middle or outer third of the head, with or without downward and outward displacement of the outer fragment.

III. Fragmentation of the head.

Pain, swelling, and tenderness over the head of the radius, with limitation of movement, especially extension, and pain on pronation and supination are usually pathognomonic. The diagnosis must always be confirmed by X-rays. It is essential that the antero-posterior X-ray should be taken in full supination, and with as much extension as possible, so that a clear joint space is visible between the humerus and radius ; otherwise the fracture may be obscured. A lateral radiograph in the mid-prone position is often useful.

Treatment

Type I.—This is usually treated by encouraging active movements from the beginning. At the end of a week, the patient is usually able to return to work. If much displacement exists, open operation is desirable so that the normal parallel alignment between the head of the radius and the capitellum is regained.

Type II (fig. 1048) (Fitzgerald's method).—A general anæsthetic is administered and a counter-traction band is fixed over the arm. An assistant exerts traction by pulling on the fingers, *with forearm fully supinated.* The medial aspect of the

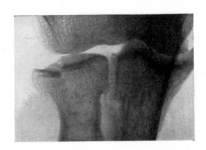

Fig. 1048.—Type II, showing downward displacement of outer segment of the head of the radius.

elbow rests on a pad on a table. A piece of adhesive felt is fixed over the region of the fracture, and, using a blunt instrument, very forcible pressure is exerted on the broken fragment in an upward and inward direction. It may even be necessary to use a broad punch and hammer to replace the fragment

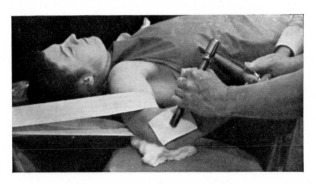

Fig. 1049.—Traction is exerted on the supinated forearm. Counter-traction by band over the upper arm. The elbow rests on a pad of wool on a table. A piece of adhesive felt prevents skin damage from the punch.

(fig. 1049). The skin is not damaged by these manipulations, provided the felt is in position. (Fig. 1050 shows the position after reduction.)

If manipulation fails, the fragment can be elevated into position after being impaled on the point of a Steinmann's pin.

Active movements are begun the next day.

Type III.—Manipulation is attempted, but in adults the

F. P. *Fitzgerald, Contemporary. Orthopœdic Surgeon, Royal Northern Hospital, London.*

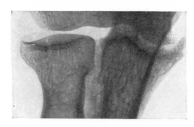

FIG. 1050.—Fragment replaced.

head will occasionally require excision by open operation.

(ii) The *shaft* of the radius is fractured either above or below the pronator radii teres muscle. If above the insertion of this muscle, the upper fragment is supinated by the biceps and supinator brevis, while the lower portion is pronated by the pronator radii teres and the pronator quadratus. If an unimpacted fracture occurs below the middle of the shaft, the upper fragment is in a position of mid-supination, as the position is influenced by both the biceps and pronator radii teres, while the lower fragment is pronated by the quadrate muscle. Therefore with a fracture above the pronator radii teres treatment consists in fixation in complete supination, whereas a fracture below the teres muscle is fixed in the mid-position. These positions are maintained by means of a plaster cast, which is applied from above the elbow to heads of the meta-carpals. This is retained for three weeks, movement of the fingers and thumb being carried out daily. A special variety of fracture of the radial shaft is a chauffeur's fracture (fig. 1051), which is due to sudden hyper-extension of the wrist, e.g. as a result of a " backfire." Some cases are possibly due to a revolution of the starting-handle, which violently strikes the back of the wrist, and are thus due to direct violence. The fracture occurs about 3 inches (7 cm.) from the lower end of the radius. Impaction does not occur, and treatment is similar to that described for Colles's fracture (fig. 1052).

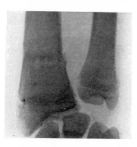

FIG. 1051.—Chauffeur's fracture, non-impacted, in an adolescent subject.

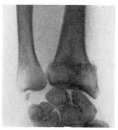

FIG. 1052.—Colles's fracture ; the ulnar sty-loid process is avulsed and on the same level as that of the radius.

Abraham Colles, 1773–1843. Professor of Surgery, Dublin, Surgeon at St. Stephen's Hospital. He journeyed on foot from Edinburgh to London, and declined a baronetcy.

(iii) Fractures of the *lower end* are common, the most important being Colles's fracture. This fracture commonly occurs in old ladies who trip and fall on the outstretched hand. The lesion occurs from $\frac{1}{2}$ to 1 inch (1·25 to 2·5 cm.) above the wrist joint, and either the styloid process of the ulna is avulsed, or the internal lateral ligament of the wrist joint is ruptured. The lower fragment of the radius is displaced backwards and outwards, and also rotated, so that the articular surface looks backwards and outwards, i.e. it is both displaced and rotated in the direction of the violence. In addition, impaction usually occurs, so that the lower fragment is also displaced upwards and a " dinner fork " deformity is produced (fig. 1053). On

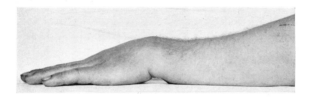

Fig. 1053.—" Dinner-fork " deformity of a Colles's fracture.
(*H. Osmond Clarke*.)

palpation the radial styloid process, instead of being $\frac{1}{2}$ inch (1·25 cm.) below that of the ulna, is on a level with it, or if marked displacement has occurred, even higher (fig. 1052). In some cases a projection is felt on the back of the wrist, caused by the upper end of the lower fragment of the radius.

Smith's fracture is due to falling with the hand behind the body, and the deformity is the reverse of that which occurs in Colles's fracture.

Treatment consists in early disimpaction and reduction. General or local anæsthesia is necessary, and either the surgeon grasps the patient's hand as for a hand-shake, or preferably applies direct pressure to the distal fragment with the ball of his thumb, the other hand firmly grasping the forearm. Counter-traction is maintained by a sling or applied by an assistant. The lower fragment is manipulated in a forward and inward direction, traction being exerted simultaneously (fig. 1054). It was formerly recommended that if disimpaction was difficult a sudden jerk in the direction of the deformity snaps some of the

Robert William Smith, 1807–1873. Professor of Surgery, Trinity College, Dublin.

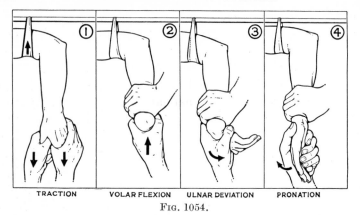

TRACTION   VOLAR FLEXION   ULNAR DEVIATION   PRONATION

Fig. 1054.

interlocking bony spicules and reduction can then be accomplished. This procedure, however, is apt to cause further
damage to soft tissues, and prolonged and adequate traction will
usually succeed in disimpacting the fragments. After disimpaction, reduction is effected by volar flexion and ulnar
deviation, and the fragments are locked in position by pronation
of the wrist joint. Early active movements of the fingers are
essential in order to prevent adhesions between tendons and
their sheaths, and a plaster slab is now the recognised method
of immobilising the fracture while permitting movements of
joints. A plaster slab is applied directly to the skin along the
back of the hand and forearm, with the hand in a position of
full ulnar deviation. It is moulded to the limb, and extends
distally to just short of the heads of the metacarpals. When
the slab has set it is fixed to the limb with a flannel bandage.
A confirmatory radiograph is taken twenty-four hours later,
and if the position is satisfactory the slab is fixed in position
with a gauze bandage (fig. 1055), which is tightened as
necessary. The delay obviates the possibility of swelling within the
plaster cast. The patient is encouraged to use the limb, and
suitable exercises of the
fingers, elbow, and shoulder
are arranged in the rehabilitation department (fig.
1056), and four or six weeks
later, according to the age
of the patient, the cast is
removed. Full return of

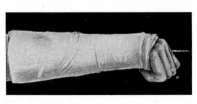

Fig. 1055.—A plaster cast applied for
Colles's fracture.

function is usually obtained after a further three or four weeks.

If after reduction it is found that the fragments are apt to slip, fixation of the hand in a partially flexed position is advisable, so that the extensor tendons can act as splints and so assist in maintaining correction. The drawback to this position is that movements of the fingers are hampered.

In the case of feeble old women disimpaction is unnecessary, all that is needed being a temporary support to the wrist and encouragement regarding movements of the fingers. In fact, medical advice is not always sought, the condition being regarded as a sprain, and the result in these cases is usually very satisfactory.

Sudeck's osteoporosis is an obscure condition which occasionally follows Colles's fracture, but which can occur after a mere sprain; it also sometimes affects the foot. As a sequela of Colles's fracture it affects the small bones in the neighbourhood of the wrist, and is supposed to be due to reflex hyperæmia occasioned by trauma. It is characterised by muscular weakness, pain, vasomotor changes, and atrophy of the bones

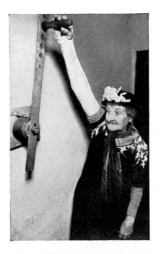

Fig. 1056.—A useful overhead exercise to prevent swelling and stiffness of shoulder.

(fig. 1057). It has been mistaken for tuberculous disease, but differs radiologically in that osteoporosis is not improved by immobilisation. Very gradual voluntary movements are indicated, but if the condition persists sympathectomy should be performed. Although ganglionectomy is the rational treatment, periarterial sympathectomy is worthy of trial, and we have obtained some good results with this simpler procedure.

Rupture of the extensor longus pollicis tendon occurs in 0·5 per cent. of Colles's fractures. It is also apt to follow a posterior marginal fracture of the radius. Rupture, due to fraying of the tendon over the ridge of the fracture, occurs during the second month following the injury. The distal end of the tendon should be sutured to the tendon of one of the extensors of the wrist, or to the extensor indicis tendon.

Average period of disability after Colles's fracture—heavy work twelve weeks, light work six weeks.

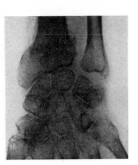

Fig. 1057.—Sudeck's osteoporosis.

Separation of the lower epiphysis of the radius can occur between the ages of two and twenty, but is seen most commonly in the early years of the second decade. The epiphysis is displaced backwards, and the deformity and treatment

Paul Sudeck, Contemporary. *Professor of Surgery, Hamburg.*

are similar to those already described in the case of Colles's fractures. If reduction is unsatisfactory operation must be performed, so that the periosteum through which the diaphysis protrudes can be divided (p. 1039).

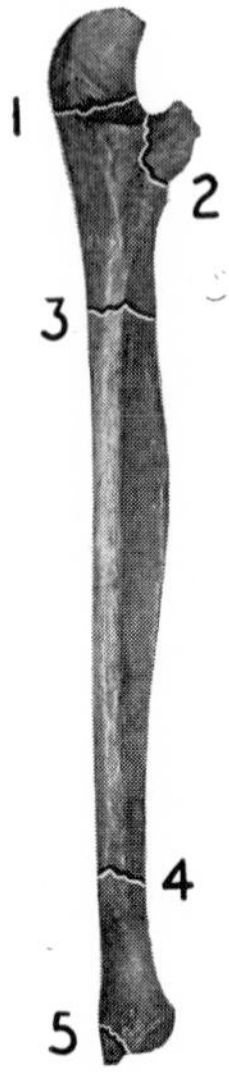

Fractures of the lower end of the radius and separation of the epiphysis, if associated with marked deformity, are liable to be accompanied by stretching, or hæmorrhage into the sheath of the median nerve. Evidence of nerve injury should be sought before reduction and immobilisation.

Fractures of the **Ulna** (fig. 1058).

(i) The *olecranon process* is usually fractured as a result of falls on the elbow. Separation commonly occurs through the constricted base of the process, and may be almost negligible if the triceps expansion remains untorn. If wide separation is present, diagnosis is easy, as the gap between the process and the shaft can be palpated, and the power of extension is lost.

If separation is sufficient to require operation, the fragment is easily fixed in position by means of a vitallium screw (fig. 1059), kangaroo tendon, or silk. No plaster fixation is necessary, and active movements are encouraged after two or three days.

FIG. 1058.—Ulna.

1. Olecranon process.
2. Coronoid process, which may complicate dislocation of the elbow joint.
3. Upper third of shaft, which may be associated with dislocation of the head of the radius.
4. Lower part of shaft, as from direct violence.
5. Styloid process.

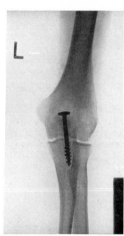

FIG. 1059. — Fracture secured by " lag " screw. (*The A.P. film also showed perfect position.*)
(*Royal Northern Operative Surgery.*)

The *coronoid process* is occasionally fractured, usually in conjunction with a posterior dislocation of the elbow joint. The condition should be suspected when the dislocation recurs after apparently successful reduction. Treatment consists in maintaining complete flexion for three weeks, in order to relax the brachialis anticus muscle. If flexion of the elbow joint is subsequently limited, removal of the process may be necessary, as accurate fixation is difficult and results in callus formation.

(ii) Fractures of the *shaft* of the ulna are due to direct or indirect violence. In the latter case they are sometimes associated with dislocation of the head of the radius (Monteggia's fracture, p. 1048). Diagnosis is easy, as the bone is subcutaneous, and displacement or localised tenderness is readily palpable.

The upper fragment is usually pulled slightly forwards by the brachialis anticus, and the lower fragment inwards by the pronator quadratus. Treatment consists in immobilising the forearm either by splints or preferably by a plaster cast, in a position of partial flexion and mid-supination. If manipulation is unsatisfactory, open reduction is easy and gives good results.

(iii) The *styloid process* of the ulna is commonly avulsed, or the ulnar carpal ligament torn, in association with a Colles's fracture (fig. 1052). The maintenance of the hand in a position of adduction, which is an integral part of the treatment of Colles's fracture, approximates the position of the ulnar styloid process or of the ruptured ligaments.

Fractures of the **Radius** and **Ulna** are due to direct or indirect violence. In the former case the bones are fractured at approximately the same level, which depends upon the site of injury. If the fractures are due to indirect violence, the radius usually fractures in its lower third, and the ulna about its centre. The position of the fragments depends on the direction of violence and the site of fracture ; some approximation of the fractured ends is common, with consequent risk of cross-union (fig. 1060). Reduction is attempted by an assistant exercising traction on the hand with counter-extension by a padded calico loop over the upper arm, while the surgeon applies interosseous pressure in order to separate

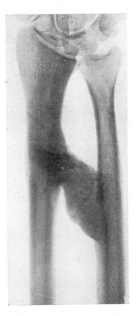

Fig. 1060.—Cross-union following fractures of the radius and ulna.

the broken bones. A posterior plaster slab is applied from the middle of the arm to the knuckles, and is moulded to the contour of the limb. An anterior slab is then applied, extending from the elbow to the wrist, and a wooden rod is pressed into the plaster so as to augment separation of the bones. A gauze bandage is then applied over the arm, forearm, and wrist. Should manipulation fail, as is sometimes the case if the bones are fractured at approximately the same level, the open reduction is performed and the bones fixed with bone plates if necessary. In some cases operation on one bone only will be sufficient, usually the radius, which suffers more displacement than the ulna. Exposure is obtained by an incision along the outer side of the forearm, between the supinator longus and the extensor tendons and muscles. If necessary, the ulna is exposed by a separate incision over the subcutaneous surface.

In 1814 Monteggia described fractures of the upper third of the ulna, associated with dislocation of the head of the radius. The condition usually occurs in young children. Most cases of Monteggia fractures can be reduced by traction. The arm is then fixed in a plaster cast with the elbow at a right angle and the forearm pronated. Failure of reduction demands fixation of the fragments of the ulna and possibly excision of the head of the radius.

Carpal bones are fractured by either direct or indirect violence. In the former case any bones may be involved, and comminution is common. The commonest bone to be fractured by indirect violence is the *scaphoid*. A " sprained wrist " after such an

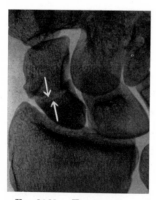

FIG. 1061.—Fracture through the waist of the scaphoid. (A doubtful fracture is often confirmed if the X-ray is taken in an oblique plane.)

incident as falling on the hand, delivering a blow with the fist, or receiving a jerk from the starting-handle of a car should arouse suspicion. If a fracture is present, inspection of the backs of the hands, with fingers and thumb fully extended, will reveal some fullness of the anatomical " snuff-box," and on palpation of that area definite local tenderness is experienced by the patient. X-rays will confirm the diagnosis (fig. 1061) and many fractures show best in an oblique X-ray. Some fractures are only visible after two or three weeks (when decal-

Giovanni Battista Monteggia, 1762–1815. Professor of Anatomy and Surgery, Milan.

cification has occurred along the fracture line). Unless treated efficiently a fracture through the waist of the bone will cause permanent weakness of the wrist and subsequent osteoarthritis. As soon as the condition is diagnosed, the hand must be fixed in 30° dorsi-flexion and abduction. A dorsal plaster cast is applied directly to the skin along the back of the forearm and hand, as far as the heads of the metacarpal bones. The plaster must not interfere with movements of fingers, and the metacarpal bone of thumb must be included. The cast embraces the sides of the forearm and wrist so as to prevent lateral movement. The wrist is immobilised absolutely and completely for about three months, or until there is X-ray evidence of bony union. If " shearing " movements are allowed to occur between the fractured surfaces, the capillaries which bridge the fracture will be ruptured and bony union is thereby discouraged. The patient is encouraged to use his fingers and thumb while awaiting union. A leather support may be worn with advantage for the ensuing three months. Cases which do not present themselves, or which are unfortunately not diagnosed until after the expiration of some weeks from the time of injury, require immobilisation for three months or longer. Removal of one or both fragments may result in permanent weakness and increases the risk of osteoarthritis ; the few cases which remain ununited after prolonged immobilisation are best treated by drilling and further immobilisation, or, as a last resort, by the insertion of a bone peg in order to fix the fragments.

Metacarpal bones and phalanges are commonly fractured, and unless adequate treatment is provided prolonged disability will result. The following principles must be observed—only the injured finger (or fingers) is immobilised, during which period other fingers must be actively exercised, the injured finger must be immobilised in flexion, and during rehabilitation passive movements are to be avoided.

A fracture of any of the four inner metacarpal bones is easily reduced by flexion and traction on the finger and manipulation of the bone. A spiral fracture of the shaft can be controlled by a dorsal plaster slab which extends to the heads of the meta-carpals, and to which the hand is firmly bandaged. Union occurs in four weeks. Transverse fractures and fractures through the neck are more difficult to control, and require a dorsal slab with which is incorporated a narrow plaster strip which immobilises the injured finger in a position of flexion of the metacarpo-phalangeal and interphalangeal joints. Movements of uninjured fingers are maintained and, following removal of the plaster in three or four weeks' time, passive movements of the injured finger are encouraged.

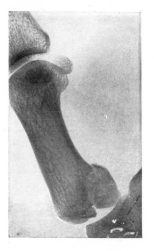

Fig. 1062.—Bennett's fracture-dislocation.

Fracture of the first metacarpal requires special mention, as a fracture of the base (Bennett's fracture), due to a blow on the point of the thumb, may be overlooked. Unless efficient treatment is instituted, permanent weakness may result. An oblique fracture occurs through the articular surface of the metacarpal, which allows subluxation of the joint. The shaft of the bone is drawn backwards and outwards by the extensors of the phalanges (fig. 1062). The fracture somewhat resembles the " stave " of musical manuscript.

The deformity is easily reduced by traction, but immediately recurs when released. Traction is best obtained by means of a plaster cast applied to the forearm, in which is incorporated a loop of thick wire. The injured digit or digits are attached to the wire by strapping, or if more than a moderate pull is required the pulp of the finger is transfixed by a metal pin. This method is desirable in the case of a Bennett's fracture, or if overlap occurs in other metacarpals.

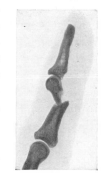

Fig. 1063.—Typical angulation in fracture of shaft of phalanx.

Phalanges are commonly fractured by direct violence, e.g. by a blow with a hammer, or crushed by a door of a car or slipping window sash. If much displacement results (fig. 1063) traction should be obtained by pushing a piece of 0·5-mm. steel wire through the pulp of the finger. A Böhler's finger splint is incorporated in a plaster cast so that traction and

Edward Hallaran Bennett, 1837–1907. Professor of Surgery, Trinity College, Dublin.

flexion can be obtained (fig. 1064). The condition known as "mallet finger" is frequently due to avulsion of the base of the terminal phalanx (p. 1172) rather than to rupture of the extensor tendon.

Ribs and Sternum.

Fractures of the **Ribs** occur as a result of direct, indirect, or muscular violence. In certain nervous diseases, e.g. tabes dorsalis, very slight trauma may cause a fracture.

(i) Fractures due to *indirect violence* may occur while struggling

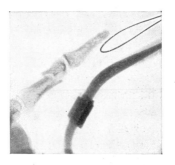

FIG. 1064.—The wire has been pushed through the pulp and fixed to the end of the splint. Finger and splint have then been flexed, thus exerting traction and reducing angulation.

in a crowd, in which dilemma the arms should be kept at the sides in order to protect the ribs (and pockets !). The fifth to the eighth ribs, which are compressed beyond their limit of elasticity, are those usually fractured.

The fracture occurs a short distance in front of the angle of the rib (fig. 1065).

The condition is suggested by the history, and localised pain on deep inspiration. Pain is referred to the site of fracture if simultaneous pressure is exerted upon the sternum and spine.

(ii) Fractures due to *direct violence* affect the ribs most exposed to injury. Thus the first and second ribs are rarely fractured, as they are protected by the clavicle, and trauma sufficiently severe to smash the clavicle and upper ribs is likely to inflict fatal injuries on adjacent structures (hence the introduction of metal epaulettes on army uniforms in bygone days).

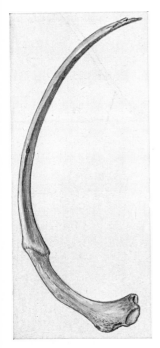

FIG. 1065.—Rib of Robert the Bruce, King of Scotland, fractured by indirect violence while jousting in England many years before his death. (*R.C.S. Museum.*)

Similarly, the lower two ribs are protected by muscles, and enjoy a degree of mobility which diminishes the risk of fracture.

Fractures due to direct injury are more serious than those due to indirect causes, as bone fragments may be driven inwards and damage the pleuræ, lungs, diaphragm, liver, kidneys, spleen, pericardium, or heart. Surgical emphysema is likely to follow laceration of the lung.

(iii) Fractures due to *muscular violence* occasionally occur, e.g. a violent sneeze, especially if partially suppressed. These fractures resemble those due to indirect violence.

The treatment of fracture of the ribs depends on whether there is risk of driving fragments into subjacent soft tissues. Fractures due to indirect violence, muscular action, or direct violence with no depression of fragments are treated by the application of strapping. Strips of adhesive strapping, from 4 to 6 inches (10–15 cm.) wide, depending upon the size of the patient, are applied around the chest, reaching from the opposite side of the spinal furrow behind to the opposite nipple line in front (fig. 1066). These strips are applied at the end of expiration, the patient is requested to emit a long-drawn whistle, and the strapping applied as this becomes tremulous. Additional support is provided by the application of a flannel bandage.

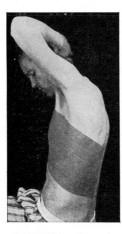

Fig. 1066.—Strapping applied for fractured ribs.

In elderly patients chest complications may endanger life. Local anæsthetic injected at the site of the fractures gives a temporary relief from pain, so that breathing and expectoration can be performed in comfort.

In cases where depression exists, further pressure is obviously dangerous. The patient is therefore propped up in bed, or, if he will tolerate the position, is kept recumbent with a sandbag in the spinal furrow. A close watch is kept for evidence of visceral injury, and operative interference may be necessary.

Ribs, in spite of lack of immobility, unite readily, and support for three weeks is usually sufficient.

The **Sternum** is occasionally fractured as a result of direct violence, e.g. by the steering-wheel of a car as the result of a collision. If displacement is gross, death is likely, owing to injury to or pressure on the heart and great vessels. In less severe cases the patient is confined to bed with a pillow or sandbag between the shoulders, and strapping applied to steady the fragments.

Fracture due to indirect violence is likely to be associated with a fracture-dislocation of the spine, and is due to excessive flexion of the trunk. Treatment is symptomatic, as the more serious injury to the spine takes precedence.

LOWER EXTREMITY

Fractures of the **Pelvis** involve the false or true pelvis, or portions of either.

(i) Fractures of the **False Pelvis** sometimes involve the ilium, but displacement is slight, as the iliacus muscle on the inner side, and gluteal muscles on the outer side, support the bone. Portions of the iliac crest may be fractured and displaced by muscles attached thereto, or the anterior superior spine may be knocked off by direct violence. The anterior superior and inferior spines may be detached by muscular contraction, the former by the sartorius, and the latter by the straight head of the rectus femoris.

If no displacement occurs a firm flannel bandage is applied to the pelvis, and the patient confined to bed until union has occurred. Small detached fragments can be pegged back into position, although no disability follows slight separation.

(ii) Fractures of the **True Pelvis** usually occur in the oblique diameter, i.e. the obturator foramen on one side is involved, and the ala of the sacrum on the opposite side, although in some cases the pelvic ring is fractured in two places on the same side. The cause is some severe crush, such as a horse rolling over its rider, or a light car passing over a pedestrian. Severe shock is common, but if the patient is sufficiently composed, and is unfortunately assisted to his feet by sympathetic but ignorant bystanders, he feels as though the pelvis was " coming to bits." Rapid extravasation of blood occurs, and crepitus may be detected when the patient is lifted.

The most important aspect of a fractured pelvis is the liability to injury of viscera—the urethra commonly, bladder occasionally, and rectum rarely. Therefore the patient should be instructed not to attempt to pass urine, and as soon as possible a detailed examination should be made.

Blood escaping from the external urinary meatus immediately suggests rupture of the urethra, and unless a soft rubber catheter can be passed into the bladder, steps must be immediately taken to suture the urethra (p. 757).   Should no blood be escaping, a catheter is passed, and a small quantity of blood-stained urine will suggest rupture of the bladder, which is usually extraperitoneal (p. 698).   A rectal examination is made, and in rare cases a fragment of jagged bone may be encountered.   In such cases the anal canal should be divided from the anus below to the rent above in order to provide drainage for the inevitable infection.   The wound is lightly packed with gauze soaked in mild antiseptic, and an iliac colostomy performed in order to divert fæces.   Wounds of the vagina are rare and can usually be sutured.

Having methodically excluded or dealt with visceral lesions, attention is directed towards the fracture.   In some instances fragments may be more or less adequately replaced; thus a finger in the rectum or vagina may exert pressure on, and improve the position of, a displaced piece of sacrum or pubic bone.   A plaster cast is then applied so as to embrace the lower part of the trunk and upper third of the thighs, and the patient sits out of bed in a few days.   The pelvic bones readily unite, but walking is prohibited for some weeks, depending on the site and nature of the fracture.

(iii) **Incomplete** fractures include those of the acetabulum, ischial tuberosity, the sacrum, and coccyx.

Fractures of the *acetabulum* occur either in connection with dislocation of the hip joint (p. 1132) or following a heavy fall on the great trochanter. In the former case the upper or posterior part of the rim is carried away with the head of the femur, and the condition is suspected if the dislocation tends to recur after reduction.   Extension is required for six weeks in an abducted position.

In the case of falls upon the trochanter, any degree of injury may occur from a fissured acetabulum to central dislocation of the head of the femur, in which case it is driven through the acetabulum into the pelvis, where it can be felt on rectal or vaginal examination.   If deformity exists, reduction must be attempted under anæsthesia, and weight extension applied for six to eight weeks, followed by the use of a walking calliper until consolidation is satisfactory.   Degenerative arthritis may ensue from injury to the articular cartilage.

The *ischial tuberosity* may be cracked as a result of a fall on the buttocks, as by withdrawal of a chair when a person is about to sit down.   The diagnosis is suggested by persistent pain and unwillingness to sit on the centre of a chair.   A radiograph may clinch the diagnosis, but displacement is slight.   Treatment is symptomatic.

The *sacrum* is fractured by either direct or indirect violence.   The latter is usually associated with fracture of the pelvis. Fracture from direct violence, e.g. a fall or kick, may result in displacement and consequent injury to sacral nerves or pressure on the rectum. The displacement can sometimes be detected and partially corrected on rectal examination. Treatment otherwise is conducted along the lines suggested for fractures of the true pelvis.

The *coccyx* may be fractured as a result of kicks, falls, or even parturition. Pain, which is often severe, occurs on walking, sitting, or actions which cause contraction of the levator ani, such as defæcation or coughing. Rectal examination reveals local tenderness and often deformity. It should be remembered that the sacrococcygeal joint usually enjoys some degree of movement until middle age is reached.

In some cases these symptoms are produced when no fracture is evident, the condition being known as *coccydynia*, which is probably due to traumatic periostitis, with possible involvement of the lowest sacral and coccygeal nerves.

If adequate rest and symptomatic treatment are of no avail, excision of the coccyx should be performed.

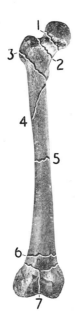

Fig. 1067.—Femur.

1. Common site for adduction fracture.
2. Abduction fracture, often comminuted.
3. Per-trochanteric fracture.
4. Spiral fracture of upper third of shaft, due to indirect violence.
5. Transverse fracture of the middle of shaft, due to direct violence.
6. Supracondylar.
7. T-shaped into joint.

Fractures of the **Femur** are of the greatest surgical importance, both on account of difficulties in treatment and also because of the disability which results if such is inefficient.

(i) Fractures of the **Upper End.** These occur near the head of the bone, near the trochanters, or through the trochanters (fig. 1067). For practical purposes, fractures of the femoral neck are divided into adduction fractures, due to indirect

In 1858 Sir James Y. Simpson, of Edinburgh, the discoverer of the anæsthetic properties of chloroform, coined the term coccydynia.

violence, and abduction fractures, which are impacted and due to a fall on to the great trochanter. In addition, separation of the epiphysis sometimes occurs, and the great or small trochanter may be separated from the femur.

(*a*) *Adduction* fractures are common in elderly people, especially females, owing to atrophic changes which occur in the bone, particularly atrophy of the strong lamina which runs in the neck of the femur from the small trochanter to the head—the calcar femorale of Merkel. The accident usually occurs as a result of indirect violence, often of a trivial nature, such as catching the toe in a mat. The line of fracture is usually sub-capital or through the neck of the bone (intracapsular).

The head of the bone may not be completely separated from the neck owing to some of the retinacular fibres remaining intact. These fibres are reflected from the under-surface of the capsule at its attachment to the neck of the femur, and pass inwards along the neck of the bone. Impaction only occurs if the patient falls on the injured limb at the time of the fracture.

The diagnosis is usually made without difficulty ; typically an elderly person suffers some slight accident, followed by inability to use the limb. On inspection the limb is everted and shortened, the eversion being due to the weight of the limb and to the pull of the psoas muscle, which becomes an external rotator when the neck of the femur is fractured. The ilio-tibial band is felt to be relaxed, but movements should not be at-tempted, as unnecessary pain is caused, and intact retinacular fibres may thereby be torn and avascular necrosis of the head thus encouraged. The great tro-chanter is above Nélaton's line, which connects the anterior superior iliac spine to the most prominent part of the ischial tuberosity. Bryant's triangle, which is formed by drawing a line backwards from the anterior superior iliac spine, a second line from the spine to the top of the great trochanter, and a third from the top of the great trochanter upwards to meet the first line, also demonstrates elevation of the great trochanter, in

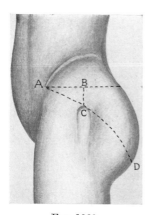

FIG. 1068.

A D = Nélaton's line.
A B C = Bryant's △.

Karl L. Merkel, 1812–1876. Professor of Oto-rhino-laryngology, Leipzig.
Auguste Nélaton, 1807–1873. Professor of Clinical Surgery in the University of Paris.
Sir Thomas Bryant, 1828–1914. Surgeon, Guy's Hospital, London.

that the base (fig. 1068 B–C) is shorter than the corresponding measurement on the normal leg.

These geometrical tests were of great practical importance in the pre-radiographic era. Modern investigation demands that every patient who, even after slight injury, complains of pain and limitation of movement of the hip *must be subjected to X-ray examination.*

Diagnosis must be made from severe bruising, in which case shortening and eversion are absent. Osteoarthritis associated with trauma may present difficulty, in that shortening and crepitus are present, but eversion, complete loss of power, and relaxation of the ilio-tibial band are absent. In cases of dislocation the head of the bone is felt in an abnormal position.

Treatment depends upon the general condition of the patient. The age of the patient is almost immaterial, and many nonagenarians have benefited by Smith-Petersen's nail.

If the patient is feeble or shocked, skeletal traction on a Braun's splint is advisable for a week or ten days. Under local anæsthesia a Steinmann's nail is hammered through the tibia, $\frac{1}{2}$ inch (1·25 cm.) behind the tuberosity, from the inner side. The puncture holes are protected with a covering of Mastisol and balsam of Peru on cottonwool. A Böhler's U-shaped stirrup is then attached to the nail. Movement can thus occur between the stirrup and nail, without any movement of the nail in the bone, which would encourage infection. The limb is then slung in a Morrison's modification of the Balkan frame (p. 1061). The direction of traction is in the line of the femur, and external rotation is overcome by a cord passing from the outer part of the nail to the horizontal part of the frame. The splint and beam are abducted as far as necessary, and the splint is then tied to the foot of the bed. Counter-traction is obtained by elevating the foot of the bed, and a firm support is placed at the end of the bed, so that

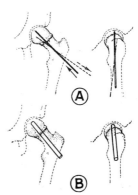

FIG. 1069.—A. Insertion of guide wires. The one in good position is retained. B. The nail is inserted and the wire withdrawn.
(*A.P. and lateral views.*)

Marius N. Smith-Petersen, Contemporary. Professor of Orthopædic Surgery, Harvard.
Heinrich Braun, 1862–1934. Professor of Surgery, Leipzig.

the patient can push against this with his sound leg so as to adjust his position to his liking.

In the majority of cases a Smith-Petersen nail is inserted through the femoral neck. In patients who are reasonably robust, skeletal traction can be dispensed with, and after a day or two the fracture is reduced and the nail inserted. Reduction is accomplished by abduction, extension, and internal rotation of the hip. Reduction is confirmed by antero-posterior and lateral X-rays, after which the pin is inserted.

Smith-Petersen's nail is of vitallium, and is sufficiently long to prevent angular displacement. The three flanges prevent rotation of the head of the bone.

Before the pin is introduced 3 Kirschner wires are inserted into the head of the bone in slightly different directions. Antero-posterior and lateral X-rays are taken and rapidly developed, and the wire which is seen to occupy the best position is left *in situ*. A pin with a hollow centre is then driven along the wire. X-ray control ensures good apposition, and the wire steadies the head of the bone so that the impact of the nail causes no displacement. Unless the blood-supply to the femoral head is impaired, bony union occurs in six months or so, with painless, free movements of the knee and hip, and negligible wasting of muscles. It is important that knee exercises are begun the day after the operation, and movements of the hip are allowed when discomfort has subsided.

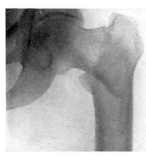

Fig.1070.—Abduction fracture of the femoral neck.

(*b*) *Abduction* fractures most commonly occur in young men as a result of a fall on the great trochanter (fig. 1070).

The deformity resembles the adduction fracture in that shortening and eversion are usually present, but in this case shortening is due to impaction rather than to muscular contraction, and eversion is due to more extensive comminution and impaction posteriorly than anteriorly, as the posterior aspect of the neck of the femur is the more brittle. In addition, marked bruising over the region of the great trochanter is present. Shortening is variable in amount, and depends on the degree of impaction. As the fracture is impacted, loss of power is not complete and limited movements of the hip are painless. Cases have occurred in which the patient has succeeded in walking after the injury, or even sought medical

Martin Kirschner, Contemporary. Professor of Surgery, Heidelberg.

advice only for the condition to be overlooked by the doctor! Nélaton's line and Bryant's triangle confirm the elevation of the great trochanter, but X-rays must be taken if the slightest doubt exists regarding the possibility of a fracture.

In some cases, owing to the direction of violence, inversion may occur instead of eversion.

Treatment usually consists in the application of a plaster spica (fig. 1071). No attempt should be made at reduction, as disimpaction will convert the fracture into the more serious adduction variety. After six to eight weeks the patient is fitted with a walking calliper, which is worn for about three months. If impaction is firm the plaster spica is unnecessary, and a walking calliper is fitted a few days after the injury.

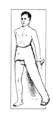

FIG. 1071.—Plaster applied by Whitman's method.

Bony union usually occurs, but some limitation of movement may result from callus formation, and the older the patient the greater is the risk of subsequent osteoarthritis.

(*c*) Fracture through the trochanters and Kocher's pertrochanteric fracture also occur as a result of direct violence. Owing to considerable bruising and tenderness, the exact diagnosis is seldom possible apart from radiography. The fracture is impacted and an adequate blood-supply exists on both sides of the fracture line, therefore adequate immobilisation should result in bony union.

Treatment.—Nailing is the ideal treatment provided that comminution does not prevent a firm bite. The nail is inserted about 2 inches (5 cm.) below the great trochanter. If the fracture is comminuted and unsuitable for nailing, a Roger Anderson's "Well leg traction" splint is applied (fig. 1072). The normal limb is encased in plaster from the sole to the upper thigh, and the splint is incorporated in the plaster. On the side of the fracture a pin is driven through the lower end of the tibia just above the ankle joint, and incorporated in a plaster from the toes to below the knee. Traction on the injured limb is obtained by means of a screw, and as the pelvis, the sound leg, and the cross-bar of the splint are stable, adequate traction will immobilise the fracture. The patient can sit up in bed, perform

Royal Whitman, Contemporary. Consulting Surgeon, Hospital for the Ruptured and Crippled, New York.
Theodore Kocher, 1841–1917. Professor of Surgery, University of Berne.

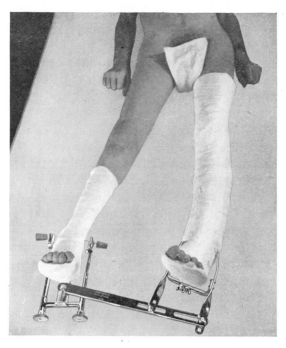

Fig. 1072.—" Well leg traction " splint. (*Watson-Jones.*)

quadriceps drill, and move his toes. The splint is removed when X-ray reveals sound union of the fracture, usually in about twelve weeks.

(*d*) Traumatic separation of the epiphysis of the head of the femur is of rare occurrence. The centre appears during the first year, and unites at the age of twenty. The clinical features resemble those of an intracapsular fracture, and treatment is conducted on similar lines; but if reduction is unsatisfactory, open operation should be performed, as irregular growth may subsequently lead to coxa vara.

(*e*) Fracture of the great trochanter occasionally results from direct violence, and pegging will be necessary if displacement is other than slight. Before the age of eighteen years this injury is a separation of the epiphysis.

(*f*) Avulsion of the small trochanter is sometimes caused by sudden contraction of the ilio-psoas. The commonest age for this accident is about puberty, in which case the epiphysis is separated. The condition is unlikely to be diagnosed without the assistance of X-rays. Treatment consists in immobilising the limb for five or six weeks in a position of flexion and eversion.

(ii) Fractures of the **Shaft** of the femur occur at any site; those in the upper part are usually due to indirect violence, and those nearer the knee joint are more commonly caused by direct injury.

Displacement depends on the direction of violence, muscular contraction, and gravity. In the upper third the upper fragment is flexed by the ilio-psoas, abducted by the gluteal muscles, and everted by the external rotators. The lower fragment is adducted by the adductor muscles, drawn upwards by the hamstrings and everted by the weight of the limb.

In the middle third fractures result from either direct or indirect violence. In the former case comminution may occur, and the line of fracture is transverse, while in the latter it is oblique. Displacement in fractures due to direct violence depends to some extent on the direction in which the violence was applied, but tends to resemble the position assumed in cases due to indirect violence. Thus the upper fragment is flexed, abducted, and slightly everted, while the lower fragment is displaced backwards, upwards, and rotated outwards.

Fractures of the lower third, being due to direct violence, are usually transverse. The lower fragment is drawn downwards and backwards by the gastrocnemius, and may cause injury to structures in the popliteal space. Eversion is present owing to the leg rolling outwards.

Restoration of alignment is essential if a satisfactory result is to be obtained, particularly in the case of the femur, which is a single, weight-bearing bone. Also alteration of direction of the lines of stress associated with malalignment throws an abnormal strain upon the hip or knee joint, and osteoarthritis is prone to develop in later life.

Many varieties and modifications of splints have been devised for the treatment of fractures of the femur ; those most commonly used are the following :

Morrison's modification of the Balkan frame is made from gas piping, and it can be assembled and dismantled easily (fig. 1073). The upper end of the tibia is transfixed by a Steinmann's nail, and a cord is fixed to the tractor or stirrup and brought over a pulley on the Balkan frame, and adequate weights are attached in order to obtain balanced traction. External rotation is prevented by a cord which connects the outer part of the nail with the overhead frame. Counter-traction can be obtained by elevating the foot of the bed.

Thomas's Knee Splint.—This consists of a ring padded with leather, which may be softened if necessary by the application

Gordon M. Morrison, Contemporary. Orthopœdic Surgeon, Boston City Hospital.
Hugh Owen Thomas, 1834–1891, of Liverpool. The son of a famous bone-setter, and the founder of orthopœdic surgery. Introduced his splint in 1886.

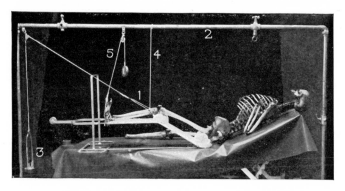

Fig. 1073.—1. U-shaped tractor or stirrup. 2. Morrison's frame. 3. Spain's type of weight-hanger and weights. 4. Cord controlling external rotation. 5. Cord and weight preventing drop-foot.

of soap, or further padded with chamois leather. Extending from the ring on either side is an iron bar, which reaches about 4 inches below the foot, the two lateral bars being joined by a cross-bar. The limb is passed through the ring, which comes to rest against the ischial tuberosity. The traction apparatus is fixed on the leg, the splint is fitted, and traction exerted either by a weight attached to a cord which runs over a pulley, or by strapping.

The limb is supported by a trough composed of pieces of soft leather, which are fixed to the splint by means of large paper-clips. Sagging of a fragment can be remedied by tightening the appropriate support, and lateral displacement corrected by passing a loop around the limb and fixing it to one of the lateral bars of the splint. The bottom of the bed is raised on blocks in order that the weight of the patient may provide counterextension. A movable leg piece can, with advantage, be attached to the splint, so as to allow movements of the knee joint and prevent stiffness.

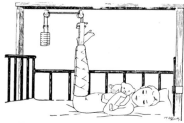

Fig. 1074.—A " gallows " splint.

A *gallows splint* (fig. 1074) is useful for children below the age of five years. Traction is applied by means of strapping, and the legs are slung up to the cross-piece, so that the pelvis is just lifted from the mattress. The child's weight acts as counter-traction, and this position is very convenient for nursing purposes.

Treatment.—(*a*) *Upper End.*—A fracture at this level must be treated in abduction, as it is impossible to manipulate the short and deep upper fragment, which is flexed and abducted. Skeletal traction is obtained by a Steinmann's pin through the tibia.

(*b*) *Shaft.*—After reduction immobilisation is maintained either by a Thomas's splint and adhesive strapping, or by skeletal traction. In the latter case, a Steinmann's pin is driven through the tibia behind the tubercle and sufficient weight is applied in order to maintain reduction without distraction. Check X-rays are taken at intervals. After about two months the pin is removed and skin traction substituted.

Interposition of muscle between the fragments may prevent reduction. Absence of crepitus on attempted reduction suggests the condition. The fracture must then be exposed by a lateral incision, so that the ends can be freed and interlocked. Skeletal traction is then applied.

(*c*) *Lower End.*—The lower fragment is flexed by the gastrocnemius, and manual reposition is impossible. Vertical traction applied to the lower fragment and skeletal traction of the limb are necessary for good alignment. A Hawley's table is used, and a pin is driven through the lower fragment close to the fracture, and a second pin behind the tibial tubercle. Vertical traction is applied to the fragment and counter-pressure by means of a sling which passes over the thigh to a bar under the table. If a check X-ray shows that backward angulation is not completely corrected a second sling is applied over the knee joint (fig. 1075). When the X-ray shows good alignment the plaster is

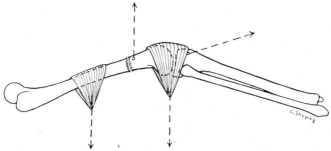

Fig. 1075.—Treatment of supracondylar fracture. (*Watson-Jones.*

applied and firmly incorporates the pins, the knee joint being flexed at about 10 degrees. The table is then adjusted so that a spica can be applied. After a month the spica is replaced and the pins are removed, and immobilisation is continued until the fracture has united.

Average period of disability after fracture of the shaft of the femur— heavy work forty weeks, light work thirty weeks.

(iii) Fractures involving the knee joint. T- or Y-shaped fractures occur as a result of direct violence. A variable degree of separation of the condyles occurs, and the joint is rapidly distended with blood. Aspiration is performed, but in some cases open operation is advisable, so that blood can be evacuated and the fragments fixed if necessary (p. 1027). Massage and active movements are commenced after the third day in order to prevent muscular atrophy and to minimise adhesions.

One or other condyle is sometimes separated, either by direct violence or as a result of a fall on the knee. Treatment is conducted as for fractures implicating joints.

Separation of the lower epiphysis was more common in the days of horse-drawn vehicles, when children enjoyed the excitement of riding on the rear axle. Entanglement of the foot in the spokes caused violent hyperextension of the leg and forward separation of the epiphysis. The lower end of the diaphysis projects backwards, and gangrene sometimes followed pressure on the popliteal vessels. The deformity is reduced by traction on the flexed knee with the patient lying on his back on the floor, the pelvis being fixed by assistants. After reduction the limb is bandaged in slight flexion, the pulsations of the dorsalis pedis artery being a guide to the circulation of the limb. After about eight weeks, active movements are commenced, and a walking calliper is worn until six months after the accident. If manipulation fails, open operation must be performed, otherwise stunted growth or deformity will result.

Fractures of the **Patella** are due to direct or indirect violence.

If due to *direct violence,* a comminuted or star-shaped fracture usually results. Separation of the fragments is not extensive, and may be absent, owing to the intact aponeurosis of the quadriceps expansion and periosteum, which hold them in position. Considerable bruising and effusion into the joint are to be expected. Aspiration of the joint is often desirable.

A posterior plaster slab is applied for a week, after which active movements are encouraged.

Fractures due to *indirect violence* occur when the knee is semi-flexed. In this position the patella is balanced on the front of the condyles, and sudden contraction of the quadriceps, as in an effort to regain balance, snaps the bone in the same manner as a stick is broken across the knee. The fracture usually occurs in the lower third of the bone, the smaller fragment being tilted forwards by contraction of the patellar ligament. The fracture may be heard by the patient, who falls to the ground, possibly on to the injured knee, in which case a vertical fracture of the patella may convert the transverse fracture into a comminuted one. Local pain and loss of power to extend the leg are prominent symptoms. The joint rapidly fills with blood, and the gap between the fragments can sometimes be seen, and in any case is readily palpable, this feature distinguishing the condition from rupture of the quadriceps tendon. Owing to separation of the fragments, and the interposition of torn aponeurosis, fibrous union will occur unless operation is undertaken. Moreover, in cases treated conservatively, the band of fibrous tissue which unites the fragments will stretch, and eventually the fragments will be widely separated (fig. 1029).

Treatment is therefore operative, unless some contraindication exists. Five or six days' confinement to bed allows œdema to absorb, otherwise anatomical structures and planes are obscured. Operation is then performed as follows :

A curved flap is turned downwards, so that the scar is not subjected to pressure, and aponeurosis and blood-clot, which cover the raw surfaces of the fragments, are carefully removed, the aponeurosis being excised with scissors, and blood-clot scraped away with a sharp spoon. The bone is drilled and approximated by kangaroo tendon or Viennese twist, size 3. Silver wire should not be used, as rarefaction of the bone subsequently occurs and the wire becomes loose, which necessitates removal. After the fragments are approximated the torn quadriceps expansion is carefully sutured, and the wound closed. Massage of the quadriceps should be commenced on the following day, active movements at the end of one week, and limited active flexion at the end of two weeks. Normal function is regained after two months.

Excision of the fragments yields good results (Brooke), and is especially indicated if the fracture is comminuted, and in order to obviate osteoarthritis in patients over forty years of

Ralph Brooke, Contemporary. Surgeon, Royal West Sussex Hospital, Chichester, England.

age. The fragments are easily dissected from the tendinous attachments, and the torn aponeurosis is sutured with chromic catgut, size 2. Care must be taken not to shorten the expansion by overlapping, otherwise full flexion of the knee will be hindered. The gap resulting from excision of the patella is closed with vertical sutures as accurately as possible, but some slight inadequacy is of no moment. As with all operations on the knee joint, a firm bandage is applied to control oozing, and it is loosened after twenty-four hours. Active contraction of the quadriceps is begun after three days, and graduated active flexion in one week. Patients are enabled to return to work in from three to eight weeks, according to the nature of their occupation. We have obtained excellent results in selected cases by this method ; there is no possibility of refracture, and however carefully the bone is sutured there is likelihood of a ridge of bone forming on the patella, which predisposes to subsequent osteoarthritis.

Cases due to muscular contraction occasionally occur, in which the bone is fractured, but the aponeurosis remains intact. Localised pain and tenderness result, and a radiograph shows a transverse crack in the bone. Diagnosis is important, as otherwise injudicious movements are liable to tear supporting soft tissues, with separation of fragments. Treatment consists in the application of a posterior plaster slab for three weeks, and restricted movements until two months have elapsed from the time of injury.

In cases in which fibrous union has been allowed to occur (fig. 1029), and which subsequently require operation on account of disability, a two-stage operation is often necessary. At the first operation the upper fragment is separated from the intercondylar notch to which it is usually adherent, and, with the leg held vertically, the two fragments are approximated as nearly as possible. During the ensuing two or three weeks the leg is gradually brought to the horizontal position, thus stretching the quadriceps muscle. At a second operation the gap is usually so narrowed that the fragments can be excised and the tendons and aponeurosis sutured.

Fracture of one patella is occasionally followed by fracture of the other at a later date, possibly owing to some congenital abnormality in the shape of the bones.

Fractures of the **Tibia** (fig. 1077).

(i) Fractures of the *upper end* are usually due to direct violence, one or other tuberosity being separated, but occasionally a Y- or T-shaped fracture is produced by a fall on to the feet. In either case the knee joint is involved, and rapidly fills with blood. A "bumper" fracture is due to a severe blow on the outer side of the joint, e.g. impact with the bumper of a car ; the external condyle of the femur impinges on and wrenches off the outer tuberosity of the tibia (fig. 1076). Accurate reduction, possibly with the help of a redresseur (fig. 1084), is essential, otherwise malalignment of the tibial plateau will eventually result in osteoarthritis.

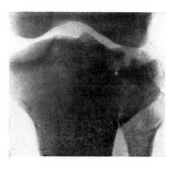

Fig. 1076.—" Bumper " fracture.

As the internal lateral and probably the cruciate ligaments are necessarily torn, the joint should be encased in plaster for three months. Systematic drill for the quadriceps muscle must be practised during the period of immobilisation, as the stability of the joint depends on the tone of muscles. Adequate reduction of the outer tuberosity is more important than that of the inner, as a greater proportion of the weight of the body is transmitted through the outer tuberosity, particularly in females and persons with a tendency to genu valgum.

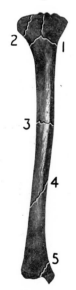

Fig. 1077.—Tibia.

1. Y-shaped fracture involving the knee joint.
2. Outer tuberosity.
3. Transverse fracture due to direct violence.
4. Oblique fracture due to indirect violence.
5. Internal malleolus.

Separation of the upper epiphysis of the tibia is a rare accident, but can occur up to the age of twenty-two years. The epiphysis includes the articular facet for the head of the fibula and the tongue-shaped prolongation in front for the tubercle of the tibia. Adequate reduction must be effected by manipulation, after which a light plaster is applied.

(ii) Fractures of the *shaft* of the tibia, without implication of the fibula, are usually due to direct violence, in which case the fracture is transverse and often comminuted. Diagnosis is readily made, as the bone is subcutaneous and irregularity or localised tenderness is readily palpable.

" Fatigue " fractures of the upper third of the tibia are spontaneous fractures, which occur in young adults, especially when abruptly subjected to strenuous exercises, e.g. military training. Similar " stress " fractures have been described occurring in the neck of the femur, spine, inferior pubic ramus, and other situations. A "march" fracture (p. 1074) is a similar condition. Especially in the case of the tibia, the boss of callus may resemble an osteogenic sarcoma.

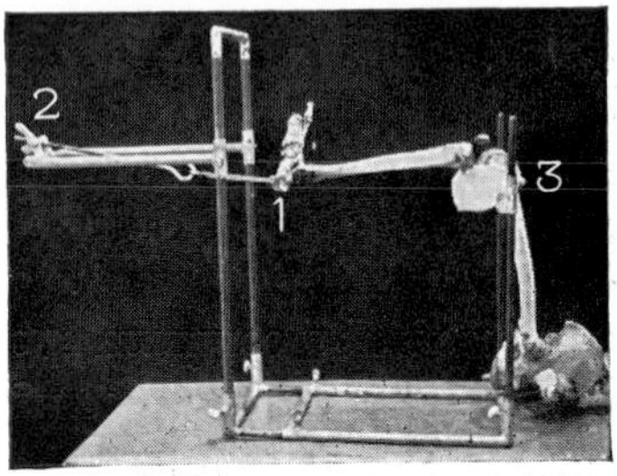

FIG. 1078.—Böhler's screw-traction apparatus. 1. Nail through lower end of tibia, attached by stirrup to hook. 2. Screw and wing nut. 3. Knee flexed to right angle over counter-traction stop and wool pad.

Treatment consists in reduction of deformity and fixation of the fragments by means of a plaster cast.

It should be remembered that in all fractures below the knee joint, correct alignment is only regained when the inner border of the patella, the internal malleolus, and the ball of the big toe are in line with one another.

If reduction is difficult to maintain, as in oblique or spiral fractures, skeletal traction, used in conjunction with Böhler's screw-traction apparatus, is necessary (fig. 1078). By means of the screw the traction is increased until the bone ends are felt in accurate apposition, and verification is obtained by screening or X-ray. The leg and foot are then incorporated in a skin-tight plaster.

Method.—A slab is made from a 6-inch (15 cm.) bandage. It extends from one tuberosity of the tibia, round the heel, to the other tuberosity. It is folded on itself to form a 3-inch (7·5 cm.) slab and applied in the form of a ∪ (fig. 1079), and is incised to fit round the Steinmann's nail. The slab is maintained in position by a 6-inch (15 cm.) gauze bandage 6 yards (6 m.) long. A second plaster slab, 6 inches (15 cm.) wide, is made so as to extend from the tips of the toes, behind the heel to the knee. The edges of the plaster at the heel are incised and folded accurately over each other. Two 6-inch (15 cm.) plaster bandages are then applied circularly. When the plaster has set, the limb is removed from the screw-traction apparatus and laid on a properly padded Braun's splint (fig. 1080). A weight of about

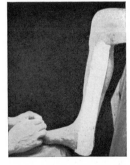

FIG. 1079.—The plaster loop made from a 3-inch slab is in position along the inner and outer aspects of the leg.

7 lb. (3 kgm.) (which is not enough to cause distraction) is attached by a cord to the U-shaped tractor. The foot of the bed is elevated on 12-inch (30 cm.) blocks. The limb is placed in the screw-traction apparatus again at the end of three weeks. The plaster is removed and a new one applied. X-rays are taken subsequently to confirm that reduction is satisfactory and slight angulation can be corrected by wedging. While the limb is in plaster, toe exercises are carried out systematically. No weight-bearing is permitted until the fracture has united clinically.

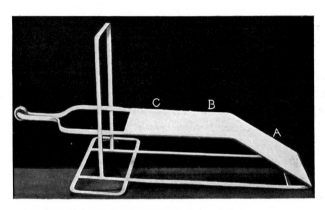

Fig. 1080.—Braun's splint. The oblique bars are bandaged very tightly at A to support the thigh. The bandage is applied loosely at B to allow for the contour of the calf. It is tightly applied again at C for the leg.

Transverse fractures involving the lower third of the tibia are commonly slow in uniting. Fractures of the tibia in children are reduced by manipulation and immobilised in a skin-tight plaster until united.

Average disability after fracture of tibial shaft—heavy work twenty-two weeks, light work eighteen weeks.

(iii) Fractures of the *lower end*. The only common fracture in this situation is a fracture of the internal malleolus. This occurs either as a result of direct injury, or the malleolus may be avulsed following a stumble or slip, which throws the weight of the body on the everted foot. Localised tenderness and ecchymosis suggest the nature of the injury. Treatment consists in reduction and the application of a plaster until union has occurred, and toe exercises in the meanwhile. The inner side of the boot should be raised when walking is resumed.

Fractures of the **Fibula** alone are usually due to direct violence, the lower end being most commonly affected. The procedure of " springing " the fibula assists in the diagnosis, and consists in compressing the fibula against the tibia, local pain being referred to the site of a fracture. A radiograph confirms the diagnosis, and treatment, if any is required, consists in the application of a plaster cast.

Fractures of the **Tibia** and **Fibula** commonly occur either as a result of direct or indirect violence. In the former case the bones are fractured at the same level, but if due to indirect violence the tibia is broken at the junction of its lower and middle thirds, and the fibula at about its centre. The upper fragment tends to be displaced forwards by the pull of the quadriceps muscle, and may pierce the skin, while the lower fragment is usually displaced backwards and upwards by the calf muscles, and is rotated outwards by the weight of the foot.

Treatment is conducted as in the case of a fractured tibia.

If reduction is unsatisfactory, operation should be considered, as malalignment predisposes to osteoarthritis of the knee joint, and fixation of the fragments permits early movements of the adjacent joints. Troublesome " fracture blisters " occasionally occur, and prevent or delay operation. They are probably due to interference with the subcutaneous lymphatic circulation by pressure of extravasated blood and exudate.

Average disability after fracture of the tibia and fibula—heavy work thirty weeks, light work twenty weeks.

Fractures involving the **Ankle Joint.**

Pott's Fracture-dislocation and modifications of this fracture constitute an important group of injuries, as inefficient treatment leads to severe disability and even permanent crippling.

This group of injuries is due to such accidents as slipping off a stair or kerb, or the foot " turning over " while walking or hurrying over rough ground. An abduction fracture follows, due to excessive abduction or eversion of the foot. In the former case the strain falls on the inner side of the foot, and either the internal malleolus is fractured or the internal lateral ligament is ruptured. The astragalus is then forced against the external malleolus, and the fibula snaps transversely or obliquely 2 or 3 inches (5–7·5 cm.) above its lower end. If due to eversion, the fracture is oblique and passes downwards and forwards. In many cases both eversion and abduction combine to cause the fracture, and the foot is then typically everted and displaced backwards and outwards. In some cases the internal malleolus projects through the skin. The ankle joint is

Percival Pott, 1714–1789, St. Bartholomew's Hospital, wrote surgical papers while recovering from a compound fracture of the tibia and fibula.

of necessity involved, and effusion occurs in the tendon sheaths surrounding the ankle joint.

Modifications of Pott's fracture-dislocation :

(i) Continuance of abduction ruptures the interosseous tibio-fibular ligament, or the flake of tibia to which it is attached may be avulsed. The astragalus is forced upwards between the two bones, resulting in marked broadening of the ankle (Dupuytren's fracture) (fig. 1081).

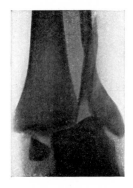

Fig. 1081.—Dupuytren's fracture.

(ii) Adduction fracture.—Inversion of the foot occurs instead of eversion, due to the patient slipping in such a manner that the fibula fractures, and the astragalus is forced against the internal malleolus.

(iii) The tibia is fractured transversely immediately above the internal malleolus, or in children the lower tibial epiphysis is separated.

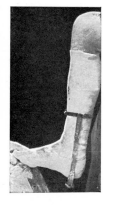

Fig. 1082. — The upright bar of the iron heel is in the line of the leg. It must not tilt backwards or forwards.

Treatment consists in the administration of a general, spinal, or local anæsthetic. The leg must be flexed in order to relax the calf muscles, and the foot is manipulated forwards and inwards in order to bring the astragalus in normal relationship with the tibia. Accuracy of replacement is important, if future arthritis is to be avoided, but a slight amount of inversion, i.e. over-correction, is desirable, and counteracts the subsequent tendency to flat-foot. A plaster cast is then applied, and the incorporation of a metal stirrup in the plaster is an additional aid to ambulatory treatment (fig. 1082). If much swelling is present, a few days' delay is advisable to allow exudates to absorb, so that the plaster (which may be replaced after a few days) will fit more accurately. A plaster cast is necessary for at least ten weeks, the actual time depending on the degree of deformity and the weight of the patient. When walking is resumed the inner side of the heel should be raised $\frac{1}{4}$ inch

Baron Guillaume Dupuytren, 1778–1835. Surgeon, Hôtel-Dieu, Paris. Very parsimonious, and died a millionaire.

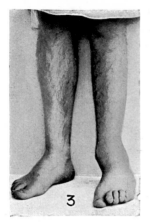

Fig.1083.—Mal-union following a Pott's fracture.
(*Macewen: Practures.*)

(0·5 cm.). In some cases of Dupuytren's fracture, or if the margins of the tibia are fractured, screw traction will be necessary.

Old-standing cases of mal-union and consequent disability occasionally require osteotomy of the tibia and fibula, or even reconstruction of the fracture with more adequate reduction and possibly fixation by screw or peg (fig. 1083).

It cannot be over-emphasised that careful reduction and constant super-vision are essential in cases of Pott's fracture-dislocation and allied injuries, if osteoarthritis of the ankle joint, flat-foot, and adhesions in the joint and surrounding tendons are to be avoided.

Average disability after Pott's fracture—heavy work thirty weeks, light work ten weeks.

Fractures of the **Tarsal** and **Metatarsal Bones.**

The **Os Calcis** may be fractured by falls from a height, a comminuted compression fracture occurring. In other cases the sustentaculum tali, to which the "spring" ligament is attached, may be broken, or a fracture may occur through the body of the bone. In the latter case displacement is usually slight on account of ligamentous attachment, but if complete separation occurs, the posterior part of the bone is drawn backwards by the calf muscles.

Rarely the epiphysis into which the tendo Achillis is inserted is avulsed (ten to fourteen years), or the portion of bone to which the tendon is inserted is separated.

Treatment depends on the degree of deformity. If this is slight, a plaster of Paris cast is applied for a few weeks and the patient is allowed to walk at once. If a portion of bone is avulsed, pegging may be necessary. Compression of the bone is best accomplished by means of a redresseur, which acts on the principle of a vice and exerts lateral pressure (fig. 1084). If flat-foot is likely to develop, e.g. as a result of fracture of the sustentaculum tali, prolonged convalescence is essential. Per-

sistent pain sometimes follows from osteoarthritis of the subastragaloid joint, curable only by arthrodesis.

The **Astragalus** is sometimes fractured as a result of a fall from
a height. If the foot is flexed and supported, as by the strut in
an airplane, the neck of the bone may be shorn through by the

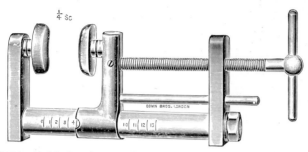

FIG. 1084.—Böhler's redresseur for reduction of fractures of the os calcis and
fractures in the region of the knee joint.

sharp anterior articular surface of the tibia; comminution is
common, and injuries to neighbouring bones are often associated.
As in the case of the os calcis, considerable swelling rapidly
develops and obscures the diagnosis, which is often only conclusive after radiography.

Treatment consists in the application of a plaster cast as soon
as swelling has diminished, and prolonged abstinence from
weight-bearing so as to avoid flat-foot.

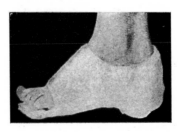

FIG. 1085.—The upper edge of
the plaster shoe follows the lines of
a walking shoe. Ankle movements
are free.

Fractures of the **Metatarsals** commonly occur, either as a
result of falls or crushes, as by a wheel passing over the dorsum
of the foot. Adequate rest is necessary, depending on the
number of bones fractured, and the weight and occupation of
the patient. If considered necessary, a plaster shoe (fig. 1085)
is applied for three weeks, after which an elastoplast bandage
is applied for a similar period.

March fractures (*syn.* pied forcé, pied de jeune soldat) occasionally occur near the necks of the second or third metatarsals. The fracture occurs spontaneously, and is predisposed to by a short first metatarsal. This common atavism causes undue strain to fall on the heads of the second and third metatarsals during such exertions as standing on the toes. The

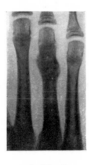

Fig. 1086. — March fracture of the third metatarsal.

fracture is also encouraged by loss of muscular tone, which is predisposed to by wearing heavy boots. Sudden pain, localised over the dorsal aspect of the bone, is characteristic. An immediate X-ray will often fail to reveal the crack, but if repeated in three weeks callus will be obvious (fig. 1086). Strapping and restricted activity only are required. A plaster shoe encourages further atrophy of muscles and renders rehabilitation necessary. Many cases are doubtless treated as " foot strain," and more or less ignored, with good results !

CHAPTER XLI

DISEASES OF BONES

ACUTE INFLAMMATION

Acute periostitis is either traumatic or infective in origin.

Traumatic periostitis is a common condition, e.g. a kick on the shin. A tender swelling follows, due to bruising of the periosteum and sub-periosteal extravasation of blood. Cold applications relieve pain and limit further extravasation, and the blood is usually absorbed. Repeated or severe trauma may result in the formation of a periosteal node of bone, as on the irregular shins of footballers. If the resistance of the patient is low, or if infective foci are present elsewhere, the subperiosteal hæmatoma, in common with hæmatomata in any part of the body, may become infected, since blood-clot is an excellent nidus for organisms circulating in the blood-stream. A subperiosteal abscess results, and unless the pus is evacuated without delay, necrosis of superficial bone may occur.

ACUTE INFECTIVE OSTEOMYELITIS

Predisposing causes of this condition are as follows :

(i) *Trauma.*—Before ossification has occurred, the weakest part of a long bone is at the diaphyseal side of the epiphyseal line. At this level loops of blood-vessels penetrate the epiphyseal cartilage, and constitute a row of perforations across the diaphysis. Any strain imposed on the bone first affects the weakest portion, and rupture of one or more capillary loops is liable to occur, with the formation of a hæmatoma (fig. 1087).

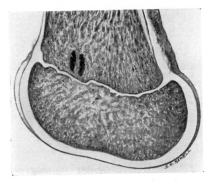

Fig. 1087.—The lower end of a femur, from a child who died of multiple injuries, showing hæmatomata on the diaphyseal side of the epiphyseal line.
(*London Hospital Museum.*)

Juxta-epiphyseal hæmatomata have been demonstrated during necropsy in children who have died from injuries. Also osteomyelitis of the lower end of the femur usually occurs at the posterior part of the epiphyseal line. The explanation is that strains of the knee joint occur when the joint is extended, when the brunt of the force is borne by the posterior ligament, and transmitted to the posterior part of the epiphysis, with consequent formation of a hæmatoma at that site.

(ii) *An Infective Focus.*—Such conditions as infected scratches, tonsillitis, impetigo, or pediculi allow organisms to enter the blood-stream. A hæmatoma in any situation then forms an excellent culture medium, in which organisms rapidly multiply and possibly increase in virulence.

(iii) *Lowered General Resistance.*—The disease is most frequent in industrial areas, where overcrowding occurs and children spend much time in ill-ventilated cinemas. In such places as naval schools, where minor injuries from games, etc., are common, and infected abrasions frequent, acute osteomyelitis is almost unknown, as the general health of the boys is excellent.

Pathology.—The causative organism in the majority of cases is the staphylococcus aureus, other organisms which are less frequently responsible being the staphylococcus albus, pneumococcus, and streptococcus.

The local effects depend upon the actual site of infection, which travels along the lines of least resistance. If infection commences near the surface of the bone, a subperiosteal abscess is likely to form. If infection occurs nearer the centre of the epiphyseal line, extension occurs along the medullary cavity. The changes associated with inflammation of bone are peculiar, in that the vessels in the unyielding bony canals become compressed by exudate and thus the circulation is impeded, with risk of necrosis of adjacent bone. This extending inflammation may affect the whole of the diaphysis, and sooner or later reaches the periosteum, which is stripped up as the collection of pus extends beneath it. Owing to the firm attachment of the periosteum to the epiphyseal cartilage and the resistance of the cartilage itself, subperiosteal pus is unlikely to invade the neighbouring joint, unless the epiphyseal line is intra-articular, as in the case of the head of the femur and olecranon process. Pus finally bursts through the periosteum, and tracks under muscles or finds its way to the surface. If the patient survives, the necrosed bone forms a sequestrum, the surrounding periosteum becoming extensively thickened to form an involucrum (fig. 1088), which is perforated by cloacæ through which pus and spicules of dead bone escape from the cavity containing the sequestrum.

Clinical Features.—The symptoms usually commence abruptly, the child complaining of severe pain near the end of a bone, the pain being aggravated by movement. Shivering or an actual rigor may occur, and the general symptoms of infection are present.

The severity of the general signs of infection depends on the virulence of the organism and the resistance of the patient. In severe cases the child may be comatose as a result of profound toxæmia ; more usually elevation of the temperature by 2°–3° F. and associated increase in pulse-rate indicate a more moderate degree of infection.

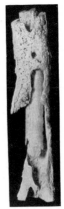

Fig. 1088.— Large sequestrum and involucrum. (*Sheffield University Museum.*)

The local signs depend to some extent on the depth of the affected bone. Thus, if the bone is well covered by muscle as in the case of the lower end of the femur, a localised area of tenderness is the most definite sign to be discovered in the early stages. In the case of a subcutaneous bone, such as the tibia, redness and œdema of the skin, in addition to local exquisite tenderness, will be present in the early stages. In both cases movements of the limb are painful, and likely to be strongly resented. At a later date thickened periosteum is palpable, and sympathetic effusion occurs into the neighbouring joint. Unless efficient treatment is adopted or a fatal issue results, the local signs of pus become increasingly obvious, a painful brawny area appears which gradually softens, and finally an abscess bursts through the skin, the resulting sinus leading down to the bone by a more or less direct route.

Radiography is of little value in the early stages, as bony changes are not usually visible until the end of the second week. Leucocytosis is to be expected, and in half the cases a blood culture is positive.

Differential Diagnosis.— *Acute Infective Arthritis.*—This is an intra-articular condition, and therefore the slightest movement of the joint is painful. In cases of osteomyelitis associated with " sympathetic " effusion, a few degrees of painless movement can usually be obtained, and the maximum pain is near the end of the bone rather than over the joint. If doubt exists, some of the fluid should be aspirated for examination.

Acute rheumatic arthritis is usually polyarticular, and associated with characteristic acid sweats. If the diagnosis is doubtful, repeated blood cultures are necessary.

Hæmarthrosis in children is mentioned on p. 1119.

Cellulitis and Erysipelas.—If the affected bone is subcutaneous, redness and œdema rapidly involve the overlying skin. Constitutional symptoms are usually more marked in the case of acute osteomyelitis, and the changes in the skin remain more localised.

Scurvy.—Subperiosteal hæmatomata are sometimes very tender, and if near an epiphysis the condition may be confused with acute osteomyelitis. If sought for, other evidence of scurvy will be found.

Acute Exanthemata and Typhoid Fever.—These conditions may be suspected on account of the profoundly toxic and even comatose condition of the patient. Careful palpation of the iliac bones and the ends of the long bones is necessary, and if pressure over a localised area induces resentful movements or moaning, then the possibility of osteomyelitis should be considered.

Acute Abdominal Conditions.—Acute osteomyelitis may occur in a vertebra or in connection with an iliac epiphysis. In the former case pain is referred to either or both sides of the abdomen, while involvement of the right iliac bone resembles acute appendicitis.

Complications.—Adequate and early treatment by penicillin and sulphonamides renders serious complications unlikely.

General.—(i) *Toxæmia.*—Some degree of toxæmia is inevitable. Before the advent of antibiotics toxæmia was sometimes fatal.

(ii) *Septicæmia.*—Should be suspected if shivering, rigors, or an intermittent temperature are present. Infection of any serous membrane is likely to occur, particularly of the pericardium.

(iii) *Pyæmia.*—In the acute stages this condition is fatal, for infected emboli are carried to the lungs. Plum-coloured, wedge-shaped infarcts occur, with a small quantity of blood-stained fibrinous fluid in the pleural cavity. Increased respiration, cyanosis, and patches of bronchial breathing are indicative of this complication. Acute pyæmia is particularly liable to occur if the bone involved consists largely of cancellous tissue, e.g. the ilium.

In addition to these acute manifestations, chronic septicæmia and pyæmia can occur and give rise to abscesses in any part of the body, particularly in other bones. These abscesses reveal themselves at any time from the first few days of the disease until after the lapse of many years.

(iv) *Brodie's Abscess.* — Abscesses which occur after a year or more cause intermittent pain near the end of a long bone, with perhaps transitory effusion into the adjacent joint during an exacerbation. The condition is often considered to be " rheumatic," but examination reveals thickening of the bone, and a radiograph is diagnostic

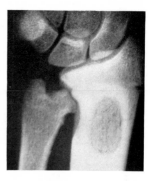

Fig. 1089.—Brodie's abscess with sclerosis and overgrowth of the lower end of the radius.

(fig. 1089). These chronic staphylococcal abscesses were first described by Brodie in connection with the head of the tibia. Free exposure, curetting, and " saucerisation " are necessary, and the cavity is found to contain jelly-like granulation tissue rather than actual pus.

Local Complications.—(i) *Bone.*—Spontaneous fracture may occur, especially if an unsupported bone, such as the femur, is extensively destroyed (fig. 1090).

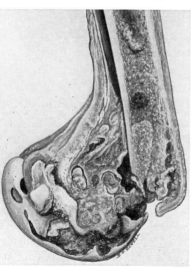

Fig. 1090.—Acute osteomyelitis, complicated by a spontaneous fracture and acute infective arthritis of the knee joint, the cartilage of which is partially destroyed. (*London Hospital Museum.*)

Deformity sometimes follows from interference with the epiphyseal line. Tissue adjacent to the focus of infection is destroyed, but around this area a zone of hyperæmia exists, which encourages increased growth. Therefore, if the destructive area is sufficiently extensive to affect the epiphyseal line, growth is arrested (fig. 1091), but if infection is more localised the hyperæmic zone will stimulate epiphyseal activity and cause growth to

Sir Benjamin Brodie, 1783–1862. Surgeon, St. George's Hospital, London.

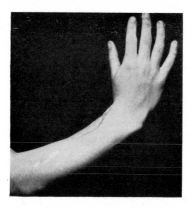

FIG. 1091.—Manus valga, following osteomyelitis of the radius, and consequent diminution of its growth.

be more rapid (fig. 1089). The whole or part of the epiphysis may be affected, and thus regular or irregular growth, or an increase or diminution of growth, results.

(ii) *Joint.* — Acute infective arthritis (p. 1139) occurs in a variety of ways :

(*a*) A subperiosteal abscess bursts into the periarticular tissues, and pus invades the joint through a weak part of the capsule, e.g. where it is pierced by a blood-vessel.

(*b*) Pus may track along a tendon which passes into the joint, such as the biceps in the arm or the popliteus.

(*c*) Very occasionally the infection destroys the epiphyseal line and so directly invades the joint. This complication may occur in young children attacked by a virulent organism.

(*d*) The epiphyseal line may be wholly or partly intra-articular, as in the case of the head of the femur, olecranon process, and inner side of the head of the humerus.

(*e*) Any joint may be affected by blood-borne infection.

(iii) *Muscles and Tendons.*—Œdema occurs in the neighbouring muscles, and effusion in the tendon sheaths. This predisposes to stiffness, which is further encouraged by the desirability of fixation of the limb during the acute stage of inflammation. Therefore, as soon as possible movements are encouraged, particularly in the case of the wrist and ankle, which are surrounded by tendons.

(iv) *Nerves.*—Are rarely involved by fibrosis.

(v) *Blood-vessels.*—Secondary hæmorrhage occasionally occurs if a large artery is adjacent to the affected bone, e.g. perforating arteries in the thigh. Thrombosis of the popliteal vein may give rise to permanent œdema.

(vi) *Special sites*—e.g. osteomyelitis of the pubic bone sometimes causes hæmaturia, owing to local inflammation causing hyperæmia of the bladder. Involvement of the skull is likely to give rise to sinus thrombosis via the emissary veins, or to meningitis by direct extension.

Treatment.—Clinical examination includes a careful search for metastatic foci, and the condition of the adjacent joint is ioted. A blood culture should be performed, and usually penicillin-sensitive staphylococci will be isolated.

Penicillin is administered immediately after the diagnosis is made, and this procedure has reduced the mortality of the disease from 25 per cent. to about 3 per cent. In cases treated within two or three days of onset resolution is to be expected. At least 200,000 units of penicillin are administered daily, either by periodical injections or a continuous intramuscular drip, for a period of three weeks. Needless to say, the limb must be immobilised, and persistent local tenderness indicates the possibility of sequestrum formation. Owing to the widespread and often unnecessary) use of penicillin, resistant strains of staphylococci are increasing in numbers. Therefore, if response to penicillin is disappointing, sulphathiazole, or some other suitable preparation, must be administered. In severe cases sulpha-therapy should be combined with penicillin at the commencement of treatment.

OPERATION is indicated in order to evacuate a subperiosteal abscess, or, in the later stages, to remove a sequestrum.

(i) *Abscess Formation.*—Aspiration is inadequate. A small incision should be made so that all the pus can be evacuated. The wound is then dusted with penicillin-sulphathiazole powder, and sutured. If constitutional disturbance is severe, or if deep-seated pain suggests intramedullary infection, drilling of the bone is advisable (fig. 1092), and the wound is then closed.

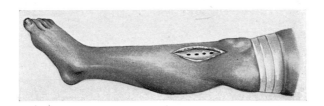

FIG. 1092.—Drilling of the tibia in a case of acute osteomyelitis. An Esmarch's tourniquet has been applied to control hæmorrhage.

If operation is necessary, the affected bone is exposed by the most convenient route, such as :

Upper End of Femur.—Between the tensor fasciæ femoris and gluteal muscles on the outer side, and sartorius and rectus femoris medially (fig. 1157).

Friedrich von Esmarch, 1823–1908. Professor of Surgery, Kiel.

Lower End of Femur.—Between the biceps and vastus externus, o alternatively between the latter muscle and the rectus femoris.

Upper End of Humerus.—Between the deltoid and pectoralis majo muscles, the cephalic vein being displaced inwards.

Lower End of Radius.—From the outer side, between the brachio radialis and the extensor muscles and tendons.

The *Tibia* and *Ulna* are exposed on their subcutaneous surfaces.

(ii) *Sequestrum Formation.*—Sequestra usually occur because treatment began too late or was discontinued too soon. X-ray examination reveals the site and size of the sequestrum, which should be removed with a minimum of exposure and separation of soft tissues. Penicillin should be readministered twenty four hours before sequestrectomy is undertaken. The wound is closed, and healing by first intention is to be expected.

Amputation is very rarely required if treatment can be conducted or modern principles. Otherwise in severely toxic cases, which occur in larg bones, such as the femur, immediate amputation may afford the onl chance of recovery. Owing to lymphangitis, infection of the stump i certain to occur, and therefore, in order to obviate further toxæmia, " guillotine " amputation is indicated. This consists of dividing skir muscles, and bone at the same level, so that no flaps are sewn over th infected stump. As a modification, skin flaps may be fashioned and stitche back over the stump, and if infection subsides they are sutured over th raw surface a few days later, but the principle must not be violated tha any discharge is free and unhindered. Retraction of skin can be limite by the method depicted in fig. 1093.

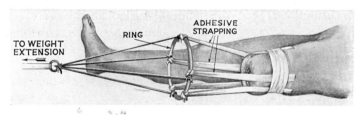

Fig. 1093.—Strapping and weight extension applied to overcome retraction skin following amputation.

Amputation is also necessary if the adjacent joint is disorganisec spontaneous fracture occurs, secondary hæmorrhage is otherwise ur controllable, or if amyloid disease (p. 5) develops.

Mention must be made of a subacute form of osteomyelitis due t *B. typhosus.* This condition occurs at any period of the disease or durin the ensuing two years. The bones most commonly affected are the skul tibia, or ribs, and the inflammation commences in the periosteum. Se ondary infection sometimes follows, and incision and scraping are usuall necessary.

ACUTE TRAUMATIC OSTEOMYELITIS

This condition arises as a result of infected wounds, e.g compound fractures, operations on bones, following amputa tions, etc. The constitutional disturbances are less severe than in cases of infective osteomyelitis, as the causative wound provides some measure of drainage. More extensive opening of the wound, removal of dead bone, or even amputation may be necessary.

CHRONIC INFLAMMATION

CHRONIC PYOGENIC OSTEOMYELITIS

In addition to Brodie's abscess (p. 1079), which is a hæmatogenous infection of a distant bone, acute osteomyelitis may persist locally, and chronic inflammation of the bone is then likely to become a lifelong disability. The risk of this condition developing is now greatly minimised by the modern treatment of the acute infection, but many cases still remain as a legacy of the pre-penicillin era, and more will probably occur if staphylococci become penicillin resistant.

Chronic osteomyelitis may remain quiescent for months or years, but from time to time acute or subacute exacerbations recur, especially if the patient's resistance is undermined by worry, overwork, or other debilitating conditions.

An exacerbation is ushered in with constitutional disturbances and local evidence of inflammation, which may culminate in discharge of pus from a pre-existing sinus. An X-ray sometimes reveals a sequestrum which has separated from the surface of the bone or which lies in a cavity (fig. 1094).

Treatment consists in immobilisation of the limb, the administration of penicillin and sulphonamide, under which régime many cases subside for a variable period. Surgical intervention is required if an X-ray indicates the presence of a sequestrum or cavitation. If a sinus is present a sequestrum may be detected with a probe, which grates on the loose fragment of dead bone. Penicillin is administered for some days prior to the operation, and access to the bone is usually gained through a previous scar. The soft tissues are stripped from the bone with a rasp-

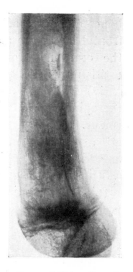

Fig. 1094.—Chronic osteomyelitis of the femur with a cavity containing a sequestrum.

atory, and the involucrum is removed as necessary in order to gain access to the sequestrum. If a cavity is present, the overhanging walls are removed with an osteotome, until it is efficiently "saucerised." The wound is dusted with penicillin-sulphathiazole powder and it is either closed or a tube or tubes are introduced for the subsequent introduction of penicillin.

Amputation is advisable if exacerbations are frequent or prolonged in order to rid the patient of recurring periods of painful disability, and to forestall the onset of amyloid disease.

SYPHILITIC DISEASES

Congenital.—(i) *Osteochondritis* of the nasal septum is the first manifestation. Necrosis of cartilage occurs at the age of about four weeks, and the resulting discharge causes " snuffles." Characteristic depression of the bridge of the nose follows destruction of its support (fig. 28).

(ii) *Craniotabes* of the vault of the skull occurs during the first six months, as a result of absorption of bone. This condition is likely to occur in any debilitating disease at this age, and is often due to concomitant rickets.

(iii) *Parrot's nodes* may appear on the skull during the early years. They consist of patches of periostitis, and if the parietal bones alone are affected, a " natiform " head results ; if the frontal bones are also involved, so that there are four bosses, the term " hot-cross bun " is applied. Similar patches of periostitis may affect the long bones.

(iv) *Epiphysitis.*—Occurs towards the end of the first year, the epiphyseal line being broader than usual and yellowish in colour. Separation may occur, and occasionally infection follows, resulting in so-called " pseudo-paralysis." Periostitis extends from the epiphysis along the shaft of the bone and forms a fusiform swelling, unlike the abrupt expansion of rickets.

(v) *Dactylitis* is a rare manifestation which occasionally occurs in severe cases. The osteitis commences centrally, and a marked periosteal reaction occurs.

(vi) *Overgrowth and Curvature of the Tibia.*—Usually appears towards puberty. The curve is only in an antero-posterior plane, and affects the whole bone. The anterior border of the tibia is rounded, and as the tibia is sclerotic and therefore stronger than a normal bone, no buttress develops in the con-

Joseph Marie Parrot, 1829–1883. Professor of Children's Diseases, Paris.

cavity. These features distinguish the curved tibia of syphilis from that of rickets (fig. 1103).

Formerly, the curvature of the tibia was considered to be due to fixation at either end of the elongating bone by the fibula, but in other cases in which increase of length of the tibia occurs, it is found that the fibula is avulsed from the tibia at its upper articulation.

(vii) *Teeth.*—Hutchinson's notched and peg-shaped teeth affect the permanent incisors (fig. 1095), and Moon's turret-teeth, so called from the absence of the central cusp, occasionally occur in the permanent molars.

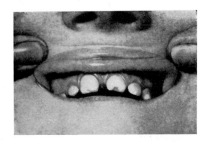

Fig. 1095.—Hutchinson's teeth, characteristic of congenital syphilis.

Acquired.—Secondary stage, osteocopic pains may occur, due to localised patches of periostitis. Permanent periosteal nodes occasionally persist.

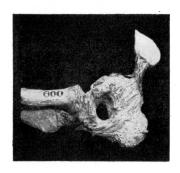

Fig. 1096.—A local periosteal gumma of the manubrium. Secondary infection and necrosis of bone supervened.

Tertiary stage, a variety of osseous changes occur; the following are those usually described, but intermediate forms exist:

(*a*) *Periosteal Gumma.* — Single gumma arising in the periosteum characteristically occurs in the tibia, clavicle, and manubrium (fig. 1096), although other bones may be affected. A firm, slightly tender swelling appears, which is obviously connected with the underlying bone. As the swelling enlarges the superficial structures are progressively involved, and the skin becomes reddened over the indurated tissues. Eventually the skin softens and sinuses form which allow the escape of necrotic material. A punched-out or serpiginous ulcer results, the floor of which is temporarily covered by a wash-leather slough. Secondary infection is probable, and necrosis of bone then follows.

The nasal septum and hard palate are not uncommonly affected. In these situations extensive necrosis of bone occurs,

Sir Jonathan Hutchinson, 1828–1913. Surgeon, London Hospital.
Henry Moon, 1845–1892. Dental Surgeon, Guy's Hospital.

commonly resulting in perforation of the septum or the hard palate.

Multiple periosteal gummata occur characteristically on the skull (fig. 1097). This condition is now uncommon in civilised

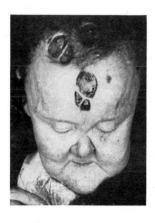

FIG. 1097.—Multiple gummata of the skull. (*A. J. King, F.R.C.S.*)

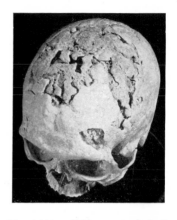

FIG. 1 098.—" Worm-eaten" skull. (*R.C.S. Museum.*)

countries, but the " worm-eaten " skulls of previous sufferers are common museum exhibits (fig. 1098). The local signs are similar to those described above, but secondary infection soon occurs owing to the depth of the hair follicles in the scalp. Necrosis of bone follows, but sequestra may require years to separate, owing to relative avascularity of the compact bone, and associated endarteritis.

TREATMENT consists, in addition to the usual antisyphilitic remedies, in local application of mercurial lotion (*lotio nigra*). Attempts to remove a sequestrum before separation is complete may result in spread of infection to the meninges, or via emissary veins to the intracranial venous sinuses.

(b) *Endosteal Gumma.*—Syphilitic osteomyelitis occurring in the tertiary period affects the shafts of long bones. It is now an uncommon condition, but when it does occur errors of diagnosis are likely, and many a limb has been sacrificed unnecessarily under the impression that the bony enlargement was malignant, e.g. osteosarcoma. Perhaps in no other situation does syphilis more justly deserve its title of " the great imitator."

The chief symptom of syphilitic osteomyelitis is an aching pain in the bone, boring in character, particularly when the limb is dependent, or at night when covered by warm bed-clothes. On examination, some local swelling may be obvious, and palpation reveals thickening of the bone, due to associated periostitis. Examination of the patient frequently reveals other signs of the disease, and the Wassermann reaction is usually positive. X-ray shows marked sclerosis and periostitis, the superficial bone being deposited in the long axis of the shaft, in distinction from right-angled spiculation sometimes to be seen in cases of periosteal sarcoma. Exploration should be undertaken in doubtful cases.

Even vigorous antisyphilitic treatment may fail to relieve the constant pain associated with an endosteal gumma, owing to the protection afforded by the surrounding zone of thickened bone, which prevents remedial substances in the blood from reaching the affected area. Hence trephining or " guttering " the bone is sometimes necessary so as to open up the medulla and allow the re-establishment of an adequate blood-supply to the interior of the bone (fig. 1099).

(c) *Diffuse Sclerosis.* — This consists of thickening of all or any of the periosteal, cancellous, or medullary elements of a bone. The skull and shafts of the long bones are those most commonly affected (fig. 27), and in long-standing cases such a degree of density occurs that the medullary cavity is obliterated.

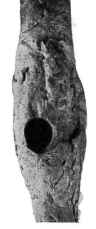

Fig. 1099.—An endosteal gumma. The bone has been trephined in order to relieve pain.

TUBERCULOUS DISEASE

Tuberculous disease of bone is secondary to some other tuberculous focus, the organisms from which reach the bone either via the blood-stream, as from deep-seated lymph nodes, or by direct invasion from an adjacent lesion, e.g. tuberculous arthritis. The disease commences either in the interior of the bone or in the periosteum. (For tuberculous disease of the spine, see p. 884.)

(a) **Endosteal tuberculosis,** other than that due to direct invasion, occurs either in an epiphysis or in the cancellous tissue of the affected bone. In the case of a long bone, infection usually appears near one end, where the nutrient vessel breaks up into capillaries in which the bacilli lodge.

Tarsal and carpal bones are commonly affected, and children are particularly susceptible to infection of the phalanges (tuberculous dactylitis) (fig. 1100).

Tuberculous osteitis is insidious in onset, and for some weeks or months the patient may be conscious only of slight weakness or aching, particularly after use. On examination, some puffiness may be noticed, and palpation reveals slight thickening of the periosteum, due to œdema. At a later stage the skin becomes shiny, the bone is thickened and tender, and muscular wasting is evident. Finally, a subperiosteal abscess forms, which erodes the periosteum and finds its way to the surface, the last stage being represented by sinuses which lead down to the bone and allow the entry of secondary infection.

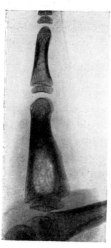

FIG. 1100.—Tuberculous dactylitis. Surrounding sclerosis indicates response to treatment.

Necrosis of bone occasionally occurs in cases of uncomplicated tuberculous osteitis, but separation of dead bone is slow, and sequestra are usually small and spiculated. With the advent of secondary infection larger sequestra are formed and bone destruction is greatly hastened.

Careful clinical examination often reveals other active or latent tuberculous foci, and X-ray examination shows rarefaction of bone, i.e. the density is diminished owing to absorption of calcium, and the pattern is blurred on account of destruction of trabeculæ.

(b) **Periosteal tuberculosis** most commonly affects the flat bones, e.g. the ribs, sternum, or skull. Infection commences in the deeper layers of the periosteum, which becomes œdematous, and is soon separated from the underlying bone by granulation tissue. Caseation and cold abscess formation follow, the superficial structures becoming progressively adherent and invaded, while the bone itself is eroded. In the case of a rib the abscess extends along the bone in a characteristic manner. Finally, the skin is involved and the abscess discharges on the surface, and secondary infection follows. X-rays show erosion of the bone if the condition has advanced sufficiently, but in some cases (notably metacarpals in children, fig. 1101) considerable periosteal reaction occurs (*syn.* spina ventosa).

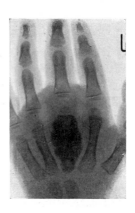

Treatment.—As with tuberculous disease in any part of the body, treatment depends upon the functional value of the part affected and the risk entailed should conservative treatment fail to arrest the disease.

Thus, tuberculous disease of a rib is treated by excision of the affected portion of bone and evacuation of pus. The loss of part of a rib is of little moment to the

FIG. 1101.—Tuberculous disease of a metacarpal, periosteal type.

patient, and speedy convalescence is probable. In the case of osteitis of a tarsal bone, with the exception of the os calcis, removal should be advised, partly to shorten convalescence, but chiefly to obviate the risk of extension of infection to the tendon sheaths and synovial membranes. This latter consideration especially applies to the bones on the inner side of the foot which are in contact with the common synovial sac, and through which infection readily spreads to adjacent bones.

Conservative measures are indicated in cases in which excision of the affected bone is impracticable or would entail grave disability. Immobilisation is essential, and counter-irritation or Bier's passive congestion may be applied. General treatment, including helio-therapy and streptomycin, receives due consideration. The success of conservative measures is indicated by an improvement in the general condition of the patient and diminution of local tenderness and swelling ; also, in the case of endosteal infection, radiography reveals increasing sclerosis around the affected area (fig. 1100). If conservative measures fail the bone should be thoroughly scraped and the wound carefully closed. If abscesses appear, aspiration is performed, and if sinuses form and persist in spite of surgical measures, excision of the bone, or even amputation, is sometimes necessary.

August Karl Gustav Bier, 1861—1949. Professor of Surgery, Berlin.

DEFICIENCY DISEASES

RICKETS

Rickets is a disease not exclusively affecting bones, but involving the body as a whole. The characteristic bony changes may be considered with advantage in this chapter.

Rickets is a deficiency disease, the essential cause being lack of vitamin D, which is a component of natural fats and oils. In addition, lack of sunshine and insufficient ingestion of calcium and phosphorus are contributory factors.

The pathological changes which occur mainly affect the epiphyses, the cartilages of which are enlarged both longitudinally and laterally. In addition, the epiphyseal line, as seen on section, is strikingly irregular. The zone of provisional calcification is either absent or represented by irregular patches, and therefore no definite line of demarcation exists between the proliferating cartilage and the medullary spaces. Instead of being composed of bone, the walls of the medullary spaces are formed of osteoid tissue, which contains no calcium salts, and is not laminated, while the medullary spaces are filled with vascular fibro-cellular tissue instead of normal bone marrow. The deformities associated with rickets are due to lack of rigidity of this osteoid tissue. As the disease is overcome, calcium salts are deposited, and the deformed bones become normal in texture, or in some cases even denser than normal.

Deformities are due to inability to bear the body weight, to the influence of posture, or to the constant pull of muscles bending the softened bones.

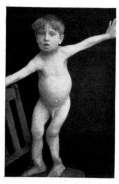

FIG. 1102.—Rickets, showing the deformed legs and pot-belly.

(*Pybus.*)

Clinical Features.—The child is usually flabby, and sweating of the head is common. It is particularly susceptible to respiratory and gastro-intestinal disturbances, and the abdomen becomes protuberant owing to enlargement of the liver and spleen, and flatulence. Umbilical hernia is common as a result of prolonged distension.

Bony developments cause restlessness and peevishness, and the child, on account of epiphyseal tenderness, resents being

1andled.   As the disease progresses deformities appear, among
which the following are typical :

Epiphyseal Enlargement.—The increased width of the epiphyses can
usually be felt.   As the child uses the limbs, compression of the softened
epiphyseal line may cause visible swelling, and as
the child crawls before it walks the enlargement is
first obvious at the wrist, and later at the ankles
(fig. 1102).   These swellings disappear as the disease
fades, and the formation of periosteal bone causes
increased width of the shaft.

Long Bones.—Bending of the long bones is more
marked in the legs on account of standing and walking.   Natural curves are exaggerated and thus the
femur shows increase of the normal anterior curve.
The linea aspera may be thickened to form a buttress.
Bending of the neck produces coxa vara.

The tibia is characteristically bent in two planes.
An abrupt kink occurs in the lower third of the
bone, the portion below this being bent backwards
and inwards (fig. 1103).   A well-marked buttress
formation occurs in the concavity, and the anterior
border of the bone is sharp, owing to lateral compression of the shaft.

Bending of the bones of the arms indicates a
severe degree of rickets.   The radius and ulna are
bent backwards, and the humerus outwards at the
site of the insertion of the deltoid.

Ribs.—The " rickety rosary," due to beading of
the costo-chondral junctions, is of the same nature
as epiphyseal enlargements.   The swelling is more
pronounced on the posterior surface.   Harrison's
sulcus is due to abdominal distension " spreading "
the lower ribs, and not to the inward pull of the
diaphragm.

The Skull.—Craniotabes occurs as a result of any
severe constitutional disturbance, and if associated
with rickets is most obvious in the region of the
lambdoid suture.   Closure of the fontanelles and
dentition are delayed.   As the skull develops it
becomes broader and flatter than normal, and the
increased width between the eyes indicates broadening of the base.

The Spine.—The child is tardy in its efforts to
sit up.   Kyphosis constitutes the first spinal deformity, which may be followed by scoliosis due to
posture or to inequality of the legs.

The Pelvis.—Two types of deformity may result.

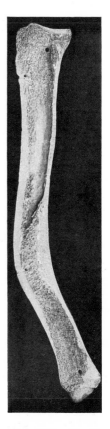

Fig. 1103.—Rachi-
tic tibia, showing
abrupt curvature in
the lower third of
the bone, and well-
marked buttress
formation.

In the flattened type the conjugate diameter is diminished, while if the
lateral walls are approximated, a tri-radiate deformity results.

Stature.—Diminution in stature is due to the following reasons:

(i) The actual growth of bone is retarded, especially that of the tibia
and femur, which may be as much as one-quarter shorter than those of a
normal child of equal size and age.

(ii) The weight of the body compresses the softened epiphyses.   This

Edward Harrison, 1766–1838.   A general practitioner, Horncastle, Lincolnshire, England.

is well marked in the case of genu valgum, as the growth of the weight-bearing external condyle is repressed.

(iii) Bending of the bones of the legs, and by spinal deformities.

Treatment.—Early recognition and appropriate treatment are rewarded by ready response. Fresh milk, cod-liver oil, and meat extracts are administered as freely as the child will digest them. Judicious exposure to natural or artificial sunlight or ultra-violet rays is beneficial, as by this means ergosterol, normally present in the skin, is converted into vitamin D. The child's activities are curbed by means of light splints, but some degree of movement is desirable, otherwise circulation is discouraged.

Early bony deformities respond to appropriate splinting. In the case of the tibia, manual osteoclasis may be necessary, and should be performed during the third or fourth year.

OSTEOCLASIS is performed by resting the leg on a rubber-covered wedge, the leg lying on its outer side. Pressure is applied so that the fibula and then the tibia snap opposite the site of maximum deformity. Care must be taken to grasp the lower end of the bone as close to the deformity as possible, as cases have occurred where the lower epiphysis has been separated. A plaster of Paris casing is applied for three weeks.

In older children or adults osteotomies, either linear or cuneiform, are sometimes necessary.

SCURVY RICKETS

Scurvy rickets is occasionally seen in children who are weaned at an early age. Most prepared foods are deficient in vitamins, and the antiscorbutic vitamin appears to be particularly susceptible to heat.

The disease commonly appears between the sixth and tenth months, and in addition to rickety changes of a variable degree, evidence of scurvy is superadded. This latter condition is evinced by subcutaneous or submucous hæmorrhage, subperiosteal extravasations which are markedly tender (they have been mistaken for acute osteomyelitis), and in more advanced cases by sponginess of the gums and even hæmaturia.

If neglected, the disease may progress to a fatal issue, preceded by separation of epiphyses, melæna, and emaciation.

Treatment consists in the administration of such antiscorbutic remedies as fresh fruit juice, cabbage water, mashed potato, and cream.

Due attention is paid to the associated rickety element.

RENAL DWARFISM

is a rare condition, due to renal insufficiency during childhood, as a result of a condition similar to chronic interstitial nephritis, or, more rarely, polycystic kidneys. Thirst and polyuria, followed by headache and vomiting, are the symptoms which should suggest renal disease, but cardiovascular changes are absent. The blood urea content may be as high as 300 mgm. or more per cent.

Bony deformities appear at any age, and in the early years separation of epiphyses may occur. After the first decade the changes somewhat resemble adolescent rickets, and deformity follows (fig. 1104). This occurs chiefly at the epiphyseal line, and is due to displacement of the epiphysis rather than to bending of the shaft of the bone, a point which distinguishes this condition from true rickets.

Death from uræmia is seldom delayed beyond puberty, and is hastened by any operative interference, such as osteotomy.

LATE RICKETS AND OSTEOMALACIA

Later in life the dietary deficiencies which are responsible for rickets, particularly when associated with unfavourable hygienic and social conditions, may be associated with important bone changes which are called late rickets, juvenile osteomalacia, or osteomalacia, according to the age at which they occur. The lesions of osteomalacia may be regarded as those of adult rickets modified by the absence of growth.

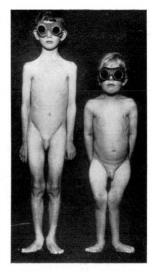

Fig. 1104.—A renal dwarf, with a normal child of the same age for comparison.
(*Dr. Schlesinger's case.*)

Late rickets is a rare disease which occurs during puberty or adolescence. In some cases careful enquiry and examination suggest that this is due to a recrudescence or relapse of the ordinary type of this disease. In a typical case of late rickets the head is not affected, and bending of the bones occurs close to the epiphyses. Severe pain occurs in the bones, which are tender on palpation, and gross deformity occurs in advanced cases. As with infantile rickets, ingestion of substances containing fat-soluble vitamin D results in rapid improvement.

Osteomalacia is rare in this country, although in some localities, e.g. the Himalayas and North China, it is by no means uncommon. In China only women with deformed feet are affected. Nine-tenths of cases occur in females, mostly during the child-bearing age. The condition often appears during pregnancy, but the actual cause is an insufficiency of vitamin D and calcium salts. Tetany may occur in advanced cases.

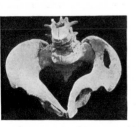

Fig. 1105.—Pelvic deformity due to osteomalacia.

The changes in the bone consist of decalcification of the osseous framework and metaplasia of the resulting matrix and medulla to fibro-cellular tissue. The compact bone may become as thin as paper, and the marrow represented by fatty fibro-cellular tissue of a vascular nature, which has been likened to liver or splenic pulp. Calcium and phosphorus contents of the blood are normal.

The main symptom is pain in the bones, which is deep-seated, and aggravated by movements or pressure. Lassitude and asthenia follow, and gross deformities (fig. 1105) and fractures become increasingly in evidence, especially with repeated pregnancies.

Treatment demands a food rich in calcium and substances containing fat-soluble vitamin D. Cæsarian section is sometimes necessary.

GENERAL DISEASES OF BONE

OSTEITIS DEFORMANS (Syn. PAGET'S DISEASE OF BONES)

This condition, first described by Sir James Paget in 1877, occurs slightly more commonly in men than in women. The generalised disease as Paget described it is uncommon, but in more recent years the detailed autopsy investigations of Schmorl show that localised forms of the disease occur in 3 per cent. of persons over forty years of age. This figure, of course, includes many sub-clinical and non-clinical forms of the disease as well as examples of the classical deforming condition that Paget described.

A peculiar modelling process, which is a special feature of the disease, allows involved bone trabeculæ to be recognised by a characteristic " mosaic " histological pattern.

These changes cause enlargement and softening of the bones. Atrophy of the compact tissue and absorption of the calcium salts weaken the bone, and at the same time spongy subperiosteal bone is deposited. The X ray appearance of the bone at this stage is aptly likened to cottonwool.

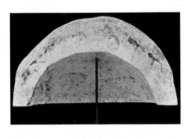

FIG. 1106.—Paget's disease of the skull.

The skull is usually enlarged although not invariably.

Three stages are described, the first being the vascular stage, in which the skull is brick-red in colour and soft in texture. Advancing sclerosis then follows, the skull being greatly thickened and deeply grooved for meningeal vessels. Finally, complete diffuse sclerosis ensues, the diploic zone being almost obliterated (fig. 1106). The cranial cavity is but slightly diminished in volume, as the increase in thickness of the skull is almost entirely eccentric.

The most striking change in the spine is the development of kyphosis, due to softening and yielding of the vertebral bodies. Cases of paraplegia have occurred owing to diminution in calibre of the spinal canal usually in the thoracic region, and improvement has been effected by laminectomy.

The long bones are affected by two processes—absorption of original, and especially the compact bone, and deposition of vascular porous bone. An eccentric enlargement and softening

Sir James Paget, 1814–1899, Surgeon to St. Bartholomew's Hospital, London, described the disease in 1877.
G. Schmorl, Contemporary. Professor of Pathology, Dresden.

follows, with consequent bending, as although the bone is more bulky, it is weaker (fig. 1107). After a period of many years the porous bone gradually becomes dense, and eventually the deformed bones are hard and heavy, i.e. a permanent state of complete sclerosis. Some degree of coxa vara is common.

The pelvic bones, spine, tibiæ, and clavicles are usually affected in the early stages. Involvement of the pelvic bones radiologically resembles secondary carcinoma. The conditions are distinguished by estimation of the acid serum phosphatase which is normal in Paget's disease (p. 1118). The facial bones, base of the skull, jaw, and ribs are involved in the minority of cases.

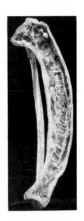

FIG. 1107.—Paget's disease of the tibia.

Chemical investigation of the blood reveals no abnormality in the calcium or phosphorus contents. The alkaline serum phosphatase is usually increased.

Clinical Features.—(i) *Pain* is the most constant symptom, and is usually complained of long before the cause is realised. The tibia is one of the first bones to be affected, and the disease may remain localised in a single bone for years. The tibia in Paget's disease differs from a syphilitic osteitis in that the whole bone bends (fig. 1107), whereas in the latter condition the curvature is mainly due to periostitis affecting the anterior part of the bone, so that the palpable inner border is comparatively straight. Pain is intermittent, and in the case of a subcutaneous bone, hyperæmia of the skin occurs during exacerbations.

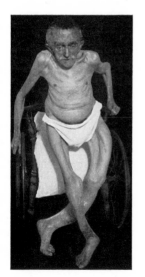

FIG. 1108.—Advanced Paget's disease, showing large head and multiple bony deformities.

(ii) *Diminution of stature*, due to kyphosis and bending of the long bones of the legs (fig. 1108). A diminution of 13 inches is recorded.

(iii) *Increased diameter of the head*, an early indication of which may be the necessity for larger hats.

(iv) *Spontaneous fracture* is common,

and may first bring the patient under supervision. Radiographs often reveal partial transverse fracture, and probably a spontaneous fracture occurs in stages.

Complications.—In about 5 per cent. of cases Paget's disease is terminated by the development of bone sarcoma ; this may be either of the bone-forming or bone-destroying type, and its behaviour is not different from bone sarcoma occurring independently of Paget's disease.

Mesial calcification of the arteries commonly occurs, and the interventricular septum occasionally calcifies, resulting in heart block.

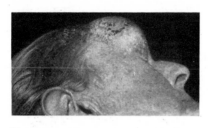

Fig. 1109.—Sarcoma of the skull associated with Paget's disease.
(*Sir Lancelot Barrington-Ward.*)

Necrosis of small areas of bone may occur in late stages following excessive sclerosis interfering with the circulation.

Osteoarthritis occurs in joints adjacent to deformed bones, owing to alteration in the mechanics of the joint. Paraplegia has already been mentioned. Some degree of deafness is common, and is probably due to changes in the bony framework of the internal ear. Death commonly results from intercurrent pulmonary complications.

Treatment.—Ultra-violet rays administered in sub-erythema doses in conjunction with calcium often arrests the disease for a long period. In some cases of Paget's disease the pain due to faulty mechanics can be relieved by osteotomy, and satisfactory union is the rule. Potassium iodide (" the morphia of bones ") often relieves pain in this condition, as with most chronic inflammations of bones.

OSTEITIS FIBROSA CYSTICA (*Syn.* RECKLINGHAUSEN'S DISEASE OF BONE)

This disease usually becomes obvious in the second decade of life, and generalised active bone resorption results in diffuse cystic changes that are widely scattered throughout the skeleton, involving particularly the long bones and the skull. The destruction of bone is associated with the development of fibrous tissue, and sometimes " brown tumours " structurally comparable with giant-cell tumours of bone develop. Fractures, pain, bending of bones, and grotesque deformities occur, so that the patient becomes bedridden.

Cases of generalised osteitis fibrosa have an unduly high calcium content

Friedrich Daniel von Recklinghausen, 1833–1910. Professor of Pathology, Strasburg.

in the blood, often as high as 16–28 mg. per 100 ml. instead of the normal 9–11 mg.,and metastatic calcification is sometimes associated with the disease.

Cases sometimes present themselves with bilateral renal calculi, treatment of which is postponed until the possibility of a parathyroid tumour has been considered.

The blood phosphorus is either normal or diminished in amount. Even when a parathyroid tumour is not palpable, i.e. 80 per cent. of cases, careful exploration is rewarded by its discovery, either embedded in the thyroid gland, or lying at a lower level in the mediastinum. Removal of the parathyroid tumour is followed by an immediate drop in the calcium content of the blood, and by rapid amelioration of the symptoms. Following such an operation reconstruction of the decalcified bones takes place.

LOCAL CYST

This condition usually appears at the end of the first decade. The condition most frequently occurs at the end of a long bone or in the skull. Coxa vara some-times follows a cyst in the femoral neck (fig. 1110). Cysts in other bones attract the patient's atten-tion because of either spontaneous fracture or swelling, depending on whether the affected bone is covered with muscle or is sub-cutaneous. Radiography shows a clear cavity in the bone, which later becomes expanded.

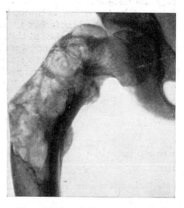

Fig. 1110.—A bone cyst of the neck and upper end of the femur resulting in coxa vara (female, aged fourteen years).

Treatment consists in exposure of the bone and curettage of the cyst, which contains straw-coloured fluid, and is lined with a fibrous wall in which giant cells have been demonstrated. Cure not infrequently follows union of a spontaneous fracture. There is no abnormality of the calcium content of the blood, nor any parathyroid derangement with local cysts of bone.

IDIOPATHIC STEATORRHŒA (Syn. GEE'S DISEASE)

This disease begins in early childhood and is characterised by the passage of offensive fatty stools, and changes in the bones similar to osteomalacia. The patient is usually ill-developed, anæmic, and in severe cases tetany may supervene. It is probably due to some gastro-intestinal disturbance which results in deficient utilisation or absorption of some essential factor. In most cases the serum calcium is below normal, and the plasma phosphatase is increased.

Rapid improvement follows if a diet is given which is rich in calcium and low in fats, together with some preparation of vitamin D. Anæmia is

Samuel J. Gee, 1839–1911. Physician to St. Bartholomew's Hospital, London.

combated with iron, and deformities require splinting pending regeneration of bones.

Thyrotoxicosis and *renal glycosuria* are sometimes associated with osteoporosis. In the former case the blood shows no chemical abnormality, but calcium excretion is increased. In cases of renal glycosuria the plasma phosphorus is below normal, and possibly the renal threshold is lowered for phosphorus as well as for sugar. The osteoporosis follows persistent deficiency of phosphorus in the plasma.

LEONTIASIS OSSEA

This condition consists in a creeping periostitis of the bones of the face and skull. The probable cause is some infection spreading from the nose, accessory sinuses, or possibly teeth. The periostitis is arrested for variable periods at the suture lines, thus the squamous portion of the temporal bone may be greatly thickened and raised above the surface of the skull, while the parietal and frontal bones remain unaffected for years. Eventually the suture line is crossed, and the periostitis creeps on over another bone. The lower jaw becomes implicated, infection presumably reaching it by way of the buccinator muscle and pterygomandibular ligament, as the periostitis commences at the attachment of these structures.

The early symptoms may be those of lachrymal duct or nasal obstruction. The facial bones then become enlarged, and adjacent bones are successively attacked. Eventually hideous deformity results (fig. 1111), and the patient's sufferings are increased by pressure on the eye, brain, and cranial nerves.

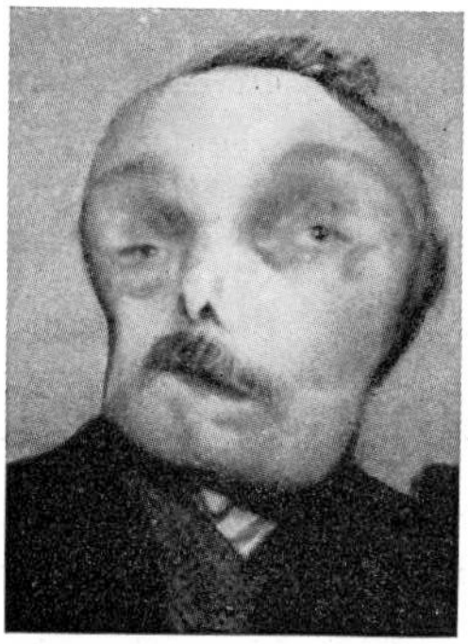

Leontiasis ossea has been mistaken for sarcoma of the maxillary antrum, osteitis fibrosa, and " frog face," due to displacement forwards of the maxillæ by naso-pharyngeal tumours (fig. 117). Treatment consists in dealing with any discoverable infection, otherwise it is symptomatic.

FIG. 1111.—Leontiasis ossea. *(G. H. Kirkland.)* *(British Journal of Surgery.)*

OSTEOGENESIS IMPERFECTA (*Syn.* FRAGILITAS OSSIUM)

This rare familial condition is due to some congenital defect in the evolution of the connective-tissue cells. Normally, some of these develop into fibrous tissue, and those in connection with the osseous system become bone-forming cells. The blue sclerotics so characteristic of this disease are not due to diminution in thickness, and no abnormality can be detected on microscopic examination. The translucency is therefore due to some peculiarity of the fibrous tissue, which suggestion is supported by the fact that another associated abnormality is a tendency to lax ligaments and sprains.

In the case of bone, the evolution of osteoblasts is interfered with, and development stops short at the formation of cartilage cells.

The main clinical feature is an abnormal tendency for bones to fracture. Thus the fœtus may be still-born, the skull being represented by a membranous bag with a few small bony plates, and evidence of antenatal fractures is common. In the infantile type the child is born alive, but the fragile limbs break with distressing ease. In less severe cases fractures begin to occur in childhood or adolescence, and Wormian bones persist in the skull. Stature is diminished, the skull is commonly flattened and

Claus Worm, 1588–1654. A Danish anatomist.

the ears pointed, so that the patient has an elf-like appearance. The fractures are less painful than those occurring in normal bones, and although union occurs readily, deformity is common owing to multiple fractures. Otosclerosis commonly develops about the third decade.

Treatment consists in dealing with fractures as they arise, and of protecting the patient from the risk of injury.

OSTEOCHONDRITIS JUVENILIS

Various lesions, the pathology of which is doubtful, are grouped under this term. Certain epiphyses are commonly involved, and also some bones which develop from a single ossific centre may be affected. The essential changes consist of partial arrest and irregularity of growth, followed by sclerosis. Interference to the blood-supply following trauma appears to be a causative factor, especially the cumulative effect of repeated minor strains. For instance Schlatter's disease has been known to follow training for cross-country running, and Sever's disease has occurred after dancing lessons.

In all cases symptoms are relatively mild, and comprise aching of the affected limb and local tenderness. Relief is afforded by rest and prevention of strain. If the affected portion is palpable, such as the tibial tubercle, enlargement can be detected.

The more important of these conditions are:

Perthes' Disease (*syn.* coxa plana, pseudo-coxalgia). This condition appears between the ages of five and ten, and is three times more common in boys than girls, and 15 per cent. of cases are bilateral. Calvé, of Paris, suggested the name " pseudo-coxalgie," in order to distinguish the condition from tuberculous arthritis, as formerly cases diagnosed as tuberculous disease, which surprised surgeons by their rapid recovery, were undoubtedly suffering from Perthes' disease. Slight pain, especially after vigorous use, and limp, are the early symptoms. On examination, wasting is slight, and movements are restricted according to the extent of bony change. Thus, as the head of the bone becomes flatter, so inversion and eversion are progressively restricted, and if coxa vara supervenes, then abduction also is limited. Flexion and extension, however, are free and painless, and this feature, combined with negligible wasting of muscles, and the robust health of the patient, should prevent an erroneous diagnosis of tuberculous disease. As with other chronic conditions, e.g. coxa vara, traumatic arthritis may be

James W. Sever, Contemporary. Orthopœdic Surgeon, Boston.
Georg Perthes, 1869–1927. Professor of Surgery at Tübingen, Germany.
Jacques Calvé, Contemporary. Surgeon, Foundation Franco-Américaine Hôpital, Berck Plage, France.

superimposed and cause painful limitation of all movements. In these cases a week in bed results in the disappearance of the recent traumatic element and its associated muscular spasm, after which the characteristic features of the underlying condition can be recognised.

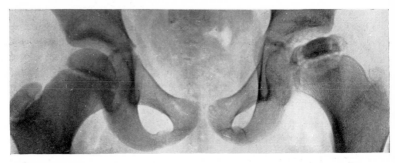

FIG. 1112.—Perthes' disease of the left femoral head.

A radiograph shows, in the early stages, slight broadening of the neck of the femur, the upper border of which is *convex*. Later the head of the bone becomes flattened (" mushroomed "), and the epiphysis is represented by two or more nuclei. Finally the neck becomes thickened, and the epiphyseal fragments fuse to form an expanded flattened head of the femur.

Surgeons were formerly content to restrict movements and limit weight-bearing, as by the application of a walking calliper. However, it is becoming increasingly appreciated that, although a deformed femoral head causes little disability for many years, osteoarthritis is prone to develop in later life. Therefore treatment by recumbency and traction is to be recommended, in a modified form from that used for a tuberculous hip.

Osgood-Schlatter's disease is much commoner in boys than girls, and appears between the ages of ten and sixteen. It is

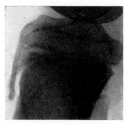

FIG. 1113. — Osgood-Schlatter's disease.

frequently preceded by some unusual strain, e.g. training for sports. The tibial tubercle becomes unduly prominent and tender on pressure. A radiograph shows partial separation of the tongue-shaped portion of the epiphysis from the shaft (fig. 1113). Vigorous activities should be curtailed, and firm strapping provides mild support. If pain persists a posterior

Robert Osgood, Contemporary, Orthopœdic Surgeon of Boston, U.S.A., and Carl Schlatter, Contemporary, Professor of Surgery, Zürich, described apophysitis of the tibia simultaneously in 1903.

plaster slab should be worn for a few weeks. Local tenderness disappears in from three to six months, but enlargement persists for a much longer period.

Sever's disease, or apophysitis of the os calcis, affects the epiphysis of the heel, which is present between the tenth and sixteenth years. This condition forms one variety of painful heel. A radiograph shows fragmentation and irregularity of the epiphysis (fig. 1114). The child should wear a boot which is cut away at the back (to relieve pressure) and the heel of which is raised (to relax the calf muscles).

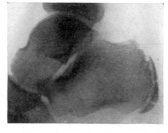

FIG. 1114.—Sever's disease.

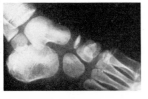

FIG. 1115.—Köhler's disease, showing disc-like scaphoid.

Köhler's disease affects the scaphoid tarsal bone and occurs between three and eight years of age. The bone is at first fragmented and tender, but later is compressed and sclerotic (fig. 1115). Strapping support is usually adequate.

Kienböck's disease of the semilunar bone of the wrist occurs in adults of any age (fig. 1116). In most cases a history of injury is obtainable, which is followed by pain, tenderness over the bone, and limitation of wrist movements. Finsterer's sign is sometimes present, and consists of sharply tapping the head of the third metacarpal when the fist is closed. If the sign is positive, pain is felt in the region of the bone. Treatment consists in immobilisation for six months in order to encourage regeneration. If sclerosis occurs, the head of the third metacarpal becomes less prominent. The opposite wrist should be X-rayed, as the condition is sometimes bilateral.

Madelung's deformity (*syn.* manus valga) may be included in this group of diseases, and occurs in girls at the period of adolescence. Deficient growth of the lower radial epiphysis results in relative elongation of the ulna, so that the hand is displaced outwards and forwards. The condition is liable to occur in typists.

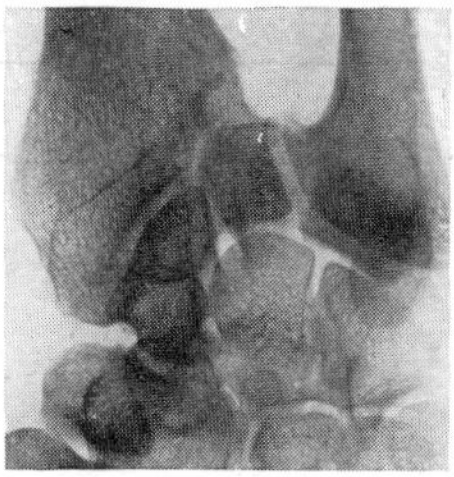

Calvé's epiphysitis affects the epiphysis of one or more vertebræ, not necessarily contiguous. It is commoner in boys than girls, and appears about puberty.

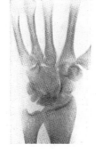

FIG. 1116.—Kienböck's disease.

FIG. 1117.—Madelung's deformity.

Scheuermann's disease involves adjacent dorsal vertebral epiphyses in adolescents. The development of a kyphosis is the first indication of the disease, which is con-

Albert Köhler, Contemporary. Professor of Surgery, Berlin.
Robert Kienböck, Contemporary. Professor of Radiology, Vienna.
Otto Madelung, 1846–1926. Professor of Surgery, Strasburg.
Holger Werfel Scheuermann, Contemporary. Director of Radiological Department, Military Hospital and Sundby-hospital, Copenhagen.

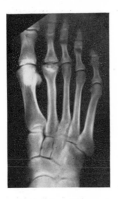

FIG. 1118.—Freiberg's disease of the head of the second metatarsal. Partial excision of the bone to relieve pain.

(*F. P. Fitzgerald.*)

firmed by radiography. In early stages remedial exercises and perhaps a spinal support improve the deformity, but often some kyphosis persists.

Freiberg's disease is uncommon and occurs in young adults. It affects the head of the second or third metatarsal, in the region of which tenderness and swelling are detected. The X-ray shows flattening of the articular surface and irregular sclerosis of the head. Treatment consists of rest, a metatarsal bar, or, if necessary, excision of the head of the bone (fig. 1118).

ACHONDROPLASIA

This familial condition is due to maldevelopment of bones arising from cartilage. Thus the stature is markedly diminished and the limbs in particular are stunted. The legs are obviously short, and the fingertips reach only to the great trochanters, the arms thus resembling flippers (fig. 1119). The fingers themselves diverge, so that they resemble the spokes of a wheel. As the fibula is less shortened than the tibia, it frequently enters into the formation of the knee joint. The base of the skull, being developed from cartilage, is small in proportion to the vertex, so that the prominent forehead causes the bridge of the nose to appear to be depressed. Mental development is normal, and sufferers often find ready employment in circuses.

ANOSTEOPLASIA (*Syn.* CRANIO-CLEIDODYSOSTOSIS)

The counterpart of achondroplasia, in that it is due to failure of development of bones arising in membrane. Thus the vertex of the skull and clavicles are ill-formed, so that the head appears flattened, and as the buttress action of the clavicles is lost, the heads of the humeri are approximated to, and may articulate with, the sternum (fig. 1020). A curious feature is delayed ossification of the pubic bones.

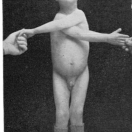

FIG. 1120.—Anosteoplasia.
(*Pybus.*)

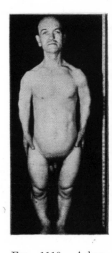

FIG. 1119.—Achondroplasia.

DIAPHYSEAL ACLASIS (*Syn.* MULTIPLE CONGENITAL OSTEOCHONDROMATA)

This rare disease is hereditary, and is characterised by cartilaginous and osseous outgrowths from the neighbourhood of the epiphyseal line. These multiple swellings first appear about puberty, and are associated with diminution of stature and deformities, such as coxa vara and genu valgum.

Albert H. Freiberg, Contemporary. Professor of Orthopœdic Surgery, Cincinnati, Ohio, U.S.A.
Statues of the Egyptian gods Bes and Phtah are accurate figurations of achondroplasia.

Bones which develop from membrane are unaffected. Sarcomatous changes have been reported in a few cases.

Dyschondroplasia (syn. Ollier's disease) is characterised by the formation of bony masses in the metaphyses, especially those of the hands and feet. The disease is not hereditary. Malignant changes may supervene.

Schuller-Christian's disease is rare, and is due to faulty lipoid metabolism. Soft swellings occur in the scalp, beneath which the skull is eroded (" map-like " skull). Exophthalmos and diabetes insipidus develop and growth is retarded. Other bones are sometimes affected, in which case differential diagnosis is often difficult. The condition responds to deep X-ray therapy.

Osteopetrosis (syn. " Albers-Schönberg's disease ") is a rare and familial condition in which the bones become progressively more dense owing to excessive deposition of calcium (fig. 1121). " Marble bones " is a misnomer, as although the bones are sclerotic they are friable, and pathological fractures occur. *Osteopoikily* (speckled bones) is a similar but less extensive condition.

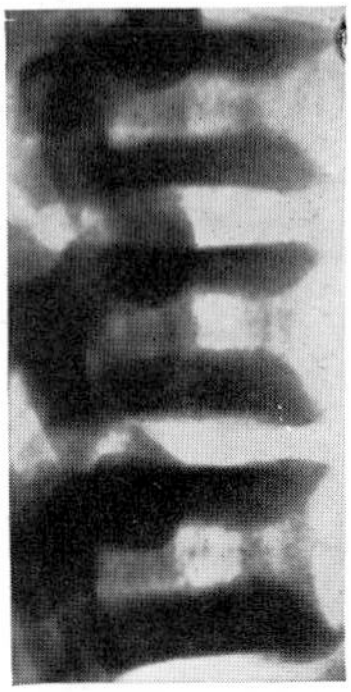

ACROMEGALY

Hunter's famous example of acromegaly, the skeleton of the Irish giant, now in the museum of the Royal College of Surgeons of England, showed an enlarged sella turcica when the skull was opened at Harvey Cushing's suggestion.

Fig. 1121. — Osteopetrosis of the lumbar verte-bræ. *(Karl Krebs Aarhus, Denmark.)*

The early signs are enlargement of the hands and feet, at first confined to the soft tissues, but later bony thickening also occurs. The jaws enlarge, especially the lower, which becomes prognathic, and separation of the teeth indicates that the enlargement is partly interstitial. Overgrowth of facial bones also occurs, especially of natural ridges and at the sites of muscular attachment. The lips, nose, and ears show a variable amount of thickening (fig. 893). When the disease is established, the spine is kyphotic.

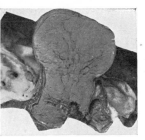

Fig. 1122.—A large pituitary tumour.

As the disease is associated with new-growth and enlargement of the pituitary gland (p. 867) symptoms of increased intracranial pressure supervene. Vision is affected, partly owing to this general increased pressure, and also as a result of local pressure of the enlarged gland on the optic chiasma giving rise to bilateral temporal hemianopia. More rarely an optic nerve is displaced, so that

Pierre Ollier, 1847–1905. Professor of Surgery, Lyons.
Arthur Schuller, Contemporary. Radiologist, St. Vincent's Hospital, Melbourne.
Henry Asbury Christian, Contemporary. Professor of Medicine, Harvard.
Heinrich Ernest Albers-Schönberg, 1865–1921. Professor of Roentgenology, Hamburg.

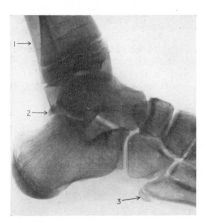

Fig. 1123.—(1) Harris's lines. Two abnormalities are also seen—(2) An os trigonum, and (3) An epiphysis at the base of the fifth metatarsal. These may be of importance in compensation cases, but an X-ray of the other foot will show a similar condition.

it is compressed by the circle of Willis, with consequent blindness of the corresponding eye. Involvement of the fifth nerve, and proptosis from pressure on the cavernous sinus, to which the ophthalmic veins pass, sometimes occur.

A radiograph will demonstrate enlargement of the sella turcica (fig. 894).

Operation should be undertaken only for intolerable headache or threatened blindness (p. 865).

Harris's Lines. — Radiographic examination of long bones in children and adolescents sometimes reveals transverse lines of compact bone near the epiphyses (fig. 1123).   These are due to arrest of growth which accompanies some severe constitutional disturbance.

TUMOURS OF BONES

The various types of bone tumours are the neoplastic counterparts of the various tissue components that go to make up bone. Thus we can relate chondroma and chondro-sarcoma to cartilage, the varieties of true osteo-sarcoma to the specific bone-forming tissue, giant-cell tumour of bone to the bone-destroying osteoclasts, fibro-sarcoma of bone to the periosteal and other collaginous connective tissues, and other tumours such as myeloma and Ewing's tumour to the hæmopoietic tissue of bone.

It is important to bear in mind that various groups of bone tumours are not to be regarded as absolutely rigid ones and that although these " labels " are the ones attached to the commoner types observed, an individual tumour may on occasions show features of more than one of these types (Sissons).

CHONDROMA

Cartilaginous tumours, usually benign, may arise in connection with the epiphyseal cartilage.

Thomas Willis, 1621–1675. Practised in St. Martin's Lane, London. Buried in West-
    minster Abbey.
H. A. Harris, Contemporary. *Professor of Anatomy, Cambridge University.*
H. A. Sissons, Contemporary. *Department of Pathology, Royal College of Surgeons.*

The tumours are composed of hyaline cartilage, the cells of which are variable in size and shape. All stages of transitional forms link non-progressive developmental abnormalities and benign chondromas to malignant chondro-sarcomata, and no sharply dividing line can be drawn between the two extremes.

Chondromata are conveniently classified according to the type of bone from which they arise :

(*a*) **Small Bones of the Hands and Feet.**—As these tumours arise within the bone they are termed *en*chondromata. They most commonly appear during childhood. The affected bone becomes gradually and painlessly expanded, and the local condition may suggest dactylitis. However, the more advanced age of the patient and the absence of evidence of local inflammation or of any general manifestation of disease should prevent an error of diagnosis. A radiograph shows a clear expansion of the bone (fig. 1124), and sometimes the presence of small specks of calcification help to distinguish it from a bone cyst. If allowed to grow, destruction of the bone is inevitable, and finally myxomatous degeneration may occur.

An X-ray sometimes reveals small en-chondromata in other digits, which have not expanded the bone sufficiently to call attention to their presence.

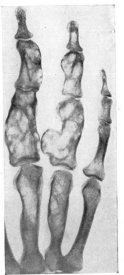

FIG. 1124.—Multiple enchondromata of phalanges.

Boeck's sarcoidosis may simulate enchondromata, in that cavitation sometimes occurs in digital bones. However, the presence of granulomatous swellings in lymph nodes, salivary and lachrymal glands and elsewhere (p. 183) should clarify the diagnosis.

Treatment consists in scraping out the tumour. In the case of a digit a posterolateral incision is made, which passes between the extensor tendon and the digital vessels and nerve. Prognosis is guarded, as enchondromata are sometimes multiple, or others may develop later.

(*b*) **Long Bones.**—Ecchondromata commence under the periosteum in the region of the epiphyseal line, but as growth proceeds and the bone lengthens they remain stranded in the shaft. Thus, if the tumour originates in a small child near the growing

Caesar Peter Moeller Boeck, 1845–1917. Professor of Dermatology, Oslo.

end of a long bone, by the time adult life is reached it may be some inches from the end of the bone. The tumour projects from the surface of the bone, to which it is attached by a pedicle, therefore the term *ec*chondroma is applied.

An ecchondroma forms a hard, fixed, and painless swelling near the end of a bone. If the tumour is ignored, it ossifies when the epiphyseal line from which it arises joins the shaft, and a cancellous osteoma results (fig. 1126). This suggests that it is not a true tumour, but is due to irregular growth of the bone.

As ecchondromata rarely undergo malignant change, and cease to grow when the bone ossifies, removal is only indicated if disabling symptoms occur, such as :

(i) Displacement of adjacent muscles or tendons, causing a sensation of weakness owing to interference with their efficient action. Occasionally a tendon becomes hitched around the tumour in certain positions of the limb, a condition known as a " snapping " tendon.

(ii) Interference with joints, or, more rarely, vessels or nerves.

(iii) Inflammation of an overlying adventitious bursa, e.g. on the inner side of the knee in a jockey.

(iv) Fracture, due to direct violence or muscular action.

(v) Cosmetic reasons, e.g. upper end of the humerus in women who desire to wear low evening dress.

If removal is indicated, care must be taken to divide the base of the tumour close to the parent bone, so that none of the cartilaginous " cap " is left, otherwise recurrence is possible.

(*c*) **Flat Bones.**—These tumours grow from such bones as the ribs, scapula, and pelvis, and form characteristically hard and painless swellings. However, they may remain unnoticed until myxomatous degeneration causes pain and increase in size, in which case errors of diagnosis are common. Thus an enchondroma of the rib resembles a simple cyst, or in other situations it may be confused with sarcoma, which condition may develop in a chondroma, particularly when the pelvic bones are affected.

Treatment consists in excision of the affected portion of a rib, but in the case of the pelvis, unless complete excision is practicable, X-ray therapy is preferable, as inadequate removal encourages sarcomatous changes.

OSTEOMA

Osteomata are of two varieties, ivory or cancellous.

Ivory osteomata are uncommon, but are occasionally found on the skull, particularly in connection with bones which form the walls of air sinuses (fig. 1125.)

Treatment.—Removal is indicated if pressure symptoms result, e.g. deafness from auditory obstruction, displacement of the eye, or involvement of nerves. Owing to the density of these tumours, removal should be effected through adjacent normal bone, as chiselling through the unyielding tumour may cause concussion.

Cancellous osteomata are comparatively common tumours, and occur as a result of ossification in an ecchondroma. Thus they are found near the ends of long bones (fig. 1126); the physical signs are identical with those of an ecchondroma, and treatment is conducted on the same lines.

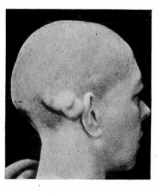

Fig. 1125.—Ivory osteoma arising from the mastoid antrum.

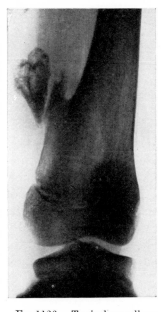

Fig.1126.—Typical cancellous osteoma, growing away from the epiphysis. A fracture has occurred near the base.

A *subungual exostosis* is an irregular bony outgrowth under the nail of the big toe, which is lifted off the underlying phalanx. It is included in this section for convenience, but it is not a neoplasm. It is due to pressure of an ill-fitting boot and consequent periosteal irritation. The nail should be removed or displaced, and the bony excrescence excised by means of a chisel or bone-cutting forceps.

Spurs on the os calcis are due to ossification of the external plantar ligament. Formerly they were a not uncommon complication of gonorrhœal flat-foot. If troublesome the spur is removed through an incision on the outer side of the heel.

GIANT-CELL TUMOUR (*Syn.* OSTEOCLASTOMA)

Giant-cell tumours occur most commonly at the end of a long bone, particularly in the vicinity of the knee joint. Tumours with similar histological structure occur in relation to tendons (p. 1176), where they arise from synovial tissue, and also on the gums, giving rise to one variety of epulis (p. 158).

Osteoclastomata usually occur during the third or fourth decades of life, and are presumed to arise from osteoclasts, which are giant cells normally engaged in absorption of bone. Clinical features depend upon whether the affected bone is

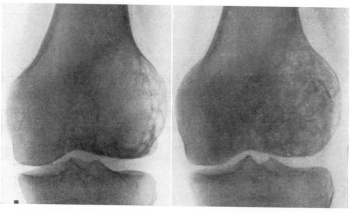

FIG. 1127.—Osteoclastoma of the   The bone has been curretted and
        internal condyle.   the cavity filled with bone chips.
                                              (*F. P. Fitzgerald.*)

subcutaneous or surrounded by muscle. In the former case a swelling is first noticed, which is somewhat abrupt and painless. Expansion of the bone follows, which process consists in destruction of the bone from within, while at the same time new periosteal bone is formed (fig. 1127). This new formation of bone occurs more slowly than the destructive process, so that the bone becomes larger but progressively thinner, and eventually " egg-shell crackling " may be detected. Finally, the growth, if ignored, erodes the compact bone, and a soft, pulsating swelling results. The final stages are rarely seen in countries where surgical amenities are available.

In the case of deep-seated bones, enlargement and consequent destruction of the bone may be unnoticed, in which case the first evidence of the tumour is either a spontaneous fracture or a pulsating swelling. A fracture is especially liable to occur in the femur or humerus, which are unsupported bones.

Owing to the slow rate of growth of these tumours, pain is not a prominent feature. When a large osteoclastoma is adjacent to a joint, e.g. the lower end of the femur, a " sympathetic " effusion may occur as a result of local hyperæmia. A radiograph confirms the abrupt expansion of the bone, and presents a stippled or mottled appearance, due to bony trabeculæ which traverse the cavity. The appearance often resembles a collection of soap bubbles.

Macroscopically, the tumour appears as a soft, maroon-coloured tumour, with localised extravasations of blood. A definite bony septum usually separates it from the medullary cavity, and bony trabeculæ intersect the softer portions (fig. 1128). Histologically, characteristic myeloplaxes are strikingly evident ; these large cells, about 120 μ in diameter, are irregular in shape, and contain from twelve to fifteen deeply staining nuclei scattered throughout the cell. The remainder of the tumour consists of spindle cells, extravasated blood, and numerous blood-vessels. " White " osteoclastomata occasionally occur, usually at the lower end of the radius.

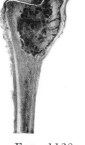

Treatment.—Until recently it was believed that osteoclastomata were only locally malignant, but a more careful " follow-up " shows that in about 8 per cent. of cases metastases occur, usually in the lungs, and they are especially prone to follow inadequate treatment. Prompt and efficient treatment is therefore indicated, and in the majority of cases the choice lies between deep X-ray therapy and curettage. X-ray therapy is advisable if adequate surgical approach is formidable or difficult, such as the upper end of the femur or the ilium, or if so much destruction has occurred that curetting might precipitate a fracture. Curetting is preferred for early cases, or if an epiphyseal line is still present and adjacent to the tumour, in which case radiation might interfere with growth of the bone. However, there is an increasing tendency, which we support, to use X-ray therapy whenever practicable, as suitable cases are thereby

Fig. 1128.— Osteoclastoma of the upper end of the tibia. (*British Journal of Surgery.*)

cured. Cases which are curetted not infrequently recur, with consequent risk of dissemination. When X-ray therapy is instituted, the early local reaction suggests that the tumour is rapidly increasing in size, but after two or three months tenderness and swelling subside, and ossification begins. Care must be taken during treatment to forestall a spontaneous fracture. Interstitial radium-therapy is apt to initiate malignant changes.

Curetting.—The bone is opened with a gouge or chisel, and the growth scraped away with a sharp spoon, care being taken not to penetrate the adjacent articular cartilage. The cavity is swabbed with pure carbolic acid, any excess being removed with spirit. If necessary, the cavity is reduced in size by compression of its walls, or bone chips may be inserted. If the cavity is small, it is sufficient to allow it to fill with blood-clot. Precautions must be taken to obviate excessive hæmorrhage, and therefore a tourniquet is applied, or vessel tied in continuity, e.g. ligation of the external carotid above its superior thyroid branch as a preliminary to curetting an osteoclastoma of the lower jaw.

In some cases one of the following procedures will be preferable to curettage or radiation :

(*a*) LOCAL EXCISION.—If removal of the bone will cause little disability, then excision is performed, e.g. rib or fibula. This method is certain in its result, and convalescence is speedy.

In the case of the upper end of the fibula the external popliteal nerve must be isolated above the swelling, as it lies under the tendon of the biceps, since its anatomical relations in the region of the tumour will be distorted. The nerve is traced downwards and held aside, and the fibula is divided and cleared of muscles from below upwards. If possible the styloid process is spared, otherwise the external lateral ligament and tendon of the biceps must be sutured to the periosteum of the outer tuberosity of the tibia.

(*b*) AMPUTATION.—In the case of extensive destruction of a bone, such as the lower end of the femur or head of the tibia, amputation is usually performed. Although bone-grafting is possible, the convalescence is tedious, and as the knee joint must of necessity be bridged by the graft, the end result is a rigid leg.

MULTIPLE MYELOMA (*Syn.* KAHLER'S DISEASE)

This is a rare condition in which multiple endosteal tumours occur and are associated with marked bone destruction. The lesions involve spine and ribs most frequently and the skull and femora are other common sites. The proliferating tumour cells are plasma-cells, and for this reason the condition is sometimes known as plasmacytoma. The involvement of bone marrow is widespread and the sternal marrow is practically always affected even in the absence of clinical evidence, thus the diagnosis can often be confirmed by examination of smears of sternal marrow. The multiple nature of the lesions and the sharply delimited bone destruction gives a radiographic appearance that is sometimes suggestive of metastatic

Otto Kahler, 1849–1893. Professor of Medicine, Prague.

carcinoma (fig. 1129). The proteose, first described by Bence-Jones, appears in the urine in most cases, but it may absent itself for a period in any patient. It precipitates on the addition of nitric acid and disappears on warming. Owing to extensive bone destruction the blood calcium is

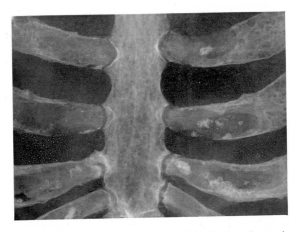

Fig.1129.—Myelo-matoses of sternum and ribs. (*Dr. L. S. Carstairs.*)

usually increased, and if renal inefficiency coexists the blood phosphorus is also raised.

In a relatively small number of cases only a single bone is involved by a myeloma lesion. Sometimes these cases remain well after X-ray therapy, but more often the development of additional lesions shows the condition to be one of generalised disease. Death may result from uræmia following obstruction of the renal tubules by protein, or some intercurrent disease in a bedridden sufferer.

SARCOMA

Periosteal fibro-sarcomata are spindle-shaped tumours which arise from the periosteum, or from the insertion of tendons or muscles, and should therefore be regarded as tumours of these structures rather than of the bone itself. Local and free excision, including the periosteum in the neighbourhood, occasionally results in cure, but, as in the case of fibro-sarcoma arising from a muscle sheath, incomplete removal will be followed by recurrence of the tumour with increased malignancy.

Osteo-sarcoma is a highly malignant tumour. The clinical presentation and the radiographic appearance each shows great variety, depending on the osteogenic or osteolytic properties of the tumour and on its site of origin. In many cases the presence of enlarged superficial veins and possibly of an effusion into a neighbouring joint indicate the vascular nature of the tumour. Dissemination occurs by the blood-stream, but the lymphatic system is involved when soft tissues are invaded.

Osteo-sarcoma most commonly occurs during puberty or adolescence, and is practically unknown after the age of fifty, except as a complication of Paget's disease. The favourite sites

Henry Bence-Jones, 1814–1873. Physician, St. George's Hospital, London.

are the ends of the shafts of long bones, and the leg is affected five times as often as the arm. The patient's general health is not affected until the final stages of the disease.

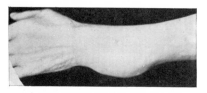

FIG. 1130.—Osteo-sarcoma of the ulna.

If the tumour arises subperiosteally pain is an early symptom, due to stretching of the periosteum. On inspection of the affected part distended veins are often seen,

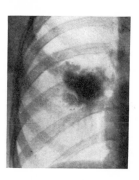

FIG. 1131. — Ossifying metastasis in the lung from osteo-sarcoma of the femur.

which indicate the vascular nature of the growth. On palpation a spindle-shaped swelling of the bone is detected (fig. 1130),

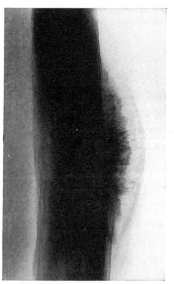

FIG. 1132.—Fusiform swelling and spiculation in a periosteal sarcoma of the tibia.

at first elastic in consistency, but pulsatile in the later stages. Eventually soft tissues are invaded, and finally the tumour involves and fungates through the skin. Dissemination occurs early, the lungs being commonly affected via the systemic veins, and if the tumour progresses slowly these deposits occasionally ossify (fig. 1131). A blood-stained pleural effusion is sometimes the first evidence of pulmonary involvement. Secondary deposits also occur via the lymphatic system, and other bones are frequently affected in the later stages.

The radiographic appearances of subperiosteal osteo-sarcoma vary according to the rate of growth of the tumour. If the tumour is rapidly destructive (osteolytic type), erosion of the bone is the principal feature, but if the tumour is of moderate malignancy, characteristic spiculation is evident (" sun-ray pattern ") (fig. 1132). This phenomenon is due to separation of the periosteum from the bone, and formation of bone by osteoblasts on the walls of the blood-vessels which pass from the bone to the uplifted periosteum. In cases which are of slow growth (osteoblastic type), fusion of the bony spicules results in the formation of an irregular osseous mass surrounding the normal bone from which the tumour originates, and erosion of the compact bone is masked by the ossifying tumour (fig. 1133).

A tumour commencing endosteally erodes and destroys the pre-existing bony tissue as it expands, and eventually spontaneous fracture may occur or the appearance of a soft pulsating swelling indicates that the bone is extensively destroyed.

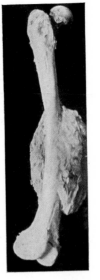

Fig. 1133. — Osteo-sarcoma of the femur—a vascular, fusiform tumour.

In both these classes of tumour a confident diagnosis is always difficult in the early stages. Besides other types of primary bone tumour such possibilities as an acute inflammatory process, an endosteal gumma, or a metastatic tumour must always be considered.

If the diagnosis is doubtful and the W.R. negative, then a biopsy must be performed, as exact diagnosis is essential for treatment and prognosis. Biopsy is alleged to encourage dissemination, but if a tourniquet and diathermy punch are employed, the slight risk is far outweighed by the importance of a positive diagnosis.

Treatment of an osteo-sarcoma depends on the site and extent of the growth :

(a) *Amputation* is the usual procedure, providing the diagnosis is accepted, and should be performed at the " site of election " above the tumour. Local recurrence does not occur, therefore there is no necessity to amputate above the joint proximal to the growth. In the case of the femur or humerus disarticulation should be performed through the hip or shoulder joint, or even by a hind- or fore-quarter amputation (fig. 1134). However, the prognosis is extremely gloomy, but

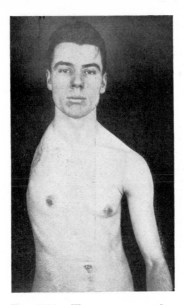

Fig. 1134.—The appearance after a fore-quarter amputation.

amputation relieves the patient of a limb which will become increasingly painful, and fungation and risk of secondary hæmorrhage are obviated. Some surgeons recommend that the patient be given a maximum dose of radiation over a period of three or four weeks prior to amputation, which is performed a fortnight later.

(b) In certain situations local excision of the affected bone and the insertion of a bone graft have been adopted. Earlier permission is likely to be given for this procedure, as compared with amputation. Also in the early stages local recurrence is unlikely, and if secondary deposits have occurred, even amputation cannot retard their progress. Hence in situations where bone grafting yields good results, such as the upper limb, the arm may be saved, and cases are on record where this line of treatment has been adopted, and the unmaimed patient has survived for many years.

X-ray therapy has little influence in retarding the progress of the tumour, but it stimulates osteogenesis, diminishes vascularity, and often relieves pain. Fractional doses are given over a period of about six weeks, and this can be repeated after six months if considered advisable.

Prognosis.—Out of 650 cases collected by the American Registry of Bone Sarcoma, only seventeen *appear* to have been cured—sixteen after amputation, and one following treatment by radium.

Recurrence within a year is likely to occur in viscera or other bones if the primary growth is situated near the trunk. In more distant tumours recurrence commonly occurs within three years, although we have known a case in which a secondary deposit appeared in the spine thirteen years after amputation through the thigh for periosteal sarcoma of the tibia. Thus the time limit for a " cure " is almost unlimited.

An X-ray of the chest may reveal secondary deposits in the lungs, which indicates that the expectation of life is, at the most, but a few months.

EWING'S TUMOUR

This rare syndrome includes the following characteristics : acute onset with pyrexia, local tenderness, a situation in the middle of the shaft of a long bone, a patient between five and sixteen years of age, a pattern of longitudinal layers of sub-periosteal ossification likened to the layers of an onion (fig. 1135)—and, finally, striking radiosensitivity. It is probable that a number of pathological entities can give rise to this syndrome, and

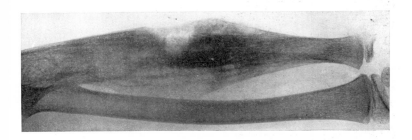

FIG. 1135.—Ewing's tumour. (*Karl Krebs, Aarhus, Denmark.*)

in addition to the " angio-endothelioma " that Ewing regarded as its corresponding pathological counterpart, there must be mentioned not only other unusual forms of primary endosteal tumour (such as sarcoma derived from reticulo-endothelial tissues) but also metastatic lesions, particularly neuroblastoma, which occur in children of this age.

The prognosis is poor, even after amputation, as secondary deposits occur in other parts of the skeleton, and eventually in lymph nodes and viscera. Deep X-ray therapy causes striking retrogression of the primary growth, which is an important point both in differential diagnosis and treatment, but secondary deposits are less radiosensitive. Local recurrence after an adequate course of radiotherapy demands amputation.

SECONDARY TUMOURS

Carcinoma.—Carcinoma of bone occurs either by direct extension, as in the case of the chest wall following carcinoma of the breast, or by metastasis.

Secondary deposits are liable to occur particularly as a result of a primary growth in the following situations :

(i) *Breast.*—Is the commonest cause of secondary carcinoma of bone. Secondary deposits occur in about 50 per cent. of fatal cases, the favourite situations being the spine, pelvis, and upper ends of the femur and humerus.

(ii) *Prostate.*—This gland is commonly associated with osseous dissemination. The usual manifestation is diffuse sclerosis of the pelvis and lumbo-sacral regions (fig. 1136). This osteo-blastic type of metastasis is peculiar to the prostate and, in

James Ewing, Contemporary. Professor of Oncology (Tumours), Cornell University Medical College, U.S.A.

the early stages, may be difficult to distinguish from Paget's disease (p. 1094).   Secondary prostatic deposits arising in other sites are osteolytic, in which the bone is irregularly destroyed

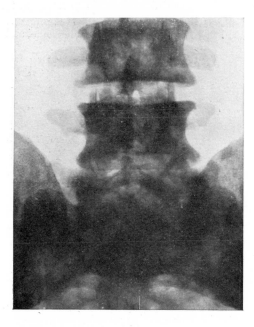

Fig. 1136.—Osteoblastic (sclerotic) carcinomatous secondaries in the verte-bræ and pelvic bones. The primary was in the prostate.

with little or no surrounding reaction.   Oestrogens are worthy of trial.

(iii) *Kidney.*—Any bone is liable to be affected, perhaps most commonly the pelvis. A bony swelling or a spontaneous fracture is sometimes the first evidence of a carcinoma of the kidney. Occasionally the deposit is single, in which case nephrectomy and resection of the affected bone is feasible.

(iv) *Bronchus.*—Carcinoma appears to be increasing in fre-quency and diagnostic methods have improved during the past decade.   Secondary deposits in bones are not uncommon.

(v) *Thyroid.*—The flat bones, especially the vertex of the skull, are likely to be affected. These tumours in particular are very vascular, and apparently are capable of function, as after complete thyroidectomy for carcinoma the post-operative myxœdema has disappeared on the appearance of secondary deposits. If the cells are sufficiently differentiated the metas-tasis becomes more opaque to radiography after the administration of radio-active iodine, which is an important point in the diagnosis of a doubtful case.

Secondary deposits in general usually cause considerable pain, and if occurring in the vertebræ pain is liable to be referred along spinal nerves. In most cases a swelling eventually becomes palpable (fig. 1137); the presence of superficial veins and possibly pulsation indicate the vascular nature of the tumour. Spontaneous fracture is common, and if immobilised, union sometimes occurs, in distinction from spontaneous fractures caused by sarcoma, which never unite.

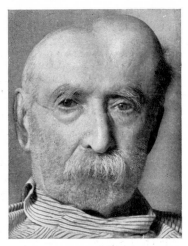

Fig. 1137.—Secondary deposit in the skull from a carcinoma of the prostate.

A radiograph (fig. 1138) shows irregular destruction of bone with little or no surrounding reaction unless fracture has occurred, in which case evidence of callus formation is sometimes seen.

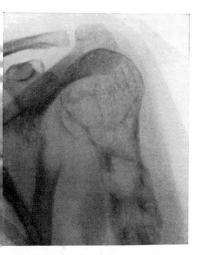

Fig. 1138.—Secondary carcinoma, showing destruction of the upper end of the humerus and the glenoid cavity. The primary was in the breast.

If a tumour in connexion with bone raises a suspicion of secondary carcinoma, then the common primary sites must be carefully examined. Carcinoma of the breast, prostate, or bronchus can usually be detected. The presence of a slowly growing carcinoma of the kidney is often difficult to diagnose in the absence of hæmorrhage, but a pyelogram will usually show a "spidery" pelvis. Primary carcinoma of the thyroid gland is sometimes so unobtrusive as to be impalpable, or a tumour which clinically appears to be a simple adenoma may actually be malignant.

Treatment.—Secondary osseous deposits are sensitive to deep X-ray therapy. Pain is relieved, and a spontaneous fracture or paraplegia may be prevented, and much suffering thereby obviated. Therefore, unless metastases are widespread, irradiation should receive consideration.

Secondary deposits arising from the prostate are often checked, and may even disappear, following the administration of œstrogen. Up to 5 mgm. of stilbœstrol is administered thrice daily, and although cure is not to be expected, palliation is often remarkable. Tenderness of the breasts and pigmentation of the nipples commonly occur during treatment.

Some surgeons recommend subcapsular castration, so as to eliminate the chief source of androgen, but œstrogen arrests secretion of androgen from the testicle by inhibiting the gonadotrophic hormone which is secreted by the anterior lobe of the pituitary. Androgens stimulate prostatic activity, and also that of the secondary deposits.

The estimation of the amount of acid phosphatase in the serum is of value in the diagnosis of prostatic secondaries, and also in prognosis. Normally $0\cdot5$–2 units of acid phosphatase is present in 100 ml. of serum. Over 5 units is very suggestive of prostatic secondaries, and 10 units or more is diagnostic. The value of treatment by œstrogen is assessed by the degree of diminution in the amount of acid phosphatase. This test is also useful in distinguishing prostatic secondaries from osteitis deformans, as in the latter case the acid phosphatase is not increased, but the alkaline phosphatase is above normal.

CHAPTER XLII

INJURIES TO JOINTS

Sprains are due to overstretching of ligaments with consequent partial or complete rupture. The ligaments commonly affected are the external lateral of the ankle and the internal lateral of the knee. Localised pain, which may be sickening in severe cases, and tenderness over the site of the torn ligament, are immediate features. Extravasation of blood occurs in the neighbourhood of the torn ligament, and if the synovial membrane is also torn, a hæmorrhagic effusion occurs into the joint.

Treatment consists in the immediate application of a bandage soaked in cold water or lead lotion. The bandage must be applied firmly so as to limit further effusion. After two or three days graduated movements are instituted, and subsequently care is taken to relax the damaged ligament, e.g. the boot raised on its inner side in order to relieve strain on a torn internal lateral ligament of the knee joint.

According to Leriche a slight injury to the sensitive nerve-endings in a ligament causes a reflex vasomotor reaction, followed by œdema, pain, and limitation of movement. An injection of local anæsthetic, e.g. 3 to 10 ml. of 2 per cent. procaine, abolishes the centripetal impulses. The injection is made in the region of maximum tenderness, and good results are obtained if the damaged ligament is relaxed for a few days, so that healing can occur without further injury. The injection should be made as soon as possible after injury, but the treatment is worthy of trial even after some weeks of disability.

HÆMARTHROSIS is not uncommon in children, as a result of a seemingly trivial or a forgotten injury. The knee joint is most commonly affected, and is rapidly distended with blood. An associated rise of temperature may suggest the diagnosis of infective arthritis or adjacent osteomyelitis, but movements are free and relatively painless, and the condition usually subsides uneventfully.

DISLOCATIONS

Dislocations are either complete or partial (subluxation). The three causes of dislocations are : congenital malformations, pathological processes, and injury.

Congenital dislocation most commonly occurs in the hip joint, and is considered in the chapter on Deformities.

Pathological dislocations are due to :

(*a*) *Destruction*, e.g. " travelling " acetabulum in advanced tuberculous arthritis of the hip joint, or subluxation of the knee in cases of triple deformity (*vide* p. 1159).

(*b*) *Distension*, which, if excessive, may cause ligaments to stretch to such an extent that the articular ends of the bones slip apart, e.g. Charcot's joint. In cases of typhoid arthritis, softening of the ligaments predisposes to stretching, and pathological dislocation is liable to occur, even in the hip joint.

(*c*) *Paralysis* of muscles which support a joint, as in the case of infantile paralysis of the shoulder girdle, or of the muscles around the hip joint.

Traumatic dislocations occur most commonly in adult life. In children separation of an epiphysis is more likely, while older people are less subject to trauma, and atrophy of bone pre-disposes to fracture. Traumatic dislocations are always accompanied by tearing of the capsule and injury to surrounding tissues, especially to muscles and ligaments which are attached to adjacent bones. Nerves and blood-vessels are occasionally injured.

The likelihood of any individual joint suffering dislocation depends upon its liability to injury, the shape of the articular surfaces, and the support given by muscles and ligaments. The shoulder joint is commonly dislocated, as the glenoid cavity is shallow, and the support given to the head of the bone by muscles and ligaments is somewhat lax. Conversely, in the case of the hip, the acetabulum is deep, and muscles closely support the joint, therefore dislocation is uncommon.

Clinical Features.—(*a*) Pain—due to local trauma, or pressure on nerves, e.g. the displaced head of the humerus may press on the brachial plexus.

(*b*) Loss of function—fixity replaces mobility.

(*c*) Deformity. The limb is shortened or lengthened, or malalignment is present.

(*d*) The end of the bone can be detected in an abnormal position. This is the *absolute* sign of a dislocation. Unless the dislocation is accompanied by a fracture, movement of the shaft of the bone causes corresponding movement of the articular end.

(*e*) Associated swelling may be so extensive as to mask the deformity. An X-ray will reveal the dislocation and also discover any concomitant fracture.

Treatment.—Reduction is obtained by manipulation, extension, or operation. Manipulation is carried out as soon as any attendant shock has subsided, and in any case all avoidable delay must be eliminated. In the case of large joints surrounded by powerful muscles, general anæsthesia is desirable in order to overcome muscular spasm. The path taken by the displaced bone should be visualised, and movements carried out so that this path is retraced without causing additional damage to soft tissues. From two to four weeks immobilisation is advisable after reduction, in order to allow healing of the soft tissues ; the larger joints require a longer period of rest than the smaller ones, e.g. interphalangeal. Extension is occasionally required if manipulation fails, and is preferable in some situations, e.g. cervical spine. Operative measures are sometimes necessary, e.g. thumb (p. 1131), and in the case of larger joints open reduction is required should manipulation fail.

In elderly patients osteoarthritis commonly supervenes following a dislocation, particularly of a large joint.

Attempts at reduction by manipulation are seldom justified after a lapse of three or four weeks. If considered advisable, late cases are treated either by open reduction or excision of part of an implicated bone.

DISLOCATIONS OF SPECIAL JOINTS

LOWER JAW

The usual cause of dislocation of the mandible is a blow on the chin when the mouth is partly open. Dental operations, particularly those performed under general anæsthesia, and excessive yawning, are other causes.

If the dislocation is unilateral, the jaw is displaced towards the opposite side, and saliva dribbles from the partially open mouth. A hollow is palpable immediately in front of the tragus, and the condyle can be seen in a slightly anterior situation (fig. 1139). In bilateral cases the mouth is fixed in a partly open position, and both condyles are displaced in front of their normal situations.

Reduction can usually be performed with ease by pressing the padded thumbs on the lower molar teeth, at the same time rotating the body of the jaw upwards with the fingers. A general anæsthetic is occasionally

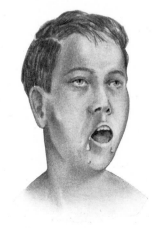

FIG. 1139.—Unilateral dislocation of the jaw.

necessary. After reduction a four-tailed bandage is worn for three weeks.

CLICKING JAW

This condition may follow excessive yawning, injury, dental extractions of lower molars, or a large bite at a hard apple. The click may embarrass the patient because it is so audible that people nearby comment on it. The condition is sometimes painful, and osteoarthritis of the affected joint, and later of the opposite one, may supervene.

The condition is predisposed to by alteration in the " bite " owing to abnormalities or absence of molar teeth. Thus the gliding movement of the condyle is interfered with, and the inter-articular cartilage may later subluxate. Consequently the advice of a dental surgeon should be sought, so that a normal bite can be restored. In intractable cases excision of the condyle is advisable, which is more promising than attempts to remove the subluxed fibro-cartilage.

STERNO-CLAVICULAR JOINT

Violence affecting this joint is transmitted along the clavicle, but in the majority of cases fracture of the clavicle occurs before force sufficient to cause dislocation reaches the sterno-clavicular joint. Moreover, the sturdy rhomboid ligament anchors the inner end of the clavicle to the first costal cartilage. When dislocation occurs the inner end of the clavicle is displaced forwards and downwards, or backwards and upwards, the first of these being the more common. Backward dislocation may cause severe dyspnœa from pressure on the trachea, or congestion of the head or arm owing to obstruction to the great veins at the root of the neck. Owing to the sub-cutaneous position of the bone, the dislocation is readily recognised.

Reduction is effected by standing behind the seated patient and placing the knee on the upper dorsal spine. The shoulders are then drawn backwards until reduction is accomplished. If necessary, further leverage in an outward direction can be obtained by means of a pad placed in the axilla. A piece of folded lint is firmly strapped over the joint in order to prevent redislocation, and the arm is supported in the same manner as for a fractured clavicle.

THE ACROMIO-CLAVICULAR JOINT

Dislocation of this joint is not uncommon, owing to the obliquity of the articular surfaces, which are separated by an inverted triangular intra-articular cartilage. The conoid and trapezoid ligaments are ruptured, and the prominence caused by the displaced clavicle is readily palpable. The dislocation is easily reduced by elevation of the shoulder, but withdrawal of support results in immediate redislocation. Treatment consists

in flexing the forearm, and applying elastoplast so that pressure is exerted on a pad
situated over the outer end of the clavicle
(fig. 1140) ; the arm is then supported by a
sling. If an unreduced dislocation causes
disability, the joint should be stabilised by
passing a fascial graft through the articular
ends of the clavicle and the acromion, or
by resection of the outer end of the clavicle.

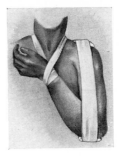

FIG. 1140.—The ap-
plication of pads and
strapping for disloca-
tion of the acromio-
clavicular joint.

SHOULDER JOINT

Owing to the wide range of movement,
the shallowness of the glenoid cavity, and
the lack of support by ligaments and
muscles, particularly on the inferior aspect, dislocations of this
joint are of common occurrence, and are caused by sudden violence
to the joint with the arm in abduction. In the majority of cases
a subglenoid dislocation occurs, as excessive abduction of the arm

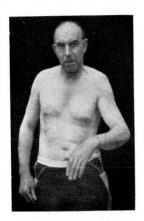

brings the neck of the humerus against
the coracoacromial arch, and the head of
the bone is forced downwards against the
weak inferior part of the capsule. Dislocation sometimes follows a trifling injury,
e.g. tossing a deck quoit, and in these
cases the condition may be overlooked.

On *inspection* of the shoulders an
alteration of contour is obvious, unless
the patient is very obese. The rounded
appearance of the shoulder is lost owing
to displacement inwards of the head of the
humerus, and consequently the " point "
of the shoulder is angular (fig. 1141).
The axis of the arm passes upwards
and inwards, and a fullness is noticed

FIG. 1141.—Subcoracoid
dislocation of the left
shoulder.

below the outer part of the clavicle. On *palpation* loss of resistance is felt beneath the acromion process, and the head of
the bone is palpable on following upwards the shaft of the
humerus. Pain and limitation of movement are complained of
by the patient. The teres minor muscle is ruptured, but this is
of no consequence.

The following academic tests are rarely necessary, provided that a careful examination is made.

Hamilton's Ruler Test.—The acromion process and the external condyle can be connected by a straight line.

Callaway's Test.—The axillary folds are lowered, and therefore the vertical measurement around the axilla is increased on the injured side.

Dugas' Test.—Owing to the abduction of the lower end of the humerus it is impossible to place the hand of the patient on the opposite shoulder while the elbow is in contact with the chest.

Varieties (fig. 1142).—With the exception of the supracoracoid dislocation, which is of necessity accompanied by fracture of the

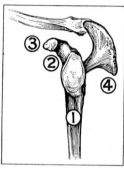

Fig. 1142. — 1. Subglenoid. 2. Subcoracoid. 3. Subclavicular. 4. Subacromial or subspinous.

overhanging coraco-acromial arch, dislocations are primarily subglenoid. The head of the humerus thus rests in a precarious manner on a narrow ridge of bone, and usually slips forward into the subcoracoid position. Should the exciting force continue to act, the head of the bone moves further inwards, and comes to rest in the subclavicular position. Occasionally the head of the bone is displaced backwards under the acromion process (subacromial). In this position it is balanced on the posterior rim of the glenoid cavity, so that it frequently slips further inwards to the subspinous position.

Luxatio erecta is a rare variety (under 1 per cent.), in which the head of the humerus is displaced into the subglenoid position, the arm being fixed in extreme abduction.

Treatment.—A general anæsthetic is usually advisable, particularly in a muscular subject, or when delay has allowed muscular spasm to supervene. Special care is taken in the administration of the anæsthetic, as the patient is often ill-prepared, and sudden changes of posture should be avoided.

Kocher's Method.—The patient may be either sitting or lying down, and the scapula is steadied by a towel, which passes round the chest. The following manipulations are then performed in a smooth and deliberate manner (fig. 1143) :

(i) The elbow is flexed and adducted.

(ii) The arm is rotated outwards, so as to stretch the subscapularis muscle, which has contracted owing to the inward

Frank Hastings Hamilton, 1813–1886.   Orthopædic surgeon at Wilmington, Vermont, U.S.A.

Thomas Callaway, 1822–1869.   English surgeon who practised in Algiers.

Louis Alexander Dugas, 1806–1884.   Professor of Surgery, Medical College of Georgia, U.S.A.

Theodore Kocher, 1841–1917.   Professor of Clinical Surgery, University of Berne.

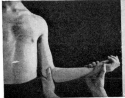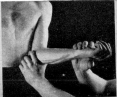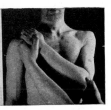

FIG. 1143.—Kocher's method for reduction of a dislocated shoulder.
(*F. P. Fitzgerald.*)

displacement of the upper end of the humerus. This manipulation must be performed gradually and to its fullest extent.

(iii) When full external rotation is obtained, the elbow is lifted upwards and forwards (in order to bring the head of the bone downwards into the axilla) and the arm is then rotated inwards, so that the elbow is carried across the chest, and the fingers sweep downwards across the opposite shoulder.

This method is successful in the majority of cases, and frequently reduction occurs during external rotation.

Traction.—If Kocher's method fails, traction can be applied by placing the unbooted foot in the axilla of the patient, who is lying supine. A steady pull is maintained on the forearm in an outward and downward direction. (*N.B.*—This method was practised by Hippocrates.)

A more scientific method of applying traction is to place the patient on a table, with a towel round the chest in order to provide a means of counter-extension. A 4-inch flannel bandage is then looped round the affected arm just below the axilla. Traction is applied in an outward direction by means of the flannel bandage, and downwards by pulling on the arm itself.

Operation.—In rare cases manipulative measures fail, and open reduction should be then considered.

After-treatment consists in supporting the arm in a sling in a partially abducted position. If the arm is kept in an adducted position, e.g. bandaged to the chest wall, the loose inferior portion of the capsule is thrown into folds which become adherent to each other, and thus return of full abduction is hindered. Finger and wrist movements are indulged in immediately, and active movements of the shoulder are commenced a few days later within the limit of pain, but abduction to more than a right angle should be prohibited for one month.

COMPLICATIONS

FRACTURE.—Dislocation of the shoulder may be complicated by fracture of the surgical neck of the humerus. Not uncommonly the great tuberosity is avulsed, but apposition occurs when the dislocation is reduced (fig. 1144).

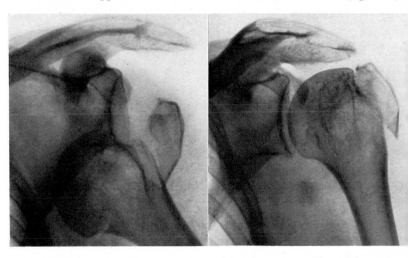

FIG. 1144.—Subcoracoid dislocation of the shoulder with avulsion of the greater tuberosity. Good apposition after reduction.

RECURRENT DISLOCATION.—*Vide infra.*

NERVES.—Any part of the brachial plexus, or adjacent nerves, may be involved. Owing to its limited mobility and proximity to the head of the humerus the circumflex nerve is most commonly injured (10 per cent. of cases), but if the deltoid is supported recovery usually ensues in from two to six months (fig. 904).

MUSCLES.—The tendon of the supraspinous muscle is occasionally ruptured, as is evinced by inability to abduct the arm. The arm should be supported in abduction for three weeks, and if this fails suture of the tendon should be considered.

VESSELS.—Damage to vessels is rare, but has occurred during attempted reduction of a long-standing dislocation.

OSTEOARTHRITIS of the shoulder joint is liable to follow dislocation in elderly subjects.

RECURRENT DISLOCATION

In cases in which after-treatment has been inadequate, or in persons who are subjected to frequent injury, e.g. epileptics, weakness of the capsule persists, and it may even happen that the patient is able to dislocate a joint voluntarily. If disability occurs, Bankart's operation gives consistently good results, and has many modifications. It postulates that recurrent dislocation is due to separation of the anterior part of the glenoid fibro-cartilage. The joint is exposed, and the coracoid process is divided and displaced downwards with the attached muscles. The subscapularis muscle and capsule are divided and the joint is thus opened. Sutures are inserted so that the detached labrum is firmly stitched to the capsule of the joint. Further stability is obtained by double-breasting the capsule, and

A. S. Blundell Bankart, 1879–1951. Consulting Surgeon, Royal National Orthopædic Hospital, London.

the subscapularis is then repaired. The coracoid process is replaced and held in position by sutures inserted into the adjacent soft tissues. External rotation is not permitted for at least a month, after which active exercises are encouraged. A simpler procedure is that devised by Nicola, and consists in exposing the joint and severing the distal end of the biceps tendon. The humeral head is drilled, the tendon is threaded through the resulting hole and stitched to the proximal end, so that it resembles the ligamentum teres in the hip joint. The results are good provided that the patient does not require to indulge in vigorous exercises. It is a curious fact, which we have personally observed, that in some epileptics the frequency of fits diminishes after an operation for recurrent dislocation.

If the patient is unsuitable for operation an appliance is fitted which supports the joint and prevents more than limited abduction.

FRACTURE—DISLOCATION

This serious accident is due to continuation of force after the shoulder has been dislocated, the fracture occurring through the surgical neck of the humerus. The condition is recognised by the fact that the head of the bone is absent from the glenoid cavity, and is palpable under the coracoid process, but rotation of the arm causes no corresponding movement of the humeral head. Crepitus is obtained on manipulation, and more pain and extravasation are present than in cases of dislocation only. In fat patients radiography is often necessary before diagnosis is possible.

Reduction by manipulation is unlikely to be successful, owing to the small size of the upper fragment and consequent difficulty in controlling it. Open reduction is therefore usually necessary, the bone being exposed by an incision which separates the deltoid and pectoralis major muscles. The upper fragment is conveniently manipulated by means of a screwdriver, which is thrust upwards through the fractured neck, and thus impales the head of the bone. Attachments of soft tissues to the head of the bone must be carefully preserved, otherwise avascular necrosis may follow. In late or neglected cases, arthrodesis of the joint gives a satisfactory result.

UNREDUCED DISLOCATION OF THE SHOULDER

If the dislocation is not reduced within a few days, the surrounding soft structures become matted together by inflammatory exudates and extravasated blood. After two or three weeks organisation occurs, and soft tissues become secondarily contracted. As time passes the articular cartilage is replaced by fibrous tissue, and a false joint may form around the end of the displaced bone. Thus reduction becomes progressively more difficult. Eventually absorption of the adjacent bony surfaces will occur (fig. 1145).

The treatment of an unreduced dislocation often presents a

Toufick Nicola, Contemporary. Clinical Professor of Orthopædics, New York Polyclinic Medical School and Hospital.

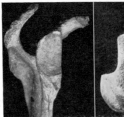
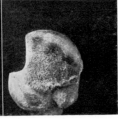

FIG. 1145.—Un-reduced dislocation of the shoulder, with absorption of the glenoid cavity.

The head of the humerus from the same case.

difficult surgical problem. It is generally conceded that reduction should be attempted up to within three weeks from the date of the injury. In healthy adults who need a full range of movement this period is extended for a further three weeks. After the lapse of six weeks surrounding fibrosis and secondary contraction render success unlikely, and the risk of injury to blood-vessels or nerves, or fracture of the bone, is increased. If manipulation fails, open reduction is sometimes indicated. If secondary contraction has occurred, excision of the articular end of the bone is sometimes preferable.

If attempts at reduction fail or are contraindicated, then massage, exercises, and movements are adopted, and the function of the limb is frequently adequate for the needs of the patient. In a few cases such sequelæ as osteoarthritis or pressure on nerves occur, e.g. the head of the displaced humerus on the brachial plexus, which may necessitate excision of the head of the bone through the anatomical neck.

ELBOW JOINT

In cases of dislocation displacement is either forwards, lateral (fig. 1146), or backwards, the last being the most common. Forward dislocation is usually accompanied by fracture of the olecranon, while lateral dislocation is seldom complete. Backward dislocation usually occurs in young adults or children, and may be associated with fracture of the coronoid process, unless the patient is under the age of fourteen, as prior to this the coronoid process is ill-developed. The condition is distinguished from separation of the lower humeral epiphysis by the fact that the normal posi-

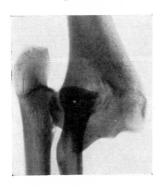

FIG. 1146.—Lateral dislocation of the elbow.

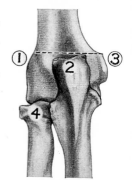

FIG. 1147.—1. External condyle. 2. Tip of olecranon process. 3. Internal condyle. 4. Head of radius.

tions of bony points around the elbow are distorted (fig. 1147). Also on inspection the forearm is apparently shortened, and the measurement between the external epicondyle and radial styloid process confirms this shortening. Examination of the bony points is best performed, when possible, with the patient facing the surgeon and clasping his hands behind his head. The two sides are then readily comparable, and the triangle formed by the olecranon process and the epicondyles can easily be palpated (fig. 1148).

Reduction is effected by flexing the arm to a right angle and applying traction to the forearm. The joint is kept at rest in a sling for three weeks unless the coronoid process is fractured, in which case immobilisation in a plaster cast is required for about two months.

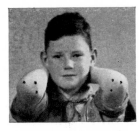

FIG. 1148.—Position for examination of elbow joints.

Anterior dislocations are associated with fracture of the olecranon process. Reduction is obtained by traction with the arm extended, and a few days later the olecranon process is exposed and mechanically fixed in position. A plaster cast is then applied for about six weeks.

Dislocation of the upper end of the **radius** occasionally occurs as a congenital abnormality. In cases due to trauma the head of the bone usually passes forwards and hinders flexion of the joint. Fracture of the shaft of the ulna (Monteggia's fracture, p. 1048) is commonly associated, and can be readily recognised by palpation of its subcutaneous border. Traction of the forearm combined with pressure on the radial head usually permits of reduction, but as the orbicular ligament is torn the dislocation tends to recur. In most cases the head of the bone can be retained in position by means of a pad, the joint then being placed in the fully flexed position. If the ulna is not fractured, attempts at reduction may fail. Osteotomy of the ulna should then be performed in order to facilitate reduction and obviate the alternative of excision of the head of the radius, which always results in permanent weakness.

WRIST JOINT

This joint is rarely dislocated, as a severe injury is more likely to separate the radial epiphysis in children, or to cause a Colles's fracture in adults. The injury is recognised by the fact that the styloid processes retain their normal relationships, i.e. the radial

Abraham Colles, 1773–1843. Professor of Surgery, Dublin.

process is $\frac{1}{2}$ inch lower than that of the ulnar. Reduction is effected by traction, and a dorsal slab is applied for six weeks. Finger movements begin on the day following reduction.

Transcarpal dislocation is due to excessive dorsiflexion of the wrist. The lunate bone remains in position and the remainder of the carpal bones are displaced backwards. Treatment is as for dislocation of the wrist.

Inferior radio-ulnar joint.—Dislocation of this joint is usually associated with a fracture of the lower half of the radius (Galeazzi's fracture). The fracture is easily reduced but is unstable, therefore plating of the radius is advisable.

CARPAL BONES

Dislocation of the **os magnum** very occasionally occurs, the bone being displaced backwards and forming an obvious swelling under the extensor tendons. The bone can sometimes be reduced by applying pressure with the wrist joint flexed. If this is unsuccessful, or the dislocation recurs, then excision is indicated.

The *lunate* bone is sometimes dislocated forwards and then interferes with movements of the wrist. The median nerve is commonly contused. If only partial dislocation occurs reduction is usually easy—traction is applied to the thumb and fingers by an assistant while the surgeon presses on the displaced bone. The wrist joint is immobilised by a plaster slab for about a month. Complete dislocation (fig. 1149) is associated with disruption of all ligamentous attachments. Reduction is impossible, therefore the bone should be excised through an anterior incision, the flexor tendons being separated and the median nerve carefully avoided.

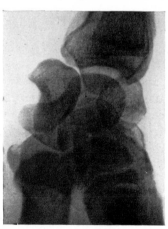

Fig. 1149.—Anterior dislocation of the lunate bone.

Metacarpo-phalangeal and **inter-phalangeal** dislocations can be reduced easily by traction and flexion, with the exception of the metacarpo-phalangeal joint of the thumb. Traction should be applied, and a bandage, placed as a clove-hitch round the thumb, may assist in securing a firm grip. Manipulation frequently fails, the commonest cause of failure being the interposition of the glenoid (anterior) ligament between the two bones. This tough ligament, firmly attached to the base of the

Ricardo Galeazzi, 1866–1950, Mailander University, Italy.

phalanx, is carried backwards, and lies like a curtain between the phalanx and the head of the metacarpal (fig. 1150A).

If manipulation is unsuccessful, the ligament should be split vertically by means of a tenotomy knife, which is inserted from the posterior aspect, and passes underneath the base of the displaced phalanx. The two halves of the ligament then separate and allow the head of the metacarpal to pass between them. We have found this to be a most successful procedure.

Other causes of failure in reduction are buttonholing of the two slips of the flexor pollicis brevis (fig. 1150B), and interposition of the long flexor tendon (fig. 1150c).

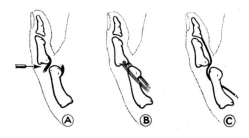

Fig. 1150.—Causes which prevent reduction of a dislocation of the metacarpophalangeal joint of the thumb.

SACRO-ILIAC STRAIN

Genuine sacro-iliac strain is an uncommon disability, frequently confused with such conditions as traumatic myositis, fibrositis of the lowest part of the sacrospinalis muscle, and prolapse of an intervertebral disc. It occurs in females of the child-bearing age. The usual symptom is a localised ache, relieved by rest and rendered worse by exercise. Pain may be referred to the lower abdomen or leg. The patient may notice that the symptoms are suddenly aggravated following a " click," which is due to subluxation, and in some cases she learns how to manipulate her pelvis so as to " unclick " the joint.

Diagnosis is confirmed if pain is produced by stretching the sacro-iliac ligaments. Thus, if the patient lies on her back, pressure exerted outwards on the anterior superior spines stretches the anterior ligaments. When the patient lies on her side, pressure applied in a downward direction over and just behind the anterior superior spine stretches the posterior ligaments. Pressure applied over the sacrum while the patient is prone tends to produce subluxation and consequent pain. Radiography is of little value except to exclude other conditions.

Treatment depends on the fact that symptoms are due to ligamentous strain. Immobilisation is therefore necessary, and is often satisfactorily obtained by adequate corsetry. As a prophylactic measure patients who have suffered from the condition should wear a corset before and after future pregnancies. If a suitable corset fails to relieve symptoms, rest in bed for three months should be prescribed, and as a last resort arthrodesis of the joint will result in permanent cure.

HIP

Owing to the depth of the acetabular cavity, and the strong support afforded by ligaments and muscles, traumatic dislocation of this joint is distinctly uncommon.

The term " irregular " dislocation is applied to cases where the Y-shaped ligament of the Bigelow is ruptured, or the rim of the acetabulum is fractured. If the head of the bone is driven through the acetabulum, a " central " dislocation results.

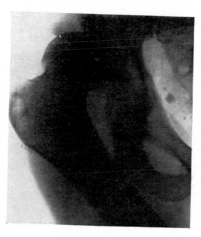

FIG. 1151.—Dislocation of hip following car collision, caused by impact of patient's leg against the dashboard. The driver was killed.

Regular dislocation usually occurs when the thigh is abducted, as in this position the head of the bone is in contact with the relatively weak undersurface of the capsule. The usual causes are stepping sideways on to an unstable object, e.g. a boat, a weight falling on the back of a person in a stooping position, machinery and car accidents (" dashboard " dislocations, fig. 1151).

Anterior dislocation is either obturator or pubic (fig. 1152), and in both cases the limb is in a position of flexion, abduction, and eversion. In obturator dislocations the head of the femur rests upon the obturator externus muscle, and pain may be referred along the obturator nerve, which is compressed as it passes through the upper part of the foramen. The limb is apparently lengthened. If the head of the bone slips upwards, it comes to rest upon the pectineus muscle, where it covers the ascending ramus of the pubis, and a pubic dislocation results. The limb is shortened, and pain is sometimes referred along the anterior crural nerve.

Posterior dislocations are more common than the anterior variety. The head of the bone escapes into the sciatic

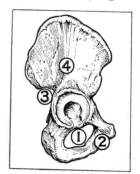

FIG. 1152.—1. Obturator. 2. Pubic.   3. Sciatic.   4. Dorsal.

Henry Bigelow, 1818–1890. Professor of Surgery, Harvard Medical School, Boston.

notch (sciatic variety), and if the tendon of the obturator internus is ruptured the femoral head passes up into the dorsum of the ilium (dorsal variety). In both cases the leg is flexed, adducted, and inverted, so that the sole rests upon the opposite instep. Pain is sometimes referred along the sciatic nerve, which may be injured, and the limb is shortened. X-rays should always be taken to confirm the dislocation and detect any associated fracture.

Reduction is usually accomplished without difficulty, provided that the anæsthetist obtains adequate relaxation of the muscles. The patient is placed on a mattress on the floor, and the iliac crests are steadied by an assistant. The surgeon stands over the limb and flexes the knee and thigh, bringing the head of the bone beneath the acetabulum. In the case of a posterior dislocation the flexed thigh is adducted and inverted. It is then externally circumducted, and rapidly straightened alongside the opposite leg. These movements were summarised by Bigelow in the phrase, " lift up, bend out, roll out." If an anterior dislocation is present, the leg and thigh are flexed as before, and the limb placed in an abducted and everted position. It is then internally circumducted and straightened.

After apparent reduction the movements of the limb must be tested, as cases have occurred in which manipulation merely converted an anterior dislocation into a posterior one or *vice versa*, owing to the head of the bone rotating underneath the acetabulum.

Should these manœuvres fail, upward traction is employed. The patient is held down by assistants, or a towel or binder is fixed firmly across the trunk by means of staples driven into the floor. The surgeon then places the patient's flexed leg against his perineum, and, folding his arms beneath the upper part of the leg, exerts vigorous upward traction, thus lifting the head of the bone upwards into the acetabulum. The method which causes least additional trauma is a combination of rotation and traction. The leg is flexed, and the thigh is rotated so that the head of the femur lies below the acetabulum. Upward traction is then applied and usually reduction follows.

Attempts at reduction in neglected cases have resulted in fracture of the neck of the femur. Following reduction a plaster spica should be applied to below the knee for two months, or longer if the rim of the acetabulum is fractured. This obviates the possibility of redislocation, and prevents further damage to blood-vessels and consequent risk of avascular necrosis. In some cases avascular necrosis of the femoral head is inevitable and osteoarthritis is a common sequela.

KNEE

Complete dislocation of this joint is rare, but subluxation occasionally occurs, following rupture of one or other cruciate ligament, or both. The diagnosis is usually obvious, although rapid effusion into the knee joint tends to render immediate recognition difficult. The most common direction of dislocation is forward, and the popliteal vessels are occasionally compressed by the lower end of the femur.

Reduction is effected by flexion and traction, and aspiration of the distended knee joint is often advisable. The joint should be immobilised in plaster in slight flexion for three months. Quadriceps drill is instituted to begin with, and weight-bearing is permitted after about a month. Instability sometimes persists owing to rupture of the cruciate ligaments (*vide* internal derangement).

PATELLA

This sesamoid bone may be dislocated inwards or outwards, or become twisted, so that its anterior surface is in contact with the condyles. By far the most common direction is outwards, often in association with some degree of genu valgum. The diagnosis is readily made on palpation, and lateral dislocation causes the joint to appear broadened. Reduction is effected by laying the patient on his back with the leg and thigh extended. The quadriceps muscle is thus relaxed, and the bone can be manipulated into position. Recurrence is common if genu valgum co-exists, and if this disables the patient operative measures may be necessary. If genu valgum is severe osteotomy is the obvious treatment. Such operations as transplantation of the sartorius muscle to the inner border of the patella, or plastic operations on the capsule, are likely to be followed by recurrence. If osteotomy is not indicated, a satisfactory procedure is to detach the patellar ligament with a portion of bone and, having prepared a suitable bed on the inner side of the tibia, fix it in this position with a bone peg. More recently excision of the patella has been performed, and this simple operation gives excellent results with no risk of subsequent osteoarthritis.

INTERNAL DERANGEMENT OF THE KNEE JOINT

This term is used to include intra-articular lesions due to trauma occurring in a previously healthy knee joint. The injuries are classified in accordance with the anatomical structure involved.

(i) **Synovial Membrane.**—Injury to the knee joint may result in traumatic synovitis, the synovial membrane becoming hyperæmic and œdematous. If movements are permitted before the swelling has disappeared, the thickened synovial fringes become nipped between the articular surfaces, and thus a vicious circle is established, i.e. frequent nipping causes increased thickening, and consequently a greater liability for nipping to occur. Pain is experienced behind and on either side of the patella (fig. 1153).

Hence, cases of synovitis should be carefully treated and flexion of the joint prevented until swelling has completely disappeared. Recurrent attacks are treated by prolonged immobilisation, and counter-irritation as with Scott's dressing. If this is unsuccessful, arthrotomy must be performed and the thickened fringes excised.

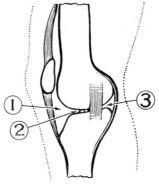

Fig. 1153.—The site of pain in various forms of internal derangement: (1) synovial fringes, (2) semilunar cartilage, (3) loose body in the joint.

(ii) **Ligaments.**—Partial tear or rupture of the lateral ligaments sometimes occurs, especially of the strap-like internal lateral ligament, owing to the normal slight degree of genu varum. Localised pain and tenderness follow, with some hæmorrhagic effusion into the joint. Treatment consists in applying cooling lotions in the early stages and later in relieving the strain by raising the boot about $\frac{1}{3}$ inch (1 cm.) on the corresponding side. In severe cases suture of the torn ligament is advisable.

The cruciate ligaments are very occasionally ruptured as a result of severe trauma, such as lateral dislocation. The anterior cruciate ligament alone may be ruptured by hyperextension. Undue mobility and subluxation of the joint indicate the nature of the injury; if the anterior ligament is torn hyperextension follows, and the tibia can be subluxated forwards on the femur. Actual suture of the torn ligament is impracticable, as the injury is in reality avulsion of the ligament at the tibial attachment. Efforts have been made to reconstruct the ligaments by drilling the bones obliquely, and threading a strip of iliotibial band as a substitute for the anterior ligament, and the tendon of semi-tendinosus for the posterior ligament. Ultimate results are, however, disappointing, as these substituted structures tend to stretch. The most satisfactory treatment, after immobilisation

John Scott, 1798–1846. Surgeon to the London Hospital. The dressing contains mercury ointment, wax, olive oil, and camphor.

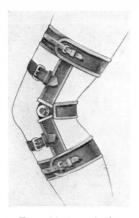

Fig. 1154. — A knee cage. The lock can be adjusted to allow the required degree of flexion.

for three months in plaster has failed, is to furnish the patient with some apparatus which steadies the knee joint, such as Howard Marsh's knee brace (fig. 1154).

(iii) **Cartilage.**—Portions of articular or interarticular cartilage may become detached ; the resulting loose body constitutes one variety of internal derangement. More commonly a semilunar cartilage becomes torn or loosened. The internal cartilage is affected twenty times more commonly than the external, because it is attached to the internal lateral ligament, and is therefore unable to accommodate itself to rotatory movements of the corresponding condyle (fig. 1155). The torn portion of cartilage becomes nipped between the articular surfaces, giving rise to sickening pain and inability to extend the joint. A rapid effusion follows, and localised tenderness is present over the interarticular groove on the inner side.

Treatment of this condition is of the utmost importance if subsequent convalescence is to be shortened and disability

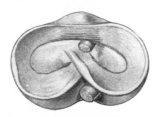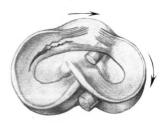

Fig. 1155.—Indicating the mechanism by which outward rotation of the femur is transmitted to the external cartilage, and, via the transverse ligament, to the internal cartilage, with consequent avulsion of its free border.

prevented. Reduction of the cartilage is essential, and should be performed without delay. The cartilage can sometimes be reduced by flexing the knee and hip and placing the leg in a position of eversion and abduction to its fullest extent. Sudden inversion of the tibia and extension of the leg, e.g. by instructing the patient to kick suddenly, often results in reduction. Should this procedure fail, a more deliberate effort must be made.

Howard Marsh, 1839–1915. Surgeon to St. Bartholomew's Hospital, London.

Technique for Reduction.—An anæsthetic is desirable ; gas and oxygen or pentothal usually afford sufficient relaxation. The thigh is supported by an assistant and flexed at the hip. The leg is slowly rotated outwards, so as to open the space between the internal condyle and tibia, and steadily flexed. The cartilage is usually felt to reduce with a click as full flexion is approached, and reduction is confirmed by ability to extend the leg completely. Should this manipulation fail the leg is suddenly extended and rotated inwards, both movements being performed at the same time. If manipulation is unsuccessful the cartilage should be removed.

After reduction lead lotion and a firm bandage discourage further effusion, and a back splint is applied so as to prevent flexion of the joint. Active contractions of the quadriceps are important, as these muscles waste rapidly. After three weeks it is hoped that the torn cartilage has united, but in many cases it is more likely that the torn portion has become fixed in such a position that subsequent movements will not again bring it between the articular surfaces. Gradual flexion is then permitted, and subsequent events awaited. In the majority of cases recurrence follows, and operation is then advised, as a repetition of conservative measures is unlikely to be successful, and repeated locking will lead to osteoarthritis.

A few days are usually allowed in order that effusion may be absorbed, and the skin is then carefully prepared prior to operation. An Esmarch's rubber bandage or a sphygmomanometer is applied as a tourniquet. The internal cartilage is exposed through either a J-shaped or transverse incision on the inner side of the joint. The torn cartilage is steadied by a blunt hook, the transverse ligament is divided anteriorly, and an incision through the coronary ligament separates the cartilage from the tibial tuberosity. The cartilage is then grasped by mosquito forceps and divided as far back as possible, but no traction is permissible, otherwise the posterior portion may be loosened and give rise to subsequent trouble. Usually about two-thirds of the cartilage is removed, and if the posterior portion is unduly mobile it should be removed through a posterior vertical incision. The synovial membrane, capsule, and skin are sutured with interrupted stitches, and a firm bandage applied before the tourniquet is removed, so as to limit bleeding into the joint. The limb is steadied between sandbags, and quadriceps drill is commenced on the following day. The inner side of the boot is raised $\frac{1}{3}$ inch (1 cm.), so that when the patient walks strain on the inner side of the capsule is relieved.

Investigation of a series of personal cases indicated that operation in 84 per cent. of cases gave perfect results (i.e. freedom from pain, freedom from stiffness, and freedom from instability), provided that the patient was under thirty-five years of age and had not suffered from more than three attacks.

(iv) **Bone.**—Small portions of bone are sometimes separated by injury, or avulsion of a tibial spine may be associated with a

Friedrich von Esmarch, 1823–1908. A famous military surgeon, and Professor at Kiel.

torn anterior crucial ligament. The features and treatment have already been indicated.

(v) **Loose Bodies.**—These are considered on p. 1165.

CYST OF SEMILUNAR CARTILAGE

A *cyst* of a semilunar cartilage occasionally occurs, and is alleged to be due to myxomatous degeneration following trauma. The external cartilage is affected more commonly than the internal, and a tense swelling appears over the interarticular groove. The cyst appears suddenly, due to some movement forcing it out from between the bones, and then steadily increases in size (fig. 1156). The cartilage from which the cyst originates should be removed.

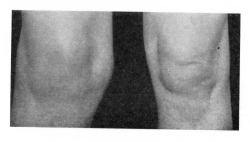

Fig. 1156.—Cyst of the right internal semilunar cartilage.

ANKLE

Owing to the deep mortise formed by the tibia and fibula, dislocation of the ankle joint, without fracture, is extremely rare. Dislocations of the astragalus are more common than formerly, as aeroplane crashes contribute a number of cases. The displacement is anterior, and the bone pushes forward the extensor tendons, or may even protrude through the skin. If reduction is impossible astragalectomy must be performed.

Subastragaloid dislocation occasionally occurs as a result of severe twists or wrenches, e.g. the patient being dragged by a horse with a foot in the stirrup. If manipulation fails, open reduction is necessary.

CHAPTER XLIII

DISEASES OF JOINTS

SYNOVITIS

INFLAMMATION of the synovial membrane occurring other than as part of a generalised arthritis is commonly due to injury. Traumatic synovitis is caused by such accidents as aseptic penetrating wounds (including operations), direct blows, sprains, or nipping of a loose body or cartilage. An effusion follows, either serous or blood-stained, according to the severity of the lesion. The joint assumes a position of ease, i.e. its greatest capacity, and palpation or movements are painful.

Treatment consists, in the early stages, in rest, combined with cold lotions and firm bandaging, in order to minimise further effusion. If effusion is excessive, aspiration is sometimes advisable, as symptoms are thereby relieved, and the time necessary for absorption is shortened. When the early symptoms have abated, muscle drill and subsequently active movements are employed in order to prevent adhesions and to maintain muscular tone.

As movements are increased, the joint should be supported by strapping or a firm bandage, and physiotherapy hastens final recovery.

ACUTE INFECTIVE ARTHRITIS

Acute infection of a joint occurs as a result of :

(i) Direct infection, as by a penetrating wound, or a compound fracture which involves the joint.

(ii) Local extension, from some neighbouring focus, such as acute arthritis of the hip joint from osteomyelitis of the femoral neck.

(iii) Blood-borne infection, the usual organisms being streptococcus, staphylococcus, and pneumococcus, and less commonly the gonococcus and B. typhosis.

The knee joint, owing to its large size and exposed position, is the commonest joint to be involved by penetrating wounds, while blood-borne infections, due to pyæmic conditions, not infrequently attack small joints, particularly the sterno-clavicular or temporo-mandibular.

Clinical Features.—*General*, as of any infection, depending on the size of the joint and virulence of the infection.

Local.—Pain, especially on attempted movement. The joint is held in the position of greatest capacity, and swelling is usually evident. Palpation reveals increased heat and tenderness. Movements are limited by muscular spasm, and attempts at either active or passive movement cause severe pain.

Joint.	Position of ease.	Site of maximum swelling.	Position for ankylosis.
Shoulder	Adducted	Under the deltoid, along the tendon of the biceps, and in the axilla	40° to 50° of abduction, and just anterior to the coronal plane.
Elbow	Flexed at a right angle and pronated	On either side of triceps tendon	130° of extension semi-pronated. If both sides, the second elbow at 75° of extension. These positions may be modified according to occupation.
Wrist	Slight flexion	Under extensor and flexor tendons	Dorsi-flexed to allow a firm grasp.
Hip	Flexed, abducted, and everted	Upper part of Scarpa's triangle	20° to 30° of flexion to allow sitting, and sufficient abduction to compensate for the resultant shortening.
Knee	Flexed	Subcrureal pouch, and either side of patellar tendon	5° to 10° of flexion to allow foot to clear ground in walking.
Ankle	Slightly extended and inverted	Anteriorly and on either side of the Achilles tendon	Just over a right angle, with slight inversion to discourage flat-foot.

It will be seen that in most cases the position of ease differs widely from the position which is most useful should ankylosis occur. As any case of arthritis may be followed by ankylosis, the first duty of the surgeon is to anticipate this possibility by immobilising the joint in the best position for ankylosis, as indicated in the preceding table.

Treatment.—Chemotherapy and penicillin are prescribed, and have greatly reduced the incidence and severity of joint infections, as a result of both prophylactic and therapeutic administration. In the early stages the limb is supported and fixed

by a suitable splint or appliance in the correct position, an anæsthetic being administered if necessary. If infection is already
established weight-extension is advisable, as by this means
muscular spasm and pain are relieved, and intra-articular pressure is prevented. The following lines of treatment are then to
be considered.

(i) *Aspiration,* which is useful for both diagnostic and therapeutic reasons. Thus the nature of the fluid can be ascertained,
and smears of cultures assist in identifying the causative organism, so that suitable chemotherapy can be instituted. Aspiration also reduces the tension within the
joint, thereby relieving pain, and obviating the stretching of ligaments and
capsule. Daily aspirations are usually
adequate.

(ii) *Aspiration and Irrigation.*—After
fluid has been aspirated 200,000 units
of penicillin may be injected into the
joint. In early cases, or when the infection is of low virulence, aspiration
and penicillin replacement, repeated if
necessary, encourage the inflammation
to subside. Penicillin is also administered parenterally, and the limb is
suitably splinted.

(iii) *Arthrotomy and Drainage.*—In
more advanced cases the joint is opened,
washed out, and drainage tubes inserted
down to the synovial membrane (fig. 1157). On no account should
tubes project into the articular cavity. The knee joint is
drained through an antero-lateral incision, combined, if necessary, with a postero-lateral incision which passes behind the
ilio-tibial band and in front of the biceps tendon. In all cases
adequate immobilisation is essential.

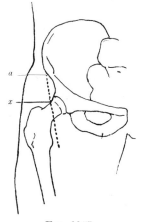

Fig. 1157.

a = incision for approach to hip
joint, which passes between the
tensor fasciæ femoris and glutei
on the outside, and the sartorius
and rectus femoris muscles on
the inner side.

x = site for puncture.

Extra-articular abscesses sometimes require to be opened and
drained. In the case of the knee joint, pus is particularly liable
to track upwards beneath the quadriceps, where its presence
may be overlooked.

(iv) *Excision.*—If in spite of treatment the condition of the
patient deteriorates, or if suppuration is prolonged, then ex-

cision of the joint may be considered, although infection of bone and delay in healing are to be expected. However, provided that the condition of the patient does not demand amputation, excision should be performed in the case of the wrist, elbow, or shoulder, as an artificial arm is a poor substitute. Excision of the ankle or knee is rarely performed, as amputation and provision of an artificial leg are likely to be followed by rapid convalescence and a satisfactory functional result. In the case of the hip joint, excision is sometimes performed in an attempt to avoid such a mutilating procedure as amputation through that joint, but the functional result, even after a successful excision, is usually poor. Needless to say, the patient's life must not be jeopardised in an endeavour to spare a limb, particularly as the affected joint will eventually be more or less disorganised.

(v) *Amputation* is indicated if at any stage the patient's life is threatened, or prolonged suppuration leads to amyloid disease (which is particularly liable to occur in connexion with infection of the hip joint). Also, in some cases a painful and disorganised joint causes such disability that an artificial limb is preferable.

PENETRATING WOUNDS OF JOINTS

Owing to its size and exposed position the knee joint is most commonly affected by penetrating wounds. For the purposes of treatment wounds are classified according to the risk of subsequent infection.

(i) *Infection is unlikely*, e.g. recent puncture by a small and comparatively clean article, such as a needle. In these cases the needle is removed and the wound is sterilised with an antiseptic. The limb is immobilised in the most useful position should ankylosis subsequently occur, and chemotherapy and penicillin are administered. Usually a mild, transitory effusion occurs, which subsides in two or three days. Should general and local symptoms or signs suggest that infection is occurring, then the joint is aspirated, and treatment continued along the lines already indicated for acute arthritis.

(ii) *Infection is probable*, such as penetration by a rusty nail, particularly if delay has already permitted infection. In these cases emergency operation must be performed, and the wound excised layer by layer until the joint is opened. Irrigation is advisable if obvious contamination has occurred, as by fragments of rust. The wound is partially or completely closed according to the risk of infection, and the limb is immobilised in the most useful position should ankylosis follow. A prophylactic course of sulphonamide and penicillin is prescribed.

(iii) *Infection is certain*, e.g. extensive laceration of the capsule, or less severe wounds which have been neglected. Recent extensive wounds, which formerly would inevitably have become infected, often do remarkably well following thorough débridement, insufflation of sulphonamide powder, encasement in plaster, and chemotherapy. If infection supervenes, or is already established, the wound is rendered as surgically clean as possible, and drainage is provided if necessary. The limb is immobilised, and further treatment conducted on the lines indicated for acute arthritis.

GONOCOCCAL ARTHRITIS

Owing to more efficient treatment of gonococcal urethritis and conjunctivitis, articular complications are now uncommon.

Joint lesions occur at any stage after infection, but are most common when the initial infection is subsiding, or during an exacerbation, e.g. after urethral manipulations.

The following types of gonococcal arthritis occur :

(i) **Rheumatism** is characterised by attacks of pain in one or more joints. The duration is variable, and pain frequently attacks different joints in succession. No physical signs are detectable, and the condition subsides gradually.

(ii) **Acute Arthritis.**—Usually a single large joint is affected, especially the ankle, elbow, or wrist, the last particularly in females. All the symptoms and signs of acute infective arthritis are present, and destruction is sometimes sufficiently extensive to cause bony ankylosis. On aspiration the fluid may be found to contain other organisms in addition to gonococci; in less acute or later cases it is sometimes sterile. Treatment is conducted on the lines already indicated.

(iii) **Chronic plastic arthritis** is a polyarticular infection, in which there is but slight effusion in the joints. Considerable œdema of the synovial membrane and periarticular structures occurs. Troublesome adhesions and stiffness are to be expected.

(iv) **Periarticular Arthritis.**—Chiefly affects tendon sheaths and ligaments, and occasionally occurs in the hands or feet. In the latter situation stretching of ligaments leads to flat-foot unless preventive measures are adopted.

(v) **Pyæmia.**—The small joints are most likely to be affected, e.g. the temporo-mandibular or sterno-clavicular. In common with other types of pyæmic abscesses, the condition is relatively painless, and swelling is sometimes the first indication of the condition.

Treatment.—Limitation of movement arising from fibrosis of extra-articular structures, or fibrous and sometimes even bony ankylosis, are characteristic features of gonococcal affections. A course of chemotherapy or antibiotics is prescribed, and as soon as the acute phase of inflammation has abated judicious physiotherapy and active movements must be instituted. Diathermy is particularly useful, as gonococci are susceptible to a degree of heat which is readily tolerated by the tissues.

SYPHILITIC DISEASES OF JOINTS

Inherited.—*Painless Effusion.*—This has been aptly described as " symmetrical, serous, syphilitic synovitis," and is associated with the name of Clutton. It is characterised by a painless effusion into a large joint, most commonly the knee (fig. 29). This condition is frequently bilateral, although the swelling of the two joints may not synchronise. The effusion causes a sensation of weakness and insecurity, and on examination the joint is seen and felt to be distended. Movements are only limited if the amount of fluid mechanically prevents the full range.

The condition occurs between the ages of ten and eighteen, and other stigmata of inherited syphilis are usually present. This condition is one of the four characteristic signs of inherited syphilis, which appear about puberty, and give rise to " the halt, the deaf, the blind, and the impotent," i.e. halt owing to Clutton's joints, deaf because of otitis interna, blind following interstitial keratitis (fig. 1158), and impotent secondary to orchitis.

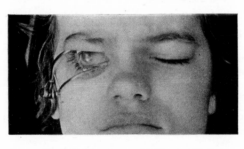

FIG. 1158.—Interstitial keratitis.

If no confirmatory clinical evidence of syphilis is discovered, then the family history is usually suggestive, and finally the W.R. of the patient and parents, or even of the fluid aspirated from the joint, should be tested.

Acquired.—During the *secondary* stage a transient or variable effusion sometimes occurs in any of the larger joints. The condition is painless, and sometimes, like most secondary lesions, symmetrical.

Henry Clutton, 1850–1909.   Surgeon to St. Thomas's Hospital, London.

Lesions of the *tertiary* stage are classified as follows :

(*a*) *Local Synovial Gumma.*—This uncommon condition commences in the synovial membrane of a large joint, e.g. on the inner side of the knee. At first firm and nodular, like all gummata it tends to infiltrate superficial tissues, and if neglected it eventually softens and discharges through the skin, giving rise to a gummatous ulcer which communicates with the joint cavity.

(*b*) *Gummatous Synovitis.*—In some respects this simulates tuberculous disease, but the synovial thickening is more irregular. Moreover, the condition is painless, therefore muscular spasm and wasting are not pronounced.

(*c*) *Chondroarthritis.*—Chiefly affects the bone and cartilage, which are eroded. It is distinguished from osteoarthritis in that pain is slight, and erosion does not necessarily occur at sites of intra-articular pressure. Moreover, lipping is absent, and the synovial membrane is sometimes palpably thickened.

Unless it is remembered that syphilitic joints do occur, the true nature of the condition is sometimes overlooked ; therefore any " tuberculous " or " osteoarthritic " joint which presents abnormal features should be considered as being possibly affected by syphilis—the " great imitator."

NEUROPATHIC JOINTS

The most important pathological conditions of joints secondary to affections of the nervous system occur in connection with :

I. Parasyphilis.

II. Syringomyelia.

III. Hysteria.

IV. Other lesions of the Nervous System.

I. PARASYPHILIS

Owing to the more efficient treatment of syphilis Charcot's joints occur with diminishing frequency. About 4 per cent. of tabetic patients develop an arthropathy, of which 85 per cent. occur in the lower limbs, the knee being the commonest joint to be affected. The " hypertrophic " type usually occurs in hinge joints, while the " atrophic " variety occurs more frequently in ball-and-socket joints. In either case, an effusion, which varies in amount, is present, and complete *absence of pain* is a striking feature. Examination of a typical case, following the routine which should be adopted for all joints, comprises :

(i) *Inspection.*—The joint is distended, and if the effusion is generous, it assumes the position of greatest capacity. In advanced cases the joint is obviously disorganised (fig. 1159).

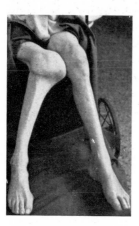

FIG. 1159.—Charcot's disease of the right knee.
(*Dr. Worster-Drought.*)

(ii) *Palpation.*—The presence of fluid is confirmed, and in hypertrophic cases irregular masses of bone are readily palpable. Bursæ which communicate with the joint, such as the psoas bursa, are sometimes distended. Synovial membrane is liable to herniate through weak parts of the distended capsule, e.g. into the popliteal fossa. These "cysts," first described by Morrant Baker, sometimes track under the muscles, and may appear some inches from the joint, e.g. in the case of the knee between the peroneal and anterior tibial groups of muscles.

(iii) *Movements.* — A characteristic soft crepitus is usually noticed, which resembles the "crunching" under the foot when walking over snow. Movements vary with the amount of restriction imposed by new bone formation, but in the absence of interlocking they are usually surprisingly free and painless.

(iv) *Measurement.*—Shortening of the limb sometimes occurs owing to absorption of bone, and some degree of muscular wasting may result from disuse.

(v) *Radiograph.*—Irregular masses of bone are seen in the hypertrophic variety. The atrophic type will show irregular and eventually almost complete absorption of the articular ends of the affected bones (fig. 1160).

(vi) *General Examination.*—It is rare for a Charcot's joint to appear as the first evidence of tabes. Lightning pains, Romberg's sign, ataxia or other symptoms are usually present, while examination commonly reveals Argyll-Robertson pupils and loss of tendon reflexes, particularly the knee and ankle jerks.

Treatment consists in supporting the joint by a suitable

William Morrant Baker, 1839–1896. Surgeon to St. Bartholomew's Hospital, London.
Moritz Romberg, 1795–1873. Professor of Medicine in Berlin.
Douglas Argyll-Robertson, 1837–1909. Ophthalmic Surgeon, Edinburgh Royal Infirmary.

appliance, e.g. a knee brace or a walking calliper.

Excision of the knee joint has been practised, but is only justifiable if ataxia has not developed, otherwise the doubtful benefit secured by stabilisation of an ataxic joint is more than offset by the risk of infection of the wound, or non-union of the atrophic bones.

II. SYRINGOMYELIA

is due to gliomatous degeneration round the central canal of the spinal cord, and usually occurs in the lower cervical region. Joint complications occur in about 15 per cent. of cases of syringomyelia, and

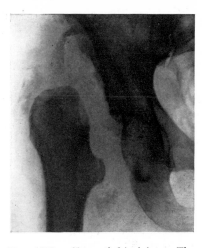

FIG. 1160.—Charcot's hip joint. The opposite knee joint was also affected.

closely resemble the Charcot's joints described above, except that the arm is more often affected than the leg (80 per cent.) (figs. 1161 and 1162). The shoulder is most frequently

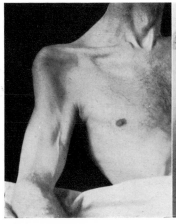
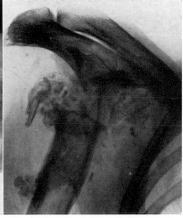

FIG. 1161.—Charcot's disease of the shoulder, due to syringomyelia.

FIG. 1162.—X-ray of the same case, showing absorption of bone, and gross disorganisation.

attacked, and being a ball-and-socket joint, the atrophic type of the disease is the more usual.

Further examination of the patient reveals other evidence of syringomyelia, such as :

(a) *Dissociation of Sensation in the Hands.*—The sensibility to pain and variations of temperature are lost, but tactile sensation and muscular sense remain. Owing to the loss of sensation, small injuries, notably cigarette burns, occur unnoticed.

(b) *Trophic Changes.*—Wasting occurs of all the muscles of the hand, and later the forearms. Also the tissues are more prone to injury, and healing is delayed. Eventually the soft tissues and finally the phalanges become absorbed (fig. 1163).

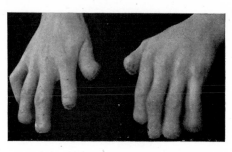

(c) *Scoliosis*, due to asymmetrical irritation of the pyramidal tracts, so that the erector spinæ on one side is more spastic than its fellow, and acts on the spinal column in the manner of a bow-string.

(d) *Unequal Pupils*, due to asymmetrical irritation of the oculo-pupillary fibres, which pass down the cervical cord, and leave it in company with the first dorsal nerve, passing thence via the rami communicantes to the inferior cervical sympathetic ganglion, and along the carotid sheath and ophthalmic artery to the ciliary ganglion.

FIG. 1163.—Trophic loss of the fingers, due to syringomyelia, Morvan type.

(e) *Spasticity of the Legs*, due to irritation of the pyramidal tracts.

Syringobulbia, as evinced by hoarseness and dysphagia, may subsequently develop.

Treatment of the joint condition entails adequate support, pressure being carefully guarded against, as owing to insensitiveness to pain pressure sores are particularly liable to occur.

III. HYSTERIA (Syn. MIMETIC JOINT)

Disability in connection with a joint sometimes occurs in patients of hysterical tendencies, and is most commonly seen in adolescent or young adult females. The history in some cases is suggestive, in that the onset follows some emotional crisis, or mimicry of some joint condition seen in another patient. The larger joints are usually affected, the commonest being the hip or knee.

The more important clinical features are as follows :

(a) *Inspection.*—The limb is often in a position which is unusual for any early pathological condition, e.g. in the case of the hip joint the thigh may be markedly flexed, adducted, and inverted. Wasting of muscles, if any, is slight, and is due to disuse.

(b) *Palpation.*—Gentle palpation may appear to cause intolerable pain, but if the attention is distracted, considerable pressure will pass unnoticed. Otherwise no abnormal features are discovered.

(c) *Movements.*—All movements are restricted, and if the patient is requested to move a joint, both the group of muscles which carry out the movement, and also the antagonistic muscles, are contracted, so that the limb is rigidly fixed. This phenomenon can easily be appreciated by pal-

Augustin Marie Morvan, 1819–1897. A physician of Lannelis, Finisterre.

pation of the muscles, while the patient attempts to carry out the desired movement.

(*d*) *Measurement.*—If the condition has persisted for a sufficient length of time, wasting will be detected owing to disuse atrophy.

(*e*) *Radiograph.*—In long-standing cases disuse atrophy of bone occurs, as is shown by thinning of the compact layer, and loss of density of the cancellous tissue owing to absorption of calcium salts.

(*f*) *General Examination.*—Other hysterical manifestations will probably be found, such as globus hystericus, anæsthesia of the palate, and glove or stocking anæsthesia.

Treatment.—Psycho-analysis might be employed in order to correct the abnormal mental outlook. Symptomatic treatment directed to the joint includes encouragement regarding movements, or an anæsthetic is given, and the position of the joint altered. In the case of the lower limb spinal anæsthesia is particularly useful, as the patient can then be impressed by the range of movements which are then obtainable.

IV. OTHER LESIONS OF THE NERVOUS SYSTEM

Long-standing impairment of the trophic innervation of a limb is followed by changes in the small joints of the hands and feet. Such causes include cerebral injury, spina bifida, and peripheral nerve lesions, e.g. injury, neuritis, or leprosy. The articular surfaces of the bones are absorbed, and ligamentous structures become contracted. Treatment consists in prevention of deformity and physiotherapy to the affected joints.

TUBERCULOUS DISEASE

Tuberculous arthritis originates either in the synovial membrane or in the bone. The factors which influence the site of origin are the age of the patient, and the individual joint which is affected, thus in children the osseous type is commoner than the synovial, as the epiphysis is frequently affected, whereas the reverse is true for adults. In the knee and elbow, the disease usually first attacks the synovial membrane, whereas in other joints, notably the hip and wrist, the initial focus of infection is generally in the adjacent bone.

Four types of tuberculous arthritis are recognised :

(i) *Synovial.*—Characterised by œdema and infiltration of the synovial membrane and periarticular tissues, giving rise to the typical " white swelling " (fig. 1164). The synovial membrane becomes thickened and succulent, and subserous tubercles appear. Gradually the structure is lost, and the membrane becomes converted into granulation tissue. These granulations creep across the articular cartilage, which

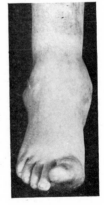

Fig. 1164.— Tuberculous disease of the ankle joint.

is eroded and destroyed, thus exposing the underlying bone to invasion. If neglected, subluxation or dislocation of the joint will follow, e.g. a " wandering " acetabulum. Tuberculous abscesses may develop, and secondary infection will follow if they are allowed to erode the skin.

(ii) *Osseous.*—The infection commences in the bone adjacent to the joint, or in the case of a child in the epiphysis, and extends into the joint by the continuous invasion of the intervening tissue. This type is more insidious than the synovial type, and symptoms are usually present before clinical signs are obvious.

(iii) *Caries Sicca.*—Is seen most commonly in the shoulder joint. Gradual destruction of the bones occurs with very little synovial œdema.

(iv) *Hydrops.*—Excess of fluid is a rare occurrence in tuberculous arthritis, but occasionally the knee joint becomes distended with fluid containing fibrin, which is later converted into flat, oval objects, referred to as " melonseed bodies " (fig. 1186).

Clinical Features.—*Symptoms.*—Tuberculous arthritis presents an insidious onset, aching after use and stiffness following rest being early symptoms. Pain is not severe, but sudden strains and twists are deliberately or subconsciously avoided. When erosion of cartilage has occurred, " starting pains " are characteristic, and occur just when the patient is dropping off to sleep. They are due to relaxation of the muscles which guard the joint, so that slight movement between the articular surfaces causes friction between the exposed and sensitive bones. Swelling of the joint is sometimes noticed by the patient, and is due to œdema of the synovial membrane and periarticular structures.

Some deterioration of the general health is to be expected, and the temperament of a small child may completely alter, so that happiness and contentment give way to peevishness and fretfulness.

Signs.—Following the routine which always should be adopted for the examination of joints, we find :

(*a*) *Inspection.*—The limbs are exposed, and the position of the affected one is observed. The opposite limb is then placed in a corresponding position. Deformity in the early stages is due to the position of ease which the joint automatically assumes ; later, deformity results from disorganisation. Swelling of and

around the joint is due to œdema ; only in the rare cases of
hydrops is it caused by distension of the joint by free fluid.   The
swelling therefore, in most cases, fades away above and below the
joint, and is characteristically spindle-shaped.   The whiteness
of the overlying skin is due to pressure of the œdema emptying
the cutaneous capillaries, which are not in a condition of reflex
hyperæmia, such as occurs in acute infection.   Muscular wasting
is a constant feature, and is due both to disuse atrophy and
trophic disturbances (fig. 1165).

Fig. 1165.—
Tuberculosis of the
left knee joint,
showing   flexion,
swelling, and wast-
ing of muscles.

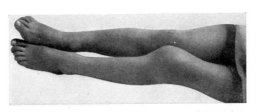

In the later stages abscesses and sinus formation are apt to
occur.

(b) *Palpation.*—Sensitive hands may detect a slight rise of
cutaneous temperature over the affected joint.   A somewhat
boggy or doughy thickening of the synovial membrane will be
detected if this structure is sufficiently superficial.   Owing to
muscular atrophy, and flabbiness of atonic muscles, the articular
ends of bones are much more easily palpable than those of the
opposite limb, and this leads the unwary into the erroneous
belief that the bone ends are enlarged, instead of merely being
" thrown into relief."

(c) *Movements.*—The patient is requested to move the joint as
far as possible in all directions, and it will be noted that all active
movements are limited.

The surgeon then puts the sound limb through its full range of
movements, in order to gain the confidence of the patient, and
also to ascertain the degree of mobility present in that individual
patient.   The movements of the affected limb are then tested, if
possible while the patient's attention is diverted.   In cases of
tuberculous arthritis movements become increasingly limited
owing to protective spasm of muscles.

(d) *Measurement.*—The presence of muscular wasting is confirmed, and the amount of shortening, due to lack of growth or
disorganisation of the joint, is estimated.

(e) *Radiograph.*—If the bone is actively affected, rarefaction is present, as shown by loss of pattern due to destruction of the bony trabeculæ, and also by diminution in density, owing to absorption of calcium salts (fig. 1166).

If the disease is limited to the synovial membrane, the bone undergoes some degree of atrophy, in common with the soft

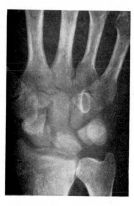

tissues. The X-ray then shows thinning of the compact bone and loss of density of the cancellous bone, the pattern of which remains unaltered, as trabeculæ are not destroyed. Invariably, it is necessary to compare the radiograph with one of the normal side in order to appreciate early bony changes.

(f) *General Examination.*—Other evidence of tuberculous trouble, either active, latent, or healed, may be discovered.

(g) *Special Tests.*—The erythrocyte sedimentation rate is increased. A negative tuberculin test is useful in excluding tuberculosis. Examination of

FIG. 1166.—Tuberculosis of the wrist joint.

pus aspirated from an associated abscess will often establish the diagnosis.

Excision and microscopical examination of a regional lymph node shows invasion by B. tuberculosis in 80 per cent. of cases. This is a valuable measure in doubtful cases, and is simpler and safer than the removal of a portion of synovial membrane for biopsy, which may result in a sinus. An inguinal node is removed in suspected disease of the knee, and one of the external iliac group in the case of the hip joint.

In suspicious cases the patient should be confined to bed and the joint immobilised. Mild toxic affections (such as may be associated with tonsillitis), or slight effusions due to injury, will rapidly respond. A tuberculous joint will improve to some extent, but relapses as soon as normal use is permitted.

Differential Diagnosis.—The diagnosis of a typical tuberculous joint causes no difficulty, but less typical cases may be confused with the following conditions: Osteochondritis juvenalis, especially Perthes' disease (p.1099), and possibly other members of this group. Hæmophilic joints (p. 1169). Osteoarthritis of a single joint, especially the knee or hip. Subacute toxic arthritis or mild traumatic synovitis, which subside with a short period of rest. Tumour at the end of a long bone (sarcoma or osteoclastoma), which may cause synovial hyperæmia before X-ray changes are obvious.

PROGNOSIS depends upon the following factors :

(i) *Age of Patient.*—Patients at the two extremes of life have less resistance to tuberculous disease than those of adolescence or middle adult life.

(ii) *Family History.*—Lack of resistance appears to be a familial characteristic, and when the disease occurs in a member of a tuberculous family, the prognosis is less bright.

(iii) *The Stage of the Disease.*—Cases which are diagnosed in the early stages and which receive appropriate treatment are more likely to make a good recovery than those which have been neglected.

(iv) *The Presence of other Tuberculous Foci.*—If the patient is otherwise healthy, the chances of a good result are materially increased.

Treatment.—GENERAL TREATMENT in a suitable centre is instituted without delay, and maintained until the condition is assumed to be cured. Fresh air, natural or artificial sunlight, suitable food, and cheerful surroundings are all of great importance. Children continue their education and adults are employed in occupational therapy. Streptomycin is worthy of trial if recovery is retarded.

LOCAL TREATMENT consists of immobilisation of the joint, with aspiration of abscesses if necessary, as the routine procedure. At a later date operative intervention is sometimes advisable.

Immobilisation.—The limb is immobilised in the optimum position until some six months after the last sign or symptom has disappeared. The actual length of time for which treatment should be continued, after the disease is apparently cured, depends on the general condition of the patient, local response to treatment, including X-ray appearances, and the actual joint affected. The hip joint in particular requires prolongation fixation, and one year's further treatment is usually advisable after the disease is apparently cured.

If the limb is in an unsuitable position when first seen, e.g. considerable flexion of the knee joint, then the deformity is usually overcome by weight extension, which is applied so that traction is exerted in the line of the bone below the affected joint. Cases with slight deformity often respond to a period of rest in bed, which results in disappearance of some of the muscular spasm, and permits the joint to be placed in the correct position. If weight extension is necessary, e.g. in the case of the knee joint, strapping is applied along either side of the leg as far as the tuberosities of the tibia.

These two lateral strips are attached to a wooden stirrup below the foot, from which a cord passes over a pulley. Sufficient weight is than applied to overcome muscular spasm ; 1 lb. for each stone of the patient's weight is usually adequate. Interosseous pressure and starting pains are thereby relieved. After a few days the muscles relax, and the pull of the weight then stretches ligaments and causes a renewed aching, so the weight is then reduced. As spasm is overcome the leg is straightened until the desired position is reached.

Immobilisation is obtained by means of some suitable appliance or apparatus. For the hip joint a Jones's abduction frame, which fixes the spine and hip joints, is commonly applied. A plaster case is adequate for most joints, although it is cumbersome and cannot be removed frequently for inspection or to permit the limb to enjoy heliotherapy. When the condition appears to be responding to treatment, a lighter and removable splint is substituted for the plaster. Such materials as poroplastic or celluloid are used for this purpose, or a light bivalve plaster is sometimes adequate and convenient. In the case of the lower limb a walking calliper forms a very suitable appliance for convalescent cases.

The last signs or symptoms to disappear are local or referred pain, abscess formation, and spasm of muscles. After a further variable period (*vide supra*) the patient is allowed to regain gradually the use of his limb.

OPERATIVE TREATMENT

Surgical intervention is only indicated when the disease is quiescent, as in the presence of active infection attempts at fixation, even if extra-articular, are unlikely to be successful. The aim of the surgeon is to obtain a bony ankylosis in good position. Briefly, the indications for operative procedures are as follows :

(i) *To Shorten the Time Necessary for Treatment.*—In some instances experience teaches that the result obtainable by operation is as good as or even better than that resulting from immobilisation, e.g. tuberculous arthritis of the wrist or knee in patients past the meridian of life. Therefore, provided that the disease is quiescent, operation is recommended in order to save time, and to rid the patient of an active tuberculous focus which may otherwise impair health, or disseminate and so endanger life.

In other cases it becomes increasingly obvious during conservative treatment that, although the disease is being overcome gradually, yet destruction of the joint is inevitable. For example, in the case of the knee joint, fixity of the patella to the intercondylar notch suggests that, *a fortiori*, the condyles are becoming fixed to the tibial plateau. Excision of the knee is then indicated, as bony ankylosis is obtainable in a comparatively short time, and is preferable to a more or less complete and possibly painful fibrous ankylosis.

(ii) *To Improve Position.*—A tuberculous joint which has been allowed to ankylose in a faulty position is usually an indication that the elementary principles of immobilisation have been ignored.

The positions of election for ankylosis have been indicated (p. 1140), and operation is sometimes desirable to improve the position and function of the limb.

(iii) *To Regain Mobility.*—Ankylosis in a good position results in adequate function as far as the majority of joints are concerned. However, in certain situations, notably the elbow and temporo-mandibular joints, excision with a view to regaining mobility is desirable. In the rare event of bilateral ankylosis of the hip joints, a successful arthroplasty of one joint will facilitate such activities as ascending or descending stairs.

Operations.—(i) *Arthrectomy.*—Consists in opening the joint freely, and dissecting away as much diseased synovial membrane as possible. Eroded or loose cartilage is removed, and any local areas of diseased bone are gouged away. If a slice of articular cartilage is removed, the procedure is then termed *erasion*, and is preferable to excision in the case of children, as the epiphyseal cartilage is not injured.

(ii) *Extra-articular Arthrodesis.*—This procedure is especially applicable to the hip joint (p. 1159).

(iii) *Excision.*—Is the most common operation to be performed. It consists of free removal of all intra-articular soft tissues, together with the articular ends of the bones, and diseased foci in the shaft. Fusion is often aided by use of a bone graft. Classical excisions are rarely performed in practice, and in the case of children every attempt should be made to spare the epiphyseal cartilage. The object of the operation is to secure firm, bony ankylosis, which yields a stable and painless arthrodesis.

(iv) *Amputation.*—In cases where other measures have failed, either for local or general reasons, amputation will be necessary in order to remove a useless encumbrance, or to terminate the debilitating effects of prolonged toxæmia.

Results.—(i) *Resolution.*—Complete resolution probably never occurs, but in a small percentage of children a considerable degree of painless movement is regained. However, some years must elapse before the risk of recurrence is past. In the large majority of cases the best result is a firmly ankylosed joint in the best functional position.

(ii) *Fibrous Ankylosis* is the commonest natural termination following the gradual organisation of granulation tissue. The presence of adhesions in the joint may still allow some degree of movement, so that the function is not necessarily much impaired. If dense adhesions form, movement is probably entirely absent, but is distinguished from bony ankylosis by the fact that vigorous attempts to move the joint cause pain if ankylosis is of the fibrous variety. Organisms may be buried in fibrous tissue for years, only to resurrect themselves should the joint be injured or the general health of the patient impaired.

(iii) *Bony Ankylosis*, apart from surgical intervention, only occurs as a result of secondary infection, which gains entry to the joint along sinuses formed by abscesses bursting through the skin (fig. 1167).

(iv) *General Dissemination.*—Acute miliary tuberculosis occasionally occurs as a result of blood-borne infection, particularly if the general resistance of the patient is undermined by any debilitating condition. This complication has also followed manipulation of tuberculous joints by osteopaths, bone-setters, and other unskilled persons.

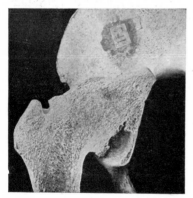

Fig. 1167.—Bony ankylosis of the hip joint with adduction of the femur, and a " travelling acetabulum."
(*London Hospital Museum.*)

(v) *Toxæmia.* — If sinuses occur and prolonged suppuration follows, subacute or chronic toxæmia is likely, and if of sufficiently long duration, amyloid disease may develop. Amyloid disease is prone to occur if the hip is involved, for such a mutilating procedure as amputation through that joint is naturally dreaded and postponed by the patient.

SPECIAL JOINTS

Sacro-iliac.—This joint is not commonly affected, and, owing to vagueness of the early symptoms and late appearances of definite signs, the correct diagnosis is often delayed. A local ache, pain referred along the great sciatic nerve, which lies in front of the joint, and a sensation of weakness of the pelvic ring are among the first symptoms. After a few weeks a boggy swelling appears over the back of the joint, which gradually enlarges to form an abscess. Rectal or vaginal examination may reveal a similar condition in the pelvis. When the disease is established, pressure on the iliac crests causes articular pain. A radiograph confirms the diagnosis.

Treatment necessitates operation as soon as the condition is quiescent, as obliteration of the joint causes no disability, and removal of diseased issue and fixation of the joint favours a cure in the shortest possible time. Access is gained by removal of the posterior superior spine and adjacent iliac crest. Tuberculous granulation tissue and diseased bone are removed with a sharp spoon and gouge, and a bone graft or peg is driven through the bones so as to bridge the joint.

Hip.—The disease usually commences in a bone, either in the under-surface of the neck of the femur or in the acetabulum. It is uncommon after the age of twenty.

Early symptoms include a limp, and pain commonly referred to the knee joint along the geniculate branch of the obturator nerve. The femoral and great sciatic nerves also send articular branches to both joints.

During the *first stage* of this condition the joint is held in the position of ease, i.e. flexed, abducted, and everted. The abduction causes the pelvis to tilt downwards, and gives rise to apparent lengthening of the limb. Flexion of the hip is usually masked by lordosis, which should be corrected by flexion of the thigh so that the true position of the limb can be assessed (fig. 1209). As the joint becomes more painful, the patient is increasingly inclined to assume a recumbent position, during which the patient lies on the sound and painless hip. Thus in the *second stage* the affected joint gradually becomes adducted and inverted, and flexion becomes more marked (fig. 1168). Owing to adduc-

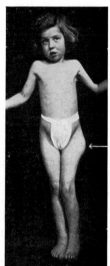

FIG. 1168.—Tuberculosis of the left hip, second stage. The arrow indicates a periarticular abscess.

tion, the limb is apparently shortened. The *third stage* corresponds with articular disorganisation, including absorption of the femoral head and acetabular cavity. The position of adduction and inversion encourages the head of the femur to slip out of the eroded acetabulum, and consequently the femoral head is displaced upwards on to the dorsum ilii. Further absorption of bone, combined with continuous pull of spastic muscles, results in a " travelling acetabulum " (fig. 1167). In a small percentage of cases complete erosion of the acetabulum is associated with the formation of a tuberculous abscess in the pelvic cavity. During the third stage the hip is in a position of flexion, inversion, and adduction, and disorganisation of the joint leads to true shortening of the limb, in addition to the apparent shortening due to adduction (fig. 1169).

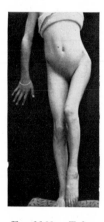

FIG. 1169.—Tuberculosis of the left hip, third stage.
(*Pybus.*)

In considering the differential diagnosis, such conditions as spasm of the psoas (which causes flexion of the joint) and tuberculosis of the gluteal bursa (which leads to abduction and eversion) must be considered. Coxa vara, with superadded traumatic arthritis, may cause confusion, but a week or so in bed results in disappearance of the arthritis, after which the typical signs of unmasked coxa vara become evident (p. 1200).

The most important feature in early tuberculosis of the hip is limitation of movement. Movements in all directions are tested, but limitation of extension, due to psoas spasm, is often the earliest and perhaps the only objective sign. To demonstrate this feature the patient must lie on his face with the knees bent. The pelvis is steadied, and the thighs are raised as far as possible. Impaired extension on the affected side is then obvious.

Treatment is conducted along the lines already prescribed. Deformity is corrected by weight extension, the limb being supported in a Thomas's knee splint, and suspended either from an upright fixed to the end of the bed, or a Balkan frame. Care must be taken that tilting of the pelvis does not mask the true position of the leg. When the disease is quiescent either arthrodesis is performed, or if for any reason operation is contraindicated, the patient is fitted with a Thomas's hip splint, a patten on the boot of the sound foot, and crutches, and so

A Balkan frame consists of four upright rods fixed to bed-posts, which are connected at the top and ends by adjustable slats.

allowed to get about (fig. 1170). Owing to the tendency for relapse to occur, and the serious disability which results should immobilisation fail, treatment is persisted in until twelve months after apparent cure.

Operative measures such as arthrectomy or excision of the head of the bone are obsolete, as excellent results are obtained by a fusion operation, e.g. extra-articular arthrodesis.

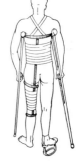

Extra-articular Arthrodesis.—As firm ankylosis in good position is the best result which can be expected, time is saved and this result obtained more certainly by extra-articular fixation. One method of obtaining this result consists in bridging the joint, by means of a bone graft inserted from a bed in the ilium to the base of the great trochanter (fig. 1171). (See also fig. 1033.)

Alternatively, a bone graft or pin is driven through a hole drilled in the great trochanter into the ilium, combined with osteotomy to correct adduction if necessary.

Fig. 1170.—
Thomas's hip
splint with a
patten on the
opposite foot.

Amputation is seldom required nowadays, but if necessary the preliminary step should be ligation of the common iliac artery by the extraperitoneal route, which effectively controls hæmorrhage from both the internal and external iliac arteries.

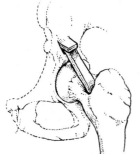

Fig. 1171.—Extra-articular arthrodesis.

Knee.—The knee joint is commonly affected by tuberculous disease, and diagnosis is as a rule not difficult. In neglected cases the position of triple deformity will occur, which consists of flexion, external rotation, and backward subluxation of the tibia, the latter occurring when the cruciate ligaments have become softened and destroyed. Excision of the knee joint yields good results provided bony ankylosis is obtained. A bone graft encourages osseous union. Flexion of the joint is unnecessary, as the limb is already shortened by removal of bone.

Ankle.—Tuberculous disease of this joint usually commences in the synovial membrane. Puffiness first appears under the extensor tendons, and later at the sides of the Achilles tendon.

Arthrodesis is performed through an incision on the outer side of the joint, and a sliding bone graft from the tibia is inserted into the talus. In advanced cases amputation is indicated, and should be performed at the modern site of election, i.e. about 7 inches below the upper end of the tibia.

Shoulder.—Tuberculous disease of this joint usually occurs in the form of caries sicca. The ends of the bones are destroyed, but very little œdema or thickening of the soft structures is evident. On examination, wasting of the deltoid muscle is obvious (fig. 1044), and the arm is held against the chest wall. Movements are all limited, and pain is produced when they are attempted. Treatment consists in fixation of the joint in abduction, and a few weeks in bed with lateral traction on the arm are usually required in order to obtain the desired position. Care must be taken to observe that true abduction is obtained, and not apparent abduction due to rotation of the scapula.

If recovery is delayed arthrodesis may be advisable, and an extra-articular arthrodesis obtained by implanting the acromion process into a groove prepared in the great tuberosity of the humerus.

Elbow.—In this joint the disease usually commences in the synovial membrane. The arm becomes weak and aches after use, and a doughy swelling appears on either side of the triceps tendon. Fixation is obtained by a plaster of Paris casing, or, if frequent inspection is desirable, a poroplastic splint can be applied. Abscesses usually appear posteriorly. Excision should, if possible, be reserved until after the age of sixteen, otherwise stunting of the limb will result. The insertion of a bone graft encourages arthrodesis.

Wrist.—This joint is not uncommonly affected in elderly patients, in whom the prognosis is gloomy. Carpal bones are readily destroyed, and abscesses appear under the extensor tendons on the back of the wrist.

If response to conservative measures is unduly delayed, arthrodesis is performed. After excision a wide tibial graft is inserted to secure fusion. If the disease has been allowed to progress to sinus formation, amputation is usually necessary.

OSTEOARTHRITIS

Various types of joint affections may be included under this heading, the predisposing factors being trauma, infection, exposure, and declining years. For practical purposes the different members of this disease may be classified as acute polyarticular, chronic polyarticular, and chronic monarticular, the latter being surgically the most important.

(i) **Acute Polyarticular.**—This variety, sometimes referred to as rheumatoid arthritis, is seen most commonly in young females, and commences in the small joints of the hands and feet. It gradually spreads to the larger joints, thus causing progressive crippling, until the patient may become almost helpless. It is apparently a toxic condition, and sometimes follows acute sinusitis or tonsillitis ; improvement often follows eradication of a focus of infection. During the earlier stages of the condition bouts of pyrexia occur periodically, associated with sweating, tachycardia, and exacerbations of pain and swelling in the affected joints. Fibrosis and contraction of ligaments gradually occur, and eventually the fingers become flexed and the hand fixed in a position of ulnar adduction. This disease is apt to run a painful course to more or less complete crippledom.

Still's disease is a similar condition occurring in children usually as they approach the second decade. In addition to joint changes, splenic and lymphatic enlargement, and a lymphocytosis are also associated.

The treatment of acute polyarticular osteoarthritis comprises an exhaustive search for any possible causative focus of infection, including the Fallopian tubes, teeth, tonsils, air sinuses, gall bladder, and bowels. Protein shock or gold injections seem to improve a few cases. Locally, deformities are prevented, and massage, warmth, electrical therapy, etc., are utilised in order to delay degenerative changes.

(ii) **Chronic Polyarticular** (*syn.* arthrosis deformans) occurs chiefly in middle-aged or elderly females. Again the smaller joints are usually the first to be affected, the changes which occur being degenerative—and atrophy of the ends of the bones and fibrosis of ligaments cause disorganisation and stiffness of the joints. Localised patches of periostitis (Heberden's nodules)

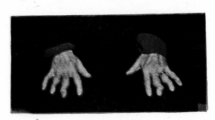

Fig. 1172.—Heberden's nodules.

may appear on the phalanges (fig. 1172). Treatment consists in the prevention of deformity and stimulation of the affected joints.

Sir Frederick Still, 1868–1941. Consulting Physician to King's College Hospital, and the Hospital for Sick Children, London.
William Heberden, 1710–1801. A practitioner in London, and a friend of Dr. Samuel Johnson.

Spondylitis deformans is a similar condition, more commonly seen in men, which occurs in the spine, and is associated with osteoarthritis of the articulations, and fibrosis or ossification of ligaments (*vide* Spine).

(iii) **Chronic Monarticular** (*syn.* Hypertrophic Arthritis).— Trauma is the causative factor, although the recuperative powers of the affected joint may be undermined by some low-grade toxic condition. As injury is the essential predisposing cause, the disease is more common in men. The injury is either of a single severe nature, e.g. following dislocation of the shoulder, or results from minor repeated traumata, such as nipping of a loose body or semilunar cartilage in the knee joint. Other factors which can be considered as " unfair wear and tear " are excessive use (fig. 1174), frequent exposure to cold or damp, alteration in the mechanics of a joint, e.g. old-standing Perthes' disease, or malalignment following a fracture.

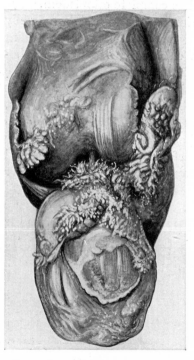

Pathological Changes.—The process first affects the soft structures, and later spreads to the cartilage and bone. Thickening of the synovial membrane occurs, and as this progresses a villiform process may develop, which on movement is nipped between the bones, and when unduly enlarged is termed a " lipoma arborescens." The matrix of the cartilage undergoes a fibrous metaplasia, and the cells multiply and become arranged at right angles to the articular surface. The superficial cells burst into the joint, sometimes in sufficient numbers to render the fluid turbid, and consequently the surface of the cartilage becomes velvety or " fibrillated." The thickened

FIG. 1173.—Osteoarthritis of the knee joint, showing thickened synovial fringes, lipping of the cartilaginous margins, and eburnation of bone on surfaces exposed to friction.

synovial membrane overlaps the edge of the articular cartilage, and under this fringe cartilage cells collect. Thus lipping or osteophytic growth occurs, as the cartilage cells subsequently ossify. Owing to the degeneration of the matrix and increase of cells, the cartilage softens, and is worn away on pressure-bearing surfaces, with resulting erosion and grating on movement. The underlying bone thus exposed reacts to pressure, and becomes dense and smooth, i.e. " eburnation " (fig. 1173).

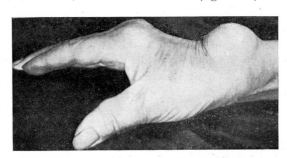

Fig. 1174.— A Baker's cyst due to osteoarthritis of the wrist joint. The patient had been digging daily for forty years.

Not infrequently exacerbations occur with synovial effusion, and as a result bursa communicating with the joint are apt to become distended, e.g. the psoas or semi-membranosus bursa, or Baker's cysts appear. The latter are protrusions of synovial membrane through weakened portions of capsule (fig. 1174). The popliteal space is a favourite site for a Baker's cyst, as the capsule here is weakened by blood-vessels supplying the joint. Occasionally chondrification or ossification occurs in the synovia, and in the case of the knee joint a solid mass sometimes appears due to chondrification of the synovial membrane lining the subcrureal pouch. Ossified synovial villi or osteophytes sometimes become detached and form loose bodies in the joint.

In the case of the shoulder joint the tendon of the long head of the biceps is liable to fray, and it eventually snaps as a result of some slight muscular effort (fig. 1175).

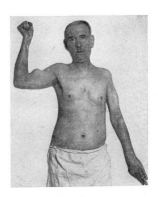

Fig. 1175.—Osteoarthritis of the right shoulder, with rupture of the biceps tendon, and "bunching" of the muscle. The patient is also suffering from left-sided Erb's palsy.

William Erb, 1840–1921. Professor of Medicine, Heidelberg.

Clinical Features.—The early symptoms of hypertrophic osteoarthritis are pain and stiffness. Pain is characteristically aggravated by changes in the weather, so that the appropriate term " barometric joint " is sometimes used. Stiffness is intensified by rest, and the joint must be " worked loose " before the range of movement is recovered. In advanced cases creaking, or locking of the joint by osteophytes, is noticed.

The signs depend upon the extent to which the disease has progressed. In the early stages some effusion, thickening of synovial membrane, and perhaps a little wasting of muscles are the only features. At a later stage lipping or osteophytes are sometimes palpable, while grating or creaking is detected on movement. Any communicating bursæ are palpated. In the case of the knee joint, the popliteal fossa must be examined for Baker's cysts or distended bursæ.

Treatment.—In the early stages, the joint should be protected from exposure and cold, and in the case of the knee joint, a knitted woollen cap should be worn. Rest to the joint should only be permitted during painful exacerbations, and movements and massage are resumed as soon as they can be tolerated. Radiant-heat baths, diathermy, and rubefacients are useful. The intramuscular injection of gold salts, although empirical, undoubtedly benefits some cases. The possibility that some chronic infection is undermining the resistance of the joint is borne in mind, and such conditions as sinusitis or pyorrhœa must receive due attention.

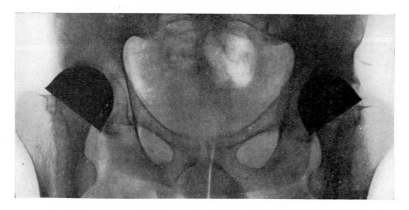

Fig. 1176.—Advanced osteoarthritis of the hips treated by vitallium cups.
(*C. H. Gray, F.R.C.S.*)

Operative treatment is sometimes necessary to remove inter-locking osteophytes or excessive lipping (cheilotomy). If pain is intolerable, excision of a stiff and painful knee may give life-long comfort to the patient. In the case of the hip joint, arthroplasty is occasionally required if the characteristic, deep-seated, boring pain interferes with sleep, and renders the sufferer's life a misery. The application of vitallium or plastic, cups preserves the movements of the joints, provided the cup fits snugly into the acetabulum. This is especially important if both hips require operative treatment, as bilateral ankylosis is a serious disability (fig. 1176).

Bifurcation osteotomy (fig. 1177) is an operation of less magni-tude, and pain is relieved at the expense of shortening of the limb. After the bone is divided the upper end of the shaft is

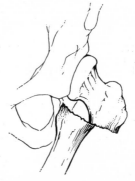

Fig. 1177. — Bifurcation osteotomy. The shaft is subsequently abducted.

then displaced so that it lies below the acetabulum, and subse-quently supports the body weight. The limb is immobilised in plaster for a few months.

A simple method of relieving pain is to immobilise the hip joint by driving a Smith-Petersen pin or bone graft through the head of the bone into the ilium.

Patients who are prone to osteoarthritis of any type should seriously consider a change of residence. Some localities un-doubtedly predispose to osteoarthritis, and a change to a warmer or drier climate may prevent or delay the onset of painful and crippling deformities.

LOOSE BODIES IN JOINTS

Loose bodies (a definition which excludes foreign bodies introduced from without), arise from the various constituents of the joint :

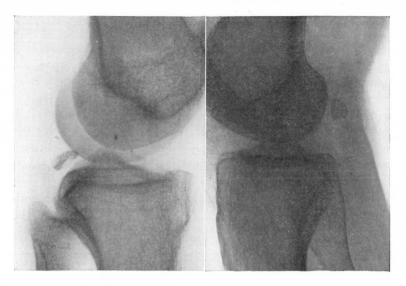

FIG. 1178.—Loose body in knee joint, flattened, and in the interarticular space. It resulted from influenzal arthritis.

FIG. 1179.—Sesamoid bone in the outer head of the gastrocnemius muscle (flabella). Oval in shape and behind the condyles.

SYNOVIAL FLUID.—A single fibrinous body sometimes results from a hæmorrhagic or inflammatory effusion (fig. 1178), or less commonly the joint contains many loose bodies (fig. 1180). In tuberculous disease flattened " melon-seed " bodies may be present in large numbers.

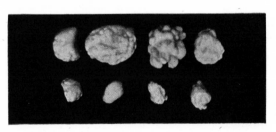

SYNOVIAL MEMBRANE.— Villous processes, such as those which occur in osteoarthritis, become detached, especi-

FIG. 1180.—Loose bodies removed from a knee joint.
(*Actual size.*)

ally if bone or cartilage develops within them.

CARTILAGE.—In the knee joint a portion of a semilunar cartilage sometimes becomes detached, and in most joints it is possible for a localised injury to chip off a portion of articular cartilage.

BONE.—Injury may cause separation of a small portion of bone, e.g. a tibial spine. Osteophytes are occasionally detached in cases of osteoarthritis. If the loose body contains living cells, growth may continue, nutriment being obtained from the synovial fluid.

Paget's quiet necrosis (*syn.* osteochondritis dessicans) is an uncommon cause of a loose body, and follows a direct injury. It most commonly occurs in the knee joint, and is probably due to violent rotation of the tibia, so that the tibial spine is driven against the internal condyle. Separation of a small sequestrum occurs without suppuration (fig. 1181).

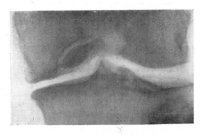

FIG. 1181.—Osteochondritis dessicans affecting the internal condyle.
(*Karl Krebs, Aarhus, Denmark.*)

Symptoms.—The commonest symptom caused by a loose body is locking of the joint. This causes severe pain and is followed by synovial effusion. Repeated attacks cause stretching of the capsule and ligaments, after which locking is often only momentary, and some slight manœuvre of the joint by the patient causes the body to slip out from between the bones and so unlock the joint. Repeated attacks of locking and synovitis eventually result in degeneration of the joint and hypertrophic osteoarthritis. Occasionally the patient learns to manipulate the joint so that the loose body becomes palpable, in which case it is felt to slip away from under the examining finger when the position of the joint is altered. This free mobility explains why loose bodies are sometimes referred to as " joint mice." A radiograph usually reveals the presence of the body. In the case of the knee, distension of the joint with 20 ml. of oxygen, followed by X-rays, will sometimes reveal the body.

Treatment.—Unless the joint is already disorganised, the loose body should be removed in order to relieve symptoms, and prevent the onset of osteoarthritic changes. In the case of the knee joint, the body should be manipulated, if possible, so that it comes to lie in the subcrureal pouch. It is then imprisoned in that situation by a firm, sterile, elastic bandage passed around the extended joint, so that a small vertical suprapatellar incision is sufficient to allow removal. Otherwise the joint is opened, and if the loose body cannot be found, it may be dislodged by a stream of sterile saline forcibly injected by a Higginson's syringe.

ANKYLOSIS

This term indicates a condition in which the normal range of movement of a joint is diminished. The cause is either outside the joint (false ankylosis) or intra-articular (true ankylosis).

False ankylosis is due to many conditions, such as :

Skin.—Scars, following burns.

Fascia.—Dupuytren's contracture.

Muscles.—Myositis fibrosa.

Tendons.—Stiffness following a Colles's fracture.

Nervous System.—Contractures due to paraplegia.

True ankylosis is either due to fibrous adhesions in the joint, or to actual bony union between the articular ends of the bones. As a rule some degree of movement can be obtained if the ankylosis is fibrous in character. However, if adhesions are so dense that no movement is possible, the two varieties are distinguished when vigorous attempts at passive movement cause pain in the case of a fibrous ankylosis. Fibrous ankylosis follows bleeding into a joint, low-grade pyogenic infection, or tuberculous disease. Bony ankylosis is due to a virulent infective arthritis, or a tuberculous infection complicated by secondary infection.

Treatment.—Many cases require no treatment, as the function of the joint is adequate. The two main indications for active interference are to increase or regain mobility, or to improve the position of the joint.

(*a*) *To Increase or Regain Mobility.*—The procedures which can be adopted include manipulations (often with the assistance of various appliances), anæsthesia and stretching or rupture of adhesions, and open operation. In connexion with forcible stretching of adhesions, care must be taken to avoid fracture of bones which are often atrophic, and it must be remembered that torn adhesions will bleed, and so predispose to re-formation. Old-standing cases of tuberculous arthritis should never be manipulated, as latent infection is thereby stimulated to activity. Open operations include wide excision of bones, as in the case of the jaw or elbow joint, and arthroplasty, e.g. the head of the femur is exposed and surrounded by a vitallium cup (fig. 1176). In either case early movements must be instituted.

Alfred Higginson, 1809–1884. Surgeon, Southern Hospital, Liverpool.

In the case of false ankylosis of the jaw, e.g. following fibrosis of the masseter muscle secondary to an alveolar abscess, the formation of a false joint may be considered when other measures have failed. The operation entails removal of a wedge-shaped piece of jaw in the region of the angle, and suturing portions of the internal pterygoid and masseter muscles together so that formation of a false joint is encouraged (Esmarch).

(*b*) *To Improve Position.*—The necessity for dealing with this contingency should, theoretically, not arise, as ankylosis should only be allowed to occur in a satisfactory position. However, if alteration in the position of the joint will result in improvement of function, then excision of the joint or osteotomy are the usual procedures. Thus, a flexed knee is excised, and arthrodesis secured in the completely extended position, with a slight degree of genu valgum. By this means a rigid leg, nearly equal in length to its fellow, is obtained, the only remote drawback being risk of fracture (p. 1022).

In some cases osteotomy is preferable to excision, e.g. in the case of a quiescent tuberculous hip joint with marked adduction. A Gant's subtrochanteric osteotomy, possibly combined with division of some of the adductor muscles close to their origins, is a simple operation which permits correction without risk of lighting up tuberculous infection.

HÆMOPHILIA

This condition is a familial disease, but only males are affected. It is due to failure of the platelets to produce thrombokinase. Consequently there is a delay in the conversion of prothrombin into thrombin, which results in a prolonged clotting time.

Extravasations of blood are characteristic of this condition, and joints are commonly affected, notably the knee joint. A rapid hæmorrhagic effusion occurs, which is followed by an inflammatory reaction, so that the joint feels hot and somewhat tender. As absorption occurs, the thickened synovial membrane remains palpable, and this feature, with its associated stiffness and wasting due to enforced rest, may simulate tuberculous disease.

If repeated hæmorrhages are allowed to take place, degenerative changes follow, similar to those seen in osteoarthritis.

Treatment consists in rest and the application of a cooling lotion to the affected joint. A small intravenous transfusion prevents further hæmorrhage, but intramuscular hæmoplastin or horse serum are suitable substitutes. Monthly injections of blood should be given until the child outgrows the tendency to bleed.

External bleeding in hæmophilics (and oozing in general) can be arrested by the local application of the venom of Russell's viper. The venom is kept in the dry state to prevent decomposition, and is applied in 1 : 10,000 dilution (stypven is one commercial preparation). In this strength the venom still possesses powerful coagulant properties, but the poison is too dilute to be harmful.

Friedrich von Esmarch, 1823–1908. Professor of Surgery, Kiel.
Frederick James Gant, 1825–1905. Surgeon, Royal Free Hospital, London.

SNAPPING HIP

This condition is usually due to the great trochanter slipping out from beneath the fascia lata as it encloses the tensor fasciæ femoris muscle. In some cases the anterior fibres of the gluteus maximus seem to be to blame. As a rule little disability ensues, but if troublesome, division or fixation of the fascia or muscle cures the condition. The operation must be performed under local anæsthesia, so that the patient can demonstrate the snap during the operation.

CHAPTER XLIV

MUSCLES, TENDONS, AND BURSÆ

INJURIES OF MUSCLES AND TENDONS

Contusion of a muscle is due to a direct injury. Localised pain follows attempts at contraction, and an extravasation of blood occurs within the muscle sheath. This extravasation often appears at a considerable distance from the actual site of injury, e.g. hæmorrhage from a torn rectus femoris in its upper part usually appears near the patella. As with all hæmatomata, blood-borne infection is a possibility, in which case the blood clot may be converted into an abscess.

Cold applications and relaxation of the muscle are required for the first two days, and, when risk of further extravasation has passed, massage and movements will expedite absorption, and prevent, or limit, subsequent stiffness.

Rupture of a muscle usually occurs at the junction of tendon and muscle itself. Thus the *quadriceps extensor* ruptures immediately above the patella. The gap is easily visible and palpable when the patient contracts the quadriceps muscle (fig. 1182). Repair with mattress or interlocking stitches is necessary. The prognosis regarding complete restoration of function is less favourable than in the case of a fractured patella, as accurate approxi-

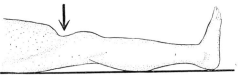

FIG. 1182.—Torn quadriceps femoris muscle.

mation of the muscle is difficult, and the fibrous union in the muscle tends to stretch.

Two varieties of " *tennis leg* " are partial rupture of the inner head of the gastrocnemius, and complete rupture of the plantaris muscle, which occurs in the middle of the muscular belly, i.e. about 3 inches below the knee joint. (Probably many cases of so-called rupture of the plantaris are actually a tear of some of the fibres of the soleus muscle.) In either case sudden pain results, which is often so severe that the sufferer imagines that he has been struck by a stone or his partner's racket. Pain on walking is relieved if the patient learns temporarily to walk on the heel, as this position inhibits contraction of the gastrocnemius and plantaris muscles. Rest and strapping relieve the pain, and recovery occurs in three weeks.

"*Tennis elbow*" is usually due to one of the following conditions:

(i) Tearing of part of the deep head of the pronator radii teres. It follows the abrupt pronation necessary to impart "top spin." Pain is localised to the antecubital fossa, and is accentuated on efforts to pronate the forearm.

(ii) Rupture of some of the fibres of the radial carpal extensors at their origin from the external condyle, over which bony prominence localised pain and tenderness are elicited. If conservative measures are disappointing, manipulation may be successful. By this means the incomplete rupture is converted into a complete one, so that healing can occur without the constant irritation caused by intermittently contracting muscle fibres.

(iii) A tear of the orbicular ligament, the frayed edge of which becomes interposed between the bones. Under manipulation the patient experiences a " click " as the torn portion is reduced, and full movements of the joint are then regained.

A " *mallet* " *finger* (*syn.* baseball finger) is due to avulsion of an extensor tendon of the finger, which often includes a small

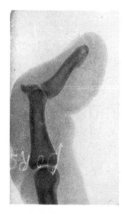

Fig. 1183.—Avulsion of a flake of bone to which the long extensor tendon is attached, resulting in a " mallet " finger.

flake of bone from the base of the distal phalanx (fig. 1183). The finger is fixed in a position of right-angled flexion of the proximal interphalangeal joint, with hyperextension of the terminal interphalangeal joint, so that the central slip of the extensor tendon is relaxed. For this purpose the patient is shown how to press the thumb against the finger-tip so that the correct position is maintained. A dry tube of plaster is then slipped over the finger, and the hand dipped in warm water. The wet plaster is then moulded by the surgeon, and the finger is retained in the correct position until the plaster dries (fig. 1184). The patient conducts his usual occupation, and the plaster is removed in six weeks.

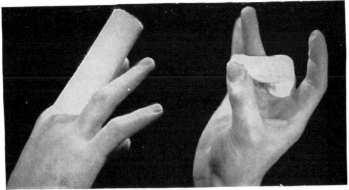

Fig. 1184.—The treatment of " mallet " finger.
(*Cellona Technique, T. J. Smith & Nephew, Ltd.*)

The *tendon of the biceps* is sometimes torn at its junction with the muscle, or, in the case of osteoarthritis of the shoulder joint, the frayed tendon may snap (fig. 1175). Recognition is easy, as on flexing the forearm the soft muscular belly is drawn downwards towards the elbow. Some hypertrophy of the short head partially compensates for the resulting deficiency. Efforts at repair, such as suture to the trans-humeral ligament, are not always successful, and are unnecessary in elderly patients.

The pubic attachment of the *adductor longus* muscle is sometimes partially avulsed when riding a frisky horse. Myositis ossificans may subsequently supervene. Tetanus or strychnine poisoning may cause such violent contractions that rupture of the *rectus abdominis* muscle has resulted (fig. 19).

Rupture of the *tendon of the supraspinatus* is a not uncommon accident in middle-aged men. Following injury the patient is unable to abduct the arm as the supraspinatus fixes the head of the humerus, and so enables the deltoid muscle to exercise a pull on the shaft. Localised tenderness is present between the outer border of the acromion process and the great tuberosity. In complete rupture suture is essential if full power is to be regained. Exposure is obtained by splitting the deltoid muscle as it covers the great tuberosity. Partial rupture will improve if the arm is fixed in 90 degrees of abduction and 60 degrees of external rotation for two months.

Rupture of the *extensor longus pollicis* tendon sometimes complicates Colles's fractures (p. 1045).

The *Achilles tendon* occasionally ruptures during dancing or a game of tennis, or sometimes as a result of a surprisingly trivial injury. The gap in the tendon may be palpable, but diagnosis can always be confirmed in that dorsi-flexion of the foot is increased on the side of the injury. Prompt suture is desirable (fig. 1185), and the limb is immobilised in plaster for six weeks.

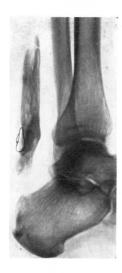

FIG. 1185.—Calcification of the tendo Achillis following rupture and suture with wire.

Hernia of a muscle sometimes follows a tear of the muscle sheath, the adductors and biceps brachii being the muscles most commonly affected. On contraction, muscular fibres protrude through the aperture in the sheath. This feature distinguishes a torn sheath from a torn muscle, as in the latter case a gap appears between the two portions on contraction. If disability ensues, the sheath is sutured.

A small rupture of the sheath of the *tibialis anticus* is not uncommon in athletes. The swelling appears over the belly of the muscle on the outer side of the tibia. Unless the clinician is aware of the condition he may be puzzled by its appearance. No disability results, and the swelling disappears as life becomes less strenuous.

Displacement of tendons occasionally occurs where these structures traverse fibro-osseous canals, e.g. in the region of the wrist or ankle, or the long head of the biceps in the arm. Sudden pain occurs, followed by a sensation of weakness and further pain on attempted movements. The displaced tendon, if superficial, e.g. the peroneus longus, can be palpated in its abnormal position. The replaced tendon should be immobilised for at least eight weeks. The condition sometimes recurs, and if disability persists, the tendon is fixed in position, e.g. a flap of periosteum is raised from the bone in order to form a tunnel for the tendon. " Snapping hip " is discussed elsewhere (p. 1170).

TENDON SHEATHS

Simple teno-synovitis follows excessive or unaccustomed use, and is commonly seen in connexion with the extensor tendons of the hand, or the Achilles tendon. Pain and local œdema are present, and a characteristic soft crepitus is palpable when the fingers are moved. An adequate period of rest, followed by counter-irritants, and massage effect a cure.

Acute infective teno-synovitis either follows wounds, e.g. extension from whitlows, or is blood-borne, as in the case of gonococcal infection. Severe pain results from any movement which causes the tendon to glide in its sheath. If due to a virulent organism, suppuration is probable, which rapidly extends along the tendon sheath. Unless early and adequate incisions are made, sloughing of tendons is likely to occur (p. 1000). If this complication is avoided by rest and antibiotics early movements discourage the organisation of exudate and consequent troublesome adhesions.

Tuberculous teno-synovitis is of two types :

(*a*) The endothelial lining of the sheath is replaced by œdematous granulation tissue containing miliary tubercles. Very little free fluid is present. A soft, elastic swelling appears, and if the disease progresses, pus may form, and track into neighbouring sheaths or joints.

(*b*) An effusion occurs in the tendon sheaths, and "melon-seed" bodies are usually present in large numbers, so that a soft, coarse crepitus is detected on pressing fluid from one part of the sheath to another. These "melon-seed" bodies may be rounded, as distinct from the flat variety found in joints, and in appearance resemble grains of boiled sago (fig. 1186). The

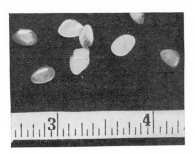

Fig. 1186.—"Melon-seed" bodies from a case of compound palmar ganglion.

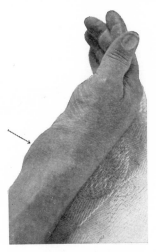

Fig. 1187.—Compound palmar ganglion, showing swelling above the anterior annular ligament.

term "compound palmar ganglion" is applied to this condition when it occurs in connexion with the flexor tendons of the fingers. A soft, painless swelling appears (fig. 1187), and fluctuation may be transmitted above and below the anterior annular ligament. As with all forms of tuberculous disease of bone, joint, or tendon, obvious wasting of adjacent muscles is present. Treatment consists in general measures and the application of a plaster cast, but if the condition progresses careful dissection and removal of the diseased tendon sheaths is indicated.

Stenosing tendovaginitis is a fibrous thickening of the sheath of a tendon, and is characterised by thickening and tenderness immediately above the radial styloid process. The extensor ossis metacarpi pollicis and extensor primi internodii pollicis (abductor pollicis longus and extensor pollicis brevis), as they lie on the lower and outer aspect of the radius, are most commonly affected, especially in workers who use their thumbs excessively (e.g. charwomen wringing cloths). The condition is cured by excision of the thickened sheath under local anæsthesia, after which suture of the skin only is sufficient.

Calcification of the supraspinatus tendon follows tendinitis. Exacerbations of localised pain suggest the condition, which is confirmed by X-rays. If physiotherapy fails to relieve, the area is exposed by splitting the deltoid, and the chalky mass is removed with a sharp spoon.

A simple ganglion appears as a localised, tense swelling in connexion with a tendon sheath, and contains clear gelatinous fluid. It is probably due to mucoid degeneration of a tendon sheath, and is predisposed to by injury. Injury to the sheath is most likely to occur where the tendon lies on bone. Thus simple ganglia are commonly found on the dorsum of the wrist and foot (fig. 1188). Rupture of the ganglion can be accomplished by pressure, or a blow, and although recurrence is likely this simple method is worth a trial. Some cases are cured by aspiration with a wide-bore needle and injection with collodion or other sclerosing agent, followed by firm pressure for a few days. If simple measures fail, excision should be performed, but even then recurrence sometimes occurs. Not infrequently, a ganglion disappears spontaneously, so unseemly haste on the part of the surgeon is unnecessary.

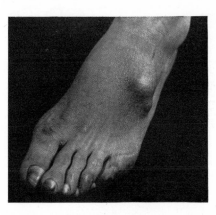

Fig. 1188.—Simple ganglion in connexion with the tendon of the peroneus brevis muscle.

Tumours of tendon sheaths occasionally occur, in the form of *tenosynoviomata*. These tumours arise from the synovial membrane lining the tendon sheath, and are either innocent or malignant. Innocent tumours are apt to undergo metaplasia, and are liable to contain fibrous tissue, cartilage, or even bone. In both the innocent and malignant types " foam " cells are characteristic, which are large and spheroidal, and contain numerous fat droplets.

Myelomata occasionally occur in tendon sheaths. They are easily excised, and usually are only recognised on microscopy.

CUT TENDONS

In a book of this nature space precludes other than an abbreviation of general principles, with a short account of some common injuries.

Cut tendons are a common cause of disability, and only too frequently receive inappropriate treatment by surgeons who have not received adequate training in this often difficult problem.

Tendons which flex joints are provided with a sheath, and consequently considerable separation occurs when such a tendon is divided; union is therefore unlikely without surgical intervention. The remaining tendons are enclosed in loose elastic and connective tissue—the paratenon. Severance of such tendons results in a minor degree of separation, and union of the ends may occur if the tendon is relaxed for an adequate period.

Immediate repair of tendons is only indicated under the following circumstances :

(1) A competent surgeon is available, and suitable instruments and sutures are to hand.

(2) The wound must be uncontaminated, and not more than six hours should have elapsed since the accident occurred.

(3) There is no loss of skin or serious damage to bones or joints. A divided nerve is not a contraindication as it may be sutured immediately or subsequently (p. 907).

Unless these conditions are fulfilled it is only permissible to attend to wound toilet, suture the skin, and administer penicillin in order to obviate infection. A formal operation and suture is performed when the wound has healed, usually within four weeks. A further lapse of time results in excessive retraction of the ends so that approximation is impracticable, and a tendon graft is then required.

Flexor Tendons.—If conditions are suitable immediate suture yields satisfactory results. If both the sublimus and profundus are divided within the digital sheath, the profundus alone is sutured, and the superficial tendon removed. Suture of both tendons inevitably results in the formation of adhesions and impairment of function. In late cases tendon grafting is usually required.

Extensor Tendons.—The condition of mallet finger is described on p. 1172. Tendons divided distal to the wrist joint do not retract to such an extent that union is unlikely with immediate adequate relaxation. The hand and fingers should be maintained in full extension by means of a plaster slab for six weeks.

Tendons divided at wrist level require suture in accordance with the principles mentioned above. Rupture of the long extensor tendon of the thumb in association with a Colles's fracture is best treated by the insertion of a graft taken from the extensor indicis tendon.

TENDON SUTURE

Some of the important points in technique are as follows : A bloodless field is obtained by means of a sphygmomanometer,

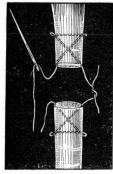

FIG. 1189.—Tendon suture.

which is deflated at hourly intervals for five minutes or so. Incisions follow the natural creases of the hand, or in the case of a digit it passes longitudinally just posterior to the digital vessels and nerve. The most suitable suture material is 40-gauge wire, which should be threaded into the end of the needle to minimise trauma. If these needles are not available the tendon can be transfixed with a hypodermic needle, along the lumen of which the wire is threaded and the needle is then withdrawn. Various stitches are used to approximate the ends of the tendon (fig. 1189). Measures to prevent adhesions by insulating tendons with flaps of fascia or artificial preparations are not recommended, and reliance is placed on covering the suture line with any local tissue available.

Larger tendons, such as the tendo Achillis, require more elaborate suture with strong material, such as kangaroo tendon. Interlocking sutures are sometimes useful in order to secure approximation.

TENDON GRAFTING

This procedure is necessary if excessive retraction has occurred, or if part of the tendon has been destroyed. Considerable skill and experience are necessary to obtain a good result. The palmaris longus or extensor indicis are most suitable in the hand, or grafts may be taken from the long extensor tendons of the toes. The paratenon is included with the graft. Free exposure is necessary. Preservation or reconstruction of the fibrous sheaths over the interphalangeal joints is important.

TENOTOMY

This operation is performed either by the open or the subcutaneous method. The latter is to be preferred in situations where there is little risk of damage to important structures. Thus the tendo Achillis is divided by the insertion of a tenotomy knife under the tendon, from the inner side, about 1 inch above its insertion. Dorsi-flexion of the foot facilitates division of the

tendon. Deformity should not be corrected until about two weeks after division, which lapse of time allows granulation tissue to form between the two ends of the tendon, and thus the risk of non-union is diminished. In children over the age of five years, open operation and lengthening of the tendon by the " Z " method is advisable (fig. 1190), as otherwise excessive retraction and non-union may result.

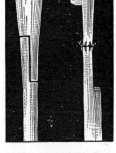

FIG. 1190.—Tendon lengthening.

Three tendons should be exposed before division :

(1) The biceps cruris, in order to avoid injury to the external popliteal nerve.

(2) The sternomastoid tendon and muscle, on account of important adjacent structures and also to allow division of fascia.

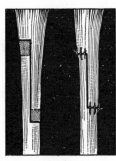

FIG. 1191.—Tendon shortening.

(3) The femoral adductors, as division of both muscle and tendon is necessary, and the femoral vessels are often displaced inwards when considerable adduction deformity is present. Moreover, the internal saphenous vein and the obturator nerve are in danger if tenotomy is performed subcutaneously.

SHORTENING of a tendon is accomplished by the " Z " method (fig. 1191). The two halves of the tendon, after separation, are shortened as required, and the tendon is then sutured.

TENDON TRANSPLANTATION is performed in order to restore muscular balance, or to supplement the action of ligaments (p. 909).

INFLAMMATION OF MUSCLES

Acute suppurative myositis follows either direct infection, or local extension from adjacent structures, e.g. osteomyelitis. " Rheumatic " myositis is a troublesome complaint, and mainly affects fascial aponeuroses, tendinous insertions, or muscular sheaths, and in these cases the term " fibrositis " is applied. The condition often arises abruptly; e.g. in the case of lumbago, on attempting to get out of bed the affected person may be seized in the midway position, and be unable to move without assistance. In some cases exposure precipitates an attack, e.g. a draught may result in a stiff neck. Some focus of infection is frequently a predisposing cause, and should always be sought. Treatment consists in local warmth and rubefacients. Radiant-heat baths, ionisation, or diathermy may be useful. In severe

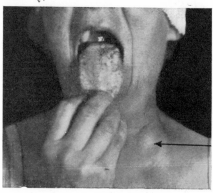

Fig. 1192.—Gumma of the left sterno-mastoid muscle. The patient exhibited extensive leucoplakia and fissuring of the tongue.

localised cases injection of procaine often results in immediate improvement. Aspirin and antirheumatic remedies are prescribed. Tuberculous myositis is due to extension from some neighbouring focus of infection, e.g. a psoas abscess in connexion with a tuberculous spine. Syphilitic myositis may occur as a localised gumma, particularly in the sternomastoid muscle or tongue (fig. 1192). An indurated swelling appears, which gradually involves the overlying skin or mucous membrane. More rarely a diffuse myositis occurs, e.g. parenchymatous glossitis, the tongue eventually becoming fibrotic.

Myositis ossificans of the generalised type is a rare condition, commencing in young adults, in which muscles are gradually transformed into bone. The condition usually commences in the flat muscles of the back (fig. 1193), and spreads to the spinal and thoracic muscles. The condition steadily progresses, and the patient gradually becomes more rigid (" poker " man), until fatal respiratory complications supervene. Congenital absence of the last phalanx of the big toes and inability to flex the thumbs are sometimes associated conditions.

Trichiniasis is an uncommon cause of myositis in this country. Nematode worms obtain access to the alimentary canal in infected pork. After a few days the embryos find their way to striated muscles via the lymphatics. The muscles become painful and indurated, and the migration of the embryos continues for from two to four weeks, during which period eosinophilia is present. The embryos become encysted, or eventually perish and calcify. The treatment is symptomatic.

Myositis fibrosa and traumatic myositis ossificans are considered in connexion with fractures.

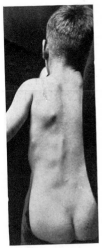

Fig. 1193.—Ossification of the flat muscles of the back. The child had characteristic deformities of the thumbs and toes.

(G. D. F. McFadden, Belfast.)

TUMOURS OF MUSCLES

Innocent.—Lipomata and fibromata occasionally occur (Chapter iii).

Malignant.—Primary fibro-sarcoma is not uncommon, and arises from the muscle sheath. This tumour was formerly considered to be a simple fibroma, and it is sometimes difficult to be dogmatic in distinguishing a fibroma from a slowly growing fibro-sarcoma. Failure to realise the sarcomatous nature of these tumours accounts for Paget's description of them as " recurrent fibroids " (fig. 36). A slowly growing swelling appears, which is firm, circumscribed, and connected with the muscle. Exploration is necessary if the tumour is deeply situated, and on confirmation the tumour is removed with a wide margin of surrounding muscle. Even then local recurrence is all too common, and dissemination by the blood-stream will already have occurred in the majority of cases.

Secondary invasion of muscles sometimes occurs, e.g. the pectoralis major, following carcinoma of the breast.

DISEASES OF BURSÆ

Injury.—Acute non-infective bursitis follows injury. Thus a blow on the shoulder may cause subdeltoid bursitis (Codman's disease). If effusion follows, the rounded shoulder suggests an effusion into the joint, but absence of swelling in the axilla

Ernest A. Codman, Contemporary. Consulting Surgeon, Massachusetts General Hospital.

excludes the latter condition, and rotary movements of the joint are painless.

Non-infective bursitis may also follow unaccustomed exercise, e.g. inflammation of the bursa under the tendo Achillis after a cross-country run.

Chronic bursitis is the result of repeated slight injuries, or constant pressure, e.g. housemaid's knee (prepatellar), parson's knee (pretubercular), student's or miner's elbow (olecranon) (fig. 1194), weaver's bottom (tuber ischii). Certain bursæ show a marked tendency to enlarge, e.g. those in the popliteal space. The bursa between the inner head of the gastrocnemius and the semimembranosus tendon is commonly affected, a rounded, painless swelling resulting (fig. 1195). Examination in *both flexion and extension* is imperative, as in extension compression by adjacent tendons renders the bursa tense, and it may even be mistaken for a bony swelling, whereas the flaccidity

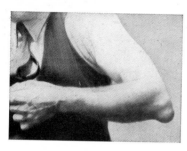

FIG. 1194.—Chronic olecranon bursitis.

which accompanies flexion indicates the cystic nature of the swelling. Enlargement of the semimembranosus bursa is common in children. If disability results aspiration is performed, but most cases disappear spontaneously. Popliteal bursæ, which communicate with the knee joint, sometimes enlarge as a result of such conditions as osteoarthritis of the joint, and similarly enlargement of the psoas bursa may follow recurrent effusions into the hip joint, e.g. Charcot's disease or osteoarthritis.

Adventitious bursæ form as a result of prolonged pressure over bony prominences, e.g. Billingsgate hump, due to pressure of a fish-basket over the seventh cervical spinous process. The common-

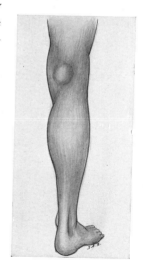

FIG. 1195.—A semimembranosus bursa, tense in extension and flaccid in flexion.

est example is over the inner side of the head of the first metatarsal bone in cases of hallux valgus, the term " bunion " being
applied when inflammation supervenes (fig. 1196). Chronically
inflamed bursæ are excised if troublesome.

Infection.—ACUTE INFECTIVE BURSITIS is
due to direct infection by penetrating
wounds, or from local extension, e.g. " gravel
rash " over the patella may cause subcutaneous infection and involvement of the
prepatellar bursa. In the case of prepatellar
bursitis, a " sympathetic " effusion into the
knee joint sometimes follows, but confusion
with infective arthritis should be avoided,
as in the latter condition any attempt to
move the joint is painful, and pain is elicited
by pressure in the popliteal space. If suppuration ensues,
excision or drainage may be necessary.

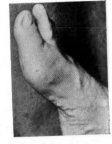

FIG. 1196.—A bunion.

CHRONIC INFECTIVE BURSITIS is either tuberculous or, rarely,
syphilitic.

Tuberculous bursitis resembles tuberculous teno-synovitis,
in that one of two varieties occurs ; either an effusion containing
" melon-seed " bodies, or a variety in which the bursa becomes
lined with granulation tissue, and which may progress to abscess
formation, and eventually fistulæ. The gluteal bursa between
the insertion of the gluteus maximus and the great trochanter
is particularly prone to tuberculous infection. A rounded swelling occurs below the great trochanter, and the limb is held
abducted and everted, in order to relax the gluteus maximus.
The condition thus resembles to some extent the first stage of a
tuberculous hip joint, but flexion deformity is absent, and movements of the hip joint are not unduly restricted.

A tuberculous bursa should be completely excised, an operation which often requires considerable patience, on account of
ramifications and lobulations of the bursa.

Syphilitic bursitis occurs during the secondary stage, and
gives rise to transitory, and often symmetrical, effusion. During
the tertiary stage, a local gumma or a diffuse gummatous
bursitis are uncommon manifestations.

New-growths.—An endothelioma from the lining membrane,
or fibro-sarcoma from the wall, occur as curiosities.

CHAPTER XLV

DEFORMITIES

DEFORMITY is due to changes in the following anatomical structures :

(i) Skin and subcutaneous tissues, such as scars from wounds or burns, or Dupuytren's contracture.

(ii) Muscles and tendons, as in the case of unbalanced muscular action in infantile paralysis, or spastic diplegia.

(iii) Ligaments, such as relaxation following distension of a joint, or fibrosis, as in rheumatoid arthritis.

(iv) Joints, e.g. congenital deformities, ankylosis following infection, or disorganisation as in Charcot's joints.

(v) Bones, e.g. irregular growth, as in partial destruction of an epiphyseal line following osteomyelitis (fig. 1090).

(vi) Nervous lesions, either peripheral, such as claw-hand following injury to the ulnar nerve, or central, as in cases of syringomyelia or hysterical manifestations.

Consideration of the above causes will suggest that deformities are often preventable, and that in some cases operations would be rendered unnecessary if care and foresight were used in the early treatment. The following summary indicates the surgical procedures which may be adopted for the correction of deformities :

(i) Manipulation, such as stretching the sternomastoid muscle in early cases of congenital torticollis.

(ii) Manipulation with retentive apparatus, as by stretching the tendo Achillis in a case of talipes equinus, and applying a metal night shoe.

(iii) Operations on soft parts, such as fasciotomy, tenotomy, or muscle-sliding operations.

(iv) Operations on joints, as by performing arthrodesis for a flail ankle joint.

(v) Operations on bones, either osteotomy, excision, or amputation.

The following are some of the factors which require con-

Baron Guillaume Dupuytren, 1777–1835. Surgeon, Hôtel Dieu, Paris.

sideration in deciding whether intervention is advisable in any given deformity. Age is of obvious importance, and, as a general rule the older the patient the less need arises for correction. Patients often adapt themselves to a long-standing deformity in a remarkable manner (fig. 1224), and in such cases anatomical correction may not improve function. Risk of sequelæ is taken into account, thus genu valgum in childhood should be rectified in order to forestall osteoarthritic degeneration of the knee and hip in later years.

TORTICOLLIS (Syn. WRY NECK)

Acquired torticollis is due to the following causes :

(i) *Rheumatic.*—This is due to fibrositis following exposure to cold or a draught, e.g. a chilly drive in a draughty car. The onset is sudden, and muscles are tender on pressure. Radiant-heat and salicylates hasten recovery.

(ii) *Spastic.*—This distressing condition, fortunately uncommon, occurs chiefly in neurotic, middle-aged females. It is characterised by clonic spasms of the sternomastoid and trapezius muscles on one side of the neck, and later the deep cervical muscles on the opposite side may be affected. The head is continually jerked downwards towards one shoulder, particularly during excitement, and mental instability may be an associated condition. Treatment is unsatisfactory, but every effort is made to discover any functional cause or source of peripheral irritation. Division of the spinal accessory nerve on one side, and of the opposite posterior primary divisions as they lie on the semispinalis colli, is sometimes necessary, but even this procedure is not always successful, owing to the presence of a cerebral lesion.

(iii) *Reflex.*—This is due to some associated source of peripheral irritation, e.g. teeth, nose, or air sinuses.

(iv) *Inflammatory.*—Parotitis, or an inflamed node adjacent to the spinal accessory nerve, is liable to cause temporary contraction of the sternomastoid muscle. The deformity is occasionally associated with Pott's disease.

(v) *Hysterical.*—Torticollis, in common with almost any deformity, is sometimes due to hysteria. Facial asymmetry is absent.

(vi) *Compensatory.*—Torticollis may develop as a result of scoliosis, in order to maintain the eyes on a horizontal level. Defective vision in one eye may cause ocular torticollis.

Congenital torticollis, unless associated with such conditions as wedge-shaped vertebræ or atlanto-occipital fusion, is due to myositis fibrosa of the sternomastoid muscle, following temporary interference with the venous return (see p. 821) or trauma during lateral flexion of the head at delivery. The condition resembles Volkmann's ischæmic contracture. That lateral flexion of the head does certainly occur in some of these cases is proved by the fact that Erb's palsy of the opposite arm is occasionally associated, and this condition is known to follow acute lateral flexion of the head to the *opposite* side, i.e. the side

Richard von Volkmann, 1830–1889. Professor of Surgery, Halle.
Wilhelm H. Erb, 1840–1921. Professor of Medicine, Heidelberg.

upon which the torticollis occurs. Hemiatrophy of the face follows, due to lack of use ; thus the nose appears flattened, the eyebrow is less arched, and the distance between the outer canthus and the angle of the mouth is less on the affected side than on the normal. The bodies of the cervical vertebræ become wedge-shaped, and a compensatory curve develops in the dorsal spine so as to maintain the eyes on a horizontal level.

The diagnosis of congenital torticollis is easily made, as the sternomastoid tendon is apparent as a rigid subcutaneous bar, and the muscle can be palpated as a tense band, postero-lateral to the tendon.

Treatment.—(i) *Manipulation.*—As soon as the condition is recognised, the mother or nurse is instructed to rotate the child's head so as to stretch the contracted muscle, i.e. the chin must be rotated to the affected side, the rotation being combined with extension of the head. An assistant is required to steady the body while the head is manipulated. In early cases patience and perseverance will correct the deformity.

(ii) In old-standing cases, or under circumstances where the child will not receive careful or intelligent attention, division of the sternomastoid muscle should be performed.

Subcutaneous division of the tendon alone is easily performed, but little improvement is likely, as contraction of the muscle and underlying fascia still persists. Open division leaves a small scar, but is devoid of danger, and permits thorough division of the whole muscle and also of contracted underlying fascia. A transverse incision is made $\frac{1}{2}$ inch (1·25 cm.) above the clavicle, and the tendon and muscle are divided. The anæsthetist rotates the head, and successive tense fascial bands are divided. Large veins, particularly the anterior jugular as it passes underneath the muscle, must be carefully avoided, as injury is liable to cause troublesome hæmorrhage. The head is subsequently fixed in plaster for about three weeks (fig. 1197) in the corrected position. The constant and intelligent performance of exercises under supervision will cure the deformity, although some degree of hemiatrophy of the face may persist as a permanent condition if treatment is delayed.

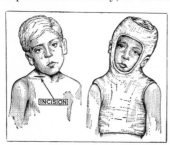

Fig. 1197.—Operative treatment of congenital torticollis.

SPINAL DEFORMITIES

Scoliosis.—This condition consists of lateral curvature of the spine, followed by rotation of the vertebræ if the deformity progresses. It occasionally occurs as a congenital deformity, and is then due to a wedge-shaped vertebral body following maldevelopment.

ACQUIRED

(i) *General disease of bone*, such as rickets, osteomalacia.

(ii) *Local disease of bone*, e.g. Pott's disease, osteomyelitis.

(iii) *Muscular imbalance*, as with infantile paralysis of one erector spinæ, the normal muscle acting as a bowstring so that the concavity of the spine is towards the sound side. Increased spasticity of one erector spinæ exerts a similar effect, e.g. in cases of syringomyelia, in which asymmetrical dilatation of the central canal of the cord irritates one pyramidal tract to a greater extent than its fellow, thus causing spasticity of the corresponding group of spinal muscles.

(iv) *Compensatory*, e.g. irregularity in the length of the legs, collapse of one side of the chest following pulmonary tuberculosis or a chronic empyema, or in association with torticollis.

(v) *Static*, by which is meant a deformity which is due to no actual disease, but to a combination of some or all of the following conditions :

(*a*) Excessive fatigue, e.g. prolonged standing.

(*b*) Habitual assumption of a faulty posture, e.g. a nurse-maid carrying a baby always on the same arm—both suffer. A patient with a prolapsed lumbar disc sometimes tilts his spine laterally in order to relieve irritation of the compressed nerve root.

(*c*) Adolescence, with its associated asthenia, rapid increase in weight, etc.

(*d*) Hygienic conditions, such as inadequate diet, working in ill-ventilated atmospheres, etc.

Static scoliosis is the most important group from the surgeon's standpoint, as early recognition and adequate treatment may prevent lifelong deformity, with its associated physical and psychical effects. Usually two curves are present, the primary being in the lumbar region and the compensatory in the dorsal. In addition to the lateral curvature and rotation of the vertebræ, changes also occur in the thoracic wall ; thus, the ribs on the side of dorsal convexity are separated, and the scapula projects or " grows out " on that side, while the chest appears flattened

Percival Pott, 1713–1787. *Surgeon, St Bartholomew's Hospital, London.*

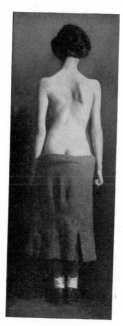

FIG. 1198.—Adolescent scoliosis, showing "growing out" of the right shoulder and left hip (Stage 2).

(*Dr. R. V. Harris.*)

in front. On the other hand, the ribs on the side of the concavity are crowded together, and the chest as seen from the front is unduly prominent, also the space between the ribs and the iliac crest on this side is narrowed, and the hip appears to project (fig. 1198).

In severe cases neuralgia occurs from pressure on spinal nerves, and osteoarthritis of the spine will eventually supervene. Right heart failure or intercurrent lung complications sometimes contribute to a fatal issue.

Treatment.—For the purpose of treatment and prognosis, static scoliosis is divided into three stages. It must be confessed that once obvious structural changes have occurred cure is unlikely, but efficient treatment should stabilise the condition.

Stage 1.—The patient is allowed to assume a postural position of ease, so that deformity is apparent. The spinous processes are marked with a skin pencil, so that the extent and situation of the curve are obvious. The curve, as indicated by the spinous processes, is less than that assumed by the bodies of the vertebræ as, owing to rotation, the spines are directed towards the concavity. The patient is still in Stage 1 if, on touching the toes, the curve is obliterated.

Stage 2.—As the condition advances, secondary contracture of ligaments and muscles occurs, and hence flexion of the spine fails to correct the deformity. X-ray examination, however, reveals no bony change.

Stage 3.—The effect of prolonged contracture of ligaments and muscles, and consequent protracted interosseous pressure, is to cause pressure absorption of vertebral bodies, which consequently become wedge-shaped (figs. 1199 and 1200).

The treatment of static scoliosis which is still in its *first stage* (i.e. postural) consists in careful attention to the patient's health and hygiene, remedial exercises well within the limit of fatigue, and adequate rest, including a definite period during the day-

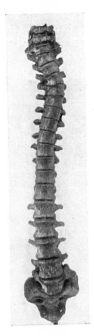

Fig. 1199. — Third degree of static scoliosis, early stage. The bodies of the vertebræ are becoming wedge-shaped.

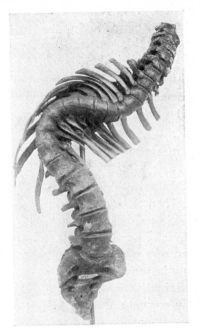

Fig. 1200.—Third degree of static scoliosis, advanced stage. The bodies of the vertebræ are excessively rotated, and ribs on the concave side are crowded together.

time, in the supine position. Care should be taken to obviate faulty posture, e.g. badly constructed school desks, or the constant twist of the body in order to view a blackboard continuously from the same angle. These measures, if practicable, are curative in the early stages. If, for economic reasons, such ideal treatment cannot be carried out, then a corset or spinal jacket should be worn, except during periods of rest, and the above general treatment is modified to the circumstances of the patient.

When the *second stage* has developed, spinal jackets prevent the condition progressing, and often effect an improvement. A poroplastic jacket should be fitted for a child, as it is cheap, and can be economically renewed as growth occurs. A hinged flap can be provided so that continuous pressure is exerted over the prominent ribs. The general principles indicated in connexion with the first stage are applied as adequately as circumstances permit. In the case of patients so situated that considerable time can be devoted to treatment, the application of Abbott's jacket should be considered.

This consists of a plaster jacket which is applied while the patient lies on a canvas frame, or is suspended in order to obliterate curves as completely as possible. Apertures are cut in the jacket over the concavity and convexity of the chest, and felt pads are inserted over the prominent ribs in order to exert continuous pressure on them, while the aperture over the concavity encourages expansion of that portion of the chest. Jackets are renewed at intervals of about three months, and the application of three or four jackets usually results in some improvement.

Alternatively, the patient is provided with a plaster bed, which is padded so as to exert pressure over suitable areas.

When the *third stage* is established, remedial treatment may still improve the condition if it is persevered with over a period of years, particularly if the patient is adolescent. The application of a poroplastic or leather jacket with proper sling straps may improve even severe cases.

Spinal fusion is of value when muscles are too weak to maintain correction, as in infantile paralysis, and also in congenital cases which tend to progress. Successful fusion obviates the necessity of prolonged treatment.

Other types of scoliosis are treated by dealing with the cause of the trouble, e.g. rickets is combated by means of hygiene and diet, while inequality in the length of the legs needs correction. Compensatory scoliosis due to collapse of a lung is readily recognised by flattening of the chest, as distinguished from the usual prominence of the ribs in front on the side of the concavity, and no treatment is necessary for this type. Scoliosis due to unbalanced muscular action should be kept in check by a spinal support, e.g. a Taylor's brace or Chance's splint, or spinal fusion may be considered.

Kyphosis (*syn.* hunchback), is a term applied to a condition of increased dorsal convexity of the spine. If only two or three vertebræ are affected the deformity is abrupt (fig. 1201), whereas more extensive involvement results in a rounded back such as occurs in osteoarthritis (fig. 1202 (1)). Its causes are similar to those of scoliosis, and are as follows :

(i) General disease of bone, such as osteitis deformans, ankylosing spondylitis, senile atrophy.

(ii) Local disease of bone, which may be associated with Pott's disease (fig. 1201), secondary carcinoma, fracture-dislocation, or Scheuermann's disease (p. 1101).

(iii) Static, especially the " round shoulders " of children,

Edville Gergardt Abbott, 1871–1938. Orthopædic Surgeon, General Hospital, Maine, U.S.A.
Charles F. Taylor, 1827–1899. Surgeon, New York Orthopædic Dispensary and Hospital.
Sir Arthur Chance, 1859–1928. P.R.C.S.I., Surgeon to Mater Misericordiæ Hospital, Dublin.

and in those whose occupation entails stooping or carrying heavy weights, e.g. porters.

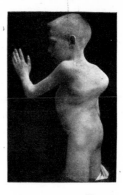

Kyphosis is divided into *three stages*, corresponding to those of scoliosis, i.e. when posture corrects the deformity ; secondly, when the deformity persists in spite of posture, but no bony change is seen in a radiograph ; and thirdly, when a lateral X-ray shows alteration in the shape of the bodies of the vertebræ.

Treatment consists in dealing with any preventable cause, attention to the general health, adequate rest, and suitable exercises. A spinal support is useful in selected cases.

FIG. 1201.—Hunch-back deformity following Pott's disease. (*Pybus.*)

SPINAL OSTEOTOMY is indicated in cases of severe kyphosis resulting from ankylosing spondylitis. A V-shaped osteotomy is performed on each side from the inter-laminar space to the

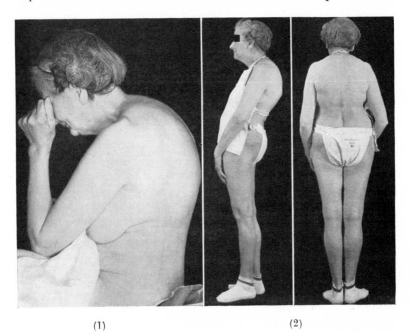

(1)   (2)

FIG. 1202.—(1) Pre-operative rigid dorsal kyphosis with flattening of lumbar curve. (2) Post-operative correction, with a re-established lumbar lordosis to compensate for the dorsal kyphosis. (*W. Alexander Law.*)

intervertebral foramen. This allows hyperextension of the back, and the resulting lumbar lordosis compensates for the dorsal and cervical kyphosis (fig. 1202). The osteotomy is performed in the lumbar region where the spinal canal is relatively commodious, and the canda equina is less likely to be compressed than the cord. The patient is immobilised in plaster for about three months.

The results of spinal osteotomy in suitable cases are dramatic (Alexander Law). Not only can the patient once again look ahead, which is of psychological as well as physical benefit, but movements of the diaphragm are increased. Increased respiratory excursions not only improve the patient's well being, but diminish the risk of pulmonary complications which are the usual cause of death in these patients.

Lordosis consists in an exaggeration of the anterior lumbar curve, and is usually compensatory. Thus it is present in cases of bilateral congenital dislocation of the hip (fig. 1211), in order that the centre of gravity of the body may pass behind the hip joints, as is normally the case. Increase of weight of the abdominal contents, e.g. fat, tumours, or pregnancy, causes lordosis for the same reason.

Spondylolisthesis is a rare deformity, in which the lower lumbar vertebræ slip forward on to the front of the sacrum. It is due to imperfect development of the pedicles of a lumbar vertebra, usually the fifth, and any tendency to lordosis, e.g. pregnancy, encourages the displacement forward of the vertebræ. Cases have also been attributed to fracture of the lumbo-sacral articular processes. Pain, local and referred, results, and on examination a hollow is seen posteriorly, and the body of the displaced vertebra is often palpable through the abdominal wall. The lower ribs descend, and sometimes rest on the iliac crests, and stature diminishes.

Treatment consists in rest and supports, so arranged that part of the body weight is transmitted from the axillæ to a pelvic band by means of lateral irons. Reinforcement of the lumbo-sacral joints by a bone graft has been adopted in some cases.

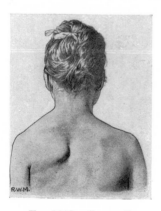

FIG. 1203.—Sprengel's shoulder. (*Sir John Fraser.*)

UPPER EXTREMITY

Congenital elevation of the shoulder (*syn.* Sprengel's shoulder) is a condition in which the scapula is smaller than normal, and situated at a higher level. The inferior angle is rotated inwards, and abduction is restricted (fig. 1203). In bilateral cases the appearance of the patient at first suggests that the neck is abnormally short. The rhomboid muscles are partially fibrous or even cartilaginous or ossified, and the trapezius and serratus muscles are sometimes deficient.

Treatment consists in exercises if such are considered necessary, but surprisingly little disability results. Operations to improve function are unsatisfactory, but the upper and inner portion of the scapula may be excised for cosmetic improvement.

Cubitus valgus or varus results from separation of the lower epiphyses of the humerus, fractures, or excessive excision of the head of the radius. Normally, the forearm is in a position of abduction as compared with the arm, this " carrying angle " being 13 degrees in men, and 15 degrees in women. Increase of this angle, or cubitus valgus, may give rise to a localised patch of neuritis in the ulnar nerve, as the groove behind the internal condyle acts as a pulley, and friction results. Anterior transposition of the nerve is indicated as soon as symptoms appear, e.g. paræsthesia or muscular weakness. The treatment of cubitus valgus or varus is largely preventive, but if disability results, supracondylar osteotomy is considered.

Congenital absence of the radius occasionally occurs, in which case growth of the ulna pushes the hand to the radial side. The lower articular surface of the ulna is expanded, and articulates with the proximal row of carpal bones.

Congenital dislocation of the head of the radius is sometimes accompanied by curvature of the ulna. If considered advisable, the head of the radius is excised, and the deformity of the ulna corrected by osteotomy.

Contraction of the palmar fascia (*syn.* Dupuytren's contracture) usually occurs in individuals whose work entails pressure on the palms, e.g. cobblers, and is consequently more frequent in men than in women (fig. 1204). However, a local patch is not uncommon in women from pressure of a plaster, e.g. after a Colles's fracture. The condition commences as an indurated area in the palm, and contraction first affects the ring finger, which becomes drawn into the palm. The little finger is usually next affected, and other fingers may follow.

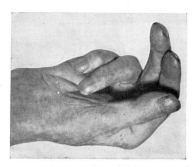

Fig. 1204.—A typical Dupuytren's contracture. The patient drove a horse and van for over thirty years.

The thumb is rarely involved. The condition is readily diagnosed by the presence of palmar induration, and the fact that the fingers cannot be extended even when the wrist is flexed (in distinction from myositis fibrosa).

In the early cases splinting, combined with energetic hyper-extension of the fingers, usually arrests progress. When the condition is established, the usual treatment is free excision of the affected palmar fascia. Splints should be applied during healing. In advanced cases excision of the heads of the first phalanges is also necessary.

Complete excision of the fascia without injury to the skin is often impossible, and we have found the following procedure to give excellent results. Skin and fascia are excised until the fingers can be completely extended. Absolute hæmostasis is obtained, and the raw area is covered with a whole-thickness skin graft from the thigh. Every particle of fat is removed from the graft, which is stitched into place. The field is dusted with sulphanilamide powder, a stent mould is applied, and firm pressure is obtained by means of a bandage over a piece of sorbo sponge. Ten days later the dressing is removed, and movements of the fingers are encouraged (fig. 1205).

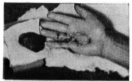

FIG. 1205.—Appearance of wound after operation for Dupuytren's contracture. The dressing has just been removed (see text).

Trigger finger is a condition in which extension of a finger or thumb is arrested, but when assistance is forthcoming with the other hand, the flexed finger extends with a jerk or snap. The condition may follow a sprain, and is usually due to a thickening of the tendon sheath as it passes under the transverse metacarpal ligament, and thus it bears a resemblance to stenosing tendovaginitis (p. 1176). Occasionally it results from a simple ganglion or a fibroma growing from the tendon sheath.

Treatment consists in division of the thickened tendon sheath, or removal of any obvious obstruction.

Congenital deformities of the fingers include the conditions of syndactylism, macrodactyly, and congenital contracture. *Syndactylism*, or webbed fingers, is a condition in which two or more fingers are joined together (fig. 1206). An X-ray should be taken, and if normal bones are present, separation of the fingers will improve the function of the hand.

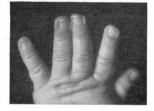

FIG. 1206.—Syndactyly.

The two-stage operation (Didot) should be performed, the first step of which consists in establishing an epithelialised tunnel at the base of the

Alphonse Didot, a surgeon of Brussels, described his operation in 1849.

web. This is obtained by dividing the base and stitching a flap of adjacent skin over the raw surface. A glass rod is inserted between the fingers and kept in position until the tunnel is covered by epithelium. The second stage consists in a plastic operation, two flaps of skin, the length of the web, being dissected from the front and back of the fingers respectively, in such a manner that when the web is divided the raw surfaces of the fingers are covered, one by the dorsal, and the other by the palmar, flap. Syndactylism of the toes needs no treatment, and may even benefit swimmers !

Macrodactyly consists in overgrowth, possibly enormous, of a digit. A plastic operation, or amputation, is occasionally necessary.

Congenital contracture of a finger most commonly affects the little finger, and is due to contraction of the central slip of palmar fascia. Hyperextension occurs at the metacarpo-phalangeal joint, and flexion at the proximal inter-phalangeal joint, and extension at the distal joint (fig. 1207). If necessary, a posterior splint is applied, or if sufficient disability

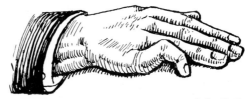

Fig. 1207.—Congenital contracture of the little finger.

exists, the central slip of fascia is excised.

DEFORMITIES OF THE LOWER EXTREMITY

Congenital dislocation of the hip

Dislocation of the posterior variety is a not uncommon condition ; about a quarter of the cases occur in boys, and about the same proportion are bilateral.

The incidence varies in different localities, e.g. it is relatively common in Northern Italy, and there is a definite familial tendency.

The condition is due to lack of development of the iliac portion of the acetabulum, and at birth the head of the bone articulates with the ill-formed articular cavity. Absence of the normal pressure on the head of the bone results in deficient growth. Walking displaces the head of the bone upwards on the dorsal surface of the ilium and the acetabulum assumes a triangular shape. The capsule of the joint stretches and is sometimes constricted about its centre, where it is crossed by the ilio-psoas tendon, thus forming an isthmus. The ligamentum teres lengthens. A slight degree of coxa valga occurs, and the

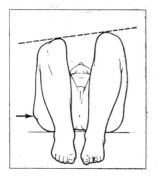

FIG. 1208. — Congenital dislocation of the right hip. The arrow indicates the prominent great trochanter.

angle of declination, or torsion of the neck of the femur on the shaft, is increased.

Clinical Features.—The early signs in a unilateral case are asymmetry of the skin creases on the inner side of the thigh, a slight hollow below Poupart's ligament, and a less obvious gluteal fold. If the child lies on its back with the knees drawn up, difference in the level of the joints indicates shortening of the thigh on the affected side (fig. 1208). Early diagnosis greatly improves the prognosis, as the sooner manipulation is performed the better are the results. Unfortunately the condition is not usually recognised until the child begins to walk, which is somewhat later than usual, e.g. sixteen to twenty-four months. If unilateral a limp is noticed, whereas in bilateral cases the child "waddles like a duck."

Examination of a unilateral case reveals the following features :

(a) *Inspection.*—Lordosis, if present, is obliterated by flexion of the hip (fig. 1209), and any obliquity of the pelvis is corrected.

FIG. 1209.—Flexion of the hip masked by lordosis. When lordosis is corrected 30 degrees of flexion is revealed.

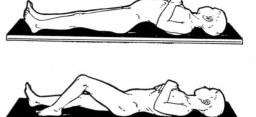

Shortening of the leg is then apparent, and some degree of flexion is present. The great trochanter appears prominent, and muscular wasting is slight.

(b) *Palpation.*—As the head of the femur is absent, there is loss of resistance in Scarpa's triangle, and the pulsation of the unsupported femoral artery is difficult to detect. The great trochanter is raised, and on palpation posteriorly the head of the

Antonio Scarpa, 1747–1832. Anatomist and surgeon, Venice.

femur is detected on the dorsum ilii as a hard, rounded, painless swelling. Confirmation is obtained by adducting the leg and rotating the femur, when the head of the bone is felt to roll beneath the fingers.

(c) *Movements.*—An abnormally wide range of movements is usually obtainable, especially in the direction of adduction. " Telescopic " movements are sometimes obtained by traction on the femur, and, if the child has walked but little, reduction of the dislocation may be possible.

(d) *Measurement.*—This confirms shortening of the limb. The tip of the great trochanter is above Nélaton's line, which connects the anterior superior spine and the most prominent part of the tuber ischii ; and the base of Bryant's triangle, i.e. the side connecting the great trochanter with the line drawn backwards from the anterior superior iliac spine, is shorter than on the normal side.

Morris's bitrochanteric measurement, which is obtained by means of a calliper, shows that the great trochanter on the affected side is nearer the mid-line than its fellow.

(e) *Trendelenburg's Test.*—The child stands on the affected limb, with the sound limb raised from the ground. The pelvis tilts downwards towards the sound limb owing to inability of

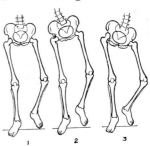

Fig. 1210.—Trendelenburg's test. 1. Normal hips : the pelvis remains level on raising one leg. 2. Coxa vara : on raising the sound leg the pelvis tilts upwards on that side. 3. Congenital dislocation : on raising the sound leg the pelvis tilts downwards.

the muscles to steady the lax joint on the affected side. In the case of a normal joint, contraction of muscles fixes the hip joint and no tilting occurs (fig. 1210).

Trendelenburg's test is positive if the ilio-femoral ligament is relaxed. In addition to congenital dislocation it may occur in late Perthes' disease, infantile paralysis of the gluteal muscles, old fractures of the femoral neck, and advanced osteoarthritis.

(f) *X-ray* shows interruption of Shenton's line, and invariably reveals shelving of the upper portion of the acetabulum.

Auguste Nélaton, 1807–1873. Professor of Clinical Surgery, Paris.
Sir Thomas Bryant, 1828–1914. Surgeon, Guy's Hospital, London.
Sir Henry Morris, 1844–1926. P.R.C.S., Surgeon, Middlesex Hospital, London.
Friedrich Trendelenburg, 1844–1924. Professor of Surgery, Leipzig.
E. W. H. Shenton, Contemporary. Consulting Radiologist, Guy's Hospital, London, and St. Bartholomew's Hospital, Rochester, Kent (the oldest hospital in England, situated on the Pilgrims' Way to Canterbury).

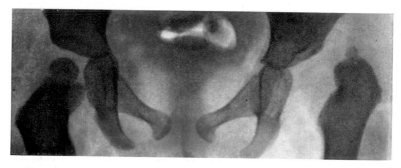

FIG. 1211.—Congenital dislocation of the left hip in a female one year old.
(*F. P. Fitzgerald.*)

The ossific centre in the femoral head is diminished in size (fig. 1211).

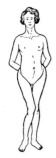

FIG. 1212.—Congenital dislocation of both hips, showing lordosis and perineal gap.

Shenton's line is an imaginary line formed by the under-surface of the neck of the femur and the upper part of the obturator foramen. It is interrupted by the ischium, and normally forms an arc. Displacement of the head of the femur, or irregularities in the neck, interrupt the continuity of the arc.

In *bilateral* cases marked lordosis is present which gives the appearance of prominent genitalia. Bilateral adduction causes a perineal gap, and in marked cases "scissors" deformity of the legs may result (fig. 1212).

Treatment.—1. *Manipulative.*—If the condition is diagnosed by the time the child is twelve months old, simple abduction without anæsthesia, gradually increased to its fullest limit, and then maintained in plaster for at least twelve months, will cure 90 per cent. of cases (fig. 1213). From the age of one year until six or seven forcible manipulation under anæsthesia is necessary, but the results are not so satisfactory.

Forcible manipulation is conducted on the lines suggested by Lorenz. General anæsthesia is necessary, and the pelvis is steadied by an assistant. The flexors, extensors, and adduc-

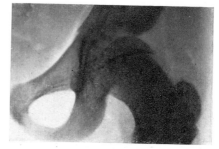

FIG. 1213.—Same case as shown in Fig. 1211, aged eight years. Shenton's line is now perfect.

Adolf Lorenz, Contemporary. Emeritus Professor of Orthopædic Surgery, Vienna.

tors are successively stretched, and the dislocation is reduced. Reduction is indicated by a "click," which can be both felt and heard, also the loss of resistance in Scarpa's triangle disappears, and the hamstring muscles become taut, i.e. the knee cannot be extended. The limb is then fixed in plaster of Paris in the fully flexed and abducted position, with perhaps slight internal rotation. The plaster reaches to the ankle on the affected side, and includes the upper part of the opposite thigh, so as to fix the pelvis. A subsequent X-ray will be sufficiently clear to confirm the reduction. The plaster is removed in about three months, and reapplied in a less abducted position, this procedure being repeated at intervals. Walking is encouraged as soon as possible in order to force the head of the femur into the acetabulum. One year or more is necessary for treatment.

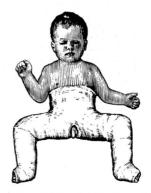

Fig. 1214.—Application of plaster of Paris for bilateral congenital dislocation of the hips.

2. *Operative.*—Open reduction is considered after the age of six years until puberty, or in cases in which manipulation has failed owing to impossibility of reduction on account of the hour-glass contraction of the capsule, or shallowness of the acetabulum.

Before open reduction is attempted, shortening of the limb must be reduced to 1 in. (2·5 cm.) or less by means of weight extension in the abducted position, supplemented, if necessary, by division of the adductors, otherwise an undue amount of muscle and other soft tissues will need division in order to bring the head of the bone down to the level of the acetabulum. The usual anterior incision is made, passing downwards and slightly inwards from the anterior superior spine between the tensor fasciæ femoris and gluteal muscles on the outside, and the sartorius and rectus femoris on the inner side. If necessary the incision is prolonged upwards and outwards under the iliac crest. The capsule of the joint is opened and the isthmus divided, and the acetabulum is deepened by means of a burr. The head of the femur is trimmed if necessary and reduction is effected. An attempt may be made to reinforce the upper lip of the acetabulum by means of a bone graft, or the periosteum can be stripped up in order to encourage bony outgrowth. The limb is fixed in abduction for some months, but walking is permitted after a few weeks. The results of open reduction are variable, and considerable limitation of movement usually results. However, stability is correspondingly obtained, and shortening is reduced.

In the adolescent a subtrochanteric or bifurcation osteotomy may be performed in order to minimise lordosis and forestall lumbar strain.

3. *Palliative.*—If reduction fails, and operation is contra-indicated on account of the condition of the patient, or if the child has reached puberty, then a high boot should be worn in order to correct shortening of the limb and prevent the develop-

ment of compensatory scoliosis. The joint can be steadied by means of a pelvic band, to which is attached a leather cap, which is situated so that it exerts pressure over the great trochanter.

Anterior dislocation of the hip is a rare deformity, and gives rise to little disability. This being the case, some surgeons perform anterior re-position of the head of the femur in cases of posterior dislocation rather than reduction by open operation. The leg is manipulated so that the head of the bone is brought to lie beneath the anterior superior spine, and it may be steadied in this position by raising a periosteal flap with a flake of bone attached, so that a false acetabulum is partially formed.

COXA VARA

This term indicates a diminution of the angle between the neck and shaft of the femur, which is, in adult males, about 135 degrees. The angle is less in females, and gradually diminishes with age in both sexes. In addition to diminution of this angle, a curvature of the neck of the femur occurs, with its convexity forwards (fig. 1215).

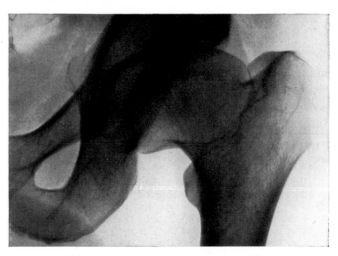

Fig. 1215.—Advanced coxa vara, due to untreated Perthes' disease (p. 1099).

Infantile coxa vara is a rare condition, and is due to maldevelopment of the head of the femur.

Acquired coxa vara is due to the following causes :

(i) General disease of bone, such as rickets, osteomalacia, or osteitis deformans.

Georg Perthes, 1869–1927. Professor of Surgery, Leipzig.

(ii) Local disease of bone, e.g. osteomyelitis, pseudocoxalgia, or a local cyst.

(iii) Trauma, as by separation of the epiphysis or fracture of the neck of the femur. A more important cause is " slipped epiphysis," which condition occurs during adolescence, and may date from a definite injury, or be due to repeated slight injuries, e.g. errand boys who repeatedly jar their right leg in dismounting from a bicycle. The clinical features of an established " slipped epiphysis," which from the surgical standpoint is the most important type of coxa vara, consist of pain, which is commonly referred to the knee, and limp, which in the early stages is due to pain, and later to actual shortening.

Examination reveals the following signs :

(i) *Inspection.*—The limb is adducted, and usually slightly everted. If definite bony change is present, a corresponding degree of shortening is apparent, and the great trochanter is prominent, owing to the fact that as it rises towards the anterior superior spine it becomes more superficial. Wasting is detectable in established cases.

(ii) *Palpation.*—No tenderness or loss of resistance can be detected in Scarpa's triangle. The prominence of the great trochanter is verified.

(iii) *Movements.*—These are characteristic, abduction and internal rotation being limited. The narrowing of the angle between the neck and shaft of the femur explains the limitation of abduction, and adduction is correspondingly increased. Limitation of internal rotation is due to the anterior curvature of the neck of the femur, which comes in contact with the anterior rim of the acetabulum when inversion is attempted.

If the limb is examined during an exacerbation of traumatic synovitis, movements of the limb in all directions are restricted. A few days' rest in bed allows the synovitis to subside, and then the above characteristics are demonstrable.

(iv) *Measurement.*—Shortening of the limb is confirmed, and Bryant's triangle and Nélaton's line indicate that the shortening is above the great trochanter.

(v) *X-ray.*—In the pre-slipping stage some blurring on the distal side of the epiphysis is noticeable. When slipping has actually occurred the deformity is obvious, especially in a lateral X-ray.

Treatment.—The treatment of slipped epiphysis depends upon the extent to which the condition has progressed. In the early stages skeletal traction is applied with a Steinmann's pin through the upper end of the tibia with both limbs in Thomas's splints, each in about 25 degrees of abduction. A weight of 15–20 lb. (7-9 kgm.) is applied to the affected limb, and counter-extension is obtained by raising the foot of the bed. Traction is usually necessary for eight weeks, and during the final period weight is gradually reduced. After a further two weeks in bed a walking calliper is applied, which is worn for six months.

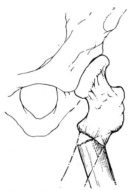

FIG. 1216.—Subtrochanteric osteotomy.

Some surgeons, in order to shorten the time necessary for treatment, insert a Smith-Petersen nail under X-ray control, in the same manner as for a fracture of the neck of the femur. Walking is permitted three months later.

In the later stages, when gross deformity is present, osteotomy provides the quickest and most certain line of treatment. Subtrochanteric osteotomy (fig. 1216) is performed through a stab wound, or a larger incision may be made in order to allow separation of the periosteum from the femoral shaft prior to division of the bone. The adductor muscles are forcibly stretched, or if necessary divided through an open wound which permits of free division and avoids injury to the saphenous vein and femoral vessels. Weight traction in abduction is then applied for six or eight weeks, after which a plaster or walking calliper is provided.

Coxa valga is the reverse deformity, and sometimes occurs in old-standing cases of infantile paralysis, or following amputations below the knee in childhood, owing to the weight of the limb dragging on the femoral neck without counter-pressure. The condition sometimes occurs in adults as a result of excessive traction on fractures involving the neck of the femur.

GENU VALGUM

Knock-knee is due to :

(i) General disease of bone, such as rickets.

(ii) Local disease of bone, as in cases of acute osteomyelitis with irregular epiphyseal growth.

Hugh Owen Thomas, 1834–1891. Orthopædic Surgeon, Liverpool.

(iii) Static causes, which are often associated with flat-feet or scoliosis. The normal angle at which the femur articulates with the tibia causes a great proportion of weight to be transmitted through the outer condyle and tuberosity. This causes a strain on the inner side of the knee joint, and explains why the internal lateral ligament is attached to the shaft of the tibia rather than to the epiphysis. When influences which predispose to a static deformity are present (*vide* scoliosis), the internal lateral ligament stretches, the outer condyle becomes atrophic from excessive transmission of weight, while the inner condyle increases in size, and thus knock-knee follows. No enlargement of the inner condyle occurs in the antero-posterior direction, and thus deformity disappears when the knee is flexed. In advanced cases outward dislocation of the patella occurs.

Treatment.—The principles of treatment are as follows :

(i) Attention to the general health, with special regard to vitamin D deficiency.

(ii) Physiotherapy to improve the tone of muscles. Moulding is simple and effective, and consists in grasping the lower third of the leg and applying as much pressure as is tolerated on the inner side of the knee. This procedure is carried out two or three times a day for ten to fifteen minutes at a sitting, and can easily be performed by a mother or nurse.

(iii) Redistribution of body weight by conservative or operative measures.

Conservative measures include wedging of the shoes, the inner border being raised up to ½ inch (1·25 cm.). This is a simple and efficient measure, provided the shoes are worn continuously. Night splints are sometimes necessary in addition to wedging. In more severe cases day splints in the form of walking irons, or plasters of Paris renewed at frequent intervals, are recommended by some surgeons.

Operative correction is seldom required in civilised communities, but if the patient is over ten years of age, and the space between the internal malleoli is over 4 inches (10 cm.) (perhaps slightly more in a female), then osteotomy is advisable, not only to correct the unsightliness, but to obviate osteoarthritis in adult life (fig. 1217).

Operation.—The leg is flexed, and lies on its outer side supported by a sandbag. A point is selected ½ inch (1·25 cm.) in front of and above the

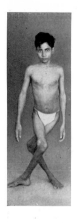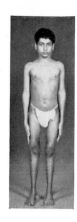

Fig. 1217. — Advanced genu valgum corrected by osteotomy. (*T. Seshcchalam.*)

adductor tubercle, and at this point a vertical stab wound is made to the bone with a broad-bladed scalpel. If gross deformity exists, these measurements do not ensure the safety of the outer part of the very oblique epiphyseal line, and in such cases the stab wound is made at the intersection of two lines—a vertical line ½ inch (1·25 cm.) in front of the adductor tubercle, i.e. over the shaft of the femur, and a transverse line ½ inch (1·25 cm.) above the upper limit of the external condyle, which indicates the outer extremity of the epiphyseal line (Macewen). An osteotome is inserted in the wound, passed down to the bone, and then rotated through a right angle. The dense posterior part of the bone is first divided, then the anterior, and after division of part of the intermediate portion the remainder is fractured. Bleeding may occur from the anastomotica magna artery, but is controlled by a firm bandage. Injury to the popliteal artery has occurred from omitting to keep the ulnar side of the hand which grasps the osteotome resting on the limb in order to prevent uncontrolled penetration of the instrument. In the event of this rare complication the artery must be exposed, and the divided ends sutured or ligated. After division of the bone the limb is splinted for ten days, i.e. until the wound has healed, and swelling due to extravasated blood has disappeared. A plaster casing is then applied for about six weeks, after which a walking calliper is worn for a few months.

Genu Varum (*syn.* bow-legs) is less common than knock-knee, and is usually

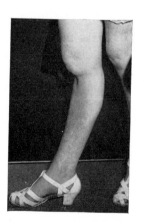

due to rickets (fig. 1218), but may follow epiphyseal derangements or excessive horse-riding in childhood. Osteotomy is performed if necessary.

Genu Recurvatum is due to abnormal hyperextension of the joint, and severe degrees are congenital in origin (fig. 1219). Minor degrees are associated with irregular epiphyseal growth and are improved by exercises which increase the tone of the quadriceps muscle. More severe degrees

Fig. 1218.—Genu varum. (*Pybus.*)

Fig. 1219.—Genu recurvatum.

are due to epiphyseal injury, or to rupture of the cruciate ligaments. In some cases a knee cage is required.

CURVATURE OF THE TIBIA

This is due to either :

(i) Weakening and consequent bending of the bone.

(ii) Change in its shape owing to deposition of new bone on its anterior aspect.

The first group includes osteitis deformans, osteomalacia, and rickets (p. 1090). The treatment of a rachitic tibia is first constitutional, combined, if necessary, with suitable splints (fig.

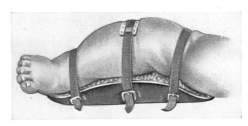

FIG. 1220.—A splint applied for a rickety tibia.

1220). If the deformity is marked and little improvement results, then manual osteoclasis is performed before the age of five years, i.e. while the bone is still comparatively soft. This simple operation consists in holding the leg, resting on its outer side, over a rubber-covered wedge (fig. 1221). Pressure, gradually increased,

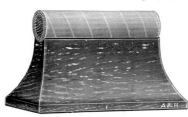

FIG. 1221.

first snaps the fibula and then the tibia. Care must be taken to grasp the leg as close to the site of curvature as possible, as pressure near the end of the bone may avulse the lower epiphysis of the tibia. A sub-periosteal fracture occurs, and the straightened limb is put in a plaster case for about a month, union readily occurring. In older children with considerable deformity, open osteotomy, either linear or cuneiform, is necessary.

Curvature of the tibia due to deposition of bone is commonly due to syphilis, either congenital or acquired. The deformity is only antero-posterior, and chiefly occurs at the centre of the bone (*vide* Syphilis of Bones).

FLAT-FOOT

The inner longitudinal arch of the foot, which extends from the inner tuberosity of the os calcis to the head of the first metatarsal bone, is supported and maintained as follows :

(i) By the plantar fascia and short muscles of the foot, which act as somewhat weak "tie beams," connecting the ends and component parts of the arch.

(ii) By ligaments, particularly the long and short plantar ligaments (calcaneo-cuboid), and the spring ligament (inferior calcaneo-navicular), which supports the head of the astragalus, and in some cases is responsible for a facet on the under-surface of that bone.

(iii) By tendons, particularly the tendon of the tibialis posterior, which is attached to all the tarsal bones, excepting the astragalus, and also to the middle three metatarsals.

(iv) By reciprocal modelling of the tarsal bones, which by their shape encourage the formation and maintenance of the arch.

The outer longitudinal arch is very shallow, and is normally in apposition with the ground when walking. The transverse arch owes its existence to the two longitudinal arches, and varies in prominence with the height of the instep. As the inner longitudinal arch sinks, so the transverse arch disappears. Interosseous ligaments and the tendon of the peroneus longus form the main supports of this arch.

Flat-foot is due to the following causes :

1. *Congenital.*—At birth the neck of the astragalus deviates inwards from the axis of the body to an extent of 30 degrees, which accounts for the apparent varus deformity in a new-born child. As the child grows, the angle of deviation diminishes, but further diminution of this normal angle predisposes to flat-foot.

2. *Acquired.*—(i) *Static.*—This is the commonest cause, and is often associated with other static deformities, e.g. genu valgum or scoliosis. The factors contributing to a static

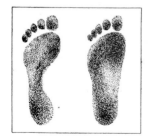

Fig. 1222.—Imprint of a normal foot as compared with a flat foot.

deformity have been mentioned (*vide* Scoliosis). Flat-feet often develop at the menopause, owing to increase in weight and decrease of muscular tone.

The patient complains of weakness and fatigue, especially in the sole and calf, and particularly during and after exertion. As the arch sinks pain is felt across the dorsum of the foot, and later the external malleolus comes into contact with the outer side of the os calcis and causes local pain at the site of pressure. Finally, osteoarthritis affects the tarsal joints, but when the arch has completely collapsed, pain diminishes and the gait becomes shuffling (fig. 1222).

(ii) *Traumatic.*—Injury to any structures which form or maintain the inner longitudinal arch is liable to result in flat-foot. Thus a fall on to the foot sometimes ruptures the spring ligament or fractures the sustentaculum tali, or a wheel passing over the foot may fracture the first (or other) metatarsal bones. Flat-foot was formerly a common sequela of Pott's fracture, due to incomplete reduction, or non-maintenance of inversion during union.

(iii) *Inflammatory.*—Disease of the bones which form the arch sometimes results in partial collapse, e.g. tuberculous disease of the scaphoid. Softening of ligaments due to periarticular gonococcal arthritis predisposes to flat-foot unless temporary supports are worn, or walking curtailed.

(iv) *Paralytic.*—Paralysis of the flexor muscles of the leg, particularly the tibialis posticus, or of the intrinsic muscles of the foot, predisposes to flat-foot by weakening a normal method of support.

(v) *Spastic.*—Spasm of the peroneal muscles is not uncommon, and usually occurs during adolescence. Eversion of the anterior part of the foot follows, and the contracted peroneal tendons are visible beneath the skin behind the external malleolus. The spasm disappears under anæsthesia and a plaster is then applied.

Treatment.—In the case of static flat-foot, treatment depends upon the stage to which the condition has advanced.

Stage 1.—The deformity can be corrected by the patient ; thus standing on the toes with the feet inverted restores the arch by the pull of the posterior tibial muscles.

Treatment of this stage consists in general treatment for debility, combined with adequate rest and suitable graduated exercises, the simplest being toe-raising on inverted feet, which strengthens the short muscles of the sole. Electrical treatment further stimulates weakened muscles. Boots or shoes must be low-heeled and not pointed. The heel should be prolonged on the inner side to support the arch, and the inner border of the sole raised $\frac{1}{4}$ inch (0·75 cm.) in order to throw the weight of the body on to the outer side of the foot.

Stage 2.—This stage can be corrected by the surgeon, who, while the leg is flexed, can forcibly invert the foot and restore the arch. Treatment is carried out on the above lines, the arch being supported by adjustments to the boot, or valgus pads. If considered advisable, manipulation may be performed under general anæsthesia.

Stage 3.—If neither the patient nor the surgeon can correct the deformity (fig. 1223), wrenching under an anæsthetic can be employed, the foot being encased in plaster in an over-corrected position. In cases in which severe pain results from osteoarthritis of tarsal joints, Dunn's arthrodesis often gives

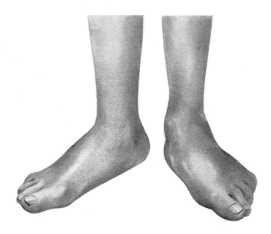

Fig. 1223.—Flat-feet, third stage, with early hallux valgus.

relief (p. 1211). However, it must also be stated that once the arch has completely dropped many sufferers shuffle through life in comparative comfort.

Cases of flat-foot, other than static, are dealt with according to the cause of the condition. Thus a spastic flat-foot is manipulated under anæsthesia, so as to stretch the peroneal muscles, and the foot put up in plaster in the over-corrected position. Traumatic flat-foot should be prevented by anticipatory measures, but if the condition has occurred following a Pott's fracture, reconstruction of the fracture is sometimes advisable.

TALIPES (*Syn.* CLUB FOOT)

Is either congenital or acquired.

1. *Congenital.*—Is rarely due to absence of one of the bones of the leg. More commonly it is associated with spina bifida, in which case it is bilateral. If no cause can be found, malposition *in utero* or a deficient amount of liquor amnii are possible explanations.

2. *Acquired.*—Talipes of the acquired variety is predisposed to by unbalanced muscular action, or the influence of gravity, particularly if prolonged or acting upon weakened muscles. The actual causes may be :

Naughton Dunn, 1884–1939. Surgeon, Royal Cripples' Hospital, Birmingham.

(i) **Paralytic**, such as infantile paralysis, or involvement of peripheral nerves by injury or severe neuritis (e.g. prolonged administration of arsenic).

(ii) **Spastic**, due to upper motor neurone lesions, especially spastic paraplegia or syringomyelia.

(iii) **Compensatory**, e.g. equinus, owing to shortening of the leg (fig. 1224).

(iv) **Muscular contractures**, as with myositis fibrosa, or infective myositis of the calf muscles.

(v) **Postural**, e.g. talipes decubitus from prolonged confinement to bed.

The four primary varieties of talipes are as follows :

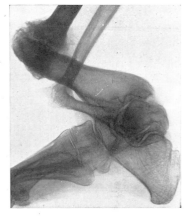

Fig. 1224.—Compensatory talipes equinus, following ununited fracture of the tibia with pseudarthrosis and gross deformity. (The fibula united, and the patient walked on his toes with little disability.)

Talipes equinus, or plantar flexion, the patient walking on the toes.

Talipes calcaneus, or dorsi-flexion, the patient walking on the heel.

Talipes valgus, produced by abduction and eversion of the anterior part of the foot.

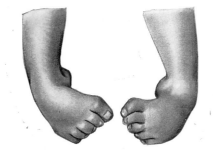

Fig. 1225.— Talipes equino-varus, bilateral and congenital.

Talipes varus—the anterior part of the foot is adducted and inverted, and the patient walks on the outer border.

Usually mixed forms of talipes occur, talipes equino-varus being the commonest (fig. 1225).

In comparing the clinical features of talipes due to congenital causes, and the acquired variety which follows infantile paralysis, the following distinctions are found :

Congenital	*Acquired*
1. From birth.	Born healthy.
2. Often bilateral.	Usually unilateral.
3. No trophic changes :	Trophic changes present :
(*a*) Skin healthy.	(*a*) Skin may be ulcerated.
(*b*) Subcutaneous fat present with creases in soles.	(*b*) Subcutaneous fat and creases disappear.
(*c*) Circulation good and limb warm.	(*c*) Circulation poor, limb blue and cold.
(*d*) Muscles little wasted and electrical reactions present.	(*d*) Marked wasting and reactions much impaired.
(*e*) Bones unaffected.	(*e*) Growth deficient.

Treatment.—*Congenital.*—Treatment is adopted according to the lines already suggested for any congenital deformity. Perseverance and patience often yield surprisingly good results.

(*a*) *Manipulation.*—A few days after birth regular manipulation should be carried out in order to correct the deformity (fig. 1226). Strapping is applied in the intervals, and in slight cases this may be sufficient to cure the condition.

(*b*) *Manipulation and Retentive Apparatus.* — Metal night shoes, malleable splints, etc., are worn and removed as often as necessary to allow manipulation to be applied. Denis Browne splints are excellent in early cases, and they allow use of the leg muscles. The limbs can be retained in any desired position, and the splints are connected by a cross-piece. They are removed at about

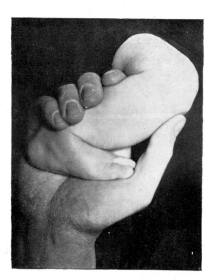

Fig. 1226.—Talipes equino-varus, showing full correction.
(*Royal Northern Operative Surgery.*)

Denis Browne, Contemporary. Surgeon, Hospital for Sick Children, London.

fortnightly intervals for manipulation of the feet and readjustment. Repeated plasters, which are applied in an overcorrected position, are required for more advanced cases, and subsequently splints are worn to maintain correction.

If a dual deformity is present, such as talipes equino-varus, the foot should first be brought in line with the leg so that dorsi-flexion of the foot will exert the maximum pull on the contracted tendo Achillis. Hence the varus deformity is first corrected, after which the plantar flexion is overcome by manipulation and suitable splints.

(c) *Anæsthesia and Forcible Correction.*—Manipulation is forcibly applied manually and after forcible correction, or overcorrection, a plaster of Paris casing, or some suitable apparatus, is applied.

(d) *Operations on Soft Parts.*—Portions of fascia or ligaments are excised, or tendons are divided or lengthened. Thus in a case of equino-varus, tenotomy of the tibialis anticus (and possibly tibialis posticus) is performed, after which the tendo Achillis is lengthened.

(e) *Operations on Joints and Bones.*—Osteotomy, tarsectomy, or even amputation are sometimes necessary.

Naughton Dunn's arthrodesis consists in excision of the subastragaloid joint, and removal of a wedge of tarsal bones. This includes, on the inner side, the scaphoid and adjacent parts of the astragalus and cuneiform bones, and on the outer side adjacent parts of the os calcis and cuboid (fig. 1227). The foot is displaced backwards, and becomes stabilised by ankylosis of the mid-tarsal and subastragaloid joints, but ankle movements are preserved.

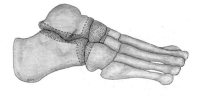

Fig. 1227.—The shaded areas indicate the bone to be removed in Naughton Dunn's arthrodesis.

Whitman's operation consists in removal of the astragalus and displacement of the foot backwards, so that the external and internal malleoli are in contact with the outer side of the os calcis and sustentaculum tali respectively. Owing to backward projection of the heel, a specially constructed boot is subsequently necessary.

INFANTILE PARALYSIS

This condition occurs most commonly in the late summer months, and is possibly associated with the seasonal consumption of fruit. The responsible organism is ultra-microscopic, passes through a porcelain filter, and can be transmitted to apes. The virus causes a meningeal reaction, the cerebro-spinal fluid being under pressure and containing an excess of cells and albumin. The anterior horn cells in the cord are then attacked and the corresponding muscles are paralysed. Anterior polio-

Royal Whitman, Contemporary. Consulting Surgeon, Hospital for Ruptured and Crippled, New York.

myelitis is a notifiable disease, and may be transmitted by the nasal secretion or fæcal contamination of " carriers."

The disease is divided in three stages :

(*a*) *Stage of Invasion.*—The onset is usually sudden, and is characterised by a rise of temperature, pain in the head and spine, and usually more or less widespread cutaneous hyper- æsthesia.   Owing to meningeal irritation stiffness of the neck or back is constant and early—the " spine sign."   Paralysis is evident after two or three days, and unless an epidemic is rife the true nature of the condition is frequently unsuspected un- til the paralysis is discovered.   Lumbar puncture shows a pre- liminary rise in polymorphonuclear cells, followed by an increase in lymphocytes.   The commonest muscles to be affected are those below the knee, but if the arm is involved the muscles above the elbow and of the shoulder girdle (particularly the pectorals) are most commonly paralysed.   Spinal and abdominal muscles are occasionally affected, the former leading to scoliosis and the latter predisposing to herniæ.   Paralysis is very variable in extent and distribution ; in severe cases the bulk of the skeletal muscles are initially affected, while in others merely one or two isolated muscle groups suffer.

(*b*) *Stage of Recovery.*—Muscle movement is noticed within about two months, and continues during the ensuing two years, or even longer.

Response to galvanic stimulation first returns, and while this reaction of degeneration is present, complete recovery is a possibility.   Continued recovery is indicated by response to faradic stimulation, and finally by voluntary movements.

(*c*) *Stationary Stage.*—This is approximately after the lapse of two years, but further slight improvement is possible.

Treatment.—(*a*) *Stage of Paralysis.*—Symptomatic treat- ment is all that can be attempted.   Diaphoretics and sedatives are given, and the affected limb or trunk is wrapped in cotton- wool and immobilised.   Local treatment, such as massage or electricity, is harmful, in that the affected muscles require absolute rest.   Lumbar puncture is indicated for meningeal irritation, and withdrawal of fluid under pressure gives relief.

Serum is of extremely doubtful value.   It is best obtained from abortive cases, and must be administered within forty-eight hours of the onset of infection, otherwise it is useless.

(*b*) *Stage of Recovery.*—During this period three principles of treatment must be observed :

(i) Relaxation of paralysed muscles. If paralysed muscles are allowed to become stretched, as by the pull of healthy antagonistic muscles or by the influence of gravity, any subsequent recovery of tone is neutralised by the " slack " which has been allowed to develop. Therefore splints, surgical boots, and other forms of apparatus must be worn to prevent overstretching of affected muscles (fig. 1228). A plaster of Paris shell is required for spinal cases, to be succeeded by a jacket.

(ii) Maintenance of nutrition. Massage, electrical baths, radiant heat, are all useful in stimulating the circulation and improving nutrition. Weak muscles must not be overstimulated, and the limb is maintained in such a position as to relax affected muscles during treatment.

(iii) Exercise. As recovery occurs, active muscular contractions are encouraged, provided that the effort is well within the powers of the weakened muscle.

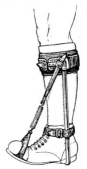

F i g. 1 2 2 8.— Surgical boot— lateral irons to the knee, a valgus strap and a toe-raising spring to correct talipes equino-valgus.

If a limb remains *completely* paralysed for four months, then paralysis is permanent, and further efforts to improve muscular tone are a waste of time. If no muscles are completely paralysed after the acute phase has subsided, then almost complete recovery may be expected (H. J. Seddon).

(*c*) *Stationary Stage.*—After a period of two years the value of the affected muscles can be assessed, although it should be remembered that, unless paralysis is stationary, some degree of improvement is still possible. The principle of treatment is to restore muscular balance, either by means of surgical apparatus or by operative procedures, which have the advantage that appliances can then be discarded or simplified.

The following procedures may therefore be adopted :

(i) Tenotomy, which has little scope in the treatment of infantile paralysis, as muscles are already weakened and contraction of stronger muscles should have been prevented.

(ii) Tendon transplantation, by which means the action of a stronger muscle is transferred to a weaker group, or the direction of muscular pull is altered so as to overcome deformity.

Herbert J. Seddon, Contemporary. Clinical Director, Royal National Orthopædic Hospital, London.

Implantation of a healthy tendon into a paralysed one yields disappointing results, as the paralysed portion gradually stretches.

The following principles should be considered in connexion with tendon transplantation :

(*a*) If possible the tendon is selected from muscles with the same innervation as those affected, so that re-education is simplified. Transplantation of antagonistic muscles is usually unsatisfactory.

(*b*) The detached tendon should be fixed to bone rather than implanted into a paralysed tendon.

(*c*) The path of the transplanted tendon should be as direct as possible.

(*d*) The limb must be relaxed before the tendon is fixed.

(iii) *Tendon fixation* has been used in order to assist in the fixation of a flail joint. Thus in the case of the ankle joint the selected tendon is fixed to the bone on either side of the joint in order to secure stabilisation. Results are disappointing, as paralysed tendons readily stretch when subjected to strain.

(iv) Arthrodesis is a useful procedure, in that it obviates the continued use of surgical apparatus devised to stabilise a flail joint. The operation consists in removal of the articular cartilage, and securing bony union between the bones which comprise the joint. Arthrodesis of the shoulder is recommended following deltoid paralysis, provided that the scapular and limb muscles are adequate.

A rare sequela which may follow arthrodesis of the knee joint is fracture of the leg, usually through the lower third of the femur, owing to the length of rigid and somewhat atrophic bone which extends from the hip to the ankle, and which is therefore subjected to severe strain even in the case of minor accidents, such as stumbling.

(v) Bone lengthening is valuable in cases of shortening. The femur is divided obliquely and continuous skeletal traction will augment the length of the limb up to 2 inches (5 cm.)

Some surgeons prefer to excise a part of the femur, in order to shorten the normal leg. Alternatively, in a growing child, staples are driven into the bone to include the epiphyseal line and so prevent further growth.

(vi) Amputation. This is sometimes necessary in the case of extensive paralysis associated with stunted growth and trophic ulceration. It may be combined with other procedures ; thus, in the case of gross paralysis of the leg, an arthrodesis of the knee and a Syme's amputation of the foot will sometimes provide the patient with a stable and adequately nourished lower extremity.

PES CAVUS (*Syn.* CLAW-FOOT)

Pes cavus is due to an increased concavity of the arch of the foot, so that the instep is unduly high. It is sometimes associated with nervous diseases, e.g. Friedreich's ataxia, or

James Syme, 1799–1870. Professor of Clinical Surgery, University of Edinburgh.
Nikolaus Friedreich 1825–1882. Professor of Pathology, Heidelberg

arises as a compensatory condition in cases of talipes equinus. In many cases the condition occurs idiopathically, and a possible explanation is a transient mild poliomyelitis affecting the extensors of the foot and toes.

Pes cavus is divided into three stages :

Stage 1.—An increase of normal arch is present. This can be remedied by the wearing of a metatarsal bar, which consists of leather about ⅓ inch (1 cm.) thickness, and is fixed obliquely across the sole of the boot just behind the heads of the metatarsal bones. The bar causes slight dorsiflexion, and tends to stretch the Achilles tendon. In long-standing cases, or if improvement is slow, then lengthening of the Achilles tendon should also be performed.

Stage 2.—The heads of the metatarsal bones, particularly the first, project into the sole of the foot, and hammer-toes develop (fig. 1229). The deformity can be remedied by firm pressure on the sole of the foot, so that the heads of the meta-

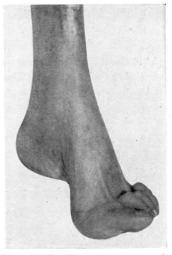

Fig. 1229.—Pes cavus, second stage.

tarsal bones are raised, and hammer-toes straightened.

Treatment of this stage usually requires excision of the plantar fascia and lengthening of the Achilles tendon, and these procedures may be combined with slinging up the head of the first metatarsal by means of the extensor longus hallucis tendon, which is detached and passed through a hole drilled in the head of the metatarsal bone. To prevent a hammer-toe deformity consequent on section of the extensor tendon, arthrodesis of the interphalangeal joint is necessary (fig. 1230). The foot is maintained in its corrected position in plaster of Paris for one month.

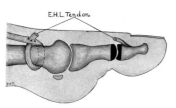

E.H.L. Tendon.

Fig. 1230.—Operation for pes cavus. The shaded portions of bone are excised.

Steindler's muscle-slide operation is advocated by some surgeons. An incision is made on the inner aspect of

Arthur Steindler, Contemporary. Professor of Orthopædic Surgery, Iowa.

the heel, and the soft structures are separated with a raspatory from the under-side of the os calcis, so that excessive arching is diminished. A plaster is applied, which is renewed after further correction in two weeks A metatarsal bar is worn subsequently for some months.

Stage 3.—Permanent hammer-toes are present, and painful callosities develop over the heads of the metatarsals on the sole of the foot, and over the hammer-toes on the dorsum. Much pain and considerable crippling result, and walking is reduced to a painful limp.

When this stage is reached excision of the head and part of the shaft of all the metatarsals is necessary. The excision is performed through dorsal incisions, and toes can then be straightened. In neglected cases amputation of the toes, including part of the metatarsals, and astragalectomy yield a serviceable foot.

CALCANEAN SPUR

is a result of plantar fasciitis following foot strain, which is perhaps aggravated by some focus of infection. Persistent local tenderness suggests the diagnosis, and an X-ray shows the bony outgrowth projecting forward from the under-surface of the bone. A horseshoe-shaped sorbo insole should be fitted in order to relieve pressure, but if disabling symptoms persist excision is performed through a lateral incision.

HALLUX VALGUS

is encouraged by wearing of boots or shoes with pointed toes. The deformity, which consists in abduction, or outward displacement, of the big toe, tends to be progressive, as the direction of pull of the extensor longus hallucis tendon further increases the deformity when once outward displacement has occurred. The following conditions are often associated :

(i) Hammer-toe, owing to the misplaced big toe exerting pressure on the adjacent toes, especially the second toe.

(ii) A bunion, which is an inflamed adventitious bursa, developing over the prominent head of the first metatarsal bone as a result of pressure. Suppuration sometimes follows, and the big toe joint may be secondarily affected.

(iii) Osteoarthritis of the big toe joint, owing to pressure, malalignment of the bones, etc. Severe pain results, varying with the weather, and X-rays frequently show osteophytic outgrowths.

Treatment consists, in the early stages, in wearing roomy boots with a straight inner border. The application of strapping often overcomes early deformity (fig. 1231). New socks or

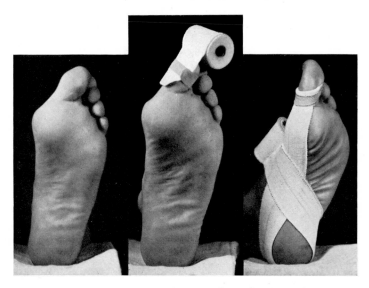

Fig. 1231.—Application of strapping for hallux valgus. (*Gordon Macdonald.*)

stockings should be washed before being worn, so as to minimise their elastic properties, which otherwise tend to crowd the toes together. If the condition is established, the stocking should be digitated so that the big toe is separated from its neighbour, and a peg is introduced into the shoe so that it is maintained in its correct position.

Operation.—Removal of the metatarsal head always weakens the arch, and throws a strain on the heads of the second and third metatarsals, under which callosities are apt to form. The most satisfactory method is to expose the joint through a dorsal incision, and elevate the capsule and periosteum. The phalanx is displaced downwards so as to expose the head of the metatarsal, and excess of bone and osteophytes are removed on either side of the head with an osteotome (fig. 1232). If

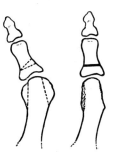

Fig. 1232.—Trimming the metatarsal head for hallux valgus. If deformity is severe, a wedge is also removed from the shaft of the proximal phalanx.

valgus deformity is severe, a wedge of bone is excised from the phalanx by means of a fine saw. No deep sutures are necessary, and the skin is closed with silkworm-gut stitches. A temporary metatarsal bar will enable the patient to walk in comparative comfort, and can be discarded in two or three months.

HALLUX RIGIDUS

occurs as two distinct varieties.

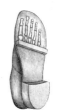

FIG. 1233.—Metatarsal bar.

(i) The adolescent type is due to synovitis of the metatarso-phalangeal joint following injury, and is associated with muscular spasm. It is relieved by wearing a metatarsal bar $\frac{3}{4}$ inch (2 cm.) wide and $\frac{1}{2}$ inch (1·25 cm.) thick (fig. 1233).

(ii) The adult type follows osteoarthritis, and is predisposed to by injury. The limitation of movement is due to interlocking of osteophytes, and also to flattening of the metatarsal head. If manipulation fails to restore movement, the head of the bone should be trimmed, and the proximal third of the adjacent phalanx removed.

HAMMER-TOE

consists in hyperextension of the first phalanx, flexion of the second, and either flexion or extension of the terminal phalanx (fig. 1234). Callosities form over the bony prominences, and in long-standing cases adventitious bursæ develop. Fascia and ligaments become secondarily contracted.

Hammer-toes sometimes develop from overcrowding, either by small or pointed shoes, or as a result of hallux valgus. Pes cavus, as an associated condition, has already been mentioned.

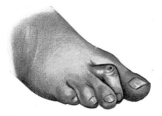

FIG. 1234.—Hammer-toe, with callosity.

Treatment consists in correcting any predisposing cause and wearing a corrective splint. If the deformity is established, operative intervention is required. The " spike " operation (Higgs) ensures bony ankylosis, and consists in sharpening the base of the middle phalanx and impaling it into the shaft of the proximal phalanx, after removal of the condyles.

S. L. Higgs, Contemporary. Orthopædic Surgeon, St. Bartholomew's Hospital, London.

GLOSSARY

OSTEOLOGY

Birmingham Revision of the B.N.A.

Chassaignac's tubercle.	Carotid tubercle (6th cervical vertebra).
Great sacro-sciatic notch.	Greater sciatic notch.
Lesser sacro-sciatic notch.	Lesser sciatic notch.
Musculo-spiral groove.	Spiral groove (radial groove).
Ascending ramus.	Superior ramus.
Astragalus.	Talus.
Maxillary antrum.	Maxillary sinus.
Os magnum.	Capitate bone (os capitatum).

NEUROLOGY

Genito-crural nerve.	Genito-femoral nerve.
Aqueduct of Sylvius.	Aqueduct of mid-brain.
Anterior crural nerve.	Femoral nerve.
Gasserian ganglion.	Trigeminal ganglion.
Nerve of Bell.	Nerve to serratus anterior.
Musculo-spiral nerve.	Radial nerve.

MYOLOGY

Serratus magnus.	Serratus anterior.
Brachialis anticus.	Brachialis.
Orbicularis palpebrarum.	Orbicularis oculi.
Adductor transversus pollicis.	Adductor pollicis (transverse head).
Tensor fasciæ femoris.	Tensor fasciæ latæ.
Supinator longus.	Brachio-radialis.
Biceps cruris.	Biceps femoris.

LIGAMENTS AND MEMBRANES

Poupart's ligament.	Inguinal ligament.
Tenon's capsule.	Fascial sheath of eyeball (B.N.A. fascia bulbi).
Astley Cooper's ligament.	Pectineal ligament.
Gimbernat's ligament.	Pectineal part of inguinal ligament (B.N.A. lacunar ligament).
Ligamentum subflavum.	Ligamentum flavum.
Costo-coracoid membrane.	Clavi-pectoral fascia.
" Spring " ligament.	Plantar calcaneo-navicular ligament.
Rhomboid ligament.	Costo-clavicular ligament.
Y-shaped ligament of Bigelow.	Ilio-femoral ligament.
Achilles' tendon.	Tendo calcaneus.

BLOOD VASCULAR SYSTEM

Birmingham Revision
of the B.N.A.

Lateral sinus.

Transverse sinus.

Anastomotica magna artery.

Artery genu suprema.

Angular vein.

Anterior facial vein.

Vasa brevia.

Short gastric branches of splenic artery.

Veins of Sappey.

Accessory portal veins.

Deep epigastric vessels.

Inferior epigastric vessels.

Superior hæmorrhoidal vein.

Superior rectal vein.

Deep epigastric artery.

Inferior epigastric artery.

DIGESTIVE SYSTEM

Sigmoid colon.

Pelvic colon.

Wharton's duct.

Submandibular duct.

Glands of Blandin and Nühn.

Anterior lingual glands.

Stensen's duct.

Parotid duct.

Veins of Mayo.

Prepyloric veins.

Ampulla of Vater.

Ampulla of bile duct.

Duct of Wirsung.

Pancreatic duct.

Spigelian lobe.

Caudate lobe.

Gerlach's valve.

Semilunar valve of appendix.

Hilton's line.

Pectinate line (white line of anal canal).

Columns of Morgagni.

Anal columns.

PERITONEUM

Gastro-splenic omentum.

Gastro-splenic ligament.

Gastro-hepatic omentum.

Lesser omentum.

Foramen of Winslow.

Opening into lesser sac.

GENITO-URINARY SYSTEM

Glands of Littré.

Urethral glands.

Bartholin's glands.

Greater vestibular glands.

Fallopian tubes.

Uterine tubes.

External abdominal ring.

Superficial inguinal ring.

Internal abdominal ring.

Deep inguinal ring.

Fascia of Zückerkandl.

Renal fascia.

Cave of Retzius.

Retro-pubic space.

Cowper's glands.

Bulbo-urethral glands.

Sinus pocularis.

Prostatic utricle.

Fossa navicularis.

Fossa terminalis.

Internal urinary meatus.

Internal urethral orifice.

Bulbous urethra.

Intrabulbar fossa of the urethra.

Colles' fascia.

Deep layer of superficial perineal fascia.

Triangular ligament.

Perineal membrane.

Compressor urethræ.

Sphincter urethræ.

Vas aberrans of Haller.

Ductulus aberrans.

SURGICAL SPACES, ETC.

Birmingham Revision
of the B.N.A.

Hunter's canal.
Fossa ovalis.
Burn's space.
Fossa of Rosenmüller.
Hesselbach's triangle.
Scarpa's triangle.
Petit's triangle.
Fascia of Scarpa.

Subsartorial canal.
Saphenous opening.
Suprasternal space.
Pharyngeal recess.
Inguinal triangle.
Femoral triangle.
Lumbar triangle.
Deep layer of the superficial fascia
of the abdominal wall.

THE METRIC SYSTEM

METRE is 39·37 inches.
LITRE is 61 cub. ins., or 1·76 pints, or ·22 of a gallon.
GRAMME is 15·43 grains.
KILOGRAMME is 2·2 pounds avoir.

To convert—	Multiply by—
Millilitres into fluid ounces	0·0352
Litres into fluid ounces	35·2
Fluid ounces into millilitres..	28·42
Pints into litres	0·568
Grammes into grains	15·432
Kilogrammes into pounds	2·2046
Grains into grammes	0·0648
Ounces avoirdupois into grammes	28·35
Ounces troy into grammes	31·104
Metres into inches	39·37
Inches into metres	0·0254

ML.s INTO ℳ, etc.

1 ml. = 17 (16·9) ℳ
5 ,, = 1ʒ 24ℳ
10 ,, = 2ʒ 49ℳ
50 ,, = 1ℨ 6ʒ 5ℳ
100 ,, = 3ℨ 4ʒ 10ℳ
1 litre = 35ℨ 1ʒ 34ℳ

ℳ INTO ML.s

1 ℳ = 0·059 ml.
5 = 0·296 ,,
10 = 0·592 ,,
50 = 2·96 ,,
120 = 7·10 ,,
480 = 28·42 ,,

25 drops of water make 1 millilitre (approx.).

GRAINS INTO GRAMMES

1 grain = 0·065 gm.
5 ,, = 0·324 ,,
10 ,, = 0·648 ,,
60 ,, = 3·89 ,,
½ oz. = 14·17 ,,
1 oz. = 28·35 ,,

GRAMMES INTO GRAINS

1 gram. = 15½ (15·432) grains
5 ,, = 77⅙ grains
10 ,, = 154⅓ grains
100 ,, = 3 oz. 230¾ grains
500 ,, = 1 lb. 1 oz. 278 grains
1 Klgr. = 2 lb. 3 oz. 120 grains

INDEX